Smith and Aitkenhead's
Textbook of Anaesthesia

Content Strategist: Jeremy Bowes
Content Development Specialists: Mike Parkinson and Alexandra Mortimer
Project Manager: Sukanthi Sukumar
Designer: Christian Bilbow
Illustration Manager: Jennifer Rose
Illustrator: Graeme Chambers
Marketing Manager: Deborah Watkins

Smith and Aitkenhead's Textbook of Anaesthesia

Sixth Edition

ALAN R. AITKENHEAD

Emeritus Professor of Anaesthesia
Division of Anaesthesia and Intensive Care
Queen's Medical Centre
Nottingham, UK

IAIN K. MOPPETT

Associate Professor and Honorary Consultant
Division of Anaesthesia and Intensive Care
Queen's Medical Centre
Nottingham, UK

JONATHAN P. THOMPSON

Senior Lecturer/Hon Consultant in Anaesthesia and Critical Care
University of Leicester and UHL NHS Trust
Leicester Royal Infirmary
Leicester, UK

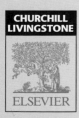

CHURCHILL LIVINGSTONE

ELSEVIER

CHURCHILL
LIVINGSTONE
ELSEVIER

First edition 1985
Second edition 1990
Third edition 1996
Fourth edition 2001
Fifth edition 2007
Sixth edition 2013

The right of A.R. Aitkenhead, I.K. Moppett and J.P. Thompson to be identified as authors of this work has been asserted by them in accordance with the Copyright, Designs and Patents Act 1988.

Notices

Knowledge and best practice in this field are constantly changing. As new research and experience broaden our understanding, changes in research methods, professional practices, or medical treatment may become necessary.

Practitioners and researchers must always rely on their own experience and knowledge in evaluating and using any information, methods, compounds, or experiments described herein. In using such information or methods they should be mindful of their own safety and the safety of others, including parties for whom they have a professional responsibility.

With respect to any drug or pharmaceutical products identified, readers are advised to check the most current information provided (i) on procedures featured or (ii) by the manufacturer of each product to be administered, to verify the recommended dose or formula, the method and duration of administration, and contraindications. It is the responsibility of practitioners, relying on their own experience and knowledge of their patients, to make diagnoses, to determine dosages and the best treatment for each individual patient, and to take all appropriate safety precautions.

To the fullest extent of the law, neither the Publisher nor the authors, contributors, or editors, assume any liability for any injury and/or damage to persons or property as a matter of products liability, negligence or otherwise, or from any use or operation of any methods, products, instructions, or ideas contained in the material herein.

ISBN: 978-0-7020-4192-1
  Reprinted 2014

International **ISBN:** 978-0-8089-2429-6
  Reprinted 2014 (twice), 2015

Ebook ISBN: 978-0-7020-5112-8

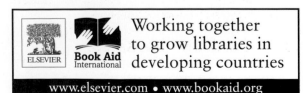

Working together to grow libraries in developing countries

www.elsevier.com • www.bookaid.org

The Publisher's policy is to use paper manufactured from sustainable forests

Printed in China

CONTENTS

PREFACE

■ ■

The objective of the sixth edition of *Textbook of Anaesthesia* remains the same as that of previous editions, namely to provide a concise, easy-to-read text for novices in anaesthesia and an essential resource for those preparing for the Primary Examinations of the Royal College of Anaesthetists. Candidates for these examinations require an extensive knowledge of the basic sciences underpinning anaesthesia, critical care and pain management, and the clinical knowledge and skills expected in those who have completed at least 12-18 months in a full-time training post.

In preparing the present edition, there have been many significant modifications. The title has been changed to '*Smith and Aitkenhead's Textbook of Anaesthesia*' to reflect the enormous contributions of Professor Graham Smith to the first five editions. Two new editors have joined the editorial team to replace Professors Smith and Rowbotham. After extensive and careful review, we felt that it was essential to continue to cover in detail the basic sciences which have direct and close clinical relevance. Indeed, without this information, it is not possible to understand the clinical material described in the book. We have introduced new chapters dealing with consent and information for patients, management of the difficult airway, management of the high-risk patient, anaesthesia for abdominal surgery and in the obese patient, anaesthetic considerations in transplant patients, safety and quality improvement, resuscitation, and education and training. We have also combined the subjects of clinical measurement and monitoring into a single chapter.

In addition, we have rearranged the order of chapters into a more logical format.

We asked a number of senior, experienced authors with expertise in their subject to modify or completely re-write their contributions. We have also recruited 25 new authors to ensure the invigoration of the text by fresh younger minds. We are grateful to all the authors for their contributions and we also thank our reviewers and readers who have made helpful suggestions, many of which have influenced the planning of the new edition. We are also grateful to the publishers who have cooperated in our desire to make fundamental changes.

We hope that the sixth edition will be as popular as previous editions and remain the book of choice for trainees embarking on a career in anaesthesia. Although this book is aimed primarily at the novice trainee, we are aware that many anaesthetists studying for the Final FRCA examinations use *Textbook of Anaesthesia* when revising the basics; we hope that this will continue. We are also aware that the book is used by trainee anaesthetists in many countries other than the UK; of course, the training needs are the same although the examination structures differ. We also believe that this is more than a book suitable for examination preparation; it continues to be a practical guide for all anaesthetists and other healthcare professionals involved in the care of patients in the perioperative period.

A.R. AITKENHEAD, NOTTINGHAM
I.K. MOPPETT, NOTTINGHAM
J.P. THOMPSON, LEICESTER

LIST OF CONTRIBUTORS

ALAN R. AITKENHEAD BSc MD FRCA
Emeritus Professor of Anaesthesia
Division of Anaesthesia and Intensive Care
Queen's Medical Centre
Nottingham, UK

JOSEPH E. ARROWSMITH MD FRCP FRCA FFICM
Consultant Anaesthetist
Papworth Hospital
Cambridge, UK

NIGEL M. BEDFORTH BM BS B MED SCI FRCA
Consultant Anaesthetist and Honorary
    Associate Professor
Division of Anaesthesia and Intensive Care
Queen's Medical Centre
Nottingham, UK

MARTIN BEED BMEDSCI BMBS FRCA FFICM DM
Consultant in Anaesthesia and Intensive Care
Nottingham University Hospitals
Nottingham, UK

ANDREW BODENHAM MB BS FRCA FICM
Consultant in Anaesthesia and Intensive Care Medicine
Leeds General Infirmary
Leeds, UK

DAVID G. BOGOD FRCA LLM
Consultant Anaesthetist
Nottingham University Hospitals NHS Trust
Nottingham, UK

MARGARET BONE MB CHB FRCA FFPMRCA
Clinical Lead for Pain Management
Consultant in Pain Medicine
University Hospitals of Leicester NHS Trust
Leicester, UK

LIAM BRENNAN BSc MBBS FRCA
Consultant Anaesthetist
Addenbrooke's Hospital
Cambridge, UK

NICHOLAS J. CHESSHIRE MB BS FRCA
Consultant Anaesthetist
Royal Derby Hospital
Derby, UK

BEVERLY J. COLLETT MBBS FRCA FFPMRCA
Consultant in Pain Medicine
Pain Management Service
University Hospitals of Leicester
Leicester General Hospital
Leicester, UK

LESLEY A. COLVIN MBCHB FRCA PHD
Consultant/Reader in Anaesthesia and Pain Medicine
Department of Anaesthesia, Critical Care and Pain
    Management
Western General Hospital
Edinburgh, UK

TIM COOK BA MBBS FRCA FFICM
Consultant in Anaesthesia and Intensive Care
    Medicine
Royal United Hospital
Bath, UK

DAVID M. COVENTRY MB CHB FRCA
Consultant Anaesthetist
Ninewells Hospital and Medical School
Dundee, UK

MELANIE DAVIES MBBS MRCP FRCA
Consultant Anaesthetist
Nottingham University Hospitals
Nottingham, UK

CHARLES D. DEAKIN MA MD FRCP FRCA FERC FFICM
Honorary Professor of Resuscitation and Prehospital
    Emergency Medicine
Consultant in Cardiac Anaesthesia and Intensive Care
Department of Anaesthetics
University Hospital Southampton
Southampton, UK

ERIC DE MELO MB CHB FRCA
Consultant Anaesthetist
Leicester Royal Infirmary
Leicester, UK

JOHN DELOUGHRY MA MB BCHIR FRCA
Consultant Anaesthetist
Peterborough City Hospital
Peterborough, UK

DAVID J.R. DUTHIE MD FRCA FFICM
Consultant Anaesthetist
Leeds General Infirmary
Leeds, UK

LORNA EYRE BSC(HONS) FRCA DICM (UK)
Consultant in Critical Care and Anaesthesia
St James's University Hospital
Leeds Teaching Hospitals NHS Trust
Leeds, UK

DAVID FELL MB CHB FRCA
Consultant Anaesthetist
Leicester Royal infirmary
Leicester, UK

SIMON FLOOD BMEDSCI BMBS MRCP FRCA DICM
Consultant in Anaesthesia and Critical Care
Leeds Teaching Hospitals NHS Trust
Leeds, UK

SATYA FRANCIS MBBS FRCA
Consultant Anaesthetist
Leicester Royal Infirmary
Leicester, UK

RICHARD GRIFFITHS MD FRCA
Consultant Anaesthetist
Peterborough District Hospital
Peterborough, UK

TIM G. HALES BSC(HONS) PHD FRCA
Professor of Anaesthesia
Institute of Academic Anaesthesia
Division of Neuroscience
Medical Research Institute
University of Dundee
Dundee, UK

SALLY HANCOCK MBCHB FRCA
Consultant Anaesthetist
Department of Anaesthesia
Queen's Medical Centre
Nottingham, UK

JONATHAN G. HARDMAN B MED SCI (HONS) BM BS FRCA FANZCA DM
Professor
Division of Anaesthesia and Intensive Care
University of Nottingham
Honorary Consultant Anaesthetist
Nottingham University Hospitals NHS Trust
Nottingham, UK

JENNIFER M. HUNTER MB CHB PHD FRCA FCARCSI (HON)
Emeritus Professor of Anaesthesia
Department of Musculoskeletal Biology
Institute of Ageing and Chronic Disease
University of Liverpool
Liverpool, UK

HANNAH KING MBBS FRCA
Division of Anaesthesia and Intensive Care
Queen's Medical Centre
Nottingham, UK

DAVID KIRKBRIDE BMED SCI (HONS) BMBS FRCA
Consultant Anaesthetist
Leicester Royal Infirmary
Leicester, UK

ANDREW KLEIN MBBS FRCA FFICM
Consultant Anaesthetist
Papworth Hospital
Cambridge, UK

CHANDRA KUMAR MBBS DA FFARCS MSc FRCA EDRA
Senior Consultant in Anaesthesia
Khoo Teck Puat Hospital
Singapore

JEREMY A. LANGTON MD FRCA
Consultant Anaesthetist
Plymouth Hospitals NHS Trust
Plymouth, UK

ANDREW LUMB MB BS FRCA
Consultant Anaesthetist
St James's University Hospital
Leeds, UK

PATRICK MAGEE MSc FRCA
Consultant Anaesthetist
Royal United Hospital
Bath, UK

RAVI P. MAHAJAN MD FRCA
Professor of Anaesthesia
Division of Anaesthesia and Intensive Care
Queen's Medical Centre
Nottingham, UK

GRAEME A. MCLEOD MBChB PGCertMedEd MRCGP FRCA FFPMRCA MD
Consultant and Reader in Anaesthesia
Institute of Academic Anaesthesia
Division of Neuroscience
College of Medicine, Dentistry and Nursing
Ninewells Hospital and Medical School
Dundee, UK

IAIN K. MOPPETT MA MRCP FRCA DM
Associate Professor and Honorary Consultant
Division of Anaesthesia and Intensive Care
Queen's Medical Centre
Nottingham, UK

MARY C. MUSHAMBI MBChB FRCA
Consultant Anaesthetist
Leicester Royal infirmary
Leicester, UK

MICHAEL H. NATHANSON MB BS MRCP FRCA
Consultant Neuroanaesthetist
Nottingham University Hospitals
Queen's Medical Centre
Nottingham, UK

GRAHAM R. NIMMO MD FRCP EDIN FFARCSI FFICM
Consultant Physician in Intensive Care Medicine
Department of Anaesthetics
Critical Care and Pain Medicine
Western General Hospital
Edinburgh, UK

SUSAN NIMMO BSc (HONS) MBChB (HONS) FRCP FRCA FFPMRCA MSc
Department of Anaesthetics
Critical Care and Pain Medicine
Western General Hospital
Edinburgh, UK

JERRY P. NOLAN FRCA FRCP FCEM FFICM
Consultant in Anaesthesia and Intensive Care
    Medicine
Royal United Hospital
Bath, UK

NICHOLAS REYNOLDS LLM FRCA FFICM
Consultant in Anaesthesia and Intensive Care
    Medicine
Royal Derby Hospital
Derby, UK

SIMON SCOTT MA BM BCH FRCA
Specialty Registrar and Honorary Lecturer in
    Anaesthesia and Critical Care
University of Leicester and UHL NHS Trust
Leicester Royal Infirmary
Leicester, UK

TOM SIMPSON MB BS FRCA
Consultant in Anaesthesia and Intensive Care
Royal United Hospital
Bath, UK

CHRISTOPHER P. SNOWDEN BMEDSCI(HONS)
FRCA MD
Consultant Anaesthetist and Senior Lecturer
Freeman Hospital
Newcastle upon Tyne, UK

JUSTIAAN C. SWANEVELDER MBCHB
MMED(ANES) FRCA
Consultant Anaesthetist
Glenfield Hospital
Leicester, UK

JONATHAN P. THOMPSON BSC (HONS) MBCHB
MD FRCA
Senior Lecturer/Hon Consultant in Anaesthesia
    and Critical Care
University of Leicester and UHL NHS Trust
Leicester Royal Infirmary
Leicester, UK

K. ELAINE TIGHE MB CHB MRCP FRCA
FFPMRCA
Consultant in Anaesthesia and Pain Management
Leicester Royal infirmary
Leicester, UK

GERRIE VAN DER WALT MBBS FRCA
Division of Anaesthesia and Intensive Care
Queen's Medical Centre
Nottingham, UK

CAMERON WEIR BSC(HONS) MBCHB
FRCA PHD
Consultant Anaesthetist
Centre for Neuroscience
Division of Medical Sciences
College of Medicine, Dentistry and Nursing
Ninewells Hospital and Medical School
Dundee, UK

MATTHEW WILES BMEDSCI MMEDSCI(CLIN ED)
BM BS MRCP FRCA FFICM
Consultant Anaesthetist
Department of Anaesthesia
Royal Hallamshire Hospital
Sheffield, UK

GARETH WILLIAMS MB BS FRCA FFICM
Consultant in Anaesthesia and Adult Critical Care
Leicester Royal Infirmary
Leicester, UK

SEAN WILLIAMSON MB CHB FRCA
MACADMED
Consultant Anaesthetist
The James Cook University Hospital
Middlesbrough, UK

JONATHAN WILSON BSC MB CHB FRCA
Consultant Anaesthetist
York Hospital
York, UK

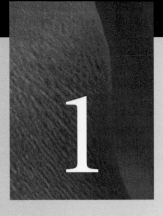

1

GENERAL PRINCIPLES OF PHARMACOLOGY

HOW DO DRUGS ACT?

Drugs produce their effects on biological systems by several mechanisms; these include physicochemical action, activity at receptors and inhibition of reactions mediated by enzymes.

Physicochemical Properties

Sodium citrate is an alkali and neutralizes acid; it is often administered orally to reduce the likelihood of pneumonitis after regurgitation of gastric contents. Chelating agents (*chel* is the Greek word for a crab's claw) combine chemically with metal ions, reducing their toxicity and enhancing elimination, usually in the urine. Such drugs include desferrioxamine (chelates iron and aluminium), dicobalt edetate (cyanide toxicity), sodium calcium edetate (lead) and penicillamine (copper and lead). Stored blood contains a citrate-based anticoagulant which prevents clotting; this chelates calcium ions and may cause hypocalcaemia after massive blood transfusion. Phenol and alcohol denature proteins; they are used occasionally to produce prolonged or permanent nerve blockade.

Action on Receptors

A receptor is a complex structure on the cell membrane which can bind selectively with endogenous compounds or drugs, resulting in changes within the cell which modify its function. These include changes in selective ion channel permeability (e.g. acetylcholine, glutamate, GABA receptors), cyclic adenosine monophosphate (e.g. opioid, β, α_2 and dopamine receptors), cyclic guanosine monophosphate (e.g. atrial natriuretic peptide receptor), inositol phosphate and diacylglycerol (e.g. α_1, angiotensin AT_1, endothelin, histamine H_1 and vasopressin V_1 receptors) and nitric oxide (e.g. muscarinic M_3 receptor).

A compound which binds to a receptor and changes intracellular function is termed an agonist. The classic dose–response relationship of an agonist is shown in Figure 1.1. As the concentration of the agonist increases, a maximum effect is reached as the receptors in the system become saturated (Fig. 1.1A). Conventionally, log dose is plotted against effect, resulting in a sigmoid curve which is approximately linear between 20 and 80% of maximum effect (Fig. 1.1B). Three agonists are shown in Figure 1.2. Agonist A produces 100% effect at a lower concentration than agonist B. Therefore, compared with A, agonist B is less potent but has similar efficacy. Drug C is termed a partial agonist as the maximum effect is less than that of A or B. Buprenorphine is a partial agonist (at the μ-opioid receptor), as are some of the β-blockers with intrinsic activity, e.g. oxprenolol, pindolol, acebutalol, celiprolol.

Antagonists combine selectively with the receptor but produce no effect. They may interact with the receptor in a competitive (reversible) or non-competitive (irreversible) fashion. In the presence of a competitive antagonist, the dose–response curve of an agonist is shifted to the right but the maximum effect remains unaltered (Fig. 1.3A). Examples of this effect include the displacement of morphine by naloxone and endogenous catecholamines by β-blockers.

A non-competitive (irreversible) antagonist also shifts the dose–response curve to the right but, with

1

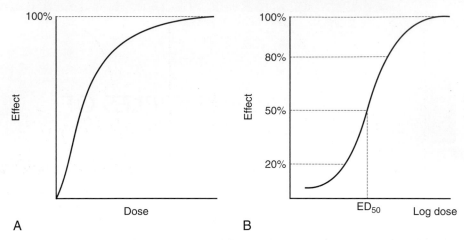

FIGURE 1.1 ■ (**A**) The effect of an agonist peaks when all the receptors are occupied. (**B**) A semilog plot produces a sigmoid curve which is linear between 20 and 80% effect. ED_{50} is the dose which produces 50% of maximum effect.

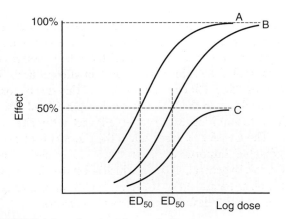

FIGURE 1.2 ■ Agonist B has a similar dose–response curve to A but is displaced to the right. A is more potent than B (smaller ED_{50}) but has the same efficacy. C is a partial agonist which is less potent than A and B and less efficacious (maximum effect 50% of A and B).

increasing concentrations, reduces the maximum effect (Fig. 1.3B). For example, the α_1-antagonist phenoxybenzamine, used in the preoperative preparation of patients with phaeochromocytoma, has a long duration of action because of the formation of stable chemical bonds between drug and receptor.

The relationship between drug dose and response is often described by a Hill plot (Fig. 1.4). A typical agonist such as that shown in Figure 1.1 produces a straight line with a slope (i.e. Hill coefficient) of +1.

Action on Enzymes

Drugs may act by inhibiting the action of an enzyme or competing for its endogenous substrate. Reversible inhibition is the mechanism of action of edrophonium (acetylcholinesterase), aminophylline (phosphodiesterase) and captopril (angiotensin-converting enzyme). Irreversible enzyme inhibition occurs when a stable chemical bond is formed between drug and enzyme, resulting in prolonged or permanent inactivity e.g. omeprazole (gastric hydrogen-potassium ATPase), aspirin (cyclo-oxygenase) and organophosphorus compounds (acetylcholinesterase).

However, the interaction between drug and enzyme may be more complex than this simple classification implies. For example, neostigmine inhibits acetylcholinesterase in a reversible manner, but the mechanism of action is more akin to that of an irreversible drug because neostigmine forms covalent chemical bonds with the enzyme.

THE BLOOD–BRAIN BARRIER AND PLACENTA

Many drugs used in anaesthetic practice must cross the blood–brain barrier in order to reach their site of action. The brain is protected from most potentially toxic agents by tightly overlapping endothelial cells which surround the capillaries and interfere with passive diffusion. In addition, enzyme systems are present

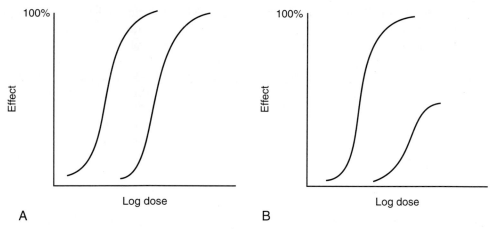

FIGURE 1.3 ■ (**A**) The dose–response curve of an agonist is displaced to the right in the presence of a reversible antagonist. There is no change in maximum effect but the ED_{50} is increased. (**B**) The dose–response curve is displaced to the right also in the presence of an irreversible antagonist but the maximum effect is reduced.

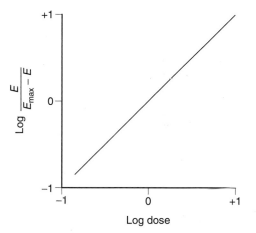

FIGURE 1.4 ■ A Hill plot. The Hill coefficient is the slope of the line (+1 for this drug). E_{max} = maximum effect, E = effect at different doses.

in the endothelium which break down many potential toxins. Consequently, only relatively small, highly lipid-soluble molecules (e.g. intravenous and volatile anaesthetic agents, opioids, local anaesthetics) have access to the central nervous system (CNS). Compared with most opioids, morphine takes some time to reach its site of action because it has a relatively low lipid solubility. Highly ionized drugs (e.g. muscle relaxants, glycopyrronium) do not cross the blood–brain barrier.

The chemoreceptor trigger zone is situated in the area postrema near the base of the fourth ventricle (see Ch 42). It is not protected by the blood–brain barrier because the capillary endothelial cells are not bound tightly in this area and allow relatively free passage of large molecules. This is an important afferent limb of the vomiting reflex and stimulation of this area by toxins or drugs in the blood or cerebrospinal fluid often leads to vomiting. Many antiemetics act at this site.

The transfer of drugs across the placenta is of considerable importance in obstetric anaesthesia (see Ch 35). In general, all drugs which affect the CNS cross the placenta and affect the fetus. Highly ionized drugs (e.g. muscle relaxants) pass across less readily.

PLASMA PROTEIN BINDING

Many drugs are bound to proteins in the plasma. This is important because only the unbound portion of the drug is available for diffusion to its site of action. Changes in protein binding may have significant effects on the active unbound concentration of a drug, and therefore its actions.

Albumin is the most important protein in this regard and is responsible mainly for the binding of acidic and neutral drugs. Globulins, especially α_1-glycoprotein, bind mainly basic drugs. If a drug is highly protein bound (>80%), any change in plasma protein concentration or displacement of the drug by another with similar binding properties may have clinically significant effects. For example, most NSAIDs displace warfarin, phenytoin and lithium from plasma binding sites, leading to potential toxicity.

Plasma albumin concentration is often decreased in the elderly, in neonates and in the presence of malnutrition, liver, renal or cardiac failure and malignancy. α_1-Glycoprotein concentration is decreased during pregnancy and in the neonate but may be increased in the postoperative period and other conditions such as infection, trauma, burns and malignancy.

METABOLISM

Most drugs are lipid-soluble and many are metabolized in the liver into more ionized compounds which are inactive pharmacologically and excreted by the kidneys. However, metabolites may be active (Table 1.1). The liver is not the only site of metabolism. For example, succinylcholine and mivacurium are metabolized by plasma cholinesterase, esmolol by erythrocyte esterases, remifentanil by tissue esterases and, in part, dopamine by the kidney and prilocaine by the lungs.

A substance is termed a *prodrug* if it is inactive in the form in which it is administered, pharmacological effects being dependent on the formation of active metabolites. Examples of this are codeine (morphine), diamorphine (6-monoacetylmorphine, morphine), chloral hydrate (trichlorethanol) and parecoxib (valdecoxib). Midazolam is ionized and

TABLE 1.1
Examples of Active Metabolites

Drug	Metabolite	Action
Morphine	Morphine-6-glucuronide	Potent opioid agonist
Diamorphine	6-Monoacetylmorphine Morphine	Opioid agonist
Meperidine (pethidine)	Normeperidine (norpethidine)	Epileptogenic
Codeine	Morphine	Opioid agonist
Diazepam	Desmethyldiazepam Temazepam Oxazepam	Sedative
Tramadol	O-desmethyltramadol	Opioid agonist
Parecoxib	Valdecoxib	COX-2 specific inhibitor

dissolved in an acidic solution in the ampoule; after intravenous injection and exposure in the blood to pH 7.4, the molecule becomes lipid-soluble.

Drugs undergo two types of reactions during metabolism: phase I and phase II. Phase I reactions include reduction, oxidation and hydrolysis. Drug oxidation occurs in the smooth endoplasmic reticulum, primarily by the cytochrome P450 enzyme system. This system and other enzymes also perform reduction reactions. Hydrolysis is a common phase I reaction in the metabolism of drugs with ester groups (e.g. remifentanil, succinylcholine, atracurium, mivacurium). Amide drugs often undergo hydrolysis and oxidative N-dealkylation (e.g. lidocaine, bupivacaine).

Phase II reactions involve conjugation of a metabolite or the drug itself with an endogenous substrate. Conjugation with glucuronic acid is a major metabolic pathway, but others include acetylation, methylation and conjugation with sulphate or glycine.

Enzyme Induction and Inhibition

Some drugs may enhance the activity of enzymes responsible for drug metabolism, particularly the cytochrome P450 enzymes and glucuronyl transferase. Such drugs include phenytoin, carbamazepine, phenylbutazone, barbiturates, ethanol, steroids and some inhalational anaesthetic agents (halothane, enflurane). Cigarette smoking also induces cytochrome P450 enzymes.

Drugs with mechanisms of action other than on enzymes may also interfere significantly with enzyme systems. For example, etomidate inhibits the synthesis of cortisol and aldosterone – an effect which may explain the increased mortality in critically ill patients which occurred when it was used as a sedative in intensive care. Cimetidine is a potent enzyme inhibitor and may prolong the elimination of drugs such as diazepam, propranolol, oral anticoagulants, phenytoin and lidocaine. Troublesome interactions with enzyme systems are less of a problem with new drugs; if significant enzyme interaction is discovered in the early stages of development, the drug is usually abandoned.

DRUG EXCRETION

Ionized compounds with a low molecular weight (MW) are excreted mainly by the kidneys. Most drugs and metabolites diffuse passively into the proximal renal tubules by the process of glomerular filtration, but some are secreted actively (e.g. penicillins, aspirin, many diuretics, morphine, lidocaine and glucuronides). Ionization is a significant barrier to reabsorption at the distal tubule. Consequently, basic drugs or metabolites are excreted more efficiently in acid urine and acidic compounds in alkaline urine.

Some drugs and metabolites, particularly those with larger molecules (MW >400 D), are excreted in the bile (e.g. glycopyrronium, vecuronium, pancuronium and the metabolites of morphine and buprenorphine). Ventilation is responsible for excretion of volatile anaesthetic agents.

PHARMACOKINETIC PRINCIPLES

Pharmacokinetics is the study of what happens to drugs after they have been administered. In contrast, pharmacodynamics is concerned with their effects on biological systems. An understanding of the basic principles of pharmacokinetics is an important aid to the safe use of drugs in anaesthesia, pain management and intensive care medicine. Pharmacokinetics is an attempt to fit observed changes in plasma concentration of drugs into mathematical equations which may then be used to predict concentrations under various circumstances.

Derived values describing volume of distribution (V), clearance (Cl) and half-life ($t_{1/2}$) give an indication of the likely properties of a drug. However, even in healthy individuals of the same sex, weight and age, there is significant variability which makes precise prediction very difficult. It is important to remember that the accepted pharmacokinetic values of drugs are usually the mean of a wide range of observations.

Volume of Distribution

Volume of distribution is a good example of the abstract nature of pharmacokinetics; it is not a real volume but merely a concept which helps us to understand what we observe. Nevertheless, it is a very useful notion which enables us to predict certain properties of a drug and also calculate other pharmacokinetic values.

Imagine that a patient receiving an intravenous dose of an anaesthetic induction agent is a bucket of water and that the drug is distributed evenly throughout the water immediately after injection. The volume of water represents the initial volume of distribution (V). It may be calculated easily:

$$C_0 = \frac{\text{dose}}{V} \tag{1}$$

where C_0 is the initial concentration. Therefore:

$$V = \frac{\text{dose}}{C_0} \tag{2}$$

A more accurate measurement of V is possible during constant rate infusion when the distribution of the drug in the tissues has time to equilibrate; this is termed volume of distribution at steady state (V_{ss}).

Drugs which remain in the plasma and do not pass easily to other tissues have a small V and therefore a large C_0. Relatively ionized drugs (e.g. muscle relaxants) or drugs highly bound to plasma proteins (e.g. NSAIDs) often have a small V. Drugs with a large V are often lipid-soluble and therefore penetrate and accumulate in tissues outside the plasma (e.g. intravenous induction agents). Some drugs accumulate outside the plasma, making values for V greater than total body volume (a reminder of the abstract nature of pharmacokinetics). Large V values are often observed for drugs highly bound to proteins outside plasma (e.g. local anaesthetics, digoxin).

Several factors may affect V and therefore C_0 on bolus injection of a drug. Patients who are dehydrated, or have lost blood, have a significantly greater plasma C_0 after a normal dose of intravenous induction agent, increasing the likelihood of severe side-effects, especially hypotension. Neonates have a proportionally greater volume of extracellular fluid compared with adults, and water-soluble drugs (e.g. muscle relaxants) tend to have a proportionally greater V. Factors affecting plasma protein binding (see above) may also affect V.

Finally, V can give some indication as to the half-life. A large V is often associated with a relatively slow decline in plasma concentration; this relationship is expressed below in a useful pharmacokinetic equation (eqn 4).

Clearance

Clearance is defined as the volume of blood or plasma from which the drug is removed completely in unit time. Drugs may be eliminated from the blood by the liver, kidney or occasionally other routes (see above). The relative proportion of hepatic and renal clearance of a drug is important. Most drugs used in anaesthetic practice are cleared predominantly by the liver, but some rely on renal or non-organ-dependent clearance. Excessive accumulation of a drug occurs in patients in renal failure if its renal clearance is significant. For example, morphine is metabolized primarily in the liver and this is not affected significantly in renal impairment. However, the active metabolite morphine-6-glucuronide is excreted predominantly by the kidney. This accumulates in renal insufficiency and is responsible for increased morphine sensitivity in these patients.

As with volume of distribution, clearance may suggest likely properties of a drug. For example, if clearance is greater than hepatic blood flow, factors other than hepatic metabolism must account for its total clearance. Values greater than cardiac output may indicate metabolism in the plasma (e.g. succinylcholine) or other tissues (e.g. remifentanil). Clearance is an important (but not the only) factor affecting $t_{1/2}$ and steady-state plasma concentrations achieved during constant rate infusions (see below).

Elimination Half-Life

Methods of administration of a drug are influenced considerably by its plasma $t_{1/2}$, as this often reflects duration of action. It is important to remember that $t_{1/2}$ is influenced not only by clearance (Cl) but also by V:

$$t_{1/2} \propto \frac{V}{Cl} \qquad (3)$$

or

$$t_{1/2} = \text{constant} \times \frac{V}{Cl}$$

The constant in this equation (elimination rate constant) is the natural logarithm of 2 (ln 2) i.e. 0.693. Therefore:

$$t_{1/2} = 0.693 \times \frac{V}{Cl} \qquad (4)$$

Half-life often reflects duration of action but not if the drug acts irreversibly (e.g. some NSAIDs, omeprazole, phenoxybenzamine) or if active metabolites are formed (Table 1.1).

So far, we have considered metabolic or elimination $t_{1/2}$ only. The initial decrease in plasma concentrations after administration of many drugs, especially if given intravenously, occurs primarily because of redistribution into tissues. Therefore, the simple relationship between elimination $t_{1/2}$ and duration of action does not apply in many situations (see below, 'Two-Compartment Models').

Calculating $t_{1/2}$, V and Clearance

It is a simple exercise to calculate these values for a drug after intravenous bolus administration. A known dose is given and regular blood samples are taken for plasma concentration measurements. In this example, we assume that the drug remains in the plasma and is removed only by metabolism; this is a called a one-compartment model. After achieving C_0, plasma concentration (C_p) declines in a simple exponential manner as shown in Figure 1.5A. If the natural logs of the concentrations are plotted against time (semilog plot), a straight line is produced (Figure 1.5B). The gradient of this line is the elimination rate constant k, which is related to $t_{1/2}$ in the following equation:

$$k = \frac{\ln 2}{t_{1/2}} \qquad (5)$$

We may calculate V using equation (2) and then clearance from equation (4). C_p may be predicted at any time from the following equation:

$$C_p = C_0 e^{-kt} \qquad (6)$$

where t is the time after administration.

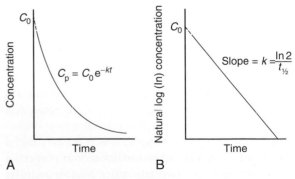

FIGURE 1.5 ■ (**A**) Exponential decline in plasma drug concentration (C_p) in a one-compartment model. The equation predicts C_p at any time (t). (**B**) Semilog plot enables easy calculation of $t_{1/2}$. Extrapolation of this line enables C_0 and AUC_∞ to be derived easily.

Clearance may be derived also by calculation of the area under the concentration-time curve extrapolated to infinity (AUC_∞) and substitution in the following equation:

$$Cl = \frac{dose}{AUC_\infty} \qquad (7)$$

Two-Compartment Models

The body is not, of course, a single homogeneous compartment; drug plasma concentrations are the result of elimination by metabolism and redistribution to and from tissues such as brain, heart, liver, muscles and fat. The mathematics describing this real situation are extremely complex. However, plasma concentrations of many drugs behave approximately as if they were distributed in two or three compartments. Applying these mathematical models is a reasonable compromise.

Let us consider a two-compartment model; one compartment may be thought of as representing the plasma and the other, the remainder of the body. When an intravenous bolus is injected into this system, C_p decreases because of an exponential decay resulting from elimination and another exponential decay resulting from redistribution into the tissues. Therefore, when C_p is plotted against time, the curve may be described by a biexponential equation. If plotted on a semilogarithmic plot (Fig. 1.6), two straight lines can be identified and derived. Their gradients are the elimination rate constants dependent on elimination (β) and redistribution (α).

Redistribution kinetics are not only of theoretical interest, because it is often the decline in C_p resulting from redistribution which is responsible for the cessation of an observed effect of a drug; intravenous induction agents and *initial* doses of intravenous fentanyl are good examples of this. Patients wake up after a bolus administration of propofol because of redistribution, not metabolism.

Calculating the separate pharmacokinetic values is easy; one curve is simply subtracted from the other. Consider Figure 1.6 in which natural log concentration is plotted against time and two slopes are seen. The second and less steep slope represents decline in plasma concentration caused by elimination of the drug by metabolism. From this, the elimination half-life ($t^\beta_{1/2}$)

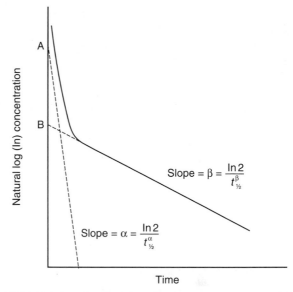

FIGURE 1.6 ■ Semilog plot of a two-compartment model: α=rate constant for exponential decay resulting from redistribution; β=rate constant for exponential decay resulting from elimination.

may be calculated. In order to calculate the half-life of the redistribution phase ($t^\alpha_{1/2}$), the elimination slope is extrapolated back to time 0. If data on this imaginary part of the elimination slope are subtracted from those on the real line above it, another imaginary line may be constructed which represents that part of the decline in plasma concentration which is the result of redistribution. From this line, the redistribution half-life ($t^\alpha_{1/2}$) may be calculated.

The equation for C_p at any time in a two-compartment model after bolus intravenous administration is therefore:

$$C_p = Ae^{-\alpha t} + Be^{-\beta t} \qquad (8)$$

where α and β are the redistribution and elimination rate constants, respectively, and A and B are values derived by back extrapolation of the redistribution and elimination slopes to the y-axis.

Some drugs, e.g. propofol, are best fitted to a triexponential, three-compartment model which reveals half-lives for two processes of redistribution (conventionally $t^\alpha_{1/2}$ and $t^\beta_{1/2}$) and one for elimination ($t^\gamma_{1/2}$). Equations developed from these basic concepts are contained in the software of target-controlled infusion pumps.

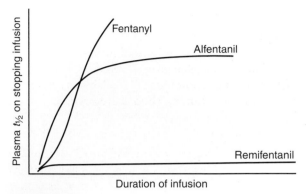

FIGURE 1.7 ■ Context-sensitive half-life. The time for plasma concentration to decline by 50% increases with duration of infusion for alfentanil and fentanyl. This is not the case for remifentanil.

Context-Sensitive Half-Life

This concept refers to plasma half-life (time for plasma concentration to decline by 50%) after an intravenous drug infusion is stopped; 'context' refers to the duration of infusion. The amount of drug accumulating in body tissues increases with duration of infusion for most drugs. Consequently, on stopping the infusion, time for the plasma concentration to decline by 50% depends on duration of infusion. The longer the infusion, the more drug accumulates and the longer the plasma half-life becomes, because there is more drug to enter the plasma on stopping the infusion.

Figure 1.7 shows the effect of infusion duration on the half-lives of alfentanil, fentanyl and remifentanil. Alfentanil, and especially fentanyl, accumulate during infusion, causing an increase in context-sensitive half-life as the duration of infusion increases. In other words, time to recovery from alfentanil- or fentanyl-based anaesthesia depends on duration of infusion. Remifentanil is metabolized by tissue esterases and does not accumulate. Therefore, time for plasma concentration of remifentanil to decline by 50% is independent of duration of infusion, i.e. recovery times after remifentanil-based anaesthesia are short and predictable, no matter how long the infusion has run.

PHARMACOGENETICS

Pharmacogenetics refers to genetic differences in metabolic pathways which can affect individual responses to drugs, both in terms of therapeutic effect as well as adverse effects. Pharmacogenetics is a rising concern in clinical oncology, because the therapeutic window of most anticancer drugs is narrow and patients with impaired ability to detoxify drugs may undergo life-threatening toxicities.

The first observations of genetic variation in drug response date from the 1950s, involving the muscle relaxant (succinylcholine [suxamethonium]). Up to 4% of patients have a less efficient variant of the enzyme butyrylcholinesterase (plasma cholinesterase), which metabolizes succinylcholine chloride. As a consequence, the drug's effect is prolonged to varying degrees (depending on the nature of the abnormal gene and whether the individual is homozygous or heterozygous), with slower recovery from paralysis (see Ch 6).

Variation in the N-acetyltransferase gene divides people into 'slow acetylators' and 'fast acetylators', with very different half-lives and blood concentrations of drugs such as isoniazid and procainamide.

As part of the inborn system for clearing the body of xenobiotics, the cytochrome P450 oxidases (CYPs) are heavily involved in drug metabolism, and genetic variations in CYPs affect large populations. One member of the CYP superfamily, CYP2D6, now has over 75 known allelic variations, some of which lead to no activity, and some to enhanced activity. An estimated 29% of people in some parts of the world may have multiple copies of the gene, and therefore may not be treated adequately with standard doses of drugs such as codeine (which is activated by the enzyme).

METHODS OF DRUG ADMINISTRATION

Oral

The oral route of drug administration is important in modern anaesthetic practice (e.g. premedication, postoperative analgesia). It is often necessary also to continue concurrent medication during the perioperative period (e.g. antihypertension therapy, anti-anginal medication). It is therefore important to appreciate the factors involved in the absorption of orally administered drugs.

The formulation of tablets or capsules is very precise, as their consistent dissolution is necessary before absorption can take place. The rate of absorption, and therefore effect of the drug, may be influenced significantly by this factor. Most preparations dissolve in the acidic gastric juices and the intact drug is absorbed in the upper intestine. However, some drugs are broken down by acids (e.g. omeprazole, benzyl-penicillin) or are irritant to the stomach (e.g. aspirin, phenylbutazone) and may be given as enteric-coated preparations. Drugs given in solution are often absorbed more rapidly but this may induce nausea or vomiting immediately after anaesthesia. Some drugs used in anaesthetic practice are available in slow-release preparations (e.g. morphine, oxycontin, tramadol).

Gastric Emptying

Most drugs are absorbed only when they have left the stomach; therefore, if gastric emptying is delayed, absorption is affected. Furthermore, if oral medication is given continuously during periods of impaired emptying, it may accumulate in the stomach, only to be delivered to the small intestine *en masse* when gastric function returns, resulting in overdose. Many factors influence the rate of gastric emptying and these are described in Chapter 42.

Any factor increasing upper intestinal motility (e.g. metoclopramide) reduces the time available for absorption and may reduce the total amount of drug absorbed.

First-Pass Effect

Before entering the systemic circulation, a drug must pass through the portal circulation and, if metabolized extensively by the liver or even the gut wall, absorption may be reduced significantly (i.e. first-pass effect). For example, compared with intramuscular administration, significantly larger doses of oral morphine are required for the same effect. In fact, most opioids, except methadone, are susceptible to significant first-pass metabolism.

Bioavailability

Bioavailability is the percentage of the oral dose of a drug which is absorbed into the systemic circulation. It is calculated by giving the same individual, on two separate occasions, the same dose of a drug orally and intravenously. The resulting plasma drug concentrations are plotted against time and the area under the curve after oral administration is compared with that after intravenous administration.

Lingual and Buccal

This is a useful method of administration if a drug is lipid-soluble and crosses the oral mucosa with relative ease. First-pass metabolism is avoided. Glyceryl trinitrate and buprenorphine are available as sublingual tablets and morphine as a buccal preparation.

Intramuscular

Intramuscular administration is still used occasionally in the perioperative period. It may avoid the problems associated with large initial plasma concentrations after rapid intravenous administration, is devoid of first-pass effects and may be administered relatively easily. However, absorption may be unpredictable, some preparations are particularly painful and irritant (e.g. diclofenac) and complications include damage to nervous and vascular tissue and inadvertent intravenous injection. It is disliked intensely by most adults and nearly all children.

Variations in absorption may be clinically relevant. For example, peak plasma concentrations of morphine may occur at any time from 5 to 60 min after intramuscular administration, an important factor in the failure of this method to produce good reliable analgesia (see Ch 41).

Subcutaneous

Absorption is very susceptible to changes in skin perfusion, and tissue irritation may be a significant problem. However, this method is used in many centres for providing postoperative pain relief, particularly in children or after intermediate surgery, and has the advantage that potentially difficult intravenous access is not required. A small cannula is placed subcutaneously during anaesthesia and can be replaced, if necessary, with relative ease. Even patient-controlled analgesia (PCA) has been used effectively by this route.

Intravenous

Bolus

The majority of drugs used in anaesthetic practice are given intravenously as boluses and the pharmacokinetics are described in some detail above. The major disadvantage of this method is that dangerously high drug concentrations may occur readily, particularly with drugs of narrow therapeutic index and large interpatient pharmacodynamic and pharmacokinetic variations (i.e. most drugs used in anaesthetic practice). Therefore, it is an important general rule that all drugs administered intravenously should be given slowly. Manufacturers' recommendations in this regard are often surprising; for example, a 10 mg dose of metoclopramide should be given over 1–2 min.

Only two factors have a major influence on the plasma concentrations achieved during a bolus intravenous injection: speed of injection and cardiac output. Therefore, an elderly, sick or hypovolaemic patient undergoing intravenous induction of anaesthesia is likely to suffer significant side-effects if the drug is given at the same rate as would be used in a normal, healthy young adult.

Infusion

Drugs may be given by constant-rate infusion, a method used frequently for propofol, neuromuscular blocking agents, opioids and many other drugs. Plasma concentrations achieved during infusions may be described by a simple wash-in exponential curve (Fig. 1.8). The only factor influencing time to reach steady-state concentration is $t_{1/2}$. Maximum concentration is achieved after approximately 4–5 half-lives. Therefore, this method of administration is best suited to drugs with short half-lives, such as remifentanil, glyceryl trinitrate, Adrenaline and dopamine. However, in practice, it is often used for drugs such as morphine. Assuming a

morphine $t_{1/2}$ of 4 h, it will be about 20 h before steady-state concentration is reached (although an effective concentration can be achieved by initial bolus doses or a more rapid infusion). Therefore, vigilant observation is required with this method of delivery, especially if active metabolites are involved – in this example, morphine-6-glucuronide.

There is a simple equation describing the concentration achieved at steady state during a constant-rate infusion; this is based on the principle that, at steady state, the amount of drug cleared from the plasma is equal to that delivered:

$$\text{Rate of infusion} = \text{Cl} \times C_{ss} \qquad (9)$$

where C_{ss} is the concentration at steady state.

Many pathological conditions reduce drug clearance and may therefore result in unexpectedly large plasma concentrations during infusions. Half-life does not influence C_{ss}, only how quickly it is achieved.

Patient-Controlled Analgesia (PCA)

The use of PCA for the treatment of postoperative pain has become widespread and is described in detail in Chapter 41. The patient titrates opioid delivery to requirements by pressing a button on a PCA device which results in the delivery of a small bolus dose. A lockout time is set which does not allow another bolus to be delivered until the previous dose has had time to have an effect. There is an enormous interpatient variability in opioid requirement after surgery; effective and closely monitored PCA is able to cope with this.

Rectal

This technique reduces the problems of first-pass metabolism and the need for injections. It is used in children and adults (paracetamol, diclofenac, ibuprofen) for postoperative analgesia. However, the proportion of drug absorbed is very variable.

Transdermal

Drugs with a high lipid solubility and potency may be given transdermally. The pharmacological properties of glyceryl trinitrate render it ideal for this technique (i.e. potent, highly lipid-soluble, short half-life). Transdermal hyoscine is used for travel and other causes of sickness. Fentanyl patches can be very

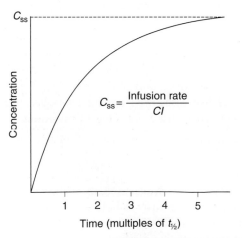

FIGURE 1.8 ■ Plasma concentrations during a constant-rate intravenous infusion against time expressed as multiples of $t_{1/2}$. C_{ss}=concentration at steady state, Cl=clearance.

effective, particularly in patients with cancer pain. Buprenorphine and lidocaine transdermal delivery systems are also available. The latter is used for post-herpetic neuralgia which has not responded to more conventional techniques.

It may take some time before a steady-state plasma concentration is achieved and many devices incorporate large amounts of drug in the adhesive layer in order to provide a loading dose which reduces this period. At steady state, transdermal delivery has several similarities to intravenous infusion. However, on removing the adhesive patch, plasma concentrations may decline relatively slowly because of a depot of drug in the surrounding skin; this occurs with transdermal fentanyl systems.

Inhalation

The delivery of inhaled volatile anaesthetics is discussed below, but other drugs may be given by this route, especially bronchodilators and steroids. Atropine and Adrenaline are absorbed if injected into the bronchial tree and this offers a route of administration in emergencies if no other method of delivery is possible. Opioids such as fentanyl and diamorphine have been given as nebulized solutions but this technique is not routine.

Epidural

This is a common route of administration in anaesthetic practice. The epidural space is very vascular and significant amounts of drug may be absorbed systemically, even if any vessels are avoided by the needle or cannula. Opioids diffuse across the dura to act on spinal opioid receptors, but much of their action when given epidurally is the result of systemic absorption. Complications include haematoma and infection, inadvertent dural puncture with consequent headache or spinal administration of the drug.

Spinal (Subarachnoid)

When given spinally, drugs have free access to the neural tissue of the spinal cord and small doses have profound, rapid effects, an advantage and also a disadvantage of the method. Protein binding is not a significant factor because CSF protein concentration is relatively low.

DRUG INTERACTIONS

There are three basic types of drug interaction; examples are listed in Table 1.2.

Pharmaceutical

In this type of interaction, drugs mixed in the same syringe or infusion bag react chemically with adverse results. For example, mixing succinylcholine with thiopental (pH 10–11) hydrolyses the former, rendering it inactive. Before mixing drugs, data should be sought on their compatibility.

Pharmacokinetic

Absorption of a drug, particularly if given orally, may be affected by other drugs because of their action on gastric emptying (see above). Interference with protein

TABLE 1.2		
Examples of Drug Interactions in Anaesthesia		
Type	*Drugs*	*Effect*
Pharmaceutical	Thiopental: succinylcholine	Hydrolysis of succinylcholine
	Ampicillin: glucose, lactate	Reduced potency
	Blood: dextrans	Rouleaux formation Cross-matching difficulties
	Plastic: glyceryl trinitrate	Adsorption to plastic
	Sevoflurane: soda lime	Compound A
Pharmacokinetic	Opioids: most drugs	Delayed oral absorption
	Warfarin: NSAIDs	↑ Free warfarin
	Barbiturates: warfarin	↑ Warfarin metabolism
	Neostigmine: succinylcholine	↓ Succinylcholine metabolism
Pharmacodynamic	Volatiles: opioids	↓ MAC
	Volatiles: benzodiazepines	↓ MAC
	Volatiles: N_2O	↓ MAC
	Volatiles: muscle relaxants	↑ Relaxation
	Morphine: naloxone	Reversal (receptor antagonism)
	Muscle relaxants: neostigmine	↑ Relaxation

binding (see above) is a common cause of drug interaction. We have discussed drug metabolism in some detail and there are many potential sites in this process where interactions can occur (e.g. competition for enzyme systems, enzyme inhibition or induction).

Pharmacodynamic

This is the most frequent type of interaction in anaesthetic practice. A typical anaesthetic is a series of pharmacodynamic interactions. These may be adverse (e.g. increased respiratory depression with opioids and volatile agents) or advantageous (e.g. reversal of muscle relaxation with neostigmine). An understanding of the many subtle pharmacodynamic interactions in modern anaesthesia accounts for much of the difference in the quality of anaesthesia and recovery associated with the experienced compared with the novice anaesthetist.

VOLATILE ANAESTHETIC AGENTS

Mechanism of Action

The exact mechanism of action of volatile anaesthetic agents is at present unknown. Potency is, in general, related to lipid solubility (Meyer-Overton relationship, Table 1.3) and this has given rise to the concept of volatile agents dissolving in the lipid cell membrane in a non-specific manner, disrupting membrane function and thereby influencing the function of proteins, e.g. ion channels. However, it is now appreciated that volatile agents affect neuronal function as a consequence of binding to specific protein sites (e.g. $GABA_A$ receptor).

Potency

The potency of volatile agents is defined in terms of minimum alveolar concentration (MAC). MAC is the alveolar concentration of a volatile agent which produces no movement in 50% of spontaneously breathing patients after skin incision. MAC is inversely related to lipid solubility (Table 1.3).

Onset of Action

When considering onset of action of volatile agents, there is a fundamental difference compared with intravenous agents. Effects of non-volatile drugs are related to plasma or tissue concentrations; this is not so with volatile agents. Partial pressure of the volatile agent is important, not concentration. If a volatile agent is highly soluble in blood, partial pressure increases slowly because large amounts dissolve in the blood. Consequently, onset of anaesthesia is slow with agents soluble in blood and rapid with agents which are relatively insoluble. The same applies to recovery from anaesthesia. Table 1.4 lists the most commonly used inhaled agents (in order of speed of onset) and their relative blood/gas solubilities.

Alveolar partial pressure (P_A) is assumed to be equivalent to cerebral artery partial pressure and therefore depth of anaesthesia. At a fixed inspired partial pressure (P_I), the rate at which P_A approaches P_I is related to speed of onset of effect (Fig. 1.9). This is rapid with agents of low blood solubility (e.g. sevoflurane) and relatively slow with more soluble agents (e.g. halothane).

Clearly, solubility of the agent in blood is a major determinant of the speed of onset of anaesthesia, but other factors can have significant effects. The rate of delivery of the agent to the alveoli is important;

TABLE 1.3		
MAC in Oxygen and Lipid Solubility (Expressed as Oil/Gas Solubility Coefficient)		
Agent	*MAC (%) in O_2*	*Oil/Gas Solubility*
N_2O	104	1.4
Desflurane	6.0	18.7
Sevoflurane	1.8	47
Isoflurane	1.17	98
Halothane	0.75	220

TABLE 1.4	
Solubility of Inhaled Anaesthetic Agents in Blood (Expressed as Blood/Gas Solubility Coefficients)	
Agent	*Blood/Gas Solubility Coefficient*
Desflurane	0.42
N_2O	0.47
Sevoflurane	0.68
Isoflurane	1.4
Halothane	2.3

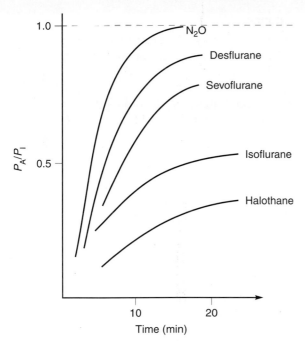

FIGURE 1.9 ■ The rate at which P_A reaches P_I is related to the speed of induction of anaesthesia. Agents insoluble in blood equilibrate more rapidly.

therefore increasing P_I by adjusting the vaporizer (a factor limited with some agents by irritant effects on the airway in spontaneously breathing patients), reducing apparatus dead space and increasing alveolar ventilation increase speed of induction of anaesthesia. If cardiac output is reduced, relatively less agent is removed from the alveolus and P_A increases towards P_I more rapidly. Consequently, induction of anaesthesia is more rapid in patients with reduced cardiac output. Both rate of delivery and cardiac output have particularly significant effects with agents that are relatively soluble in blood but less so with insoluble agents.

Ventilation/perfusion mismatch may reduce the speed of induction, an effect more significant in agents of low solubility. For example, if one lung is collapsed (i.e. perfused but not ventilated) increasing ventilation or inspired concentration of agents such as halothane helps to compensate. However, this is not the case for agents such as sevoflurane.

FURTHER READING

Calvey, N., Williams, N., 2008. Principles and practice of pharmacology for anaesthetists, fifth ed. Wiley-Blackwell, Oxford.

2 INHALATIONAL ANAESTHETIC AGENTS

■ ■ ■ ■ ■ ■ ■ ■ ■ ■ ■ ■

V olatile and gaseous anaesthetic agents are used widely for maintenance of anaesthesia and, under some circumstances, for induction of anaesthesia. In many situations, it is appropriate to use a mixture of 66% N_2O in oxygen and a small concentration of a volatile agent to maintain anaesthesia, although for reasons discussed below there are occasions when an anaesthetist might wish actively to avoid the use of nitrous oxide.

PROPERTIES OF THE IDEAL INHALATIONAL ANAESTHETIC AGENT

- It should have a pleasant odour, be non-irritant to the respiratory tract and allow pleasant and rapid induction of anaesthesia.
- It should possess a low blood/gas solubility, which permits rapid induction of and rapid recovery from anaesthesia.
- It should be chemically stable in storage and should not interact with the material of anaesthetic circuits or with soda lime.
- It should be neither flammable nor explosive.
- It should be capable of producing unconsciousness with analgesia and preferably some degree of muscle relaxation.
- It should be sufficiently potent to allow the use of high inspired oxygen concentrations when necessary.
- It should not be metabolized in the body, be non-toxic and not provoke allergic reactions.
- It should produce minimal depression of the cardiovascular and respiratory systems and should not interact with other drugs used commonly during anaesthesia, e.g. pressor agents or catecholamines.
- It should be completely inert and eliminated completely and rapidly in an unchanged form via the lungs.
- It should be easy to administer using standard vaporizers.
- It should not be epileptogenic or raise intracranial pressure.

None of the inhalational anaesthetic agents approaches the standards required of the ideal agent.

Minimum Alveolar Concentration (MAC)

MAC is the minimum alveolar concentration (in volumes per cent) of an anaesthetic at 1 atmosphere absolute (ata) which prevents movement to a standard surgical stimulus in 50% of the population. Anaesthesia is related to the partial pressure of an inhalational agent in the brain rather than its percentage concentration in alveoli, but the term MAC has gained widespread acceptance as an index of anaesthetic potency because it can be measured. It may be applied to all inhalational anaesthetics and it permits comparison of different agents. However, it represents only one point on a dose–response curve; 1 MAC of one agent is equivalent in anaesthetic potency to 1 MAC of another, but it does not follow that the agents are equipotent at 2 MAC. Nevertheless, in general terms, 0.5 MAC of one agent in combination with 0.5 MAC of another approximates to 1 MAC in total.

The MAC values for the anaesthetic agents quoted in Table 2.1 were determined experimentally in humans (volunteers) breathing a mixture of the agent in oxygen. MAC values vary under the following circumstances:

TABLE 2.1 Comparison of Modern Volatile Anaesthetic Agents					
	Halothane	Enflurane	Isoflurane	Desflurane	Sevoflurane
Molecular weight (Da)	197	184.5	184.5	168	200
Boiling point (°C)	50	56	49	23.5	58.5
Blood/gas partition coefficient	2.5	1.9	1.4	0.42	0.68
Oil/gas partition coefficient	224	98	98	18.7	47
MAC (in oxygen) %	0.75	1.68	1.15	6.0	1.7–2.0
Preservative	Thymol	None	None	None	None
Stability in CO_2 absorbers	?Unstable	Stable	Stable	Stable	Unstable

Factors Which Lead to a Reduction in MAC

- Sedative drugs such as premedication agents, analgesics
- Nitrous oxide
- Increasing age
- Drugs which affect neurotransmitter release such as methyldopa, pancuronium and clonidine
- Higher atmospheric pressure, as anaesthetic potency is related to partial pressure – e.g. MAC for sevoflurane is 2.0% (2.03 kPa) at a pressure of 1 ata, but 1.0% (still 2.03 kPa) at 2 ata
- Hypotension
- Hypothermia
- Myxoedema
- Pregnancy.

Factors Which Increase MAC

- Decreasing age
- Pyrexia
- Induced sympathoadrenal stimulation, e.g. hypercapnia
- The presence of ephedrine, or amphetamine
- Thyrotoxicosis
- Chronic alcohol ingestion.

Mechanisms of Action

General anaesthetics act by the potentiation of inhibitory neurotransmitter pathways in the CNS, in particular by potentiation of $GABA_A$ and glycine receptors, and inhibition of excitatory pathways such as NMDA. Both $GABA_A$ and glycine receptors are associated with chloride channels, and binding of the ligand allows entry of chloride into the neurone causing membrane hyperpolarization. General anaesthetics (volatile agents, propofol, etomidate and thiopental) bind to the β subunit of the $GABA_A$-chloride receptor complex. Central nicotinic acetylcholine receptors, potassium and sodium channels are also activated by clinically relevant concentrations of volatile anaesthetic agents. This can reduce presynaptic action potentials and reduce neurotransmitter release, and may also contribute to their mechanism of action.

Individual Anaesthetic Agents

Physical properties of the inhalational anaesthetic agents are summarized in Appendix B, II. The structural formulae of the agents discussed in this chapter are shown in Figure 2.1.

AGENTS IN COMMON CLINICAL USE

In Western countries, it is customary to use one of the four modern volatile anaesthetic agents – isoflurane, desflurane, sevoflurane or halothane – vaporized in a mixture of nitrous oxide in oxygen or air and oxygen. The use of halothane has declined because of medicolegal pressure relating to the very rare occurrence of hepatotoxicity. The use of sevoflurane has increased rapidly, particularly in paediatric anaesthesia because of its superior quality as an inhalational induction agent. Desflurane produces rapid recovery from anaesthesia, but it is very irritant to the airway and is therefore not used as an inhalational induction agent.

Ethers

Diethyl ether

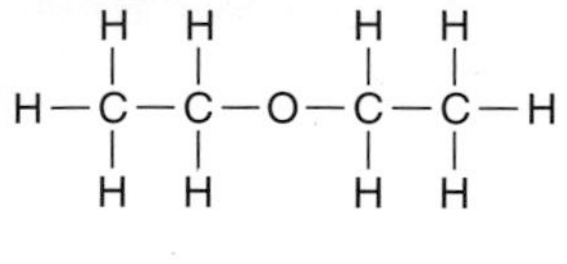

$$H-\overset{\displaystyle H}{\underset{\displaystyle H}{C}}-\overset{\displaystyle H}{\underset{\displaystyle H}{C}}-O-\overset{\displaystyle H}{\underset{\displaystyle H}{C}}-\overset{\displaystyle H}{\underset{\displaystyle H}{C}}-H$$

Desflurane

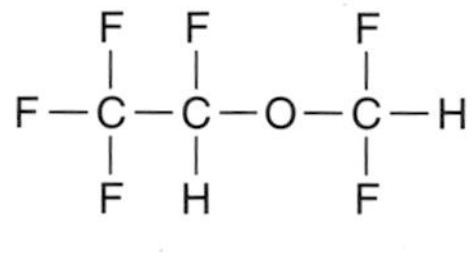

$$F-\overset{\displaystyle F}{\underset{\displaystyle F}{C}}-\overset{\displaystyle F}{\underset{\displaystyle H}{C}}-O-\overset{\displaystyle F}{\underset{\displaystyle F}{C}}-H$$

Enflurane

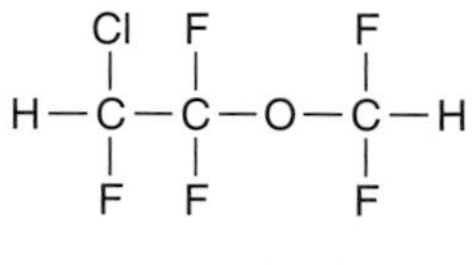

$$H-\overset{\displaystyle Cl}{\underset{\displaystyle F}{C}}-\overset{\displaystyle F}{\underset{\displaystyle F}{C}}-O-\overset{\displaystyle F}{\underset{\displaystyle F}{C}}-H$$

Isoflurane

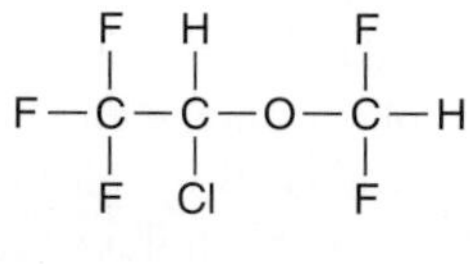

$$F-\overset{\displaystyle F}{\underset{\displaystyle F}{C}}-\overset{\displaystyle H}{\underset{\displaystyle Cl}{C}}-O-\overset{\displaystyle F}{\underset{\displaystyle F}{C}}-H$$

Sevoflurane

$$\begin{array}{c} F \\ | \\ F-C-F \quad H \\ | \quad\quad | \\ H-C-O-C-F \\ | \quad\quad | \\ F-C-F \quad H \\ | \\ F \end{array}$$

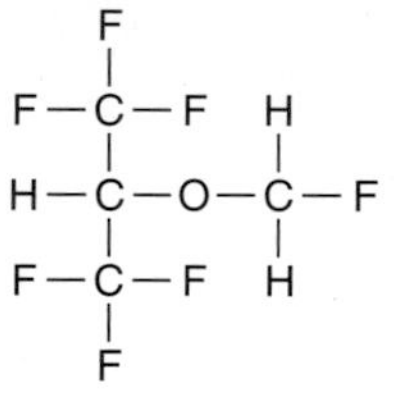

Halogenated hydrocarbons

Halothane

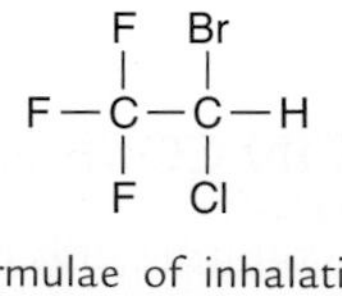

$$F-\overset{\displaystyle F}{\underset{\displaystyle F}{C}}-\overset{\displaystyle Br}{\underset{\displaystyle Cl}{C}}-H$$

FIGURE 2.1 ■ Structural formulae of inhalational anaesthetic agents.

The following account of these agents, with a comparison of their pharmacological properties, may tend to exaggerate the differences between them. However, an equally satisfactory anaesthetic may be administered in the majority of patients with any of the four agents.

Isoflurane

Isoflurane (1-chloro-2,2,2-trifluoroethyl difluoromethyl ether) is an isomer of enflurane and was synthesized in 1965. Clinical studies were undertaken in 1970, but because of early laboratory reports of carcinogenesis (which were not confirmed subsequently) it was not approved by the Food and Drug Administration in the United States until 1980.

Physical Properties

Isoflurane is a colourless, volatile liquid with a slightly pungent odour. It is stable and does not react with metal or other substances. It does not require preservatives. Isoflurane is non-flammable in clinical concentrations. The MAC of isoflurane is 1.15% in oxygen and 0.56% in 70% nitrous oxide.

Uptake and Distribution

Isoflurane has a low blood/gas solubility of 1.4 and thus alveolar concentrations equilibrate fairly rapidly with inspired concentrations. The alveolar (or arterial) partial pressure of isoflurane increases to 50% of the inspired partial pressure within 4–8 min, and to 60% by 15 min (Fig. 2.2). However, the rate of induction is limited by the pungency of the vapour and in clinical practice may be no faster than that achieved with halothane. The incidence of coughing or breath-holding on induction is significantly greater with isoflurane than with halothane. It is not an ideal agent to use for inhalational induction. The rate of recovery is slower than that associated with desflurane or sevoflurane, but more rapid than after administration of halothane (Fig. 2.3).

Metabolism

Approximately 0.17% of the absorbed dose is metabolized. Metabolism takes place predominantly in the form of oxidation to produce difluoromethanol and trifluoroacetic acid; the former breaks down to formic acid and fluoride. Because of the minimal metabolism, only very small concentrations of serum fluoride ions are found, even after prolonged administration. The minimal metabolism renders hepatic and renal toxicity most unlikely.

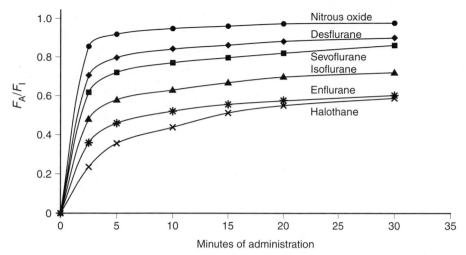

FIGURE 2.2 ■ Ratio of alveolar (F_A) to inspired (F_I) fractional concentration of nitrous oxide, desflurane, sevoflurane, isoflurane, enflurane and halothane in the first 30 min of anaesthesia. The plot of F_A/F_I expresses the rapidity with which alveolar concentration equilibrates with inspired concentration. It is most rapid for agents with a low blood/gas partition coefficient.

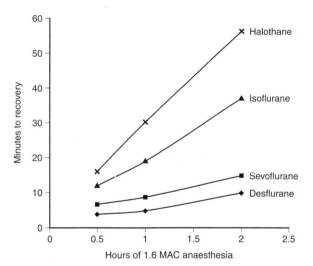

FIGURE 2.3 ■ Rapidity of recovery from anaesthesia is inversely proportional to the solubility of the anaesthetic: the most rapid recovery is with the least soluble anaesthetic (desflurane). The difference is amplified by duration of anaesthesia. Note that the difference in time of recovery between the least (desflurane) and most soluble anaesthetic (halothane) is greater after 2 h of anaesthesia than after 0.5 h of anaesthesia.

Respiratory System

In common with other modern volatile agents, it causes dose-dependent depression of ventilation (Fig. 2.4); there is a decrease in tidal volume but an increase in ventilatory rate in the absence of opioid drugs. Isoflurane causes some respiratory irritation. This makes inhalational induction with isoflurane difficult.

Cardiovascular System

In vitro, isoflurane is a myocardial depressant, but in clinical use there is less depression of cardiac output than with halothane or enflurane (Fig. 2.5). Systemic hypotension occurs predominantly as a result of a reduction in systemic vascular resistance (Figs 2.6, 2.7). Arrhythmias are uncommon and there is little sensitization of the myocardium to catecholamines (Fig. 2.8).

In addition to dilating systemic arterioles, isoflurane causes coronary vasodilatation. In the past there has been some controversy regarding the safety of isoflurane in patients with coronary artery disease because of the possibility that the coronary steal syndrome may be induced; dilatation in normal coronary arteries offers a low resistance to flow and may reduce perfusion through stenosed neighbouring vessels. It has been shown that isoflurane affects small arterioles (which makes coronary steal a theoretical possibility), but this does not appear to be of any clinical significance. Production of myocardial ischaemia in clinical practice may be a result of many factors in addition to coronary vasodilatation, including tachycardia, hypotension,

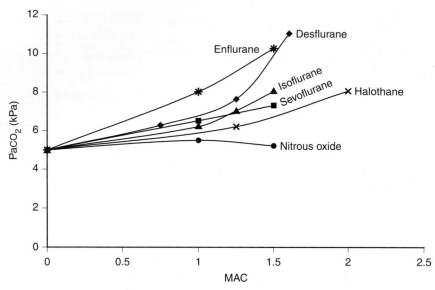

FIGURE 2.4 ■ Effects on PaCO$_2$ of halothane, enflurane, isoflurane, sevoflurane, desflurane and nitrous oxide at equivalent MAC during spontaneous ventilation by healthy volunteers. (Nitrous oxide was administered in a hyperbaric chamber.)

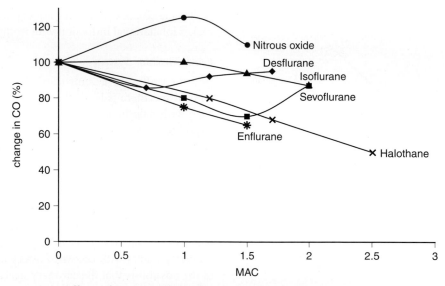

FIGURE 2.5 ■ Comparative effects of nitrous oxide, isoflurane, halothane, enflurane, desflurane and sevoflurane on cardiac output (CO) in healthy volunteers.

increase in left ventricular end-diastolic pressure and reduced ventricular compliance. Attention should be directed to these factors before a diagnosis of isoflurane-induced coronary steal is considered.

Uterus

Isoflurane has an effect on the pregnant uterus similar to that of halothane.

Central Nervous System

Low concentrations of isoflurane do not cause any change in cerebral blood flow at normocapnia. In this respect, the drug is superior to halothane, which causes cerebral vasodilatation. However, higher inspired concentrations of isoflurane cause vasodilatation and increase cerebral blood flow. It does not cause seizure activity on the EEG.

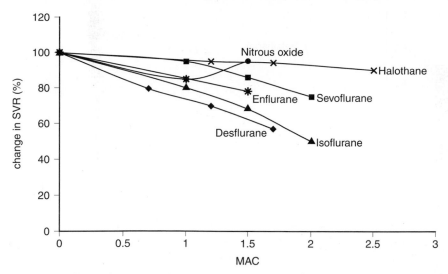

FIGURE 2.6 ■ Comparative effects of nitrous oxide, halothane, enflurane, isoflurane, sevoflurane and desflurane on systemic vascular resistance (SVR) in healthy volunteers.

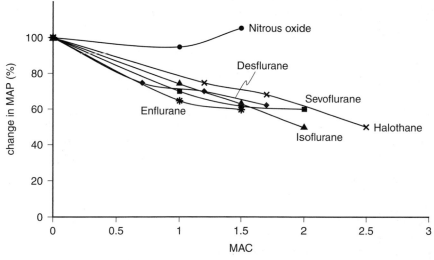

FIGURE 2.7 ■ Comparative effects of nitrous oxide, halothane, enflurane, isoflurane, sevoflurane and desflurane on mean arterial pressure (MAP) in healthy volunteers.

Muscle Relaxation

Isoflurane causes dose-dependent depression of neuro-muscular transmission with potentiation of non-depolarizing neuromuscular blocking drugs.

In summary, the advantages of isoflurane are:

- rapid recovery
- minimal biotransformation with little risk of he-patic or renal toxicity
- very low risk of arrhythmias

- muscle relaxation.

Its disadvantage is:

- a pungent odour which makes inhalational induc-tion relatively unpleasant, particularly in children.

Desflurane

Between 1959 and 1966, Terrell and his associates at Ohio Medical Products synthesized more than 700 compounds to try to produce improved inhalational

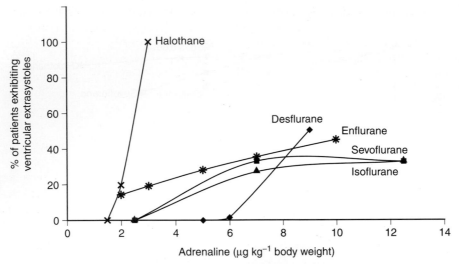

FIGURE 2.8 ■ Cumulative plots representing dose of subcutaneous adrenaline required to produce ventricular extrasystoles in normocapnic patients receiving 1.25 MAC of halothane, enflurane, isoflurane, sevoflurane or desflurane.

anaesthetic agents. Two of these products were the halogenated methyl ethyl ethers, isoflurane and enflurane, which became widely used. Some of the original 700 products were re-examined many years later. Many were discarded for a variety of reasons. One of these (the 653rd) was difficult to synthesize because of a potentially explosive step using elemental fluorine and it had a vapour pressure close to 1 atmosphere. However, because it was predicted to have a low solubility in blood and hence would allow rapid recovery, it was re-examined with heightened interest. This product became known as desflurane. Desflurane was first used in humans in 1988 and it became available for general clinical use in the UK in 1993. Its structure (CHF_2–O–CHF–CF_3) differs from that of isoflurane (CHF_2–O–CHCl–CF_3) only in the substitution of fluorine for chlorine.

Physical Properties

It is a colourless agent, which is stored in amber-coloured bottles without preservative. It is not broken down by soda lime, light or metals. It is non-flammable.

Desflurane has a boiling point of 23.5 °C and a vapour pressure of 88.5 kPa (664 mmHg) at 20 °C and therefore it cannot be used in a standard vaporizer. A special vaporizer (the TEC-6) has been developed which requires a source of electric power to heat and pressurize it.

The MAC of desflurane is approximately 6% in oxygen (3% in 60% nitrous oxide). As with all volatile

agents, its MAC is higher in children (9–10% in the neonate in oxygen, 7% in 60% nitrous oxide).

It has an ethereal and pungent odour.

Uptake and Distribution

Desflurane has a blood/gas partition coefficient of 0.42, almost the same as that of nitrous oxide. The rate of equilibration of alveolar with inspired concentrations of desflurane is virtually identical to that for nitrous oxide (Fig. 2.2). Induction of anaesthesia is therefore extremely rapid in theory but limited somewhat by its pungent nature. However, it is possible to alter the depth of anaesthesia very rapidly and the rate of recovery of anaesthesia is faster than that following any other volatile anaesthetic agent (Fig. 2.3).

Metabolism

There is very little defluorination of desflurane, and after prolonged anaesthesia there is only a very small increase in serum and urine trifluoroacetic acid concentrations. Approximately 0.02% of inhaled desflurane is metabolized in the body.

Respiratory System

Desflurane causes respiratory depression to a degree similar to that of isoflurane up to a MAC of 1.5. It increases $PaCO_2$ (Fig. 2.4) and decreases the ventilatory response to imposed increases in $PaCO_2$. It is irritant to the upper respiratory tract, particularly at concentrations greater than 6%. It is therefore not recommended for gaseous induction of anaesthesia because it causes coughing, breath-holding and laryngospasm.

Cardiovascular Effects

Desflurane appears to have two distinct actions on the cardiovascular system. Firstly, its main actions are those which are similar to isoflurane: dose-related decreases in systemic vascular resistance, myocardial contractility and mean arterial pressure (Figs 2.5–2.7). Heart rate is unchanged at lower steady-state concentrations, but increases with higher concentrations (Fig. 2.9). Addition of nitrous oxide maintains heart rate unchanged. Cardiac output tends to be maintained as with isoflurane. The second cardiovascular action occurs when its inspired concentration is increased rapidly to greater than 1 MAC. In the absence of premedicant drugs, this increases sympathetic activity, leading to increased heart rate and arterial pressure. Experimental studies in animals have not detected a coronary steal phenomenon. Desflurane, in common with isoflurane and sevoflurane, does not sensitize the myocardium to catecholamines (Fig. 2.8).

Central Nervous System

The effects of desflurane are similar to those of isoflurane. It depresses the EEG in a dose-related manner. It does not cause seizure activity at any level of anaesthesia, with or without hypocapnia. Desflurane decreases cerebrovascular resistance and increases intracranial pressure in a dose-related manner. In dogs, it increases cerebral blood flow at deep levels of anaesthesia if systemic arterial pressure is maintained.

Musculoskeletal System

Desflurane causes muscle relaxation in a dose-related manner. Concentrations exceeding 1 MAC produce fade in response to tetanic stimulation of the ulnar nerve. It enhances the effect of muscle relaxants. Studies in susceptible swine indicate that desflurane may trigger malignant hyperthermia.

Therefore, in summary, desflurane offers some advantages over other agents:

- it has a low blood solubility; therefore it offers more precise control of maintenance of anaesthesia and rapid recovery.
- it is minimally biodegradable and therefore non-toxic to the liver and kidney.
- it does not cause convulsive activity on EEG.

However, it has some significant drawbacks:

- it cannot be used for inhalational induction because of its irritant effects on the airway.
- it causes tachycardia at higher concentrations.
- it requires a special vaporizer. Although the TEC-6 vaporizer is reasonably easy to use, it is more

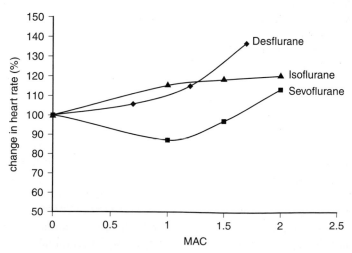

FIGURE 2.9 ■ Comparative effects of isoflurane, sevoflurane and desflurane on heart rate in healthy volunteers.

complex than the more conventional vaporizers and the potential for failure may be higher.

■ it is expensive.

Sevoflurane

Sevoflurane (fluoromethyl-2,2,2-trifluoro-1-ethyl ether) was first synthesized in 1968 and its clinical use reported in 1971. The initial development was slow because of some apparent toxic effects, which were found later to be caused by flawed experimental design. After its first use in volunteers in 1981, further work was delayed again because of problems of biotransformation and stability with soda lime. The drug has been available for general clinical use since 1990.

Physical Properties

It is non-flammable and has a pleasant smell. The blood/gas partition coefficient of sevoflurane is 0.69, which is about half that of isoflurane (1.43) and closer to those of desflurane (0.42) and nitrous oxide (0.44). The MAC value of sevoflurane in adults is between 1.7 and 2% in oxygen and 0.66% in 60% nitrous oxide. The MAC, in common with other volatile agents, is higher in children (2.6% in oxygen and 2.0% in nitrous oxide) and neonates (3.3%) and it is reduced in the elderly (1.48%). It is stable and is stored in amber-coloured bottles. In the presence of water, it undergoes some hydrolysis and this reaction also occurs with soda lime.

Uptake and Distribution

Sevoflurane has a low blood/gas partition coefficient and therefore the rate of equilibration between alveolar and inspired concentrations is faster than that for halothane or isoflurane but slower than that for desflurane (Fig. 2.2). It is non-irritant to the upper respiratory tract and therefore the rate of induction of anaesthesia should be faster than that with any of the other agents.

Because of its higher partition coefficients in vessel-rich tissues, muscle and fat than corresponding values for desflurane, the rate of recovery is slower than that after desflurane anaesthesia (Fig. 2.3).

Metabolism

Approximately 5% of the absorbed dose is metabolized in the liver to two main metabolites. The major breakdown product is hexafluoroisopropanol, an organic fluoride molecule which is excreted in the urine as a glucuronide conjugate. Although this molecule is potentially hepatotoxic, conjugation of hexafluoroisopropanol occurs so rapidly that clinically significant liver damage seems theoretically impossible. The second breakdown product is inorganic fluoride ion. The mean peak fluoride ion concentration after 60 min of anaesthesia at 1 MAC is $22\,\mu mol\,L^{-1}$, which is significantly higher than that after an equivalent dose of isoflurane. The metabolism of sevoflurane is catalysed by the 2E1 isoform of cytochrome P450 which may be induced by phenobarbital, isoniazid and ethanol and inhibited by disulfiram.

Respiratory System

The drug is non-irritant to the upper respiratory tract. It produces dose-dependent ventilatory depression, reduces respiratory drive in response to hypoxaemia and increases carbon dioxide partial pressure to a similar degree to other volatile agents (Fig. 2.4). The ventilatory depression associated with sevoflurane may result from a combination of central depression of medullary respiratory neurones and depression of diaphragmatic function and contractility. It relaxes bronchial smooth muscle but not as effectively as halothane.

Cardiovascular System

The properties of sevoflurane are similar to those of isoflurane, with slightly smaller effects on heart rate (Fig. 2.9) and less coronary vasodilatation. It decreases arterial pressure (Fig. 2.7) mainly by reducing peripheral vascular resistance (Fig. 2.6), but cardiac output is well maintained over the normal anaesthetic maintenance doses (Fig. 2.5). There is mild myocardial depression resulting from its effect on calcium channels. Sevoflurane does not differ from isoflurane in its sensitization of the myocardium to exogenous catecholamines (Fig. 2.8). It is a less potent coronary arteriolar dilator and does not appear to cause coronary steal. Sevoflurane is associated with a lower heart rate and therefore helps to reduce myocardial oxygen consumption.

Central Nervous System

CNS effects are similar to those of isoflurane and desflurane. Intracranial pressure increases at high inspired concentrations of sevoflurane but this effect is minimal over the 0.5–1.0 MAC range. It decreases cerebral vascular resistance and cerebral metabolic rate. It does not cause excitatory effects on the EEG.

Renal System

The peak concentration of inorganic fluoride after sevoflurane is similar to that after enflurane anaesthesia and there is a positive correlation between duration of exposure and the peak concentration of fluoride ions. Serum fluoride concentrations greater than $50 \mu mol L^{-1}$ have been reported. However, renal toxicity following anaesthesia with sevoflurane does not appear to be related to inorganic fluoride concentrations as opposed to that associated with methoxyflurane. The apparent lack of renal toxicity with sevoflurane may be related to its rapid elimination from the body. This reduces the total amount of drug available for *in vivo* metabolism.

Renal blood flow is well preserved with sevoflurane.

Musculoskeletal System

Sevoflurane potentiates non-depolarizing muscle relaxants to a similar extent to isoflurane. Sevoflurane may trigger malignant hyperthermia in susceptible patients.

Obstetric Use

There are limited data on the use of sevoflurane in the obstetric population.

Interaction with Carbon Dioxide Absorbers

Sevoflurane is absorbed and degraded by both soda lime and Baralyme. When mixed with soda lime in artificial situations, five breakdown products are identified, which are termed compounds A, B, C, D and E. These products are thought to be toxic in rats, primarily causing renal, hepatic and cerebral damage. However, in clinical situations, it is mainly compound A and, to a lesser extent, compound B that are produced. The evidence suggests that the concentration of compound A produced is well below the level that is toxic to animals. The use of Baralyme is associated with production of higher concentrations of compound A and this may be related to the higher temperature which is attained when Baralyme is used. The presence of moisture reduces compound A formation. The concentration of compound A is highest during low-flow anaesthesia ($<2 L min^{-1}$) and is reduced by increasing fresh gas flow rate. The toxicity of sevoflurane in combination with carbon dioxide absorbers is probably more a theoretical than a clinical problem.

In summary, sevoflurane is a newer inhalational anaesthetic agent which offers many advantages over other volatile agents. These are:

- smooth, fast induction
- rapid recovery
- ease of use, requiring conventional vaporizers (particularly when compared with desflurane).

Its disadvantages are:

- production of potentially toxic metabolites in the body (more a theoretical problem)
- instability with carbon dioxide absorbers
- relative expense.

Halothane

Halothane (2-bromo-2-chloro-1,1,1-trifluoroethane) was synthesized in 1951 and introduced into clinical practice in the UK in 1956. It is a colourless liquid with a relatively pleasant smell. It is decomposed by light. The addition of 0.01% thymol and storage in amber-coloured bottles renders it stable. Although it is decomposed by soda lime, it may be used safely with this mixture. It corrodes metals in vaporizers and breathing systems. In the presence of moisture, it corrodes aluminium, tin, lead, magnesium and alloys. It should be stored in a closed container away from light and heat.

Uptake and Distribution

Halothane has a blood/gas solubility coefficient of 2.5, which is the highest of all the modern agents. It is not irritant to the airway and therefore inhalational induction with halothane is relatively fast compared with either desflurane or isoflurane. However, it may take at least 30 min for the alveolar inspired concentration to reach 50% of the inspired concentration (Fig. 2.2); this is slower than for the other agents. As with all the volatile agents, it is customary to use the technique of 'over-pressure' and induce halothane anaesthesia with concentrations two to three times higher than the MAC value; the inspired concentration is reduced when a stable level of anaesthesia has been achieved. The MAC of halothane in oxygen is approximately 1.1% in the neonate, 0.95% in the infant, 0.9% at 1–2 years, 0.75% at 40 years (0.29 in 70% nitrous oxide) and 0.65% at 80 years.

Recovery from halothane anaesthesia is slower than with the other agents because of its high blood/gas solubility, and recovery is prolonged with increasing duration of anaesthesia (Fig. 2.3).

Metabolism

Approximately 20% of halothane is metabolized in the liver, usually by oxidative pathways. The end products are excreted in the urine. The major metabolites are bromine, chlorine, trifluoroacetic acid and trifluoro-acetylethanol amide.

A small proportion of halothane may undergo reductive metabolism, particularly in the presence of hypoxaemia and when the hepatic microsomal enzymes have been stimulated by enzyme-inducing agents such as phenobarbital. Reductive metabolism may result in the formation of reactive metabolites and fluoride, although normally serum fluoride ion concentrations are considerably lower than those likely to induce renal dysfunction.

Respiratory System

Halothane is non-irritant and pleasant to breathe during induction of anaesthesia. There is rapid loss of pharyngeal and laryngeal reflexes and inhibition of salivary and bronchial secretions. In the unpremedicated subject, halothane anaesthesia is associated with an increase in ventilatory rate and reduction in tidal volume. $PaCO_2$ increases as the depth of halothane anaesthesia increases (Fig. 2.4).

Halothane causes a dose-dependent decrease in mucociliary function, which may persist for several hours after anaesthesia. This may contribute to postoperative sputum retention.

Halothane antagonizes bronchospasm and reduces airway resistance in patients with bronchoconstriction, possibly by central inhibition of reflex bronchoconstriction and relaxation of bronchial smooth muscle. It has been suggested that halothane exerts a β-mimetic effect on bronchial muscle.

Cardiovascular System

Halothane is a potent depressant of myocardial contractility and myocardial metabolic activity as a result of inhibition of glucose uptake by myocardial cells. During controlled ventilation, halothane anaesthesia is associated with dose-related depression of cardiac output (by decrease in myocardial contractility) with little effect on peripheral resistance (Figs 2.5, 2.6). Thus, there is a reduction in arterial pressure (Fig. 2.7) and an increase in right atrial pressure. In spontaneously breathing patients, some of these effects may be offset by a small increase in $PaCO_2$ which leads to a reduction in systemic vascular resistance and a shift in cardiac output back towards baseline values as a result of indirect sympatho-adrenal stimulation.

The hypotensive effect of halothane is augmented by a reduction in heart rate, which commonly accompanies halothane anaesthesia. Antagonism of the bradycardia by administration of atropine frequently leads to an increase in arterial pressure.

The reduction in myocardial contractility is associated with reductions in myocardial oxygen demand and coronary blood flow. Provided that undue elevations in left ventricular diastolic pressure and undue hypotension do not occur, halothane may be advantageous in patients with coronary artery disease because of the reduced oxygen demand caused by a low heart rate and decreased contractility.

The depressant effects of halothane on cardiac output are augmented in the presence of β-blockade.

Arrhythmias are very common during halothane anaesthesia and far more frequent than with any of the other agents. Arrhythmias are produced by:

- increased myocardial excitability augmented by the presence of hypercapnia, hypoxaemia or increased circulating catecholamines
- bradycardia caused by central vagal stimulation.

During local infiltration with local anaesthetic solutions containing Adrenaline, multifocal ventricular extrasystoles and sinus tachycardia have been observed and cardiac arrest has been reported. Thus, caution should be exercised when these solutions are used. The following recommendations have been made:

- avoid hypoxaemia and hypercapnia
- avoid concentrations of Adrenaline greater than 1 in 100 000
- avoid a dosage in adults exceeding 10 ml of 1 in 100 000 Adrenaline in 10 min (i.e. 100 μg) or 30 mL h^{-1} (300 μg).

Approximately 20% of patients breathing 1.25 MAC of halothane and who receive subcutaneous infiltration of $2\,\mu g\,kg^{-1}$ Adrenaline exhibit ventricular ectopics. This increases to 100% of patients receiving $2.5–3\,\mu g\,kg^{-1}$ (Fig. 2.8).

Patients undergoing dental surgery with halothane anaesthesia are particularly prone to developing arrhythmias.

Central Nervous System

Halothane produces anaesthesia without analgesia. Cerebral blood flow and intracranial pressure are raised. It does not cause seizure activity on EEG.

Gastrointestinal Tract

Gastrointestinal motility is inhibited. Postoperative nausea and vomiting are seldom severe.

Uterus

Halothane relaxes uterine muscle and may cause postpartum haemorrhage. It is said that a concentration of less than 0.5% is not associated with increased blood loss during anaesthesia for Caesarean section, but this concentration causes increased blood loss during therapeutic abortion.

Skeletal Muscle

Halothane causes skeletal muscle relaxation and potentiates non-depolarizing relaxants. Postoperative shivering is common; this increases oxygen requirements and results in hypoxaemia unless oxygen is administered. Halothane may trigger malignant hyperthermia in susceptible patients.

Halothane-Associated Hepatic Dysfunction

There are two types of dysfunction which may occur after halothane anaesthesia. The first is mild and is associated with derangement in liver function tests. These changes are transient and generally resolve within a few days. Similar changes in liver function tests have also been reported after enflurane anaesthesia and, to a lesser extent, isoflurane anaesthesia.

This subclinical type of hepatic dysfunction, evidenced by an increase in glutathione-*S*-transferase (GST) concentrations, probably occurs as a result of metabolism of halothane in the liver, where it reacts with hepatic macromolecules, resulting in tissue necrosis, which is worsened by hypoxaemia.

The second type of hepatic dysfunction is extremely uncommon and takes the form of severe jaundice, progressing to fulminating hepatic necrosis. The mortality of this condition varies between 30 and 70%. The likelihood of this type of hepatic dysfunction is increased by repeated exposure to the drug. The mechanism of these changes is probably the formation of a hapten-protein complex. The hapten is probably one of the metabolites of halothane, notably trifluoroacetyl (TFA) halide, as antibodies to TFA proteins have been detected in patients who develop jaundice after halothane anaesthesia.

The incidence of type 2 liver dysfunction after halothane anaesthesia is extremely low – so low that it is extremely difficult to mount well-controlled studies of the condition, and consequently this whole subject has been an area of great controversy in the past. Nonetheless, as a result of this concern, the UK Committee on Safety of Medicines made the following recommendations in respect of halothane anaesthesia:

- a careful anaesthetic history should be taken to determine previous exposure and any previous reaction to halothane.
- repeated exposure to halothane within a period of 3 months should be avoided unless there are overriding clinical circumstances.
- a history of unexplained jaundice or pyrexia after previous exposure to halothane is an absolute contraindication to its future use in that patient.

The incidence of halothane hepatotoxicity in paediatric practice is extremely low, although there have been case reports in children. Nevertheless, halothane is still used in paediatric anaesthesia

In summary, halothane is a useful inhalational anaesthetic agent. Its main advantages are:

- smooth induction
- minimal stimulation of salivary and bronchial secretions
- bronchodilatation.

The disadvantages are:

- arrhythmias
- possibility of liver toxicity especially with repeated administrations
- slow recovery compared with newer agents (see Fig. 2.3).

Comparison of Isoflurane, Desflurane, Sevoflurane and Halothane

Pharmacokinetics

The rate of equilibration of alveolar with inspired concentrations is related to blood/gas solubility. The rate of uptake of desflurane is faster than that of any of the other volatile agents and similar to that of nitrous oxide (Fig. 2.2). Despite its low blood/gas solubility, the rate of induction of anaesthesia with desflurane (and isoflurane) may be reduced because of the pungent odour compared with the more pleasant odours of sevoflurane and halothane. Sevoflurane provides a smooth rapid induction and it has largely replaced halothane for induction in children. Potency, on the other hand, is related to the lower oil/water solubility. Sevoflurane and desflurane are less potent than the older agents, as reflected by their higher MAC values.

On recovery from anaesthesia, the rate of elimination of desflurane is faster than that for the other agents (Fig. 2.3).

Respiratory System

All inhalational agents cause dose-related respiratory depression. This results in reduced tidal volume, increased respiratory rate and reduced minute ventilation. $PaCO_2$ increases (Fig. 2.4). In unstimulated volunteers, desflurane causes greater ventilatory depression than isoflurane, halothane or sevoflurane. Nitrous oxide does not cause hypercapnia. Thus the reduction in inspired volatile anaesthetic concentration permitted by addition of nitrous oxide is associated with less ventilatory depression. In addition, surgical stimulation is responsible for considerable antagonism of ventilatory depression during anaesthesia and $PaCO_2$ does not normally reach the values shown in Figure 2.4 during surgery.

With all agents, depression of ventilation is associated with depression of whole body oxygen consumption and carbon dioxide production.

Halothane and, to a lesser extent, sevoflurane, causes bronchodilation.

Cardiovascular System

All the agents reduce arterial pressure because of reduced systemic vascular resistance and myocardial depression to varying degrees. Desflurane and isoflurane tend to maintain cardiac output, decreasing arterial pressure mainly by decreasing systemic vascular resistance. Halothane reduces arterial pressure principally by decreasing cardiac output with little effect on systemic vascular resistance.

Isoflurane and desflurane increase heart rate as a result of sympathetic stimulation, whereas halothane and sevoflurane reduce heart rate.

The data in Figures 2.5–2.7 and 2.9 were derived from studies in volunteers who were not subjected to surgical stimulation and in whom artificial ventilation was used to achieve normocapnia.

Some of the cardiovascular effects of these volatile agents are antagonized by the addition of nitrous oxide. In addition, during spontaneous ventilation, the modest hypercapnia which occurs with all agents also offsets some of the changes. With isoflurane, for example, cardiac output may be increased compared with pre-anaesthesia levels, although there is little effect on systemic arterial pressure.

Desflurane, isoflurane and sevoflurane do not sensitize the myocardium to exogenous catecholamines, but halothane predisposes to arrhythmias.

Isoflurane causes coronary vasodilatation and experimentally this was found to cause coronary steal syndrome but this has now been demonstrated to be of no clinical significance. Sevoflurane causes some coronary vasodilatation but does not appear to cause coronary steal syndrome. The other two agents do not cause any coronary vasodilatation.

Central Nervous System

All agents cause dose-related depression of cerebral activity. All the agents decrease cerebrovascular resistance and increase intracranial pressure in a dose-related manner.

Neuromuscular Junction

All agents produce muscle relaxation sufficient to perform lower abdominal surgery in spontaneously breathing thin subjects. In addition, there is potentiation of non-depolarizing muscle relaxants. In this respect, isoflurane, sevoflurane and desflurane are similar and cause markedly greater potentiation than that produced by halothane.

Uterus

Halothane and isoflurane relax uterine muscle in a dose-related manner. There is limited experience with desflurane and sevoflurane in the obstetric population. Sevoflurane appears to have similar uterine effects to isoflurane. In practice, isoflurane seems to be the standard volatile anaesthetic agent used for obstetric anaesthesia in the UK.

Metabolism

Halothane and sevoflurane are metabolized to potentially toxic metabolites and desflurane is the most resistant to metabolism. Halothane is associated with liver toxicity while sevoflurane is associated with production of inorganic fluoride ions.

Carbon Dioxide Absorbers

Sevoflurane and halothane react with soda lime, while the other two do not.

A comparison of other characteristics of the agents is shown in Tables 2.1 and 2.2.

TABLE 2.2
Systemic Effects of Volatile Agents

	Halothane	Enflurane	Isoflurane	Desflurane	Sevoflurane
Alveolar equilibration	Slow	Moderate	Moderate	Fast	Fast
Recovery	Slow	Moderate	Fast	Very fast	Fast
Cardiovascular system					
Heart rate	Reduced	Increased	Increased	Increased	Stable
Cardiac output	Reduced	Reduced	Slightly reduced	Stable to slightly reduced	Stable to slightly reduced
SVR	Stable	Slightly reduced	Reduced	Reduced	Reduced
MAP	Reduced	Reduced	Reduced	Reduced	Reduced
Sensitization of myocardium	Yes	Slight	No	No	No
Respiratory system					
Respiratory irritation	Nil	Minimal	Significant	Significant	Nil
Respiratory depression	Yes	Marked	Yes	Marked	Yes
Central nervous system					
Seizure activity on EEG	No	Yes	No	No	No
Renal system					
Renal toxic metabolites	No	Yes	No	No	Yes
Liver					
Hepatotoxicity	Yes	Yes	No	No	?Yes
Metabolism (%)	20	2.5	0.2	0.02	3–5
Musculoskeletal system					
Muscle weakness	Moderate	Moderate	Significant	Significant	Significant

SVR=systemic vascular resistance, MAP=mean arterial pressure.

AGENTS IN OCCASIONAL USE

Enflurane

Enflurane (2-chloro-1,1,2-trifluoroethyl difluoromethyl ether) was synthesized in 1963 and first evaluated clinically in 1966. It was introduced into clinical practice in the USA in 1971 but it is now used uncommonly in Western countries.

Physical Properties

Enflurane is a clear, colourless, volatile anaesthetic agent with a pleasant ethereal smell. It is non-flammable in clinical concentrations, stable with soda lime and metals and does not require preservatives. The MAC of enflurane is 1.68% in oxygen and 0.57% in 70% nitrous oxide.

Uptake and Distribution

Enflurane has a blood/gas solubility coefficient of 1.9, which is between that of halothane and isoflurane. Thus, induction of and recovery from anaesthesia are faster than halothane but slower than isoflurane, desflurane and sevoflurane (Fig. 2.2).

Metabolism

Approximately 2.5% of the absorbed dose is metabolized, predominantly to fluoride. In common with other ether anaesthetic agents, the presence of the ether bond imparts stability to the molecule.

Defluorination of enflurane is increased in patients treated with isoniazid, but not with a classic enzyme-inducing agent such as phenobarbital. Serum fluoride ion concentrations are greater after administration of enflurane to obese patients. Extensive studies have failed to demonstrate that the serum concentrations of fluoride ion reach toxic levels after enflurane anaesthesia. The plasma fluoride ion concentrations attained after enflurane anaesthesia are approximately $20\,\mu mol\,L^{-1}$ (which is below the $50\,\mu mol\,L^{-1}$ thought to be associated with renal damage after anaesthesia with methoxyflurane).

Respiratory System

Enflurane is non-irritant and does not increase salivary or bronchial secretions; thus inhalational induction is relatively pleasant and rapid.

In common with all other volatile anaesthetic agents, enflurane causes dose-dependent depression of alveolar ventilation with a reduction in tidal volume and an increase in ventilatory rate in the unpremedicated subject. This results in an increase in arterial PCO_2 (Fig. 2.4).

Cardiovascular System

Enflurane causes dose-dependent depression of myocardial contractility, leading to a reduction in cardiac output (Fig. 2.5). In association with a small reduction in systemic vascular resistance, this leads to a dose-dependent reduction in arterial pressure (Figs 2.6, 2.7). Because enflurane (unlike halothane) has no central vagal effects, hypotension leads to reflex tachycardia.

Enflurane anaesthesia is associated with a much smaller incidence of arrhythmias than halothane and much less sensitization of the myocardium to catecholamines, either endogenous or exogenous (Fig. 2.8).

Uterus

Enflurane relaxes uterine muscle in a dose-related manner.

Central Nervous System

Enflurane produces a dose-dependent depression of EEG activity, but at moderate to high concentrations (more than 3%) it produces epileptiform paroxysmal spike activity and burst suppression. These are accentuated by hypocapnia. Twitching of the face and arm muscles may occur occasionally. Enflurane should be avoided in the epileptic patient.

Muscle Relaxation

Enflurane produces dose-dependent muscle relaxation with potentiation of non-depolarizing neuromuscular blocking drugs to a greater extent than that produced by halothane. It may trigger malignant hyperthermia.

Hepatotoxicity

There have been several case reports of jaundice attributable to the use of enflurane, and derangement of liver enzymes also occurs after enflurane anaesthesia, although to a lesser extent than after halothane.

In summary, the advantages of enflurane are:

- low risk of hepatic dysfunction
- low incidence of arrhythmias.

Its disadvantages are:

- seizure activity on EEG
- its use in patients with pre-existing renal disease or in those taking enzyme-inducing drugs may be unwise.

Diethyl Ether

Because of its flammability, the use of ether has been abandoned in Western countries, but it is used widely in other parts of the world. It therefore warrants a brief description in this text.

It is a colourless, highly volatile liquid with a characteristic smell. It is flammable in air and explosive in oxygen. Ether is decomposed by air, light and heat, the most important products being acetaldehyde and ether peroxide. It should be stored in a cool environment in opaque containers.

Uptake and Distribution

Ether has a high blood/gas solubility coefficient of 12 and thus the rate of equilibration of alveolar with inspired concentrations is slow. Therefore induction and recovery with ether are slow.

Central Nervous System

In common with all general anaesthetic agents, there is depression of cortical activity. Because induction of anaesthesia with ether is so slow, the classical stages of anaesthesia are seen; these are described in detail on page 448 and in Figure 21.2.

Ether anaesthesia is associated with stimulation of the sympathoadrenal system and increased levels of circulating catecholamines, which offset the direct myocardial depressant effect of the drug.

Respiratory System

Ether is irritant to the respiratory tract and provokes coughing, breath-holding and profuse secretions from all mucus-secreting glands. Premedication with an anticholinergic agent is therefore essential.

Ether stimulates ventilation and minute volume is maintained with increasing depth of anaesthesia until surgical anaesthesia is achieved; thereafter, there is a gradual diminution in alveolar ventilation as plane 4 of stage 3 is approached (see Chapter 21).

Because ether is irritant to the respiratory tract, laryngeal spasm is not uncommon during induction with ether, but during established anaesthesia there is dilatation of the bronchi and bronchioles; at one time, the drug was recommended for the treatment of bronchospasm.

Cardiovascular System

In vitro, ether is a direct myocardial depressant. However, during light planes of clinical anaesthesia, there is sympathetic nervous stimulation and this often results in little change in cardiac output, arterial pressure or peripheral resistance. In deep planes of anaesthesia, cardiac output decreases as a result of myocardial depression.

Cardiac arrhythmias occur rarely with ether and there is no sensitization of the myocardium to circulating catecholamines.

Alimentary System

Salivary and gastric secretions are increased during light anaesthesia but decreased during deep anaesthesia. Ether causes a very high incidence of postoperative nausea and vomiting.

Skeletal Muscle

Ether potentiates the effects of non-depolarizing muscle relaxants.

Uterus and Placenta

The pregnant uterus is not affected during light anaesthesia, but relaxation occurs during deep anaesthesia.

Metabolism

At least 15% of ether is metabolized to carbon dioxide and water; approximately 4% is metabolized in the liver to acetaldehyde and ethanol.

Ether stimulates gluconeogenesis and therefore causes hyperglycaemia.

Clinical Use of Ether

Ether has a much higher therapeutic ratio than other volatile anaesthetic agents and is therefore safer for administration in the hands of unskilled individuals or from an uncalibrated vaporizer. Because of its high blood/gas solubility coefficient and irritant properties to the respiratory tract, induction of anaesthesia is very slow.

Administration of ether may be undertaken using an anaesthetic breathing system with a non-calibrated vaporizer (Boyle's bottle) or calibrated vaporizer (the EMO, which may be used as a draw-over or as a plenum vaporizer). It may be used safely in a closed circuit with soda lime absorption.

Vapour strengths of up to 20% are required for induction; light anaesthesia may be maintained with 3–5% and deep anaesthesia with 5–6% inspired concentrations.

ANAESTHETIC GASES

Nitrous Oxide (N_2O)

Manufacture

Nitrous oxide is prepared commercially by heating ammonium nitrate to a temperature of 245–270 °C. Various impurities are produced in this process, including ammonia, nitric acid, nitrogen, nitric oxide and nitrogen dioxide.

After cooling, ammonia and nitric acid are reconstituted to ammonium nitrate, which is returned to the beginning of the process. The remaining gases then pass through a series of scrubbers. The purified gases are compressed and dried in an aluminium dryer. The resultant gases are expanded in a liquefier, with the nitrogen escaping as gas. Nitrous oxide is then evaporated, compressed and passed through another aluminium dryer before being stored in cylinders.

The higher oxides of nitrogen dissolve in water to form nitrous and nitric acids. These substances are toxic and produce methaemoglobinaemia and pulmonary oedema if inhaled. There have been several reports of death occurring during anaesthesia as a result of the inhalation of nitrous oxide contaminated with higher oxides of nitrogen.

Storage

Nitrous oxide is stored in compressed form as a liquid in cylinders at a pressure of 44 bar (4400 kPa; 638 lb in^{-2}). In the UK, the cylinders are painted blue.

Because the cylinder contains liquid and vapour, the total quantity of nitrous oxide contained in a cylinder may be ascertained only by weighing. Thus, the cylinder weights, full and empty, are stamped on the shoulder. Nitrous oxide cylinders should be kept in a vertical position during use so that the liquid phase remains at the bottom of the cylinder. During continuous use, the cylinder may cool as a result of the latent heat of vaporization of liquid anaesthetic and ice may form on the lower part of the cylinder. Large institutions use a pipeline supply of nitrous oxide. The nitrous oxide is delivered from a large central bank of cylinders to the pipeline.

Physical Properties

Nitrous oxide is a sweet-smelling, non-irritant colourless gas, with a molecular weight of 44, boiling point of −88 °C, critical temperature of 36.5 °C and critical pressure of 72.6 bar.

Nitrous oxide is not flammable but it supports combustion of fuels in the absence of oxygen.

Pharmacology

Nitrous oxide is often said to be a good analgesic but a weak anaesthetic. The latter refers to the fact that its MAC value is 105%. This value was calculated theoretically from its low oil/water solubility coefficient of 3.2 and has been confirmed experimentally in volunteers anaesthetized in a pressure chamber compressed to 2 ata, where the MAC value was found to be 52.5% in N_2O. As it is essential to administer a minimum F_IO_2 of 0.3 during anaesthesia, nitrous oxide alone is insufficient to produce an adequate depth of anaesthesia. Therefore, nitrous oxide is used usually in combination with other agents. When using nitrous oxide in a relaxant technique, the inspired gas mixture should be supplemented with a low concentration of a volatile agent to eliminate the risk of awareness, which occurs in 1–2% of patients if nitrous oxide anaesthesia is supplemented only by the administration of opioids.

Nitrous oxide has a low blood/gas solubility coefficient (0.47 at 37 °C) and therefore the rate of equilibration of alveolar with inspired concentrations is very fast (Fig. 2.2).

Nitrous oxide does not undergo metabolism in the body and is excreted unchanged.

Nitrous oxide appears to exert its activity at different types of receptors. It has an inhibitory action on N-methyl-D-aspartate (NMDA) glutamate receptors and stimulatory activity at dopamine, α_1 and α_2-adrenergic and opioid receptors. The analgesic action of nitrous oxide is thought to be mediated by activation of opioid receptors in the periaqueductal area of the midbrain. This leads to modulation of nociceptive pathways through the release of noradrenaline and activation of the α_2-adrenoreceptors in the dorsal horn of the spinal cord. Because of its analgesic properties, nitrous oxide is used in combination with volatile agents as part of a general anaesthetic, which reduces the dose of volatile agent required. It is used in obstetrics and in acute pain management as pre-mixed nitrous oxide 50% and oxygen 50% via a demand valve.

The Concentration Effect

The inspired concentration of nitrous oxide affects its rate of equilibration; the higher the inspired concentration, the faster is the rate of equilibration between alveolar and inspired concentrations. Nitrous oxide is more soluble in blood than is nitrogen. Thus, the volume of nitrous oxide entering pulmonary capillary blood from the alveolus is greater than the volume of nitrogen moving in the opposite direction. As a result, the total volume of gas in the alveolus diminishes and the fractional concentrations of the remaining gases increase. This has two consequences:

- the higher the inspired concentration of nitrous oxide, the greater is the concentrating effect on the nitrous oxide remaining in the alveolus.
- at high inspired concentrations of nitrous oxide, the reduction in alveolar gas volume causes an increase in $PaCO_2$. Equilibration with pulmonary capillary blood results in an increase in $PaCO_2$.

The result of the concentration effect on equilibration of nitrous oxide is illustrated in Figure 2.10.

The Second Gas Effect

When nitrous oxide is administered in a high concentration with a second anaesthetic agent, e.g. sevoflurane, the reduction in gas volume in the alveoli caused by absorption of nitrous oxide increases the alveolar concentration of sevoflurane, thereby augmenting the

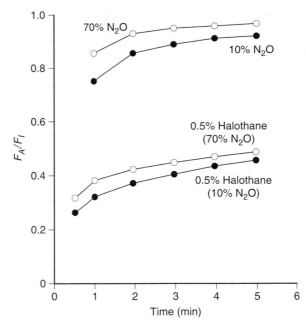

FIGURE 2.10 ■ The concentration and second gas effects. High concentrations of nitrous oxide increase the F_A/F_I ratio for nitrous oxide (the concentration effect) and for a volatile agent administered with nitrous oxide (the second gas effect). See text for details.

rate of equilibration with inspired gas. This is illustrated in the lower part of Figure 2.10. The second gas effect results also in small increases in PaO_2 and PaO_2.

Systemic Effects

Respiratory System. Nitrous oxide decreases tidal volume and increases respiratory rate and hence maintains minute ventilation. It reduces the ventilatory response to hypoxaemia and hypercapnia. It depresses tracheal mucociliary flow and neutrophil chemotaxis and may increase the incidence of post-operative respiratory complications.

Cardiovascular System. Nitrous oxide is a direct myocardial depressant, but in the normal individual this effect is antagonized by indirectly mediated sympathoadrenal stimulation (effects similar to those produced by carbon dioxide). Thus, healthy patients exhibit little change in the cardiovascular system during nitrous oxide anaesthesia. However, in patients with pre-existing high levels of sympathoadrenal activity and poor myocardial contractility, the administration of nitrous oxide may cause reductions in cardiac output and arterial pressure. For this reason (in addition to avoidance of the risk of doubling the size of air emboli), nitrous oxide is avoided in some centres during anaesthesia for cardiac surgery. Pulmonary vascular resistance is increased due to constriction of the pulmonary vascular smooth muscles and this may lead to increased right atrial pressure. For this reason, nitrous oxide is best avoided in patients with pulmonary hypertension.

Central Nervous System. Nitrous oxide increases cerebral blood flow, cerebral metabolism and intracranial pressure. These changes are more marked in patients with abnormal cerebral autoregulation and may result in reduced cerebral perfusion.

Neuromuscular Junction. Nitrous oxide does not appear to potentiate the action of non-depolarizing muscle relaxants.

Side-Effects of Nitrous Oxide

Postoperative Nausea and Vomiting. Nitrous oxide has been implicated in the aetiology of postoperative nausea and vomiting. The underlying mechanism for this is not well understood but it may be multifactorial involving changes in middle ear pressures, bowel distension and activation of dopaminergic neurones.

Diffusion Hypoxia. At the end of an anaesthetic, when the inspired gas mixture is changed from nitrous oxide/oxygen to nitrogen/oxygen, hypoxaemia may occur as the volume of nitrous oxide diffusing from mixed venous blood into the alveolus is greater than the volume of nitrogen taken up from the alveolus into pulmonary capillary blood (the opposite of the concentration effect). Thus, the concentration of gases in the alveolus is diluted by nitrous oxide, leading to reductions in PaO_2 and $PaCO_2$. In the healthy individual, diffusion hypoxia is relatively transient, but may last for up to 10 min at the end of anaesthesia; the extent of reduction in PaO_2 may be of the order of 0.5–1.5 kPa. Administration of oxygen during this period is essential in order to avoid desaturation.

Effect on Closed Gas Spaces. When blood containing nitrous oxide equilibrates with closed air-containing spaces inside the body, the volume of nitrous oxide that diffuses into the cavity exceeds the volume of nitrogen diffusing out. Thus, in compliant spaces, such as the bowel lumen or the pleural or peritoneal cavities, there is an increase in volume of the space. If the space cannot expand (e.g. sinuses, middle ear) there is an increase in pressure. In the middle ear, this may cause problems with surgery on the tympanic membrane. When nitrous oxide is administered in a concentration of 75%, the volume of a cavity may increase to as much as three to four times the original volume within 30 min. If an air embolus occurs in a patient who is breathing nitrous oxide, equilibration with the gas bubble leads to expansion of the embolus within seconds; the volume of the embolus may double within a very short period of time. A similar problem arises during prolonged procedures where nitrous oxide diffuses into the cuff of the tracheal tube and may increase the pressure exerted on the tracheal mucosa. Either avoiding the use of nitrous oxide or inflating the cuff with saline or nitrous oxide may prevent this.

A complication of the effect of nitrous oxide on closed gas spaces which has been described is the loss of vision caused by expansion of intraocular perfluoropropane gas during nitrous oxide anaesthesia. Perfluoropropane is used in vitreoretinal surgery to provide long-acting gas tamponade. The visual loss is caused possibly by central retinal artery occlusion as a result of expansion of the gas by nitrous oxide, resulting in increased intraocular pressure. Therefore the use of nitrous oxide in these patients should be avoided. In order to aid identification of these patients by anaesthetists preoperatively, it is recommended that the patients should be aware of this risk in order to warn the anaesthetist and also it may be prudent for them to wear an intraocular gas identity bracelet.

Effects on Blood and the Nervous System. Nitrous oxide inhibits the enzyme methionine synthetase which results in interference with DNA synthesis in both leucocytes and erythrocytes. It oxidizes the cobalt atom in vitamin B_{12} and interferes with folic acid metabolism. Prolonged exposure may cause agranulocytosis and bone marrow aplasia. Exposure of patients to nitrous oxide for 6 h or longer may result in megaloblastic anaemia. Occupational exposure to nitrous oxide may result in myeloneuropathy. This condition is similar to subacute combined degeneration of the spinal cord and has been reported in some dentists and also in individuals addicted to inhalation of nitrous oxide. Inhibition of methionine synthesis prevents production of methionine and tetrahydrofolate. Methionine is a precursor of S-adenosylmethionine which is incorporated into myelin and its absence leads to subacute combined degeneration of the cord.

Teratogenic Changes. Teratogenic changes have been observed in pregnant rats exposed to nitrous oxide for prolonged periods. The mechanism of this teratogenicity is not clear but it is thought to be multifactorial and may partially involve activation of the α_1-adrenergic neurones. There is no evidence that similar effects occur in humans, but it has been suggested that nitrous oxide should be avoided in the first trimester of pregnancy.

Environment. Nitrous oxide is a greenhouse gas and it is 200–300 times more effective in trapping heat than carbon dioxide and therefore may contribute to global warming. However the contribution to the greenhouse effect of anaesthetic use of nitrous oxide is very small as anaesthesia only accounts for <1% of total nitrous oxide emission.

Other Gases Used During Anaesthesia

Oxygen

Manufacture. Oxygen is manufactured commercially by fractional distillation of liquid air. Before liquefaction of air, carbon dioxide is removed and liquid oxygen and nitrogen separated by means of their different boiling points (oxygen, −183 °C; nitrogen, −195 °C).

Oxygen is supplied in cylinders at a pressure of 137 bar (approximately 2000 lb in⁻²) at 15 °C. In the UK, the cylinders are painted black with a white shoulder.

Many institutions use piped oxygen and this is supplied either by a bank of oxygen cylinders, ensuring a continuous supply, or from liquid oxygen. Premises using in excess of 150 000 L of oxygen per week find the latter more economical. The pressure of oxygen in a hospital pipeline is approximately 4 bar (60 lb in⁻²), which is the same as the pressure distal to the reducing valves of gas cylinders attached to anaesthetic machines.

Oxygen is tasteless, colourless and odourless, with a specific gravity of 1.105 and a molecular weight of 32. At atmospheric pressure, it liquefies at −183 °C, but at 50 ata the liquefaction temperature increases to −119 °C.

Oxygen supports combustion, although the gas itself is not flammable.

Oxygen Concentrators. Oxygen concentrators produce oxygen from ambient air by absorption of nitrogen onto some types of alumina silicates. Oxygen concentrators are useful both in hospitals and in long-term domestic use in remote areas, in developing countries and in military surgery. The gas produced by oxygen concentrators contains small quantities of inert gases (e.g. argon) which are harmless.

Adverse Effects of Oxygen.

FIRE. Oxygen supports combustion of fuels. An increase in the concentration of oxygen from 21% up to 100% causes a progressive increase in the rate of combustion with the production of either conflagrations or explosions with appropriate fuels.

CARDIOVASCULAR DEPRESSION. An increase in PaO_2 leads to direct vasoconstriction, which occurs in peripheral vasculature and also in the cerebral, coronary, hepatic and renal circulations. This effect is not manifest at a PaO_2 of less than 30 kPa and assumes clinical importance only at hyperbaric pressures of oxygen. Hyperbaric pressures of oxygen also cause direct myocardial depression. In patients with severe cardiovascular disease, elevation of PaO_2 from the normal physiological range to 80 kPa may produce clinically evident cardiovascular depression.

ABSORPTION ATELECTASIS. Because oxygen is highly soluble in blood, the use of 100% oxygen as the inspired gas may lead to absorption atelectasis in lung units distal to the site of airway closure. Absorption collapse may occur in as short a time as 6 min with 100% oxygen, and 60 min with 85% oxygen. Thus, even small concentrations of nitrogen exert an important splinting effect and this accounts for current avoidance of 100% oxygen in estimation of pulmonary shunt ratio ($\dot{Q}_s/\dot{Q}_t$) in patients with lung pathology, in whom a greater degree of airway closure would result in greater areas of alveolar atelectasis. Absorption atelectasis has been demonstrated in volunteers breathing 100% oxygen at FRC; atelectasis is evident on chest radiography for a period of at least 24 h after exposure.

PULMONARY OXYGEN TOXICITY. Chronic inhalation of a high inspired concentration of oxygen may result in the condition termed pulmonary oxygen toxicity (Lorrain-Smith effect), which is manifest by hyaline membranes, thickening of the interlobular and alveolar septa by oedema and fibroplastic proliferation. The clinical and radiological appearance of these changes is almost identical to that of the acute respiratory distress syndrome. The biochemical mechanisms underlying pulmonary oxygen toxicity probably include:

- oxidation of SH groups on essential enzymes such as coenzyme A
- peroxidation of lipids; the resulting lipid peroxides inhibit the function of the cell
- inhibition of the pathway of reversed electron transport, possibly by inhibition of iron and SH-containing flavoproteins.

These changes lead to loss of synthesis of pulmonary surfactant, encouraging the development of absorption collapse and alveolar oedema. The onset of oxygen-induced lung pathology occurs after approximately 30 h exposure to a $P_{I}O_2$ of 100 kPa.

CENTRAL NERVOUS SYSTEM OXYGEN TOXICITY. Convulsions, similar to those of grand mal epilepsy, occur during exposure to hyperbaric pressures of oxygen.

RETROLENTAL FIBROPLASIA. Retrolental fibroplasia (RLF) is the result of oxygen-induced retinal vasoconstriction, with obliteration of the most immature retinal vessels and subsequent new vessel formation at the site of damage in the form of a proliferative retinopathy. Leakage of intravascular fluid leads to vitreoretinal adhesions and even retinal detachment. Retrolental

fibroplasia occurs in infants exposed to hyperoxia in the paediatric intensive care unit and is related not to the $F_{I}O_2$ per se, but to an elevated retinal artery PO_2. It is not known what the threshold of PaO_2 is for the development of retinal damage, but an umbilical arterial PO_2 of 8–12 kPa (60–90 mmHg) is associated with a very low incidence of RLF and no signs of systemic hypoxia. It should be stressed, however, that there are many factors involved in the development of RLF in addition to arterial hyperoxia.

DEPRESSED HAEMOPOIESIS. Long-term exposure to elevated $F_{I}O_2$ leads to depression of haemopoiesis and anaemia.

Carbon Dioxide

Carbon dioxide is a colourless gas with a pungent odour. It has a molecular weight of 44, a critical temperature of −31°C and a critical pressure of 73.8 bar.

Carbon dioxide is obtained commercially from four sources:

- as a byproduct of fermentation in brewing of beer
- as a byproduct of the manufacture of hydrogen
- by heating magnesium and calcium carbonate in the presence of their oxides
- as a combustion gas from burning fuel.

In the UK, carbon dioxide is supplied in a liquid state in grey cylinders at a pressure of 50 bar. The liquid phase occupies approximately 90–95% of the cylinder capacity.

Physiological Data. Variations in cardiovascular state induced by alterations in $PaCO_2$ may be similar to those induced by pain or lightness of anaesthesia and the differential diagnosis is described in Table 40.2. The cardiovascular effects of CO_2 are summarized in Table 2.3.

Uses of Carbon Dioxide in anaesthesia. The use of carbon dioxide in anaesthetic practice has declined as appreciation of its disadvantages has increased. Because of reports of accidental administration of high concentrations of CO_2, it is not available on most modern anaesthetic machines. Carbon dioxide is used mainly by surgeons for insufflation during laparoscopic procedures.

TABLE 2.3	
Cardiovascular Effects of CO_2	
Arterial pressure Cardiac output Heart rate	Biphasic response. Progressive increases in these variables with increase in $PaCO_2$ up to approximately 10 kPa as a result of indirect sympathetic stimulation. At very high $PaCO_2$, these variables decrease as a result of myocardial depression
Skin Coronary circulation Cerebral circulation Gastrointestinal circulation	Dilatation with hypercapnia Constriction with hypocapnia

Medical Air

Nitrous oxide is still commonly used in combination with a volatile agent to maintain anaesthesia. However, there is growing concern regarding its toxic effects and its cost. Consequently, medical air is being used more frequently in combination with oxygen during anaesthesia.

Medical air is obtained from the atmosphere near to the site of compression. Great care is taken to position the air intake in order to avoid contamination with pollutants such as carbon monoxide from car exhausts. Air is compressed to 137 bar and then passed through columns of activated alumina to remove water.

Air for medical purposes is supplied in cylinders (grey body and black and white shoulders in the UK) or as a piped system. A pressure of 4 bar is available for attachment to anaesthetic machines, and 7 bar for orthopaedic tools. Its composition varies slightly depending on location of compression and moisture content.

Uses of Medical Air.

- Driving gas for ventilators
- To operate power tools, e.g. orthopaedic drills
- Together with oxygen and a volatile or intravenous agent to maintain anaesthesia.

Advantages of Air.

- Readily available
- Non-toxic.

Xenon

Inert gases such as argon, krypton and xenon, which form crystalline hydrates, have been reported to exert anaesthetic actions. Cullen and Gross first reported the anaesthetic properties of xenon in humans in 1951. Xenon offers many advantages over nitrous oxide, for which it could theoretically be a suitable replacement. The reasons that it is not routinely available are that it is expensive, there are no commercially available anaesthetic machines in which to use xenon, its concentration in inspired gas cannot be measured with conventional anaesthetic gas analysers and there is still limited clinical experience with its use. Xenon, in common with nitrous oxide and ketamine, acts by non-competitive inhibition of NMDA receptors in the CNS.

Physical Properties. Xenon is a non-explosive, colourless and odourless gas. It is non-flammable and does not support combustion. Its blood/gas partition coefficient of 0.14–0.2 is lower than that of nitrous oxide (0.47). It therefore provides rapid induction of and recovery from anaesthesia. Xenon is more potent than nitrous oxide, with a MAC of 70%. It does not undergo biotransformation and it is harmless to the ozone layer.

Systemic Effects. Studies so far have shown no cardiorespiratory side-effects or reduction in local organ perfusion. It is non-irritant to the respiratory tract. However, in common with nitrous oxide, xenon appears to be associated with postoperative nausea and vomiting.

Helium

Helium is a light inert gas which is present in air and natural gas. It is the second most abundant element after hydrogen. It is presented as either Heliox (79% helium and 21% oxygen) in white cylinders with white/brown shoulders or as 100% helium in brown cylinders at 137 bar. Helium has a lower density than air, nitrogen and oxygen. During turbulent flow, velocity is higher when Heliox is used. The low density of gas results in a lowering of the Reynolds' number and thus a return to laminar flow. By increasing laminar flow, the efficiency of breathing is increased. This physical characteristic is used to treat patients with upper airway obstruction to reduce the work of breathing and improve oxygenation.

Because of the lower density, patients receiving helium have a typical squeaky voice due to the higher frequency vocal sounds. Helium is used in the measurement of lung volumes because of its very low solubility. Helium/oxygen mixtures are also used for deep water diving to avoid nitrogen narcosis.

FURTHER READING

Calvey, N., Williams, N., 2008. Principles and practice of pharmacology for anaesthetists, fifth ed. Wiley-Blackwell, Oxford.

3 INTRAVENOUS ANAESTHETIC AGENTS

■ ■ ■ ■ ■ ■ ■ ■ ■ ■

General anaesthesia may be produced by many drugs which depress the CNS, including sedatives, tranquillizers and hypnotic agents. However, for some drugs, the doses required to produce surgical anaesthesia are so large that cardiovascular and respiratory depression commonly occur, and recovery is delayed for hours or even days. Only a few drugs are suitable for use routinely to produce anaesthesia after intravenous (i.v.) injection.

Intravenous anaesthetic agents are used commonly to induce anaesthesia, as induction is usually smoother and more rapid than that associated with most of the inhalational agents. Intravenous anaesthetics may also be used for maintenance, either alone or in combination with nitrous oxide; they may be administered as repeated bolus doses or by continuous i.v. infusion. Other uses include sedation during regional anaesthesia, sedation in the intensive care unit (ICU) and treatment of status epilepticus.

Properties of the Ideal Intravenous Anaesthetic Agent

- Rapid onset – this is achieved by an agent which is mainly un-ionized at blood pH and which is highly soluble in lipid; these properties permit penetration of the blood–brain barrier
- Rapid recovery – early recovery of consciousness is usually produced by rapid redistribution of the drug from the brain into other well-perfused tissues, particularly muscle. The plasma concentration of the drug decreases, and the drug diffuses out of the brain along a concentration gradient. The quality of the later recovery period

is related more to the rate of metabolism of the drug; drugs with slow metabolism are associated with a more prolonged 'hangover' effect and accumulate if used in repeated doses or by infusion for maintenance of anaesthesia
- Analgesia at subanaesthetic concentrations
- Minimal cardiovascular and respiratory depression
- No emetic effects
- No excitatory phenomena (e.g. coughing, hiccup, involuntary movement) on induction
- No emergence phenomena (e.g. nightmares)
- No interaction with neuromuscular blocking drugs
- No pain on injection
- No venous sequelae
- Safe if injected inadvertently into an artery
- No toxic effects on other organs
- No release of histamine
- No hypersensitivity reactions
- Water-soluble formulation
- Long shelf-life
- No stimulation of porphyria.

None of the agents available at present meets all these requirements. Features of the commonly used i.v. anaesthetic agents are compared in Table 3.1, and a classification of i.v. anaesthetic drugs is shown in Table 3.2.

Mechanism of Action of Intravenous Anaesthetic Drugs

In common with inhalational agents, all intravenous anaesthetics, with the exception of ketamine, potentiate GABA$_A$ receptors to inhibit CNS neurotransmission. Benzodiazepines act at a different binding site on the

TABLE 3.1
Main Properties of Intravenous Anaesthetics

	Thiopental	Methohexital	Propofol	Ketamine	Etomidate
Physical Properties					
Water-soluble	+	+	–	+	+[a]
Stable in solution	–	–	+	+	+
Long shelf-life	–	–	+	+	+
Pain on i.v. injection	–	+	++[b]	–	++[b]
Non-irritant on s.c. injection	–	±	+	+	
Painful on arterial injection	+	+	–		
No sequelae from intra-arterial injection	–	±	+		
Low incidence of venous thrombosis	+	+	+	+	–
Effects on Body					
Rapid onset	+	+	+	+	+
Recovery due to:					
Redistribution	+	+	+	+	
Detoxification	+	+			
Cumulation	++	+	–	–	–
Induction					
Excitatory effects	–	++	+	+	+++
Respiratory complications	–	+	+	–	–
Cardiovascular					
Hypotension	+	+	++	–	+
Analgesic	–	–		++	–
Antanalgesic	+	+	–	–	?
Interaction with relaxants	–	–	–	–	–
Postoperative vomiting	–	–	–	++	+
Emergence delirium		–	–	++	–
Safe in porphyria	–	–	+	+	–

[a] Aqueous solution not commercially available.
[b] Pain may be reduced when emulsion with medium-chain triglycerides is used.

GABA$_A$ receptor, the α/γ subunit interface, to increase chloride conductance. Propofol and barbiturates also potentiate the inhibitory effects of glycine at glycine receptors in the brain and, to a lesser extent, the spinal cord. In addition to effects on GABA$_A$ and glycine receptors, propofol has inhibitory actions on sodium channels and 5HT$_3$ receptors. The latter may explain its antiemetic effects.

Ketamine, in common with nitrous oxide and xenon, has its predominant effect at NMDA receptors. These CNS receptors usually bind glutamate and are excitatory. Binding by ketamine to the NMDA receptor in a non-competitive manner reduces transmission. Ketamine appears to have no effect at GABA or glycine receptors.

TABLE 3.2

Classification of Intravenous Anaesthetics

Rapidly Acting (Primary Induction) Agents

Barbiturates:
 Methohexital
 Thiobarbiturates – thiopental, thiamylal

Imidazole compounds – etomidate

Sterically hindered alkyl phenols – propofol

Steroids – eltanolone, althesin, minaxolone (none currently available)

Eugenols – propanidid (not currently available)

Slower-Acting (Basal Narcotic) Agents

Ketamine

Benzodiazepines – diazepam, flunitrazepam, midazolam

Large-dose opioids – fentanyl, alfentanil, sufentanil, remifentanil

Neuroleptic combination – opioid + neuroleptic

Pharmacokinetics of Intravenous Anaesthetic Drugs

After i.v. administration of a drug, there is an immediate rapid increase in plasma concentration followed by a slower decline. Anaesthesia is produced by diffusion of drug from arterial blood across the blood–brain barrier into the brain. The rate of transfer into the brain, and therefore the anaesthetic effect, is regulated by the following factors:

Protein binding. Only unbound drug is free to cross the blood–brain barrier. Protein binding may be reduced by low plasma protein concentrations or displacement by other drugs, resulting in higher concentrations of free drug and an exaggerated anaesthetic effect. Protein binding is also affected by changes in blood pH. Hyperventilation decreases protein binding and increases the anaesthetic effect.

Blood flow to the brain. Reduced cerebral blood flow (CBF), e.g. carotid artery stenosis, results in reduced delivery of drug to the brain. However, if CBF is reduced because of low cardiac output, initial blood concentrations are higher than normal after i.v. administration, and the anaesthetic effect may be delayed but enhanced.

Extracellular pH and pKa of the drug. Only the un-ionized fraction of the drug penetrates the lipid blood–brain barrier; thus, the potency of the drug depends on the degree of ionization at the pH of extracellular fluid and the pK_a of the drug.

The relative solubilities of the drug in lipid and water. High lipid solubility enhances transfer into the brain.

Speed of injection. Rapid i.v. administration results in high initial concentrations of drug. This increases the speed of induction, but also the extent of cardiovascular and respiratory side-effects.

In general, any factor which increases the blood concentration of free drug, e.g. reduced protein binding or low cardiac output, also increases the intensity of side-effects.

Distribution to Other Tissues

The anaesthetic effect of all i.v. anaesthetic drugs in current use is terminated predominantly by distribution to other tissues. Figure 3.1 shows this distribution for thiopental. The percentage of the injected dose in each of four body compartments as time elapses is shown after i.v. injection. A large proportion of the drug is distributed initially into well-perfused organs (termed the vessel-rich group, or viscera – predominantly brain, liver and kidneys). Distribution into muscle (lean) is slower because of its low lipid content, but it is quantitatively important because of its relatively good blood supply and large mass. Despite their high lipid solubility, i.v. anaesthetic

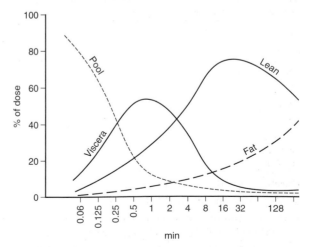

FIGURE 3.1 ■ Distribution of thiopental after intravenous bolus administration.

drugs distribute slowly to adipose tissue (fat) because of its poor blood supply. Fat contributes little to the initial redistribution or termination of action of i.v. anaesthetic agents, but fat depots contain a large proportion of the injected dose of thiopental at 90 min, and 65–75% of the total remaining in the body at 24 h. There is also a small amount of redistribution to areas with a very poor blood supply, e.g. bone. Table 3.3 indicates some of the properties of the body compartments in respect of the distribution of i.v. anaesthetic agents.

After a single i.v. dose, the concentration of drug in blood decreases as distribution occurs into viscera, and particularly muscle. Drug diffuses from the brain into blood along the changing concentration gradient, and recovery of consciousness occurs. Metabolism of most i.v. anaesthetic drugs occurs predominantly in the liver. If metabolism is rapid (indicated by a short elimination half-life), it may contribute to some extent to the recovery of consciousness. However, because of the large distribution volume of i.v. anaesthetic drugs, total elimination takes many hours, or, in some instances, days. A small proportion of drug may be excreted unchanged in the urine; the amount depends on the degree of ionization and the pH of urine.

TABLE 3.3
Factors Influencing the Distribution of Thiopental in the Body

	Viscera	Muscle	Fat	Others
Relative blood flow	Rich	Good	Poor	Very poor
Blood flow (Lmin⁻¹)	4.5	1.1	0.32	0.08
Tissue volume (L; A)	6	33	15	13
Tissue/blood partition coefficient (B)	1.5	1.5	11.0	1.5
Potential capacity (L; A×B)	9	50	165	20
Time constant (capacity/flow; min)	2	45	500	250

BARBITURATES

Amobarbital and pentobarbital were used i.v. to induce anaesthesia in the late 1920s, but their actions were unpredictable and recovery was prolonged. Manipulation of the barbituric acid ring (Fig. 3.2) enabled a short duration of action to be achieved by:

- substitution of a sulphur atom for oxygen at position 2
- substitution of a methyl group at position 1; this also confers potential convulsive activity and increases the incidence of excitatory phenomena.

An increased number of carbon atoms in the side chains at position 5 increases the potency of the agent. The presence of an aromatic nucleus in an alkyl group at position 5 produces compounds with convulsant properties; direct substitution with a phenyl group confers anticonvulsant activity.

The anaesthetically active barbiturates are classified chemically into four groups (Table 3.4). The methylated oxybarbiturate hexobarbital was moderately successful as an i.v. anaesthetic agent, but was superseded by the development in 1932 of thiopental. Although propofol has become very popular in a number of countries, thiopental remains one of the most commonly used i.v. anaesthetic agents throughout the world. Its pharmacology is therefore described fully in this chapter. Many of its effects are shared by other i.v. anaesthetic agents and consequently the pharmacology of these drugs is described more briefly.

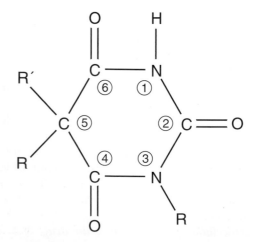

FIGURE 3.2 ■ Structure of barbiturate ring.

TABLE 3.4
Relation of Chemical Grouping to Clinical Action of Barbiturates

| Group | SUBSTITUENTS | | Group Characteristics when Given Intravenously |
	Position 1	Position 2	
Oxybarbiturates	H	O	Delay in onset of action depending on 5 and 5' side chain. Useful as basal hypnotics. Prolonged action
Methyl barbiturates	CH_3	O	Usually rapid-acting with fairly rapid recovery. High incidence of excitatory phenomena
Thiobarbiturates	H	S	Rapid-acting, usually smooth onset of sleep and fairly prompt recovery
Methyl thiobarbiturates	CH_3	S	Rapid onset of action and very rapid recovery but with so high an incidence of excitatory phenomena as to preclude use in clinical practice

Thiopental Sodium

Chemical Structure

Sodium 5-ethyl-5-(1-methylbutyl)-2-thiobarbiturate.

Physical Properties and Presentation

Thiopental sodium, the sulphur analogue of pento-barbital, is a yellowish powder with a bitter taste and a faint smell of garlic. It is stored in nitrogen to prevent chemical reaction with atmospheric carbon dioxide, and mixed with 6% anhydrous sodium carbonate to increase its solubility in water. It is available in single-dose ampoules of 500 mg and is dissolved in distilled water to produce 2.5% (25 mg ml^{-1}) solution with a pH of 10.8; this solution is slightly hypotonic. Freshly prepared solution may be kept for 24 h. The oil/water partition coefficient of thiopental is 4.7, and the pKa 7.6.

Central Nervous System.
Thiopental produces anaesthesia usually less than 30 s after i.v. injection, although there may be some delay in patients with a low cardiac output. There is progressive depression of the CNS, including spinal cord reflexes. The hypnotic action of thiopental is potent, but its analgesic effect is poor, and surgical anaesthesia is difficult to achieve unless large doses are used; these are associated with cardiorespiratory depression. The cerebral metabolic rate is reduced and there are secondary decreases in CBF, cerebral blood volume and intracranial pressure. Recovery of consciousness occurs at a higher blood concentration if a large dose is given, or if the drug is injected rapidly; this has been attributed to acute tolerance, but may represent only altered redistribution. Consciousness is usually regained in 5–10 min. At subanaesthetic blood concentrations (i.e. at low doses or during recovery), thiopental has an antanalgesic effect and reduces the pain threshold; this may result in restlessness in the postoperative period. Thiopental is a very potent anticonvulsant.

Sympathetic nervous system activity is depressed to a greater extent than parasympathetic; this may occasionally result in bradycardia. However, it is more usual for tachycardia to develop after induction of anaesthesia, partly because of baroreceptor inhibition caused by modest hypotension and partly because of loss of vagal tone which may predominate normally in young healthy adults.

Cardiovascular System.
Myocardial contractility is depressed and peripheral vasodilatation occurs, particularly when large doses are administered or if injection is rapid. Arterial pressure decreases, and profound hypotension may occur in the patient with hypovolaemia or cardiac disease. Heart rate may decrease, but there is often a reflex tachycardia (see above).

Respiratory System.
Ventilatory drive is decreased by thiopental as a result of reduced sensitivity of the respiratory centre to carbon dioxide. A short period of apnoea is common, frequently preceded by a few deep breaths. Respiratory depression is influenced by premedication and is more pronounced if opioids have been administered; assisted or controlled ventilation may be required. When spontaneous ventilation is resumed, ventilatory rate and tidal volume are usually lower than normal, but they increase in response

to surgical stimulation. There is an increase in bronchial muscle tone, although frank bronchospasm is uncommon.

Laryngeal spasm may be precipitated by surgical stimulation or the presence of secretions, blood or foreign bodies (e.g. an oropharyngeal airway or supraglottic airway device) in the region of the pharynx or larynx. Thiopental is less satisfactory than propofol in this respect, and appears to depress the parasympathetic laryngeal reflex arc to a lesser extent than other areas of the CNS.

Skeletal Muscle. Skeletal muscle tone is reduced at high blood concentrations, partly as a result of suppression of spinal cord reflexes. There is no significant direct effect on the neuromuscular junction. When thiopental is used as the sole anaesthetic agent, there is poor muscle relaxation, and movement in response to surgical stimulation is common.

Uterus and Placenta. There is little effect on resting uterine tone, but uterine contractions are suppressed at high doses. Thiopental crosses the placenta readily, although fetal blood concentrations do not reach the same levels as those observed in the mother.

Eye. Intraocular pressure is reduced by approximately 40%. The pupil dilates first, and then constricts; the light reflex remains present until surgical anaesthesia has been attained. The corneal, conjunctival, eyelash and eyelid reflexes are abolished.

Hepatorenal Function. The functions of the liver and kidneys are impaired transiently after administration of thiopental. Hepatic microsomal enzymes are induced and this may increase the metabolism and elimination of other drugs.

Pharmacokinetics

Blood concentrations of thiopental increase rapidly after i.v. administration. Between 75 and 85% of the drug is bound to protein, mostly albumin; thus, more free drug is available if plasma protein concentrations are reduced by malnutrition or disease. Protein binding is affected by pH and is decreased by alkalaemia; thus the concentration of free drug is increased during hyperventilation. Some drugs, e.g. phenylbutazone,

occupy the same binding sites, and protein binding of thiopental may be reduced in their presence.

Thiopental diffuses readily into the CNS because of its lipid solubility and predominantly un-ionized state (61%) at body pH. Consciousness returns when the brain concentration decreases to a threshold value, dependent on the individual patient, the dose of drug and its rate of administration, but at this time nearly all of the injected dose is still present in the body.

Metabolism of thiopental occurs predominantly in the liver, and the metabolites are excreted by the kidneys; a small proportion is excreted unchanged in the urine. The terminal elimination half-life is approximately 11.5 h. Metabolism is a zero-order process; 10–15% of the remaining drug is metabolized each hour. Thus, up to 30% of the original dose may remain in the body at 24 h. Consequently, a 'hangover' effect is common; in addition, further doses of thiopental administered within 1–2 days may result in cumulation. Elimination is impaired in the elderly. In obese patients, dosage should be based on an estimate of lean body mass, as distribution to fat is slow. However, elimination may be delayed in obese patients because of increased retention of the drug by adipose tissue.

Dosage and Administration

Thiopental is administered i.v. as a 2.5% solution; the use of a 5% solution increases the likelihood of serious complications and is *not* recommended. A small volume, e.g. 1–2 mL in adults, should be administered initially; the patient should be asked if any pain is experienced in case of inadvertent intra-arterial injection (see below) before the remainder of the induction dose is given.

The dose required to produce anaesthesia varies, and the response of each patient must be assessed carefully; cardiovascular depression is exaggerated if excessive doses are given. In healthy adults, an initial dose of 4 mg kg^{-1} should be administered over 15–20 s; if loss of the eyelash reflex does not occur within 30 s, supplementary doses of 50–100 mg should be given slowly until consciousness is lost. In young children, a dose of 6 mg kg^{-1} is usually necessary. Elderly patients often require smaller doses (e.g. 2.5–3 mg kg^{-1}) than young adults.

Induction is usually smooth and may be preceded by a taste of garlic. Adverse effects are related to peak blood concentrations, and in patients in whom cardiovascular depression may occur the drug should be administered more slowly; in very frail patients, as little as 50 mg may be sufficient to induce sleep.

No other drug should be mixed with thiopental. Neuromuscular blocking drugs should *not* be given until it is certain that anaesthesia has been induced. The i.v. cannula should be flushed with saline before vecuronium or atracurium is administered, to obviate precipitation.

Supplementary doses of 25–100 mg may be given to augment nitrous oxide/oxygen anaesthesia during short surgical procedures. However, recovery may be prolonged considerably if large total doses are used ($>10\,mg\,kg^{-1}$).

Adverse Effects

Hypotension. The risk is increased if excessive doses are used, or if thiopental is administered to hypovolaemic, shocked or previously hypertensive patients. Hypotension is minimized by administering the drug slowly. Thiopental should not be administered to patients in the sitting position.

Respiratory depression. The risk is increased if excessive doses are used, or if opioid drugs have also been administered. Facilities must be available to provide artificial ventilation.

Tissue necrosis. Local necrosis may follow perivenous injection. Median nerve damage may occur after extravasation in the antecubital fossa, and this site is *not* recommended. If perivenous injection occurs, the needle should be left in place and hyaluronidase injected.

Intra-arterial injection. This is usually the result of inadvertent injection into the brachial artery or an aberrant ulnar artery in the antecubital fossa but has occurred occasionally into aberrant arteries at the wrist. The patient usually complains of intense, burning pain, and drug injection should be stopped immediately. The forearm and hand may become blanched and blisters may appear distally. Intra-arterial thiopental causes profound constriction of the artery accompanied by local release of norepinephrine. In addition, crystals of thiopental form in arterioles. Thrombosis caused by endarteritis, adenosine triphosphate release from damaged red cells and aggregation of platelets

result in emboli and may cause ischaemia or gangrene in parts of the forearm, hand or fingers.

The needle should be left in the artery and a vasodilator (e.g. papaverine 20 mg) administered. Stellate ganglion or brachial plexus block may reduce arterial spasm. Heparin should be given i.v. and oral anticoagulants should be prescribed after operation.

The risk of ischaemic damage after intra-arterial injection is much greater if a 5% solution of thiopental is used.

Laryngeal spasm. The causes have been discussed above.

Bronchospasm. This is unusual, but may be precipitated in asthmatic patients.

Allergic reactions. These range from cutaneous rashes to severe or fatal anaphylactic or anaphylactoid reactions with cardiovascular collapse. Severe reactions are rare (approximately 1 in 14 000–20 000). Hypersensitivity reactions to drugs administered during anaesthesia are discussed on pages 54–55.

Thrombophlebitis. This is uncommon (Table 3.5) when the 2.5% solution is used.

Indications

- Induction of anaesthesia
- Maintenance of anaesthesia – thiopental is suitable only for short procedures because cumulation occurs with repeated doses
- Treatment of status epilepticus
- Reduction of intracranial pressure (see Ch 32).

Absolute Contraindications

- Airway obstruction – intravenous anaesthesia should not be used if there is anticipated difficulty in maintaining an adequate airway e.g. epiglottitis, oral or pharyngeal tumours.
- Porphyria – barbiturates may precipitate lower motor neurone paralysis or severe cardiovascular collapse in patients with porphyria.
- Previous hypersensitivity reaction to a barbiturate.

Precautions

Special care is needed when thiopental is administered in the following circumstances:

Cardiovascular disease. Patients with hypovolaemia, myocardial disease, cardiac valvular stenosis or

TABLE 3.5

Percentage Incidences of Pain on Injection and Thrombophlebitis After Intravenous Administration of Anaesthetic Drugs into a Large Vein in the Antecubital Fossa or a Small Vein in the Dorsum of the Hand or Wrist

Agent	PAIN		THROMBOPHLEBITIS	
	Large	Small	Large	Small
Saline 0.9%	0	0	0	0
Thiopental 2.5%	0	12	1	0
Methohexital 1%	8	21	0	0
Propofol – LCT emulsion	10	40	0	0
Propofol – MCT emulsion	n/a	15	0	0
Etomidate – propylene glycol	8	80	15	20
Etomidate – MCT emulsion	n/a	4	0	0

MCT=medium-chain triglyceride, LCT=long-chain triglyceride.

constrictive pericarditis are particularly sensitive to the hypotensive effects of thiopental. However, if the drug is administered with extreme caution, it is probably no more hazardous than other i.v. anaesthetic agents. Myocardial depression may be severe in patients with right-to-left intracardiac shunt because of high coronary artery concentrations of thiopental.

Severe hepatic disease. Reduced protein binding results in higher concentrations of free drug. Metabolism may be impaired, but this has little effect on early recovery. A normal dose may be administered, but very slowly.

Renal disease. In chronic renal failure, protein binding is reduced, but elimination is unaltered. A normal dose may be administered, but very slowly.

Muscle disease. Respiratory depression is exaggerated in patients with myasthenia gravis or dystrophia myotonica.

Reduced metabolic rate. Patients with myxoedema are exquisitely sensitive to the effects of thiopental.

Obstetrics. An adequate dose must be given to ensure that the mother is anaesthetized. However, excessive doses may result in respiratory or cardiovascular depression in the fetus, particularly if the interval between induction and delivery is short.

Outpatient anaesthesia. Early recovery is slow in comparison with other agents. This is seldom important unless rapid return of airway reflexes is essential,

e.g. after oral or dental surgery. However, slow elimination of thiopental may result in persistent drowsiness for 24–36h, and this impairs the ability to drive or use machinery. There is also potentiation of the effect of alcohol or sedative drugs ingested during that period. It is preferable to use a drug with more rapid elimination for patients who are ambulant within a few hours.

Adrenocortical insufficiency.
Extremes of age.
Asthma.

Methohexital Sodium

Chemical Structure

Sodium α-*dl*-5-allyl-1-methyl-5-(1-methyl-2-pentynyl) barbiturate.

Physical Properties and Presentation

Although no longer available in the United Kingdom, methohexital is still used in a number of other countries. The drug has two asymmetrical carbon atoms, and therefore four isomers. The α-*dl* isomers are clinically useful. The drug is presented as a white powder mixed with 6% anhydrous sodium carbonate and is readily soluble in distilled water. The resulting 1% (10 mg mL^{-1}) solution has a pH of 11.1 and pKa of 7.9. Single-dose vials of 100 mg and multidose bottles containing 500 mg or 2.5 g are available in some countries. Although the solution is chemically stable for up to

6 weeks, the manufacturers recommend that it should not be stored for longer than 24 h because it does not contain antibacterial preservative.

Pharmacology

Central Nervous System. Unconsciousness is usually induced in 15–30 s. Recovery is more rapid with methohexital than with thiopental, and occurs after 2–3 min; it is caused predominantly by redistribution. Drowsiness may persist for several hours until blood concentrations are decreased further by metabolism. Epileptiform activity has been demonstrated by EEG in epileptic patients. However, in sufficient doses, methohexital acts as an anticonvulsant.

Cardiovascular System. In general, there is less hypotension in otherwise healthy patients than occurs after thiopental; the decrease in arterial pressure is mediated predominantly by vasodilatation. Heart rate may increase slightly because of a decrease in baroreceptor activity. The cardiovascular effects are more pronounced in patients with cardiac disease or hypovolaemia.

Respiratory System. Moderate hypoventilation occurs. There may be a short period of apnoea after i.v. injection.

Pharmacokinetics

A greater proportion of methohexital than thiopental is in the un-ionized state at body pH (approximately 75%), although the drug is less lipid-soluble than the thiobarbiturate. Binding to plasma protein occurs to a similar degree. Clearance from plasma is higher than that of thiopental, and the elimination half-life is considerably shorter (approximately 4 h). Thus, cumulation is less likely to occur after repeated doses.

Dosage and Administration

Methohexital is administered i.v. in a dose of 1–1.5 mg kg^{-1} to induce anaesthesia in healthy young adult patients; smaller doses are required in the elderly and infirm.

Adverse Effects

Cardiovascular and respiratory depression. This is probably less than that associated with thiopental.

Excitatory phenomena during induction, including dyskinetic muscle movements, coughing and hiccups. Muscle movements are reduced by administration of an opioid; the incidence of cough and hiccups is reduced by premedication with an anticholinergic agent. The incidence of excitatory effects is dose-related.

Epileptiform activity on EEG in epileptic subjects.

Pain on injection (Table 3.5).

Tissue damage after perivenous injection is rare with 1% solution.

Intra-arterial injection may cause gangrene, but the risk with 1% solution is considerably less than with 2.5% thiopental.

Allergic reactions occur, but are uncommon.

Thrombophlebitis is a rare complication.

Indications

Induction of anaesthesia, particularly when a rapid recovery is desirable. Methohexital was used commonly as the anaesthetic agent for electroconvulsive therapy (ECT) and for induction of anaesthesia for outpatient dental and other minor procedures.

Absolute Contraindications

These are the same as for thiopental.

Precautions

These are similar to the precautions listed for thiopental. However, methohexital is a suitable agent for outpatients. It should not be used to induce anaesthesia in patients who are known to be epileptic.

NON-BARBITURATE INTRAVENOUS ANAESTHETIC AGENTS

Propofol

This phenol derivative was identified as a potentially useful intravenous anaesthetic agent in 1980, and became available commercially in 1986. It has achieved great popularity because of its favourable recovery characteristics and its antiemetic effect.

Chemical Structure

2,6-Di-isopropylphenol (Fig. 3.3).

Physical Properties and Presentation

Propofol is extremely lipid-soluble, but almost insoluble in water. The drug was formulated initially in Cremophor EL. However, several other drugs formulated in this solubilizing agent were associated with

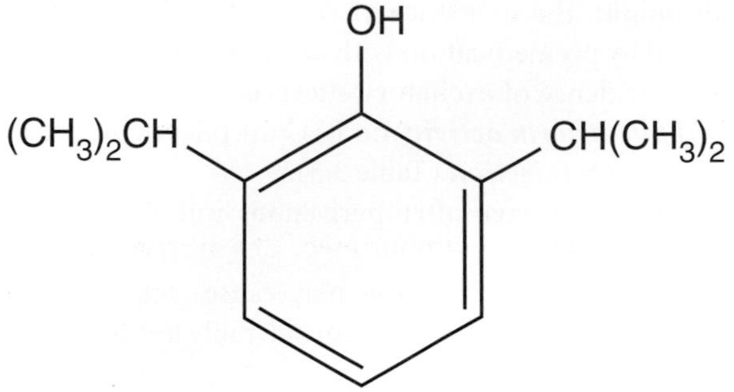

FIGURE 3.3 ■ Chemical structure of propofol (2,6-di-isopropylphenol).

release of histamine and an unacceptably high incidence of anaphylactoid reactions, and similar reactions occurred with this formulation of propofol. Consequently, the drug was reformulated in a white, aqueous emulsion containing soyabean oil and purified egg phosphatide. Ampoules of the drug contain 200 mg of propofol in 20 mL (10 mg mL⁻¹), and 50 mL bottles containing 1% (10 mg mL⁻¹) or 2% (20 mg mL⁻¹) solution, and 100 mL bottles containing 1% solution, are available for infusion. In addition, 50 mL prefilled syringes of 1 and 2% solution are available and are designed for use in target-controlled infusion techniques (see below). Recently, a 0.5% solution has been made available (5 mg mL⁻¹ in 20 mL). This produces less pain on injection, and is intended primarily for use in children.

Pharmacology

Central Nervous System. Anaesthesia is induced within 20–40 s after i.v. administration in otherwise healthy young adults. Transfer from blood to the sites of action in the brain is slower than with thiopental, and there is a delay in disappearance of the eyelash reflex, normally used as a sign of unconsciousness after administration of barbiturate anaesthetic agents. Overdosage of propofol, with exaggerated side-effects, may result if this clinical sign is used; loss of verbal contact is a better end-point. EEG frequency decreases, and amplitude increases. Propofol reduces the duration of seizures induced by ECT in humans. However, there have been reports of convulsions following the use of propofol and it is recommended that caution be exercised in the administration of propofol to epileptic patients. Normally cerebral metabolic rate, CBF and intracranial pressure are reduced.

Recovery of consciousness is rapid and there is a minimal 'hangover' effect even in the immediate post-anaesthetic period.

Cardiovascular System. In healthy patients, arterial pressure decreases to a greater degree after induction of anaesthesia with propofol than with thiopental; the reduction results predominantly from vasodilatation although there is a slight negative inotropic effect. In some patients, large decreases (>40%) occur. The degree of hypotension is substantially reduced by decreasing the rate of administration of the drug and by appreciation of the kinetics of transfer from blood to brain (see above). The pressor response to tracheal intubation is attenuated to a greater degree by propofol than thiopental. Heart rate may increase slightly after induction of anaesthesia with propofol. However, there have been occasional reports of severe bradycardia and asystole during or shortly after administration of propofol, and it is recommended that a vagolytic agent (e.g. glycopyrronium or atropine) should be considered in patients with a pre-existing bradycardia or when propofol is used in conjunction with other drugs which are likely to cause bradycardia.

Respiratory System. After induction, apnoea occurs more commonly, and for a longer duration, than after thiopental. During infusion of propofol, tidal volume is lower and respiratory rate higher than in the conscious state. There is decreased ventilatory response to carbon dioxide. As with other agents, ventilatory depression is more marked if opioids are administered.

Propofol has no effect on bronchial muscle tone and laryngospasm is particularly uncommon. The suppression of laryngeal reflexes results in a low incidence of coughing or laryngospasm when a laryngeal mask airway or other supraglottic airway device (SAD) is introduced, and propofol is regarded by most anaesthetists as the drug of choice for induction of anaesthesia when a SAD is to be used.

Skeletal Muscle. Tone is reduced, but movements may occur in response to surgical stimulation.

Gastrointestinal System. Propofol has no effect on gastrointestinal motility in animals. Its use is associated with a low incidence of postoperative nausea and vomiting.

Uterus and Placenta. Propofol has been used extensively in patients undergoing gynaecological surgery, and it does not appear to have any clinically significant effect on uterine tone. Propofol crosses the placenta. Its safety to the neonate has not been established and its use in pregnancy (except for termination), in obstetric practice and in breast-feeding mothers is not recommended by the manufacturers.

Hepatorenal. There is a transient decrease in renal function, but the impairment is less than that associated with thiopental. Hepatic blood flow is decreased by the reductions in arterial pressure and cardiac output. Liver function tests are not deranged after infusion of propofol for 24 h.

Endocrine. Plasma concentrations of cortisol are decreased after administration of propofol, but a normal response occurs to the administration of Synacthen.

Pharmacokinetics

In common with other i.v. anaesthetic drugs, propofol is distributed rapidly, and blood concentrations decline exponentially. Clearance of the drug from plasma is greater than would be expected if the drug was metabolized only in the liver, and it is believed that extrahepatic sites of metabolism exist. The kidneys excrete the metabolites of propofol (mainly glucuronides); only 0.3% of the administered dose of propofol is excreted unchanged. The terminal elimination half-life of propofol is 3–4.8 h, although its effective half-life is much shorter (30–60 min). The distribution and clearance of propofol are altered by concomitant administration of fentanyl. Elimination of propofol remains relatively constant even after infusions lasting for several days.

Dosage and Administration

In healthy, unpremedicated adults, a dose of 1.5–2.5 mg kg^{-1} is required to induce anaesthesia. The dose should be reduced in the elderly; an initial dose of 1.25 mg kg^{-1} is appropriate, with subsequent additional doses of 10 mg until consciousness is lost. In children, a dose of 3–3.5 mg kg^{-1} is usually required; the drug is not recommended for use in children less than 1 month of age. Cardiovascular side-effects are reduced if the drug is injected slowly. Lower doses are required for induction in premedicated patients. Sedation during regional analgesia or endoscopy may be achieved with infusion rates of 1.5–4.5 mg kg^{-1} h^{-1}. Infusion rates of up to 15 mg kg^{-1} h^{-1} are required to supplement nitrous oxide/oxygen for surgical anaesthesia, although these may be reduced substantially if an opioid drug is administered. The average infusion rate is approximately 2 mg kg^{-1} h^{-1} in conjunction with a slow infusion of morphine (2 mg h^{-1}) for sedation of patients in ICU.

Adverse Effects

Cardiovascular depression. Unless the drug is given very slowly, cardiovascular depression following a bolus dose of propofol is greater than that associated with a bolus dose of a barbiturate and is likely to cause profound hypotension in hypovolaemic or untreated hypertensive patients and in those with cardiac disease. Cardiovascular depression is modest if the drug is administered slowly or by infusion.

Respiratory depression. Apnoea is more common and of longer duration than after barbiturate administration.

Excitatory phenomena. These are more frequent on induction than with thiopental, but less than with methohexital. There have been occasional reports of convulsions and myoclonus during recovery from anaesthesia in which propofol has been used. Some of these reactions are delayed.

Pain on injection. This occurs in up to 40% of patients (Table 3.5). The incidence is greatly reduced if a large vein is used, if a small dose (10 mg) of lidocaine is injected shortly before propofol, or if lidocaine is mixed with propofol in the syringe (10–20 mg, i.e. 1–2 mL of 1% lidocaine per 20 mL of propofol). A preparation of propofol in an emulsion of medium-chain triglycerides and soya (Propofol-Lipuro®) causes a lower incidence of pain, and less severe pain in those who still experience it, than other formulations (which use long-chain triglycerides) and may obviate the need for lidocaine. Propofol 0.5% causes less pain than higher concentrations. Accidental extravasation or intra-arterial injection of propofol does not appear to result in adverse effects.

Allergic reactions. Skin rashes occur occasionally. Anaphylactic reactions have also been reported, but appear to be less common than with thiopental.

Indications

Induction of anaesthesia. Propofol is indicated particularly when rapid early recovery of consciousness is required. Two hours after anaesthesia, there is no difference in psychomotor function between patients who have received propofol and those given thiopental or methohexital, but the former experience less drowsiness in the ensuing 12 h. The rapid recovery characteristics are lost if induction is followed by maintenance with inhalational agents for longer than 10–15 min. The rapid redistribution and metabolism of propofol may increase the risks of awareness during tracheal intubation after the administration of non-depolarizing muscle relaxants, or at the start of surgery, unless the lungs are ventilated with an appropriate mixture of inhaled anaesthetics, or additional doses or an infusion of propofol administered.

Sedation during surgery. Propofol has been used successfully for sedation during regional analgesic techniques and during endoscopy. Control of the airway may be lost at any time, and patients must be supervised continuously by an anaesthetist.

Total i.v. anaesthesia (see below). Propofol is the most suitable of the agents currently available. Recovery time is increased after infusion of propofol compared with that after a single bolus dose, but cumulation is significantly less than with the barbiturates.

Sedation in ICU. Propofol has been used successfully by infusion to sedate adult patients for up to several days in ICU. The level of sedation is controlled easily, and recovery is rapid (usually <30 min).

Absolute Contraindications

Airway obstruction and known hypersensitivity to the drug are probably the only absolute contraindications. Propofol appears to be safe in porphyric patients. Propofol infusion syndrome is a rare reaction to prolonged, high-dose infusion of propofol. It is characterized by bradycardia, metabolic acidosis, hyperlipidaemia, fatty liver enlargement, rhabdomyolysis and/or heart failure. It is more common in children or adolescents, is associated with head injury or the use of vasopressors and is often fatal. Therefore, propofol should not be used for long-term sedation of children (under 16 years of age) in ICU.

Precautions

These are similar to those listed for thiopental. The side-effects of propofol make it less suitable than thiopental or etomidate for patients with existing cardiovascular compromise unless it is administered with great care. Propofol is more suitable than thiopental for outpatient anaesthesia, but its use does not obviate the need for an adequate period of recovery before discharge.

Solutions of propofol do not possess any antibacterial properties, and they support the growth of microorganisms. The drug must be drawn aseptically into a syringe and any unused solution should be discarded if not administered promptly. Propofol must not be drawn up or administered via a microbiological filter.

Etomidate

This carboxylated imidazole compound was introduced in 1972.

Chemical Structure

D-Ethyl-1-(α-methylbenzyl)-imidazole-5-carboxylate.

Physical Characteristics and Presentation

Etomidate is soluble but unstable in water. It is presented as a clear aqueous solution containing 35% propylene glycol, or in an emulsion preparation with medium-chain triglycerides and soya-bean oil (Etomidate-Lipuro®). Ampoules contain 20 mg of etomidate in 10 mL ($2\,mg\,mL^{-1}$). The pH of the propylene glycol solution is 8.1.

Pharmacology

Etomidate is a rapidly acting general anaesthetic agent with a short duration of action (2–3 min) resulting predominantly from redistribution, although it is also eliminated rapidly from the body. In healthy patients, it produces less cardiovascular depression than does thiopental; however, there is little evidence that this benefit is retained if the cardiovascular system is compromised (e.g. by severe hypovolaemia). Large doses may produce tachycardia. Respiratory depression is less than with other agents.

Etomidate inhibits the 11β-hydroxylase enzyme involved in adrenal cortisol synthesis, resulting in reduced synthesis of cortisol by the adrenal gland and an impaired response to adrenocorticotrophic hormone.

At much higher doses, adrenal 18β-hydroxylase and other enzymes are inhibited, thus reducing aldosterone and other steroid hormone synthesis. Long-term infusions of the drug in the ICU are associated with increased infection and mortality, probably related to reduced immunological competence. Its effects on the adrenal gland occur also after a single bolus, and last for several hours.

Pharmacokinetics

Etomidate redistributes rapidly in the body. Approximately 76% is bound to protein. It is metabolized in the plasma and liver, mainly by esterase hydrolysis, and the metabolites are excreted in the urine; 2% is excreted unchanged. The terminal elimination half-life is 2.4–5 h. There is little cumulation when repeated doses are given. The distribution and clearance of etomidate may be altered by concomitant administration of fentanyl.

Dosage and Administration

An average dose of 0.3 mg kg^{-1} i.v. induces anaesthesia. The propylene glycol preparation of the drug should be administered into a large vein to reduce the incidence of pain on injection.

Adverse Effects

Suppression of synthesis of cortisol. See above.

Excitatory phenomena. Moderate or severe involuntary movements occur in up to 40% of patients during induction of anaesthesia. This incidence is reduced in patients premedicated with an opioid. Cough and hiccups occur in up to 10% of patients.

Pain on injection. This occurs in up to 80% of patients if the propylene glycol preparation is injected into a small vein, but in less than 10% when the drug is injected into a large vein in the antecubital fossa (Table 3.5). The incidence is reduced by prior injection of lidocaine 10 mg. The incidence of pain on injection has been reported to be as low as 4% when the emulsion formulation is injected.

Nausea and vomiting. The incidence of nausea and vomiting is approximately 30%. This is very much higher than after propofol.

Emergence phenomena. The incidence of severe restlessness and delirium during recovery is greater with etomidate than barbiturates or propofol.

Venous thrombosis is more common than with other agents if the propylene glycol preparation is used.

Indications

Etomidate is used usually for patients with a compromised cardiovascular system. It is suitable for outpatient anaesthesia. The high incidence of pain on injection of the propylene glycol preparation of etomidate limited its use to patients in whom depression of the cardiovascular system was undesirable, but the preparation as an emulsion with medium-chain triglycerides has greatly reduced the incidence of pain on injection.

Absolute Contraindications

- Airway obstruction
- Porphyria
- Adrenal insufficiency
- Long-term infusion in ICU.

Precautions

These are similar to the precautions listed for thiopental. Etomidate is suitable for outpatient anaesthesia. However, the incidence of excitatory phenomena is unacceptably high unless an opioid is administered; this delays recovery and is unsuitable for most outpatients.

Ketamine Hydrochloride

This is a phencyclidine derivative and was introduced in 1965. It differs from other i.v. anaesthetic agents in many respects, and produces dissociative anaesthesia rather than generalized depression of the CNS.

Chemical Structure

2-(*o*-Chlorophenyl)-2-(methylamino)-cyclohexanone hydrochloride.

Physical Characteristics and Presentation

Ketamine is soluble in water and is presented as solutions of 10 mg mL^{-1} containing sodium chloride to produce isotonicity and 50 or 100 mg mL^{-1} in multidose vials which contain benzethonium chloride 0.1 mg mL^{-1} as preservative. The pH of the solutions is 3.5–5.5. The pKa of ketamine is 7.5.

Pharmacology

Central Nervous System. Ketamine is extremely lipid-soluble. After i.v injection, it induces anaesthesia in 30–60 s. A single i.v. dose produces unconsciousness for 10–15 min. Ketamine is also effective within 3–4 min after i.m. injection and has a duration of action of 15–25 min. It is a potent somatic analgesic at subanaesthetic blood concentrations. Amnesia often persists for up to 1 h after recovery of consciousness. Induction of anaesthesia is smooth, but emergence delirium may occur, with restlessness, disorientation and agitation. Vivid and often unpleasant nightmares or hallucinations may occur during recovery and for up to 24 h. The incidences of emergence delirium and hallucinations are reduced by avoidance of verbal and tactile stimulation during the recovery period, or by concomitant administration of opioids, butyrophenones, benzodiazepines or physostigmine; however, unpleasant dreams may persist. Nightmares are reported less commonly by children and elderly patients.

The EEG changes associated with ketamine are unlike those seen with other i.v. anaesthetics, and consist of loss of alpha rhythm and predominant theta activity. Cerebral metabolic rate is increased in several regions of the brain, and CBF, cerebral blood volume and intracranial pressure increase.

Cardiovascular System. Arterial pressure increases by up to 25% and heart rate by approximately 20%. Cardiac output may increase, and myocardial oxygen consumption increases; the positive inotropic effect may be related to increased calcium influx mediated by cyclic adenosine monophosphate. There is increased myocardial sensitivity to adrenaline. Sympathetic stimulation of the peripheral circulation is decreased, resulting in vasodilatation in tissues innervated predominantly by α-adrenergic receptors, and vasoconstriction in those with β-receptors.

Respiratory System. Transient apnoea may occur after i.v. injection, but ventilation is well maintained thereafter and may increase slightly unless high doses are given. Pharyngeal and laryngeal reflexes and a patent airway are maintained well in comparison with other i.v. agents; however, their presence cannot be guaranteed, and normal precautions must be taken to protect the airway and prevent aspiration. Bronchial muscle is dilated.

Skeletal Muscle. Muscle tone is usually increased. Spontaneous movements may occur, but reflex movement in response to surgery is uncommon.

Gastrointestinal System. Salivation is increased.

Uterus and Placenta. Ketamine crosses the placenta readily. Fetal concentrations are approximately equal to those in the mother.

The Eye. Intraocular pressure increases, although this effect is often transient. Eye movements often persist during surgical anaesthesia.

Pharmacokinetics

Only approximately 12% of ketamine is bound to protein. The initial peak concentration after i.v. injection decreases as the drug is distributed, but this occurs more slowly than with other i.v. anaesthetic agents. Metabolism occurs predominantly in the liver by demethylation and hydroxylation of the cyclohexanone ring; among the metabolites is norketamine, which is pharmacologically active. Approximately 80% of the injected dose is excreted renally as glucuronides; only 2.5% is excreted unchanged. The elimination half-life is approximately 2.5 h. Distribution and elimination are slower if halothane, benzodiazepines or barbiturates are administered concurrently.

After i.m. injection, peak concentrations are achieved after approximately 20 min.

Dosage and Administration

Induction of anaesthesia is achieved with an average dose of 2 mg kg^{-1} i.v; larger doses may be required in some patients, and smaller doses in the elderly or shocked patient. In all cases, the drug should be administered slowly. Additional doses of 1–1.5 mg kg^{-1} are required every 5–10 min. Between 8 and 10 mg kg^{-1} is used i.m. A dose of 0.25–0.5 mg kg^{-1} or an infusion of 50 μg kg^{-1} min^{-1} may be used to produce analgesia without loss of consciousness.

Adverse Effects

- Emergence delirium, nightmares and hallucinations
- Hypertension and tachycardia – this may be harmful in previously hypertensive patients and in those with ischaemic heart disease

- Prolonged recovery
- Salivation – anticholinergic premedication is essential
- Increased intracranial pressure
- Allergic reactions – skin rashes have been reported.

Indications

The high-risk patient. Ketamine is useful in the shocked patient. Arterial pressure may decrease if hypovolaemia is present, and the drug must be given cautiously. These patients are usually heavily sedated in the postoperative period, and the risk of nightmares is therefore minimized.

Paediatric anaesthesia. Children undergoing minor surgery, investigations (e.g. cardiac catheterization), ophthalmic examinations or radiotherapy may be managed successfully with ketamine administered either i.m. or i.v.

Difficult locations. Ketamine has been used successfully at the site of accidents, and for analgesia and anaesthesia in casualties of war.

Analgesia and sedation. The analgesic action of ketamine may be used when wound dressings are changed, or while positioning patients with pain before performing regional anaesthesia (e.g. fractured neck of femur). Ketamine has been used to sedate asthmatic patients in the ICU.

Developing countries. Ketamine is used extensively in countries where anaesthetic equipment and trained staff are in short supply.

Absolute Contraindications

- Airway obstruction – although the airway is maintained better with ketamine than with other agents, its patency cannot be guaranteed. Inhalational agents should be used for induction of anaesthesia if airway obstruction is anticipated.
- Raised intracranial pressure.

Precautions

Cardiovascular disease. Ketamine is unsuitable for patients with pre-existing hypertension, ischaemic heart disease or severe cardiac decompensation.

Repeated administration. Because of the prolonged recovery period, ketamine is not the most suitable drug for frequent procedures, e.g. prolonged courses of radiotherapy, as it disrupts sleep and eating patterns.

Visceral stimulation. Ketamine suppresses poorly the response to visceral stimulation; supplementation, e.g. with an opioid, is indicated if visceral stimulation is anticipated.

Outpatient anaesthesia. The prolonged recovery period and emergence phenomena make ketamine unsuitable for adult outpatients.

Other Drugs

Opioids and benzodiazepines may also be used to induce general anaesthesia. However, very large doses are required, and recovery is prolonged. Their use is confined to specialist areas, e.g. cardiac anaesthesia. The pharmacology of these drugs is described in Chapters 5 and 7, respectively.

INTRAVENOUS MAINTENANCE OF ANAESTHESIA

Indications for Intravenous Maintenance of Anaesthesia

There are several situations in which i.v. anaesthesia (IVA; the use of an i.v. anaesthetic to supplement nitrous oxide) or total i.v. anaesthesia (TIVA) may offer advantages over the traditional inhalational techniques. In the doses required to maintain clinical anaesthesia, i.v. agents cause minimal cardiovascular depression. In comparison with the most commonly used volatile anaesthetic agents, IVA with propofol (the only currently available i.v. anaesthetic with an appropriate pharmacokinetic profile) offers rapid recovery of consciousness and good recovery of psychomotor function, although desflurane and sevoflurane are also associated with rapid recovery and minimal hangover effects.

The use of TIVA allows a high inspired oxygen concentration in situations where hypoxaemia may otherwise occur, such as one-lung anaesthesia or in severely ill or traumatized patients, and has obvious advantages in procedures such as laryngoscopy or bronchoscopy, when delivery of inhaled anaesthetic agents to the lungs may be difficult. TIVA may also be used to provide anaesthesia in circumstances in which there are clinical reasons to avoid nitrous oxide, such as middle-ear surgery, prolonged bowel surgery and in patients with raised intracranial pressure. There are few contra-indications to the use of IVA, provided that the anaesthetist is aware of the wide variability in response (see below). For surgical anaesthesia, it is desirable either to use nitrous oxide supplemented by IVA or to infuse an opioid in addition to the i.v. anaesthetic.

Principles of IVA

The calibrated vaporizer allows the anaesthetist to establish stable conditions, usually with relatively few changes in delivered concentration of volatile anaesthetic agents during an operation. This is largely because the patient tends to come into equilibrium with the delivered concentration, irrespective of body size or physiological variations; the total dose of drug taken up by the body is variable, but is relatively unimportant, and is determined by the characteristics of the patient and the drug rather than by the anaesthetist. The task of achieving equilibrium with i.v. anaesthetic agents is more complex, as delivery must be matched to the size of the patient and also to the expected rates of distribution and metabolism of the drug. Conventional methods of delivering i.v. agents result in the total dose of drug being determined by the anaesthetist, and the concentration achieved in the brain depends on the volume and rate of distribution, the relative solubility of the agent in various tissues and the rate of elimination of the drug in the individual patient. Consequently, there is considerably more variability among patients in the infusion rate of an i.v. anaesthetic required to produce satisfactory anaesthesia than there is in the inspired concentration of an inhaled agent.

Techniques of Administration

Intermittent Injection

Although some anaesthetists are skilled in the delivery of i.v. anaesthetic agents by intermittent bolus injection, the plasma concentrations of drug and the anaesthetic effect fluctuate widely, and the technique is acceptable only for procedures of short duration in unparalysed patients.

Manual Infusion Techniques

The infusion rate required to achieve a predetermined concentration of an i.v. drug can be calculated if the clearance of the drug from plasma is known [infusion rate (μg min^{-1})=steady-state plasma concentration (μg mL^{-1})×clearance (mL min^{-1})]. One of the difficulties is that clearance is variable, and it is possible only to estimate the value by using population kinetics; depending on the patient's clearance in relation to the population average, the actual plasma concentration achieved may be higher or lower than the intended concentration.

A fixed-rate infusion is inappropriate because the serum concentration of the drug increases only slowly, taking four to five times the elimination half-life of the drug to reach steady state (Fig. 3.4). A bolus injection followed by a continuous infusion results initially in achievement of an excessive concentration (with an increased incidence of side-effects), and this is followed by a prolonged dip below the intended plasma concentration (Fig. 3.5). In order to achieve a reasonably constant plasma concentration (other than in very long procedures), it is necessary to use a multistep infusion regimen, a concept similar to that of overpressure for inhaled agents. A commonly used scheme for propofol is injection of a bolus dose of 1 mg kg^{-1} followed by infusion initially at a rate of 10 mg kg^{-1} h^{1} for 10 min, then 8 mg kg^{-1} h^{1} for the next 10 min, and a maintenance infusion rate of 6 mg kg^{-1} h^{1} thereafter. This achieves, on average, a plasma concentration of propofol of 3 μg mL^{-1}, and this is effective in achieving satisfactory anaesthesia in unparalysed patients who *also* receive nitrous oxide and fentanyl; higher infusion rates are required if nitrous oxide and fentanyl are not

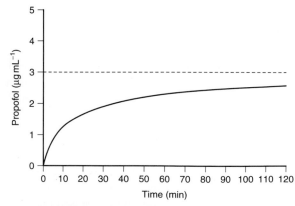

FIGURE 3.4 ■ Average blood concentration during the first 2 h of a continuous infusion of propofol at a rate of 6 mg kg^{-1} h^{-1}. Note that, even after 2 h, the equilibrium concentration of 3 μg mL^{-1} has not been achieved.

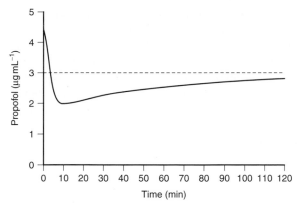

FIGURE 3.5 ■ Average blood propofol concentration following a bolus dose of propofol followed by a continuous infusion of 6 mg kg^{-1} h^{-1}. Note that the target concentration is initially exceeded, but that the blood concentration then decreases below the target concentration, which is not achieved within 2 h.

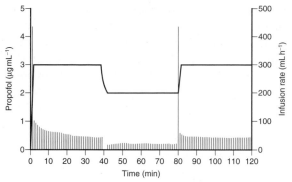

FIGURE 3.6 ■ Average blood concentrations of propofol achieved using a target-controlled infusion system. The narrow vertical lines represent the infusion rate calculated by the computer to achieve, and then to maintain, the target concentration in blood. A target concentration of 3 μg mL^{-1} was programmed initially. When the target concentration is reset to 2 μg mL^{-1}, the infusion is stopped and then restarted at a rate calculated to maintain that concentration. The target concentration is then increased to 3 μg mL^{-1}; the infusion pump delivers a rapid infusion rate to achieve the target concentration, and then gradually decreases the infusion rate to maintain a constant blood concentration.

administered. These infusion rates must be regarded only as a guide and must be adjusted as necessary according to clinical signs of anaesthesia.

Target-Controlled Infusion (TCI) Techniques

By programming a computer with appropriate pharmacokinetic data and equations, it is possible at frequent intervals (several times a minute) to calculate the appropriate infusion rate required to produce a preset target plasma concentration of drug. The drug is infused by a syringe driver. To produce a step increase in plasma concentration, the syringe driver infuses drug very rapidly (a slow bolus) and then delivers drug at a progressively decreasing infusion rate (Fig. 3.6). To decrease the plasma concentration, the syringe driver stops infusing until the computer calculates that the target concentration has been achieved, and then infuses drug at an appropriate rate to maintain a constant level. The anaesthetist is required only to enter the desired target concentration and to change it when clinically indicated, in the same way as a vaporizer might be manipulated according to clinical signs of anaesthesia.

The potential advantages of such a system are its simplicity, the speed with which plasma concentration can be changed (particularly upwards) and avoidance of the need for the anaesthetist to undertake any calculations (resulting in less potential for error). The actual concentration achieved may be >50% greater than or less than the predicted concentration, although this is

not a major practical disadvantage provided that the anaesthetist adjusts the target concentration according to clinical signs relating to adequacy of anaesthesia, rather than assuming that a specific target concentration always results in the desired effect.

Using a TCI system in female patients, the target concentration of propofol required to prevent movement in response to surgical incision in 50% of subjects (the equivalent of minimum alveolar concentration; MAC) was 6 μg mL^{-1} when patients breathed oxygen, and 4.5 μg mL^{-1} when 67% nitrous oxide was administered simultaneously.

A TCI system for administration of propofol is available in many countries. The anaesthetist is required to input the weight and age of the patient, and then to select the desired target concentration. These devices can be used only with prefilled syringes, which contain an electronic tag that is recognized by the infusion pump. These TCI systems are currently suitable for use only in patients over the age of 16 years. Target concentrations selected for elderly patients should be lower than those for younger adults, in order to minimize the risk of side-effects.

The TCI infusion pumps assume that the patient is conscious when the infusion is started. Consequently it is inappropriate to connect and start a TCI system in a patient who is already unconscious, as this results in an initial overdose.

In adult patients under 55 years of age, anaesthesia may be induced usually with a target propofol concentration of 4–8 µg mL^{-1}. An initial target concentration at the lower end of that range is suitable for premedicated patients. Induction time is usually between 1 and 2 min. The brain concentration of propofol increases more slowly than the blood concentration, and following induction it is usually appropriate to reduce the target concentration; target propofol concentrations in the range of 3–6 µg mL^{-1} usually maintain satisfactory anaesthesia in patients who are also receiving an analgesic drug.

Later versions of the TCI infusion pumps show the predicted brain concentration, which may be used as a guide to the timing of alterations in the blood target concentration.

Closed-Loop Systems

Target-controlled infusion systems may be used as part of a closed-loop system to control depth of anaesthesia. Because there is no method of measuring blood concentrations of i.v. anaesthetics on-line, it is necessary to use some type of monitor of depth of anaesthesia (such as the auditory evoked response; see Chapter 16) on the input side of the system.

Adverse Reactions to Intravenous Anaesthetic Agents

These may take the form of pain on injection, venous thrombosis, involuntary muscle movement, hiccup, hypotension and postoperative delirium. All of these reactions may be modified by the anaesthetic technique.

Hypersensitivity reactions, which resemble the effects of histamine release, are more rare and less predictable. Other vasoactive agents may also be released. Reactions to i.v. anaesthetic agents are caused usually by one of the following mechanisms:

Type I hypersensitivity response. The drug interacts with specific immunoglobulin E (IgE) antibodies, which are often bound to the surface of mast cells; these become granulated, releasing histamine and other vasoactive amines.

Classic complement-mediated reaction. The classic complement pathway may be activated by type II (cell surface antigen) or type III (immune complex formation) hypersensitivity reactions. IgG or IgM antibodies are involved.

Alternate complement pathway activation. Preformed antibodies to an antigen are not necessary for activation of this pathway; these reactions may therefore occur without prior exposure to the drug.

Direct pharmacological effects of the drug. These anaphylactoid reactions result from a direct effect on mast cells and basophils. There may be local cutaneous signs only. In more severe reactions, there are signs of systemic release of histamine.

Clinical Features

In a severe hypersensitivity reaction, a flush may develop over the upper part of the body. There is usually hypotension, which may be profound. Cutaneous and glottic oedema may develop and may result in hypovolaemia because of loss of fluid from the circulation. Very severe bronchospasm may also occur, although it is a feature in less than 50% of reactions. Diarrhoea often occurs some hours after the initial reaction.

Predisposing Factors

Age. In general, adverse reactions are less common in children than in adults.

Pregnancy. There is an increased incidence of adverse reactions in pregnancy.

Gender. Anaphylactic reactions are more common in women.

Atopy. There may be an increased incidence of type IV (delayed hypersensitivity) reactions in non-atopic individuals, and a higher incidence of type I reactions in those with a history of extrinsic asthma, hay fever or penicillin allergy.

Previous exposure. Previous exposure to the drug, or to a drug with similar constituents, exerts a much greater influence on the incidence of reactions than does a history of atopy.

Solvents. Cremophor EL, which was used as a solvent for several i.v. anaesthetic agents, was associated with a high incidence of hypersensitivity reactions.

Incidence

The incidences of hypersensitivity reactions associated with i.v. anaesthetic agents are shown in Table 3.6.

Treatment

This is summarized in Table 3.7. Appropriate investigations should be undertaken after recovery to identify the drug responsible for the reaction.

TABLE 3.6
Incidences of Adverse Reactions to Intravenous Anaesthetic Agents

Drug	Incidence
Thiopental	1:14 000–1:20 000
Methohexital	1:1600–1:7000
Etomidate	1:450 000
Propofol	1:50 000–100 000 (estimated)

FURTHER READING

Association of Anaesthetists of Great Britain and Ireland, 2009. Suspected anaphylactic reactions associated with anaesthesia. Anaesthesia 64, 199–211.

Calvey, N., Williams, N., 2008. Principles and practice of pharmacology for anaesthetists, fifth ed. Wiley-Blackwell, Oxford.

Sneyd, J.R., 2004. Recent advances in intravenous anaesthesia. Br. J. Anaesth. 93, 725–736.

TABLE 3.7
Suggested Management of Suspected Anaphylaxis During Anaesthesia

Aims

- Correct arterial hypoxaemia

- Restore intravascular fluid volume

- Inhibit further release of chemical mediators

Immediate Management

1. Stop administration of all agents likely to have caused the anaphylaxis

2. Call for help

3. Maintain airway, give 100% oxygen and lie patient supine with legs elevated

4. Give adrenaline (adrenaline). This may be given intramuscularly in a dose of 0.5–1 mg (0.5–1 mL of 1:1000) and may be repeated every 10 min according to the arterial pressure and pulse until improvement occurs

   Alternatively, 50–100 μg intravenously (0.5–1 mL of 1:10 000) over 1 min has been recommended for hypotension with titration of further doses as required

   Never give undiluted adrenaline 1:1000 intravenously

   In a patient with cardiovascular collapse, 0.5–1 mg (5–10 mL of 1:10 000) may be required intravenously in divided doses by titration. This should be given at a rate of 0.1 mg min⁻¹ stopping when a response has been obtained

   Paediatric doses of adrenaline depend on the age of the child. Intramuscular adrenaline 1:1000 should be administered as follows:

>12 years	500 μg i.m. (0.5 mL)
6–12 years	250 μg i.m. (0.25 mL)
6 months – 6 years	120 μg i.m. (0.12 mL)
<6 months	50 μg i.m. (0.05 mL)

5. Start rapid intravenous infusion of colloids or crystalloids. Adult patients may require 2–4 L of crystalloid

Secondary Management

1. Give antihistamines (chlorpheniramine 10–20 mg by slow i.v. infusion)

2. Give corticosteroids (100–500 mg hydrocortisone slowly i.v.)

3. Bronchodilators may be required for persistent bronchospasm

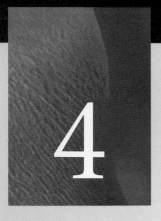

4

LOCAL ANAESTHETIC AGENTS

L ocal anaesthetics are analgesic drugs that suppress action potentials by blocking voltage-activated sodium ion (Na^+) channels in excitable tissues. Examples include the anaesthetic amides (e.g. lidocaine, bupivacaine, ropivacaine) and esters (e.g. cocaine and procaine) (Table 4.1). Other drugs which can inhibit voltage-activated Na^+ channels, such as diphenhydramine (a first-generation histamine H1 receptor antagonist) and amitriptyline (a tricyclic antidepressant) also have local anaesthetic properties. The blockade of voltage-activated Na^+ channels accounts for both their analgesic effects, mediated through inhibition of action potentials in nociceptive neurones, and their systemic effects. The inhibition of action potentials in the heart contributes to local anaesthetic toxicity and also accounts for the antiarrhythmic actions of intravenous lidocaine (a class 1b antiarrhythmic). Unlike general anaesthetics (the pharmacology of which is described in Chs 1 and 2), local anaesthetics do not diminish consciousness when administered correctly.

Local anaesthetics block sensation at the site of administration by inhibiting action potentials in all nociceptive fibres and therefore do not discriminate between pain modalities, unlike other analgesic drugs, such as the anti-inflammatory agents and opioids. Opioid analgesics (morphine, fentanyl, hydrocodone, etc.) and other central analgesic drugs such as the α_2-adrenergic agents (clonidine, dexmedetomidine) activate metabotropic (G protein-coupled) receptors within the membranes of specific neurones located within the pain pathway. A component of the actions of these drugs is centrally mediated (as described in Ch 5).

This chapter describes the pharmacology of local anaesthetics: their molecular mechanism of action, pharmacokinetics, systemic toxicity and recent developments which may improve their efficacy and safety.

MECHANISM OF ACTION OF LOCAL ANAESTHETICS

The primary target of local anaesthetics, the voltage-activated Na^+ channel (VASC) is one of numerous membrane proteins which reside in the phospholipid bilayers encapsulating neurones (Fig. 4.1). VASCs provide selective permeability to Na^+ when the cell becomes depolarized from the resting potential (approximately −70 mV), which is maintained in quiescent neurones by the tonic activity of potassium ion (K^+) channels. Local anaesthetics applied either topically to the skin or by infiltration inhibit action potentials in primary afferent nociceptive neurones, the pain-sensing neurones which transmit to the dorsal horn of the spinal cord (Fig. 4.2).

Pain transmission begins as a depolarization in the nerve ending of the primary afferent neurone initiated by the activation of cation channels. When the depolarization reaches the threshold for activation of VASCs (approximately −45 mV), action potentials are generated, resulting in rapid depolarization to approximately +20 mV (Fig. 4.3). Each action potential is brief (approximately 2 ms) because VASCs rapidly inactivate, leading to closure of their inactivation gates, and at the same time voltage-activated K^+ channels activate, leading to an increase in the permeability of the cell membrane to K^+. As a result,

The Features of Individual Local Anaesthetic Drugs

Proper Name/ Formula	% Equivalent Concentration[a]	Relative Duration[a]	Toxicity	pK$_a$	Partition Coefficient at 36°C	% Protein Bound	Main use by Anaesthetists in the UK
Cocaine	1	0.5	Very high	8.7	?	?	Nil
Benzocaine	NA	2	Low	NA	132	?	Topical
Procaine	2	0.75	Low	8.9	3.1	5.8	Nil
Chloroprocaine	1	0.75	Low	9.1	17	?	Not available
Tetracaine	0.25	2	High	8.4	541	76	Topical
Lidocaine	1	1	Medium	7.8	110	64	Infiltration Nerve block Epidural
Mepivacaine	1	1	Medium	7.7	42	77	Not available
Prilocaine	1	1.5	Low	7.7	50	55	Infiltration Nerve block IVRA
Ropivacaine	0.25	2–4	Medium	8.1	230	94	Epidural Nerve block
Bupivacaine	0.25	2–4	Medium	8.1	560	95	Epidural Spinal Nerve block

[a]Lidocaine = 1, NA = not applicable (not used in solution), ? = information not available.

NB: Published figures vary. Strichartz, G.R., Sanchez, V., Arthur, G.R., et al. 1990. Fundamental properties of local anesthetics. II. Measured octanol: buffer partition coefficients and pKa values of clinically used drugs. Anesth. Analg. 71, 158–170.

the membrane potential travels rapidly back towards the K$^+$ equilibrium potential and this period is known as the after-hyperpolarization, a phenomenon which contributes to the refractory period during which it is unlikely that another action potential will be generated (Fig. 4.3).

Mechanism of Local Anaesthetic Inhibition of the Voltage-Activated Na$^+$ Channel

Local anaesthetics inhibit VASC activity by gaining access to the open channel from the inside of the cell and binding to specific amino acids lining the channel lumen (Fig. 4.1). They bind preferentially to the open channel and are therefore said to be use-dependent (or open channel) blockers. First, the local anaesthetic must cross the cell membrane, a passage which requires lipid solubility. The molecule must then diffuse into the aqueous environment within the ion channel. Amide and ester local anaesthetics posses both lipophilic and hydrophilic properties and are described as amphipathic (Fig. 4.4). They exist in basic (uncharged) and cationic (charged) forms and the relative proportion of each (determined using the Henderson–Hasselbalch equation) is dependent upon the pH of the solution and the pK$_a$ of the local anaesthetic:

$$pK_a = pH + \log\frac{[\text{Cationic LA}]}{[\text{Uncharged LA}]}$$

$$\log\frac{[\text{Cationic LA}]}{[\text{Uncharged LA}]} = pK_a - pH$$

Local anaesthetics are weak bases and most have a pK$_a$ of approximately 8.5. Therefore there is

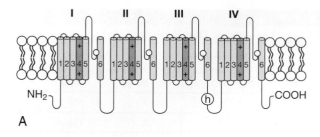

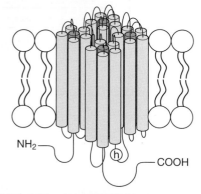

FIGURE 4.1 ■ The topology of the VASC α-subunit. (**A**) The subunit has 24 membrane-spanning segments arranged in four domains with positively charged amino acid residues in the fourth segment of each domain providing voltage-sensitivity. Pore loops between segments five and six line the channel and have negatively charged amino acids which attract Na$^+$ into the channel's outer vestibule. The intracellular loop between domains three and four contains the inactivation gate (or h gate). (**B**) The four domains come together to form a channel. The ancillary β-subunits, which modulate channel function, are not shown.

approximately 10-fold more charged than uncharged molecule at physiological pH ($\sim$7.5):

$$\log\frac{[\text{Cationic LA}]}{[\text{Uncharged LA}]} = 1$$

$$\frac{[\text{Cationic LA}]}{[\text{Uncharged LA}]} = 10$$

An alkaline solution speeds the onset of analgesia by increasing the proportion of uncharged local anaesthetic on the outside of the nerve, resulting in more rapid access to the inside of the cell where the balance of isoforms re-establishes on the basis of the intracellular pH. By contrast, infected and inflamed tissue has a relatively low (acidic) pH leading to an increase in the proportion of the membrane-impermeant cationic local anaesthetic component and the requirement for higher doses to achieve analgesia.

THE VOLTAGE-ACTIVATED Na$^+$ CHANNEL

Local anaesthetics gain access to their binding site within the inner lumen of the VASC when the activation gate opens in response to depolarization. The VASC is formed by a large protein (the α-subunit) consisting of 24 membrane-spanning segments arranged in four repetitive motifs (Fig. 4.1). The fourth segment of each motif is a voltage sensor, a series of positively charged amino acids (arginine and lysine residues) lying within the membrane. Depolarization causes electrostatic repulsion of the voltage sensors, providing the energy required to open the activation gate (Fig. 4.3). Na$^+$ ions, selected by the filter formed by the four pore loops (between the 5th and 6th segments) lining the outer vestibule of the channel, are then free to pass down their concentration gradient into the cell, generating a depolarizing electrical current. However, Na$^+$ current is inhibited by local anaesthetic bound within the inner vestibule of the channel. The inactivation gate, formed by intracellular components of the channel, closes rapidly following depolarization (Fig. 4.3) and local anaesthetics stabilize the inactivated state.

There are multiple subtypes of VASCs, named after the identity of their α-subunit (Na$_V$1.1–Na$_V$1.9) encoded by one of nine different genes (SCN1A–SCN5A, SCN8A–SCN11A) which are differentially expressed in tissues throughout the body and which have differing pharmacological and biophysical properties. This heterogeneity provides the potential (to date unmet) for selectively targeting VASCs in pain-sensing neurones. Nociceptive neurones predominantly express Na$_V$1.7, Na$_V$1.8 and/or Na$_V$1.9 α-subunits. Mutations in the SCN9A gene, which encodes Na$_V$1.7, are associated with several pain pathologies. Aspects of systemic toxicity relate to the ability of local anaesthetics to block VASCs outside the pain pathway. Cardiac VASCs are of the Na$_V$1.5 subtype and local anaesthetics such as ropivacaine and levobupivacaine are thought to have less systemic toxicity due to their lower affinity for cardiac channels. Additional VASC heterogeneity is conferred by four genes which encode ancillary β-subunits.

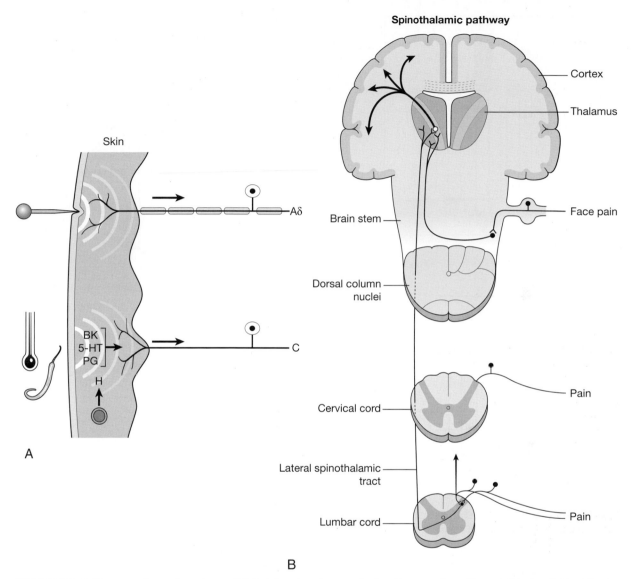

FIGURE 4.2 ■ The ascending pain pathway. (**A**) Peripheral nociceptors in the skin are activated by painful stimuli. Rapid stabbing pain is transmitted by myelinated Aδ fibres. Unmyelinated C fibres, activated by inflammatory mediators (e.g. bradykinin (BK), serotonin (5-HT), prostoglandins (PG) and histamine (H)) transmit aching pain more slowly. These fibres express TRPV1 channels activated by both noxious heat and capsaicin. (**B**) Primary afferent fibres synapse on neurones in the dorsal horn of the spinal cord, which transmit pain stimuli to the thalamus. Thalamic neurones project to the cortex.

PAIN FIBRES

Different peripheral nerve fibres have differing sensitivities to block by local anaesthetics and are classified as A, B and C according to their conduction velocities, A being the fastest conductors and C the slowest. Aδ and C fibres both conduct pain (Fig. 4.2). Other subtypes of A fibre supply skeletal muscles (α and γ) and conduct tactile sensation (β), while type B are preganglionic autonomic fibres. Aδ fibres are heavily myelinated and rapidly conduct acute stabbing pain. Myelination enables a remarkably high velocity of transmission

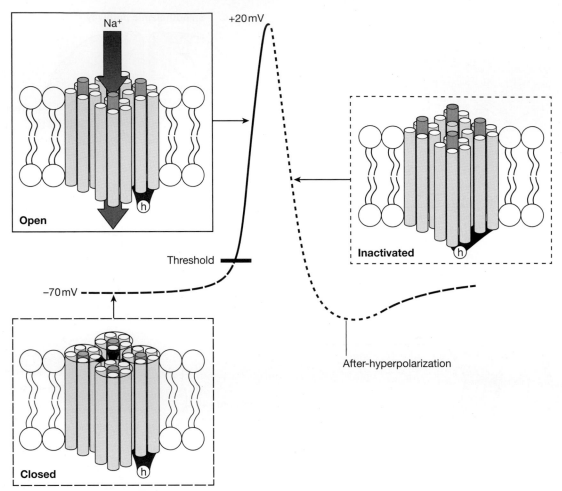

FIGURE 4.3 ■ Most VASCs are closed at resting membrane potential (−70 mV). Depolarization activates VASCs once the threshold potential is reached. Open VASCs enable greater depolarization until channels become inactivated and no longer support Na⁺ influx due to closure of the h-gate. Voltage-activated K⁺ channels (not shown) enable K⁺ efflux leading to hyperpolarization.

(approximately $20\,m\,s^{-1}$) through a mechanism known as saltatory conduction. VASCs are segregated within the neuronal membrane of Aδ fibres at gaps in the myelin sheaths (nodes of Ranvier), enabling action potentials effectively to 'jump' from one node to the next. Aδ fibres are of small diameter and therefore have little ability to conduct changes in membrane potential once VASC activity has been inhibited. This makes them particularly sensitive to local anaesthetic block. Unlike Aδ fibres, C fibres are unmyelinated and their velocity

of conduction from the skin to the spinal cord is relatively slow (approximately $1\,m\,s^{-1}$). Local anaesthetics effectively block the transmission of dull, aching pain mediated by C fibres. The fibre diameter is very small (approximately $1\,\mu m$) and therefore there is little passive conduction, making transmission reliant on the activity of VASCs. C fibres are activated by inflammatory mediators and therefore the pain resulting from their stimulation can also be treated by anti-inflammatory agents.

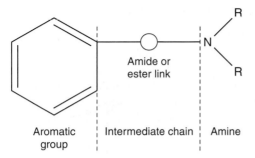

Amide or ester link

Aromatic group | Intermediate chain | Amine

FIGURE 4.4 ■ General formula for local anaesthetic drugs.

LOCAL ANAESTHETIC STRUCTURE

Local anaesthetics of the amide and ester classes share three structural moieties: an aromatic portion, an intermediate chain and an amine group (Fig. 4.4). The aromatic portion is lipophilic, and lipid solubility is further enhanced in local anaesthetics with lengthy intermediate chains. The amine group is a proton acceptor, providing the potential for both charged and uncharged isoforms (i.e. the source of the amphipathic nature of local anaesthetics). Amide and ester anaesthetics are so named because of their distinctive bonds within the intermediate chain. Examples of esters are cocaine, procaine, chloroprocaine and amethocaine; examples of amides are lidocaine, prilocaine, mepivacaine, etidocaine, bupivacaine, ropivacaine and levobupivacaine. A convenient mnemonic is that the names of esters contain one letter *i* while those of amides contain two letters *i*'s. The presence of either an amide or an ester bond dictates the pathway through which the local anaesthetic is metabolized and this has important implications regarding allergy potential and pharmacokinetic profile (described below). Since the introduction of cocaine into clinical practice by Koller in 1884, numerous local anaesthetics have been synthesized, beginning with procaine in 1905. Structural modifications influence pharmacokinetics. For example, replacement of the tertiary amine by a piperidine ring increased local anaesthetic lipid solubility and duration of action; addition of an ethyl group to lidocaine on the α-carbon of the amide link created etidocaine; and addition of a propyl group or butyl group to the amine end of mepivacaine resulted in [p]ropivacaine and bupivacaine

respectively. Halogenation of the aromatic ring of procaine created chloroprocaine, an ester with faster hydrolysis and shorter duration of action.

PHARMACOLOGICAL PROPERTIES OF LOCAL ANAESTHETICS

A number of important factors influence the pharmacological profile of local anaesthetic drugs (Table 4.1). The pK_a, molecular weight, lipid solubility, protein binding and vasoactivity influence speed of onset, potency and duration of action.

- pK_a is the pH at which the ionized and non-ionized form of a compound is present in equal amounts. For basic drugs such as local anaesthetics, the greater the pK_a, the greater the ionized fraction. As diffusion across the nerve sheath and nerve membrane requires non-ionized drug, a local anaesthetic with a low pK_a has a fast onset of action while a high pK_a causes a slow onset of action. For example, lidocaine (pK_a 7.6) has a fast onset in comparison with bupivacaine (pK_a 8.2), because, at pH 7.4, 35% of lidocaine exists in the non-ionized base form compared to only 20% of bupivacaine.

- *Molecular weight* influences the rate of transfer of drug across nerve membranes and through the dura mater. The lower the molecular weight the more rapid is the transfer.

- *Lipid solubility*, often expressed as the partition coefficient, influences potency. The partition coefficient is the ratio of aqueous and lipid concentrations when a local anaesthetic is introduced into a mixture of oil- and water-based solvents.

- *Protein binding*, including local anaesthetic attachment to protein components of the nerve membrane, increases the duration of action of a local anaesthetic. In plasma, amide anaesthetics bind predominantly to α-acid glycoprotein (AAG), a high-affinity limited capacity protein, and albumin, a low-affinity large capacity protein. The bioavailability of anaesthetic is determined by the availability of plasma proteins; the greater the AAG availability, the greater the binding of anaesthetic, and the lower the free plasma concentration. After surgery, trauma or malignancy, AAG concentrations increase significantly and protect patients receiving local anaesthetic epidural or perineural infusions from anaesthetic toxicity by curbing increases in the free fraction of local anaesthetics.

■ *Vasoactivity* influences potency and duration of action. The vasoactivity of commonly used local anaesthetics is biphasic with dilatation occurring with anaesthetic concentrations ≥0.25% and vasoconstriction at concentrations <0.25%. When measured by Laser Doppler flowmetry in the forearm, the vasoactive potencies occur in the order: lidocaine>bupivacaine>levobupivacaine>ropivacaine. Adrenaline at a dose of 1.25 µg provides significant vasoconstriction when administered with bupivacaine and levobupivacaine.

DIFFERENTIAL SENSORY AND MOTOR BLOCKADE

Local anaesthetics provide differential sensory and motor block dependent on fibre size. For example epidural administration of 0.5% bupivacaine provides excellent motor block for Caesarean section, yet administration of 0.1% bupivacaine, often with fentanyl 2 µg ml⁻¹, can provide analgesia during labour but with full lower limb movement.

PHARMACOKINETICS

Absorption

The site, dose and rate of injection, and pharmacological properties, with or without addition of adrenaline, determine the absorption of a local anaesthetic drug from its site of injection. The maximum recommended clinical doses are shown in Table 4.2. The rank order of plasma concentration after injection at various sites is: intrapleural>intercostal>lumbar epidural>brachial plexus>sciatic>femoral, which reflects the vascular supply to these tissues. First-pass pulmonary metabolism limits the concentration of local anaesthetic which reaches the systemic circulation.

Distribution

Tissue distribution of local anaesthetics is proportional to the lipid solubility of the drug and the blood supply. Local anaesthetic drugs are distributed rapidly to brain, heart, liver and lungs but more slowly to muscle and fat, which have a lower blood supply. The patient's age, cardiovascular status and hepatic function influence tissue blood flow.

Metabolism

Amide metabolism is dependent on hepatic blood flow. Toxicity of amides is more likely with prolonged infusions in sick, elderly patients, although the

TABLE 4.2
Maximum Doses of Local Anaesthetics Administered as a Bolus

	Plain (mg)	Plain per kg (mg kg⁻¹)	With Adrenaline (mg)	With Adrenaline (mg kg⁻¹)	Maximum Dose Over 24h (mg)
2-Chloroprocaine	800	11	1000 mg	13	
Prilocaine	600	8	600 mg	8	
Lidocaine	200	3	500 mg	7	
Mepivacaine	400	6	500 mg	7	
Bupivacaine	150	2	225 mg	3	400
Levobupivacaine	150	2			400
Ropivacaine	225	3			800

Adapted from McLeod GA, Butterworth JF, Wildsmith JAW (2008) Local anesthetic systemic toxicity. In: Cousins, Bridenbaugh, Horlecker, Carr (eds) Neural blockade. Lippincott, Williams & Wilkins, Ch 5 pp 114–132.

postoperative increase in AAG attenuates the rise in plasma concentrations. Esters are hydrolysed rapidly in plasma by pseudocholinesterase to the metabolite para-aminobenzoic acid (PABA), which can generate an allergic reaction. Amides are not metabolized to PABA and so allergic reactions are very rare.

Clearance

Clearance of amide local anaesthetics is dependent on hepatic metabolism, and metabolites may accumulate in renal failure. Metabolism is fastest in the rank order: prilocaine>lidocaine>bupivacaine.

Placental Transfer

Protein binding determines the rate and degree of diffusion of local anaesthetics across the placenta. The relative concentration of bupivacaine between umbilical vein and maternal circulation is 0.3, but fetal toxicity is dependent primarily on the free fraction of local anaesthetic, which is the same in mother and fetus.

CLINICAL PREPARATION OF LOCAL ANAESTHETICS

Local anaesthetics are presented clinically as hydrochloride salts with pH 5–6 because an alkaline pH destabilizes local anaesthetic solutions. Alteration of pH influences the rate of onset. For example, carbonated lidocaine favours the un-ionized molecule and has a faster onset of action whereas acidic tissue enhances ionization and reduces the onset and efficacy of local anaesthetics.

ENANTIOMER PHARMACOLOGY

Bupivacaine is a chiral molecule consisting of two structurally similar, non-superimposable, mirror images called enantiomers (Table 4.3). The nomenclature of enantiomers is based on the Cahn-Ingold-Prelog priority rules whereby the smallest atom is placed to the rear of the central atom about which the molecule rotates, and the sequence of the remaining three atoms is determined. For example, an increase in atomic mass in a clockwise direction is indicative of an S (sinistra) or laevo enantiomer whereas an increase in atomic mass in an anticlockwise direction is indicative of an R (rectus) or dextro enantiomer. Levobupivacaine is

TABLE 4.3	
Chiral Terminology	
Chirality	Spatial arrangement of atoms, non-superimposable on each other
Isomer	Molecule with the same atomic composition but different stereochemical formulae and hence different physical or chemical properties
Stereoisomers	Identical isomers which differ in the arrangement of their atoms in space
Enantiomer	One of a pair of molecules which are mirror images of each other and non-superimposable
Racemate	An equimolar mixture of a pair of enantiomers

the S (−) or laevo enantiomer of bupivacaine whereas ropivacaine is a single enantiomer from the same series as bupivacaine, but with a propyl rather than a butyl group.

INDIVIDUAL LOCAL ANAESTHETIC PHARMACOLOGY

Bupivacaine

Bupivacaine is a chiral compound, used clinically for 50 years. Initial benefits of bupivacaine were sensory-motor separation and minimal tachyphylaxis, unlike repeated doses of lidocaine. However, inadvertent intravenous administration of bupivacaine may result in systemic toxicity (see Local Anaesthetic Toxicity below) although addition of adrenaline may reduce this.

Levobupivacaine

The laevo enantiomer of bupivacaine with the same molecular structure. Potency is less than bupivacaine but greater than ropivacaine. Both single enantiomers are less toxic than racemic bupivacaine.

Ropivacaine

A single enantiomer. Substitution of a propyl for the butyl side chain of levobupivacaine confers less lipid solubility and greater sensory motor separation.

Lidocaine

This is the most popular local anaesthetic as it is safe, rapidly metabolized, and has a short duration of action. Efficacy is enhanced markedly by addition of adrenaline. A testament to the relative safety of the use of lidocaine is the fact that the drug is used systemically as a class 1b antiarrhythmic and in the treatment of chronic pain that is refractory to alternative approaches.

Prilocaine

This is less toxic than lidocaine, with a high clearance, attributable to metabolism in lung and kidneys and liver. It is associated with methemoglobinaemia at doses greater than 600 mg. The best application of prilocaine is as a 0.5% concentration, the provision of Bier's block for manipulation of wrist fractures. Prilocaine is contained in a eutectic mixture with lidoacaine (EMLA) for topical anaesthesia. A 2% formulation is also available for spinal anaesthesia.

LOCAL ANAESTHETIC TOXICITY

Early Clinical Reports

In 1979, Albright reported six cases of cardiac arrest without prodromal symptoms secondary to local anaesthetic toxicity. Four years later, he presented to the U.S. Food and Drug Administration (FDA) 53 cases of inadvertent intravascular injection of bupivacaine or etidocaine associated with prolonged and difficult resuscitation, 35 during pregnancy, and resulting in 24 deaths. The overriding clinical impression at that time was that toxicity secondary to bupivacaine appeared to be considerably out of proportion to its clinical potency relative to lidocaine, and, indeed, changes in anaesthetic practice such as needle aspiration, slow incremental injection and catheter insertion did much to reduce subsequent mortality.

Scientific Investigations

Animal studies indicated that the dextro enantiomer of bupivacaine was considerably more toxic than the laevo enantiomer. In electrophysiology experiments, dextro-bupivacaine attenuated the maximum upstroke velocity of the action potential (V_{max}) and lengthened action potential duration (APD), and in isolated small animal hearts it induced QRS widening, increasing both atrioventricular (AV) conduction time and arrhythmias.

In order to mimic inadvertent intravascular injection, lidocaine, bupivacaine, ropivacaine and levobupivacaine were infused into instrumented, conscious sheep in several studies designed to measure the cardiac and cerebral responses to systemic toxicity. The rank order of local anaesthetic dose needed to induce convulsions, arrhythmias, cardiac arrest and death was consistently: lidocaine>ropivacaine>levobupivacaine>bupivacaine. Importantly, arrhythmias induced by ropivacaine and levobupivacaine were more likely to revert to sinus rhythm, indicating that resuscitation may be easier in patients receiving these drugs.

Human Volunteer Studies

Results from animal studies cannot necessarily be translated to humans. Therefore, in order to measure the cardiovascular effects of local anaesthetics, bupivacaine, ropivacaine and levobupivacaine were infused into human volunteers in a series of studies using cardiac output monitoring until prodromal symptoms such as paraesthesiae, visual impairment, light-headedness or tinnitus occurred. The rank order of reduced ejection fraction was bupivacaine>levobupivacaine=ropivacaine. Thus, data from animal and human volunteer studies suggest that levobupivacaine and ropivacaine both exhibit a stereospecific effect on cardiac arrhythmogenesis, cardiac mechanical function and resuscitation.

Systemic Toxicity

Levobupivacaine and ropivacaine were introduced into clinical practice because both drugs showed equivalent potency for nerve block compared to bupivacaine but a greater therapeutic index from animal studies. However, systemic toxicity still remains a problem in clinical practice. Reasons for this include an increase in the practice of upper limb block, increased surgical use of local anaesthetics in high volumes for procedures such as tissue infiltration and tumescent anaesthesia, use of high-concentration compound local anaesthetic mixtures in the United States, inappropriate use of medical devices and administration of levobupivacaine and ropivacaine at doses greater than those recommended by the manufacturers.

Upper limb block is associated with a greater incidence of toxicity than lower limb or neuraxial block. For example, the incidence of convulsions secondary to epidural anaesthesia has been estimated at 1 in 8435, compared to 1 in 827 for axillary block, and 1 in 130 for supraclavicular and interscalene block. Tumescent anaesthesia for liposuction using doses of lidocaine >50 mg kg^{-1} has been associated with a mortality rate between 1 in 5000 to 10 000. Deaths have also been reported after application of 6–10% lidocaine and tetracaine compound local anaesthetic cream with cellophane wrapping to the legs before laser hair removal. In the UK, three patients died after unintentional connection of epidural infusions to intravenous lines, also between January 2005 and May 2006, the National Patient Safety Agency (NPSA) identified more than 346 incidents with epidural infusions which resulted in harm to patients. Most importantly, introduction of new 'safer' local anaesthetic drugs has encouraged some practitioners to administer higher doses of local anaesthetics than those recommended by drug manufacturers, narrowing the therapeutic window, and paradoxically increasing the risk of systemic toxicity.

Mechanisms of Systemic Toxicity

Direct injection into the vasculature (especially arterial injection in the head and neck) can lead to blindness, aphasia, hemiparesis, ventricular arrhythmias including fibrillation, convulsions, respiratory depression, coma or cardiac arrest. The most potent local anaesthetics have the highest tendency to cause systemic toxicity. For example, bupivacaine is more toxic than lidocaine. Cardiovascular effects are caused by blockade of cardiac VASCs and K$^+$ channels. Levobupivacaine and ropivacaine are thought less likely to interact with cardiac VASCs. Convulsions may be caused by the blockade of GABA$_A$ receptors in the CNS and respond to positive modulators of GABA$_A$ receptor

function (barbiturates, propofol and benzodiazepines). Involvement of mitochondria in local anaesthetic toxicity was proposed when a patient with carnitine deficiency showed marked sensitivity to a low dose of bupivacaine, suggesting that local anaesthetics interfere with mitochondrial energy functions. Animal experiments and many case reports have shown the benefits of Intralipid infusion during resuscitation following local anaesthetic-induced cardiac arrest.

MANAGEMENT OF SEVERE LOCAL ANAESTHETIC TOXICITY

Treatment of systemic toxicity is outlined in the guidelines produced by the Association of Anaesthetists of Great Britain and Ireland (AAGBI) (Table 4.4).

Recognition of the prodromal symptoms, such as agitation and disruption of sensory perception, is essential in order to instigate full life support measures. Immediate management should follow the Airway, Breathing, Circulation (ABC) mnemonic of resuscitation as outlined by the UK Resuscitation Council. Seizures should be controlled with small doses of thiopental, propofol or midazolam, depending on what is at hand. Hypoxaemia, hypercapnia and acidosis should be avoided because they all suppress myocardial function. If cardiac arrest occurs, cardiopulmonary resuscitation (CPR) should be started using standard protocols, but it should be recognized that arrhythmias may be very refractory. If so, consideration should be given to using an intravenous bolus dose of 20% Intralipid 1.5 mL kg^{-1} over 1 min followed by an infusion of 15 mL kg h^{-1}. If still unresponsive, a further two boluses may be given and the infusion rate doubled (Table 4.5). The role of adrenaline in lipid-based resuscitation from local anaesthetic-induced cardiac arrest is the subject of debate and is still to be resolved. Several case reports now allude to the success of Intralipid in both paediatric and adult resuscitation.

Prevention of Severe Local Anaesthetic Toxicity

- Regional blocks should always be performed in an area equipped to deal with cardiorespiratory collapse, such as an anaesthetic room or block room within the theatre suite.

TABLE 4.4

Management of Severe Local Anaesthetic Toxicity: AAGBI Safety Guideline

| 1 | Recognition | Sudden alteration in mental status, severe agitation or loss of consciousness, with or without tonic-clonic convulsions |
| | | Cardiovascular collapse: sinus bradycardia, conduction blocks, asystole and ventricular tachyarrhythmias |

2	Immediate management	Stop injecting the LA
		Call for help
		Maintain the airway and, if necessary, secure it with a tracheal tube
		Give 100% oxygen and ensure adequate lung ventilation (hyperventilation may help by increasing plasma pH in the presence of metabolic acidosis)
		Confirm or establish intravenous access
		Control seizures: give a benzodiazepine, thiopental or propofol in small incremental doses
		Assess cardiovascular status throughout
		Consider drawing blood for analysis, but do not delay definitive treatment to do this

3	Treatment	**In circulatory arrest**	**Without circulatory arrest**
		Start cardiopulmonary resuscitation (CPR) using standard protocols	Use conventional therapies to treat: hypotension, bradycardia, tachyarrhythmia
		Manage arrhythmias using the same protocols, recognising that arrhythmias may be very refractory	**Consider lipid emulsion**
		Consider the use of cardiopulmonary bypass if available	Propofol is not a suitable substitute for lipid emulsion
		Consider lipid emulsion	
		Continue CPR with lipid emulsion	
		Recovery may be >1 hour	

4	Follow-up	Arrange safe transfer to a clinical area with appropriate equipment and suitable staff until sustained recovery is achieved
		Exclude pancreatitis by regular clinical review, including daily amylase or lipase assays for two days
		Report cases as follows:
		in the United Kingdom to the National Patient Safety Agency (via www.npsa.nhs.uk)
		in the Republic of Ireland to the Irish Medicines Board (via www.imb.ie)
		If lipid has been given, please also report its use to the international registry at www.lipidregistry.org. Details may also be posted at www.lipidrescue.org

Reproduced with permission from AAGBI Safety Guideline Management of severe local anaesthetic toxicity http://www.aagbi.org/publications/guidelines/docs/la_toxicity_ 2010.pdf.

TABLE 4.5

Intralipid Doses

Immediately

Give an initial intravenous bolus injection of 20% lipid emulsion $1.5\,mL\,kg^{-1}$ over 1 min	**and**	Start an intravenous infusion of 20% lipid emulsion at $15\,mL\,kg^{-1}\,h^{-1}$

After 5 min

Give **a maximum of two** repeat boluses (same dose) if: cardiovascular stability has not been restored **or** an adequate circulation deteriorates Leave **5 min** between boluses A maximum of **three** boluses can be given (including the initial bolus)	**and**	Continue infusion at same rate, but **double** the rate to $30\,mL\,kg^{-1}\,h^{-1}$ at any time after 5 min, if: cardiovascular stability has not been restored **or** an adequate circulation deteriorates Continue infusion until stable and adequate circulation restored or maximum dose of lipid emulsion given

Do not exceed a maximum cumulative dose of $12\,mL\,kg^{-1}$.
Reproduced with permission from AAGBI Safety Guideline Management of severe local anaesthetic toxicity http://www.aagbi.org/publications/guidelines/docs/la_toxicity_ 2010.pdf.

- The age, weight and infirmity of the patient should be taken into account, and doses adjusted accordingly.
- Syringes of local anaesthetics and perineural and epidural infusions should be labelled clearly. Use of premixed sterile solutions is encouraged.
- Gentle aspiration of the syringe should precede every injection, but anaesthetists should be aware that negative aspiration does not guarantee extravascular positioning of the needle tip – false negatives do occur.
- Both during and after drug administration, the anaesthetist must keep talking to the patient.
- An appropriate test dose should be given depending on the situation. For example, a test dose of 3 mL of 'epidural' bupivacaine 0.5% (15 mg) injected accidentally into the intrathecal space will provide a definitive outcome – spinal anaesthesia. In contrast, injection of 0.5 to 1 mL during a perineural block under ultrasound is usually sufficient to differentiate between intraneural and extraneural injection.
- Examples of alternative epidural test doses are lidocaine 2% or adrenaline 15 µg, but neither test is specific or sensitive
- Ultrasound allows visualization of the position of the needle or catheter, their relationship to other structures – both nerves and large blood vessels – and the spread of local anaesthetic solution, although no definitive evidence exists yet that its use reduces overall complication rates.

EMERGING LOCAL ANAESTHETIC APPROACHES

Imaging and Local Anaesthesia

Ultrasound has become an important 2-D technique for guiding regional anaesthesia. Direct visualization of peripheral nerves, blood vessels and muscle is now possible during needle insertion both in-plane and out-of-plane of the ultrasonic beam. Local anaesthetic is deposited precisely around nerves using the hydrolocation technique whereby 1-mL boluses of local anaesthetic are used to distend connective tissue. The spread of local anaesthetic on a standard 'B-Mode' image is relatively easy to see and is quite distinct from the intraneural swelling characteristic of direct intraneural injection in laboratory preparations. However, despite undoubted improvements in block efficacy, no evidence as yet exists to demonstrate that the incidences of inadvertent intraneural or intravascular injection have declined.

TRP Channels and Pain

There has been a great deal of recent interest in targeting ion channels of the transient receptor potential (TRP) family to produce analgesia. Noxious heat activates TRP channels of the TRPV1 subtype in primary afferent nociceptive neurones. TRPV1 channel activation triggers the influx of Na^+ and Ca^{2+} ions, leading to depolarization and activation of VASCs. The resulting action potentials in pain fibres trigger the burning pain stimulus (Fig. 4.2). TRPV1 channels are also activated by the vanilloid capsaicin, a pungent substance extracted from chilli peppers. Other subtypes of TRP channel (TRPM8 and TRPA1) appear to be stimulated by noxious cold. There is interest in antagonists of TRP channels as potential analgesic drugs. Recent studies also demonstrate that TRPV1 channels can flux the positively charged quaternary lidocaine molecule QX-314. The drug is permanently charged and therefore cannot pass across the membrane of nociceptive neurones without an aqueous passage. Stimulation of TRPV1 channels by capsaicin provides a conduit for entry of QX-314 into pain fibres. Once inside neurones, the charged molecule binds to the local anaesthetic binding site within VASCs and inhibits action potentials. There is interest in this approach for targeting local anaesthesia to nociceptive neurones, thereby increasing the selectivity of block. Animal studies demonstrate that this method provides prolonged analgesia with much less motor block than is caused by equivalent analgesia using lidocaine.

FURTHER READING

AAGBI Safety Guideline. Management of severe local anaesthetic toxicity. http://www.aagbi.org/publications/guidelines/docs/la_toxicity_2010.pdf.

Binshtok, A.M., Bean, B.P., Woolf, C.J., 2007. Inhibition of nociceptors by TRPV1-mediated entry of impermeant sodium channel blockers. Nature 449, 607–610.

Catterall, W.A., Dib-Hajj, S., Meisler, M.H., Pietrobon, D., 2008. Inherited neuronal ion channelopathies: new windows on complex neurological diseases. J. Neurosci. 28, 11768–11777.

Chang, D.H., Ladd, L.A., Wilson, K.A., Gelgor, L., Mather, L.E., 2000. Tolerability of large-dose intravenous laevo-bupivacaine in sheep. Anesth. Analg. 91, 671–679.

McLeod, G.A., Burke, D., 2001. Levobupivacaine. Anaesthesia 56, 331–341.

Rao, R.B., Ely, S.F., Hoffman, R.S., 1999. Deaths related to liposuction. N. Engl. J. Med. 340, 1471–1475.

Rosenblatt, M.A., Abel, M., Fischer, G.W., Itzkovich, C.J., Eisenkraft, J.B., 2006. Successful use of a 20% lipid emulsion to resuscitate a patient after a presumed bupivacaine-related cardiac arrest. Anesthesiology 105, 217–218.

Strichartz, G.R., Sanchez, V., Arthur, G.R., Chafetz, R., Martin, D., 1990. Fundamental properties of local anesthetics. II. Measured octanol: buffer partition coefficients and pKa values of clinically used drugs. Anesth. Analg. 71, 158–170.

Weinberg, G., Ripper, R., Feinstein, D.L., Hoffman, W., 2003. Lipid emulsion infusion rescues dogs from bupivacaine-induced cardiac toxicity. Reg. Anesth. Pain Med. 28, 198–202.

Yanagidate, F., Strichartz, G.R., 2007. Local anesthetics. Handb. Exp. Pharmacol. 177, 95–127.

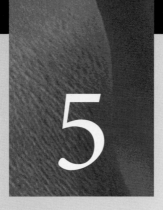

5 ANALGESIC DRUGS

T he ideal analgesic should relieve pain with a minimum of side-effects. When formulating a management plan, it is worth considering what contributes to pain perception and associated distress. The International Association for the Study of Pain (IASP) defines pain as 'an unpleasant sensory and emotional experience associated with actual or potential tissue damage or described in terms of such damage'. It is clear from this definition that the degree of tissue damage and perception of pain are not necessarily correlated. Pain perception is a complex phenomenon, involving sensory, emotional and cognitive processes. Thus, while analgesic drugs can be effective in relieving both acute and chronic pain, other factors may also need to be addressed.

There is considerable evidence that patients continue to suffer pain, despite a wide range of available analgesic drugs. When devising a management plan for both acute and chronic settings, using 'balanced' or 'multimodal analgesia' may be helpful. These terms refer to the use of combinations of drugs acting by different mechanisms or at different sites within the pain pathway. Analgesic combinations may be additive or synergistic in their mode of action, with resultant dose-sparing effects and a reduction in side-effects. Effective and repeated assessment of patients is essential in determining optimal analgesic management.

OPIOIDS

Opioids are the most frequently used analgesics for the treatment of moderate to severe pain. Despite this, there are still major gaps in our knowledge of their clinical pharmacology, with the choice of drug and dose being largely empirical. Although they may be highly effective, control of dynamic (pain on movement) or incident (breakthrough) pain may be poor and side-effects may be a significant problem. The term opioid refers to all drugs, both synthetic and natural, that act on opioid receptors. Opiates are naturally occurring opioids derived from the opium poppy *Papaver somniferum*. The most widely used opioid is morphine, although a variety of different opioids are available. Incomplete cross-tolerance occurs between them, so an alternative should be tried if morphine is poorly tolerated. There is increasing evidence that in any one individual both analgesic response and side effect profile will be, at least partly, due to that person's genetic make up. Differences in Single Nucleotide Polymorphisms (SNPs) almost certainly contribute to this variability in response between different opioids, with potential candidate genes including ABCB1 (encoding p-glycoprotein, a membrane transporter), STAT6 (signal transducer and activator of transcription 6) and beta-arrestin (intracellular protein involved in receptor internalization).

Dose conversion between different opioids is an inexact science, with equi-analgesic doses being based on relative potencies, often derived from studies that are not designed for dose equivalence calculation. Table 5.1 shows suggested equi-analgesic doses for some opioids.

Mechanism of Action

Opioid receptors belong to the G-protein coupled family of receptors with seven transmembrane domains, an extracellular N-terminal and intracellular

69

TABLE 5.1
Equi-Analgesic Doses of Opioids

| Opioid | ~ EQUI-ANALGESIC DOSE | |
	Parenteral	Oral
Morphine	10 mg	20–30 mg
Meperidine (pethidine)	100 mg	300 mg
Oxycodone	15 mg	20–30 mg
Fentanyl	100 µg	NA
Hydromorphone	1.5 mg	7.5 mg
Methadone	1–10 mg	20 mg
Codeine	NA	200 mg

C-terminal. Activation results in changes in enzyme activity such as adenylate cyclase or alterations in calcium and potassium ion channel permeability.

Opioid receptors were originally classified by pharmacological activity in animal preparations, and later by molecular sequence. The three main receptors were classified as µ (mu) or OP3, κ (kappa) or OP1 and δ (delta) or OP2. Another opioid-like receptor has been identified recently; it is termed the nociceptin orphanin FQ peptide receptor. Receptor nomenclature has changed several times in the last few years; the current International Union of Pharmacology (IUPHAR) classification is MOP (mu), KOP (kappa), DOP (delta) and NOP for the nociceptin orphanin FQ peptide receptor (Table 5.2).

Opioid receptors are distributed widely in both central and peripheral nervous systems. The different effects of currently available opioids are dependent on complex interactions at various receptors. There is a range of endogenous neuropeptide ligands active at these receptors (Table 5.2); they function as neurotransmitters, neuromodulators and neurohormones. The endogenous tetrapeptide endomorphins 1 and 2 are potent agonists acting specifically at the MOP receptor; they play a role in modulating inflammatory pain.

The analgesic action of morphine and most other opioids is related mainly to agonist activity at the MOP receptor. Unfortunately, many of the unwanted effects of opioids are also related to activity at this receptor. At a cellular level, MOP receptor activation has an overall inhibitory effect via: (i) inhibition of adenylate cyclase; (ii) increased opening of potassium channels (hyperpolarization of postsynaptic neurones, reduced synaptic transmission); and (iii) inhibition of calcium channels (decreases presynaptic neurotransmitter release).

Pharmacodynamic Effects of Opioids

The ubiquitous nature of opioid receptors implies that agents acting at them have wide-ranging effects, some of which may be problematic. Some opioids or their metabolites also have activity at other receptors, e.g. methadone acts at the N-methyl-D-aspartate (NMDA) receptor. These particular actions are discussed for

TABLE 5.2
Classification of Opioid Receptors as Defined by the International Union of Pharmacology

Receptor	Previous Classifications	Endogenous Ligand	Site
MOP	Mu; OP3	Endomorphin 1 and 2; met-enkephalin; dynorphin A and B	Peripheral inflammation, pre- and postsynaptic neurones in spinal cord, periaqueduct grey matter, limbic system, caudate putamen, thalamus, cerebral cortex
KOP	Kappa; OP1	Dynorphin A and B; β-endorphin	Nucleus raphe magnus (midbrain), hypothalamus, spinal cord
DOP	Delta; OP2	Leu- and met-enkephalins; β-endorphin	Olfactory centres, cerebral cortex, nucleus accumbens, caudate putamen, spinal cord
NOP	Orphan; ORL-1	Orphanin FQ (nociceptin)	Nucleus raphe magnus, spinal cord, afferent neurones

individual agents below. The more general effects of opioids are described in this section.

Analgesic Action

Opioids with agonist activity mainly at the MOP receptor, and to a lesser extent at the KOP receptor, have analgesic effects. Analgesic effects have also been demonstrated for the spinal DOP receptor in certain situations.

Opioids should be titrated against pain; if higher than necessary doses are given, respiratory depression and excessive sedation may result. If the pain is incompletely opioid-responsive, as may occur with neuropathic pain, then care must be taken with dose titration and a detailed reassessment of analgesic response is essential. Opioids exert their analgesic effect by:

- supraspinal effects in the brainstem, thalamus and cortex, in addition to modulating descending systems in the midbrain periaqueductal grey matter, nucleus raphe magnus and the rostral ventral medulla
- inhibitory effects within the dorsal horn of the spinal cord both pre- and postsynaptically
- a peripheral action in inflammatory states, where MOP receptors modulate immune function and nociceptors are important in regulating peripheral sensitization.

Central Nervous System

In addition to analgesia there are several potential central nervous system (CNS) effects of opioids:

Sedation and sleep. Opioids interfere with rapid-eye-movement sleep with changes in the EEG including a progressive decrease in EEG frequency and production of delta waves. However, burst suppression is not seen, even with large doses. Opioid-related ventilatory depression is more common during sleep. Opioid-induced sedation may be used therapeutically, e.g. critical care setting. There is a dose-related reduction in minimum alveolar concentration (MAC) for volatile anaesthetics, though there is a floor to this effect. Opioids alone do not act as reliable anaesthetic agents.

Mood. Significant euphoria is uncommon when opioids are used to treat pain but it occurs frequently when they are used inappropriately. Dysphoria

(possibly via a KOP receptor action) and hallucinations can occur. Commonly, the hallucinations are visual in nature and may only affect part of the visual field.

Miosis. This is mediated via a KOP receptor effect on the Edinger-Westphal nucleus of the oculomotor nerve.

Tolerance (i.e. requirement of increasing doses to achieve the same effect) is important clinically because a significant number of patients are receiving long-term opioid therapy for malignant and chronic non-malignant pain; it is also relevant in illicit drug use. Additionally, tolerance may develop much more acutely, e.g. when opioids are used for pain control before surgery or when given intrathecally. However, after initial dose titration, the majority of patients on long-term opioids are usually maintained on a stable dose.

At a cellular level, tolerance is caused by a progressive loss of active receptor sites combined with uncoupling of the receptor from the guanosine triphosphate (GTP)-binding subunit. There is also some evidence that the NMDA receptor may play a role in acute tolerance, via protein kinase C activity lifting the magnesium block at the NMDA site. There may therefore be a rationale for using ketamine in situations of acute tolerance, for example in the postoperative period. Interactions with the NOP receptor may also be important.

The incomplete cross-tolerance between different types of opioids may result from differential activity at opioid receptor subtypes. Withdrawal may occur if there is abrupt cessation of opioids or if an antagonist is given.

Opioid-induced hyperalgesia. This is a paradoxical response where an increase in opioid dose results in hyperalgesia. There is good basic science evidence of underlying mechanisms, but its importance in clinical practice is unclear. It may be part of the spectrum of opioid toxicity, or can occur in isolation. It has been shown to occur after systemic administration of potent short acting opioids such as remifentanil.

Addiction. This is defined as the compulsive use of opioids to the detriment of the patient in terms of physical, psychological or social function. Drug-seeking behaviour is not usually a problem if opioids are used appropriately for pain relief in both acute and chronic situations.

Respiratory

Opioids may cause respiratory depression, particularly in the elderly, neonates and when given without titrating effect to analgesic response. Tolerance does develop to this phenomenon, so it is less of a problem in chronic use. However, care must be taken if nociceptive input is reduced or removed, e.g. after a nerve block. Sensitivity to CO_2 is reduced, even with small doses of MOP agonists. This is caused by depression of sensitivity of neurones on the ventral surface of the medulla.

Opioids, given at sufficient dose, are effective at suppressing the stress response to laryngoscopy and airway manipulation. They may reduce the plasma concentrations of catecholamines, cortisol and other stress hormones by inhibiting the pituitary-adrenal axis, reducing central sympathetic outflow and influencing central neuroendocrine responses. Opioids also suppress cough activity and mucociliary function. This may cause inadequate clearing of secretions and hypostatic pneumonia, especially if there is associated sedation and respiratory depression. This antitussive activity is, at least in part, mediated peripherally.

Gastrointestinal

All opioids may cause nausea and vomiting, although tolerance develops. This may be mediated both centrally and peripherally, with a direct effect on the chemoreceptor trigger zone in addition to a delay in gastric emptying. Opioids increase gastrointestinal muscle tone and decrease motility. An increase in biliary pressure with gallbladder contraction may also occur. Constipation occurs commonly via a direct action on opioid receptors in the smooth muscle of the gut; many patients do not become tolerant to this when receiving long-term opioids.

Cardiovascular

In normovolaemic patients, the majority of opioids have no significant cardiovascular depressant effect. However, if histamine is released, then there may be tachycardia, decrease in systemic vascular resistance and a reduction in arterial pressure. Bradycardia may occur in response to some opioids. There is no direct action on baroreceptors but a minimal reduction in preload and afterload may occur. There is no effect on cerebral autoregulation. However, if respiratory depression is present, then the resultant increase in $PaCO_2$ may increase cerebral blood flow.

Opioids decrease central sympathetic outflow. Therefore, in patients who are relying on increased sympathetic tone to maintain cardiovascular stability, opioids may lead to haemodynamic compromise. This may be severe, particularly if potent opioids are given by rapid intravenous bolus.

Other Effects

Myoclonic jerks may occur if there is opioid toxicity and may be associated with sedation and hallucinations. *Urinary retention* and urgency may occur, probably related to a centrally mediated mechanism as these problems are much more common when neuraxial opioids are used. *Pruritus* is relatively common after neuraxial administration. The nose, face and torso are particularly affected and this may be reversed by a low dose of a MOP antagonist. *Muscle rigidity* is a recognized complication, particularly after intravenous bolus administration of potent phenylpiperidines. This may cause significant problems with ventilation because of chest wall rigidity and decreased respiratory compliance. It may be minimized by co-administration of opioids with intravenous anaesthetic agents and benzodiazepines, reversed by naloxone or prevented by neuromuscular blocking agents. *Thermoregulation* is impaired to a similar extent as that seen with volatile agents. With long-term use, *depression of the immune system* may occur. *Endocrine problems* include impaired adrenal and sexual function, and infertility.

Opioid Structure

The structures of opioid analgesics are diverse, although for most opioids it is usually the laevorotatory (*laevo*) stereoisomer that is the active compound. The structures of some of the common agents are shown in Figures 5.1 and 5.2. Agents in current use include phenanthrenes (e.g. morphine – Fig. 5.1), phenylpiperidines (e.g. meperidine (pethidine), fentanyl – Fig. 5.2) and diphenylpropylamines (e.g. methadone, dextropropoxyphene). Structural modification affects agonist activity and alters physicochemical properties such as lipid solubility. A tertiary nitrogen is necessary for activity separated from a quaternary carbon by an

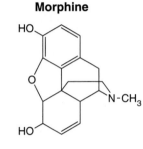

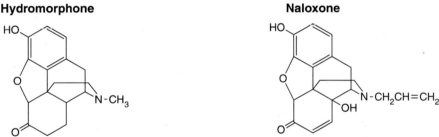

FIGURE 5.1 ■ The structure of morphine and the phenanthrenes.

ethylene chain. Chemical modifications that produce a quaternary nitrogen significantly reduce potency as a result of decreased CNS penetration. If the methyl group on the nitrogen is changed, antagonism of analgesia may be produced.

Other important positions for activity and metabolism, as seen on the morphine molecule (Fig. 5.1), include the C-3 phenol group (the distance of this from the nitrogen affects activity) and the C-6 alcohol group. Potency may be increased by hydroxylation of the C-3 phenol; oxidation of C-6 (e.g. hydromorphone); double acetylation at C-3 and C-6 (e.g. diamorphine); hydroxylation of C-14 and reducing the double bond at C-7/8. Further additions at the C-3 OH group reduce activity. A short-chain alkyl substitution is found in mixed agonist-antagonists, hydroxylation or bromination of C-14 produces full antagonists and removal or substitution of the methyl group reduces agonist activity.

Pharmacokinetics and Physicochemical Properties

Knowledge of the specific physicochemical properties and pharmacokinetics of individual agents is important in determining the optimal route of drug delivery in order to achieve an effective receptor site concentration for an appropriate duration of action. All opioids are weak bases. The relative proportion of free and ionized fractions is dependent on plasma pH and the pK_a of the particular opioid. The amount of

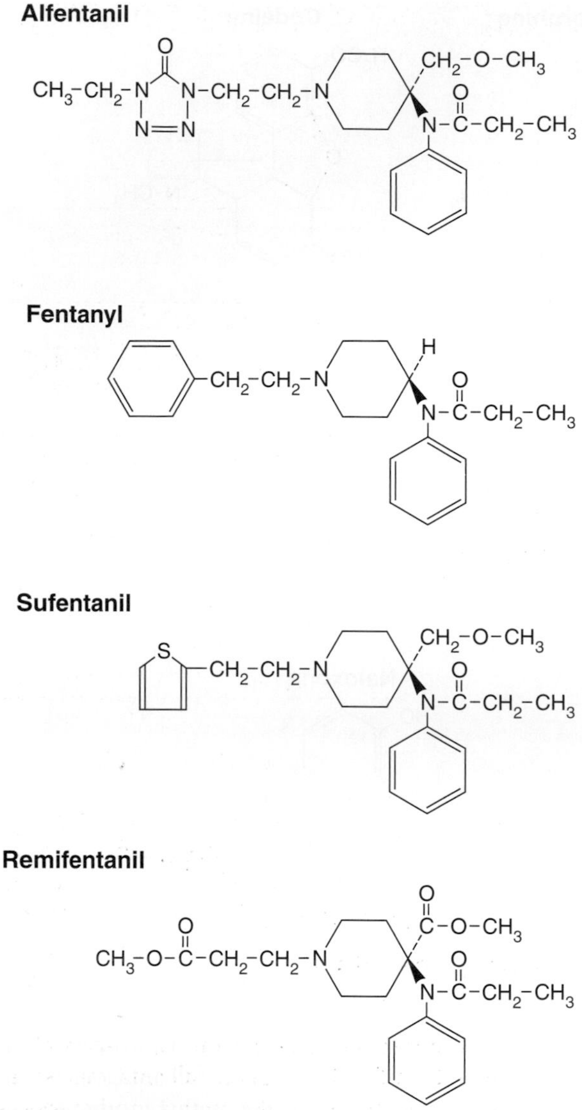

Alfentanil

Fentanyl

Sufentanil

Remifentanil

FIGURE 5.2 ■ The structures of phenylpiperidine opioids.

opioid diffusing to the site of action (diffusible fraction) is dependent on lipid solubility, concentration gradient and degree of binding. Plasma concentrations of albumin and α_1-acid glycoprotein as well as tissue binding determine the availability of the unbound, unionized fraction. This diffusible fraction moves into tissue sites in the brain and elsewhere; the amount reaching receptors is dependent not only on lipophilicity but also on the amount of non-specific tissue binding, e.g. CNS lipids.

The ionized, protonated form is active at the receptor site. This has important implications for speed and duration of activity. For example, morphine is relatively hydrophilic and penetrates the blood–brain barrier slowly. However, a large mass of any given dose eventually reaches the receptor site because of low levels of nonspecific tissue binding. This effect-site equilibration time $(t_{1/2}k_{eo})$ is measured by assessing the effect of opioids on the EEG. The offset time may also be prolonged, resulting in a longer duration of action than would be expected from the plasma half-life. Most opioids have a very steep dose-response curve. Therefore, if the dose is near the minimum effective analgesic concentration (MEAC), very small fluctuations in plasma or effect-site concentrations may lead to large changes in the level of analgesia.

Opioids tend to have a large volume of distribution (V_D) because of their high lipid solubility. A consequence of this can be that redistribution, particularly after a bolus dose or short infusion, can have significant effects on plasma concentrations. In addition, first-pass effects in the lung may remove significant amounts of drug from the circulation, reducing the initial peak plasma concentration. However, the drug re-enters the plasma several minutes later. Plasma concentrations of opioids such as fentanyl, sufentanil and meperidine (pethidine) are affected by this; the effect is negligible for remifentanil. Other lipophilic amines such as lidocaine and propranolol are affected similarly and may reduce pulmonary uptake of co-administered opioids.

After prolonged infusion, significant sequestration in fat stores and other body tissues occurs for highly lipid-soluble opioids. This is reflected in the 'context-sensitive $t_{1/2}$' i.e. the time taken for the plasma concentration to reduce by 50% after an infusion designed to maintain constant plasma concentrations has been stopped (see Chapter 1). The context-sensitive $t_{1/2}$ is increased after prolonged infusion for most opioids apart from remifentanil. For example, the elimination $t_{1/2}$ for fentanyl after bolus administration is 3–5 h, but increases to 7–12 h after prolonged infusion.

Most opioid metabolism occurs in the liver (phase I and II reactions) with the hydrophilic metabolites predominantly excreted renally, although a small amount may be excreted in the bile or unchanged in the urine. As a result, hepatic blood flow is one of the major

TABLE 5.3
Metabolism and Excretion of Some Opioids

Drug	Metabolism	Faeces	Urine
Morphine	Glucuronidation, sulphation N-dealkylation	Trace	90% in 24 h (10% morphine; 70% glucuronides; 10% 3-sulphate; 1% normorphine; 3% normorphine glucuronide)
Codeine	O-demethylation, glucuronidation	Trace	86% in 24 h (5–10% codeine; 60% codeine glucuronide; 5–15% morphine (mainly conjugated); trace normorphine)
Diamorphine	O-deacetylation, glucuronidation	Trace	80% in 24 h (5–7% morphine; 90% morphine glucuronides; 1% 6-acetylmorphine; 0.1% diamorphine)
Buprenorphine	Glucuronidation, N-dealkylation	70% mainly unchanged	2–13% in 7 days; mainly N-dealkylbuprenorphine (and glucuronide); buprenorphine-3-glucuronide
Meperidine (pethidine)	N-demethylation, hydrolysis		70% in 24 h (10% meperidine; 10% normeperidine; 20% meperidinic acid; 16% meperidinic acid glucuronide; 8% normeperidinic acid; 10% normeperidinic acid glucuronide; plus small amounts of other metabolites)
Methadone	N-dealkylation	30%	60% in 24 h (33% methadone; 43% EDDP; 10% EMDP plus small amounts of other metabolites)
Fentanyl	N-dealkylation, hydroxylation	9%	70% in 4 days (5–25% fentanyl; 50% 4-N-(N-propionylanilino-piperidine) plus other metabolites)

EDDP; 2-ethylidine-1,5-dimethyl 3,3 diphenylpyrrolidine
EMDP; 2-ethyl-5-methyl-3,3-diphenylpyraline

determinants of plasma clearance. Metabolism of individual drugs is shown in Table 5.3. Enterohepatic recirculation may occur when water-soluble metabolites excreted in the gut may be metabolized by gut flora to the parent opioid and then reabsorbed. Lipid-soluble opioids may diffuse into the stomach, become ionized because of the low pH and then be reabsorbed in the small intestine; this results in a secondary peak in plasma concentration.

A summary of physicochemical and pharmacokinetic properties of some opioids is shown in Table 5.4. Metabolism (including production of active metabolites), distribution between different tissues and elimination all interact within individual subjects to produce clinically important actions at receptor sites.

Factors affecting pharmacokinetics include:

- *Age.* Systemic dose is often calculated on body weight, although there is little evidence to support this in adult clinical practice. Age is often more important because of both pharmacokinetic and pharmacodynamic factors. Metabolism and volume of distribution are often reduced in the elderly, leading to increased free drug concentrations in the plasma. Hepatic blood flow may have declined by 40–50% by age 75 years, with reduced clearance of opioids. Increased CNS sensitivity to opioid effects is also found in the elderly.

- *Hepatic disease* has unpredictable effects, although there may be little clinical difference unless there is coexisting encephalopathy. Reductions in plasma protein concentrations also have effects on plasma concentrations of free unbound drug.

- *Renal failure* may have significant effects for opioids with renally excreted active metabolites such as morphine, diamorphine and meperidine.

- *Obesity* will result in a larger V_D and prolonged elimination $t_{1/2}$. This may be a particular problem if infusions are being used.

- *Hypothermia, hypotension and hypovolaemia* may also result in variable absorption and altered distribution and metabolism.

TABLE 5.4							
Pharmacokinetic and Physicochemical Properties of Some Opioids							
Opioid	pK$_a$	Protein Binding (%)	Octanol:Water Partition Coefficient	Terminal Half-Life (h)	Clearance (mL kg^{-1} min^{-1})	Volume of Distribution (L kg^{-1})	Duration of Action (h)
Morphine	7.9	30	6	1.7–3.0	15–20	3–5	3–5
Oxycodone	8.5	45		3–4	13	2–3	2–4
Codeine	8.2	20	0.6	2–4		2.5–3.5	
Meperidine (pethidine)	8.5	70	39	3–5	8–18	3–5	2–4
Fentanyl	8.4	90	813	2–4	10–20	3–5	1–1.5
Alfentanil	6.5	91	128	1–2	4–9	0.4–1	0.25–0.4
Remifentanil	7.3	70	18	0.1–0.2	40–60	0.3–0.4	2–5 min
Sufentanil	8.0	93	1778	2–3.5	10–15	2.5–3	0.8–1.3
Methadone	8.3	90	26–57	15–20	2	5	4–8

Routes of Administration

Opioids given parenterally have 100% bioavailability (see Chapter 1), although peak plasma concentrations may be affected by site of administration and haemodynamic status. Opioids may be given by many routes; variations between specific agents are discussed below. It is unclear how much cross-tolerance exists for different routes of administration, e.g. intravenous versus epidural.

The choice of route is dependent on the clinical situation and several factors may need to be considered:

- If there is delayed gastrointestinal transit time, the biological half-life may be prolonged with orally administered agents. Similarly, if there is rapid GI transit time or reduced area for absorption, then there may be reduced absorption, particularly of long acting agents.
- Intrathecal administration is associated with fewer supraspinal effects, although both urinary retention and pruritus may be more common. Highly lipid-soluble opioids (e.g. fentanyl) do not spread readily in cerebrospinal fluid (CSF). It is claimed that they are less likely than water-soluble opioids (e.g. morphine) to cause late respiratory depression due to rostral spread.
- Dural penetration from epidural administration is dependent on molecular size and lipophilicity

For example, only 3–5% of morphine crosses into the CSF, with a peak concentration after 60–240 min; fentanyl peaks at approximately 20 min.

MOP Agonists

Morphine is the standard opioid against which other agents are compared. Other MOP agonists have a similar pharmacodynamic profile but differ in relative potency, pharmacokinetics and biotransformation to other active metabolites.

Phenylpiperidine opioids (Fig. 5.2) are potent MOP receptor agonists with moderate (alfentanil) to high (sufentanil) lipid solubility and good diffusion through membranes. Both potency and time to reach the effect site vary considerably. In contrast to morphine, these agents do not cause histamine release. All except remifentanil may cause postoperative respiratory depression as a result of secondary peaks in plasma concentrations. This may be caused by release from body stores if large doses have been infused intra-operatively. Fentanyl, alfentanil and sufentanil are metabolized mainly in the liver to inactive metabolites. Very little is excreted unchanged in the urine (Table 5.3).

Morphine

Morphine is a relatively hydrophilic phenanthrene derivative. It may be given orally, rectally, topically, parenterally and via the neuraxial route. The standard parenteral dose for adults is 10 mg, although many factors affect this and the dose should be titrated to effect. Its oral bioavailability is dependent on first-pass hepatic metabolism and may be unpredictable (35–75%). Oral morphine is available either as immediate-release liquid, simple tablet or as a modified-release preparation. Single-dose studies of morphine bioavailability indicate that the relative potency of oral:intramuscular morphine is 1:6 although, with repeated regular administration, this ratio becomes approximately 1:3. The dose of short-acting morphine for breakthrough pain should be approximately one-sixth of the total daily dose. Morphine has a plasma half-life of approximately 3 h and a duration of analgesia of 4–6 h.

Morphine is metabolized, at least in part, by microsomal UDP glucuronyl transferases (UDPGT) found in the liver, kidney and intestines. Several of these metabolites may have clinically significant effects (see below). Although morphine conjugation occurs in the liver, there is evidence that extrahepatic sites may also be important, e.g. kidney, gastrointestinal tract. The site of conjugation on the molecule also varies, leading to a variety of metabolites (Table 5.3). After glucuronidation, metabolites are excreted in urine or bile, dependent on molecular weight and polarity; more than 90% of morphine metabolites are excreted in the urine. The main metabolite in humans is morphine-3-glucuronide (60–80%) and this may have an excitatory effect via CNS actions not related to opioid receptor activation. Morphine-6-glucuronide (M-6-G) is active at the MOP receptor, producing analgesia and other MOP-related effects. It is significantly more potent than morphine. Therefore, M-6-G produces significant clinical effects despite only 10% of morphine being metabolized in this way. As it is renally excreted, it may accumulate in patients with impaired renal function, causing respiratory depression. Current evidence indicates that accumulation of morphine metabolites, especially M-6-G, becomes significant when creatinine clearance declines to 50 mL min^{-1} or less.

Diamorphine

Diamorphine is a prodrug; it is inactive at opioid receptors. However, it is converted rapidly to the active metabolites 6-monoacetylmorphine, morphine and M-6-G. Further metabolism is similar to that of morphine (Table 5.3) and similar problems may arise if there is renal impairment.

It is available for parenteral and oral use. Diamorphine is more lipid soluble than morphine, affecting distribution and tissue penetration. One advantage over morphine is in settings where high concentrations are required in relatively low volumes, such as palliative care. Additionally, when lipid solubility is important in regulating site of action (e.g. epidural, intrathecal use), some practitioners believe that diamorphine has specific advantages over morphine.

Papaveretum

This naturally occurring opioid is rarely used now. It is a mixture of morphine hydrochloride (253 parts), codeine hydrochloride (20 parts) and papaverine hydrochloride (23 parts). There is no oral preparation. A dose of 15.4 mg is approximately equivalent to 10 mg of anhydrous morphine.

Hydromorphone

This potent opioid is used mainly in the palliative care setting or in patients who are not opioid naive. It can be useful if considering opioid rotation. Hydromorphone 1.3 mg is ~equi-analgesic to morphine 10 mg. Both immediate- and sustained-release preparations are available.

Meperidine (Pethidine)

Meperidine (pethidine) is available as parenteral and oral preparations. There is no evidence that this opioid provides any advantage over morphine, e.g. treatment of colic-type pain. It is fairly short acting in terms of analgesia, and if repeated doses are given, the metabolite normeperidine can accumulate ($t_{1/2}$ ~15 h). This is a CNS stimulant and can cause seizures, especially if there is renal dysfunction. Its clearance is significantly reduced in hepatic disease. Chronic use may result in enzyme induction and an increase in normeperidine plasma concentrations. Its metabolism is decreased by the oral contraceptive pill.

Meperidine has other significant effects related to activity at non-opioid receptors. For example, its atropine-like action may cause a tachycardia, in addition to direct myocardial depression at high doses. It was used originally as a bronchodilator. It can also reduce shivering related to hypothermia or epidurals, although the mechanism for this is not fully understood. Meperidine also has a local anaesthetic-like membrane stabilizing action.

Fentanyl

Fentanyl is available in a variety of preparations for parenteral, transdermal and transmucosal (including buccal) administration. Due to high first-pass metabolism (~70%) it is not given orally. It is approx. 80–100 times more potent than morphine in the acute setting, although it is approx. 30–40 times as potent when given chronically e.g. slow-release transdermal patches. With transdermal administration, the patch and underlying dermis act as a reservoir and plasma concentration does not reach steady state until approx. 15 h after initial application. Plasma concentration also declines slowly after removal ($t_{1/2}$ ~15–20 h).

Fentanyl is very lipophilic with a relatively short duration of action. There are several new buccal/transmucosal preparations developed for rapid onset breakthrough pain. These aim to have a very rapid onset in ~10 minutes, although this may not be the case in clinical practice. Fentanyl has a large V_D with rapid peripheral tissue uptake limiting initial hepatic metabolism. This may result in significant variability in plasma concentrations and secondary plasma peaks. It binds to α_1-acid glycoprotein and albumin; 40% of the protein-bound fraction is taken up by erythrocytes. The lung may be important in exerting a first-pass effect on fentanyl (up to 75% of the dose), thus buffering the plasma from high peak drug concentrations.

Alfentanil

The low pK_a of alfentanil (6.9) results in it being largely unionized at plasma pH, allowing rapid diffusion to the effect site ($t_{1/2}k_{eo}$ ~1 min) and rapid onset of action. Although less lipid-soluble than some opioids, it has the most rapid onset time. It does not bind strongly to opioid receptors and the effect-site concentration also decreases rapidly as plasma concentrations decrease. It is metabolized by one of the most abundantly expressed isoforms of hepatic P450 (CYP3 A3/4). Genetic variability in the activity of this enzyme may result in two- to three-fold variations in pharmacokinetic values when given by infusion. Low, medium or high metabolizers have been identified; this has implications for duration of action when prolonged use is contemplated.

Sufentanil

Sufentanil is one of the most potent opioids; it has a rapid onset of action after intravenous administration and peak analgesic effect is at approximately 8 min. It is 625 times more potent than morphine and 12 times more potent than fentanyl. However, diffusion to tissues is slower than alfentanil because, although sufentanil is highly lipid soluble, it is also highly protein bound, resulting in low unbound plasma fractions at body pH. It has very low levels of non-specific binding that may increase potential effect-site concentrations. The speed of onset of a large dose is caused by saturation of receptors and non-specific sites, with potential for overdose. One of its metabolites (desmethylsufentanil) is active at the MOP receptor (10% of sufentanil's potency).

Remifentanil

Remifentanil is available for parenteral use as a lyophilized white crystalline powder containing glycine. It should not be administered epidurally or spinally. After being made up in solution, it is stable for 24 h. This MOP receptor agonist has a similar potency to fentanyl and is ~20 times more potent than alfentanil. It differs from other opioids in that it has an ester linkage, resulting in degradation by tissue and non-specific plasma esterases. This process is non-saturable and clearance is significantly greater than hepatic blood flow. Plasma cholinesterase deficiency does not affect clearance. Hepatic and renal dysfunction have no effect on clearance also, although increased opioid sensitivity in hepatic disease may result in a lower dosage requirement. Other situations requiring a reduction in dose include haemorrhage or shock. Hydrolysis produces a carboxylic acid metabolite with limited action at the MOP receptor (~1000 times<remifentanil). It is not thought to be clinically significant, even in renal dysfunction.

Remifentanil has a rapid blood–brain equilibration time of just over 1 min, with a short context-sensitive half-time of 3–5 min which is unaffected by duration of infusion. This makes it ideally suited for infusion during anaesthesia and in the critical care setting. It may be titrated rapidly to achieve the desired effect. The high clearance and low V_D imply that the offset of effect is caused by metabolism rather then redistribution. Hypothermia, such as may occur in cardiac surgery, may reduce clearance by up to 20%.

There is some evidence to suggest that acute opioid tolerance and hyperalgesia may occur after remifentanil infusions. If high doses are used without neuromuscular blockade, muscle rigidity may be a problem. It is unlikely to be a problem when using a concentration of $100 \mu g\, mL^{-1}$ or less and an infusion rate of $0.2–0.5\, \mu g\, kg^{-1}\, min^{-1}$. Bradycardia has also been reported.

Oxycodone

This potent semi-synthetic opioid has been in use for many years. In addition to actions at the MOP receptor, it may also have analgesic effects mediated via the KOP receptor, resulting in incomplete cross-tolerance with morphine. It has a good oral bioavailability, and its plasma concentrations are more predictable than those of morphine after oral administration. It is available in both long- and short-acting oral preparations and, more recently, in a parenteral formulation. Oral oxycodone is roughly 1.5 times more potent than oral morphine.

Methadone

Methadone is a diphenylpropylamine. It has very good oral bioavailability (~85%) with an oral to parenteral ratio of 1:2. Its plasma half-life can be very variable (3–50 h, average 24 h) but its duration of action is relatively short. With repeated dosing, problems with accumulation can occur because of this discrepancy between half-life and analgesic effect. Careful monitoring is therefore required when converting patients to long-term methadone. Also, there is incomplete cross-tolerance with morphine. The racemic mixture in common use has agonist actions at the MOP receptor (mainly the *laevo*-isomer) as well as antagonist activity at the NMDA receptor (*dextro*-isomer). Given the importance of this receptor in central sensitization in a variety of pain states, there may be cases where methadone offers particular advantages over and above other opioids, e.g. neuropathic pain.

Plasma concentrations of methadone can be reduced by carbamazepine and its metabolism is accelerated by phenytoin.

Codeine

Codeine is a constituent of opium. Up to 10% of a dose of codeine is metabolized by the hepatic microsomal enzyme CYP2D6 to morphine, which contributes significantly to its analgesic effect. The rest is metabolized in the liver to norcodeine and then conjugated to produce glucuronide conjugates of codeine, norcodeine and morphine. Codeine is considerably less potent than morphine. Around 8% of Western Europeans are deficient in the CYP2D6 enzyme due to genetic polymorphism and such individuals may not experience adequate analgesia with codeine. Similarly, with "super-metabolizers", there may be problems with opioid toxicity. It can cause significant histamine release and its intravenous administration should be avoided. It has marked antitussive effects and also causes significant constipation. It is often combined with paracetamol.

Dihydrocodeine

Dihydrocodeine is a synthetic opioid developed in the early 1900s. Its structure and pharmacokinetics are similar to codeine and it is used for the treatment of postoperative and chronic pain. Both immediate- and sustained-release preparations are available. Despite its common use, there are very few clinical trials demonstrating efficacy. It has significant abuse potential.

Tramadol

Tramadol is thought to produce analgesia by two distinct actions. Firstly, it has agonist activity at the MOP and KOP receptors. Most of its analgesia is mediated by a metabolite - O-desmethyltramadol - that has a 200 fold higher affinity for the MOP receptor. Secondly, it enhances the descending inhibitory systems in the spinal cord by inhibiting noradrenaline (norepinephrine) reuptake and releasing serotonin from nerve endings. It is available in immediate- and sustained-release oral preparations and for parenteral administration. Its use is contraindicated in patients receiving monoamine oxidase inhibitors (MAOIs). Caution must also be exercised in hepatic impairment as its clearance is reduced to a much greater extent than morphine and related agents.

Mixed Agonist–Antagonist Opioids

These agents have a ceiling effect for analgesia and possibly respiratory depression. They have agonist effects at the KOP receptor and weak antagonist effects at the MOP receptor. Dysphoria and hallucinations are relatively common and withdrawal effects may occur if given to patients taking MOP agonists. Pentazocine may be given orally or parenterally but is now rarely used. It may increase pulmonary and aortic blood pressure and myocardial oxygen demand. Hallucinations and dysphoria occur less commonly with nalbuphine.

Partial Agonists

These agents have high affinity for the MOP receptor but limited efficacy (see Chapter 1). A ceiling effect is seen in the dose-response curve at less than the maximal analgesic effect of full MOP agonists. If given with a full MOP agonist, there may be a reduction in the maximal analgesic effect.

Buprenorphine

This is the only partial agonist in common use. It binds to the MOP receptor and dissociates very slowly from it. Consequently, although significant respiratory depression is less likely compared with morphine, it may be more difficult to reverse. It has poor oral bioavailability and parenteral, sublingual or transdermal formulations are used. In addition to it having a partial agonist effect at the MOP receptor, it is also a partial agonist at the NOP receptor, as well as being an antagonist at the KOP receptor. This may contribute to some of its analgesic effects. Increasingly it is also used (usually in relatively large does up to 24 mg day^{-1}) for the management of opioid use, instead of methadone.

Opioid Antagonists

Naloxone is a short-acting opioid antagonist that is relatively selective for the MOP receptor. It is structurally similar to morphine, with some modifications resulting in antagonist activity including an OH group at C-14. It can reverse opioid-induced respiratory depression but repeated administration may be required because of its short duration of action; it can be given by continuous infusion. However, sudden and complete reversal of the analgesic effects of opioids may be accompanied by major cardiovascular and sympathetic responses. Naloxone has a very low oral bioavailability (~3%), allowing its use in combination with oxycodone (see below) to reduce gastrointestinal effects.

Naltrexone is a long-acting opioid antagonist used in the management of opioid dependence. It is available only in oral formulation.

New Developments in Opioid Pharmacology

There is considerable interest in developing opioid analgesics with an improved side effect profile, and there are some promising recent developments in this area. It has been recognized that by using agents which act on more than one type of opioid receptor there may be beneficial effects (see Fig. 5.3) Some recently developed agents include:

- **Oxycodone/Naloxone (Targinact®).** This drug combination utilizes a fixed ratio of oxycodone and naloxone (2:1). The oral naloxone has a greater affinity for opioid receptors in the gut than oxycodone and therefore preferentially binds to these receptors. As a result, gastrointestinal side effects may be reduced, without any effect on the central analgesic effect of oxycodone.
- **Tapentadol.** The analgesic effect of this agent is due to actions at several receptors, including the MOP receptor. It is much more potent at the MOP receptor than tramadol and also has a strong action in inhibiting noradrenaline reuptake. Preliminary evidence is that it is equianalgesic to oxycodone, but has reduced gastrointestinal side effects.
- **MoxDuo®** is a novel opioid combination of morphine and oxycodone in a 3:2 ratio, with promising evidence of at least 50% decrease in clinically significant side effects such as nausea, vomiting, and dizziness when compared to either opioid alone. This seems to be achieved by the need to use lower doses of both morphine and oxycodone to reach an equivalent analgesic effect.

PARACETAMOL

Paracetamol (acetaminophen) was first used in 1893 and is the only remaining *p*-aminophenol available in clinical practice. It is the active metabolite of the earlier, more toxic drugs acetanilide and phenacetin.

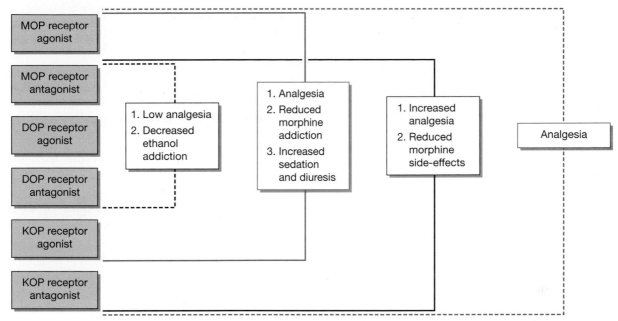

FIGURE 5.3 ■ Schemtic representation of the potential clinical advantages of using bivalent ligands, with the various combinations of pharmacophores (antagonists and agonists). *(Adapted from Dietis N, et al. British Journal of Anaesthesia 2009;103:38-49.)*

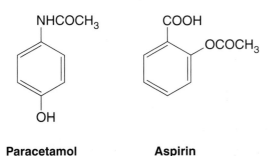

Paracetamol   **Aspirin**

FIGURE 5.4 ■ The structures of paracetamol and aspirin.

Its structure is shown in Figure 5.4. Paracetamol is an effective analgesic and antipyretic but has no anti-inflammatory activity. In recommended doses, it is safe and has remarkably few side-effects.

Mechanism of Action

The mechanism of action of paracetamol is not well understood but it may act by inhibiting prostaglandin synthesis in the central nervous system with limited effect on the peripheral nervous system. Unlike opioids, paracetamol has no well-defined endogenous binding sites. There is however some recent evidence that paracetamol has an inhibitory action on peripheral prostaglandin synthesizing cyclo-oxygenase enzymes, inhibiting both isoforms in certain tissues. In some circumstances it may exhibit a preferential effect on cyclo-oxygenase 2 (COX-2) inhibition. There is growing evidence of a central antinociceptive effect of paracetamol. It has also been shown to prevent prostaglandin production at cellular transcriptional level, independent of COX activity.

Pharmacokinetics

Paracetamol is absorbed rapidly from the small intestine after oral administration; peak plasma concentrations are reached after 30–60 min. It may also be given rectally and intravenously (either as paracetamol or the prodrug proparacetamol). It has good oral bioavailability (70–90%); rectal absorption is more variable (bioavailability ~50–80%) with a longer time to reach peak plasma concentration. The plasma half-life is approx. 2–3 h.

Paracetamol is metabolized by hepatic microsomal enzymes mainly to the glucuronide, sulphate and cysteine conjugates. None of these metabolites is pharmacologically active. A minimal amount of the metabolite N-acetyl-p-amino-benzoquinone imine is normally produced by cytochrome P450-mediated hydroxylation. This reactive toxic metabolite is rendered harmless by conjugation with liver glutathione, then excreted renally as mercapturic derivatives. With larger doses of paracetamol, the rate of formation of the reactive metabolite exceeds that of glutathione conjugation, and the reactive metabolite combines with hepatocellular macromolecules, resulting in cell death and potentially fatal hepatic failure. The formation of this metabolite is increased by drugs inducing cytochrome P450 enzymes, such as barbiturates or carbamazepine.

Pharmacodynamics

Paracetamol has been shown to be effective in both acute and chronic settings and is available for oral or intravenous use. It is an effective postoperative analgesic but probably less effective than NSAIDs in many situations. It may reduce postoperative opioid requirements by up to 30%. The combination of paracetamol with an NSAID also improves efficacy. Paracetamol is also a very effective antipyretic. This is a centrally mediated effect.

Overdose and Hepatic Toxicity

In overdose, there is the potential for the toxic metabolite described above to cause centrilobular hepatocellular necrosis, occasionally with acute renal tubular necrosis. The threshold dose in adults is ~10–15 g. Accidental overdosage can occur if combined preparations such as co-codamol are used together with paracetamol. Doses of more than 150 mg kg^{-1} taken within 24 h may result in severe liver damage, hypoglycaemia and acute tubular necrosis. Individuals taking enzyme-inducing agents are more likely to develop hepatotoxicity.

Early signs include nausea and vomiting, followed by right subcostal pain and tenderness. Hepatic damage is maximal 3–4 days after ingestion, and may lead to liver failure and death. Treatment consists of gastric emptying and the specific antidotes methionine and acetylcysteine. The former offers effective protection up to 10–12 h after ingestion. Acetylcysteine is effective within 24 h and perhaps beyond. The plasma paracetamol concentration related to time

from ingestion indicates the risk of liver damage. Acetylcysteine is given if the plasma paracetamol concentration is >200 mg L^{-1} at 4 h and 6.25 mg L^{-1} at 24 h after ingestion.

NON-STEROIDAL ANTI-INFLAMMATORY DRUGS

The analgesic, anti-inflammatory and antipyretic effects of salicylates, derived from the bark of the willow tree, were described as early as 1763. Acetylsalicylic acid (aspirin) was first produced in 1853 (Fig. 5.4). More recently, many other NSAIDs have been developed with actions similar to aspirin. Perioperative analgesia using NSAIDs is free from many of the adverse effects of opioids, such as respiratory depression, sedation, nausea and vomiting and gastrointestinal stasis. NSAIDs have been shown to be effective analgesics in acute and chronic conditions, although significant contraindications and adverse effects limit their use.

Mechanism of Action

The mechanism of action of aspirin was discovered in the 1970s. It was shown to irreversibly inhibit the production of prostanoids (i.e. prostaglandins and thromboxanes) from arachidonic acid released from phospholipids in cell membranes (Fig. 5.5). The basal rate of prostaglandin production is low and regulated by tissue stimuli or trauma that activate phospholipases to release arachidonic acid. Prostaglandins are then produced by the enzyme prostaglandin endoperoxide synthase which has both cyclo-oxygenase and hydroperoxidase sites. At least two subtypes of cyclo-oxygenase enzyme have been identified in humans: COX-1 and COX-2. The prostanoids produced by COX-1 are functionally active in many areas, including the gastrointestinal tract, kidney, lung and cardiovascular systems. By contrast, the functional COX-2 enzyme is normally found less widely, e.g. brain, spinal cord, renal cortex, tracheal epithelium and vascular endothelium. However, COX-2 mRNA is widely distributed. In response to specific stimuli, especially those associated with inflammation, the expression of COX-2 isoenzyme is induced or upregulated, leading to increased local production of prostaglandins. A range of specific prostanoid receptors (e.g. EP1-4)

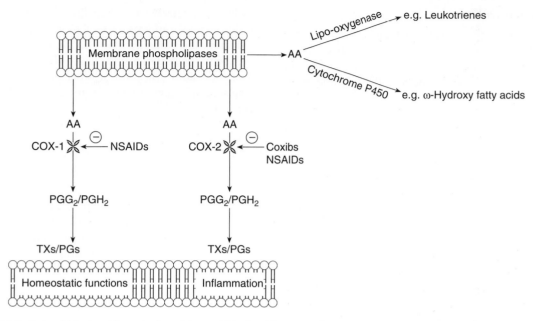

FIGURE 5.5 ■ Arachidonic acid metabolism. AA=arachidonic acid, COX=cyclo-oxygenase, PG=prostaglandin, TXs=thromboxanes.

are involved in peripheral sensitization associated with inflammation.

NSAIDs also have central effects as cyclo-oxygenases are widely distributed in both the peripheral and central nervous systems. NSAIDs may also have other mechanisms of action independent of any effect on prostaglandins, including effects on basic cellular and neuronal processes. NSAIDs are 'non-selective'; they inhibit both COX-1 and COX-2.

Pharmacokinetics

All NSAIDs are rapidly absorbed. They are weak acids and are therefore mainly unionized in the stomach where absorption can occur. When given orally, most absorption occurs in the small intestine because the absorptive area of the microvilli of the small intestine is much more extensive. Most have pK_a values lower than 5 and are therefore 99% ionized at a pH value greater than 7. Most are almost insoluble in water at body pH, although the sodium salt (diclofenac sodium, naproxen sodium) is more soluble. Ketorolac trometamol is the most soluble and can be given intravenously as a bolus and intramuscularly with less chance of significant irritation.

Most NSAIDs are highly protein bound (90–99%), with low volumes of distribution (approx. 0.1–0.2 L kg^{-1}). The unbound fraction is active. NSAIDs may potentiate the effects of other highly protein-bound drugs by displacing them from protein-binding sites (e.g. oral anticoagulants, oral hypoglycaemics, sulphonamides, anticonvulsants).

NSAIDs are mostly oxidized or hydroxylated and then conjugated and excreted in the urine. A few have active metabolites. For example, nabumetone is metabolized to 6-methoxy-2-naphthyl acetic acid, which is more active than the parent drug.

The interaction between NSAID and cyclo-oxygenase enzyme is often complex and plasma half-life may not reflect pharmacodynamic half-life. Diclofenac has a terminal half-life of 1–2 h. It is conjugated to glucuronides and sulphates, with 65% being excreted in the urine and 35% in the bile. The metabolites are less active than the parent compound. Ketorolac trometamol has a terminal half-life of 5 h and more than 90% is excreted renally. Naproxen has a terminal half-life of 12–15 h and is excreted almost entirely through the kidney as the conjugate. Tenoxicam is cleared mainly through the urine as the inactive hydroxypyridyl metabolite, although approximately 30% is via biliary excretion as the glucuronide.

Pharmacodynamics

NSAIDs are very effective analgesics, although their use is limited by adverse effects due to their general effect on prostanoid synthesis and the ubiquitous nature of prostanoids. Generally, the risk and severity of NSAID-associated side-effects is increased in the elderly population or those with other significant co-morbidity.

Analgesia

NSAIDs have well-demonstrated efficacy both as postoperative analgesics and in chronic conditions such as rheumatoid and osteoarthritis. They can have significant opioid-sparing effects. NSAIDs are insufficient alone for severe pain after major surgery but are valuable as part of a multimodal analgesic regimen.

Gastrointestinal System

The gastric and duodenal epithelia have various protective mechanisms against acid and enzyme attack, and many of these involve prostaglandin production via a COX-1 pathway. Acute and particularly chronic NSAID administration can result in gastroduodenal ulceration and bleeding; the latter is exacerbated by the antiplatelet effect.

Platelet Function

Platelet COX-1 is essential for the production of the cyclic endoperoxides and thromboxane A_2 that mediate the primary haemostatic response to vessel injury by producing vasoconstriction and platelet aggregation. Aspirin acetylates COX-1 irreversibly, whereas other NSAIDs do so in a reversible fashion. This can result in prolonged bleeding times and increased perioperative blood loss has been reported in some studies. The presence of a bleeding diathesis or co-administration of anticoagulants may increase the risk of significant surgical blood loss.

Renal Function

Renal prostaglandins have many physiological roles, including the maintenance of renal blood flow and glomerular filtration rate in the presence of circulating vasoconstrictors, regulation of tubular electrolyte handling and modulation of the actions of renal hormones. NSAIDs can adversely affect renal function. High circulating concentrations of the vasoconstrictors renin, angiotensin, noradrenaline (norepinephrine) and vasopressin increase production of intrarenal vasodilators including prostacyclin, and renal function may be particularly sensitive to NSAIDs in these situations. Co-administration of other potential nephrotoxins, such as gentamicin, may increase the likelihood of renal toxicity.

Aspirin-Induced Asthma

Aspirin-induced asthma may affect up to 20% of asthmatics; it may be severe and there is often cross-sensitivity with other NSAIDs. Patients with coexisting chronic rhinitis and nasal polyps appear to be at most risk. A history of aspirin-induced asthma is a contraindication to NSAID use after surgery. There is no reason to avoid NSAIDs in other asthmatics if previous exposure has not been associated with bronchospasm. However, patients should be warned of potential problems and advised to stop taking them if their asthma worsens. The mechanism of this problem is unclear; it may be that cyclo-oxygenase inhibition increases arachidonic acid availability for production of inflammatory leukotrienes by lipo-oxygenase pathways.

Contraindications

Specific contraindications to NSAID administration include a history of a bleeding diathesis, peptic ulceration, significant renal impairment or aspirin-induced asthma. Care should be taken in high-risk groups, such as the elderly, those with cardiovascular disease and the dehydrated.

COX-2-SPECIFIC INHIBITORS

These drugs are anti-inflammatory analgesics that reduce prostaglandin synthesis by specifically inhibiting COX-2 with little or no effect on COX-1 (relative specificity varies between drugs). They were developed as an alternative to traditional NSAIDs with the aim of avoiding COX-1-mediated side-effects, primarily gastric ulceration and platelet effects.

Mechanism of Action

The mechanism of action is similar to that of NSAIDs (Fig. 5.4). Both COX-1 and COX-2 enzymes have very similar active sites and catalytic properties, although COX-2 has a larger potential binding site because of a secondary internal pocket. This has allowed design of drugs to target predominantly COX-2. COX-2 is induced at sites of inflammation and trauma, producing prostaglandins, and these drugs, inhibit this process. However, COX-2 is an important constitutive enzyme in the CNS, including the spinal cord, and inhibition at this site is thought to be an important mechanism also.

Pharmacodynamics

Analgesia

Systematic reviews and meta-analyses indicate similar efficacy to NSAIDs in both acute postoperative pain and for chronic conditions such as osteoarthritis. Agents are available orally (e.g. celecoxib, etoricoxib, valdecoxib) and parenterally (parecoxib).

Gastrointestinal

One of the commonest side-effects of NSAIDs is gastrointestinal toxicity. Approximately 1 in 1200 patients receiving chronic NSAID treatment (>2 months) die from related gastroduodenal complications. COX-1 isoenzyme is the predominant cyclo-oxygenase found in the gastric mucosa. The prostanoids produced here help to protect the gastric mucosa by reducing acid secretion, stimulating mucus secretion, increasing production of mucosal phospholipids and bicarbonate and regulating mucosal blood flow. Specific COX-2 inhibitors have less effect on these processes.

Short- to medium-term treatment with specific COX-2 inhibitors (up to 3 months) is associated with a significant reduction in the incidence of gastroduodenal ulceration. However, this effect is reduced during prolonged treatment and in patients taking low-dose aspirin. It is likely that the degree of COX-2 specificity is related to the efficacy of gastric protection.

Haematological

COX-2-specific agents have very little adverse effect on platelet function. This is potentially advantageous when compared with NSAIDs with respect to perioperative or gastrointestinal bleeding.

Cardiovascular

Some large long-term studies of COX-2 inhibitors have found an increased risk of cardiovascular events (e.g. myocardial infarction, stroke) compared with traditional NSAIDs and placebo. This has led to the recommendation that they should not be used in patients with ischaemic heart or cerebrovascular disease and that their use in others should be guided by individual risk assessments for each patient. Some drugs have been withdrawn. A similar phenomenon has been reported when some of these drugs have been used after coronary artery bypass surgery. An increased risk of myocardial events may not be confined to COX-2 inhibitors – there is some evidence for increased risk with general NSAIDs.

The mechanism of this adverse outcome is under investigation. However, it may be that COX-2 specificity itself is the cause. COX-2 is present in vessel endothelium where it produces prostacyclins which inhibit platelet function and cause vasodilatation. Inhibition of COX-2 at this site may increase the likelihood of thrombus formation and occlusion, and therefore myocardial infarction and stroke. NSAIDs inhibit COX-2 in addition but they also inhibit COX-1 which causes significant impairment of platelet function. Therefore, the combined effect of NSAIDs is such that the risk of adverse cardiovascular and cerebrovascular events is not increased; in fact, the incidence may be decreased (certainly true for low-dose aspirin).

Renal

COX-2 is normally found in the renal cortex and is therefore inhibited both by conventional NSAIDs and COX-2 inhibitors. There is the potential both for peripheral oedema and hypertension, as well as direct effects on renal excretory function with oliguria and decreased creatinine clearance.

KETAMINE

Ketamine (2-chlorophenyl-2-methylaminocyclohexanone hydrochloride) is an anaesthetic agent that has analgesic actions at low doses. It is structurally similar to phencyclidine. It is available in parenteral formulation in a variety of concentrations ($10–100\,mg\,mL^{-1}$). It is normally presented as a racemic mixture, although the S(+) isomer is available in some countries and may have an improved therapeutic index. This isomer may be administered orally but bioavailability is relatively low and unpredictable. If given by the epidural route, the preservative-free formulation must be used.

Mechanism of Action

The main analgesic effect of ketamine is likely to be mediated via antagonism at a specific glutamate receptor, the NMDA receptor. This receptor plays a role in central sensitization of the spinal cord, although its ubiquitous distribution in the CNS accounts for side-effects that often limit its use. The NMDA receptor is important in the mechanisms of neuropathic pain, both acutely and chronically, and may be involved in opioid tolerance.

Pharmacokinetics

Ketamine is water soluble, forming an acidic solution (pH=3.5–5.5). It is ~45% unionized at body pH and rapidly distributed across the blood–brain barrier. It is mainly metabolized in the liver by mixed function oxidases, and has an elimination half-life of ~200 min. Its main metabolite is norketamine, which is excreted renally and has some limited activity. Other metabolites include hydroxynorketamine and hydroxyketamine glucuronide. Ketamine has a volume of distribution of 2.9–3.1 L kg^{-1} and clearance of ~20 mL kg^{-1} min^{-1}.

Pharmacodynamics

Low-dose ketamine has analgesic effects in both acute and chronic pain. It appears to have an opioid-sparing effect in the postoperative setting, and there is evidence from systematic reviews of its efficacy for neuropathic pain. Its use may be limited by side-effects, although a Cochrane review of its use in the perioperative period did not find this to be a major problem. It is unclear what the optimal route of administration is. Given parenterally either intravenously or subcutaneously, bolus doses of 0.25–0.5 mg kg^{-1} or infusion rates of 0.125–0.25 mg kg^{-1} h^{-1} can provide analgesia.

Psychotomimetic effects can often limit use. Hallucinations and nightmares may be troublesome. In large doses, or in susceptible individuals, excess sedation can occur. Ketamine can cause hypertension, increased heart rate and cardiac output, and increased intracranial pressure.

FURTHER READING

Bell, R.F., Dahl, J.B., Moore, R.A., Kalso, E.A., 2006. Perioperative ketamine for acute postoperative pain. Cochrane Database Syst. Rev. 2006 (1). Art. No.:CD004603. DOI:10.1002/14651858. CD004603.pub2.

Christo, P.J., 2003. Opioid effectiveness and side effects in chronic pain. Anesthesiol. Clin. North America 21, 699–713.

Colvin, L.A., Fallon, M.T., 2010. Opioid-induced hyperalgesia – a clinical challenge. Br. J. Anaesth. 104, 125–127.

Dietis, N., Guerrini, R., Calo, G., et al., 2009. Simultaneous targeting of multiple opioid receptors: a strategy to improve side-effect profile. Br. J. Anaesth. 103, 38–49.

Hinz, B., Brune, K., 2012. Paracetamol and cyclooxygenase inhibition: is there a cause for concern? Ann. Rheum. Dis. 71 (1), 20–25.

Hocking, G., Cousins, M.J., 2003. Ketamine in chronic pain management: an evidence-based review. Anesth. Analg. 97, 1730–1739.

Mather, L.E., 2001. Trends in the pharmacology of opioids: implications for the pharmacotherapy of pain. Eur. J. Pain 5 (Suppl. A), 49–57.

McDonald, J., Lambert, D.G., 2005. Opioid receptors. Continuing Education in Anaesthesia, Critical Care and Pain 5, 22–25.

Yaksh, T.L., 1997. Pharmacology and mechanisms of opioid analgesic activity. Acta Anaesthesiol. Scand. 41, 94–111.

6 MUSCLE FUNCTION AND NEUROMUSCULAR BLOCKADE

I n the last 70 years, neuromuscular blocking drugs have become an established part of anaesthetic practice. They were first administered in 1942, when Griffith and Johnson in Montreal used Intocostrin, a biologically standardized mixture of the alkaloids of the Indian rubber plant *Chondrodendron tomentosum,* to facilitate relaxation during cyclopropane anaesthesia. Previously, only inhalational agents (nitrous oxide, diethyl ether, cyclopropane and chloroform) had been used during general anaesthesia, making surgical access for some procedures difficult because of lack of muscle relaxation. To achieve significant muscle relaxation, it was necessary to deepen anaesthesia, which often had adverse cardiac and respiratory effects. Local analgesia was the only alternative.

At first, muscle relaxants were used only occasionally, in small doses, as an adjuvant to aid in the management of a difficult case; they were not used routinely. A tracheal tube was not always used, the lungs were not ventilated artificially and residual block was not routinely reversed; all of these caused significant morbidity and mortality, as demonstrated in the retrospective study by Beecher & Todd (1954). By 1946, however, it was appreciated that using drugs such as curare in larger doses allowed the depth of anaesthesia to be lightened, and it was suggested that incremental doses should also be used during prolonged surgery, rather than deepening anaesthesia – an entirely new concept at that time. The use of routine tracheal intubation and artificial ventilation then evolved.

In 1946, Gray & Halton in Liverpool reported their experience of using the pure alkaloid tubocurarine in more than 1000 patients receiving various anaesthetic agents. Over the following 6 years, they developed a concise description of the necessary ingredients of any anaesthetic technique; narcosis, analgesia and muscle relaxation were essential – the *triad* of anaesthesia. A fourth ingredient, controlled apnoea, was added at a later stage to emphasize the need for fully controlled ventilation, reducing the amount of relaxant required.

This concept is the basis of the use of neuromuscular blocking drugs in modern anaesthetic practice. In particular, it has allowed seriously ill patients undergoing complex surgery to be anaesthetized safely and to be cared for postoperatively in the intensive therapy unit.

PHYSIOLOGY OF NEUROMUSCULAR TRANSMISSION

Acetylcholine, the neurotransmitter at the neuromuscular junction, is released from presynaptic nerve endings on passage of a nerve impulse (an action potential) down the axon to the nerve terminal. The neurotransmitter is synthesized from choline and acetyl-coenzyme A by the enzyme *choline acetyltransferase* and stored in vesicles in the nerve terminal. The action potential depolarizes the nerve terminal to release the neurotransmitter; entry of Ca^{2+} ions into the nerve terminal is a necessary part of this process, promoting further acetylcholine release. On the arrival of an action potential, the storage vesicles are transferred to the active zones on the edge of the axonal membrane, where they fuse with the terminal wall to release the acetylcholine (Fig. 6.1). Three proteins, synaptobrevin, syntaxin and synaptosome-associated protein SNAP-25, are involved in this process. These proteins along

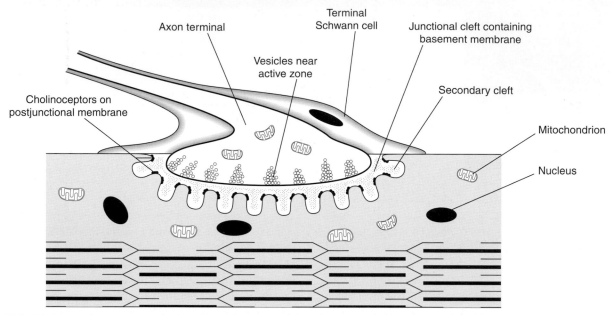

FIGURE 6.1 ■ The neuromuscular junction with an axon terminal, containing vesicles of acetylcholine. The neurotransmitter is released on arrival of an action potential and crosses the junctional cleft to stimulate the postjunctional receptors on the shoulders of the secondary clefts. *(Reproduced with kind permission of Professor WC Bowman.)*

with vesicle membrane-associated synaptotagmins cause the docking, fusion and release (exocytosis) of acetylcholine from the vesicles. There are about 1000 active sites at each nerve ending and any one nerve action potential leads to the release of 200–300 vesicles. In addition, small *quanta* of acetylcholine, equivalent to the contents of one vesicle, are released at the neuromuscular junction spontaneously, causing miniature end-plate potentials (MEPPs) on the postsynaptic membrane, but these are insufficient to generate a muscle action potential.

The active sites of release are aligned directly opposite the acetylcholine receptors on the junctional folds of the postsynaptic membrane, lying on the muscle surface. The junctional cleft, the gap between the nerve terminal and the muscle membrane, has a width of only 60 nm. It contains the enzyme *acetylcholinesterase,* which is responsible for the ultimate breakdown of acetylcholine. This enzyme is also present, in higher concentrations, in the junctional folds in the postsynaptic membrane (Fig. 6.1). The choline produced by the breakdown of acetylcholine is taken up across the nerve membrane to be reused in the synthesis of the transmitter.

The nicotinic acetylcholine receptors on the postsynaptic membrane are organized in discrete clusters on the shoulders of the junctional folds (Fig. 6.1). Each cluster is about $0.1\,\mu m$ in diameter and contains a few hundred receptors. Each receptor consists of five subunits, two of which, the alpha (α; MW$=40000$ Da), are identical. The other three, slightly larger subunits, are the beta (β), delta (δ) and epsilon (ε). In fetal muscle, the epsilon is replaced by a gamma (γ) subunit. Each subunit of the receptor is a glycosated protein – a chain of amino acids – coded by a different gene. The receptors are arranged as a cylinder which spans the membrane, with a central, normally closed, channel – the ionophore (Fig. 6.2). Each of the α subunits carries a single acetylcholine binding region on its extracellular surface. They also bind neuromuscular blocking drugs.

Activation of the receptor requires both α sites to be occupied, producing a structural change in the receptor complex that opens the central channel running between the receptors for a very short period, about 1 ms (Fig. 6.2). This allows movement of cations such as Na^+, K^+, Ca^{2+} and Mg^{2+} along their concentration gradients. The main change is influx of Na^+ ions, the *end-plate current,* followed by efflux of K^+ ions. The

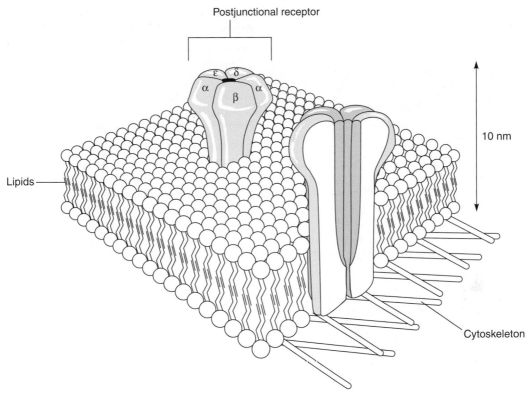

FIGURE 6.2 ■ Two postjunctional receptors, embedded in the lipid layer of the postsynaptic muscle membrane. The α, β, ε and δ subunits are demonstrated on the surface of one receptor and the ionophore is seen in cross-section on the other receptor. On stimulation of the two α subunits by two molecules of acetylcholine, the ionophore opens to allow the passage of the end-plate current. *(Reproduced with kind permission of Professor WC Bowman.)*

summation of this current through a large number of receptor channels lowers the transmembrane potential of the end-plate region sufficiently to depolarize it and generate a muscle action potential sufficient to allow muscle contraction.

At rest, the transmembrane potential is about −90 mV (inside negative). Under normal physiological conditions, a depolarization of about 40 mV occurs, lowering the potential from −90 to −50 mV. When the *end-plate potential* reaches this critical threshold, it triggers an *all-or-nothing* action potential that passes around the sarcolemma to activate muscle contraction via a mechanism involving Ca^{2+} release from the sarcoplasmic reticulum.

Each acetylcholine molecule is involved in opening one ion channel only before it is broken down rapidly by acetylcholinesterase; it does not interact with any of the other receptors. There is a large safety factor in the transmission process, in respect of both the amount of acetylcholine released and the number of postsynaptic receptors. Much more acetylcholine is released than is necessary to trigger the action potential. The end-plate region is depolarized for only a very short period (a few milliseconds) before it rapidly repolarizes and is ready to transmit another impulse.

Acetylcholine receptors are also present on the presynaptic area of the nerve terminal. These are of a slightly different structure to the postsynaptic nicotinic receptors (α3β2). It is thought that a positive feedback mechanism exists for the further release of acetylcholine, such that some of the released molecules of acetylcholine stimulate these presynaptic receptors, producing further mobilization of the neurotransmitter to the readily releasable sites, ready for the arrival of the next nerve stimulus (Fig. 6.3). Acetylcholine activates sodium channels on the prejunctional nerve

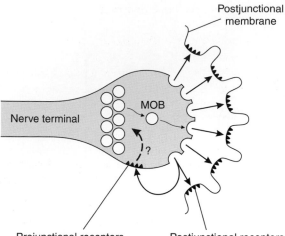

FIGURE 6.3 ■ Acetylcholine receptors are present on the shoulders of the axon terminal, as well as on the postjunctional membrane. Stimulation of the prejunctional receptors mobilizes (MOB) the vesicles of acetylcholine to move into the active zone, ready for release on arrival of another nerve impulse. The mechanism requires Ca^{2+} ions. *(Reproduced with kind permission of Professor WC Bowman.)*

membrane, which in turn activate voltage-dependent calcium channels (P-type fast channels) on the motor neurone causing an influx of calcium into the nerve cytoplasm to promote further acetylcholine release.

In health, postsynaptic acetylcholine receptors are restricted to the neuromuscular junction by a mechanism involving the presence of an active nerve terminal. In many disease states affecting the neuromuscular junction, this control is lost and acetylcholine receptors of the fetal type develop on the adjacent muscle surface. The excessive release of K^+ ions from diseased or swollen muscle on administration of succinylcholine is probably the result of stimulation of these *extrajunctional receptors*. They develop in many conditions, including polyneuropathies, severe burns and muscle disorders.

PHARMACOLOGY OF NEUROMUSCULAR TRANSMISSION

Neuromuscular blocking agents used regularly by anaesthetists are classified into *depolarizing* (or *non-competitive)* and *non-depolarizing* (or *competitive)* agents.

Depolarizing Neuromuscular Blocking Agents

The only depolarizing relaxant now available in clinical practice is succinylcholine. Decamethonium was used clinically in the UK for many years, but it is now available only for research purposes.

Succinylcholine Chloride (Suxamethonium)

This quaternary ammonium compound is comparable to two molecules of acetylcholine linked together (Fig. 6.4). The two quaternary ammonium radicals, $N^+(CH_3)_3$ have the capacity to cling to each of the α units of the postsynaptic acetylcholine receptor, altering its structural conformation and opening the ion channel, but for a longer period than does a molecule of acetylcholine. Administration of succinylcholine therefore results in an initial depolarization and muscle contraction, termed *fasciculation*. As this effect

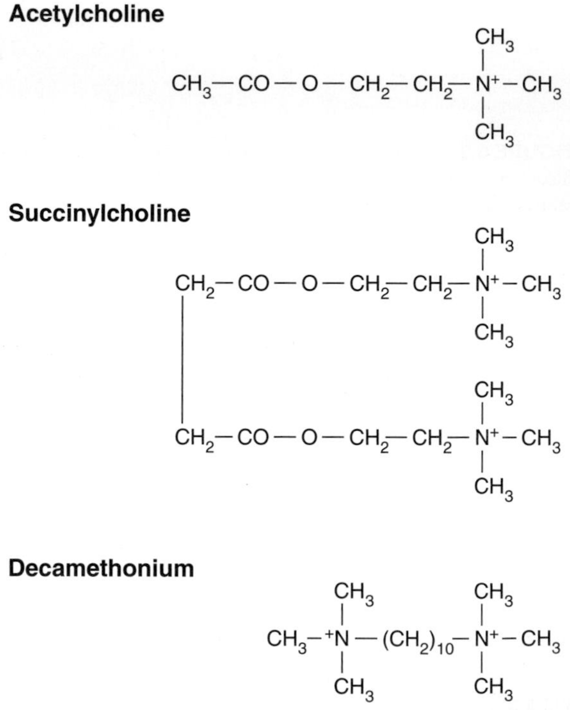

Acetylcholine

$$CH_3-CO-O-CH_2-CH_2-\overset{\overset{\displaystyle CH_3}{|}}{\underset{\underset{\displaystyle CH_3}{|}}{N^+}}-CH_3$$

Succinylcholine

$$CH_2-CO-O-CH_2-CH_2-\overset{\overset{\displaystyle CH_3}{|}}{\underset{\underset{\displaystyle CH_3}{|}}{N^+}}-CH_3$$

$$CH_2-CO-O-CH_2-CH_2-\overset{\overset{\displaystyle CH_3}{|}}{\underset{\underset{\displaystyle CH_3}{|}}{N^+}}-CH_3$$

Decamethonium

$$CH_3-\overset{\overset{\displaystyle CH_3}{|}}{\underset{\underset{\displaystyle CH_3}{|}}{{}^+N}}-(CH_2)_{10}-\overset{\overset{\displaystyle CH_3}{|}}{\underset{\underset{\displaystyle CH_3}{|}}{N^+}}-CH_3$$

FIGURE 6.4 ■ The chemical structures of acetylcholine and succinylcholine. The similarity between the structure of succinylcholine and two molecules of acetylcholine can be seen. The structure of decamethonium is also shown. The quaternary ammonium radicals $N^+(CH_3)_3$ cling to the α subunits of the postsynaptic receptor.

persists, however, further action potentials cannot pass down the ion channels and the muscle becomes flaccid; repolarization does not occur.

The dose of succinylcholine necessary for tracheal intubation in adults is $1.0-1.5\,mg\,kg^{-1}$. This dose has the most rapid and reliable onset of action of any of the muscle relaxants presently available, producing profound block within 1 min. Succinylcholine is therefore of particular benefit when it is essential to achieve tracheal intubation rapidly, e.g. in a patient with a full stomach or an obstetric patient. It is also indicated if tracheal intubation is expected to be difficult for anatomical reasons, because it produces optimal intubating conditions.

The drug is metabolized predominantly in the plasma by the enzyme *plasma cholinesterase,* at one time termed pseudocholinesterase, at a very rapid rate. Recovery from neuromuscular block may start to occur within 3 min and is complete within 12–15 min. The use of an anticholinesterase such as neostigmine, which would inhibit such enzyme activity, is contraindicated (see below). About 10% of the drug is excreted in the urine; there is very little metabolism in the liver although some breakdown by non-specific esterases occurs in the plasma.

If plasma cholinesterase is structurally abnormal because of inherited factors, or if its concentration is reduced by acquired factors, then the duration of action of the drug may be altered significantly.

Inherited Factors. The exact structure of plasma cholinesterase is determined genetically, by autosomal genes, and this has been completely defined. Several abnormalities in the amino acid sequence of the normal enzyme, usually designated E_1^u, are recognized. The most common is produced by the atypical gene, E_1^a, which occurs in about 4% of the Caucasian population. Thus a patient who is a *heterozygote* for the atypical gene $\left(E_1^u, E_1^a\right)$ demonstrates a longer effect from a standard dose of succinylcholine (about 30 min). If the individual is a *homozygote* for the atypical gene $\left(E_1^a, E_1^a\right)$, the duration of action of succinylcholine may exceed 2 h. Other, rarer, abnormalities in the structure of plasma cholinesterase are also recognized, e.g. the fluoride $\left(E_1^f\right)$ and silent $\left(E_1^s\right)$ genes. The latter has very little capacity to metabolize succinylcholine and thus neuromuscular block in the homozygous state $\left(E_1^s, E_1^s\right)$ lasts for at least 3 h. In such patients, non-specific esterases gradually clear the drug from plasma.

It has been suggested that a source of cholinesterase, such as fresh frozen plasma, should be administered in such cases, or an anticholinesterase such as neostigmine be used to reverse what has usually developed into a *dual block* (see below). However, it is wiser to:

- keep the patient anaesthetized and the lungs ventilated artificially, and
- monitor neuromuscular transmission accurately, until full recovery from residual neuromuscular block.

This condition is not life-threatening, but the risk of awareness is considerable, especially after the end of surgery, when the anaesthetist, who may not yet have made the diagnosis, is attempting to waken the patient. Anaesthesia must be continued until full recovery from neuromuscular block is demonstrable.

As plasma cholinesterase activity is reduced by the presence of succinylcholine, a plasma sample to measure the patient's cholinesterase activity should not be taken for several days after prolonged block has been experienced, by which time new enzyme has been synthesized. A patient who is found to have reduced enzyme activity and structurally abnormal enzyme should be given a warning card or alarm bracelet, detailing his or her genetic status. Examining the genetic status of the patient's immediate relatives should be considered.

In 1957, Kalow & Genest first described a method for detecting structurally abnormal cholinesterase. If plasma from a patient of normal genotype is added to a water bath containing a substrate such as benzoylcholine, a chemical reaction occurs with plasma cholinesterase, emitting light of a given wavelength, which may be detected spectrophotometrically. If dibucaine is also added to the water bath, this reaction is inhibited; no light is produced. The percentage inhibition is referred to as the *dibucaine number*. A patient with normal plasma cholinesterase has a high dibucaine number of 77–83. A heterozygote for the atypical gene has a dibucaine number of 45–68; in a homozygote, the dibucaine number is less than 30.

If fluoride is added to the solution instead of dibucaine, the fluoride gene may be detected. If there is no reaction in the presence of the substrate only, the silent gene is present.

Acquired Factors. In these instances, the structure of plasma cholinesterase is normal but its activity is reduced. Thus, neuromuscular block is prolonged by only minutes rather than hours. Causes of reduced plasma cholinesterase activity include:

- liver disease, because of reduced enzyme synthesis.
- carcinomatosis and starvation, also because of reduced enzyme synthesis.
- pregnancy, for two reasons: an increased circulating volume (dilutional effect) and decreased enzyme synthesis.
- anticholinesterases, including those used to reverse residual neuromuscular block after a non-depolarizing muscle relaxant (e.g. neostigmine or edrophonium); these drugs inhibit plasma cholinesterase in addition to acetylcholinesterase. The organophosphorus compound *ecothiopate*, once used topically as a miotic in ophthalmology, is also an anticholinesterase.
- other drugs which are metabolized by plasma cholinesterase, and which therefore decrease its availability, include etomidate, propanidid, ester local anaesthetics, anti-cancer drugs such as methotrexate, monoamine oxidase inhibitors and esmolol (the short-acting β-blocker).
- hypothyroidism.
- cardiopulmonary bypass, plasmapheresis.
- renal disease.

Side-Effects of Succinylcholine

Although succinylcholine is a very useful drug for achieving tracheal intubation rapidly, it has several undesirable side-effects which may limit its use.

Muscle Pains. These occur especially in the patient who is ambulant soon after surgery, such as the day-case patient. The pains, thought possibly to be caused by the initial fasciculations, are more common in young, healthy patients with a large muscle mass. They occur in unusual sites, such as the diaphragm and between the scapulae, and are not relieved easily by conventional analgesics. The incidence and severity may be reduced by the use of a small dose of a non-depolarizing muscle relaxant given immediately before administration of succinylcholine, e.g. gallamine 10 mg (which is thought to be most efficacious

in this respect) or atracurium 2.5 mg. However, this technique, termed *pre-curarization* or *pretreatment*, reduces the potency of succinylcholine, necessitating administration of a larger dose to produce the same effect. Many other drugs have been used in an attempt to reduce the muscle pains, including lidocaine, calcium, magnesium and repeated doses of thiopental, but none is completely reliable.

Increased Intraocular Pressure. This is thought to be caused partly by the initial contraction of the external ocular muscles and contracture of the internal ocular muscles after administration of succinylcholine. It is not reduced by pre-curarization. The effect lasts for as long as the neuromuscular block and concern has been expressed that it may be sufficient to cause expulsion of the vitreal contents in the patient with an open eye injury. This is unlikely. Protection of the airway from gastric contents must take priority in the patient with a full stomach in addition to an eye injury, as inhalation of gastric contents may threaten life.

It is also possible that succinylcholine may increase intracranial pressure, although this is less certain.

Increased Intragastric Pressure. In the presence of a normal lower oesophageal sphincter, the increase in intragastric pressure produced by succinylcholine should be insufficient to produce regurgitation of gastric contents. However, in the patient with incompetence of this sphincter from, for example, hiatus hernia, regurgitation may occur.

Hyperkalaemia. It has long been recognized that administration of succinylcholine during halothane anaesthesia increases the serum potassium concentration by 0.5 mmol L^{-1}. This effect is thought to be caused by muscle fasciculation. It is probable that the effect is less marked with the newer potent inhalational agents, e.g. isoflurane, sevoflurane. A similar increase occurs in patients with renal failure, but as these patients may already have an elevated serum potassium concentration, such an increase may precipitate cardiac irregularities and even cardiac arrest.

In some conditions in which the muscle cells are swollen or damaged, or in which there is proliferation of extrajunctional receptors, this release of potassium may be exaggerated. This is most marked in the burned patient, in whom potassium concentrations up to 13 mmol L^{-1} have been reported. In such patients, precurarization is of no benefit. Succinylcholine should be avoided in this condition. In diseases of the muscle cell, or its nerve supply, hyperkalaemia after succinylcholine may also be exaggerated. These include the muscular dystrophies, dystrophia myotonica and paraplegia. Hyperkalaemia has been reported to cause death in such patients. Succinylcholine may also precipitate prolonged contracture of the masseter muscles in patients with these disorders, making tracheal intubation impossible. The drug should be avoided in any patient with a neuromuscular disorder, including the patient with *malignant hyperthermia,* in whom the drug is a recognized trigger factor (see p. 879).

Hyperkalaemia after succinylcholine has also been reported, albeit rarely, in patients with widespread intra-abdominal infection, severe trauma and closed head injury.

Cardiovascular Effects. Succinylcholine has muscarinic in addition to nicotinic effects, as does acetylcholine. The direct vagal effect (muscarinic) produces sinus bradycardia, especially in patients with high vagal tone, such as children and the physically fit. It is also more common in the patient who has not received an anticholinergic agent (such as glycopyrrolate) or who is given repeated increments of succinylcholine. It is advisable to use an anticholinergic routinely if it is planned to administer more than one dose of succinylcholine. Nodal or ventricular escape beats may develop in extreme circumstances.

Anaphylactic Reactions. Anaphylactic reactions to succinylcholine are rare, but may occur, especially after repeated exposure to the drug. They are more common after succinylcholine than any other neuromuscular blocking agent.

Characteristics of Depolarizing Neuromuscular Block

If neuromuscular block is monitored (see below), several differences between depolarizing and non-depolarizing block may be defined. In the presence of a small dose of succinylcholine:

- a decreased response to a single, low-voltage (1 Hz) twitch stimulus applied to a peripheral nerve is detected. Tetanic stimulation (e.g. at 50 Hz) produces a small, but sustained, response.
- if four twitch stimuli are applied at 2 Hz over 2 s (train-of-four stimulus), followed by a 10-s interval before the next train-of-four, no decrease in the height of successive stimuli is noted (Fig. 6.5).
- the application of a 5-s burst of tetanic stimulation after the application of single twitch stimuli, followed 3 s later by a further run of twitch stimuli, produces no potentiation of the twitch height; there is no *post-tetanic potentiation* (sometimes termed *facilitation*).
- neuromuscular block is *potentiated* by the administration of an anticholinesterase such as neostigmine or edrophonium.
- if repeated doses of succinylcholine are given, the characteristics of this depolarizing block alter; signs typical of a non-depolarizing block develop (see below). Initially, such changes are demonstrable only at fast rates of stimulation, but with further increments of succinylcholine they may occur at slower rates. This phenomenon is termed 'dual block'.
- muscle fasciculation is typical of a depolarizing block.

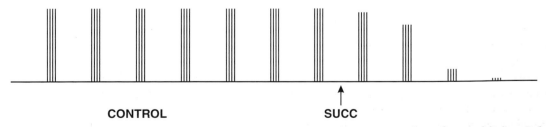

CONTROL   **SUCC**

FIGURE 6.5 ■ The train-of-four twitch response recorded before (CONTROL) and after a dose of succinylcholine. Before administration of succinylcholine 1 mg kg^{-1}, four twitches of equal height are visible. After giving the drug (SUCC), the height of all four twitches decreases equally; no 'fade' of the train-of-four is seen. Within 1 min, the trace has been ablated.

Decamethonium

This depolarizing neuromuscular blocking agent has as rapid an onset of action as succinylcholine, but a longer duration of effect (about 20 min), as it is not metabolized by plasma cholinesterase, but mainly excreted unchanged through the kidneys. It is prone to produce *tachyphylaxis* – a rapid increase in the dose required incrementally to produce the same effect – which, together with its route of excretion, limits its use. It is no longer available for clinical use.

Non-Depolarizing Neuromuscular Blocking Agents

Unlike succinylcholine, these drugs do not alter the structural conformity of the postsynaptic acetylcholine receptor and therefore do not produce an initial contraction. Instead, they compete with the neurotransmitter at this site, binding reversibly to one or two of the α-receptors, whenever these are not occupied by acetylcholine. The end-plate potential produced in the presence of a non-depolarizing agent is therefore smaller; it does not reach the threshold necessary to initiate a propagating action potential to activate the sarcolemma and produce an initial muscle contraction. More than 75% of the postsynaptic receptors have to be blocked in this way before there is failure of muscle contraction – a large safety factor. However, in large doses, non-depolarizing muscle relaxants impair neuromuscular transmission sufficiently to produce profound neuromuscular block.

Metabolism of neuromuscular blocking agents does not occur at the neuromuscular junction. By the end of surgery, the end-plate concentration of the relaxant is decreasing as the drug diffuses down a concentration gradient back into the plasma, from which it is cleared. Thus, more receptors are stimulated by the neurotransmitter, allowing recovery from block. An anticholinesterase given at this time increases the half-life of acetylcholine at the neuromuscular junction, facilitating recovery.

Non-depolarizing muscle relaxants are highly ionized, water-soluble drugs, which are distributed mainly in plasma and extracellular fluid. Thus, they have a relatively small volume of distribution. They are of two main types of chemical structure: either *benzylisoquinolinium compounds*, such as tubocurarine, alcuronium, atracurium, mivacurium and

cisatracurium, or *aminosteroid compounds*, such as pancuronium, vecuronium, pipecuronium and rocuronium. All these drugs possess at least one quaternary ammonium group, $N^+(CH_3)_3$, to bind to an α subunit on the postsynaptic receptor. Their structural type determines many of their chemical properties. Some benzylisoquinolinium compounds consist of quaternary ammonium groups joined by a thin chain of methyl groups. They are therefore more liable to breakdown in the plasma than are the aminosteroids. They are also more likely to release histamine.

Non-depolarizing muscle relaxants are administered usually in multiples of the effective dose (ED) required to produce 95% neuromuscular block (ED_{95}). A dose of at least $2 \times ED_{95}$ is required to produce adequate conditions for reliable tracheal intubation in all patients.

Benzylisoquinolinium Compounds

Tubocurarine Chloride. This is the only naturally occurring muscle relaxant. It is derived from the bark of the South American plant *Chondrodendron tomentosum* which has been used for centuries by South American Indians as an arrow poison. It was the first non-depolarizing neuromuscular blocking agent to be used in humans, by Griffith and Johnson in Montreal, in 1942. The intubating dose is $0.5–0.6\,mg\,kg^{-1}$. It has a slow onset of action and a prolonged duration of effect (Table 6.1), and its effects are potentiated by inhalational agents and prior administration of succinylcholine. It has a marked propensity to produce histamine release and thus hypotension, with possibly a compensatory tachycardia. In large doses, it may also produce ganglion blockade, which potentiates these cardiovascular effects. It is excreted unchanged through the kidneys, with some biliary excretion. It is no longer available in the UK.

Alcuronium Chloride. This drug is a semi-synthetic derivative of toxiferin, an alkaloid of calabash curare. It has less histamine-releasing properties, and therefore cardiovascular effect, than tubocurarine, although it may have some vagolytic effect, producing a mild tachycardia. It also has a slow onset time and nearly as long a duration of effect as tubocurarine (Table 6.1). It is almost entirely excreted unchanged through the kidneys. The intubating dose is $0.2–0.25\,mg\,kg^{-1}$. Before

TABLE 6.1

Time to 95% Depression of the Twitch Response, After a Dose of $2\times ED_{95}$ of a Neuromuscular Blocking Drug (When Tracheal Intubation Should be Possible), and Time to 20–25% Recovery, When an Anti-Cholinesterase May be Used Reliably to Reverse Residual Block Produced by a Non-Depolarizing Drug

	95% Twitch Depression (s)	*20–25% Recovery (min)*
Succinylcholine	60	10
Tubocurarine	220	80+
Alcuronium	420	70
Gallamine	300	80
Atracurium	110	43
Cisatracurium	150	45
Doxacurium	250	83
Mivacurium	170	16
Pancuronium	220	75
Vecuronium	180	33
Pipecuronium	300	95
Rocuronium	75	33
Rapacuronium	<75	15

the advent of atracurium and vecuronium, this inexpensive agent was used widely, but now its popularity has declined and it is no longer available commercially in the UK.

Gallamine Triethiodide. This synthetic substance is a trisquaternary amine. It was first used in France in 1948. The intubating dose in adults is of the order of 160 mg. It has a similar onset to, but slightly shorter duration of action than, tubocurarine, and is excreted almost entirely by the kidneys. Consequently, it should not be used in patients with renal impairment. Being more lipid-soluble than bisquaternary amines, it crosses the placenta to a significant degree and should not be used in obstetric practice. Gallamine has potent vagolytic properties and produces some direct sympathomimetic stimulation. Thus, it increases pulse rate and arterial pressure.

The only recent use of gallamine in the UK has been as a small pretreatment dose (10 mg) prior to succinylcholine, when it seems to be more efficacious than any other non-depolarizing muscle relaxant in minimizing muscle pains.

Atracurium Besylate. This drug, introduced into clinical practice in 1982, was developed by Stenlake at Strathclyde University. Quaternary ammonium compounds break down spontaneously at varying temperature and pH, a phenomenon recognized for over 100 years and known as *Hofmann degradation.* Many such substances also have neuromuscular blocking properties, and atracurium was developed in the search for such an agent which broke down at body temperature and pH. Hofmann degradation may be considered as a 'safety net' in the sick patient with impaired liver or renal function, because atracurium is still cleared from the body. Some renal excretion occurs in the healthy patient (10%), as does ester hydrolysis in the plasma; probably only about 45% of the drug is eliminated by Hofmann degradation in the normal patient.

Atracurium (and vecuronium) was developed in an attempt to obtain a non-depolarizing agent which had a more rapid onset, was shorter-acting and had fewer cardiovascular effects than the older agents. Atracurium $0.5\,mg\,kg^{-1}$ does not produce neuromuscular block as rapidly as succinylcholine; the onset time is 2.0–2.5 min, depending on the dose used (Table 6.1). However, recovery occurs more rapidly from it than after use of the older non-depolarizing agents and atracurium may be reversed easily 20–25 min after administration of a dose of $2\times ED_{95}$ (0.45 mg kg^{-1}). The drug does not have any direct cardiovascular effect, but may release histamine (about a third of that released by tubocurarine) and may therefore produce a local wheal and flare around the injection site, especially if a small vein is used. This may be accompanied by a slight reduction in arterial pressure. It can produce anaphylaxis, but to a lesser degree than succinylcholine.

A metabolite of Hofmann degradation, *laudanosine*, has epileptogenic properties, although fits have never been reported in humans. The plasma concentrations of laudanosine required to make animals convulse are much higher than those occurring during general anaesthesia, even if large doses of atracurium are given during a prolonged procedure, and there is little cause for concern about this metabolite in clinical practice. In patients in the ITU with multiple organ failure, who may receive atracurium for several days, laudanosine concentrations are higher, but as yet no reports of cerebral toxicity have occurred.

Cisatracurium. This is the most recently introduced benzylisoquinolinium neuromuscular blocker. It is of particular interest because it is an example of the development of a specific isomer of a drug to produce a 'clean' substance with the desired clinical actions but with reduced side-effects. Cisatracurium is the 1R-*cis* 1'R-*cis* isomer of atracurium, and one of 10 isomers of the parent compound. It is three to four times more potent than atracurium ($ED_{95}=0.05$ mg kg^{-1}) and has a slightly slower onset and longer duration of action. Its main advantage is that it does not release histamine and therefore is associated with greater cardiovascular stability. It undergoes even more Hofmann degradation than atracurium. Because a lower dose of this more potent drug is given, it produces less laudanosine than an equipotent dose of atracurium. It is therefore particularly useful in the critically ill patient requiring prolonged infusion of a neuromuscular blocking drug.

Doxacurium Chloride. This bisquaternary ammonium compound is only available in the USA. It undergoes a small amount of metabolism in the plasma by cholinesterase (6%), but is excreted mainly through the kidneys. It is the most potent non-depolarizing neuromuscular blocking agent available; an intubating dose is only 0.05 mg kg^{-1}. It has a very slow onset of action (Table 6.1) and a prolonged and unpredictable duration of effect. However, it has no cardiovascular effects and may therefore be of use during long surgical procedures in which cardiovascular stability is required, e.g. cardiac surgery.

Mivacurium Chloride. This drug is metabolized by plasma cholinesterase at 88% of the rate of succinylcholine. An intubating dose ($2\times ED_{95}=0.15$ mg kg^{-1}) has a similar onset of action to an equipotent dose of atracurium, but in the presence of normal plasma cholinesterase, recovery after mivacurium is much faster (Table 6.1) and administration of an anticholinesterase may not be necessary (if neuromuscular function is being monitored and good recovery can be demonstrated). Full recovery in such circumstances takes about 20–25 min, but the drug may be antagonized easily within 15 min. Mivacurium is useful particularly for surgical procedures requiring muscle relaxation in which even atracurium and vecuronium seem too long-acting, and when it is desirable to avoid the side-effects of succinylcholine, e.g. for bronchoscopy, oesophagoscopy, laparoscopy or tonsillectomy. The drug produces a similar amount of histamine release to atracurium.

In the presence of reduced plasma cholinesterase activity, because of either inherited or acquired factors, the duration of action of mivacurium may be increased. In patients heterozygous for the atypical cholinesterase gene, the duration of action of mivacurium is comparable to that of atracurium, negating its advantages. The action of the drug may also be prolonged in patients with hepatic or renal disease, in whom plasma cholinesterase activity may be reduced.

Aminosteroid Compounds

These non-depolarizing neuromuscular blocking agents possess at least one quaternary ammonium group, attached to a steroid nucleus. They produce fewer adverse cardiovascular effects than do the benzylisoquinolinium compounds and do not stimulate histamine release from mast cells to the same degree. They are excreted unchanged through the kidneys and also undergo deacetylation in the liver. The deacetylated metabolites may possess weak neuromuscular blocking properties. The parent compound may also be excreted unchanged in the bile.

Pancuronium Bromide. This bisquaternary amine, the first steroid muscle relaxant used clinically, was developed by Savege and Hewitt and marketed in 1964. The intubating dose is 0.1 mg kg^{-1}, which takes 3–4 min to reach its maximum effect (Table 6.1). The clinical duration of action of the drug is long, especially in the presence of potent inhalational agents or renal dysfunction, as 60% of a dose of the drug is excreted unchanged through the kidneys. It is also deacetylated in the liver; some of the metabolites have neuromuscular blocking properties.

Pancuronium does not stimulate histamine release and is therefore useful in patients with a history of allergy. However, it has direct vagolytic and sympathomimetic effects which may cause tachycardia and hypertension. It slightly inhibits plasma cholinesterase and therefore potentiates any drug metabolized by this enzyme, e.g. succinylcholine and mivacurium.

Vecuronium Bromide. This steroidal agent was developed in an attempt to reduce the cardiovascular effects of pancuronium. It is similar in structure to the older drug, differing only in the loss of a methyl group from one quaternary ammonium radical. Thus it is a monoquaternary amine. An intubating dose of 0.1 mg kg^{-1} produces profound neuromuscular block within 3 min, which is slightly longer than the onset time of atracurium, but shorter than those of tubocurarine and pancuronium. This dose produces clinical block for about 30 min. Vecuronium rarely produces histamine release, nor does it have any direct cardiovascular effects, although it allows the cardiac effects of other anaesthetic agents, such as bradycardia produced by the opioids, to go unchallenged. Vecuronium is excreted through the kidneys (30%), although to a lesser extent than pancuronium, and undergoes hepatic deacetylation; the deacetylated metabolites have neuromuscular blocking properties. Repeated doses should be used with care in patients with renal or hepatic disease because they accumulate.

Pipecuronium Bromide. This analogue of pancuronium was developed in Hungary in 1980 and is marketed in Eastern Europe and the USA. The intubating dose is 0.07 mg kg^{-1}. The onset time and time to recovery from block are similar to those of pancuronium (Table 6.1), and excretion of the drug through the kidneys is significant (66%). In contrast to pancuronium, pipecuronium possesses marked cardiovascular stability, having no vagolytic or sympathomimetic effects. It may therefore be useful during major surgery in patients with cardiac disease.

Rocuronium Bromide. This monoquaternary amine has a very rapid onset of action for a non-depolarizing muscle relaxant. It is six to eight times less potent than vecuronium but has approximately the same molecular weight; consequently, a greater number of drug molecules may reach the postjunctional receptors within the first few circulations, enabling faster development of neuromuscular block. In a dose of 0.6 mg kg^{-1}, good or excellent intubating conditions are achieved within 60–90 s; this is only slightly slower than the onset time of succinylcholine. The clinical duration is 30–45 min. At higher doses, such as 0.9 mg kg^{-1}, rocuronium has an onset time similar to succinylcholine, albeit with a greater range of effect. In such doses, however, rocuronium is a very long-acting drug, lasting about 90 min.

In most other respects, rocuronium resembles vecuronium. The drug stimulates little histamine release or cardiovascular disturbance, although in high doses it has a mild vagolytic property which sometimes results in an increase in heart rate. The drug is excreted unchanged in the urine and in the bile, and thus the duration of action may be increased by severe renal or hepatic dysfunction. Rocuronium has no metabolites with significant neuromuscular blocking activity.

Anaphylactic reactions are more common after rocuronium than after any other aminosteroid neuromuscular blocking drug. They occur at a similar rate to anaphylactic reactions to atracurium and mivacurium.

Rapacuronium Bromide. This was the last aminosteroid to become available. It is less potent than rocuronium ($2 \times ED_{90} = 1.15$ mg kg^{-1}) and in equipotent doses has an even more rapid onset of action (<75 s). It is cleared rapidly from the plasma by hepatic uptake and deacetylation and thus has a shorter duration of effect than rocuronium, 12–15 min (Table 6.1). As with the deacetylation of pancuronium and vecuronium, a metabolite of rapacuronium has neuromuscular blocking properties (Org 9488). This may prolong the effect of incremental doses of the drug.

Rapacuronium has similar cardiovascular effects to rocuronium but it may also produce bronchospasm, possibly because of the release of histamine or leukotrienes. After several reports to the US Food and Drug Administration of bronchospasm and hypoxaemia following administration of rapacuronium, especially in small children, the manufacturers voluntarily withdrew the drug from release in the USA in 2002. It has never been commercially available in the UK.

Factors Affecting Duration of Non-Depolarizing Neuromuscular Block

The duration of action of non-depolarizing muscle relaxants is affected by several factors. Effects are most marked with the longer-acting agents, such as tubocurarine and pancuronium. Prior administration of succinylcholine potentiates the effect and prolongs the duration of action of non-depolarizing drugs. Concomitant administration of a potent inhalational agent increases the duration of block. This is most marked with the ether anaesthetic agents such as isoflurane, enflurane and sevoflurane, but occurs to a lesser extent with halothane.

pH changes. Metabolic and, to a lesser extent, respiratory acidosis extend the duration of block. With monoquaternary amines such as tubocurarine and vecuronium, this effect is produced probably by the ionization, under acidic conditions, of a second nitrogen atom in the molecule, making the drug more potent.

Body temperature. Hypothermia potentiates block because impairment of organ function delays metabolism and excretion of these drugs. Enzyme activity is also reduced. This may occur in patients undergoing cardiac surgery; reduced doses of muscle relaxants are required during cardiopulmonary bypass.

Age. Non-depolarizing muscle relaxants which depend on organ metabolism and excretion may be expected to have a prolonged effect in old age, as organ function deteriorates. In healthy neonates, who have a higher extracellular volume than adults, resistance may occur, but if the baby is sick or immature then, because of underdevelopment of the neuromuscular junction and other organ function, increased sensitivity may be encountered. Children of school age tend to be relatively resistant to non-depolarizing muscle relaxants, when given on a weight basis.

Electrolyte changes. A low serum potassium concentration potentiates neuromuscular block by changing the value of the resting membrane potential of the postsynaptic membrane. A reduced ionized calcium concentration also potentiates block by impairing presynaptic acetylcholine release.

Myasthenia gravis. In this disease, the number and half-life of the postsynaptic receptors are reduced by autoantibodies produced in the thymus gland. Thus, the patient is more sensitive to the effects of nondepolarizing muscle relaxants. Resistance to succinylcholine may be encountered.

Other disease states. Due to the altered pharmacokinetics of muscle relaxants in hepatic and renal disease, prolongation of action may be found in these conditions, especially if excretion of the drug is dependent upon these organs.

Characteristics of Non-Depolarizing Neuromuscular Block

If a small, subparalysing dose of a non-depolarizing neuromuscular blocking drug is administered, the following characteristics are recognized:

- decreased response to a low-voltage twitch stimulus (e.g. 1 Hz) which, if repeated, decreases further in amplitude. This effect, which is in contrast to that produced by a depolarizing drug, also occurs to a greater degree when the train-of-four (TOF) twitch response is applied, and even more so with higher, tetanic rates of stimulation. It is referred to as 'fade' or decrement.
- post-tetanic potentiation (PTP) or facilitation (PTF) of the twitch response may be demonstrated (Fig. 6.6).
- neuromuscular block is reversed by administration of an anticholinesterase.
- no muscle fasciculation is visible.

REVERSAL AGENTS

Anticholinesterases

These agents are used in clinical practice to inhibit the action of acetylcholinesterase at the neuromuscular junction, thus prolonging the half-life of acetylcholine

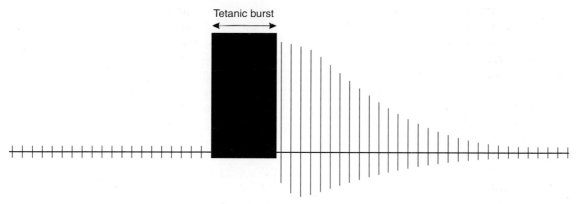

Tetanic burst

FIGURE 6.6 ■ A 5-s burst of tetanus (50 Hz), applied after a run of single twitch stimuli, causes a transient increase in the height of subsequent twitches, although they gradually decrease to their former height; this is post-tetanic potentiation (PTP) or facilitation (PTF). The number of twitches detectable after the burst of tetanus is referred to as the 'post-tetanic count'.

and potentiating its effect, especially in the presence of residual amounts of non-depolarizing muscle relaxant at the end of surgery. The most commonly used anticholinesterase during anaesthesia is neostigmine, but edrophonium and pyridostigmine are also available. These carbamate esters are water-soluble, quaternary ammonium compounds which are absorbed poorly from the gastrointestinal tract. The more lipid-soluble tertiary amine, physostigmine, has a similar effect and is more suitable for oral administration, but crosses the blood–brain barrier. Organophosphorus compounds which are used as poisons in farming and in nerve gas, also inhibit acetylcholinesterase, but unlike other agents, their effect is irreversible; recovery occurs only on generation of more enzyme, which takes some weeks.

Anticholinesterases are given orally to patients with *myasthenia gravis*. In this disease, the patient possesses antibodies to the postsynaptic nicotinic receptor, reducing the efficacy of acetylcholine. The use of these drugs is thought to increase the amount and duration of action of acetylcholine at the neuromuscular junction, thus enhancing neuromuscular transmission.

Neostigmine. This drug combines reversibly with acetylcholinesterase by formation of an ester linkage. Neostigmine is excreted largely unchanged through the kidneys and has a half-life of about 45 min. It is presented in brown vials because it breaks down on exposure to light. Neostigmine potentiates the action of acetylcholine wherever it is a neurotransmitter, including all cholinergic nerve endings; thus, it produces

bradycardia, salivation, sweating, bronchospasm, increased intestinal motility and blurred vision. These cholinergic effects may be reduced by simultaneous administration of an anticholinergic agent such as atropine or glycopyrrolate. The usual dose of neostigmine is of the order of 0.035 mg kg^{-1}, in combination with either atropine 0.015 mg kg^{-1} or glycopyrrolate 0.01 mg kg^{-1}. Neostigmine takes at least 2 min to have an initial effect, and recovery from neuromuscular block is maximally enhanced by 10 min.

Edrophonium. This anticholinesterase forms an ionic bond with the enzyme but does not undergo a chemical reaction with it. The effect is therefore more short-lived than with neostigmine, of the order of only a few minutes. Edrophonium has a quicker onset of action than neostigmine, producing signs of recovery within 1 min. However, its effects are more evanescent; when edrophonium is given in the presence of profound neuromuscular block, the degree of neuromuscular block may *increase* after an initial period of recovery. The dose of edrophonium is 0.5–1.0 mg kg^{-1}.

Pyridostigmine. This drug has a slower onset time than neostigmine or edrophonium, and also a longer duration of action. It is used more frequently as oral therapy in patients with myasthenia gravis than in anaesthesia.

Physostigmine. This anticholinesterase, also known as *eserine*, is a tertiary amine and is more lipid-soluble than the other carbamate esters. It is therefore absorbed more easily from the gastrointestinal tract, and also crosses the blood–brain barrier.

Organophosphorus Compounds. These substances are irreversible inhibitors of acetylcholinesterase; by phosphorylation of the enzyme, they produce a very stable complex which is resistant to reactivation or hydrolysis. Synthesis of new enzyme must occur before recovery. These agents, which include di-isopropylfluorophosphonate (DFP) and tetraethylpyrophosphate (TEPP), are used as insecticides and chemical warfare agents. They are absorbed readily through the lungs and skin. Poisoning is not uncommon among farm workers. Muscarinic effects such as salivation, sweating and bronchospasm are combined with nicotinic effects, such as muscle weakness. Central nervous effects such as tremor and convulsions may occur, as may unconsciousness and respiratory failure. Reactivators of acetylcholinesterase are used to treat this form of poisoning: they include *pralidoxime* and *obidoxime*. Atropine, anticonvulsants and artificial ventilation may be necessary. Chronic exposure may produce polyneuritis. Carbamates such as pyridostigmine are used prophylactically in those threatened by chemical warfare with these compounds.

Ecothiopate is an organophosphorus compound with a quaternary amine group; it was used as an eye drop preparation in ophthalmology to produce miosis in narrow-angle glaucoma. It inhibits cholinesterase by phosphorylation and thus potentiates all esters metabolized by this enzyme. It has now been withdrawn from the UK market.

A new generation of organophosphorus compounds may be beneficial in Alzheimer's disease, and clinical trials are in progress. Neuromuscular blockers must be used with caution if such patients require anaesthesia.

Cyclodextrins

Sugammadex

Anticholinesterases, although used routinely in anaesthetic practice, are recognized to have disadvantages. The most important is that recovery from block must be established before they are given (see below). Their muscarinic effects may be disadvantageous in patients with a history of nausea and vomiting, or in the presence of cardiac arrhythmias or bronchospasm.

A novel approach to reversal of neuromuscular block was therefore developed. Sugammadex (Org 25969), a γ-cyclodextrin, was designed to chelate or encapsulate rocuronium (and to a lesser extent vecuronium) in the plasma, preventing its access to the nicotinic receptor and encouraging dissociation from it. Sugammadex consists of eight oligosaccharides arranged in a cylindrical structure to encapsulate all four steroidal rings of rocuronium completely (Fig. 6.7). This cylindrical structure is known as a toroid. The hydrophilic external tails on the toroid are negatively charged, attracting the quaternary nitrogen group on the muscle relaxant and drawing it into the lipophilic core of sugammadex. The complex of sugammadex and rocuronium is excreted in the urine and has no muscarinic effect: the use of anticholinergic agents is unnecessary. Sugammadex seems to be devoid of adverse cardiovascular effects, although prolongation of the QT interval has been reported anecdotally. It acts three times as rapidly as neostigmine in reversing neuromuscular block produced by rocuronium.

Dose: The dose is adjusted according to the degree of residual block. If at least two twitches of the TOF response are detectable (when anticholinesterases can be used), $2\,mg\,kg^{-1}$ should be given. If block is still profound, with no response to the TOF and a post-tetanic count (PTC) of 1–2, 4–$8\,mg\,kg^{-1}$ should be used. If it is necessary to reverse block immediately in the case of, for instance, a 'cannot intubate, cannot ventilate' scenario, sugammadex $16\,mg\,kg^{-1}$ should be used.

This chelating agent is drug-specific and will not reverse residual block produced by other muscle relaxants. Sugammadex does not antagonize neuromuscular block produced by the benzylisoquinoliniums and has only a limited effect in reversing pancuronium. Sugammadex has been used in the management of anaphylaxis to rocuronium when conventional ALS treatment has failed, although this is not recommended on the drug's data sheet. In contrast, there have already been a few reports of anaphylaxis to sugammadex.

Sugammadex became available in the UK in 2008. Its high cost has limited its use.

NEUROMUSCULAR MONITORING

There is no clinical tool available to measure neuromuscular transmission accurately in a muscle group. Thus, neither the amount of acetylcholine released in

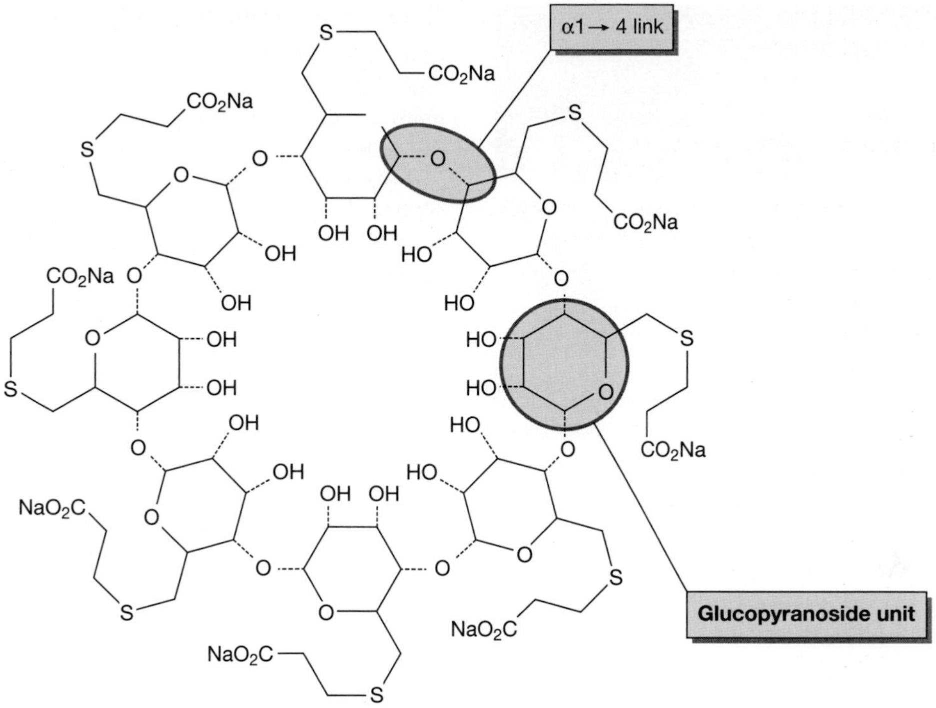

FIGURE 6.7 ■ The cyclical structure of sugammadex consisting of eight glucopyranoside units linked by oxygen radicals (example marked by circle). The negatively charged hydrophilic chains on the outside of the molecule attract rocuronium to the core of the toroid. *(Downloaded from Wikipedia, freely accessible.)*

response to a given stimulus nor the number of post-synaptic receptors blocked by a non-depolarizing muscle relaxant may be assessed. However, it is possible to obtain a crude estimate of muscle contraction during anaesthesia using a variety of techniques. All require the application to a peripheral nerve of a current of up to 60 mA, for a fraction of a millisecond (often 0.2 ms), necessitating a voltage of up to 300 mV. Usually, a nerve which is readily accessible to the anaesthetist, such as the ulnar, facial or common peroneal nerve, is used. The muscle response to the nerve stimulus may then be assessed by either *visual* or *tactile* means, or it may be recorded by more sophisticated methods.

Mechanomyography

A strain-gauge transducer may be used to measure the force of contraction of, for instance, the thumb, in response to stimulation of the ulnar nerve at the wrist. This measurement may then be charted using a recording device. Accurate measurements of the twitch or tetanic response may be made, although the hand must be splinted firmly for reproducible results. This technique is primarily a research tool.

Electromyography

The electromyographic response of a muscle is measured in response to the same electrical stimulus, using recording electrodes similar to ECG pads placed over the motor point of the stimulated muscle. For instance, if the ulnar nerve is stimulated, the recording electrodes are placed over the motor point of adductor pollicis in the thumb (Fig. 6.8). A compound muscle action potential may be recorded. Although primarily a research tool, there are several simple clinical instruments, such as the Datex Relaxograph, which give a less accurate, but similar recording. Maintaining the exact position of the hand is not as essential with electromyography as with mechanomyography.

Accelerography

With this technique, the acceleration of the thumb is measured in response to the nerve stimulus and the force

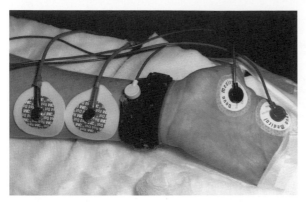

FIGURE 6.8 ■ Positioning of the hand necessary to obtain an electromyographic recording of the response of the adductor pollicis muscle to stimulation of the ulnar nerve is demonstrated. An earth electrode is placed round the wrist. Two recording electrodes are placed over the muscle on the hand; the distal one lies over the motor point.

of contraction may be derived (force = mass × acceleration). Clinical equipment is available (e.g. the TOF Watch, which is an accelerograph) which provides a quantitative assessment of, for instance, the twitch height in comparison with a control reading. The TOF Watch SX in addition gives a read-out of the train-of-four ratio (TOFR). This is essential to determine if an anticholinesterase is to be avoided. The TOFR must have reached 0.9 before extubation can be effected safely.

Modes of Stimulation

Several different rates of stimulation can be applied to the nerve in an attempt to produce a sensitive index of neuromuscular function. It is considered essential always to apply a *supramaximal* stimulus to the nerve, i.e. the strength of the electrical stimulus (V) should be increased until the response no longer increases. It is then increased by an additional 25%.

Twitch

A square-wave stimulus of short duration (0.1–0.2 ms) is applied to a peripheral nerve. In isolation, such a stimulus is of limited value, although if applied repeatedly, before and after a dose of a muscle relaxant, it may be possible to assess crudely the effects of the drug. Such rates of stimulation have the benefit of being less painful than tetanic stimulation, with no untoward effects after recovery from anaesthesia.

Train-of-Four (TOF) Twitch Response

In an attempt to assess the degree of neuromuscular block clinically, Ali et al (1971) described a development of the twitch response which, it was hoped, would be more sensitive than repeated single twitches and did not require a control response. Four stimuli (at 2 Hz) are applied over 2 s, with at least a 10-s gap between each TOF. On administration of a small dose of a non-depolarizing muscle relaxant, *fade* of the amplitude of the TOF may be visible. The ratio of the amplitude of the fourth to the first twitch is called the *train-of-four ratio* (TOFR). In the presence of a larger dose of such a drug, the fourth twitch disappears first, then the third, followed by the second and, finally, the first twitch (Fig. 6.9A). On recovery from neuromuscular block, the first twitch appears first, then the second (when the first twitch has recovered to about 20% of control), then the third, and finally the fourth (Fig. 6.9B).

It is generally thought that at least three of the four twitches must be absent to obtain adequate surgical access for upper abdominal surgery. Full reversal can only be relied upon if at least the second twitch is visible when an anticholinesterase is given. After reversal, good muscle tone – as assessed clinically by the patient being able to cough, raise his or her head from the pillow for at least 5 s, protrude the tongue and have good grip strength – may be anticipated when the TOFR has reached at least 0.7. However, recovery to a TOFR of 0.9 has now been shown to be necessary prior to extubation if the airway is to be protected completely.

It is recognized that, although the number of twitches present in the TOF during neuromuscular block is easily counted by visual or tactile means, it is impossible, even for the expert, to assess the value of the TOFR accurately by these methods. Visual or tactile evaluation fails to detect any fade of the TOF when the ratio is in excess of 40%. Thus, failure to detect fade with a nerve stimulator does not always guarantee adequate reversal. Recording of the TOFR is essential for this purpose.

Tetanic Stimulation

This is the most sensitive form of neuromuscular stimulation. Frequencies of 50–100 Hz are applied to a peripheral nerve to detect even minor degrees of residual neuromuscular block; thus, tetanic fade

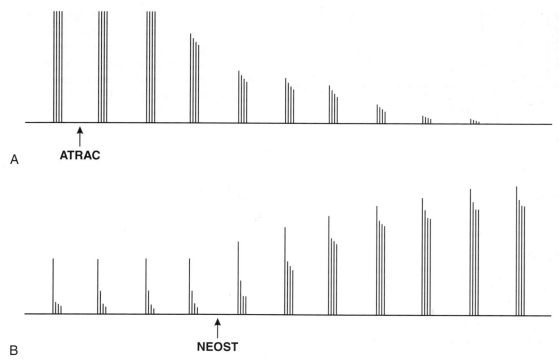

A   ↑ **ATRAC**

B   ↑ **NEOST**

FIGURE 6.9 ■ (**A**) After administration of a non-depolarizing muscle relaxant (in this instance, atracurium (ATRAC), the decrease in height of the fourth twitch of the TOF response is more marked than the decrease in height of the third twitch, which is more marked than the decrease in the second, which is greater than the decrease in the first. The effect is known as 'fade'. Within 2 min, the TOF response has been ablated completely. (**B**) On recovery, the first twitch response appears first, then the second, the third and finally the fourth. Marked fade is present, but after administration of an anticholinesterase (neostigmine (NEOST)) recovery of all four twitches occurs rapidly.

may be present when the twitch response is normal. Tetanic rates of stimulation may be applied under anaesthesia, but in the awake patient they are intolerably painful. Indeed, on recovery from anaesthesia in which tetanic stimulation has been applied, the patient may be aware of some discomfort in the area of application.

Post-Tetanic Potentiation or Facilitation

This method of monitoring was developed in an attempt to assess more profound degrees of neuromuscular block produced by non-depolarizing neuromuscular blocking agents. If a single twitch stimulus is applied to the nerve with little or no neuromuscular response, but after a 5 s delay a burst of 50-Hz tetanus is given for 5 s, the effect of a further twitch stimulus 3 s later is enhanced (Fig. 6.6). In the presence of profound block, the effect of repeated single twitches applied after the tetanus until the

response disappears can be counted; this is termed the *post-tetanic count*. The augmentation of the twitch is thought to be caused by presynaptic mobilization of acetylcholine as a result of the positive feedback effect of the run of tetanus.

Double-Burst Stimulation (DBS)

In an attempt to develop a clinical tool which would allow more accurate assessment of residual block by visual or tactile means than fade of the TOF response, Viby-Mogensen suggested the application of two or three short bursts of 50-Hz tetanus, each comprising two or three impulses separated by a 750-ms interval. Each square-wave impulse lasts for 0.2 ms (Fig. 6.10). If records of the fade of the DBS and the TOF response are compared, they are very similar, but there is evidence to suggest that visual assessment of DBS in the later stages of recovery (TOFR <0.6), is more accurate.

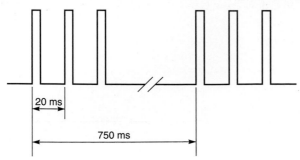

FIGURE 6.10 ■ The pattern of double-burst stimulation. Three bursts of 50-Hz tetanus, at 20-ms intervals, separated by a 750-ms gap, are shown.

Indications for Neuromuscular Monitoring

It is preferable always to monitor neuromuscular function when a muscle relaxant is used during anaesthesia, but it is especially indicated in the following circumstances:

- during prolonged anaesthesia, when repeated increments of neuromuscular blocking agents are required
- when infusions of muscle relaxants are given (including in the ITU)

- in the presence of renal or hepatic dysfunction
- in patients with neuromuscular disorders
- in patients with a history of sensitivity to a muscle relaxant or poor recovery from block
- when poor reversal of neuromuscular block is encountered unexpectedly.

REFERENCE

Beecher, H.K., Todd, D.P., 1954. A study of the deaths associated with anesthesia and surgery. Ann. Surg. 140, 2–34.

FURTHER READING

Ali, H.H., Utting, J.E., Gray, T.C., 1971. Quantitative assessment of residual antidepolarizing block. II. Br. J. Anaesth. 43, 478–485.

Appiah-Ankam, J., Hunter, J.M., 2004. Pharmacology of neuromuscular blocking drugs. Continuing Education in Anaesthesia Critical Care and Pain 4, 2–7.

Khirwadkar, R., Hunter, J.M., 2012. Neuromuscular physiology and pharmacology: an update. Continuing Education in Anaesthesia Critical Care and Pain 12, 237–244.

King, J.M., Hunter, J.M., 2002. Physiology of the neuromuscular junction. Continuing Education in Anaesthesia Critical Care and Pain 2, 129–133.

Srivastava, A., Hunter, J.M., 2009. Reversal of neuromuscular block. Br. J. Anaesth. 103, 115–129.

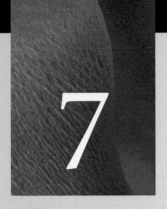

7 SEDATIVE AND ANXIOLYTIC DRUGS

■ ■ ■ ■ ■ ■ ■ ■ ■ ■ ■ ■ ■ ■

S edation is best considered as a continuum between normal consciousness and general anaesthesia. The most frequently cited description of the varying levels of sedation utilized in clinical practice is that from the American Society of Anesthesiologists (Table 7.1).

There is a seamless progression from minimal sedation to deep sedation, in which verbal contact and protective airway reflexes may be lost. It is very difficult to predict how an individual patient will respond to a sedative agent. The ability of the patient to maintain a patent airway independently is one characteristic of moderate or conscious sedation, but even at this level of sedation it cannot be assumed that protective airway reflexes are intact. Deep sedation may progress easily to be indistinguishable from general anaesthesia, and a higher level of skill is needed to ensure the safe management of the patient. The degree of apparent sedation is related to the stimulation from the procedure, and patients can move rapidly between levels of sedation due to procedural effects without any change in drug dosage. It is therefore important that healthcare professionals delivering sedation have the necessary skill set to cope with sedation which is deeper than intended. Similarly, patients having sedation should be fasted in an identical manner to patients having a general anaesthetic.

The difference between sedative and anaesthetic drugs is largely one of usage. Many anaesthetic drugs may be used at reduced dosage to produce sedation and, similarly, agents used primarily as sedatives will produce a form of anaesthesia if given in sufficiently high doses. The usual target is to produce conscious sedation, i.e. to titrate drug therapy so the patient is free of anxiety, free of pain and responding purposefully to command. In adults, this corresponds to the levels of sedation from anxiolysis to moderate sedation as described in Table 7.1.

Over recent years, there has been an increased focus of safe sedation practice by regulatory agencies. When sedation is used in areas outside the operating theatre environment, and by non-anaesthetic personnel, there is a particular need to ensure adequate provision of facilities, equipment and competent personnel. An audit of sedation for over 14 000 upper gastrointestinal endoscopies published in 1995 demonstrated a 30-day mortality of 1:2000 and a morbidity rate of 1:2003, primarily due to respiratory and cardiovascular problems. As a result, several practice guidelines have been published to address these issues. Examples include guidance on sedation for upper gastrointestinal endoscopy, procedures in the emergency department and dental surgery, and the sedation of children. Many of these documents share key messages: the requirement of a trained individual solely responsible for monitoring the patient during sedation; the mandatory use of pulse oximetry; the importance of supplementary oxygen therapy during sedation; the need for comprehensive resuscitation equipment which must be immediately available; and the need for personnel who are trained to recognize, and are competent to manage, cardiorespiratory complications. This guidance relates solely to conscious sedation. If deep sedation is required, the patient requires a level of care identical to that needed for general anaesthesia.

	Minimal Sedation	Moderate Sedation	Deep Sedation	General Anaesthesia
		TABLE 7.1		
	Continuum of Depth of Sedation: Definition of General Anaesthesia and Levels of Sedation/ Analgesia. American Society of Anesthesiologists, 2009			
Responsiveness	Normal response to verbal stimulation	Purposeful response to verbal or tactile stimulation	Purposeful response following repeated or painful stimulation	Unrousable even with painful stimulation
Airway	Unaffected	Maintained without intervention	Intervention may be required	Intervention often required
Ventilation	Unaffected	Adequate	May be inadequate	Frequently inadequate
Cardiovascular	Unaffected	Usually maintained	Usually maintained	May be impaired

INDICATIONS FOR THE USE OF SEDATIVE DRUGS

Procedural Sedation

This is defined as the administration of sedative(s) (with or without analgesics) to induce a state which allows a patient to tolerate unpleasant procedures whilst maintaining cardiorespiratory function and the ability to maintain airway control independently and continuously. Procedural sedation may be used for a variety of interventions including radiological investigations, gastrointestinal endoscopy and transoesophageal echocardiography. However, there is no absolute indication for the use of sedation and many procedures for which sedation was felt previously to be mandatory can now be undertaken without the need for systemic drug therapy. The requirement for procedural sedation should be determined by a combination of patient, procedural and operator factors. It is always important to ensure that the benefits of procedural sedation (such as greater patient satisfaction and better tolerance of the procedure) outweigh the associated risks. Sedation should never be used for the convenience of the individual performing the procedure.

The commonest reasons for the use of procedural sedation are to provide anxiolysis for the concerned patient, analgesia for painful procedures and to allow longer procedures (e.g. interventional radiology) to be better tolerated. In individuals with significant cardiac comorbidity, sedation may also attenuate the cardiovascular stimulation (and increase in myocardial oxygen demand) associated with some procedures.

It is important that the sedative agent used will target the specific undesirable symptom. For example, sedatives such as benzodiazepines have no analgesic action and will not provide effective sedation for painful procedures. Great care must be taken when co-administering sedative drugs and systemic opioids. The synergism between these two groups of drugs significantly increases the risks of airway obstruction and respiratory depression.

Premedication

Sedative drugs may be given in the preoperative period to reduce the apprehension experienced before undergoing anaesthesia and surgery. Sedation may be particularly useful in young children, patients with learning difficulties and individuals who are very anxious. Sedative drugs given in this way augment the actions of anaesthetic agents. The choice of drug depends on the patient, the proposed surgery and the prevailing circumstances; for example, requirements for patients undergoing ambulatory surgery are different from those scheduled for major surgery as an inpatient. The oral route of administration is preferred and benzodiazepines are the drugs used most commonly for this purpose. Nasal administration may be useful in children.

Supplementation of General or Regional Anaesthesia

The synergy between sedative drugs and intravenous induction agents is used in the technique of co-induction. The administration of a small dose of sedative may result in a significant reduction in the dose of induction agent required, and therefore in the frequency and severity of side-effects. Patients undergoing regional anaesthetic techniques (e.g. for joint arthroplasty) may also receive supplemental sedation to help alleviate anxieties regarding hearing or seeing parts of the surgery, or to help maintain comfort for prolonged surgery. A target-controlled infusion of propofol is used increasingly for this purpose. Studies in the elderly have found that sedation regimens can relatively frequently produce a deeper level of sedation than intended, resulting in unplanned general anaesthesia.

Awake Fibreoptic Tracheal Intubation

Sedation is often used to supplement the use of topical local anaesthesia when awake fibreoptic intubation is necessary. Because mask ventilation or tracheal intubation may be difficult or indeed impossible in some of these cases, great caution must be taken not to depress consciousness or respiratory drive. For this reason, an infusion of remifentanil (either manual or target-controlled) is used frequently for sedo-analgesia.

Critical Care

Most critically ill patients require sedation to facilitate mechanical ventilation and other therapeutic interventions in the intensive care unit (ICU). With the increasing sophistication of mechanical ventilators, the modern approach is to titrate adequate analgesia with sufficient sedation to maintain the patient in a tranquil but rousable state. The pharmacokinetic profiles of individual drugs should be considered because sedatives are inevitably given by infusion for prolonged periods in patients with potential organ dysfunction and impaired ability to metabolize or excrete drugs. Many different drugs and regimens have been used to provide short-term and long-term sedation in the ICU, including benzodiazepines, anaesthetic agents such as propofol, opioids, and most recently, α_2-adrenergic agonists. There is no evidence supporting the use of any particular regimen or combination of agents.

The value of sedation titration by such measures as the Ramsay Sedation Score or Richmond Agitation Sedation Scale during critical care has been recognized for many years, but more attention has focused recently on the importance of daily sedation 'holds'. These daily interruptions in the sedative and analgesic infusions of selected patients help avoid the accumulation of these agents and this now forms part of the ventilator care bundle package. This has been shown to decrease the incidence of some complications associated with mechanical ventilation during critical illness, such as ventilator-associated pneumonia. In addition, sedation 'holds' may facilitate weaning from mechanical ventilation, thereby decreasing the length of stay in critical care and the need for tracheostomy.

Administration Techniques

The administration of sedative drugs requires skill and vigilance, not least because of the seamless progression from light sedation to general anaesthesia. Traditionally, sedative drugs have been administered by intermittent intravenous bolus doses titrated to effect. There is considerable variability in the individual response to a given dose and there are many circumstances in which medical practitioners without anaesthetic training administer sedatives. Recent technological advances in microprocessor-controlled infusion pumps have improved the safety of administration of sedatives. Patient-controlled analgesia systems have been programmed for patient-controlled sedation, usually to maintain sedation after an initial bolus dose administered by the physician. When the system is wholly patient-controlled, the mean dose of sedative drug decreases while the range increases. In target-controlled infusion (TCI), an adapted syringe driver is programmed with the pharmacokinetic model of a drug and designed to rapidly achieve (and subsequently maintain) a prescribed 'target' plasma concentration. The individual using a TCI system is able to set (and alter) the desired concentration based on the clinical assessment of the patient. There are several different pharmacological models, each specific for an individual drug. Examples include Marsh and Schnider (propofol), Minto (remifentanil) and Maitre (alfentanil). All these models adjust for variations in pharmacokinetics due to gender, age and weight.

Sedative Drugs

Most sedative drugs may be categorized into one of three main groups: benzodiazepines, antipsychotics and α_2-adrenoceptor agonists. Drugs classified more usually as intravenous anaesthetic agents, particularly propofol and ketamine, are also used as sedatives in subanaesthetic doses; the pharmacology of these drugs is discussed in Chapter 3. Similarly, remifentanil, which is used increasingly as part of a sedative regimen, is described fully in Chapter 5. Inhaled anaesthetics (see Ch 2) are also used occasionally as sedatives (e.g. sevoflurane to an end-tidal concentration of 0.3–0.5 kPa, or nitrous oxide).

BENZODIAZEPINES

The term benzodiazepine originates from the structure of the molecule, which consists of the fusion of a benzene and diazepine ring. These drugs were developed initially for their anxiolytic and hypnotic properties and largely replaced oral barbiturates in the 1960s due to their favourable pharmacological profile: minimal cardiorespiratory effects, the production of anterograde amnesia and a lower incidence of physical dependence. As parenteral preparations became available, they rapidly became established in anaesthesia and intensive care. All benzodiazepines have similar pharmacological effects; their therapeutic use is determined largely by their potency and the available pharmaceutical preparations. Benzodiazepines are often classified by their duration of action as long-acting (e.g. diazepam), medium-acting (e.g. temazepam) or short-acting (e.g. midazolam).

Pharmacology

Benzodiazepines exert their actions by high-affinity binding to a specific benzodiazepine binding site, which is part of the γ-aminobutyric acid (GABA) receptor complex. GABA is the major inhibitory neurotransmitter in the central nervous system (CNS), with most neurones undergoing GABA-ergic modulation. The benzodiazepine site is an integral part of the $GABA_A$ receptor subtype. Binding of the agonist increases the affinity of the $GABA_A$ receptor to GABA, producing an increased frequency of the opening of the chloride ion channel, and thus an increase in intracellular chloride transmission. This causes hyperpolarization of the postsynaptic membrane, which makes the neurone resistant to excitation. Benzodiazepine binding sites are found throughout the brain and spinal cord, with the highest density in the cerebral cortex, cerebellum and hippocampus, and with a lower density in the medulla. The absence of $GABA_A$ receptors outside the CNS is consistent with the good cardiovascular safety profile of these drugs.

The $GABA_A$ receptor is a large structure which also contains separate binding sites for other drugs including barbiturates, alcohol and propofol. The binding of other compounds to the benzodiazepine binding site explains the synergistic effects seen with some other drugs. This synergy may lead to dangerous depression of the CNS if drugs are used in combination and also results in pharmacological cross-tolerance, e.g. with alcohol. It is also consistent with the use of benzodiazepines to manage the symptoms associated with acute withdrawal or detoxification from alcohol or other drugs. Elderly patients are particularly sensitive to the effects of benzodiazepines and dosage should be reduced accordingly.

The benzodiazepine antagonist flumazenil occupies the benzodiazepine binding site but produces no activity. Benzodiazepine compounds have been developed which are ligands at the benzodiazepine binding site but have inverse agonist activity, resulting in cerebral excitement. These compounds are also antagonized by flumazenil. This mirrors the way in which paradoxical reactions to benzodiazepines in the elderly are reversed by flumazenil and exacerbated by increasing the dose of the original drug. Other more sinister causes of restlessness, such as hypoxaemia and local anaesthetic toxicity, should always be excluded first.

Physical Properties

Benzodiazepines are relatively small lipid-soluble molecules. Unlike diazepam and lorazepam, which are dissolved in solvents (polyethylene and propylene glycol previously, now lipid emulsions), midazolam is water-soluble. This is due to the presence of an imidazole ring in its structure, which allows midazolam to act as a structural isomer demonstrating tautomerism (isomerism triggered by a change in the physical environment). Midazolam is prepared in a solution buffered to a pH of <4. At this pH, the imidazole ring is open and the molecule is ionized and therefore water-soluble. When the molecule is exposed to the higher pH of the body, the molecule forms the unionized ring, resulting in high lipid solubility.

Systemic Effects

CNS Effects

The characteristic CNS effects seen with all benzodiazepines are anxiolysis, sedation, anterograde amnesia and antiepileptic activity. The degree to which individual benzodiazepines produce these effects is variable, and is thought to be related to their affinity for particular subunits of the $GABA_A$ receptor. For example, benzodiazepines with high activity at the α_1 and/or α_5 subunits tend to have more sedative and amnesic effects, whilst those with activity at α_2 and/or α_3 subunits produce more anxiolysis.

Anxiolysis occurs at low dosage and these drugs are used extensively for the treatment of acute and chronic anxiety states. It is these anxiolytic properties which make benzodiazepines so useful in premedication and during unfamiliar or unpleasant procedures. Longer-acting oral drugs such as diazepam and chlordiazepoxide have a place in the management of acute alcohol withdrawal states.

Chronic administration of benzodiazepines results in benzodiazepine site downregulation, with decreased binding affinity and function, explaining, at least in part, the development of tolerance. Chronic administration also leads to physical and psychological dependence, although these drugs are less addictive than opioids and barbiturates. Abrupt withdrawal may lead to a clinical syndrome similar to that seen in acute alcohol withdrawal; consequently, doses of benzodiazepines should be reduced gradually after chronic administration.

Sedation occurs as a dose-dependent depression of cerebral activity with mild sedation at low receptor occupancy progressing to a state similar to general anaesthesia when most receptor sites are occupied (Table 7.2). Benzodiazepines have a high therapeutic index (ratio of effective to lethal dose) because, in overdose, the differences in receptor density result in greater sensitivity to cortical than to medullary depression. However, upper airway obstruction and loss of protective reflexes occur before profound sedation ensues, and are a major hazard following inadvertent oversedation or self-poisoning.

Amnesia is a common sequel to intravenous administration of benzodiazepines and is useful for patients undergoing unpleasant or repeated procedures. Amnesia is anterograde, affecting the acquisition of new information; retrograde amnesia has not been demonstrated following administration of benzodiazepines.

Antiepileptic activity is the result of prevention of the subcortical spread of seizure activity. Intravenous lorazepam and diazepam may be used to terminate seizures and clonazepam is used as an adjunct in chronic antiepileptic therapy. Benzodiazepines increase the threshold to seizure activity in local anaesthetic toxicity but may also mask the early signs.

Benzodiazepines have enjoyed wide use as a treatment for insomnia and are effective particularly for acute insomnia. However, chronic use is not recommended because of problems with tolerance and dependence, leading to difficulty in withdrawal of treatment. The use of benzodiazepines as hypnotics has now been partly superseded by more modern non-benzodiazepine hypnotics such as zopiclone, which also acts at the benzodiazepine site, and dependence can still occur.

Benzodiazepines decrease cerebral metabolic oxygen requirement and cerebral blood flow in a dose-dependent fashion, and the cerebrovascular response

TABLE 7.2
Relationship Between the Effects Seen with Benzodiazepines and Receptor Occupancy

Midazolam Dose	Effect	Receptor Occupancy(%)	Flumazenil Dose to Reverse
Low dose	Antiepileptic	20–25	Low dose
	Anxiolysis	20–30	
	Slight sedation		
	Reduced attention	25–50	
	Amnesia		
	Intense sedation	60–90	
	Muscle relaxation		
High dose	Anaesthesia		High dose

to carbon dioxide is preserved; consequently, they are suitable for use in selected patients with intracranial pathology. However, it should be noted that benzodiazepines do not prevent the increase in intracranial pressure associated with laryngoscopy and tracheal intubation. In addition, depression of ventilation caused by benzodiazepines in the spontaneously breathing patient results in an increase in arterial $PaCO_2$, which is undesirable if intracranial compliance is reduced.

Unwanted CNS side-effects include drowsiness and impaired psychomotor performance. Even when residual sedative effects are minimal, there may be impaired cognitive function and motor coordination, which should be taken into consideration when assessing fitness for discharge in ambulatory surgery.

Muscle Relaxation

Benzodiazepines produce a mild reduction in muscle tone, which may be advantageous, e.g. during mechanical ventilation in the ICU, when reducing articular dislocations or during endoscopy. However, muscle relaxation is partly responsible for the airway obstruction which may occur during intravenous sedation. The muscle relaxation is not related to any effect at the neuromuscular junction, but results from suppression of the internuncial neurones of the spinal cord and depression of polysynaptic transmission in the brain.

Respiratory Effects

Benzodiazepines produce dose-related central depression of ventilation. The ventilatory response to carbon dioxide is impaired and hypoxic ventilatory responses are markedly depressed. It follows that patients with hypoventilation syndromes and type 2 respiratory failure are particularly sensitive to the respiratory depressant effects of benzodiazepines. Ventilatory depression is exacerbated by airway obstruction and is more common in the elderly. Synergism occurs when both opioids and benzodiazepines are administered. If both types of drug are to be given intravenously, the opioid should be given first and its effect assessed. A reduction of up to 75% in the dose requirement of the benzodiazepine should be anticipated. It should be standard practice to provide supplemental oxygen and to monitor oxygen saturation continuously by pulse oximetry during intravenous sedation.

Cardiovascular Effects

Benzodiazepines produce modest haemodynamic effects, with good preservation of homeostatic reflex mechanisms and a much wider margin of safety than intravenous anaesthetic agents. A decrease in systemic vascular resistance results in a small decrease in arterial pressure. Significant hypotension may occur in the hypovolaemic patient.

Pharmacokinetics

Benzodiazepines are relatively small lipid-soluble molecules, which are readily absorbed orally and which pass rapidly into the CNS. Midazolam undergoes significant first-pass hepatic metabolism with only around 50% of an oral dose reaching the systemic circulation. Volume of distribution is large, as would be expected from such a highly lipid soluble compound. All benzodiazepines are extensively protein bound (>96%).

After intravenous bolus administration, termination of action occurs largely by redistribution and hepatic metabolism. Compared with drugs such as propofol, benzodiazepines have a slower effect site equilibration time. This suggests that time should be allowed to assess the full clinical effect before administering a further intravenous incremental dose. Elimination takes place by hepatic metabolism followed by renal excretion of the metabolites. There are two main pathways of metabolism involving either microsomal oxidation or conjugation with glucuronide. The significance of this is that oxidation is much more likely to be affected by age, hepatic disease, drug interactions and other factors which alter the concentration of cytochrome P450. Some of the benzodiazepines, including diazepam, have active metabolites which greatly prolong their clinical effects. Renal dysfunction results in the accumulation of these metabolites, and this is an important factor in delayed recovery from prolonged sedation in the ICU. Benzodiazepines do not induce hepatic enzyme metabolism pathways.

Diazepam

Diazepam was the first benzodiazepine available for parenteral use. It is insoluble in water and was formulated initially in propylene glycol, which is very irritant to veins and which is associated with a high incidence of thrombophlebitis. A lipid emulsion (Diazemuls) was developed later. Both formulations are presented in 2-mL ampoules containing 5 mg mL^{-1}. Diazepam is also available orally as tablets or a syrup with a bioavailability of 100% and as a rectal solution and suppositories. The elimination half-life is 20–70 h, but active metabolites are produced, including desmethyldiazepam (half-life 36–200 h) and nordiazepam (half-life >100 h). Clearance is reduced in the presence of hepatic dysfunction. Although diazepam can be given by the intramuscular route, absorption is unpredictable, and the injection is very painful.

Dosage

- Premedication: 10–20 mg orally 1–1.5 h preoperatively.
- Sedation: 5–10 mg i.v. slowly; incremental boluses of 1–2 mg.
- Status epilepticus: 2 mg, repeated every minute until seizure ends; maximum dose 20 mg.
- Intensive care: not suitable for infusion; i.v. bolus dose 5–10 mg may be used 4–hourly. However, the long half-life of the active metabolites makes diazepam undesirable for sedation in critical care patients.

Temazepam

This benzodiazepine is only available orally but is used widely as a premedicant because of its anxiolytic properties. Oral absorption is complete but it may take up to 2 h to reach peak plasma concentrations. Metabolism takes place in the liver by conjugation with glucuronide and there are no significant active metabolites. Elimination half-life is shorter than diazepam (8–15 h) and onset of action more rapid (45–60 min). Tolerance and dependence are less likely to occur with chronic use of temazepam and it has been prescribed widely as a hypnotic.

Dosage

- Premedication: 10–30 mg orally 60-120 min preoperatively.

Lorazepam

This drug is available for parenteral, oral and intramuscular administration but is not used routinely as an intravenous sedative because it is limited by a slow onset of action. The intramuscular route should be used only when no other route is available. Intravenous

lorazepam is currently the drug of choice in the management of status epilepticus, because it has a longer duration of antiepileptic action than diazepam (see below). It can also be used in the management of severe acute panic attacks. Metabolism is by glucuronidation, with an elimination half-life of 12–15 h. Amnesia is a marked feature of this drug.

Dosage

- Premediciation: 1–4 mg orally 1–2 h preoperatively.
- Panic attacks: 25–30 µg kg^{-1} i.v. or i.m. (maximum 4 mg).
- Status epilepticus: 4 mg i.v., repeated after 10 min.

Midazolam

Midazolam is available for intravenous, intramuscular, oral, rectal and buccal administration. The drug becomes highly lipid-soluble and penetrates the brain rapidly with the onset of sedation in less than 90 s and peak effect at 2–5 min. Oral bioavailability is 40–50%. Unlike diazepam, intramuscular absorption is rapid. Midazolam undergoes hepatic oxidative metabolism and has an elimination half-life of 2 h. The major metabolite, hydroxymidazolam, has a half-life of around 1 h, and although it is biologically active, it is clinically important only after prolonged infusion in patients with renal impairment. Midazolam is 1.5–2 times more potent than diazepam and has much more favourable pharmacokinetics for use as a short-term intravenous sedative.

Dosage

- Premedication: 0.5 mg kg^{-1} orally (maximum 30 mg) or 70–100 µg kg^{-1} i.m. 30–60 min preoperatively.
- Sedation: 25–50 µg kg^{-1} i.v., then incremental boluses of 0.5–1 mg to a maximum of 7.5 mg. Reduce dose by at least 50% in the elderly.
- ICU sedation: loading dose of 30–300 µg kg^{-1} i.v., then infusion of 30–200 µg kg^{-1} h^{-1}.

Flumazenil

Flumazenil is a very high-affinity competitive antagonist for all other ligands at the benzodiazepine binding site. It rapidly reverses all the CNS effects of benzodiazepines and also the other potentially dangerous adverse physiological effects, including respiratory and cardiovascular depression, and airway obstruction. It is used to reverse excessive sedation following benzodiazepine administration, either by iatrogenic overdose, following prolonged periods of sedation in ICU or by deliberate ingestion to cause self-harm. Flumazenil has only very slight intrinsic activity at high doses and is very well tolerated, with minimal adverse effects. It has no effect on benzodiazepine metabolism. Flumazenil is rapidly cleared from plasma and metabolized by the liver. It has a very short elimination half-life of less than 1 h. Its duration of action depends on the dose administered and the identity and dose of the agonist. It ranges from 20 min to 2 h and the potential exists for resedation if the agonist has a long half-life, necessitating a period of close observation. Repeated administration may be necessary.

Dosage

- The usual clinically effective dose is 300–600 μg i.v. given as 100–200 μg boluses and repeated at 1-min intervals to a maximum of 1 mg. When used in ICU, a total dose of up to 2 mg may be necessary. Flumazenil may also be given as an infusion (100–400 μg h^{-1}).

Cautions

- Epileptic patients: there is a risk of seizures, especially if a benzodiazepine has been prescribed as antiepileptic therapy.
- Benzodiazepine dependence: withdrawal symptoms may be precipitated.
- Anxiety reactions: these may occur after rapid reversal of heavy sedation.
- Patients with severe head injury: flumazenil may precipitate a sudden increase in intracranial pressure.

NEUROLEPTICS

This group of sedative drugs includes the phenothiazines and the butyrophenones, which are structurally similar drugs. These drugs are used primarily as antipsychotics in psychiatry. Both classes of drug have a high therapeutic index and a flat dose-response curve which result in a good safety profile with a low incidence of respiratory depression even when taken in overdose. Neurolepsis describes a characteristic drug-induced change in behaviour. There is an altered state of awareness, with suppression of spontaneous movement and a placid compliant affect. Loss of consciousness does not occur, and spinal and central reflexes remain intact. The combination of a neuroleptic drug with an opioid, usually fentanyl, is termed neuroleptanalgesia. This was a popular means of providing sedation before the advent of intravenous benzodiazepines. There is no amnesia and the patient may subsequently report unpleasant mental agitation despite a calm demeanour. The opioid obtunds the unpleasant mental experience but may result in respiratory depression. The addition of nitrous oxide may be used to produce neuroleptanaesthesia, in which consciousness is lost.

Pharmacology

Neuroleptics interfere with dopaminergic transmission in the brain by blocking dopamine receptors. At some synapses, dopamine is the stimulatory transmitter and GABA the inhibitory transmitter, so in common with other sedatives, neuroleptics enhance the effects of GABA. Dopamine blockade results in useful antiemetic activity but also carries the inevitable potential for extrapyramidal side-effects. These include tardive dyskinesia (involuntary movements of tongue, face and jaw), Parkinsonian symptoms, akathisia (restlessness) and dystonia (abnormal face and body movements).

All neuroleptic agents have been reported as a cause of the neuroleptic malignant syndrome, a rare but potentially fatal reaction. The syndrome is characterized by hyperthermia, muscle hypertonicity, autonomic instability and fluctuating levels of consciousness. It has some features in common with malignant hyperthermia associated with anaesthesia. Treatment includes supportive measures, dopamine agonists (e.g. bromocriptine) and dantrolene.

Neuroleptic drugs also have actions at cholinergic, α-adrenergic, histaminergic and serotonergic receptors, and these properties influence their side-effects and the degree of sedation produced. The antiadrenergic effect is responsible for inducing hypotension, which can result in syncope in the elderly. The elderly are also most at risk of hypo- and hyperthermia due to the drugs' interference with temperature regulation.

Haloperidol

Haloperidol is a butyrophenone with a long duration of action. It has almost no α-adrenoceptor blocking activity and so has a minimal effect on the cardiovascular system. It is a potent antiemetic but has a high incidence of extrapyramidal side-effects. Haloperidol has fewer antimuscarinic side-effects, but also produces less sedation than that seen with chlorpromazine. Haloperidol may be used in the short-term management of the acutely agitated patient after sinister causes of confusion such as hypoxaemia and sepsis have been excluded and is used increasingly in the management of ICU psychosis. The duration of action of haloperidol is in the region of 24–48 h.

Dosage

- Sedation: 2–10 mg i.v. or i.m. (max. 18 mg per 24 h).
- Anxiolysis: 500 μg orally every 12 h.
- Antiemesis: 1.25 mg i.v. is effective in the prevention of postoperative nausea and vomiting.

Chlorpromazine

Chlorpromazine is a phenothiazine which is prescribed commonly as an antipsychotic but no longer used as an adjunct in anaesthesia. It may be used in the same way as haloperidol in the acutely confused or agitated patient. It has pronounced sedative properties and potentiates the actions of anaesthetic drugs. There is also marked antiemetic activity. A mild anticholinergic action moderates the incidence of extrapyramidal effects. α-Adrenoceptor blockade produces vasodilatation and may result in hypotension which is exacerbated by direct cardiac depression and depression of vasomotor reflexes. Central temperature control mechanisms are affected by chlorpromazine, with a reduced shivering response.

Dosage

- Sedation for acute agitation: 25–50 mg orally or i.m. The drug must be diluted and given slowly if used intravenously (unlicensed for i.v. use) to avoid thrombophlebitis.

Droperidol

Droperidol is a butyrophenone with potent antidopaminergic activity. It is a powerful antiemetic, acting at the chemoreceptor trigger zone. Large doses may produce dystonic reactions. Droperidol has mild α-adrenoceptor blocking actions, which may cause vasodilatation after intravenous administration, resulting in hypotension. Droperidol was widely used for premedication and in neuroleptanaesthesia but its availability was discontinued in the UK in 2001 due to cases of prolonged QT syndrome. It has recently been reintroduced with a licence for the prevention of postoperative nausea and vomiting. Droperidol has an onset time of 3–10 min after intravenous injection, with a duration of action of 6–12 h. It undergoes hepatic metabolism, but approximately 10% of the drug is excreted unchanged in the urine.

Dosage

- Prophylaxis for PONV: 0.625–1.25 mg i.v. 20 min prior to the end of surgery.

Olanzapine

Olanzapine is a second generation antipsychotic (or atypical antipsychotic) drug. Although not considered a classical neuroleptic, it has a similar mechanism of action, with antidopaminergic, antihistaminergic and antimuscarinic actions. Olanzapine rarely produces hypotension and is being used increasingly in the management of ICU psychoses.

Dosage

- Sedation: 5–10 mg orally (maximum 20 mg daily).

α₂-ADRENOCEPTOR AGONISTS

α₂-Adrenergic receptors are involved in the regulation of the release of the neurotransmitter noradrenaline (norepinephrine). These receptors were initially classified anatomically as presynaptic, but α₂-adrenoceptors are also found postsynaptically and extrasynaptically. The more correct pharmacological classification is based on the predominantly α₂-selectivity of the antagonist yohimbine. α₂-Adrenoceptors are located peripherally and centrally, with the centrally mediated effects of particular relevance in anaesthesia.

The characteristic central effects of α₂-adrenoceptor agonists are sedation, anxiolysis and hypnosis. The locus coeruleus is a small neuronal nucleus in the upper brainstem which contains the major noradrenergic cell group in the brain. This nucleus is an important modulator of wakefulness. Activation of α_2-adrenoceptors results in inhibition of transmitter release. The locus coeruleus also has connections to the cortex, thalamus and vasomotor centre.

α_2-Adrenoceptor agonists have analgesic properties. Descending fibres from the locus coeruleus decrease nociceptive transmission at the spinal level. In addition, α_2-adrenoceptors occur in primary sensory neurones and the dorsal horn of the spinal cord.

Many ligands at α_2-adrenoceptors are substituted imidazoles. Non-adrenergic imidazole binding sites exist in some tissues, including the brain: the imidazoline receptors. I_1 imidazoline receptors are found in the medulla and are involved in the regulation of arterial pressure. This may explain the hypotension and bradycardia which may accompany administration of α_2-adrenoceptor agonists. Similarly, the I_2 imidazoline receptor may interact with opioid receptors and may contribute to the analgesic effect of α_2-adrenoceptor agonists.

Clonidine

Clonidine is an imidazoline compound and a selective α_2-adrenoceptor agonist with an $\alpha_2:\alpha_1$ ratio of 200:1. Clonidine has proved effective in the treatment of patients with severe hypertension but it is recognized that abrupt discontinuation of therapy can result in rebound hypertension. Clonidine is lipid-soluble and is absorbed rapidly and almost completely after oral administration, with peak plasma concentrations occurring in 60–90 min. It may be administered transdermally and is also available as a solution for intravenous, intramuscular, epidural and intrathecal use. The elimination half-life is 9–13 h and this is prolonged in renal failure. Fifty percent of an administered dose is excreted unchanged by the kidneys and 50% is metabolized in the liver to inactive metabolites.

Systemic Effects

CNS Effects. Clonidine produces sedation and anxiolysis. It also reduces requirements for both intravenous and volatile anaesthetic agents. There is a ceiling to the reduction of MAC effect, because of the potential for activity at α_1-receptors at high dose. More selective α_2-adrenoceptor agonists reduce MAC to a much greater extent.

Clonidine is a potent analgesic, acting centrally and on the α_2-adrenoceptors of the dorsal horn. It may be administered intravenously, intrathecally or epidurally to produce an analgesic response. Synergism exists with opioids, and the actions of local anaesthetics are also potentiated. Clonidine is used to provide analgesia in the perioperative period and also in chronic pain syndromes.

CVS Effects. The cardiovascular effects of clonidine probably involve both α_2-adrenoceptors and imidazoline receptors. Administration leads to decreases in heart rate and arterial pressure. Clonidine is known to lower the 'set point' around which arterial pressure is regulated. The α_2-agonist effects are a reduction in sympathetic tone and an increase in parasympathetic tone. The resulting decreases in heart rate, myocardial contractility and systemic vascular resistance lead to a reduction in myocardial oxygen requirements. This may be advantageous in attenuating stress-induced haemodynamic responses. However, undesirable cardiovascular depression has been the major limiting factor in developing the use of clonidine as a sedative.

Respiratory Effects. Clonidine has minor respiratory effects, causing only a small reduction in minute ventilation.

Dosage
- Premedication: 150–300 μg orally given 1–2 h preoperatively.
- Analgesia: used as an adjunct to local anaesthetics in both central and peripheral nerve blocks.
- Critical care: $0–2\,\mu g\,kg^{-1}\,h^{-1}$ i.v. as a sedative, especially for agitation in drug-dependent individuals.

Dexmedetomidine

Dexmedetomidine is a selective α_2-adrenoceptor agonist (1600:1, $\alpha_2: \alpha_1$) with eight times more affinity for α_2-adrenoceptors than clonidine. It has similar sedative, analgesic and anxiolytic properties to clonidine but has a more rapid elimination half-life (2 h). The reduction in α_1-activity also results in a MAC-sparing effect of up to 90%. Like clonidine, it is metabolized in the liver with >90% excreted in the urine. The side-effect profile is also similar to that of clonidine, with hypotension and bradycardia the most frequent problems. Dexmedetomidine has recently been approved for use in the UK for sedation in the ICU, although it is also being used off-licence for procedural sedation, e.g. awake craniotomy.

Dosage

- ICU sedation: infusion at an average of $0.7\,\mu g\,kg^{-1}\,h^{-1}$ (normal range $0.2–1.4\,\mu g\,kg^{-1}\,h^{-1}$).
- Procedural sedation: $1\,\mu g\,kg^{-1}$ over 10 min, then infusion at an average of $0.6\,\mu g\,kg^{-1}\,h^{-1}$ (normal range $0.2–1.0\,\mu g\,kg^{-1}\,h^{-1}$).

OTHER DRUGS

Paraldehyde

Paraldehyde is the cyclic trimer of acetaldehyde molecules and was used widely as a sedative in psychiatry up to the 1960s. Paraldehyde undergoes hepatic metabolism but 10-30% is excreted by the lungs, giving the patient's breath a characteristic odour. It is now used for sedation in paediatrics (e.g. for MRI scanning). Paraldehyde is contraindicated in gastric disorders.

Dosage

- Sedation: $0.3\,mL\,kg^{-1}$ rectally (maximum 10 mL) 20–30 min pre-procedure. It is usually diluted 1:1 with olive oil. Paraldehyde dissolves plastic, so if given using a plastic syringe, it must be injected immediately. Alternatively, feeding tubes or glass syringes can be used for administration.

Chloral Hydrate

Chloral hydrate is a sedative drug used in the treatment of insomnia and may be used for the sedation of children for brief procedures. Chloral hydrate may be given by mouth or per rectum although it is corrosive to mucous membranes unless well diluted with water. It has an unpleasant taste which can be disguised with sweet juice. Onset is within 15 min and duration can be as long as 2 h. It is metabolized to trichloroethanol, which has a half-life of 8–10 h. Chloral hydrate is contraindicated in gastric disease, and in patients with cardiac, hepatic or renal impairment.

Dosage

- Sedation: $50–75\,mg\,kg^{-1}$ orally (maximum 2 g) 20–30 min pre-procedure

Barbiturates

These drugs are derived from barbituric acid and are now used primarily for induction of anaesthesia and in the treatment of epilepsy. They have largely been superseded as sedative agents by benzodiazepines but some barbiturates are still used for paediatric sedation in specialist centres, e.g. pentobarbital $2\,mg\,kg^{-1}$ i.v. (short-acting, effective for 1 h) or quinalbarbitone $7.5–10\,mg\,kg^{-1}$ orally (to a maximum dose of 200 mg) (intermediate-acting, effective for around 2 h).

Melatonin

Melatonin is a hormone secreted by the pineal gland and has a role in controlling circadian rhythms. It is used primarily in the treatment of sleep disorders, but has also been used as a sedative agent in both adults and children (typical oral dose 3–10 mg). The mechanism by which melatonin causes sedation has not been fully elucidated, but it may be due to an enhancement of GABA activity.

FURTHER READING

American Society of Anesthesiologists, 2009. Continuum of depth of sedation: definition of general anesthesia and levels of sedation/analgesia.

Calvey, N., Williams, N., 2008. Principles and practice of pharmacology for anaesthetists, fifth ed. Wiley-Blackwell, Oxford.

8 DRUGS ACTING ON THE CARDIOVASCULAR SYSTEM

■ ■ ■ ■ ■ ■ ■ ■ ■ ■

Many drugs have either primary or secondary effects on the cardiovascular and autonomic nervous systems. Several of the drugs discussed in this chapter have more than one clinical indication and the drugs are considered according to their mechanism of action. An understanding of drugs acting on the cardiovascular and autonomic nervous systems requires an understanding of autonomic physiology and pharmacology.

THE AUTONOMIC NERVOUS SYSTEM

The term autonomic nervous system (ANS) refers to the nervous and humoral mechanisms which modify the function of the autonomous or automatic organs. These include heart rate and force of contraction, calibre of blood vessels, contraction and relaxation of smooth muscle in gut, bladder and bronchi, visual accommodation and pupillary size. Other functions include regulation of secretion from exocrine and other glands and aspects of metabolism (e.g. glycogenolysis and lipolysis) (Table 8.1). There is constant activity of both the sympathetic and parasympathetic nervous systems even at rest. This is termed sympathetic or parasympathetic tone and allows alterations in autonomic activity to produce rapid two-way regulation of physiological effect. The ANS is controlled by centres in the spinal cord, brainstem and hypothalamus, which are in turn influenced by higher centres in the cerebral and particularly the limbic cortex. The ANS is also influenced by visceral reflexes whereby afferent signals

enter the autonomic ganglia, spinal cord, hypothalamus or brainstem and directly elicit appropriate reflex responses via the visceral organs. The efferent autonomic signals are transmitted through the body to two major subdivisions (separated by anatomical, physiological and pharmacological criteria), the sympathetic and the parasympathetic nervous systems.

The Sympathetic Nervous System

The sympathetic nervous system includes nerves which originate in the spinal cord between the first thoracic and second lumbar segments (T1 to L2). Fibres leave the spinal cord with the anterior nerve roots and then branch off as white rami communicantes to synapse in the bilateral paravertebral sympathetic ganglionic chains, although some preganglionic fibres synapse instead in the paravertebral ganglia (e.g. coeliac, mesenteric and hypogastric) in the abdomen before travelling to their effector organ with the relevant arteries. Postganglionic fibres travel from paravertebral ganglia in sympathetic nerves (to supply the internal viscera, including the heart) and spinal nerves (which innervate the peripheral vasculature and sweat glands). Sympathetic nerves throughout the circulation contain vasoconstrictor fibres, particularly in the kidneys, spleen, gut and skin; however, sympathetic vasodilator fibres predominate in skeletal muscle, and coronary and cerebral vessels. Sympathetic stimulation therefore causes predominantly vasoconstriction but also a redistribution of blood flow to skeletal muscle; constriction of venous capacitance vessels may decrease their volume and thereby increase venous

TABLE 8.1
Effects of the Sympathetic and Parasympathetic Nervous Systems on Peripheral Effector Organs, and Receptor Subtypes Mediating these Functions (Where Known)

	SYMPATHETIC		PARASYMPATHETIC	
Organ	*Receptor Subtype*	*Effect*	*Receptor Subtype*	*Effect*
Heart	β_1, also β_2, ? also α and DA_1	↑ Heart rate ↑ Force of contraction ↑ Conduction velocity ↑ Automaticity (β_2) ↑ Excitability	M_2	↓ Heart rate ↓ Force of contraction Slight ↓ conduction velocity
	α_1	↑ Force of contraction		
Arteries	β_1 β_2 α_1, α_2 DA_1, β_2	Coronary vasodilatation Vasodilatation (skeletal muscle) Vasoconstriction (coronary, pulmonary, renal and splanchnic circulations, skin and skeletal muscle) Splanchnic and renal vasodilatation	M[a]	Vasodilatation in skin, skeletal muscle, pulmonary and coronary circulations
Veins	α_1, also α_2 β_2	Vasoconstriction Vasodilatation		
Lung	β_2 α_1	Bronchodilation Inhibition of secretions Bronchoconstriction	M_1, M_3	Bronchoconstriction Stimulation of secretions
GI tract	α_1, α_2, β_2 α_1, α_2	Decreased motility Contraction of sphincters Inhibition of secretions	M_2, M_3	Increased motility Relaxation of sphincters Stimulation of secretions
Pancreas	β_2 α_1, α_2	Increased insulin release Decreased insulin release		
Kidney	β	Renin secretion		
Liver	β_2, α β_2, ?α	Glycogenolysis Gluconeogenesis	M	Glycogen synthesis
Bladder	β_2 α	Detrusor relaxation Sphincter contraction	M	Detrusor contraction Sphincter relaxation
Uterus	α_1 β_2	Myometrial contraction Myometrial relaxation		
Adipocytes	β_3	Lipolysis		
Eye	α_1	Mydriasis (radial muscle contraction) Ciliary muscle relaxation for far vision	M	Miosis Ciliary muscle contraction for near vision
Platelets	α_2	Promote platelet aggregation		
Sweat glands	M[b]	Sweating		

[a] Muscarinic receptors are present on vascular smooth muscle, but they are independent of parasympathetic innervation and have little or no physiological role in the control of vasomotor tone.
[b] Sympathetic cholinergic fibres supply sweat glands and arterioles in some sites.
All postganglionic parasympathetic fibres are muscarinic (M), but in many sites the subtype has not been identified.

return. The effects of sympathetic stimulation at different receptors and effector organs are summarized in Table 8.1. The distribution of sympathetic nerve fibres to an organ or region may differ from the sensory or motor supply, according to its embryonic origin. For example, sympathetic fibres to the heart arise from T1 to T5 (but predominantly from T1 to T4), the neck is supplied by fibres from T2, the chest by fibres from T3 to T6 and the abdomen by fibres from T7 to T11.

Sympathetic Neurotransmitters

The neurotransmitter present in preganglionic neurones is acetylcholine (ACh). These and other neurones containing ACh are termed *cholinergic*. However, the activity of preganglionic neurones is modulated by several other neuropeptides including enkephalin, neurotensin, substance P, somatostatin, nitric oxide, serotonin and catecholamines. ACh is the transmitter at all preganglionic synapses, acting via nicotinic receptors. Postganglionic sympathetic neurones secrete noradrenaline and are termed *adrenergic* (except for postganglionic sympathetic nerve fibres to sweat glands, pilo-erector muscles and some blood vessels, which are cholinergic).

Activation of preganglionic nicotinic fibres to the adrenal medulla causes the release of adrenaline (adrenaline), which is released primarily as a circulating hormone and is only found in insignificant amounts in the nerve endings. Endogenous catecholamines (adrenaline, noradrenaline (norepinephrine) and dopamine) are synthesized from the essential amino acid phenylalanine. Their structure is based on a catechol ring (i.e. a benzene ring with -OH groups in the 3 and 4 positions), and an ethylamine side chain (Figs 8.1 and 8.2); substitutions in the side chain produce the different compounds. Dopamine may act as a precursor for both adrenaline and noradrenaline when administered exogenously (see below).

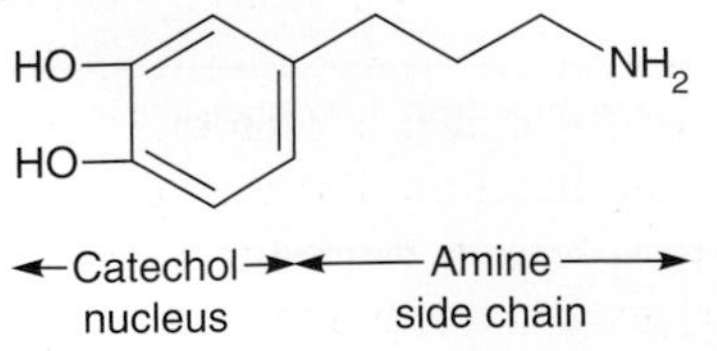

FIGURE 8.1 ■ Standard molecular structure of catecholamines.

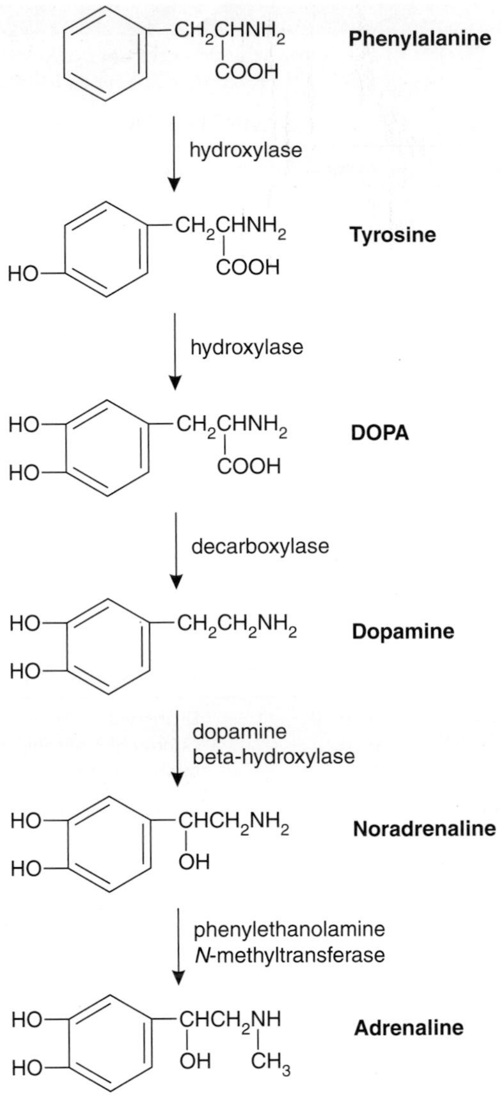

FIGURE 8.2 ■ Synthesis of endogenous catecholamines.

The action of noradrenaline released from sympathetic nerve endings is terminated in one of three ways:

- re-uptake into the nerve terminal
- diffusion into the circulation
- enzymatic destruction.

Most noradrenaline released from sympathetic nerves is taken back into the presynaptic nerve ending for storage and subsequent reuse. Re-uptake is by active transport back into the nerve terminal cytoplasm and then into cytoplasmic vesicles. This mechanism of

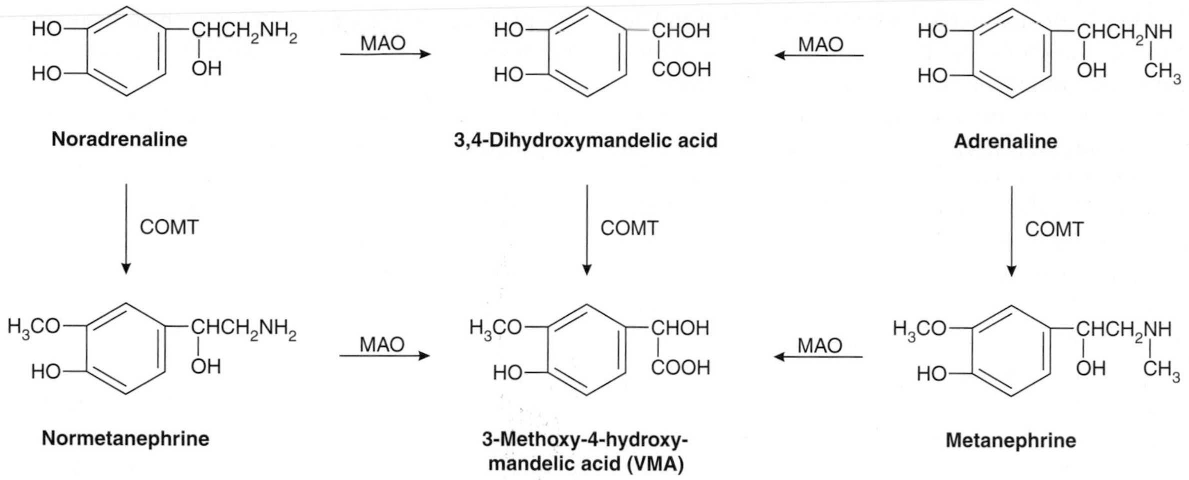

FIGURE 8.3 ■ Catecholamine metabolites. MAO=monoamine oxidase; COMT=catechol O-methyltransferase.

presynaptic re-uptake, termed *uptake*$_1$, is dependent on adenosine triphosphate (ATP) and Mg^{2+}, is enhanced by Li^+ and may be blocked by cocaine and tricyclic antidepressants. Endogenous catecholamines entering the circulation by diffusion from sympathetic nerve endings or by release from the adrenal gland are metabolized rapidly by the enzymes monamine oxidase (MAO) and catechol O-methyltransferase (COMT) in the liver, kidneys, gut and many other tissues. The metabolites are conjugated before being excreted in urine as 3-methoxy-4-hydroxymandelic acid, metanephrine (from adrenaline) and normetanephrine (from noradrenaline) (Fig. 8.3). Noradrenaline taken up into the nerve terminal may also be deaminated by cytoplasmic MAO.

Another mechanism for the postsynaptic cellular re-uptake of catecholamines, termed *uptake*$_2$, is present predominantly at the membrane of smooth muscle cells. It may be responsible for the termination of action of catecholamines released from the adrenal medulla.

Adrenergic Receptor Pharmacology

The actions of catecholamines are mediated by specific postsynaptic cell surface receptors. The original classification of these receptors into α- and β-adrenergic receptors was based upon the effects of adrenaline at peripheral sympathetic sites, α-receptors being responsible for vasoconstriction and β-receptors mediating effects on the heart, and bronchial and intestinal smooth muscle. However, several subtypes of α- and β-receptors exist in addition to receptors specific for dopamine (DA_1 and DA_2 subtypes). Two α- and β-receptor subtypes are well defined on functional, anatomical and pharmacological grounds (α_1 and α_2, β_1 and β_2). A third β-receptor subtype, β_3, is found in adipocytes, skeletal and ventricular muscle, and the vasculature. At least three further subtypes of both α_1- and α_2-receptors and five subtypes of DA-receptor have also been identified, although their precise functions are unclear. Differentiation of receptor subtypes is now based more directly on the effects of various catecholamine agonist compounds (including endogenous catecholamines). Noradrenaline and adrenaline are agonists at both α_1- and α_2-receptors; noradrenaline is slightly more potent at α_1-receptors, and more potent at α_2-receptors. Adrenaline has a more potent action at β_1-receptors, and also acts at β_2-receptors, whereas noradrenaline has no β_2-effects.

Until recently, it was thought that β_1-receptors predominated in the heart, mediating increases in force and rate of contraction, and β_2-receptors existed in bronchial, uterine and vascular smooth muscle, mediating relaxation. In fact, most organs and tissues contain both β_1- and β_2-receptors, which may even serve the same function. For example, up to 25% of cardiac β-receptors in the normal individual are of the β_2 subtype, and this proportion may be increased in patients with heart failure. It is now apparent that β_1-receptors in tissues are situated on the postsynaptic membrane of adrenergic neurones and respond to released noradrenaline. β_2-Receptors are presynaptic and, when stimulated (principally by circulating catecholamines), they modulate autonomic activity by promoting neuronal noradrenaline release. β_3-Receptors mediate thermogenesis and lipolysis in adipocytes but antagonize the effects of β_1- and β_2-receptors on the heart, and also mediate vasodilatation. Similarly, α_1-receptors are present on the postsynaptic membrane, whereas α_2-receptors are predominantly presynaptic, responding to circulating adrenaline but also mediating feedback inhibition of sympathetic nerve activity. Central α_2 stimulation causes decreases in arterial pressure, peripheral resistance, venous return, myocardial contractility, cardiac output and heart rate by inhibition of sympathetic outflow. Postsynaptic α_2-receptors present on platelets and in the CNS mediate platelet aggregation and membrane hyperpolarization, respectively.

Postsynaptic dopamine receptors (DA_1) are present in vascular smooth muscle of the renal, splanchnic, coronary and cerebral circulations, where they mediate vasodilatation. They are also situated on renal tubules, where they inhibit sodium reabsorption, causing natriuresis and diuresis. Postsynaptic DA_2-receptors are widespread in the CNS and occur on the presynaptic membrane of sympathetic nerves and in the adrenal gland. Stimulation of presynaptic DA_2-receptors inhibits dopamine release by negative feedback.

Postganglionic sympathetic fibres supplying sweat glands and arterioles in some areas of skin and skeletal muscle are cholinergic. Vascular smooth muscle also contains non-innervated cholinergic receptors which mediate vasodilatation in response to circulating agonists. Cholinergic effects on vascular smooth muscle are usually minimal but may be involved in the mechanism of vasovagal attacks.

These subdivisions and the functions of the autonomic nervous system are summarized in Table 8.1.

Structure of Adrenergic Receptors

Both α- and β-adrenergic receptors are proteins with a similar basic structure, comprising seven hydrophobic transmembrane domains and an intracellular chain. Differences in amino acid sequences of the intracellular chain differentiate α- and β-receptors. Both are linked to guanine nucleotide binding proteins

(G-proteins) in the cell membrane which mediate the generation of second messengers that activate intracellular events. These second messenger systems include enzymes (adenylate cyclase, phospholipases) and ion channels (for calcium and potassium).

Second and Third Messenger Systems

In addition to functional differences, α- and β-receptors differ in the intracellular mechanisms by which they act. Stimulation of β_1- and β_2-receptors activates G_s-proteins, which activate adenylate cyclase and cause the generation of intracellular cyclic adenosine monophosphate (cAMP). cAMP activates intracellular enzyme pathways (the third messengers) to produce the associated alteration in cell function (e.g. increased force of cardiac muscle contraction, liver glycogenolysis, bronchial smooth muscle relaxation). In cardiac myocytes, the intracellular pathway involves the activation of protein kinases to phosphorylate intracellular proteins and increase intracellular Ca^{2+} concentrations. Intracellular cAMP concentration is modulated by the enzyme phosphodiesterase, which breaks down cAMP to inactive 5' AMP. This is the site of action of phosphodiesterase inhibitor drugs. The balance between production and degradation of cAMP is an important regulatory system for cell function. α_2-Receptors interact with G_i-proteins to *inhibit* adenylate cyclase and Ca^{2+} channels, but activate K^+ channels, phospholipase C and phospholipase A_2. Cholinergic M_2-receptors and somatostatin affect G_i-proteins in the same way.

In contrast, α_1-receptor stimulation does not directly affect intracellular cAMP levels, but causes coupling with another G-protein, G_q, to activate membrane-bound phospholipase C. This in turn hydrolyses phosphatidylinositol biphosphate (PIP_2) to inositol triphosphate (IP_3), which produces changes in intracellular Ca^{2+} concentration and binding. These lead, for example, to smooth muscle contraction.

The Parasympathetic Nervous System

The parasympathetic nervous system controls vegetative functions, e.g. the digestion and absorption of nutrients, excretion of waste products and the conservation and restoration of energy. Parasympathetic neurones arise from cell bodies of the motor nuclei of cranial nerves III, VII, IX and X in the brainstem, and from the sacral segments of the spinal cord ('the craniosacral outflow'). Preganglionic fibres run almost to the organ innervated and synapse in ganglia within the organ, giving rise to postganglionic fibres which then supply the relevant tissues. The ganglion cells may be well organized (e.g. the myenteric plexus of the intestine) or diffuse (e.g. in the bladder or vasculature). As the majority of all parasympathetic nerves are contained in branches of the vagus nerve, which innervates the viscera of the thorax and abdomen, increased parasympathetic activity is characterized by signs of vagal overactivity. Parasympathetic fibres also pass to the eye via the oculomotor (third cranial) nerve, and to the lacrimal, nasal and salivary glands via the facial (fifth) and glossopharyngeal (ninth) nerves. Fibres originating in the sacral portion of the spinal cord pass to the distal GI tract, bladder and reproductive organs. The effects of parasympathetic stimulation at different receptors and effector organs are summarized in Table 8.1

Parasympathetic Neurotransmitters

The chemical neurotransmitter at both pre- and postganglionic synapses is ACh, although transmission at postganglionic synapses may be modulated by other substances, including GABA, serotonin and opioid peptides. ACh is synthesized in the cytoplasm of cholinergic nerve terminals by the combination of choline and acetate (in the form of acetyl-CoA, which is synthesized in the mitochondria as a product of normal cellular metabolism). ACh is stored in specific agranular vesicles and released from the presynaptic terminal in response to neuronal depolarization to act at specific receptor sites on the postsynaptic membrane. It is rapidly metabolized by the enzyme acetylcholinesterase (AChE) to produce acetate and choline. Choline is then taken up into the presynaptic nerve ending for the regeneration of ACh. AChE is synthesized locally at cholinergic synapses, but is also present in erythrocytes and parts of the CNS. Butyryl cholinesterase (also termed plasma cholinesterase or pseudocholinesterase) is synthesized in the liver and is found in the plasma, skin, GI tract and parts of the CNS, but not at cholinergic synapses or the neuromuscular junction. It may metabolize ACh, in addition to some neuromuscular blockers (e.g. succinylcholine and mivacurium), but its physiological role probably involves the breakdown of other choline esters which may be present in the intestine.

Parasympathetic Receptor Pharmacology

Parasympathetic receptors have been classified according to the actions of the alkaloids muscarine and nicotine. The actions of ACh at the postganglionic membrane are mimicked by muscarine and are termed muscarinic, whereas preganglionic transmission is termed nicotinic. ACh is also the neurotransmitter at the neuromuscular junction, via nicotinic receptor sites. Five subtypes of muscarinic receptors (M_1–M_5) have been characterized; all five subtypes exist in the CNS, but there are differences in their peripheral distribution and function (Table 8.2). M_1-receptors are

TABLE 8.2					
Properties of Muscarinic (M_1–M_5) Receptors					
	M_1	M_2	M_3	M_4	M_5
Second messenger	IP_3	cAMP	IP_3	cAMP	IP_3
Location	CNS, parasympathetic ganglia, stomach, vascular smooth muscle, inflammatory cells	Heart, CNS, GI smooth muscle	CNS, salivary glands, stomach, pancreas, GI bronchial and vascular smooth muscle	CNS, Heart	CNS, ?vascular epithelium
Important clinical effects	Gastric acid production, bronchial secretions and inflammation	Bradycardia, GI motility	GI secretion & motility, bronchoconstriction and mucus secretion	?	?
Clinically selective agent	Pirenzepine	None	None	None	None

IP_3 stimulates inositol triphosphate production.
cAMP inhibits adenylate cyclase to decrease cAMP formation.

found in the stomach, where they mediate acid secretion, and in inflammatory cells in the lung (including mast cells and eosinophils) where they may have a role in airway inflammation. M_2-receptors predominate in the myocardium, where they modulate heart rate and impulse conduction. Prejunctional M_2-receptors are also involved in the regulation of synaptic noradrenaline and postganglionic ACh release. M_3-receptors are present in classic postsynaptic sites in glandular tissue (of the GI and respiratory tract) and bronchial smooth muscle, where they mediate most of the postjunctional effects of ACh. M_4-receptors have been isolated in cardiac and lung tissue in animal models and may have inhibitory effects, but the distribution and functions of M_5-receptors are not yet defined. In common with adrenergic receptors, muscarinic receptors are coupled to membrane-bound G-proteins although the subtypes differ in the second messenger system with which they interact. Currently available anticholinergics probably act at all muscarinic receptor subtypes but their clinical spectra differ, which suggests that they may have differential effects at different subtypes.

DRUGS ACTING ON THE SYMPATHETIC NERVOUS SYSTEM

Sympathomimetic Drugs

Sympathomimetic drugs partially or completely mimic the effects of sympathetic nerve stimulation or adrenal medullary discharge. They may act:

- directly on the adrenergic receptor, e.g. the catecholamines, phenylephrine, methoxamine
- indirectly causing release of noradrenaline from the adrenergic nerve ending, e.g. amphetamine
- by both mechanisms, e.g. dopamine, ephedrine, metaraminol.

The drugs may be classified according to their structure (catecholamine/non-catecholamine), their origin (endogenous/synthetic) and their mechanism of action (via adrenergic receptors or via a non-adrenergic mechanism) (Table 8.3). Drugs which affect myocardial contractility are termed inotropes, although this term is usually applied to those drugs that increase cardiac contractility (strictly 'positive inotropes'). Myocardial contractility may be increased by:

- increasing intracellular cAMP by activation of the adenylate cyclase system (e.g. catecholamines and other drugs acting via the adrenergic receptor)
- decreasing breakdown of cAMP (e.g. phosphodiesterase inhibitors)
- increasing intracellular calcium availability (e.g. digoxin, calcium salts, glucagon)
- increasing the response of contractile proteins to calcium (e.g. levosimendan) (Fig. 8.4).

Inotropes may also be classified into positive inotropic drugs which also produce systemic vasoconstriction ('inoconstrictors') and those which also produce systemic vasodilatation ('inodilators'). Inoconstrictors include noradrenaline, adrenaline and ephedrine. Inodilators are dobutamine, dopexamine, isoprenaline and phosphodiesterase inhibitors. Dopamine is an inodilator at low dose, and an inoconstrictor at higher doses.

TABLE 8.3			
Classification of Sympathomimetic Drugs			
CATECHOLAMINES		**NON-CATECHOLAMINES**	
Endogenous	*Synthetic*	*Acting Via Adrenergic Receptors*	*Acting Via Non-Adrenergic Mechanisms*
Adrenaline	Isoprenaline	Ephedrine	Phosphodiesterase inhibitors
Noradrenaline	Dobutamine	Phenylephrine	Digoxin
Dopamine	Dopexamine	Methoxamine	Glucagon
		Metaraminol	Calcium salts
			Calcium sensitizers

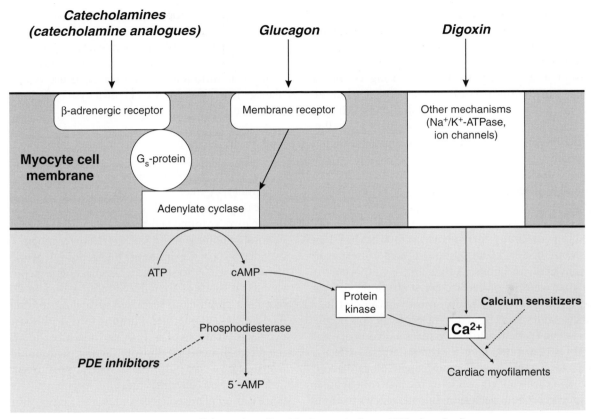

FIGURE 8.4 ■ Intracellular action of positive inotropic drugs. PDE; phosphodiesterase.

Catecholamines

Catecholamine drugs may be endogenous (adrenaline, noradrenaline and dopamine) or synthetic (dobutamine, dopexamine and isoprenaline). Several other drugs with a non-catecholamine structure produce sympathomimetic effects via adrenergic receptors, e.g. ephedrine and phenylephrine. All catecholamine drugs are inactivated in the gut by MAO and are usually only administered parenterally. They all have very short half-lives *in vivo*, and so when given by intravenous infusion, their effects may be controlled by altering the infusion rate. The comparative effects of different inotropes and vasopressors are outlined below.

Endogenous Catecholamines

Adrenaline. Adrenaline comprises 80–90% of adrenal medullary catecholamine content and is also an important CNS neurotransmitter. It is a powerful agonist at both α- and β-adrenergic receptors, being slightly less potent than noradrenaline at α_1-receptors but more potent at β-receptors. It is the treatment of choice in acute allergic (anaphylactic) reactions and is used in the management of cardiac arrest and shock, and occasionally as a bronchodilator. Except in emergency situations, i.v. injection is avoided because of the risk of inducing cardiac arrhythmias. Subcutaneous administration produces local vasoconstriction and so smoothes out its own effect by slowing absorption.

The effects of adrenaline on arterial pressure and cardiac output are dose-dependent. Although both α- and β-receptors are stimulated, β_2-vasodilator effects are most sensitive. β_1-Mediated effects cause marked increases in heart rate and contractility, cardiac output and systolic pressure. In low dosage, vasodilatation in skeletal muscle and splanchnic arterioles (β_2) may predominate over α-mediated vasoconstriction in skin and renal vasculature; systemic vascular resistance and diastolic pressure may decrease, pulse pressure widens, but mean arterial pressure remains stable. At higher doses, α-mediated vasoconstriction becomes more prominent in venous capacitance vessels (increasing venous return) and the precapillary resistance vessels of skin, mucosa and kidney (increasing peripheral resistance). Systolic pressure increases further, but cardiac output may decrease. Adrenaline causes marked decreases in renal blood flow, but coronary blood flow is increased. In contrast to other sympathomimetics, adrenaline has significant metabolic effects. Hepatic glycogenolysis and lipolysis in adipose tissue increase (β_1 and β_3 effects), and insulin secretion is inhibited (α_1 effect) so that hyperglycaemia occurs.

Adrenaline 0.5–1 mg i.m. (0.5–1.0 mL of 1:1000 solution) or 100 μg increments i.v. to a dose of 1 mg (1–10 mL of a 1:10 000 solution) is used to treat acute anaphylactic reactions. Adrenaline is important in the management of cardiac arrest (in doses of 1 mg i.v., repeated every 3–5 min), mostly because of its α effects; widespread systemic vasoconstriction occurs, increasing aortic diastolic pressure, and coronary and cerebral perfusion. Pure α-agonists are less effective than adrenaline in the management of cardiac arrest, and the β_2 effects of adrenaline may contribute to improved cerebral perfusion. In emergency situations, it may also be administered via the tracheal route, in doses of 2–3 mg diluted to a volume of 10 mL. It is effective by aerosol inhalation in bronchial asthma but has been superseded by selective β_2-agonists (see below). Unlike indirect-acting sympathomimetics which cause release of noradrenaline, tachyphylaxis should not occur with adrenaline. Adrenaline is also used as a topical vasoconstrictor to aid haemostasis and is incorporated into local anaesthetic solutions to decrease systemic absorption and prolong the duration of local anaesthesia.

Noradrenaline. Noradrenaline acts as a potent arteriolar and venous vasoconstrictor, acting predominantly at α-receptors, with a slightly greater potency there than adrenaline. It is also an agonist at β-receptors, but β_2 effects are not apparent in clinical use. Infusions of noradrenaline increase venous return, systolic and diastolic systemic and pulmonary arterial pressures, and central venous pressure. Cardiac output increases but heart rate decreases because of baroreflex activity. At higher doses, the α-mediated effects of widespread

intense vasoconstriction overcome β_1 effects on cardiac contractility, leading to a decrease in cardiac output at the cost of increased myocardial oxygen demand in conjunction with reductions in renal blood flow and glomerular filtration rate. Its principal use is in the management of septic shock when systemic vascular resistance is low.

Dopamine. Dopamine is the natural precursor of adrenaline and noradrenaline. It stimulates both α- and β-adrenergic receptors in addition to specific dopamine DA_1-receptors in renal and mesenteric arteries. Dopamine has a direct positive inotropic action on the myocardium via β-receptors and also by release of noradrenaline from adrenergic nerve terminals. The overall effects of dopamine are highly dose-dependent. In low dosage ($<3\ \mu g\,kg^{-1}\,min^{-1}$), renal and mesenteric vascular resistances are reduced by an action on DA_1-receptors, resulting in increased splanchnic and renal blood flows, glomerular filtration rate and sodium excretion. At doses of $5–10\ \mu g\,kg^{-1}\,min^{-1}$, the increasing direct β-mediated inotropic action predominates, increasing cardiac output and systolic pressure with little effect on diastolic pressure; peripheral resistance is usually unchanged. At doses $>15\ \mu g\,kg^{-1}\,min^{-1}$, α-receptor activity predominates, with direct vasoconstriction and increased cardiac stimulation (similar to noradrenaline). Renal and splanchnic blood flows decrease, and arrhythmias may occur. Dopamine receptors are widely present in the CNS, particularly in the basal ganglia, pituitary (where they mediate prolactin secretion) and the chemoreceptor trigger zone on the floor of the fourth ventricle (where they mediate nausea and vomiting). Recently, dopamine infusions have been associated with decreased prolactin secretion, and the use of 'prophylactic' dopamine infusions in an attempt to preserve renal function in perioperative or critically ill patients has declined.

Synthetic Catecholamines

Isoprenaline. Isoprenaline is a potent β_1- and β_2-agonist, with virtually no activity at α-receptors. It acts via cardiac β_1-receptors, and at β_2-receptors in the smooth muscle of bronchi, the vasculature of skeletal muscle and the gut. After intravenous infusion, heart rate increases and peripheral resistance is reduced. Cardiac output may increase because of increased heart rate and contractility but effects on arterial pressure are variable. Isoprenaline also reduces coronary perfusion pressure, increases myocardial oxygen consumption and causes arrhythmias. Other β_2-mediated effects include relaxation of bronchial smooth muscle and stabilization of mast cells. It has been superseded for use in the treatment of severe asthma by newer specific β_2-agonists with fewer cardiac effects. Its current indication is as an infusion in the treatment of bradyarrhythmias or atrioventricular heart block associated with low cardiac output (e.g. following acute myocardial infarction) because it increases heart rate and conduction by a direct action on the subsidiary pacemaker. This indication is usually an interim measure before insertion of a temporary pacing wire.

Dobutamine. Dobutamine is primarily a β_1-agonist, with moderate β_2- and mild α_1-agonist activity, and no action at DA-receptors. Its primary effect is an increase in cardiac output via increased contractility (β_1 effect) augmented by a reduction in afterload. Heart rate also increases (β_2 effect). Systolic arterial pressure may increase but peripheral resistance is reduced or unchanged. There is no direct effect on venous tone or renal blood flow but preload may decrease and urine output and sodium excretion increase as a consequence of the increased cardiac output. Dobutamine increases SA node automaticity and conduction velocity in the atria, ventricles and AV node, but to a lesser extent than isoprenaline. Dobutamine infusion produces a progressive increase in cardiac output which is greater than with comparable doses of dopamine, although arterial pressure may remain unchanged. At higher doses, tachycardia and arrhythmias may occur, but dobutamine has less effect on myocardial oxygen consumption compared with other catecholamines. Dobutamine is widely used to optimize cardiac output in septic shock, often in combination with noradrenaline. It is also used alone or in combination with vasodilator drugs in heart failure when peripheral resistance is high, and to increase heart rate and cardiac output in myocardial stress testing.

Dopexamine. Dopexamine is a synthetic dopamine analogue which is an agonist at β_2- and DA$_1$-receptors. It is also a weak DA$_2$-agonist and it inhibits the neuronal re-uptake of noradrenaline (*uptake$_1$*), but has no direct effects at β_1- or α-receptors. Its principal effect is β_2-agonism, producing vasodilatation in skeletal muscle; it is less potent at DA$_1$-receptors, but a more potent β_2-agonist than dopamine. It produces mild increases in heart rate, contractility and cardiac output (effects on β_2-receptors and noradrenaline uptake), renal and mesenteric vasodilatation (β_2 and DA$_1$ effects), and natriuresis (DA$_1$ effect). Coronary and cerebral blood flows are also increased. Systemic vascular resistance decreases and arterial pressure may decrease if intravascular volume is not maintained. Dopexamine has theoretical advantages in maintaining cardiac output and splanchnic blood flow in patients with systemic sepsis or heart failure. It is also used for this purpose in patients undergoing major abdominal surgery. Dopexamine also has anti-inflammatory effects (in common with other β-agonists) which are independent of its effects on gut mucosal perfusion. It is metabolized by hepatic methylation and conjugation and is eliminated mostly via the kidneys.

Fenoldopam is a dopamine (DA$_1$) agonist available in the USA which causes peripheral vasodilatation and increases renal blood flow and sodium and water excretion. It has been used in the treatment of hypertensive emergencies. Unlike some other vasodilators (e.g. sodium nitroprusside) it does not cause rebound hypertension after stopping the infusion.

Non-Catecholamine Sympathomimetics

Synthetic sympathomimetic drugs may mimic the effect of adrenaline at adrenergic receptors (direct-acting) or may produce effects by causing release of endogenous noradrenaline from postganglionic sympathetic nerve terminals (indirect-acting). Some drugs have direct and indirect sympathomimetic effects (e.g. ephedrine, metaraminol). Direct-acting compounds may affect α- or β-receptors selectively, whereas indirect-acting compounds have predominantly α- and β_1-agonist effects (as noradrenaline is only a weak β_2-agonist). Indirect-acting compounds are taken up into the nerve terminal via the noradrenaline re-uptake pathway, and so their effect is reduced by drugs which block noradrenaline re-uptake (e.g. tricyclic antidepressants). Conversely, the effect of direct-acting drugs is enhanced. In patients treated with drugs which decrease sympathetic nervous system activity (e.g. clonidine, reserpine), the cardiovascular response to indirect-acting drugs is diminished; however, up-regulation of adrenergic receptors occurs and an increased response to direct-acting sympathomimetics is seen. Drugs with selective α-adrenergic receptor effects (e.g. phenylephrine, methoxamine) are potent vasoconstrictors.

Ephedrine. Ephedrine is a naturally occurring sympathomimetic amine which is now produced synthetically. It acts directly and indirectly as an agonist at α-, β_1- and β_2-receptors. The indirect actions are increased endogenous noradrenaline release and inhibition of MAO. Its cardiovascular effects are similar to those of adrenaline, but the duration of action is up to 10 times longer. It causes increases in heart rate, contractility, cardiac output and arterial pressure (systolic > diastolic). It may predispose to arrhythmias. Systemic vascular resistance is usually unchanged because α-mediated vasoconstriction in some vascular beds is balanced by β-mediated vasodilatation in others, but renal and splanchnic blood flows decrease. It relaxes bronchial and other smooth muscle, and is occasionally used as a bronchodilator. It is active orally because it is not metabolized by MAO in the gut, and is useful by intramuscular injection because muscle blood flow is preserved. Ephedrine undergoes hepatic deamination and conjugation but significant amounts are excreted unchanged in urine. This accounts for its long duration of action and elimination half-life (3–6 h). Tachyphylaxis (a decreased response to repeated doses of the drug) occurs because of persistent occupation of adrenergic receptors and depletion of noradrenaline stores.

Ephedrine is often used to prevent or treat hypotension resulting from sympathetic blockade during regional anaesthesia or from the effects of general anaesthesia. Although widely used to prevent hypotension during regional anaesthesia in obstetric patients, it has largely been superseded for this indication by an infusion of phenylephrine, which has better effects on maternal and fetal haemodynamics. Oral or topical ephedrine is also useful as a nasal decongestant.

Phenylephrine. Phenylephrine is a potent synthetic direct-acting α_1-agonist, which has minimal agonist effects at α_2- and β-receptors. It has effects similar to those of noradrenaline, causing widespread vasoconstriction, increased arterial pressure, bradycardia (as a result of baroreflex activation) and a decrease in cardiac output. Venoconstriction predominates and diastolic pressure increases more than systolic pressure, so that coronary blood flow may increase. It is used as intermittent boluses (50-100 µg by slow injection) or an infusion (50–150 µg min^{-1}) to maintain arterial pressure during general or regional anaesthesia, and also topically as a nasal decongestant and mydriatic. Absorption of phenylephrine from mucous membranes may occasionally produce systemic side-effects.

Methoxamine. Methoxamine is a direct-acting α_1-agonist which also has a weak β-antagonist action. It produces vasoconstriction, increased diastolic arterial pressure and decreases in cardiac output and heart rate from baroreflex activation and the mild β-blocking effect. It is no longer available in the UK.

Metaraminol. Metaraminol is a direct- and indirect-acting α- and β-agonist, which acts partly by being taken up into sympathetic nerve terminals and acting as a false transmitter for noradrenaline. Its α effects predominate, causing pronounced vasoconstriction; arterial pressure increases and a reflex bradycardia may occur.

Vasopressin. Arginine vasopressin (AVP) (formerly termed antidiuretic hormone) is a peptide hormone secreted by the hypothalamus. Its primary role is the regulation of body fluid balance. It is secreted in response to hypotension and promotes retention of water by action on specific cAMP-coupled V_2-receptors. It causes vasoconstriction by stimulating V_1-receptors in vascular smooth muscle and is particularly potent in hypotensive patients. It is increasingly used in the treatment of refractory vasodilatory shock which is resistant to catecholamines, although it can cause peripheral or splanchnic ischaemia. The vasopressin analogue desmopressin is used to treat diabetes insipidus. Another analogue, terlipressin, is used to limit bleeding from oesophageal varices in patients with portal hypertension as an adjunct to definitive treatment.

Phosphodiesterase Inhibitors. Phosphodiesterase inhibitors increase intracellular cAMP concentrations by inhibition of the enzyme responsible for cAMP breakdown (Fig. 8.4). Increased intracellular cAMP concentrations promote the activation of protein kinases, which lead to an increase in intracellular Ca^{2+}. In cardiac muscle cells, this causes a positive inotropic effect and also facilitates diastolic relaxation and cardiac filling (termed 'positive lusitropy'). In vascular smooth muscle, increased cAMP decreases intracellular Ca^{2+} and causes marked vasodilatation. Several subtypes of phosphodiesterase (PDE) isoenzyme exist in different tissues. Theophylline is a non-specific PDE inhibitor, but the newer drugs (e.g. enoximone and milrinone) are selective for the PDE type III isoenzyme present in the myocardium, vascular smooth muscle and platelets. PDE III inhibitors are positive inotropes and potent arterial, coronary and venodilators. They decrease preload, afterload, pulmonary vascular resistance and pulmonary capillary wedge pressure (PCWP), and increase cardiac index. Heart rate may increase or remain unchanged. In contrast to sympathomimetics, they improve myocardial function *without* increasing oxygen demand or causing tachyphylaxis. Their effects are augmented by the co-administration of β_1-agonists (i.e. increases in cAMP production are synergistic with decreased cAMP breakdown). They have particular advantages in patients with chronic heart failure, in whom downregulation of myocardial β-adrenergic receptors occurs, so that there is a decreased inotropic response to β-sympathomimetic drugs. A similar phenomenon occurs with advanced age, prolonged (>72 h) catecholamine therapy and possibly with surgical stress.

PDE III inhibitors are indicated for acute refractory heart failure, e.g. cardiogenic shock, or pre- or postcardiac surgery. However, long-term oral treatment is associated with increased mortality in patients with congestive heart failure. All may cause hypotension, and tachyarrhythmias may occur. Other adverse effects include nausea, vomiting and fever. Their half-life is prolonged markedly in patients with heart or renal failure and they are commonly administered as an i.v. loading dose over 5 min with or without a subsequent i.v. infusion. *Milrinone* is a bipyridine derivative whereas *enoximone* is an imidazole derivative. Enoximone undergoes substantial first-pass metabolism, and is rapidly metabolized to an active sulphoxide metabolite which is excreted via the kidneys and which may accumulate in renal failure.

The elimination $t_{1/2}$ of enoximone is 1–2 h in healthy individuals but up to 20 h in patients with heart failure.

Glucagon. Glucagon is a polypeptide secreted by the α cells of the pancreatic islets. Its physiological actions include stimulation of hepatic gluconeogenesis in response to hypoglycaemia, amino acids and as part of the stress response. These effects are mediated by increasing adenylate cyclase activity and intracellular cAMP, by a mechanism independent of the β-adrenergic receptor (Fig. 8.4). It increases cAMP in myocardial cells and so increases cardiac contractility. Glucagon causes nausea and vomiting, hyperglycaemia and hyperkalaemia and is not used as an inotrope except in the management of β-blocker poisoning.

Calcium. Calcium ions are involved in cellular excitation, excitation-contraction coupling and muscle contraction in cardiac, skeletal and smooth muscle cells. Increased extracellular Ca^{2+} increases intracellular Ca^{2+} concentrations and consequently the force of contraction of cardiac myocytes and vascular smooth muscle cells. Massive blood loss and replacement with large volumes of calcium-free fluids or citrated blood (which chelates Ca^{2+}) may cause a decrease in serum Ca^{2+} concentration, especially in the critically ill. Therefore, Ca^{2+} salts (e.g. calcium chloride or gluconate) may be administered, particularly during and after cardiopulmonary bypass. Intravenous calcium 5 mg kg^{-1} may increase mean arterial pressure, but the effects on cardiac output and systemic vascular resistance are variable and there is little good evidence for the efficacy of Ca^{2+} salts. Moreover, high Ca^{2+} concentrations may cause cardiac arrhythmias and vasoconstriction, may be cytotoxic and may worsen the cellular effects of ischaemia. Calcium salts may be indicated for the treatment of hypocalcaemia (ionized Ca^{2+} <0.8 mmol L^{-1}), hyperkalaemia and calcium channel blocker toxicity.

Calcium Sensitizers. Levosimendan and pimobendan are positive inotropic drugs which act by stabilizing the troponin molecule in cardiac myocytes (by a cAMP-independent mechanism) and so increase myocyte Ca^{2+} sensitivity without increasing Ca^{2+} influx. Contractility is increased without an increase in oxygen consumption or a tendency to arrhythmias. Levosimendan also causes vasodilatation by opening K^+ channels via an ATP-dependent mechanism and may be used as a second line agent in acute heart failure. It is available in Europe and South America. Pimobendan also inhibits phosphodiesterase-III and has been investigated for use in chronic heart failure. It is available in Japan.

Selective β_2-Agonists

Selective β_2-receptor agonists (e.g. salbutamol, terbutaline, formoterol and salmeterol) relax bronchial, uterine and vascular smooth muscle while having much less effect on the heart than isoprenaline. These drugs are partial agonists (their maximal effect at β_2-receptors is less than that of isoprenaline) and are only partially selective for β_2-receptors. They are used widely in the treatment of bronchospasm (see Ch 9). Although less cardiotoxic than isoprenaline, dose-related tremor, tachyarrhythmias, hyperglycaemia, hypokalaemia and hypomagnesaemia may occur. β_2-Agonists are resistant to metabolism by COMT and therefore have a prolonged duration of action (mostly 3–5 h). Salmeterol is highly lipophilic, has a strong affinity for the β_2-adrenergic receptor, is longer acting than the other β_2-agonists and so is used for maintenance therapy in chronic asthma in combination with inhaled steroids. β_2-Agonists are usually administered by the inhaled (metered dose inhaler or nebulizer) or intravenous routes because of unpredictable oral absorption and a high hepatic extraction ratio. When inhaled, only 10–20% of the administered dose reaches the lower airways; this proportion is reduced further when administered via a tracheal tube. Nevertheless, systemic absorption does occur, although adverse effects are less common during long-term therapy.

Salbutamol. Salbutamol is the β_2-agonist used most commonly for the prevention and treatment of bronchospasm. When administered by metered dose inhaler (1 or 2 puffs, each delivering $100 \mu g$), it acts within a few minutes, with a peak action at 30–60 min. In severe cases, it may be given by nebulizer (2.5–5.0 mg), repeated if required, or intravenously (either $250 \mu g$ by slow i.v. injection or as an infusion starting at $5 \mu g \, min^{-1}$ and titrated to response). It is metabolized in the liver and excreted in urine both as metabolites and as unchanged drug; the proportions are dependent on the route of administration.

Sympatholytic Drugs

Sympatholytic drugs antagonize the effects of the sympathetic nervous system either at central adrenergic neurones, peripheral autonomic ganglia or neurones, or at postsynaptic α- or β-receptors. Most are hypotensive drugs, although they have other effects and indications.

Centrally Acting Sympatholytic Drugs

Centrally acting drugs act by stimulation of central α_2-receptors to decrease sympathetic tone. They were used as antihypertensive drugs, but have been superseded for this purpose by newer drugs with fewer adverse effects. They are also agonists at central imidazoline (I_1) receptors, which contributes to their hypotensive action. I_1 receptors are present in several peripheral tissues, including the kidney. Central α_2-stimulation causes decreases in arterial pressure, peripheral resistance, venous return, myocardial contractility, cardiac output and heart rate, but baroreceptor reflexes are preserved and the pressor response to ephedrine or phenylephrine may be exaggerated. Stimulation of peripheral α_2-receptors on vascular smooth muscle causes direct arteriolar vasoconstriction, although the central effects of these drugs predominate overall. However, severe rebound hypertension may occur on stopping chronic oral therapy. α_2-Receptors in the dorsal horn of the spinal cord modulate upward transmission of nociceptive signals by modifying local release of substance P and CGRP. Centrally acting α_2-agonists produce analgesia by activation of descending spinal and supraspinal inhibitory pathways, and clonidine is now used mostly for its analgesic effects. These are greatest when administered by the epidural or spinal route. Other effects include dry mouth, sedation and anxiolysis.

Clonidine is a partial agonist at central and peripheral α_2-receptors, and a central imidazoline (I_1) receptor agonist. Clonidine has some effects at α_1-receptors $(\alpha_2:\alpha_1 > 200:1)$; dexmedetomidine and azepexole are more α_2-selective alternatives. Transient hypertension and bradycardia may occur after i.v. injection, caused by direct stimulation of peripheral vascular α_2-receptors though an α_1-agonist effect may also contribute. Clonidine potentiates the MAC of inhalational anaesthetic agents by up to 50%. It has a synergistic analgesic effect with opioids which may be partly pharmacokinetic because the elimination half-life of opioids is also increased. Clonidine is well absorbed orally, with peak plasma concentrations after 60–90 min. It is highly lipid-soluble and approximately 50% is metabolized in the liver to inactive metabolites; the rest is excreted unchanged via the kidneys, with an elimination half-life of 9–12 h. Clonidine $5 \mu g kg^{-1}$ as premedication attenuates reflex sympathetic responses and may reduce cardiac complications after non-cardiac surgery in patients at high risk of cardiovascular events. It is also used in the treatment of opioid withdrawal and postoperative shivering. Epidural clonidine $1–2 \mu g kg^{-1}$ increases the duration and potency of analgesia provided by epidural opioid or local anaesthetic drugs. α_2-Agonists also have some antiarrhythmic effects, decreasing both the incidence of catecholamine-related arrhythmias and the toxicity of bupivacaine and cocaine.

Methyldopa crosses the blood-brain barrier easily and is converted to α-methyl noradrenaline, the active molecule, which is a full agonist at α_2-receptors (α_2:α_1 selectivity = 10:1). Adverse effects include peripheral oedema, hepatotoxicity, depression and a positive direct Coombs' test; some patients develop haemolytic anaemia. Its use is largely restricted to the management of pregnancy-associated hypertension.

Moxonidine is a moderately selective imidazoline I_1-receptor agonist ($I_1 > \alpha_2$) which reduces central sympathetic activity by stimulation of medullary I_1-receptors. It is used in the treatment of hypertension. Systemic vascular resistance is reduced but heart rate and stroke volume are unchanged. Moxonidine has few α_2-related adverse effects but it may potentiate bradycardia and is contraindicated in sinoatrial block, and second- or third-degree AV block.

Peripherally Acting Sympatholytic Drugs

Ganglion Blocking Drugs. Nicotinic receptor antagonists (e.g. hexamethonium, pentolinium, trimetaphan) competitively inhibit the effects of ACh at autonomic ganglia and block both parasympathetic and sympathetic transmission. Sympathetic blockade produces venodilatation, decreased myocardial contractility and hypotension, but the effects vary depending on pre-existing sympathetic tone. Tachyphylaxis develops rapidly and these drugs have now been superseded.

Adrenergic Neurone Blocking Drugs. Guanethidine decreases peripheral sympathetic nervous system activity by competitively binding to noradrenaline binding sites in storage vesicles in the cytoplasm of postganglionic sympathetic nerve terminals. Further uptake of noradrenaline into the vesicles is inhibited and it is metabolized by cytoplasmic MAO, so the nerve terminals become depleted of noradrenaline. Guanethidine has local anaesthetic properties and does not cross the blood–brain barrier. It is sometimes used to produce intravenous regional sympathetic blockade in the treatment of chronic limb pain associated with excessive autonomic activity (reflex sympathetic dystrophy or complex regional pain syndromes). Bretylium has a similar mode of action; it is used in the treatment of resistant ventricular arrhythmias (see below).

α-Adrenergic Receptor Antagonists. α-Adrenergic antagonists (α-blockers) selectively inhibit the action of catecholamines at α-adrenergic receptors. They are used mainly as vasodilators for the second-line treatment of hypertension or as urinary tract smooth muscle relaxants in patients with benign prostatic hyperplasia. They also have an important role in the preoperative management of phaeochromocytoma (see Ch 37).

α-Blockers diminish vasoconstrictor tone, causing venous pooling and a decrease in peripheral vascular resistance. In common with other vasodilators, they may have indirect positive inotropic actions as a result of reductions in afterload and preload, so cardiac output may increase. They may be classified according to their relative selectivity for α_1- and α_2-receptors. Non-selective α-blockers commonly induce postural hypotension and reflex tachycardia, partly because α_2-blockade prevents the feedback inhibition of noradrenaline on its own release at presynaptic α_2-receptors, and neuronal noradrenaline concentrations increase. The action of noradrenaline at cardiac β-receptors then limits the hypotensive effects of non-selective α-blockers. In addition, the proportions of pre- and postsynaptic α_2-receptors in the arterial and venous smooth muscle may differ, so that α_1-selective drugs have a more balanced effect on venous and arterial circulations. The co-administration of a β-blocker may attenuate reflex tachycardia and produces a synergistic effect on arterial pressure.

α₁-Selective Antagonists. Selective α₁-blockers include prazosin, doxazosin, indoramin, and urapidil. *Doxazosin* has largely succeeded prazosin as it has a more prolonged duration of action. Reflex tachycardia and postural hypotension are less common than with direct-acting vasodilators (e.g. hydralazine) and the non-selective α-blockers, but may still occur on initiating therapy. Nasal congestion, sedation and inhibition of ejaculation may occur.

Labetalol (see below) is a competitive α₁-, β₁- and β₂-antagonist, which is more active at β- than at α-receptors. At low doses (5–10 mg i.v.), it decreases arterial pressure without producing a tachycardia. At higher doses, the β effect becomes more prominent, with negative inotropic and chronotropic effects. *Carvedilol* is an α₁- and β-receptor antagonist which also has direct vasodilator effects (see below).

α₂-Selective Antagonists. Drugs of this type, e.g. yohimbine, are not used because of the unacceptable incidence of adverse effects.

Non-Selective α-Antagonists. Non-selective α-blockers, e.g. phentolamine and phenoxybenzamine, produce more postural hypotension, reflex tachycardia and adverse gastrointestinal effects (e.g. abdominal cramps, diarrhoea) than α₁-selective drugs. *Phentolamine* 2–5 mg i.v. produces a rapid decrease in arterial pressure lasting 10–15 min and is used for the treatment of hypertensive crises.

Phenoxybenzamine binds covalently (i.e. irreversibly and non-competitively) to α-receptors so that its effects last up to several days, and may be cumulative on repeated dosing. It also reduces central sympathetic activity, which enhances vasodilatation, and has antagonist effects at 5-HT receptors. It is used for the preoperative preparation of patients with phaeochromocytoma (see Ch 37).

β-Adrenergic Receptor Antagonists

β-adrenergic receptor antagonists (β-blockers) are structurally similar to the β-agonists, e.g. isoprenaline. Variations in the molecular structure (primarily of the catechol ring) have produced compounds which do not activate adenylate cyclase and the second messenger system despite binding avidly to the β-adrenergic receptor. Most are stereoisomers and the L-form is generally more potent (as an agonist or antagonist) than the D-form. β-Blockers are competitive antagonists with high receptor affinity, although their effects are attenuated by high concentrations of endogenous or exogenous agonists. They may be classified according to:

- their relative affinity for β₁- or β₂-receptors
- agonist/antagonist activity
- membrane-stabilizing effect
- ancillary effects (e.g. action at other receptors).

β₁- or β₂-Adrenergic Receptor Affinity. The relative potency of β-blockers is less important than their relative effects on the different β-receptor subtypes. Compounds are available which block preferentially either β₁- or β₂-receptors, although in clinical practice the β₁-selective drugs are more important. The first generation of β-blockers (e.g. propranolol, timolol) were non-selective; second-generation drugs (e.g. atenolol, metoprolol, bisoprolol) are selective for β₁-receptors but have no ancillary effects. The third generation of β-blockers are β₁-selective, but also have effects on other receptors (e.g. labetalol and carvedilol are antagonists at α₁-adrenergic receptors, and celiprolol produces vasodilatation by a mechanism involving endothelial nitric oxide). β₁-Selective (or 'cardioselective') drugs have theoretical advantages because some of the adverse effects of β-blockers are related to β₂-antagonism, but the selectivity of both drugs and tissues is only relative: all β₁-selective drugs antagonize β₂-receptors at higher doses, and 25% of cardiac β-receptors are of the β₂ subtype. However β₁-selective drugs appear to have fewer adverse effects on blood glucose control in diabetics, less effect on serum lipids and less effect on bronchial tone in patients with chronic obstructive pulmonary disease.

Partial Agonist Activity. Some β-blockers have intrinsic sympathomimetic activity (ISA), i.e. they are partial agonists. This stimulant effect is apparent at low levels of sympathetic activity, but at high levels of sympathetic discharge, blockade of endogenously released catecholamines is the major clinical effect. Partial agonists may be advantageous in patients with a low resting heart rate because they reduce the risk of AV conduction disturbance, and have theoretical advantages in patients with peripheral vascular disease or hyperlipidaemia. However, only β-blockers *without* partial agonist activity have been shown to be beneficial after myocardial infarction.

Membrane-Stabilizing Effect. Some β-blockers have a quinidine-like action, inhibiting Na^+ transport in nerve and cardiac conducting tissue ('membrane-stabilizing effect'). This may be demonstrated *in vivo* as a stabilizing effect on the cardiac action potential, reducing the slope of phase 4 noticeably, thus decreasing excitability and automaticity of the myocardium (see below). However, the membrane-stabilizing activity probably has little clinical significance because it occurs only at plasma concentrations above the therapeutic range, and the antiarrhythmic effect of β-blockade occurs via inhibition of the effects of catecholamines.

Ancillary Effects. Some of the newer β-blockers drugs have additional effects, e.g. action at α-receptors, vasodilatation, antioxidant effects and other actions. The relevance of these properties is discussed below.

Pharmacological Properties of β-Blockers. The pharmacological properties of β-blockers are summarized in Table 8.4. All are weak bases and most are well absorbed to produce peak plasma concentrations 1–3h after oral administration. The more lipid-soluble drugs are almost completely absorbed, but are metabolized to a greater extent and tend to have a marked first-pass effect through the liver. This reduces their bioavailability, but is offset by the fact that the 4-hydroxylated metabolites so formed are also active. These active metabolites are excreted via the kidneys and may accumulate in patients with renal failure. Propranolol decreases both the clearance of amide local anaesthetics (by decreasing hepatic blood flow and inhibiting metabolism) and the pulmonary first-pass uptake of fentanyl. The first-pass metabolic pathways may also become saturated, so that proportionately higher plasma concentrations of the parent drug occur at higher oral doses. The first-pass effect is also a source of wide interindividual variation in plasma concentrations achieved from the same dose of primarily metabolized drugs, although β-blockers have a flat dose-response curve and large changes in plasma concentration may give rise to only a small change in degree of β-blockade. However, differences in individual plasma concentration–response relationships may occur, possibly as a result of variations in sympathetic tone or the formation of active metabolites. All β-blockers are distributed widely throughout the body and significant concentrations occur in the CNS, particularly for the more lipid-soluble drugs (e.g. propranolol).

The less lipid-soluble drugs (e.g. atenolol) are less well absorbed, are metabolized to a lesser extent, are excreted via the kidneys and tend to have longer half-lives. Atenolol, nadolol and sotalol are excreted largely unchanged in urine and so are little affected by impairment of liver function.

Indications for β-Blockade. See Tables 8.5 and 8.6 for indications for β-blockade.

Hypertension. β-Blockers have been regarded as first-line therapy for the treatment of hypertension for many years, either alone or in combination with other drugs. They are of proven benefit in reducing the incidence of stroke and the morbidity and mortality from coronary artery disease in younger hypertensive patients, although the effectiveness of β-blockade in patients aged >60 years has been questioned recently. The antihypertensive effect results from a combination of factors.

- Reductions in heart rate, cardiac output and myocardial contractility.
- A reduction in central sympathetic nervous activity. The significance of this is uncertain because different drugs vary widely in their CNS penetration, but have similar effects on arterial pressure.
- Decreased plasma renin concentration. β-Blockers decrease resting and orthostatic release of renin to a variable extent. The non-selective drugs propranolol and timolol cause the greatest reduction, while partial agonists (oxprenolol, pindolol) or $β_1$-selective drugs are less effective. However, no correlation has been found between renin-lowering effect and antihypertensive activity or dosage of β-blocker used.
- *Effects on peripheral resistance.* β-Blockade does not reduce peripheral resistance directly and may even cause an increase by allowing unopposed

TABLE 8.4

Pharmacological Properties of β-Blockers

Drug	β_1 Selectivity	Partial Agonist Activity	Membrane Stabilizing Effect	Lipid Solubility	Absorption (%)	Bioavail- ability (%)	Protein Binding (%)	Terminal Half-Life (h)	Significant Active Metabolites	Elimination
Acebutolol	±	+	+	Medium	90	50	20	8-10	Yes	Hepatic, renal
Atenolol	+	−	−	Low	50	40	5	6-8	No	Renal
Bisoprolol	++	−	−	Low	>90	90		10-12	No	Hepatic, renal
Carvedilol	−	−	?	High	>90	25	98	6-10	Yes	Hepatic
Celiprolol	+	+	?	Low	30	30-70		5-6	No	Renal
Esmolol	+	−	−	High			55	0.15	No	Plasma hydrolysis
Labetalol	−	±	+	High	70	30	50	4	No	Hepatic
Metoprolol	+	−	±	High	90	50	10-20	4	No	Hepatic
Nadolol	−	−	−	Low	30	30	20	20-24	No	Renal
Oxprenolol	−	+	+	High	80	50	80	2	No	Hepatic
Pindolol	−	++	±	Medium	90	90	50	4	No	Hepatic
Propranolol	−	−	++	High	90	30	90	5	Yes	Hepatic
Sotalol	−	+	+	Low	80	90		8-15	No	Renal
Timolol	−	+	±	High	90	50	10	4	No	Hepatic, renal

TABLE 8.5
Clinical Indications for β-Blockade

Hypertension

Ischaemic heart disease

Secondary prevention of myocardial infarction

Obstructive cardiomyopathy

Congestive heart failure

Arrhythmias

Miscellaneous

TABLE 8.6
Specific Perioperative Indications for β-Blockers

Prevention or treatment of intraoperative hypertension, tachycardia and supraventricular tachyarrhythmias associated with excessive sympathetic activity

Treatment of postoperative hypertension

Controlled hypotension

Prophylaxis or treatment of perioperative myocardial ischaemia

Pre- and perioperative management of phaeochromocytoma

Pre- and perioperative management of thyrotoxic patients

α-stimulation. As the vasodilating effect of catecholamines on skeletal muscle is β_2-mediated, unopposed α stimulation would be expected to be lower with cardioselective drugs or partial agonists. However, cardioselectivity decreases with dosage and, because hypertensive patients often require a large dose of β-blocker, little real advantage is offered. Drugs with partial agonist activity may not increase peripheral resistance as much as those without.

Arterial pressure reduction begins within an hour of β-blocker administration, but several days may elapse before the plateau is reached and the full hypotensive effect of oral β-blockers takes about 2 weeks. This suggests the involvement of several mechanisms including readjustment of central and peripheral cardiovascular reflexes. During chronic administration, the hypotensive effects of β-blockers last longer than the pharmacological half-life, so that single daily dosage is adequate therapeutically. However, upregulation of

receptors may occur, leading to adverse effects (tachycardia, hypertension, myocardial ischaemia) on abrupt withdrawal of β-blockers. This is important in surgical patients, and patients receiving long-term β-blockade should continue therapy throughout the perioperative period. There is some evidence that perioperative β-blockade reduces cardiac complications in high-risk patients undergoing major vascular surgery, but the data are conflicting. All β-blockers are equally effective as hypotensive drugs; patients unresponsive to one β-blocker are generally unresponsive to all.

Ischaemic heart disease. β-Blockers improve symptoms and decrease the frequency and severity of silent myocardial ischaemia in patients with ischaemic heart disease. The incidence of myocardial ischaemia in high-risk patients is reduced by perioperative β-blockade and long-term outcome may be improved. β-Blockers reduce heart rate and contractility, with consequent decreases in wall tension and myocardial oxygen demand. A slower heart rate also permits longer diastolic filling time and hence potentially greater coronary perfusion. The perfusion of ischaemic regions may be improved by redistribution of myocardial blood flow, and other additional mechanisms may be involved.

β-Blockade also reduces exercise-induced increases in arterial pressure, velocity of cardiac contraction and oxygen consumption at any workload. Partial agonists have less effect on the resting heart rate and theoretically increase the metabolic demand of the myocardium; they may be less effective in patients with angina at rest or at very low levels of exercise. In contrast to effects on arterial pressure, there is a more direct relationship between plasma concentration and anti-anginal effect. To achieve effective plasma concentrations over a sustained period as a single daily dosage, either the long half-life drugs (e.g. atenolol, nadolol) or slow-release preparations (e.g. oxprenolol-SR, propranolol-LA, metoprolol-SR) are required.

Secondary prevention of myocardial infarction. Early i.v. administration after acute myocardial infarction can decrease infarct size, the incidence of ventricular and supraventricular arrhythmias and mortality in both lower- and higher-risk groups (e.g. elderly patients or those with left ventricular dysfunction). Mortality is reduced by 20–40%, and the risk of re-infarction is reduced if oral therapy is continued for 2–3 years.

Obstructive cardiomyopathy. β-Blockers improve exercise tolerance and alleviate symptoms in hypertrophic obstructive cardiomyopathy by decreasing heart rate, myocardial work, contractility and, thus, outflow tract obstruction. However, the incidence of sudden death in this condition is not affected. The incidence of cyanotic episodes caused by pulmonary outflow obstruction in patients with Fallot's tetralogy is reduced by a similar mechanism.

Congestive heart failure. Congestive heart failure is accompanied by a compensatory increase in sympathetic nervous stimulation with increased plasma and cardiac noradrenaline concentrations, leading to increases in cardiac output, systemic vascular resistance and afterload. Plasma renin concentration also increases. Although beneficial as an acute response in the short term, high circulating catecholamine concentrations are directly toxic to the myocardium. Desensitization of myocardial β_1-adrenergic receptors occurs via downregulation and altered signal transduction. In combination with chronically increased peripheral resistance, this leads to ventricular remodelling with progressively worsening myocardial function and a propensity to arrhythmias. Some second- and third-generation β-blockers (bisoprolol, metoprolol and carvedilol) have been shown to decrease morbidity and mortality in heart failure by improving ventricular function. The mechanism is primarily by upregulation of β-receptor density or function, although other factors may contribute, including slowing of heart rate or an antiarrhythmic effect. Bisoprolol and metoprolol are β_1-selective antagonists but carvedilol also has β_2- and α_1-antagonist and antioxidant effects which may contribute to its action. They must be introduced cautiously in heart failure because symptoms may initially worsen, and ventricular function improves only after 1 month of therapy.

Arrhythmias (see below). β-Blockers are effective in the treatment of arrhythmias caused by sympathetic nervous overactivity or after myocardial infarction. The mechanisms are related to β-blockade itself rather than any membrane-stabilizing effect, e.g. antagonism of catecholamine effects on the cardiac action potential and muscle contractility. The result is a slowing of rate of discharge from the sinus and any ectopic pacemaker, and slowing of conduction and increased refractoriness of the AV node. β-Blockers also slow conduction in anomalous pathways. They may

be used i.v. to terminate an attack of supraventricular tachycardia or decrease the ventricular rate in atrial fibrillation and flutter; conversion to sinus rhythm may also be achieved. If given within 30 min of i.v. verapamil, there is a danger of severe bradycardia or asystole. Most β-blockers have similar antiarrhythmic effects in adequate dosage, but esmolol has the advantage of a short half-life (see below) so that adverse effects are limited. They are also useful as second-line alternatives for the treatment of ventricular tachycardia. Sotalol has both class 2 and class 3 antiarrhythmic activity (see below) and is licensed for use only for its antiarrhythmic action, in particular for the treatment of supraventricular and ventricular tachycardias.

Miscellaneous. β-Blockers are prescribed for migraine prophylaxis, essential tremor and anxiety states. They are useful for glaucoma because they decrease intraocular pressure, probably by reducing the production of aqueous humour. Topical preparations (e.g. timolol, betaxolol, carteolol) are used in an attempt to decrease adverse effects but significant systemic absorption may still take place; bradycardia, hypotension and bronchospasm may occur, particularly during anaesthesia. β-Blockers diminish the symptoms of thyrotoxicosis and are used as part of preoperative preparation before thyroidectomy. They may be used also as part of a hypotensive anaesthetic technique.

Adverse Reactions to β-Blockers. All available β-blockers have similar adverse effects, although their magnitude depends on β_1-selectivity and the presence or absence of partial agonist activity. The reactions may be classified as follows.

Reactions Resulting from β-Blockade
CARDIOVASCULAR EFFECTS. β-Blockers may precipitate heart failure in patients with poor LV function, and accentuate AV block. Their negative inotropic and chronotropic effects may be additive with other drugs affecting cardiac conduction or drugs used during anaesthesia. They prevent the compensatory tachycardia which accompanies hypovolaemia so that severe hypotension may occur if intravascular replacement is delayed. Bradycardia caused by excessive β-blockade may be treated by atropine, β-agonists (e.g. dobutamine or isoprenaline), glucagon or calcium chloride. Occasionally cardiac pacing may be required.

INDUCTION OF BRONCHOSPASM. This occurs in patients with asthma or chronic bronchitis who rely on sympathetically (β_2) mediated bronchodilation. Theoretically, β_1-selective drugs are less likely to aggravate bronchospasm in asthmatics, but because their selectivity is only relative, they should not be considered completely safe.

RAYNAUD'S PHENOMENON. Raynaud's phenomenon and peripheral vascular disease are relative contraindications to the use of β-blockers because symptoms of cold extremities may be exacerbated.

DIABETES MELLITUS. Cardiovascular (tachycardia-β_1) and metabolic (hepatic glycogenolysis-β_2) responses to insulin-induced hypoglycaemia are impaired. These effects may be more marked with non-selective drugs.

OTHER. Increased muscle fatigue can occur, possibly resulting from blockade of β_2-mediated vasodilatation in muscles during exercise. A withdrawal phenomenon may occur after abrupt cessation of long-term therapy for angina, causing rebound tachycardia, worsening angina or precipitation of myocardial infarction. Impotence occurs commonly during chronic β-blocker therapy.

Idiosyncratic Reactions. Central nervous system effects occur with some β-blockers, including nightmares, hallucinations, insomnia and depression. These effects are more common with the lipophilic drugs (e.g. propranolol, acebutolol, oxprenolol and metoprolol). Gastrointestinal reactions include nausea, vomiting and diarrhoea.

Newer β-Blockers. Recently introduced third-generation β-blockers (e.g. labetalol, celiprolol, nevibolol and carvedilol) are mostly non-selective ($\beta_1 > \beta_2$) antagonists which also produce vasodilatation by several mechanisms. Labetalol and carvedilol are also α_1-antagonists; bucindolol produces direct vasodilatation by a cAMP-dependent mechanism. The severity of some of the adverse effects of β-blockade may be less with those drugs with vasodilating properties.

Labetalol is a competitive α_1-, β_1- and β_2-antagonist, which is a partial agonist at β_2-receptors. It is four to seven times more potent at β- than at α-receptors and is useful for the prevention and treatment of perioperative hypertension, or to produce controlled

hypotension (see Ch 21). It is also available as an oral preparation for the treatment of chronic hypertension or the preoperative management of phaeochromocytoma (see Ch 37). Intravenous labetalol in small increments (e.g. 5–10 mg) produces a controlled decrease in arterial pressure over 5–10 min with no change in cardiac output or reflex tachycardia, suggesting that at this dose the vasodilating action predominates. At higher doses, the β-effect becomes more prominent, with negative inotropic and chronotropic effects.

Carvedilol is an antagonist at α_1- and β-receptors (with relative β:α_1 selectivity of 10:1 and no partial agonist activity), but it has other effects including significant antioxidant activity, inhibition of endothelin synthesis and possibly calcium channel blockade in higher doses; these may account for some of its beneficial activity in patients with heart failure. Carvedilol is a stereoisomer which undergoes extensive first-pass metabolism with the production of active metabolites.

Nebivolol is a lipophilic β_1-selective blocker which is administered as a racemic mixture of equal proportions of D- and L-enantiomers. It has no membrane-stabilizing activity but has vasodilatory effects probably mediated by endothelial nitric oxide.

Celiprolol is a β_1-selective blocker which is a weak β_2-agonist and has α_2-antagonist activity. It also has direct vasodilator effects which may be mediated by endothelial nitric oxide release. Celiprolol is excreted unchanged.

Esmolol is a rapid-onset, short-acting β_1-selective blocker with no membrane-stabilizing or partial agonist activity and is only available for i.v. use. It has an onset time of 1–2 min and is metabolized rapidly by red cell esterases (distinct from plasma cholinesterases); its elimination half-life is 9 min. The rapid onset and offset of effect are an advantage in the perioperative period because any effects such as bradycardia or hypotension are short-lived. It is effective in preventing or controlling intraoperative tachycardia and hypertension, and is also useful for the treatment of supraventricular tachyarrhythmias, e.g. atrial fibrillation or flutter. It may be given as a slow i.v. bolus of 0.5–2.0 mg kg^{-1} or an infusion of 25–500 μg kg^{-1} min^{-1}; its effects terminate within 10–20 min of stopping the infusion.

DRUGS ACTING ON THE PARASYMPATHETIC NERVOUS SYSTEM

The major drugs in use which act on the parasympathetic nervous system are muscarinic antagonists (e.g. atropine, hyoscine and propantheline), and parasympathetic agonists (e.g. the anticholinesterases neostigmine and pyridostigmine). Neuromuscular blocking drugs act at nicotinic receptors, and are described in Chapter 6.

Parasympathetic Antagonists

Parasympathetic antagonists block muscarinic ACh receptors and are either tertiary or quaternary amine compounds. Tertiary amines, e.g. atropine and hyoscine, are more lipid-soluble and cross biological membranes, e.g. the blood–brain barrier, to affect central ACh receptors and produce sedative or stimulatory effects. Similar antimuscarinic drugs, e.g. orphenadrine, procyclidine, are useful in drug-induced Parkinson's disease because of their predominant central action; procyclidine is also used for the reversal of acute dystonic reactions to dopaminergic drugs (e.g. phenothiazines, droperidol). Other muscarinic antagonists used as gastrointestinal or urinary antispasmodics are quaternary amines; they are poorly absorbed after oral administration and produce minimal central effects.

Atropine

Atropine has widespread, dose-dependent antimuscarinic effects on parasympathetic functions. Salivary secretion, micturition, bradycardia and visual accommodation are impaired sequentially. CNS effects (sedation or excitation, hallucinations and hyperthermia) may occur at high doses. Atropine is administered in doses of 0.6–3.0 mg i.v. to counteract bradycardia in the presence of hypotension and to prevent the bradycardia associated with vagal stimulation or the use of anticholinesterase drugs. Adverse cardiac effects of atropine include an increase in cardiac work and ventricular arrhythmias. Occasionally, atropine may produce an initial transient bradycardia, thought to be caused by increased ACh release mediated by M_2-receptor antagonism. In therapeutic dosage, effects mediated by M_3-receptors (tachycardia, bronchodilation, dry mouth, mydriasis) predominate.

Hyoscine

Hyoscine hydrobromide has less effect on heart rate than atropine but crosses the blood–brain barrier more readily and may cause confusion, sedation and ataxia, particularly in the elderly. This may result in the 'central anticholinergic syndrome' (see p. 375). It has greater antisialagogue and mydriatic effects than atropine. It is also useful as an antiemetic, particularly for the prophylaxis of motion sickness, and is available as a transdermal patch for this purpose. Hyoscine butyl-bromide is used as a gastrointestinal or genitourinary antispasmodic.

Glycopyrronium Bromide (Glycopyrrolate)

This is a quaternary amine which has similar anticholinergic actions to those of atropine. It is used as an alternative to atropine during the reversal of neuromuscular blockade or for its antisecretory actions. Some other quaternary amines, e.g. propantheline and dicycloverine, have a mainly peripheral parasympathetic antagonist action and are used as gastrointestinal and urinary antispasmodics.

Ipratropium bromide and *tiotropium* are used as inhaled anticholinergic bronchodilators. Tiotropium is longer acting and used for the management of chronic obstructive pulmonary disease.

Antimuscarinic Drugs in Premedication

Subcutaneous or oral atropine and hyoscine have long been used as premedicant drugs, usually in combination with an opioid or sedative, to decrease salivary and respiratory secretions and counteract vagal reflexes. Their use declined with the decreased use of ether, and many patients find the associated dry mouth and blurred vision unpleasant. However, if an antisialagogue is particularly indicated, glycopyrrolate is effective in a dose of 0.2 mg i.m. or i.v. with minimal central or cardiovascular effects.

Parasympathetic Agonists

Pilocarpine is a muscarinic agonist used as a topical miotic in the treatment of glaucoma. Other parasympathetic agonists used historically as gastrointestinal tract and bladder smooth muscle stimulants have been superseded.

Anticholinesterase Drugs

Neostigmine and *pyridostigmine* antagonize acetyl-cholinesterase, thereby decreasing the breakdown of released ACh. They exert both nicotinic and muscarinic effects and are used in anaesthesia to reverse non-depolarizing neuromuscular blockade (see Ch 6), accompanied by an antimuscarinic drug to minimize the adverse vagal effects. Other anticholinesterases include *edrophonium* (short-acting) and *pyridostigmine* (long-acting), used for the diagnosis and symptomatic management of myasthenia gravis, respectively.

VASODILATORS

Vasodilators dilate arteries or veins and may reduce afterload, preload or both. Acute and chronic heart failure are both associated with a reflex increase in sympathetic tone and an increase in systemic vascular resistance. By lowering this resistance (afterload), myocardial work and oxygen requirements are reduced. Vasodilators acting on the venous side of the circulation (e.g. nitrates) increase venous capacitance, reduce venous return to the heart and so decrease left ventricular filling pressure (preload), myocardial fibre length and myocardial oxygen consumption for the same degree of cardiac work performed. They have several clinical indications (Table 8.7).

Vasodilators may be classified into those acting directly on vascular smooth muscle (nitroprusside, nitrates, hydralazine, diazoxide, minoxidil, calcium channel blockers) and neurohumoral antagonists (α-blockers and ACE inhibitors). They may also be classified according to which side of the heart they act on preferentially. Hydralazine, calcium channel blockers, and minoxidil act mainly on afterload. Nitrates principally affect

TABLE 8.7
Indications for Vasodilators
Acute and chronic left ventricular failure
Prophylaxis and treatment of unstable and stable angina
Treatment of acute myocardial ischaemia and infarction
Chronic hypertension
Acute hypertensive episodes
Elective controlled hypotensive anaesthesia

preload. Nitroprusside, α-blockers and ACE inhibitors have a balanced effect on arteries and veins.

Nitrates

The organic nitrates (*glyceryl trinitrate* and *isosorbide mononitrate and dinitrate*) cause systemic and coronary vasodilatation. They act primarily on systemic veins, causing venodilatation, sequestration of blood in venous capacitance beds and a reduction in preload. Arteriolar dilatation occurs at higher doses and afterload is reduced; tachycardia, hypotension and headaches may occur. Systolic pressure decreases more than diastolic pressure, so coronary perfusion pressure is preserved. In left ventricular failure, venodilatation is beneficial, reducing pulmonary congestion; cardiac dynamics may be improved so that stroke volume and cardiac output increase. Nitrates are used widely for the prevention and treatment of angina and myocardial infarction because they cause vasodilatation in stenotic coronary arteries and redistribution of myocardial blood flow. Glyceryl trinitrate (GTN) is a powerful myometrial relaxant. Nitrates also inhibit platelet aggregation *in vitro*.

Nitrates are converted to the active compounds nitric oxide (NO) and nitrosothiols by a denitration mechanism involving reduced sulphydryl groups. NO and nitrosothiols activate guanylate cyclase in the cytoplasm of vascular smooth muscle cells to increase intracellular cGMP. This leads to protein kinase phosphorylation and decreased intracellular calcium, causing vascular smooth muscle relaxation and vasodilatation. Tolerance to nitrates develops rapidly during continuous therapy (within 24 h), caused by depletion of reduced sulphydryl groups or activation of neurohormonal countermechanisms, and a daily nitrate-free interval of 8–12 h is required. Nitrates may be administered by oral, buccal, transdermal and intravenous routes. Intravenous nitrates may be used for the treatment of perioperative hypertension or myocardial ischaemia or as part of a deliberate hypotensive anaesthetic technique. They are absorbed by rubber and plastics (especially PVC infusion bags), so are best administered by syringe pump.

Sodium Nitroprusside

Sodium nitroprusside (SNP) is reduced to NO on exposure to reducing agents and in tissues, including vascular smooth muscle cell membranes. The process is non-enzymatic but SNP has a similar ultimate mechanism of action to nitrates (increased intracellular cGMP). SNP produces similar effects on capacitance and resistance vessels so that preload and afterload are equally reduced, and it is useful in the management of acute left ventricular failure. Systolic and diastolic pressures decrease equally in a dose-dependent manner. In larger doses (as used for hypotensive anaesthesia), heart rate increases.

Release of NO from nitroprusside is accompanied by release of cyanide ions, which are detoxified by the liver and kidney to thiocyanate (requiring thiosulphate, vitamin B_{12} and the enzyme rhodanase), which is excreted slowly in urine. It has an immediate, short-lived effect (lasting only for a few minutes) so it must be given by intravenous infusion. SNP is photodegraded to cyanide ions, so that infusion solutions should be protected from light and not used if they have turned dark brown or blue. Also, if the total dose of SNP exceeds $1.5\,\text{mg}\,\text{kg}^{-1}$ or the infusion rate exceeds $1.5\,\mu\text{g}\,\text{kg}^{-1}\,\text{min}^{-1}$, cyanide and thiocyanate may accumulate, with the risk of metabolic acidosis; plasma bicarbonate concentration should be monitored. The risks of cyanide toxicity are increased in the presence of impaired renal or hepatic function, and symptoms may be delayed until after the SNP infusion has been discontinued. Plasma cyanide or thiocyanate concentrations should also be monitored if the drug is used for more than 2 days. Thiocyanate is potentially neurotoxic and may cause hypothyroidism. In cases of suspected cyanide toxicity, sodium thiosulphate (which promotes conversion to thiocyanate), dicobalt edetate (which chelates cyanide ions) and hydroxocobalamin (which combines with cyanide to form cyanocobalamin) may be given. In practice, nitroprusside is usually well tolerated and most symptoms are associated with too rapid a decrease in arterial pressure.

Potassium Channel Activators

Hydralazine, minoxidil and diazoxide are direct-acting arteriolar vasodilators which have largely been superseded. Minoxidil and diazoxide activate ATP-sensitive K^+ channels in vascular smooth muscle cells, causing K^+ efflux and membrane hyperpolarization. This leads to closure of calcium channels, reduced intracellular calcium availability and consequently smooth muscle relaxation and arterial vasodilatation. Hydralazine may

act via a similar mechanism. All these drugs reduce afterload, with little or no effect on preload. Their effects are limited by reflex tachycardia and a tendency to cause sodium and water retention (by activation of the renin-angiotensin system and a direct renal mechanism). Consequently, they are usually administered during long-term therapy with a β-blocker and a diuretic.

Hydralazine is the most widely used of these drugs. Its half-life is short (approximately 2.5 h) but its antihypertensive effect is relatively prolonged. It may be given as a slow i.v. bolus of 5–10 mg, with appropriate monitoring, for the treatment of hypertensive emergencies.

Minoxidil is only available orally. It has a long duration of action (12–24 h) unrelated to its plasma half-life, and it causes hypertrichosis. T-wave abnormalities on ECG are observed in 60% of patients.

Diazoxide has a similar structure to thiazide diuretics. It is occasionally used for the treatment of hypertensive emergencies; $1-3\,\text{mg}\,\text{kg}^{-1}$ i.v. may be given rapidly (over 30 s) for effects lasting 4–24 h. However, it is difficult to control the action or duration of action of repeated doses.

Nicorandil

Nicorandil activates K^+ channels in vascular smooth muscle, but also causes NO release and increases intracellular cGMP in vascular endothelium, causing venous dilatation. It therefore reduces preload as well as afterload and is a potent coronary vasodilator with no effect on heart rate or contractility. It is metabolized in the liver, excreted via the kidneys and does not cause tolerance. Nicorandil is used for the treatment of angina, e.g. in nitrate-tolerant patients or those unresponsive to β-blockers.

CALCIUM CHANNEL BLOCKERS

Mechanism of Action

The normal function of cardiac myocytes and conducting tissues, skeletal muscle, vascular and other smooth muscle, and neurones depends on the availability of intracellular calcium ions. Under physiological conditions, calcium entry into the cell induces further calcium release from the sarcoplasmic reticulum, which facilitates conduction of the cardiac action potential and excitation–contraction coupling by interaction with calmodulin (in smooth muscle) or troponin (within cardiac muscle). Calcium enters the cell via several ion channels situated on the plasma membrane, the most important being voltage-gated calcium channels which are activated by nerve impulses or membrane depolarization. Other types of calcium channels are receptor-operated and stretch-activated channels. Calcium channel blockers (CCBs) are a diverse group of compounds which decrease calcium entry into cardiac and vascular smooth muscle cells through the L-subtype (long-lasting inward calcium current) of voltage-gated calcium channels. CCBs bind in several ways to the α_1 subunit of L-type channels to impede calcium entry. Phenylalkylamines (e.g. verapamil) bind to the intracellular portion of the channel and physically occlude it, whereas dihydropyridines modify the extracellular allosteric structure of the channel. Benzothiazepines (e.g. diltiazem) act on the α_1 subunit, although the mechanism has not been fully elucidated, and may have further actions on sodium-potassium exchange and calcium–calmodulin binding.

Cardiac cells in the SA and AV nodes depend on the slow inward calcium current for depolarization. CCBs which act here decrease calcium entry during phase 0 of the action potential of SA node and AV node cells, decreasing heart rate and AV node conduction. Calcium entry during phase 2 of the action potential of ventricular myocytes may be decreased (Fig. 8.5) and excitation–contraction coupling inhibited, causing decreased myocardial contractility. Some CCBs may also have favourable effects on endothelial function.

Clinical Effects

CCBs differ in their selectivity for cardiac muscle cells, conducting tissue and vascular smooth muscle, but they all decrease myocardial contractility and produce coronary and systemic vasodilatation with a consequent decrease in arterial pressure. They have been used widely for the treatment of hypertension and angina, but have been partly superseded by newer drugs. Other current indications include prevention of vasospasm in subarachnoid haemorrhage or Raynaud's disease. Verapamil and diltiazem also decrease SA node activity, AV node conduction and heart rate, and they are useful in the treatment of paroxysmal supraventricular tachyarrhythmias. CCBs may also inhibit

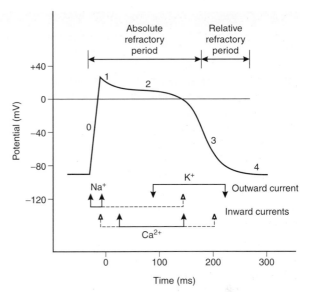

FIGURE 8.5 ■ The cardiac action potential.

platelet aggregation, protect against bronchospasm and improve lower oesophageal sphincter function. The non-dihydropyridines are contraindicated in the presence of second- or third-degree heart block and should not be combined with β-blockers because they may cause bradycardia or heart block. With the exception of amlodipine and felodipine, calcium channel blockers should not be used in patients with heart failure. In some patients, sudden cessation of CCBs may lead to an exacerbation of angina symptoms.

Classification

CCBs are a diverse group of compounds which have been classified in several ways, according to their structure, mechanism of action and specificity for slow calcium channels. They are classified here by their chemical structure, tissue selectivity and pharmacokinetic properties (Table 8.8).

First-Generation Calcium Channel Blockers

The first-generation CCBs (verapamil, diltiazem and nifedipine) have a rapid onset of action which may reduce arterial pressure acutely and produce reflex sympathetic activation. They have marked negative dromotropic and inotropic effects (especially verapamil and diltiazem). Their intrinsic duration of action is short, but slow-release formulations have

TABLE 8.8
Classification of Calcium Channel Blockers

Group	Prototype/ First-Generation Drugs	Second-and Third-Generation Drugs	EFFECTS ON				
			SA Node	AV Node Conduction	Myocardial Contractility	Peripheral Arteries	Coronary Arteries
Benzothiazepine	Diltiazem		−/+	+	+	+	++
Phenylalkylamine	Verapamil		++	++	+	+	+
Dihydropyridine	Nifedipine		−	−	+	++	++
		Nicardipine	−	−	+/−	++	+++
		Nimodipine	−	−	+/-	++	+/−
		Felodipine	−	−	−	+++	+
		Isradipine	−	−	−	+++	+
		Amlodipine[a]	−	−	−	+++	++
		Lacidipine[a]	−	−	−	++++	+/−

[a]Third-generation calcium antagonists.

been developed (see below). All are well absorbed but undergo a significant first-pass effect, leading to low bioavailability. They are highly protein-bound and metabolized extensively by hepatic demethylation and dealkylation, with wide individual pharmacokinetic variability (Table 8.9). Most CCBs possess one or more chiral centres, and the different enantiomeric forms have different pharmacokinetic and pharmacodynamic properties. For example, L-verapamil undergoes higher first-pass metabolism than the D-form, so that plasma concentrations of L-verapamil are relatively higher after intravenous administration, producing more pronounced negative inotropic and chronotropic effects.

Nifedipine is a dihydropyridine derivative which is a systemic and coronary arterial vasodilator. It is effective in countering coronary artery spasm, thought to be an important component of all forms of angina, and it may bring symptomatic relief in patients with peripheral vasospastic (e.g. Raynaud's) disease. Its anti-anginal effect is additive with that of β-adrenergic blocking drugs and nitrates. Adverse effects include flushing, headaches, ankle oedema, dizziness, tiredness and palpitations. Nifedipine is absorbed rapidly, particularly when the stomach is empty, with an onset of action of 20 min. This may produce reflex tachycardia and increased myocardial contractility.

Verapamil is a phenylalkylamine which has more pronounced effects on the SA and AV nodes compared with other CCBs, and is used mainly as an anti-arrhythmic (see below). It has vasodilator and negative

TABLE 8.9
Pharmacokinetic Properties of some Commonly used Calcium Channel Blockers

Drug	Nifedipine	Verapamil	Diltiazem	Nicardipine	Felodipine	Amlodipine	Lacidipine
Bioavailability (%)	50	20	25–50	30	15	65–80	10
Elimination half-life (h)	3–5	5–8	2–6	3–8	25	35–50	13–19
Route of elimination	Renal, hepatic	Renal, hepatic	Hepatic	Renal, hepatic	Renal, hepatic	Renal	Hepatic, renal
Time to peak plasma concentration (h)	1–2	4–8	3–4	1	12–24	6–12	1–3

inotropic properties and is also used for the treatment of angina, hypertension and hypertrophic obstructive cardiomyopathy. Verapamil has a marked negative inotropic action and may cause bradycardia, hypotension, AV block or heart failure when combined with β-blockers or other cardiodepressant drugs (including volatile anaesthetic agents). It may also potentiate the effects of neuromuscular blocking drugs. Both verapamil and diltiazem inhibit the hepatic metabolism of several drugs; plasma concentrations of digoxin, carbamazepine and theophyllines are increased by verapamil.

Diltiazem is a benzothiazepine whose predominant effect is on coronary arteries rather than conducting tissue, and is used mainly in the treatment of hypertension and angina. It can cause myocardial depression, especially when combined with β-blockers. It is metabolized in the liver, producing active metabolites, and is excreted via the kidneys.

Second- and Third-Generation CCBs

The second-generation CCBs are dihydropyridine derivatives (either sustained-release formulations or new compounds) which have a slower onset and longer duration of action, and greater vascular smooth muscle selectivity. The slow onset results in less sympathetic activation and reflex tachycardia. The new compounds (e.g. felodipine, nisoldipine, nicardipine) have less effect on AV conduction and less negative inotropic and chronotropic effects. All have little effect on lipid or glucose metabolism and may be used in patients with renal dysfunction. Some have special features.

Nimodipine is selective for cerebral vasculature and is used to prevent vasospasm after subarachnoid haemorrhage. *Nicardipine* causes less reduction in myocardial contractility than other CCBs. *Felodipine* acts predominantly on peripheral vascular smooth muscle and has negligible effects on myocardial contractility, although it does produce coronary vasodilatation. It also has a mild diuretic and natriuretic effect. It is indicated for the treatment of hypertension, but has been used in patients with impaired LV function.

The third generation of CCBs (lacidipine, amlodipine) bind to specific high-affinity sites in the calcium channel complex. They have a particularly slow onset and long duration of action, and so reflex sympathetic

stimulation is not evident but adverse effects related to vasodilatation (headache, flushing, ankle oedema) do occur. Both are extensively metabolized in the liver to inactive metabolites which are excreted via the kidneys and liver. *Lacidipine* is highly lipophilic, so that it is sequestered in the lipid bilayer of vascular smooth muscle cells and may delay the development of atherosclerosis via effects on modulators of vascular smooth muscle and platelet function. Lacidipine may augment the action of endothelium-derived relaxing factors (e.g. NO – which has vasodilator, antiplatelet and antiproliferative effects) and antagonize endothelin-1, a potent vasoconstrictor which also stimulates endothelial proliferation.

Anaesthesia and Calcium Channel Blockers

Both intravenous and volatile anaesthetic agents block conduction through L-type calcium channels in neuronal and cardiac tissues, and may therefore interact with CCBs through pharmacokinetic and pharmacodynamic mechanisms. In general, CCBs potentiate the hypotensive effects of volatile anaesthetics; verapamil (and to a lesser extent diltiazem) has additive effects with halothane on cardiac conduction and contractility, with the potential for bradycardia and myocardial depression. Verapamil decreases the MAC of halothane, and, in an animal model, nifedipine enhances the analgesic effects of morphine by stimulation of spinal 5-HT$_3$ receptors. Plasma concentrations of verapamil are increased during anaesthesia with volatile agents, possibly because of decreased hepatic blood flow.

CCBs also potentiate the effects of depolarizing and non-depolarizing neuromuscular blockers in experimental conditions, although the clinical relevance of this is uncertain.

DRUGS ACTING VIA THE RENIN–ANGIOTENSIN–ALDOSTERONE SYSTEM

The renin–angiotensin–aldosterone system (RAS) is intimately involved with cardiovascular and body fluid homeostasis. Angiotensin II (AT-II) is the major regulator of the renin-angiotensin system and is a potent vasoconstrictor with several renal and extrarenal effects. AT-II has an important role in the maintenance

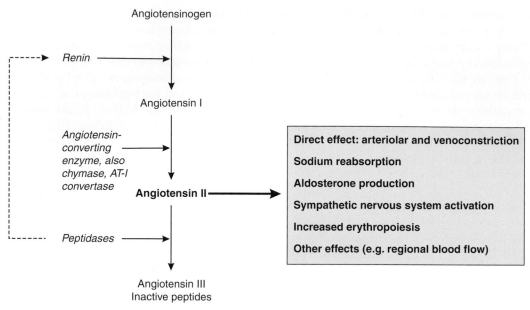

FIGURE 8.6 ■ The renin–angiotensin system.

of circulating volume in response to several stressors, while direct renal effects are mostly responsible for long-term regulation of body fluid volume and blood pressure.

The production of AT-II from angiotensinogen occurs in the walls of small blood vessels in the lungs, kidneys and other organs, and in the plasma. The rate-limiting step for this cascade is the plasma concentration of renin (Fig. 8.6). AT-II is metabolized by several peptidases to several breakdown products including angiotensin III (AT-III), which has some activity at angiotensin receptors. Four subtypes of angiotensin receptor have been defined (AT_{1-4}). AT_1-receptors are found principally in vascular smooth muscle, adrenal cortex, kidney, liver and some areas of the brain, and mediate all the known physiological functions of AT-II. AT_2-receptors are present in the kidney, adrenal medulla, uterus, ovary and the brain; they may play a role in cell growth and differentiation. The roles of AT_3- and AT_4-receptors are unclear.

AT_1-receptors are typical G-protein-coupled receptors which activate phospholipase C with the production of DAG and IP_3. IP_3 causes the release of intracellular Ca^{2+}, which activates enzymes to cause the phosphorylation of intracellular proteins. AT-II also increases Ca^{2+} entry through membrane channels.

AT-II (see Fig. 8.6) is a potent vasoconstrictor (by direct action on vascular smooth muscle of arterioles and veins) and it promotes sodium reabsorption both by direct action at the proximal tubules and by stimulating aldosterone secretion. AT-II produces preglomerular vasoconstriction and efferent arteriolar vasoconstriction, and so maintains glomerular filtration rate in response to a decrease in renal blood flow. It also affects the local regulation of blood flow in other vascular beds, e.g. the splanchnic circulation, and stimulates the sympathetic nervous system via direct and indirect methods to increase noradrenaline and adrenaline release; it may also inhibit cardiac vagal activity. AT-II stimulates erythropoiesis and has direct trophic effects on vascular smooth muscle and cardiac muscle, promoting cellular proliferation, migration and hypertrophy. There is some evidence for relative downregulation of AT_1-receptors and upregulation of AT_2-receptors in heart failure, with AT_2-receptors being responsible for some cardioprotective effects.

RAS activity tends to be low in the resting state but renin production (the rate-limiting step in the production of AT-II) is activated by several stimuli, e.g. depletion of circulating volume, haemorrhage or sodium depletion. This increases AT-II production and causes vasoconstriction, increased sympathetic activity (with increased cardiac output and arterial pressure) and sodium retention. The RAS may be involved in the pathogenesis of hypertension but the relationship is complex; RAS activity may be high (e.g. in renal artery stenosis), low (as in primary aldosteronism) or variable (essential hypertension).

Drugs Acting on the Renin–Angiotensin System

The activity of the RAS may be inhibited by several mechanisms:

- *Suppression of renin release or inhibition of renin activity.* Sympatholytic drugs (e.g. β-blockers or central α-antagonists) directly inhibit renin secretion. Renin inhibitors competitively inhibit the reaction between renin and angiotensinogen, preventing the production of AT-II. Because renin release still occurs, the consequent reduction of plasma AT-II concentrations leads to a secondary increase in renin secretion, limiting the effect of such drugs.
- *Inhibition of angiotensin-converting enzyme (ACE).* The primary mechanism of action of ACE inhibitors is to block the conversion of angiotensin I (AT-I) to AT-II, although effects on kinin and prostaglandin metabolism also contribute.
- *Blockade of AT-II receptors.* AT_1-receptor blockers (ARBs) non-competitively block AT_1-receptors and inhibit the RAS independently of the source of AT-II. They block any effects of AT-II resulting from compensatory stimulation of renin, such as reflex activation of the sympathetic nervous system.
- *Aldosterone antagonism.* Spironolactone and eplerenone are competitive antagonists of aldosterone at renal nuclear mineralocorticoid receptors (see Ch 10).

ACE Inhibitors

ACE inhibitors act principally by inhibition of AT-II formation, but effects on the kallikrein-kinin system are also important. All ACE inhibitors reduce arteriolar tone, peripheral resistance and arterial pressure by decreasing both AT-II-mediated vasoconstriction and sympathetic nervous system activity. Renal blood flow increases, further inhibiting aldosterone

and antidiuretic hormone secretion and promoting sodium excretion. ACE inhibitors are useful in patients with heart failure because preload and afterload decrease without an increase in heart rate, and cardiac output increases.

ACE is the same enzyme as kininase II and is involved in the metabolism of both kinins and prostaglandins. ACE inhibitors therefore block the degradation of kinins, substance P and endorphins, and increase prostaglandin concentrations. Bradykinin and other kinins are highly potent arterial and venous dilators which stimulate the production of arachidonic acid metabolites, NO and endothelial-derived hyperpolarization factor via specific bradykinin $β_2$-receptors in vascular endothelium. Bradykinin also enhances the uptake of circulating glucose into skeletal muscle and has a protective effect on cardiac myocytes by a mechanism involving prostacyclin stimulation. Kinins have no major effect on arterial pressure regulation in normotensive individuals or those with low-renin hypertension, but they account for up to 30% of the effects of ACE inhibitors in renovascular hypertension. The adverse effects of dry cough and angioneurotic oedema sometimes associated with ACE inhibitors may be kinin-dependent. ACE is widely distributed in tissues and plasma; ACE inhibitors may differ in their affinity for ACE at different sites. Other tissue enzymes (AT-I convertase and chymase) may also produce AT-II, from AT-I or directly from angiotensinogen, so that ACE inhibitors do not completely block RAS activity.

Clinical Applications of ACE Inhibitors. ACE inhibitors are established in the treatment of hypertension and congestive heart failure. They improve left ventricular dysfunction after myocardial infarction, delay the progression of diabetic nephropathy and have a protective effect in non-diabetic chronic renal failure. ACE inhibitors improve vascular endothelial function by their effects on AT-II and bradykinin, and improve long-term cardiovascular outcome in patients with established vascular disease. ACE inhibitors have a common mechanism of action, differing in the chemical structure of their active moieties in potency, bioavailability, plasma half-life, route of elimination, distribution and affinity for tissue-bound ACE (Table 8.10). Most of the newer compounds are prodrugs, converted to an active metabolite by the

TABLE 8.10
Pharmacology of ACE Inhibitors

	Captopril	Lisinopril	Enalapril	Perindopril	Quinapril	Trandolapril	Ramipril	Fosino
Zinc ligand	Sulphydryl	Carboxyl	Carboxyl	Carboxyl	Carboxyl	Carboxyl	Carboxyl	Phosphinyl
Prodrug	No	No	Yes	Yes	Yes	Yes	Yes	Yes
Bioavailability (%)	75	25	60	65	40	70	50	35
t_{max} (h)[b]	0.8	6–8	3–4	3–4	2	4–6	2–3	3–6
$t_{1/2e}$ (h)	2	12	11	25[a]	20–25[a]	16–24[a]	4–50[a]	12
Metabolism	Oxidation (50%)	Minimal	Minimal	Prodrug	Prodrug	Prodrug	Prodrug	Prodrug
Elimination	Renal	Renal	Renal	Renal	Renal	Renal, hepatic	Renal	Renal, hepatic

[a]These drugs have polyphasic pharmacokinetics, with a dose-dependent prolonged terminal elimination phase from plasma of over 24 h.
[b]The prodrugs are metabolized in the gut mucosa and liver to active compounds. Pharmacokinetic data refer to the active compounds.

liver, and have a prolonged duration of action. Most are excreted via the kidneys, and dosage should be reduced in the elderly and those with impaired renal or cardiac function. Enalapril is also available as the active drug, enalaprilat, and may be administered i.v. for the treatment of hypertensive emergencies.

ACE inhibitors are generally well tolerated, with no rebound hypertension after stopping therapy and few metabolic effects. Symptomatic first-dose hypotension may occur, particularly in hypovolaemic or sodium-depleted patients with high plasma renin concentrations. Symptomatic hypotension was more common with the higher doses originally used. ACE inhibitors have a synergistic effect with diuretics (which increase the activity of the renin-angiotensin system) but are less effective in patients taking NSAIDs.

Adverse effects of ACE inhibitors are classified into those that are class-specific (related to inhibition of ACE) and those which relate to specific drugs. Class-specific effects include hypotension, renal insufficiency, hyperkalaemia, cough (10%) and angioneurotic oedema (0.1–0.2%). ACE inhibitors may cause renal impairment, particularly if renal perfusion is decreased (e.g. because of renal artery stenosis, congestive heart failure or hypovolaemia) or if there is pre-existing renal disease. Renal impairment is also more likely in the elderly or those receiving NSAIDs, and renal function should be checked before starting ACE inhibitor therapy, and monitored subsequently.

Hyperkalaemia (plasma K^+ concentration usually increases by 0.1–0.2 mmol L^{-1} because of decreased aldosterone concentrations) may be more marked in those with impaired renal function or in patients taking potassium supplements or potassium-sparing diuretics. The mechanism of cough is not known but is mediated by C fibres and may be related to bradykinin or substance P production. It is reversible on stopping the ACE inhibitor. Other adverse effects include upper respiratory congestion, rhinorrhoea, gastrointestinal disturbances, and increased insulin sensitivity and hyperglycaemia in diabetic patients.

Some adverse effects, e.g. skin rashes (1%), taste disturbances, proteinuria (1%) and neutropenia (0.05%), are related to the presence of a sulphydryl group (e.g. captopril). ACE inhibitors are contraindicated in pregnancy.

Although anaesthesia *per se* has no direct effect on the RAS or ACE inhibitors, the RAS is activated by several stimuli which may occur during the perioperative period. These include blood or fluid losses and the stress response to surgical stimulation. RAS activation contributes to the maintenance of arterial pressure after haemorrhage, or during anaesthesia. Refractory hypotension during anaesthesia has been reported in patients receiving long-term antihypertensive treatment with ACE inhibitors, and it has been recommended that they are stopped 24 h before surgery if significant blood loss or fluid shifts are likely. ACE inhibitors improve ventricular function in patients with heart failure or after myocardial infarction but it is not known whether acute cessation before surgery is harmful. Conversely, they may have beneficial effects on regional blood flow and have been associated with improved renal function in patients undergoing aortic surgery.

Angiotensin-II Receptor Blockers

Angiotensin-II receptor blockers (ARBs) specifically and non-competitively block the AT_1-receptor, inhibiting the RAS independently and blocking any effects of AT-II resulting from compensatory stimulation of renin. Hence, they reduce afterload and increase cardiac output without causing tachycardia and are used in the treatment of hypertension, diabetic nephropathy and heart failure. As they have no effect on bradykinin metabolism or prostaglandin synthesis, ARBs do not produce the cough or rash associated with ACE inhibitors, though angio-oedema has been reported. However, plasma renin, AT-I and AT-II concentrations increase, and aldosterone concentrations decrease, during long-term therapy: hyperkalaemia may occur if potassium-sparing diuretics are also administered. Losartan is also uricosuric. All available ARBs are non-peptide imidazole compounds and are highly protein bound, with a prolonged duration of action exceeding their plasma half-life, and a maximum antihypertensive effect 2–4 weeks after starting therapy. In common with ACE inhibitors, they are contraindicated in pregnancy and are likely to have an adverse effect in patients with renal artery stenosis or those taking NSAIDs. The pharmacological properties of some ARBs are shown in Table 8.11. There are few data describing the effects of ARBs in the perioperative period, but caution would be appropriate when large fluid or blood losses are expected.

ANTIARRHYTHMIC DRUGS

Cardiac arrhythmias are irregular or abnormal heart rhythms and include bradycardias or tachycardias outside the physiological range. Patients may present for surgery with a pre-existing arrhythmia; alternatively, arrhythmias may be precipitated or accentuated during anaesthesia by several surgical, pharmacological or physiological factors (Table 8.12). Although several drugs (including anaesthetic drugs) have effects on heart rate and rhythm, the term antiarrhythmic is applied to drugs which primarily affect ionic currents within myocardial conducting tissue. Therapy for long-term arrhythmias has changed during the last two decades with the development of non-pharmacological techniques, e.g. DC cardioversion, implantable cardioverter-defibrillator (ICD) devices or radiofrequency ablation of ectopic foci. Most forms of supraventricular tachycardia may be controlled by radiofrequency ablation and ICDs are increasingly used in patients who have suffered an episode of ventricular tachycardia. Long-term drug therapy has therefore declined and is now largely confined to patients with atrial fibrillation, or as an adjunct in patients with

TABLE 8.11						
Pharmacology of Angiotensin Receptor Blockers						
Drug	*Losartan*	*Candesartan*	*Irbesartan*	*Valsartan*	*Eprosartan*	*Telmisartan*
Prodrug	Yes	Yes	No	No	No	No
Bioavailability (%)	33	14–40	60–80	23	10–15	40
Peak effect (h)	1[a]	3–4	1.5–2	2–4	1–3	0.5–1
$t_{1/2e}$ (h)	2[a]	9	11–15	9	5–9	24
Metabolism	Hepatic	Minimal	Hepatic	Minimal	Hepatic (most excreted unchanged)	Minimal
Elimination	Renal, hepatic	Renal, hepatic	Renal, hepatic	Bile, urine	Bile	Bile

[a]Undergoes significant first-pass metabolism, producing an active metabolite EXP 3174, which is 10–40 times more potent than the parent drug. Time to peak concentration and elimination half-life of EXP 3174 are 3–4 h and 6–9 h, respectively.

TABLE 8.12
Precipitants of Arrhythmias During Anaesthesia

Myocardial ischaemia

Hypoxia

Hypercapnia

Halogenated hydrocarbons (volatile anaesthetic agents, e.g. trichloroethylene, cyclopropane, halothane)

Catecholamines (endogenous or exogenous)

Electrolyte abnormalities (hypo- or hyperkalaemia, hypocalcaemia, hypomagnesaemia)

Hypotension

Autonomic effects (e.g. reflex vagal stimulation, brain tumours or trauma)

Acid–base abnormalities

Mechanical stimuli (e.g. during CVP or PAFC catheter insertion)

Drugs (toxicity or adverse reactions)

Medical conditions (e.g. sepsis, myocarditis, pneumonia, alcohol abuse, thyrotoxicosis)

ICDs or benign arrhythmias resistant to catheter ablation. However, owing to the frequency of arrhythmias during anaesthesia, knowledge of the available drugs and their interactions is important for the anaesthetist. Antiarrhythmic drugs are classified according to their effects on the action potential (see below).

The Cardiac Action Potential

The cardiac action potential (AP) is generated by movement of charged ions across the cell membrane and comprises five phases (see Fig. 8.5). At rest, the cells are polarized and the resting membrane potential is negative (-50 to $-60\,mV$ in sinus node pacemaker cells and -80 to $-90\,mV$ in Purkinje, atrial and ventricular muscle fibres). The AP is triggered by a low intra-cellular leak of Na^+ ions (and Ca^{2+} ions at the AV node) until a threshold point is reached, when sudden rapid influx of Na^+ ions causes an increase in positive charge within the cell and generates an impulse (phase 0, depolarization). The AP starts to reverse (phase 1), but is sustained because of slower inward movement of Ca^{2+} ions (phase 2). Efflux of K^+ ions brings about repolarization (phase 3) and the gradual termination of the AP. Thereafter, re-equilibration of Na^+ and K^+ takes

place and the resting membrane potential is restored (phase 4). The AP spreads between adjacent cells and is transmitted through the specialized conducting system from the AV node to the bundle of His and ventricular muscle fibres via the Purkinje fibres. The SA node pacemaker cells have the fastest spontaneous discharge rate and usually initiate the coordinated action potential. However, action potentials may also be generated by the AV node and other cells in the conducting system.

Mechanisms of Arrhythmias

Arrhythmias are caused by abnormalities of impulse generation or conduction, or both, via a number of mechanisms:

- *Altered automaticity.* Increased pacemaker activity in the SA node (e.g. caused by increased sympathetic tone) may cause sinus tachycardia, or atrial or ventricular tachyarrhythmias. Decreased SA node automaticity (e.g. as a result of enhanced vagal activity) may allow the emergence of latent pacemaker activity in distal conducting tissues, e.g. AV node or the bundle of His–Purkinje system, causing sinus bradycardia, AV nodal or idioventricular escape rhythms. These rhythms are common during halothane anaesthesia.
- *Unidirectional conduction block.* Interruption of the normal conduction pathways caused by anatomical defects, alterations in refractory period or excitability may cause heart block and favours arrhythmias caused by abnormal re-entry or automaticity.
- *Ectopic foci.* Ectopic foci may give rise to arrhythmias in a variety of circumstances. In the presence of bradycardia or SA node block, pathological damage in cardiac muscle cells or conducting tissues may augment the generation of arrhythmias from ectopic foci, via:
  - increased automaticity
  - re-entry phenomena
  - pathological afterdepolarizations.

Other factors may contribute. Increased automaticity in atrial, ventricular or conducting tissues caused by ischaemia or electrolyte disturbances (e.g. hypokalaemia) may trigger depolarization before the SA node and cause an arrhythmia. Re-entrant arrhythmias arise when forward conduction of impulses in a branch of the conduction pathway is blocked by disease and retrograde conduction occurs. If there is a discrepancy in the refractory periods of the two branches, retrograde conduction may occur in cells which have already discharged and repolarized, triggering a further AP which is both premature and ectopic. These premature APs become self-sustaining (circus movements), leading to atrial or ventricular tachycardia or fibrillation. Pathological afterdepolarizations are spontaneous impulses arising just after the normal AP and occur mostly in ischaemic myocardium (e.g. after myocardial infarction), especially in the presence of hypoxaemia, increased catecholamine concentrations, digoxin toxicity or electrolyte abnormalities.

Arrhythmias and Anaesthesia

Arrhythmias are common during anaesthesia and in intensive care, especially in patients with preoperative arrhythmia, cardiomyopathy, ischaemia or valvular or pericardial disease. They may be precipitated by several factors (see Table 8.13). Some arrhythmias are immediately life-threatening but all warrant attention because they usually imply the presence of other disturbances, and the effects of specific therapy (e.g. drugs, electrical cardioversion or cardiac pacing) are enhanced by prior corrective measures. Specific antiarrhythmic treatment is usually reserved for those arrhythmias affecting cardiac output or those which may progress to dangerous tachyarrhythmias.

In addition to volatile agents, several drugs used during anaesthesia may facilitate arrhythmias by direct toxicity (e.g. local anaesthetics), autonomic effects (e.g. succinylcholine, pancuronium), by enhancing the effects of catecholamines (e.g. nitrous oxide, thiopental,

cocaine) or as a result of histamine release. Opioids potentiate central vagal activity, decrease sympathetic tone and have direct negative chronotropic effects on the SA node. They may therefore cause bradycardia but decrease the incidence of ventricular arrhythmias.

Mechanisms of Action of Antiarrhythmic Drugs

An arrhythmia may be controlled either by slowing the primary mechanism or, in the case of supraventricular arrhythmias, by reducing the proportion of impulses transmitted through the AV node to the ventricular conducting system. The cardiac action potential may be pharmacologically manipulated in three ways:

- The *automaticity* (tendency to spontaneous discharge) of cells may be reduced. This result can be achieved by reducing the rate of leakage of sodium (reducing the slope of phase 4), by increasing the electronegativity of the resulting membrane potential or by decreasing the electronegativity of the threshold potential.
- The *speed of conduction* of the action potential may be suppressed as reflected by a lowering of the height and slope of the phase 0 discharge. A reduction in the electronegativity of the membrane potential at the onset of phase 0 reduces both the amplitude and the slope of the phase 0 depolarization. This situation occurs if the cell discharges before it has been completely repolarized.
- The *rate of repolarization* may be reduced, which prolongs the refractory period of the discharging cell.

TABLE 8.13					
Drug Treatments for Specific Arrhythmias					
Atrial Fibrillation	*Paroxysmal Atrial Fibrillation*	*Atrial Flutter*	*Paroxysmal SVT*	*WPW*	*Ventricular Arrhythmias*
Digoxin	Amiodarone	Digoxin	Adenosine	Amiodarone	Amiodarone
β-Blockers	Propafenone	Amiodarone	Verapamil	Disopyramide	Lidocaine
Verapamil	Flecainide	Sotalol	β-Blockers	Flecainide	Disopyramide
Amiodarone	Dronaderone	Propafenone		β-Blockers	Flecainide
Dronaderone					Propafenone
					Magnesium (torsade de pointes)

WPW: Wolff–Parkinson–White syndrome

All antiarrhythmic drugs may themselves induce arrhythmias. Many (particularly class 1 antiarrhythmics) have a narrow therapeutic index and some have been associated with an increase in mortality in large-scale studies. Antiarrhythmic agents may be classified empirically on the basis of their effectiveness in supraventricular tachycardias (e.g. digoxin, β-blockers and verapamil) or in ventricular arrhythmias (lidocaine, mexiletine, magnesium, phenytoin). Many drugs (disopyramide, amiodarone, quinidine and procainamide) are effective in both supraventricular and ventricular arrhythmias (Table 8.13). The Vaughan Williams classification (Table 8.14) is based on electrophysiological mechanisms. This classification has

TABLE 8.14				
Vaughan Williams Classification of Antiarrhythmic Drugs				
Class	*Examples*	*Mechanism*	*Effects*	*Indication*
1a	Quinidine Disopyramide	Na^+ channel blockade (moderate) ↓ Conduction velocity Prolonged polarization	Moderate ↓ V_{max} ↑ Action potential duration ↑ Refractory period QRS widened	Prevention of SVT, VT, atrial tachycardia WPW
1b	Lidocaine Mexiletine	Na^+ channel blockade (mild) ↓ Conduction velocity Shortened repolarization	Mild ↓ V_{max} ↓ Action potential duration ↓ Refractory period QRS unchanged	Prevention of VT/VF during ischaemia
1c	Flecainide Propafenone	Na^+ channel blockade (marked) ↓ Conduction velocity No change in repolarization	Marked ↓ V_{max} Minimal change in action potential duration and refractory period QRS widened	Conversion/prevention of SVT/VT/VF
2	β-Blockers	β-Adrenergic receptor blockade	Decreased automaticity (SA and AV nodes)	Prevention of sympathetic-induced tachyarrhythmias, rate control in AF, 2° prevention after MI, prevention of AV node re-entrant tachycardia
3	Amiodarone Bretylium Sotalol	Inhibition of inward K^+ current	Markedly prolonged repolarization ↑ Action potential duration ↑ Refractory period QRS unchanged	Prevention of SVT/VT/VF
4	Diltiazem	Calcium channel blockade	↓ Depolarization and V_{max} of slow response cells in SA and AV nodes ↓ Action potential duration ↓ Refractory period of AV node	Rate control in AF Prevention of AV node re-entrant tachycardias
Other*	Digoxin	Inhibition of Na^+/K^+ ATPase pump ↑ Intracellular Ca^{2+}, vagal and sympathetic effects	Slows AV node conduction Positive inotropy	Rate control and treatment of AF and atrial flutter
	Adenosine	Agonist at A_1- & A_2-receptors	Suppresses SA and AV node conduction ↓ Automaticity	Conversion of paroxysmal SVT Diagnosis of conduction defects
	Magnesium	Blockade of atrial calcium channels Blocks K^+ channels	↑ Refractory period Prolongs atrial conduction	Treatment of ventricular dysrhythmias including torsade de pointes

* The original Vaughan Williams classification included Classes 1-4 only. Digoxin, adenosine and other drugs which do not fit into this classification are sometimes termed 'Class 5' but are included here as 'Other'.

limitations (some drugs belong to more than one class, some arrhythmias may be caused by several mechanisms, some drugs, e.g. digoxin and adenosine, do not fit into the classification) but it remains in use and is therefore described below.

Class 1 antiarrhythmic drugs (Table 8.15) inhibit the fast Na$^+$ influx during depolarization; they inhibit arrhythmias caused by abnormal automaticity or re-entry. All class 1 drugs decrease the maximum rate of rise of phase 0, and decrease conduction velocity, excitability and automaticity to varying degrees. In addition to these local anaesthetic properties, some have membrane-stabilizing effects. Class 1a drugs antagonize primarily the fast influx of Na$^+$ ions and so reduce conduction velocity through the AV node and His–Purkinje system, whilst prolonging the duration of the action potential and the refractory period. They also have varying antimuscarinic and sympathomimetic effects. Class 1b drugs have much less effect on conduction velocity in usual therapeutic doses and they shorten the refractory period. Agents in class 1c affect conduction profoundly without altering the refractory period.

β-Blockers (class 2) depress automaticity in the SA and AV nodes, and attenuate the effects of catecholamines on automaticity and conduction velocity in the sinus and AV nodes. Class 3 drugs prolong the AP and so lengthen the refractory period. Verapamil (class 4) also prolongs the AP, in addition to depressing automaticity (especially in the AV node).

Class 1 Antiarrhythmics

Class 1a. These drugs (see Tables 8.14 and 8.15) are used for the treatment and prevention of ventricular and supraventricular arrhythmias. Their use in the prevention of atrial fibrillation has declined because of proarrhythmic effects causing increased mortality, especially in patients with ischaemic heart disease or poor LV function. They may induce torsades de pointes (a form of polymorphic ventricular tachycardia) even in patients without structural heart disease.

Quinidine is an isomer of quinine with antimuscarinic and α-blocking properties. It was formerly used in the treatment of atrial and supraventricular tachycardias. *Disopyramide* is useful in supraventricular tachycardias and as a second-line agent to lidocaine in ventricular arrhythmias. It has less action on the His–Purkinje system than quinidine, but greater antimuscarinic and negative inotropic effects.

Procainamide has similar effects to quinidine and may cause hypotension after i.v. administration. It may be used i.v. to terminate ventricular arrhythmias or as an oral antiarrhythmic, although it has a short half-life and requires frequent administration or the use of a sustained-release oral preparation.

Ajmalin is a quinidine-like drug used for the treatment of Wolff–Parkinson–White (WPW) syndrome. It inhibits intraventricular conduction and prolongs AV conduction time, and is available in Europe.

Class 1b. Class 1b drugs are useful for the prevention and treatment of premature ventricular contractions, ventricular tachycardia and ventricular fibrillation, particularly associated with ischaemia.

Lidocaine is the first-choice drug for ventricular arrhythmias resistant to DC cardioversion. It decreases normal and abnormal automaticity and decreases action potential and refractory period durations. The threshold for ventricular fibrillation is raised but it has minimal haemodynamic effects. The antiarrhythmic properties of lidocaine are enhanced by hypoxaemia, acidosis and hyperkalaemia, so that it is particularly effective in ischaemic cells, e.g. after acute myocardial infarction, during cardiac surgery or in arrhythmias associated with digitalis toxicity. Lidocaine may cause CNS toxicity. Cardiotoxic effects (hypotension, bradycardia or heart block) occur at higher doses and are potentiated by hypoxaemia, acidosis and hypercapnia. Clearance is decreased if hepatic blood flow is decreased (e.g. in the elderly, those with congestive heart failure, after myocardial infarction), and also by β-blockers, cimetidine and liver disease. In these circumstances, the dose should be reduced by 50%. It is less effective in the presence of hypokalaemia.

Mexiletine is a lidocaine analogue which is well absorbed orally with high bioavailability. Adverse effects are similar to those of lidocaine; nausea and vomiting are also common during oral treatment.

Class 1c. Class 1c drugs are used for the prevention and treatment of supraventricular and ventricular tachyarrhythmias and junctional tachycardias with or without an accessory pathway. They are proarrhythmogenic, particularly in patients with myocardial

TABLE 8.15

Pharmacology of Some Class 1 Antiarrhythmic Drugs

DRUG	QUINIDINE	DISOPYRAMIDE	PROCAINAMIDE	MEXILETINE	FLECAINIDE
Class	Ia	Ia	Ia	Ib	Ic
Indications	Supraventricular tachyarrhythmias	Supraventricular and ventricular tachyarrhythmias	Supraventricular tachyarrhythmias	Ventricular tachyarrhythmias	Supraventricular and ventricular tachyarrhythmias
Metabolism and elimination	80% metabolized in liver, 20% excreted unchanged via kidneys	Renal; 50–80% excreted unchanged	15–30% by hepatic acetylation, 40–70% excreted unchanged by kidneys	85% hepatic, 15% excreted unchanged by kidneys	Renal 80–90% excreted unchanged
Elimination $t_{1/2}$	5–8 h	4–6 h	3–5 h	6–10 h	7–15 h
Active metabolites?	Yes	One of metabolites has marked anticholinergic effects	Yes (N-acetyl procainamide)	No	Weakly active metabolites
Adverse effects	Ventricular arrhythmias; visual and auditory disturbances with vertigo; gastrointestinal symptoms; rashes; thrombocytopaenia and agranulocytosis	Arrhythmias (ventricular tachycardia, AV block); hypotension; dry mouth, blurred vision, urinary retention, GI irritation	Nausea; myocardial depression; drug-induced systemic lupus erythematosis; agranulocytosis	Nausea, vomiting; cardiotoxicity (bradycardia, hypotension, conduction defects); CNS toxicity (confusion, dysarthria, paraesthesiae, dizziness and convulsions)	Arrhythmias (ventricular tachycardia, AV block); myocardial depression; nausea, vomiting
Notes	Additive with other cardiodepressant drugs (e.g. disopyramide, β-blockers and calcium channel blockers); potentiates non-depolarizing neuromuscular blockers; enhances digoxin toxicity by displacing digoxin from binding sites and reducing its clearance	Negative inotropic effects more marked in combination with β-blockers or verapamil	Metabolism to N-acetyl procainamide dependent on hepatic N-acetyl transferase; usually only administered i.v.	Elimination enhanced by hepatic enzyme induction (e.g. by rifampicin or phenytoin); elimination reduced in cardiac or hepatic disease	Polymorphic metabolism; elimination prolonged in renal or heart failure; increases digoxin and propranolol concentrations

ischaemia, poor left ventricular function or after myocardial infarction, and although effective in chronic atrial fibrillation, they are reserved for life-threatening arrhythmias.

Flecainide is a procainamide derivative with little effect on repolarization, the refractory period or AP duration, but unlike other drugs in this class, it decreases automaticity and produces dose-dependent widening of the QRS complex. In acute atrial fibrillation, intravenous flecainide usually restores sinus rhythm and is useful prophylaxis against further episodes of atrial fibrillation. However, it increases the risk of ventricular arrhythmias after myocardial infarction, especially in patients with structural cardiac disease.

Propafenone has a complex pharmacology including weak antimuscarinic, β-adrenergic receptor and calcium channel blocking effects. It should be used with caution in patients with reactive airways disease. Interaction with digoxin may increase plasma digoxin concentrations.

Class 2 Antiarrhythmic Drugs

β-Blockers are used mainly for the treatment of sinus and supraventricular tachycardias, especially those provoked by endogenous or exogenous catecholamines, emotion or exercise. Their antiarrhythmic effects are an intrinsic property of β-blockade, i.e. reduced automaticity in ectopic pacemakers, prolonged AV node conduction and refractory period, although some β-blockers have class 1 activity in high doses ('membrane-stabilizing activity'). Although beneficial in chronic heart failure, their negative inotropic effects may be disadvantageous in patients with acute left ventricular dysfunction.

Class 3 Antiarrhythmic Drugs

Class 3 antiarrhythmics prolong the AP in conducting tissues and myocardial muscle. They prolong repolarization by K^+ channel blockade, and decrease outward K^+ conduction in the bundle of His, atrial and ventricular muscle, and accessory pathways. They are used for the treatment of supraventricular and ventricular tachyarrhythmias, including those associated with accessory conduction pathways. Some drugs have other actions (e.g. sotalol also produces β-blockade, and disopyramide has class 1 effects). All may prolong the QT interval and precipitate torsades de pointes,

especially in high doses or in the presence of electrolyte disturbance.

Sotalol is a non-selective β-blocker with class 3 antiarrhythmic effects. Action potential duration and refractory period are lengthened, and it is effective in the treatment of supraventricular tachyarrhythmias, especially atrial flutter and fibrillation, which may be converted to sinus rhythm. It also suppresses ventricular tachyarrhythmias and ventricular ectopic beats. However, sotalol may cause torsades de pointes and other life-threatening arrhythmias, particularly in the presence of hypokalaemia.

Amiodarone is primarily a class 3 drug; it acts by inhibition of inward K^+ current. It also blocks sodium and calcium channels, and has competitive inhibitory actions at α- and β-adrenoceptors, and may therefore be considered to have class 1, 2 and 4 antiarrhythmic activity. It prolongs AP duration, repolarization and refractory periods in the atria and ventricles. In addition, AV node conduction is markedly slowed and refractory period increased. Ventricular conduction velocity is slowed. Amiodarone is effective against a wide variety of supraventricular and ventricular arrhythmias, including WPW syndrome, and is preferred to other drugs in the presence of left ventricular dysfunction. Intravenous amiodarone is contraindicated in the presence of bradycardia or AV block but is less likely than other agents to cause arrhythmias. Bradycardia unresponsive to atropine, and hypotension, have been reported during general anaesthesia in patients receiving amiodarone therapy. Long-term oral therapy may produce a number of adverse effects. Amiodarone is an iodinated compound, which explains its effects on the thyroid (Table 8.16).

Bretylium is a quaternary ammonium compound which prevents noradrenaline uptake into sympathetic nerve endings. It prolongs AP duration and refractory period with no effect on automaticity, and was used as second-line therapy to lidocaine for resistant life-threatening ventricular tachyarrhythmias, but is no longer available in the UK.

Dronaderone and *dofetilide* are new class 3 antiarrhythmics which selectively inhibit inward K^+ currents and so prolong repolarization, effective refractory period and the QT interval. Dofetilide has high bioavailability and is excreted mostly unchanged by the kidney but may cause torsades de pointes. Dronaderone is an

TABLE 8.16

Pharmacological Properties of some Commonly used Intravenous Antiarrhythmic Drugs

Drug (class)	Lidocaine (1b)	Adenosine	Digoxin	Amiodarone (3)	Magnesium Sulphate
Typical i.v. dose	50–100 mg, repeated after 5–10 min or followed by continuous infusion	3 mg, repeated up to 6 mg and 12 mg after 1–2 min	Loading dose 250–500 µg i.v. over 10–20 min, repeated after 6–12 h	5 mg kg^{-1} over at least 5–10 min, followed by infusion of 900 mg over 24 h	8 mmol over 10–15 min followed by continuous i.v. infusion of 4–72 mmol over 24 h
Metabolism and elimination	Extensive first-pass hepatic metabolism	Vascular endothelium	Mostly excreted unchanged via kidneys	Hepatic; drug and active metabolite accumulate in tissues	Redistributed or excreted unchanged via kidneys
Elimination t$_{1/2}$	< 2 h	< 10 s	36 h	35–40 days	< 1 h
Active metabolites?	Monoethylglycine-xylidide (MEGX), glycine xylidide (GX)	No	No	Desethylamiodarone	No
Adverse effects	CNS toxicity (confusion, dysarthria, tremor, paraesthesiae, dizziness and convulsions). Cardiotoxicity (bradycardia, hypotension, asystole)	Dyspnoea, flushing, bronchospasm, bradycardia and, occasionally, ventricular standstill or malignant tachyarrhythmias	Cardiac arrhythmias (especially ventricular arrhythmias, heart block), CNS toxicity (fatigue, agitation, nightmares, visual disturbances), anorexia and nausea or abdominal pain	Bradycardia, hypotension, thrombophlebitis. With long-term therapy, corneal microdeposits, cutaneous rash, hypothyroidism, confounding of thyroid function tests	Vasodilatation, hyporeflexia, neuromuscular blockade, cardiac conduction changes, cardiac arrest and electrolyte disturbances.
Notes			Toxicity increased by hypokalaemia; plasma concentrations increased by quinidine, amiodarone, verapamil; specific digoxin antibody available for treatment of toxicity. Plasma concentrations should be monitored	Avoid co-administration with other drugs which prolong QT interval (e.g. diltiazem, verapamil, phenothiazines, sotalol or class 1a antiarrhythmics); significant drug interactions, including increasing plasma digoxin concentrations and potentiation of warfarin and heparin	Plasma concentrations should be monitored

analogue of amiodarone which also blocks multiple channels including L-type Ca^{2+} and inward Na^+ currents. Both are used for the long-term treatment of atrial fibrillation.

Class 4 Antiarrhythmic Drugs

Class 4 drugs (calcium channel blockers) prevent voltage-dependent calcium influx during depolarization, particularly in the SA and AV nodes. Verapamil is more selective for cardiac cells than other calcium channel blockers but it is also a coronary and peripheral vasodilator, and decreases myocardial contractility. It depresses AV conduction, is effective in supraventricular or re-entrant tachycardia and controls the ventricular rate in atrial fibrillation. However, it is contraindicated in WPW syndrome because conduction through the accessory pathway may be encouraged, leading to ventricular fibrillation. Intravenous administration may cause hypotension (by vasodilatation), and caution is necessary in low-output states and in patients treated with negative inotropic drugs, e.g. β-blockers, disopyramide, quinidine or procainamide. Verapamil and diltiazem are effective by both i.v. and oral routes.

Other Antiarrhythmics

Adenosine is an endogenous purine nucleoside which mediates a variety of natural cellular functions via membrane-bound adenosine receptors, of which several subtypes (A_1–A_4) have been identified. Myocardial A_1-receptors activate potassium channels and decrease cAMP by activating inhibitory G_i-proteins; A_2-receptors mediate coronary vasodilatation by stimulating endothelial-derived relaxing factor and increasing intracellular cAMP. Increased potassium conductance induces membrane hyperpolarization in the SA and AV nodes, reducing automaticity and blocking AV node conduction. Adenosine also has an antiadrenergic effect in calcium-dependent ventricular tissue. It effectively converts paroxysmal supraventricular tachyarrhythmias (including those associated with WPW syndrome) to sinus rhythm, is used in the diagnosis of broad complex tachycardias when the origin (ventricular or supraventricular) is uncertain but is ineffective in the conversion of atrial flutter or fibrillation. In patients unable to exercise, adenosine is used as a coronary vasodilator in combination with myocardial perfusion scanning to diagnose coronary artery disease. Adenosine is metabolized to AMP or inosine by erythrocytes and vascular endothelial cells, so that it has a very short duration of action and is given as a rapid i.v. bolus.

Magnesium sulphate. Magnesium is a cofactor for many enzyme systems, including myocardial Na^+/K^+ ATPase. It antagonizes atrial L and T type Ca^{2+} channels, so that it prolongs both atrial refractory periods and conduction, and also inhibits K^+ entry and suppresses ventricular afterdepolarizations. Intravenous magnesium sulphate is the treatment of choice for torsades de pointes, a type of ventricular tachycardia occasionally induced by class 1a or class 3 antiarrhythmic drugs which prolong the QT interval. It is a second-line treatment for supraventricular and ventricular arrhythmias, particularly those associated with digoxin toxicity or hypokalaemia, and is used as an anticonvulsant in patients with pre-eclampsia. Magnesium is redistributed rapidly into bone (50%) and intracellular fluid (45%), with the remainder excreted via the kidneys. It is therefore administered as an i.v. infusion.

Cardiac Glycosides

Digoxin and digitoxin are cardiac glycosides derived from plant sources, principally *Digitalis purpura* and *Digitalis lanata*. Their structure comprises a cyclopentanophenanthrene nucleus, an aglycone ring (responsible for the pharmacological activity) and a carbohydrate chain made up of sugar molecules (which aid solubility). Digitalis compounds have been used for over 200 years for the treatment of heart failure but have been largely superseded and are now principally indicated for the control of ventricular rate in supraventricular arrhythmias, particularly atrial fibrillation. They have several actions, including direct effects on the myocardium and both direct and indirect actions on the ANS. They increase myocardial contractility and decrease conduction in the AV node and bundle of His. Action potential and refractory period durations in atrial cells are reduced, and the rate of phase 4 depolarization in the SA node (automaticity) is decreased. The refractory periods of the AV node and bundle of His are increased, but in the ventricles, refractory period is decreased and spontaneous depolarization rate increases. This increased ventricular excitability is more marked in the presence of hypokalaemia and may lead to the appearance of ectopic pacemaker foci. The principal direct cardiac action is inhibition of membrane Na^+/K^+-ATPase activity. Intracellular Na^+ concentration and Na^+/Ca^{2+} exchange increase, leading to increased availability of intracellular Ca^{2+} and increased myocardial contractility. Increased local catecholamine concentrations as a result of decreased neuronal re-uptake and increased central sympathetic drive may also contribute to this positive inotropic action. In addition to direct cardiac actions, digitalis compounds have direct and indirect vagal effects. Central vagal tone, cardiac sensitivity to vagal stimulation, and local myocardial concentrations of acetylcholine are all increased and these effects may be partly antagonized by atropine.

Digoxin has a large apparent volume of distribution and a long half-life, so that effective plasma concentrations occur after approximately 5–7 days unless a loading dose is given. Doses should be reduced in renal impairment or elderly patients. The therapeutic index is low and toxicity is likely at plasma concentrations $>2.5\,\text{ng}\,\text{mL}^{-1}$. However, plasma concentrations are a poor guide to toxicity because the drug is concentrated in cardiac and other tissues. Even at therapeutic plasma concentrations, digitalis affects the ECG, causing repolarization abnormalities. The classic 'digoxin effect' on ECG is of downsloping ('reverse tick') ST-segment depression with T wave inversion which may be wrongly interpreted as ischaemia. These changes are usually widespread, are not confined to the territory of one coronary artery and do not indicate toxicity. Digoxin toxicity usually causes cardiac, CNS, visual and gastrointestinal disturbances, including almost any arrhythmia, although ventricular arrhythmias (extrasystoles, bigeminy and trigeminy) and various degrees of heart block are commonest. Supraventricular arrhythmias also occur, often with some degree of conduction block. Digoxin should be avoided in the presence of second-degree heart block, ventricular tachycardia or aberrant conduction pathways (e.g. WPW syndrome) because arrhythmias may be precipitated, and should be used with caution after myocardial infarction. Sensitivity to digoxin is increased by hypokalaemia, hypomagnesaemia, hypercalcaemia, renal impairment, chronic pulmonary or heart disease, myxoedema and hypoxaemia. β-Blockers and verapamil have combined effects on the AV node and digoxin should be administered cautiously. Treatment of serious arrhythmias involves careful administration of KCl under ECG monitoring (especially in the presence of heart block or renal impairment). Lidocaine and phenytoin are useful for ventricular arrhythmias, β-blockade for supraventricular arrhythmias, and bradyarrhythmias may be treated with atropine. Digoxin should be stopped for at least 48 h before elective DC cardioversion, otherwise ventricular fibrillation may be precipitated. If cardioversion is required, the initial energy level should be low (e.g. 10–25 J) and increased if necessary.

Digitoxin is metabolized by the liver, and is less dependent upon renal function for its elimination. It has a very long half-life (4–6 days), so maintenance doses may be required only on alternate days, but this is also a disadvantage as toxic effects are very persistent.

FURTHER READING

Calvey, T.N., Williams, N.E., 2008. Principles and practice of pharmacology for anaesthetists, fifth ed. Blackwell Science, Oxford.
Stoelting, R.K., 2005. Pharmacology and physiology in anesthetic practice, fourth ed. Lippincott, Williams & Wilkins, Philadelphia.
Sweetman, S.C. (Ed.), 2011. Martindale: the complete drug reference, thirty-seventh ed. Pharmaceutical Press, London.

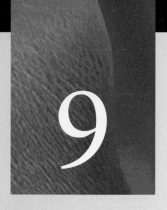

9 DRUGS ACTING ON THE RESPIRATORY SYSTEM

■ ■ ■ ■ ■ ■ ■ ■ ■ ■ ■

An understanding of how drugs interact with the respiratory system is vital for anaesthetists and those working in critical care. Knowledge of the drugs discussed in this chapter will facilitate effective management of common, potentially life-threatening medical emergencies. An appreciation of the steps in the British Thoracic Society guidelines on asthma management may help risk-stratify and optimize asthmatic patients in the perioperative period. Oxygen is increasingly being considered as a therapeutic agent or drug requiring a written prescription. Nearly 300 serious incidents associated with oxygen misuse, including nine deaths, were reported to the National Patient Safety Agency (NPSA) over a 5-year period. Anaesthetists are well placed to lead implementation of the NPSA's recent guidance and assist in the education of other healthcare staff regarding the safe use of oxygen.

DRUGS AFFECTING AIRWAY CALIBRE

Airway smooth muscle tone results from a balance between opposing sympathetic and parasympathetic influences (Fig. 9.1). Sympathetic activity causes bronchodilatation while cholinergic parasympathetic activity from the vagus nerve causes bronchoconstriction. Drugs which increase sympathetic influence or decrease cholinergic parasympathetic activity generally cause bronchodilatation by relaxation of airway smooth muscle, and so may be used in the management of asthma and chronic obstructive pulmonary disease (COPD). Sympathetic control is mediated at a cellular level by β_2-receptors. Agonists such as adrenaline

that bind to these G-protein coupled receptors (G_s) stimulate adenylate cyclase. This enzyme catalyses the conversion, within the cell, of adenosine triphosphate (ATP) to cyclic adenosine monophosphate (cAMP). Through kinase enzyme systems, cAMP relaxes airway smooth muscle. Cyclic AMP is degraded to inactive 5'-AMP by the enzyme phosphodiesterase. Drugs that increase the concentration of cAMP within the cell relax airway smooth muscle (e.g. β_2-agonists, phosphodiesterase inhibitors). Conversely, drugs which reduce the level of cAMP (e.g. β_2-antagonists) may cause bronchoconstriction.

The cholinergic parasympathetic system is mediated through several subtypes of muscarinic receptor. The most common subtype found in pulmonary tissue is the M_3 receptor. This is also a G-protein coupled receptor (G_q) but one which, when activated, stimulates phospholipase C to produce inositol triphosphate, which then binds to sarcoplasmic reticulum receptors causing release of calcium from intracellular stores, and so results in smooth muscle contraction and bronchoconstriction. Therefore muscarinic agonists cause bronchoconstriction and anticholinergic drugs cause bronchodilatation.

A third, minor, neural pathway also exists, referred to as the non-cholinergic parasympathetic system. This is a bronchodilator pathway which has vasoactive intestinal peptide (VIP) as its neurotransmitter and nitric oxide (NO) as the second messenger. The physiological significance of this in humans is unknown.

Histamine and other mediators also play an important role in promoting bronchial constriction via H_1-receptors, especially during anaphylaxis, drug

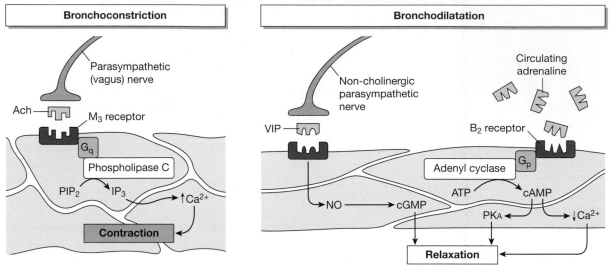

FIGURE 9.1 ■ Summary of the three physiological systems that control airway smooth muscle contraction. See text for details. ACh, acetylcholine; G_q and G_s, G-proteins; PIP_2, phosphatidylinositol biphosphate; IP_3, inositol triphosphate; VIP, vasoactive intestinal peptide; NO, nitric oxide; cGMP, cyclic guanosine monophosphate; ATP, adenosine triphosphate; PKA, phosphokinase; cAMP, cyclic adenosine monophosphate.

reactions, allergy, asthma and respiratory infections. Anti-inflammatory agents (e.g. steroids) and membrane stabilizers (e.g. sodium cromoglicate) may reduce or prevent bronchoconstriction in these conditions.

Bronchodilators

Bronchodilators are used commonly in the management of acute asthma or an exacerbation of COPD with the aim of reversing the abnormal bronchospasm that occurs in these potentially life-threatening conditions. All doctors working in acute specialties need to be familiar with their use. Anaesthetists, by ensuring optimal bronchodilator therapy, may avoid the need for invasive ventilation in some patients. In addition to alleviating the symptoms of wheeze and dyspnoea, bronchodilators improve the adequacy of ventilation and decrease the work of breathing.

β-Adrenergic Agonists

β-Adrenergic agonists are usually the first-line treatment for relieving bronchospasm in asthma and COPD. These drugs have additional beneficial effects in the management of asthma (Table 9.1). There are at least three subtypes of β-receptor in the body: β_1 is found in cardiac tissue, β_2 in pulmonary tissue and peripheral

TABLE 9.1
Effects of β-Agonist Drugs on the Airways

Specific
Increase in intracellular cAMP and bronchodilatation

Non-Specific but Complementary
Inhibition of mast cell mediator release
Inhibition of plasma exudation and microvascular leakage
Prevention of airway oedema
Increased mucous secretion
Increased mucociliary clearance
Prevention of tissue damage mediated by oxygen free radicals
Decreased acetylcholine release in cholinergic nerves by an action on prejunctional β_2-receptors

vasculature and β_3 in adipose tissue. Although nonselective β-agonists such as adrenaline and ephedrine can be used as bronchodilators, their unwanted β_1 action (e.g. tachycardia) has meant that β_2-specific agonists are preferred. Salbutamol, a synthetic sympathomimetic amine, is the most commonly used selective β_2-agonist. Although developed as a selective β_2-agonist, salbutamol may have β_1 side-effects in high doses or in the presence of hypoxaemia or hypercapnia. Salbutamol is a short-acting bronchodilator with a fast onset of action used for the relief of acute symptoms.

Indications

- Asthma
- COPD
- Hyper-reactive airways in patients undergoing mechanical ventilation
- Bronchospasm caused by allergic reactions and anaphylaxis
- Bronchospasm following aspiration or inhalation of toxins.

Route of Administration and Dose. Inhalation is usually the most appropriate route of administration of β_2-agonists in order to minimize systemic side-effects. An inhaled drug may also be more effective, because it easily reaches the mast and epithelial cells of the airway which are relatively inaccessible to a drug administered systemically. Salbutamol is administered from a pressurized aerosol (100 µg per puff; 1 or 2 puffs four times daily). The effect lasts for 4–6 h. The drug may also be nebulized in inspired gases and inhaled via a face mask or added to the breathing system in patients undergoing artificial ventilation. For this purpose, a dose of 2.5–5 mg up to four times daily is used. In severe bronchospasm, up to 5 mg may be given as frequently as every 30 min initially. Side-effects are more likely when these drugs are nebulized as they deliver a larger dose of which a significant proportion is absorbed systemically.

Oral administration has no advantage over the inhalational route and is associated with a greater incidence of adverse-effects. Intravenous administration is used occasionally, as a last resort, when bronchospasm is so severe that an aerosol or nebulizer is unlikely to deliver the drug to the narrowed airways or when inhalational therapy has failed. Intravenous administration is associated with more frequent systemic side-effects and should be used only when the patient is appropriately monitored.

Salmeterol is a more potent, longer acting β_2-agonist than salbutamol. Its effects last up to 12 h, allowing twice daily administration for the prevention of asthma attacks. It is available as an aerosol inhaler (dose: 50–100 µg twice daily).

Adverse Effects. Adverse effects of β-agonists include the following:

- tachycardia/tachyarrhythmias (β_1 effect)
- decreased peripheral vascular resistance and postural hypotension (β_2 effect)
- muscle tremor – resulting from a direct effect on β_2-receptors in skeletal muscle
- hypokalaemia caused by increased uptake of potassium ions by skeletal muscles (β_2 effect)
- metabolic effects – increases in the plasma concentrations of free fatty acids, insulin, glucose, pyruvate and lactate (β_3 effects)
- potentiation of non-depolarizing muscle relaxants.

Bronchodilatation may lead to transient hypoxaemia due to increased $\dot{V}/\dot{Q}$ mismatch and inhibition of the normal hypoxic pulmonary vasoconstriction mechanism. This may be overcome easily by supplying supplementary oxygen. β_2-agonists also cause relaxation of the gravid uterus and may be used in the management of pre-term labour.

Anticholinergic Drugs

The use of anticholinergic agents for their bronchodilator properties dates back two centuries when *Datura* plants were smoked for the relief of asthma. As an anticholinergic, atropine does cause bronchodilatation but side-effects such as tachycardia and dry mucous membranes limit its usefulness. Anticholinergic drugs are usually used as second-line agents in the management of acute bronchospasm and are very effective in reducing the frequency of acute exacerbations of COPD when taken regularly. One of the most commonly used drugs is ipratropium bromide. It is a synthetic quaternary ammonium compound derived from atropine. Ipratropium is active topically and there is little systemic absorption from the respiratory tract. Mast cell stabilization has also been proposed as a complementary mechanism of action. Maximum effect occurs 30–60 min after inhalation and may continue for up to 8 h. Tiotropium is a more recently introduced antimuscarinic bronchodilator with a longer duration of action that allows once daily administration.

Indications. Ipratropium is used as a second-line bronchodilator in acute exacerbations of asthma and COPD. It has an additive effect when used in combination with β-agonists. It is particularly effective in older patients with COPD. Tiotropium is prescribed to COPD patients with the aim of decreasing frequency of exacerbations; it is not useful in the treatment of acute bronchospasm.

Route of Administration and Dose. Ipratropium can be delivered from a metered dose inhaler (20–40 µg) or as a nebulizer (250–500 µg) up to four times daily. Tiotropium is delivered as a dry powder by a 'Spiriva HandiHaler' device; the dose is 18 µg once daily.

Adverse Effects. Dry mouth is the most commonly reported adverse effect of the antimuscarinic bronchodilators. Other less frequent side-effects include nausea, constipation and palpitations. The drugs are well known to precipitate acute urinary retention and so should be used with caution in patients with benign prostatic hypertrophy. They may also cause acute angle-closure glaucoma, particularly when given as a nebulizer (accidental instillation into the eye) with salbutamol.

Methylxanthines

The bronchodilator effect of strong coffee was first described in the 19th century. Methylxanthines, which are chemically related to caffeine, have been used to manage obstructive airways disease since the 1930s. Theophylline is the most commonly used methylxanthine and is available as an oral modified-release preparation. Aminophylline is a water-soluble salt which is used as an injectable form of theophylline. Methylxanthines have widespread effects involving multiple organ systems. With regard to their bronchodilator effects, the following mechanisms have been proposed:

- phosphodiesterase inhibition, leading to increased intracellular cAMP
- adenosine receptor antagonism, preventing mast cell degranulation
- endogenous catecholamine release
- prostaglandin inhibition
- interference with calcium mobilization
- potentiation of β_2-agonists.

Methylxanthines also increase cardiac output and the efficiency of the respiratory muscles, including improved diaphragmatic contractility. Aminophylline has been used occasionally in the management of heart failure and is known to reduce the frequency of apnoea in the premature neonate.

Indications. Methylxanthines are usually prescribed when inhaled therapies have failed or have been only partly effective. They are particularly useful in COPD.

Recently, they have been shown to improve exercise tolerance in intensive care patients on a weaning programme.

Route of Administration and Dose. Theophylline may be used as a sustained release oral preparation for the prevention of acute exacerbations of COPD. The dose depends on the preparation being used and is given twice daily. Aminophylline is an intravenous preparation used for the relief of acute episodes of bronchospasm. It is a strong alkaline solution and should not be given intramuscularly or subcutaneously. A loading dose of 5 mg kg^{-1} should be given slowly over 20 min followed by an infusion of 0.5-0.7 mg kg^{-1} h^{-1}. If the patient is already taking an oral theophylline, then the loading dose should be omitted.

There is a close relationship between the degree of bronchial dilatation and the plasma concentration of theophylline. A concentration of <10 mg L^{-1} is associated with a mild effect and a concentration of >25 mg L^{-1} with frequent side-effects. Consequently, the therapeutic window is narrow and the plasma concentration should be maintained within the range 10–20 mg L^{-1} (55–110 µmol L^{-1}). Plasma assays should be performed 6 h after commencing an infusion or following a rate change and then every 24 h. Approximately 40% of the drug is protein-bound. Theophylline is metabolized mainly in the liver by cytochrome P450 microenzymes; 10% is excreted unchanged in urine. Factors which affect the activity of hepatic enzymes and thus the clearance of the drug are summarized in Table 9.2. The infusion rate

---

TABLE 9.2

Factors Affecting the Plasma Concentration of Methylxanthines for a Given Dose

Factors Which Lower the Plasma Concentration:
Children
Smoking
Enzyme induction – rifampicin, chronic ethanol use, phenytoin, carbamazepine, barbiturates
High protein diet
Low carbohydrate diet

Factors Which Increase the Plasma Concentration:
Old age
Congestive heart failure
Enzyme inhibition – erythromycin, omeprazole, valproate, isoniazid, ciprofloxacin
High carbohydrate diet

of aminophylline should be adjusted accordingly (e.g. 1.6 times for smokers, 0.5 times for patients receiving erythromycin). The dose for obese patients should be based on ideal body weight and frequent estimation of plasma concentration is required to prevent ineffective therapy or toxicity.

Adverse Effects. Adverse effects of methylxanthines may be severe and are more likely to occur in patients also receiving a β-agonist bronchodilator or other sympathomimetic drugs.

- *Central nervous system effects:* stimulation of the CNS may lead to nausea, restlessness, agitation, insomnia, tremor and seizures. Some CNS effects (e.g. tremor) may occur even with therapeutic plasma concentrations of the drug.
- *Cardiovascular effects:* methylxanthines have positive chronotropic and inotropic effects on the heart. Tachyarrhythmias may occur with therapeutic doses, especially in the presence of halothane.
- *Renal effects:* methylxanthines cause increased urine output which may be related to an effect on tubular function or may be an indirect effect of the increased cardiac output. They may also lead to hypokalaemia.
- *Miscellaneous effects:* methylxanthines are known to increase gastric acid secretion and promote gastro-oesophageal reflux.

Extreme care should be exercised when administering aminophylline in the presence of hypoxaemia, hypercapnia, dehydration, hypokalaemia or cardiac arrhythmias. Patients must be monitored closely. Deaths caused by gross hypokalaemia and cardiac arrhythmias have been reported. If toxic symptoms develop, administration of the drug should be discontinued and symptomatic treatment provided. Serum potassium concentration should be measured and corrected if necessary. In extreme cases, haemodialysis may be required to hasten elimination of the drug.

Anti-Inflammatory Agents

Steroids

Steroids are used commonly as anti-inflammatory agents. Synthetic glucocorticoids have metabolic, anti-inflammatory and immunosuppressive effects (Table 9.3). They are able to penetrate the cell membrane

TABLE 9.3
Sites of Action for the Anti-Inflammatory Effects of Steroids

Site of Action	Mechanism
Intracellular steroid receptors	Steroid–receptor complex alters the transcription of genes leading to altered protein synthesis
Lipocortin	Increased lipocortin production inhibits release of arachidonic acid metabolites and platelet-activating factor from lung and macrophages
Eosinophils	Decrease in the number of eosinophils and inhibition of degranulation
T lymphocytes	Reduction in the number of T lymphocytes and the production of cytokines
Macrophages	Reduced secretion of leukotrienes and prostaglandin
Endothelial cells	Reduction of the leak between cells
Airway smooth muscle β$_2$-adrenoceptors	Increased agonist sensitivity, augmenting the effect of agonists; increase in receptor density and prevention of tachyphylaxis
Mucous glands	Reduced mucous secretion

and interact with intracellular steroid receptors, influencing transcription of genes and protein synthesis. Steroid administration leads to reduced numbers of lymphocytes and eosinophils, reduced secretion of prostaglandins from macrophages and a reduction in endothelial permeability. Steroids also increase the sensitivity of β$_2$-adrenoceptors to both endogenous and inhaled agonists and help prevent tachyphylaxis to adrenoceptor agonists such as salbutamol. There is some evidence that high-dose inhaled steroids help to slow the airway remodelling that results from chronic inflammation in asthma. Remodelling consists of airway smooth muscle hypertrophy, excess mucous glands and thickening of the basement membrane. It is thought to be one cause for the airway hyper-responsiveness that is characteristic of asthma.

Indications. Inhaled steroids are used commonly in the management of chronic asthma to reduce the frequency of attacks. They are usually considered when

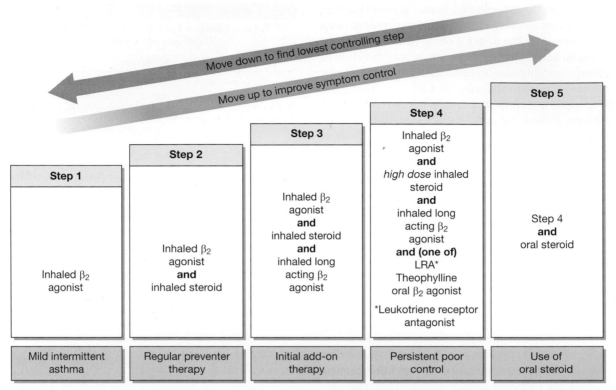

FIGURE 9.2 ■ Summary of the British Thoracic Society asthma management guidelines. *(Adapted from British Thoracic Society Scottish Intercollegiate Guidelines Network (2011): British Guideline on the Management of Asthma.)*

patients require a β_2-agonist more than twice a week, if symptoms disturb sleep more than once a week or if the patient has suffered exacerbations in the last 2 years which required a systemic corticosteroid. The addition of an inhaled steroid constitutes 'Step 2' of the British Thoracic Society (BTS) guidelines for the management of asthma (Fig. 9.2). Some patients with COPD may have steroid-responsive disease. Inhaled steroids are unlicensed for COPD but may be considered in patients with an FEV_1 <50% of predicted, or for patients having more than two acute exacerbations requiring oral steroids per year. Oral and intravenous steroids are useful in the management of acute asthma or COPD. They may also have a role in the treatment of sarcoidosis, interstitial lung disease and pulmonary eosinophilia.

Route of Administration and Dose. The three most commonly used inhaled steroids are shown in Table 9.4. Standard doses are those used in Step 2 of the BTS

TABLE 9.4
Doses of Inhaled Steroids. Step 2 and Step 4 Refer to British Thoracic Society Asthma Guidelines (Fig. 9.2)

Steroid	Standard (Step 2) Dose	High (Step 4) Dose
Beclometasone dipropionate	100–400 µg twice daily	0.4–1.0 mg twice daily
Fluticasone dipropionate	50–200 µg twice daily	200–500 µg twice daily
Mometasone furoate	200 µg twice daily	400 µg twice daily

guidelines. If symptom control is still poor on Step 3 of the protocol (steroid+long acting β_2-receptor agonist) then high-dose inhaled steroid constitutes Step 4.

Systemic steroids are part of the standard treatment for acute asthma or COPD. In moderate acute attacks, prednisolone 40–50 mg per day may be given orally. In acute severe or acute life-threatening asthma, intravenous hydrocortisone 100 mg every 6 h may be required until oral prednisolone can be taken. Therapy is usually continued for 5–7 days. Long-term or high doses of steroids may cause adrenal suppression and if stopped abruptly may precipitate an Addisonian crisis. Courses of steroids lasting less than 3 weeks may usually be stopped abruptly without the risk of precipitating a crisis. Caution should be exercised in patients who have received repeated short courses, recently stopped long-term steroid therapy, those receiving evening doses, or patients receiving >40 mg (or equivalent) of prednisolone per day.

Adverse Effects. Steroids have many local and systemic side-effects which commonly limit their use. Inhaled drugs are less likely than oral or intravenous steroids to cause systemic side-effects but may cause local irritation and predisposition to oral candidiasis. Some of the recognized side-effects of steroids are listed in Table 9.5.

Other Drugs

Sodium Cromoglicate

This is a derivative of khellin, an Egyptian herbal remedy which was found to protect bronchi against allergens. The mechanism of action is not fully understood but is thought to involve the stabilization of mast cell membranes. By blocking calcium channels, the drug is able to prevent mast cell degranulation with its subsequent histamine release. It has traditionally been used in patients with asthma in whom exercise is a trigger. Exercise-induced asthma may, however, just be a marker of poorly controlled asthma. A 4–6 week trial is useful to assess responsiveness. It is given by inhaler in a dose of 5–10 mg (1 or 2 puffs) four times a day. Side-effects are rare but include coughing, transient bronchospasm and throat irritation. Very rarely, angioedema may be precipitated. Sodium cromoglicate can also be used topically for allergic conjunctivitis and orally for the prevention of food allergy.

Leukotriene Receptor Antagonists

The leukotriene receptor antagonists are an additional therapy useful in the management of chronic asthma. They may be used in addition to, or in place of, a long acting β_2-receptor agonist such as salmeterol in Step 3 of the BTS guidelines (Fig. 9.2). There are two drugs in this class in common clinical use: montelukast and zafirlukast. They may be particularly beneficial in exercise-induced asthma and may also be used in patients with seasonal allergic rhinitis who have concomitant asthma. Two oral drugs in this class are prescribed commonly; montelukast 10 mg is given once a day, usually in the evening, or zafirlukast 20 mg can be given twice a day. The most common adverse effects are gastrointestinal upset and abdominal pain, with headache and insomnia also reported. These drugs have been associated rarely with the development of Churg-Strauss vasculitis and patients should be told to report any rash or worsening of pulmonary symptoms.

Antihistamines

Antihistamines are not used in the management of COPD or asthma but are used commonly for symptom control in hay fever and have a role in the management of anaphylaxis. Antihistamines may be classified as sedating (older compounds which easily cross the blood–brain barrier) and non-sedating (newer drugs which do not cross into the CNS). Indications for antihistamines include hay fever, urticaria, insect bites, pruritus, nausea and anaphylaxis.

TABLE 9.5

Common Adverse Effects of Steroids

Local Effects (Inhaled Steroids)
Hoarse voice
Oral/pharyngeal candidiasis
Throat irritation and cough

Systemic Effects (from Inhaled or Systemic Steroids)
Adrenergic suppression
Fluid retention
Hypertension
Peptic ulceration
Diabetes mellitus
Increased appetite
Weight gain
Bruising and skin thinning
Osteoporosis
Cataracts
Psychosis

Many individual preparations exist but two of the most commonly used drugs are chlorphenamine (chlorpheniramine) and loratadine. Chlorphenamine is a sedating antihistamine given in a dose of 4 mg every 4–6 h to a maximum of 24 mg daily. For anaphylaxis, 10 mg can be given i.v. and may be repeated to a maximum of four doses daily. Loratadine is a nonsedating antihistamine taken as a 10-mg tablet once a day. Adverse effects from antihistamines are more commonly encountered with the older drugs and include sedation, headache and antimuscarinic effects such as urinary retention and dry mouth. Other rare adverse effects include liver dysfunction and angle-closure glaucoma.

DRUGS ACTING ON THE PULMONARY VASCULATURE

Physiological control of pulmonary vascular tone is mediated by neural and humoral influences. Many of these control mechanisms have mixed actions. Sympathetic nerves originating from T1–5 release noradrenaline, causing vasoconstriction via α-receptors. Parasympathetic nerves from the vagus cause vasodilatation via the action of acetylcholine on M_3 receptors by a nitric oxide (NO) dependent mechanism. There are also non-adrenergic non-cholinergic (NANC) nerves which cause vasodilation via NO release. Circulating catecholamines act on both α- and β_2-receptors within the pulmonary vasculature, with the former vasoconstrictor effect predominating. Arachidonic acid metabolites such as thromboxane and most prostaglandins produce vasoconstriction. However, prostacyclin (PGI_2) is a potent vasodilator. Other humoral influences include amines, peptides and nucleosides which have variable effects dependent upon resting vascular tone. Hypoxaemia and acidosis are well recognized to cause vasoconstriction and an increase in pulmonary vascular resistance.

The main therapeutic benefit of modifying pulmonary vascular tone is in reducing pulmonary vascular resistance (PVR) in disease states associated with pulmonary hypertension. Pulmonary hypertension is most commonly secondary to connective tissue disorders, chronic thrombotic disease, left heart failure or chronic hypoxaemia. It may rarely be due to idiopathic pulmonary arterial hypertension (IPAH), formerly known as primary pulmonary hypertension. With the exception of chronic thrombotic disease which may be successfully treated with by pulmonary artery embolectomy and lifelong anticoagulation, the other causes of pulmonary hypertension are managed by long-term manipulation of pulmonary vascular resistance.

Inhaled Agents

Nitric Oxide

Nitric oxide is a colourless and highly reactive gas, first studied by the English chemist Joseph Priestley in 1772. It is presented in grey/green cylinders, is highly lipid soluble, and easily crosses biological membranes.

Indications. Inhaled nitric oxide may be used in the management of critically ill patients with pulmonary hypertension or severe $\dot{V}/\dot{Q}$ mismatch. It may also form part of the management of persistent pulmonary hypertension of the newborn. Given as an inhaled preparation, it only vasodilates vessels close to well ventilated areas, thereby improving $\dot{V}/\dot{Q}$ matching (Fig. 9.3). It has negligible systemic effects because of its rapid inactivation by haemoglobin after diffusing into the pulmonary circulation.

Route of Administration and Dose. NO in nitrogen is available in concentrations between 400 and 1000 ppm. It is usually administered in doses between 20 and 80 ppm. Most studies suggest that the maximum effect occurs at the lower end of this dose range and that higher doses risk toxicity. NO can be administered safely only to a patient whose trachea is intubated and whose lungs are ventilated using a closed circuit system. The usual apparatus for delivery involves placing an injector device in the inspiratory limb between the gas outlet of the ventilator and the humidifier. The device detects gas flow going to the patient and injects an appropriate quantity of NO to achieve the desired inspired concentration.

Adverse Effects. One of the risks of NO therapy is its oxidation to nitrogen dioxide (NO_2). The rate of oxidation is directly proportional to the concentration of oxygen in the gas mixture, duration of mixing and the square of the concentration of NO. These higher oxides may react with water to form nitric and nitrous acids which can lead to lipid peroxidation, impaired

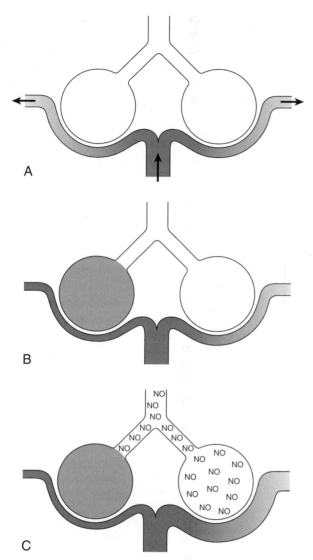

FIGURE 9.3 ■ Schematic diagram of two alveoli representing regions of lung with different V̇/Q̇ ratios. (**A**) Normal situation – all areas ventilated and equally perfused. (**B**) A region of lung is not ventilated, e.g. due to pulmonary oedema. Hypoxic pulmonary vasoconstriction reduces blood flow through this lung region; blood flow to the area which is still ventilated is unchanged, and pulmonary vascular resistance may increase. (**C**) Inhaled nitric oxide (NO) therapy – the NO reaches blood vessels only in the ventilated areas of lung and so vasodilates only these areas, resulting in better matching of ventilation and perfusion and reduced pulmonary vascular resistance.

mitochondrial function, prolonged bleeding time and mutagenesis. Therefore all delivery systems should measure levels of NO_2. NO therapy, especially in the newborn, may lead to methaemoglobinaemia. All patients receiving NO should have the methaemoglobin concentration monitored by arterial blood gas analysis; concentrations greater than 2% should be avoided. Some patients may display a rebound phenomenon on withdrawal of NO therapy, with worsening hypoxaemia and increased pulmonary vascular resistance. For this reason, NO therapy should be reduced gradually to allow endogenous production to restart.

Iloprost

Iloprost is a prostacyclin analogue which, unlike the parent drug, may be administered by nebulizer, avoiding the requirement for an indwelling tunnelled central venous catheter. Unfortunately, the drug has a short half-life, requiring administration 6–9 times daily. It is contraindicated in patients with unstable angina or those recovering from a recent myocardial infarction.

Oral Agents

Calcium Channel Antagonists

These agents may be used in the 10% of patients who have pulmonary hypertension responsive to vasodilator agents at cardiac catheterization. They are inexpensive and widely available. These drugs have negative inotropic effects and should be used cautiously in patients with severe right heart dysfunction.

Endothelin Receptor Antagonists

Endothelin is thought to play a role in the remodelling of pulmonary vessels which occurs in response to chronic hypoxaemia and leads to irreversible pulmonary hypertension. Endothelin antagonists such as bosentan prevent this remodelling by blocking the action of endothelin at ET_A and ET_B receptors. Bosentan is taken twice daily and liver function tests should be monitored monthly.

Phosphodiesterase Inhibitors

Sildenafil is an oral phosphodiesterase inhibitor better known as a treatment for erectile dysfunction. It is also effective when used to treat pulmonary arterial hypertension. Sildenafil inhibits the breakdown of secondary messengers cAMP and cGMP, leading to enhanced physiological vasodilatation. This class of drugs may also be administered by inhaled and intravenous routes.

Angiotensin-Converting Enzyme Inhibitors

These drugs are useful in patients with pulmonary hypertension secondary to chronic lung disease. Both traditional ACE inhibitors and the newer angiotensin II receptor antagonists can be used to reduce pulmonary artery pressure.

Intravenous Agents

Epoprostanol

Epoprostanol or prostacyclin has been shown to improve exercise tolerance and quality of life in patients with IPAH. Unfortunately, the drug has a short half-life of approximately 3 min and must therefore be administered as a continuous i.v. infusion. In practice, this requires the patient to have an indwelling, tunnelled central venous catheter such as a Hickman line. These long-term catheters are associated with infection risks and body image issues. The treatment was originally designed as a bridge to lung transplantation but data suggest that use of the drug may be associated with a similar improvement in life expectancy as lung transplantation. Adverse effects include flushing, headache and hypotension. Epoprostanol is also used commonly as a platelet inhibitor in renal replacement therapy.

DRUGS MODERATING VENTILATORY CONTROL

Respiratory Stimulants

Several classes of drug stimulate ventilation and may be used when ventilatory drive is inadequate. These agents increase respiratory drive through a variety of mechanisms. For example, strychnine blocks central inhibitory pathways, acetazolamide increases hydrogen ion concentration in the extracellular fluid around the respiratory centre and doxapram stimulates the respiratory centre directly. Only doxapram is now used commonly in clinical practice. Non-invasive ventilation (NIV) has now largely replaced respiratory stimulants in the management of respiratory failure. They may be used in the short-term if NIV is contraindicated or unavailable. Stimulants should not be used if muscle fatigue is thought to be contributing to respiratory failure.

Doxapram

Doxapram is the only specific respiratory stimulant available for use in anaesthesia and critical care.

Indications. Doxapram is used mostly to reverse postoperative respiratory depression following general anaesthesia. It may rarely be used in the management of acute respiratory failure or exacerbations of COPD. It is also used off-licence in the treatment of neonatal apnoea.

Route of Administration and Dose. When reversing postoperative respiratory depression, a dose of 1–$1.5\,mg\,kg^{-1}$ is given intravenously over 30 s and repeated if necessary after an hour. In exceptional cases, an intravenous infusion may be required. Up to $4\,mg\,kg^{-1}$ may be used in the treatment of acute respiratory failure, alongside oxygen therapy and frequent blood gas monitoring.

Adverse Effects. Intravenous injection of doxapram may cause perianal warmth, dizziness and sweating. The drug can lead to hypertension and tachycardia. It may rarely precipitate muscle fasciculation, laryngospasm, confusion and seizures. Administration should therefore be avoided in patients with uncontrolled hypertension, ischaemic heart disease or epilepsy. There is no role for doxapram in the management of laryngospasm or other causes of complete mechanical airway obstruction.

OXYGEN THERAPY

Oxygen therapy may be regarded as a therapeutic intervention with indications, benefits and adverse effects. It is increasingly being considered to be a pharmacological agent or drug. Oxygen is a colourless, odourless gas which forms 20.93% (by volume) of the Earth's atmosphere. It was first recognized as a distinct gas by Joseph Priestley in 1774 and was identified subsequently as the final universal oxidant in metabolic reactions. Atmospheric pressure at sea level is approximately 100 kPa and the partial pressure of oxygen which we breathe in air at sea level is 21 kPa. Alveolar oxygen partial pressure is reduced to 14.7 kPa by the addition of water vapour and carbon dioxide. Oxygen therapy is administered to hypoxaemic patients to increase alveolar oxygen partial pressure. The concentration of inspired oxygen administered depends on the condition being treated but should in most cases be titrated against either peripheral oxygen saturation or arterial oxygen tension. Administration of an excessive concentration of oxygen may be detrimental and, rarely, fatal. In patients with type 2 respiratory failure who rely on a hypoxic drive to breathe, sudden increases in inspired oxygen concentration may lead to apnoea.

Indications

The clinical indications for oxygen therapy are too numerous to list but it is useful to consider the causes of tissue hypoxia. There are four main classes of tissue hypoxia and oxygen therapy is likely to be of greatest benefit in the first.

1. Hypoxaemic hypoxia
   - reduced inspired partial pressure of oxygen, e.g. altitude
   - hypoventilation, e.g. caused by narcotics
   - diffusion impairment, e.g. pulmonary oedema
   - ventilation/perfusion mismatch or shunt, e.g. pulmonary embolus
2. Anaemic hypoxia
3. Ischaemic hypoxia
   - generalized ischaemia caused by inadequate cardiac output, e.g. hypovolaemia
   - local ischaemia and hypoxia, e.g. cerebral vascular accident
4. Cytotoxic hypoxia
   - inhibition of the final oxidative pathway, e.g. cyanide poisoning

Acute Oxygen Therapy

High-Concentration Oxygen Therapy

In most medical emergencies, oxygen therapy should be given quickly and in a high concentration because the avoidance of tissue hypoxia is of paramount importance. When managing patients with uncomplicated pneumonia, pulmonary embolism, sepsis, shock, trauma or anaphylaxis, up to 60% oxygen may be delivered via a simple oxygen mask (e.g. Hudson mask). Therapy should be titrated against peripheral oxygen saturations and in most patients a saturation of 94–98% is adequate. If higher concentrations are required, up to 80% oxygen may be given via a non-rebreathing or trauma mask in spontaneously breathing patients. During the management of cardiac arrest, 100% oxygen may be delivered via a closed circuit to an intubated patient. In severe carbon monoxide poisoning, hyperbaric oxygen therapy (HBOT) may be used

to increase the partial pressure of alveolar oxygen to >100 kPa.

Low-Concentration Oxygen Therapy

Low-concentration or controlled oxygen therapy is reserved for patients at risk of type 2 (hypercapnic) respiratory failure who may be harmed by uncontrolled high concentrations of oxygen. Patients with severe COPD, bronchiectasis, cystic fibrosis, severe kyphoscoliosis or ankylosing spondylitis are included in this group, as are patients with chronic musculoskeletal weakness on home ventilation therapy. Each case must be considered in the light of clinical findings but, as a general rule, oxygen therapy should be started at 24 or 28% and gradually titrated against oxygen saturation (SpO_2) or preferably arterial oxygen tension. An SpO_2 of 88–92% is often acceptable in these patients and may avoid pronounced hypercapnia and respiratory arrest. Patients are advised to carry an 'oxygen alert card' (Fig. 9.4) which, together with previous blood gas analysis results, may help to guide therapy.

Prescribing

The British Thoracic Society recommended in its 2008 publication 'Guideline for Emergency Oxygen Use in Adult Patients' that oxygen therapy should be prescribed by a doctor in common with other medical drugs. Both under-administration (e.g. postoperatively) and over-administration (e.g. in the COPD patient) of oxygen can cause harm. A prescription which includes target peripheral oxygen saturation (as described above) allows nursing staff to titrate the inspired oxygen concentration via various devices to

---

Oxygen alert card

Name: _____

I am at risk of type II respiratory failure with a raised CO_2 level.

Please use my _____ % Venturi mask to achieve an

oxygen saturation of _____ % to _____% during exacerbations

Use compressed air to drive nebulizers (with nasal oxygen at 2 l min⁻¹).
If compressed air not available, limit oxygen-driven nebulizers to 6 minutes.

FIGURE 9.4 ■ An oxygen alert card which may be carried by a patient who is known to be vulnerable to the respiratory depressant effects of inhaled oxygen therapy. *(Adapted from O'Driscoll, Howard and Davison (2008) BTS guideline for emergency oxygen use in adult patients. Thorax 63: Suppl 6.)*

achieve a measurable therapeutic end-point. The prescription should be signed when appropriate titration has occurred. Specialist prescription charts have improved patient safety with drugs such as theophylline and heparin, which require special monitoring; many centres are now introducing a similar chart with useful guidelines and flow charts for titrated oxygen therapy.

Long-Term Oxygen Therapy

Domiciliary or long-term oxygen therapy (LTOT) is prescribed for patients with severe COPD or a small number of other pulmonary diseases which lead to chronic hypoxaemia. Two studies in the 1980s suggested that using oxygen continuously for at least 15 h per day reduced mortality in patients with severe COPD. Other benefits of LTOT include a stabilization or small reduction in pulmonary arterial pressure, reduced polycythaemia and improved exercise tolerance. Some studies have shown that LTOT leads to an improved quality of life. The indications for LTOT are based on arterial oxygen tension measured by arterial blood gas analysis on two separate occasions, three weeks apart and at least four weeks after an acute exacerbation. COPD patients with a PaO_2 <7.3 kPa or a PaO_2 <8.0 kPa with secondary polycythaemia, peripheral oedema or pulmonary hypertension should be considered for home oxygen. Other conditions for which LTOT is considered, depending on the PaO_2, include pulmonary hypertension, cystic fibrosis, interstitial lung disease, chronic asthma and heart failure. Oxygen is usually prescribed at 2 or 4 L min^{-1} and can be supplied from either cylinders or an oxygen concentrator. Concentrators are provided for patients using oxygen for more than 8 h a day or consuming more than 21 cylinders a month. The oxygen is usually delivered via nasal cannulae, allowing the patient to talk, eat and drink. The patient should be advised to stop smoking and all smoking cessation therapy options should be explored. The prescriber should request the patient's permission to pass their details on to the local fire brigade. Ambulatory oxygen may also be provided for LTOT patients who frequently travel or spend nights away from home. The benefits of ambulatory oxygen therapy include improved compliance with LTOT (aiming for a minimum of 15 h per day) and increased exercise capacity.

Oxygen Toxicity

Oxygen, an element essential to life, may under certain circumstances produce toxic effects. Breathing high concentrations of oxygen at atmospheric pressure may lead to pulmonary toxicity. After inspiring 100% oxygen for as little as 12 h, healthy subjects have reported retrosternal discomfort, coughing and the urge to breathe deeply. Tracheobronchitis quickly supervenes and continued oxygen exposure may lead to neutrophil recruitment, impairment of surfactant and acute lung injury (ALI). Exposure to high concentrations of oxygen for a week may lead to pulmonary fibrosis. This process occurs at much lower oxygen concentrations in patients taking some chemotherapeutic agents. Cancer patients recently treated with bleomycin or mitomycin C may develop accelerated ALI and respiratory failure after exposure to only 40–50% oxygen. Neonates are also thought to be particularly sensitive to the damaging effects of hyperoxia. Babies are at risk of developing retrolental fibroplasias if the eyes are exposed to a PO_2 >10.6 kPa for longer than 3 h while under the age of 44 post-conceptual weeks. Hyperbaric conditions may cause pulmonary, optic and central nervous system toxicity. Oxygen at 2 bar causes a decrease in vital capacity of healthy volunteers after only 8 h, which persists after exposure has ceased. Hyperbaric oxygen causes narrowing of the visual fields and myopia in adults. Eventually, symptoms and signs of central nervous system toxicity ensue with nausea, facial twitching, olfactory/gustatory disturbances and ultimately tonic-clonic seizures. The underlying pathophysiology of toxicity is not well understood but may involve reactive oxygen species such as singlet oxygen interfering with enzyme systems containing sulphydryl groups.

DRUGS AFFECTING MUCOCILIARY FUNCTION

The mucous found in the airways is a non-homogeneous viscoelastic substance consisting of two phases separated by a thin film of surfactant. A superficial gel-like layer lies on a more liquid or aqueous layer in contact with the epithelial cells. Secretions from goblet cells and bronchial glands maintain the normal airway surface liquid (ASL). Goblet cells secrete mucopolysaccharides which form the gel-like layer and are stimulated by irritant factors. Epithelial cells and bronchial glands secrete the low-viscosity aqueous layer and are under vagal control. Two mechanisms exist to clear mucous from the respiratory tract: mucociliary clearance and cough clearance. The former is the dominant mechanism in health and relies on the forward propulsion of the gel layer on the aqueous layer by epithelial cell cilia. The efficiency of mucociliary clearance is affected by ciliary and ASL factors. Ciliary factors include beat frequency, amplitude and cilia spacing, while ASL factors include the depth of both layers of ASL, and the elasticity of the gel layer. Optimal aqueous layer depth is essential to ensure that the tips of the cilia interact with the gel layer only on their forward stroke. Cough clearance becomes more important in various disease states associated with impaired mucociliary clearance such as cystic fibrosis. A high-velocity interaction at the air–mucous layer boundary causes wave formation in the mucous layer, leading to forward propulsion. Many physical factors influence mucociliary function (Table 9.6) and several pharmacological agents have been developed to optimise sputum clearance.

Mucolytics

N-Acetylcysteine Derivatives

N-Acetylcysteine (NAC) is a cysteine derivative used commonly as a mucolytic. It is thought to induce physical changes in the structure of glycoproteins

present in mucous. It reduces the disulfide bond (S–S) to a sulphydryl bond (–SH) which discourages cross-linking, thereby reducing the viscosity of the mucous. It may be used in patients with COPD or bronchiectasis, including patients with cystic fibrosis, to reduce the viscosity of sputum. Carbocisteine is an oral derivative of NAC; 2.25 g may be taken initially, reducing to 1.5 g daily as symptoms improve. Nacystelyn is an inhaled lysine derivative of NAC which has been shown to reduce the viscoelasticity of mucus in patients with cystic fibrosis. Adverse effects of NAC derivatives include gastric erosion and bleeding secondary to disruption of the normal gastric mucosal barrier.

Dornase Alfa

High concentrations of undegraded DNA have been found in abnormally viscous sputum associated with poor sputum clearance. Dornase alfa is a genetically engineered version of a naturally occurring enzyme which is capable of cleaving DNA into smaller fragments. It acts only on extracellular DNA. The enzyme has an established role in the management of cystic fibrosis. Administration to cystic fibrosis patients with stable lung disease has been shown to improve FEV_1 by 5–7% and decrease the frequency of acute exacerbations. The dose is 2500 units or 2.5 mg by jet nebulizer once a day. Side-effects may include voice changes, laryngitis and chest pain.

Hypertonic Saline

Nebulized hypertonic saline has two mechanisms of action as a mucolytic. It disrupts the ionic bonds within the gel phase, reducing cross-linking and therefore mucous viscosity. It also causes water to shift from inside to outside the epithelial cells of the respiratory tract, thereby increasing the water content of the mucous. Hypertonic saline is used in patients with cystic fibrosis to enhance the removal of sputum and secretions. The usual dose is 4 mL of 6% sodium chloride nebulized twice a day. Excessive administration, especially in patients with renal impairment, may cause hypernatraemia.

TABLE 9.6

Factors Affecting Mucociliary Function

Factors that Depress Mucociliary Function:
Extremes of temperature
Acidic environment
Smoking
Dehydration
Alcohol
Anaesthetics
Dry Gases

Factors that Optimize Mucociliary Function:
Temperature range 29–34 °C
Hydration
Humidification

10

DRUGS USED IN RENAL DISEASE

DRUG CONSIDERATIONS IN PATIENTS WITH RENAL DYSFUNCTION

Influence of Renal Disease on Pharmacokinetics

Renal disease may affect drug pharmacokinetics through several mechanisms, especially effects on drug binding, distribution and elimination. Acidic drugs bind mainly to albumin. In renal failure, a decrease in serum albumin, an increase in serum urea, and the competition of endogenous substrates and drug metabolites for plasma protein binding sites lead to a decrease in the plasma protein binding of drugs. Highly protein-bound drugs have an increased unbound, active, free fraction. Under these circumstances, there may be an increase in the volume of distribution. Drugs are metabolized in the liver to water-soluble, inactive metabolites. Although uraemia has an effect on the intermediary metabolism of the liver, it does not seem to affect hepatic drug metabolism in humans.

The duration of action of most drugs administered by bolus or short-term infusion is dependent on redistribution and not elimination. It is usually not necessary to decrease the initial loading dose in patients with renal dysfunction, but subsequent maintenance doses may cause drug accumulation and should be reduced appropriately. The inactive water-soluble metabolites of drugs are eliminated by passive filtration at the glomerulus. A reduction in glomerular filtration in renal disease patients may lead to accumulation of these metabolites.

Influence of Drugs on Renal Function

All anaesthetic agents may cause a generalized depression of renal function which is transient and clinically insignificant. However, nephrotoxic drugs can impair renal function permanently. For example, they may lead to severe sodium and water depletion, reduction in renal blood supply, direct renal damage or renal obstruction (Table 10.1). Some drugs impair renal function by more than one mechanism.

Some of the fluorinated inhalation agents have well-recognized nephrotoxic effects, because they increase the serum inorganic fluoride concentration. Prolonged exposure of the renal tubules to fluoride ions impairs their ability to concentrate urine, leading to dehydration, hypernatraemia and increased plasma osmolarity. Experience with methoxyflurane (no longer in clinical use) has suggested that a plasma fluoride level of $50 \, \mu mol \, L^{-1}$ is potentially nephrotoxic. Although halothane and isoflurane do not seem to have a significant effect, prolonged administration of enflurane may lead to potentially nephrotoxic fluoride ion concentrations.

Sevoflurane undergoes approximately 5% metabolism and one of the primary metabolites is fluoride. There were initial concerns that sevoflurane may be similar to methoxyflurane and impair the ability of the kidneys to concentrate urine. However, after sevoflurane administration is stopped, there is a rapid decrease in plasma fluoride concentration because of its insolubility and rapid pulmonary elimination. Also, the metabolic production of fluoride within the kidney is much less with sevoflurane than with methoxyflurane. Though it would appear that sevoflurane

TABLE 10.1
Mechanisms of Drug-Induced Renal Damage
Sodium and water depletion
Reduced renal perfusion
Direct renal toxicity
Urinary obstruction

renal toxicity is not a problem in clinical practice, prolonged administration of sevoflurane is not recommended in patients with significantly impaired renal function.

Aprotinin is a serine-protease inhibitor and an antifibrinolytic agent occasionally administered during major surgery to improve haemostasis. It undergoes active reabsorption by the proximal tubules and is metabolized by enzymes in the kidney. There is some controversy about its effect on renal function. Although some studies have shown a low incidence of reversible renal dysfunction, others have shown changes in biochemical markers of tubular damage without evidence of renal impairment.

Other drugs with potential for impairing renal function include aminoglycosides, NSAIDs, radiocontrast agents and various chemotherapeutic drugs. The potential for renal damage with these drugs is increased in the presence of hypovolaemia, dehydration and sepsis.

Several drugs have been investigated for protection against renal damage or dysfunction in patients at risk, for example those undergoing cardiac or aortic surgery, or ICU patients with sepsis. However, there is little convincing evidence that any specific drug effectively prevents perioperative renal dysfunction, and some of the drugs used may be harmful. These are discussed below.

VASOACTIVE DRUGS USED IN RENAL DYSFUNCTION

Dopamine

Dopamine is an endogenous catecholamine precursor of noradrenaline and adrenaline, and is a neurotransmitter in its own right. It has complicated dose-dependent pharmacodynamic effects, including positive inotropy, chronotropy, vasoconstriction, and renal and splanchnic vasodilatation. Dopamine is inactive orally and has to be administered as an intravenous infusion, because it is metabolized within minutes by the enzymes dopamine β-hydroxylase and monoamine oxidase ($t_{1/2}$ <2 min). Dopamine must be diluted before infusion.

Mechanism of Action

Dopamine acts on dopaminergic and adrenergic receptors in a dose-related fashion. Dopaminergic receptors are present in various sites in the body and have been classified into five subtypes. The two most important receptors in the peripheral cardiovascular and renal systems are DA_1 and DA_2.

The infusion of relatively low doses ($<2\mu g\,kg^{-1}\,min^{-1}$) of dopamine activates postsynaptic DA_1 receptors in splanchnic blood vessels and the renal tubules. Stimulation leads to vasodilatation and increases cortical renal blood flow, glomerular filtration rate (GFR), sodium excretion and urine output. There is also an increase in mesenteric blood flow. Activation of presynaptic DA_2 receptors decreases intrarenal noradrenaline release, which leads to vasodilatation. It also causes inhibition of aldosterone secretion from the adrenal glands and a consequent decrease in sodium reabsorption. Theoretically, this should decrease renal oxygen consumption and improve the renal oxygen supply/demand relationship. At low infusion rates there is little change in cardiac output or heart rate. A reduction in arterial pressure may occur because of inhibition of the sympathetic nervous system by stimulation of the DA_2 receptors, and by DA_1-induced vasodilatation.

Increased infusion rates ($2–5\mu g\,kg^{-1}\,min^{-1}$) stimulate cardiac β_1- and β_2-adrenergic receptors, which causes an increase in myocardial contractility, stroke volume and cardiac output. At this infusion rate, the heart rate usually does not change.

Higher doses of dopamine ($>10\mu g\,kg^{-1}\,min^{-1}$) lead to stimulation of the α-adrenergic receptors, causing vasoconstriction, an increase in peripheral vascular resistance and decreases in renal and splanchnic blood flow.

The dopamine infusion rates given above are guidelines and there is considerable intra- and inter-patient variation. The maximum dose at which dopamine affects only dopamine receptors is debatable. In addition, up- and downregulation of receptors occurs so the appropriate dose for a required effect may vary from hour to hour and doses must be individually titrated.

Clinical Uses

Dopamine has been used widely in ICU and surgical patients at risk of renal dysfunction, because of its effects on renal blood flow, diuretic and natriuretic effects and also because urine output is used as a surrogate marker of tissue perfusion. However, clinical studies have not demonstrated any benefit of 'low-dose' dopamine for the prevention and treatment of acute kidney injury in critically ill or surgical patients. In fact, it reduces regional redistribution of blood flow within the kidney by shunting blood away from the outer medulla to the cortex. This is potentially detrimental in acute kidney injury given that the outer medulla is very susceptible to ischaemic injury.

The use of higher doses of dopamine as a positive inotrope during cardiac failure, or a vasopressor during hypotension, is well established. Under these circumstances, it probably has a beneficial effect on renal function, but it is important to ensure that there is an adequate circulating blood volume.

Side-Effects

Side-effects of dopamine include tachyarrhythmias, vasoconstriction with acute hypertension, and nausea and vomiting because of a direct effect on receptors within the chemoreceptor trigger zone. Intravenous administration of dopamine does not result in central nervous system effects as dopamine does not cross the blood–brain barrier. Other potentially detrimental effects of low-dose dopamine in the critically ill patient include the following.

- A decrease in splanchnic oxygen consumption in septic patients despite an increase in splanchnic blood flow
- A possible decrease in gastric motility compromising gastric feeding and absorption
- Impairment of regional ventilation-perfusion matching of the lung and the ventilatory drive in response to hypoxaemia and hypercapnia
- Reduced output of anterior pituitary hormones including prolactin, growth hormone, TSH and thyroid hormones
- Ideally, dopamine should be administered through a central venous catheter because extravasation may cause sloughing and necrosis of local surrounding tissues.

Dopexamine

Dopexamine is a synthetic catecholamine with structural and pharmacological similarities to dopamine; it is used for its increase in cardiac output and renal and splanchnic vasodilator effects. It is inactive orally and, because of its short half-life (~ 6 min), it is administered i.v. as an infusion. Infusion rate starts at $0.5\,\mu g\,kg^{-1}\,min^{-1}$ and is titrated to a therapeutic response (up to $6\,\mu g\,kg^{-1}\,min^{-1}$). Tolerance can occur and is usually associated with receptor downregulation. It is metabolized by the recognized pathways for all the catecholamines.

Dopexamine is an agonist at vascular and renal dopaminergic DA_1 and DA_2 receptors. It also stimulates cardiac and vascular β_2-receptors, and has a limited indirect β_1 effect. It therefore combines vasodilator, chronotropic and mild inotropic activity and is used in low cardiac output states where specific renal and hepatosplanchnic vasodilatation is considered beneficial. The heart rate is increased in a dose-related manner and it produces a natriuresis and diuresis. The protective effect of dopexamine on the kidneys is theoretical and an effect on outcome still has to be proven.

The most common side-effect is a tachycardia and ventricular ectopic beats when higher doses are used. Nausea and vomiting, probably caused by stimulation of DA_2 receptors in the chemoreceptor trigger zone, have been reported.

Fenoldopam

Fenoldopam is a selective DA_1 agonist. It may be administered orally or intravenously and has been used for the management of congestive cardiac failure, hypertension and renal protection after cardiac surgery, though current data are inconclusive. Its effects are slightly different to dopamine because of its DA_1 selectivity: fenoldopam may preferentially increase flow to the outer renal medulla, but it may also have anti-inflammatory effects.

Adenosine

Adenosine is a natural purine and is an important mediator in the control of renal blood flow and glomerular filtration. After i.v. administration it causes peripheral vasodilatation and decreased arterial pressure. Adenosine-induced arterial hypotension inhibits renin release by the juxtaglomerular cells and has an interesting effect on the renal vasculature, causing transient vasoconstriction of the afferent arterioles, combined with vasodilatation of the efferent arterioles. This results in decreases in renal blood flow and glomerular filtration pressure and rate. Adenosine A1 receptor antagonists increase GFR, urine production and sodium excretion without immediate effects on cardiac haemodynamics, and are being investigated for use in heart failure.

Adenosine also slows the heart rate and impairs atrioventricular conduction and is used in the treatment of supraventricular tachycardias (Ch 47).

Calcium Channel Blockers

Calcium channel blockers (CCBs) (Ch 8) are predominantly used in the treatment of hypertension. They act selectively on calcium channels in the cellular membrane of cardiac and vascular smooth muscle (VSM) cells. Free calcium within the VSM enhances vascular tone and contributes to vasoconstriction. CCBs reduce the transmembrane calcium influx in VSM cells, causing vasodilatation. In addition, CCBs have a direct diuretic effect that contributes to their long-term antihypertensive action. Nifedipine increases the urine volume and sodium excretion, and may inhibit aldosterone release. This diuretic action is independent of any change in renal blood flow or GFR.

Because of their vasodilator effects, CCBs are used in the management of conditions associated with pathological vasoconstriction, such as Prinzmetal's angina, migraine and Raynaud's disease.

In addition to renal vasodilatation, CCBs decrease calcium influx and production of oxygen free radicals in renal ischaemia. They therefore have theoretical benefits in patients undergoing renal transplantation. In transplant recipients, CCBs have been shown to improve intrarenal circulation, decrease the incidence of post-transplant acute tubular necrosis, and they may reduce the vasoconstrictive action of ciclosporin. However, despite these apparent benefits, CCBs have failed to improve graft survival. They may also cause hypotension and thereby decrease renal perfusion and there is no good clinical evidence that they have significant renal protective effects. CCBs may also enhance the effects of depolarizing and non-depolarizing neuromuscular blocking agents and this combination should be used with caution in patients with renal dysfunction.

Angiotensin-Converting Enzyme (ACE) Inhibitors

Most patients with heart failure and many with hypertension have increased activity of the renin–angiotensin–aldosterone system (RAAS). This leads to increased systemic vascular resistance, further decreases in cardiac output and renal perfusion, and more sodium and fluid retention. These patients are often receiving diuretics, which in itself triggers the RAAS. Angiotensin-converting enzyme (ACE) inhibitors (e.g. captopril, enalapril, lisinopril) are being used increasingly in this scenario, in place of, or in combination with, diuretics.

ACE inhibitors have a much greater affinity for the active site on the ACE than the natural substrate, angiotensin I. Consequently, the conversion of angiotensin I to angiotensin II is blocked. ACE is also responsible for the breakdown of bradykinin, a potent vasodilator. Therefore, ACE inhibitors lead not only to vasodilatation but, because of the decreases in aldosterone formation and sodium re-uptake, also have an indirect potassium-retaining diuretic effect. The combination of ACE inhibitors and the potassium-saving diuretics should be avoided because of the risk of hyperkalaemia.

Angiotensin II is important for the maintenance of an adequate glomerular filtration pressure in patients with decreased renal perfusion. In the presence of renal artery stenosis, the use of ACE inhibitors may lead to an impairment of renal function by decreasing renal perfusion pressure, caused by the decrease in arterial pressure together with dilatation of the efferent arteriole of the glomerulus. Underlying renal impairment should therefore always be excluded before using ACE inhibitors, and patients receiving these agents should be monitored carefully.

Noradrenaline/Adrenaline/Phenylephrine

Although noradrenaline and adrenaline also have β-receptor effects, all three of these drugs are very potent vasoconstrictors acting on the vascular α-receptors (Ch 8). Their use is often accompanied by fear of inducing decreases in renal blood flow, GFR and renal function.

The efferent arterioles are the major sites of flow resistance in the kidney and determine renal blood flow, perfusion pressure and GFR. In hypotension or septic shock, restoring the perfusion pressure of the kidney is of the utmost importance. An infusion of one of these vasoconstrictors may improve renal perfusion pressure, provided fluid resuscitation has been adequate. In septic shock, noradrenaline is preferred.

Antidiuretic Hormone (Vasopressin) and Desmopressin (DDAVP)

Antidiuretic hormone (ADH) is a naturally occurring hormone, produced in the hypothalamus, transported by nerve axons down to the posterior pituitary gland and thence secreted into the blood. The release of ADH is regulated by the osmolarity of the extracellular body fluids, changes in arterial pressure and intravascular volume, and the sympathetic nervous system. An increase in blood osmolarity and hypovolaemia stimulate the hypothalamic osmoreceptors and arterial baroreceptors as part of the stress response. ADH is released and acts primarily on receptors in the distal convoluted tubule and collecting ducts of the nephron to increase free water reabsorption and restore the plasma volume. The presence or absence of ADH determines to a large extent whether the kidney excretes a dilute or a concentrated urine. ADH is also termed vasopressin, because it has a very potent vasoconstrictor effect, even more powerful than that of angiotensin.

Vasopressin decreases splanchnic and renal blood flow and is sometimes used to treat bleeding oesophageal varices. There is some evidence that vasopressin may reduce progression to renal failure and mortality in ICU patients with septic shock.

Desmopressin (DDAVP, 1-desamino-8-D-arginine vasopressin) is a synthetic form of vasopressin that does not cause vasoconstriction. It is used in cases of central diabetes insipidus (i.e. spontaneous diuresis with a urine osmolarity $<200\,\mathrm{mosm\,L^{-1}}$).

DDAVP also has an influence on the coagulation system by increasing factor VIII von Willebrand (VIII:vWF), factor VIII coagulant (VIII:C), and factor VIII-related antigen (VIIIr:Ag) activity by stimulating their release from the storage sites. A dose of $0.3\,\mu\mathrm{g\,kg^{-1}}$ is often used in the treatment of haemorrhage in haemophiliacs.

Platelet dysfunction often occurs in renal disease when plasma urea concentrations are high. The increase in bleeding time ($>15\,\mathrm{min}$), despite a normal platelet count ($>100\times10^9\,\mathrm{L^{-1}}$), can be corrected before

major surgery. The most appropriate treatment currently is the administration of DDAVP in the same dose as above. It has also been used prophylactically to reduce bleeding after cardiac surgery.

DDAVP cannot be used repeatedly because the endothelial storage sites of factor VIII:C become depleted, resulting in tachyphylaxis. Because it also seems to release tissue plasminogen activator, DDAVP enhances fibrinolysis and the simultaneous use of an antifibrinolytic agent has to be considered. Although vasopressin is a vasoconstrictor, rapid injection of DDAVP may cause acute hypotension as a result of vasodilatation.

DIURETICS

Diuretics increase the excretion of both water and sodium. They are widely prescribed for hypertension, heart failure and clinical situations associated with fluid overload. When used on a long-term basis, they not only change the body's sodium and fluid balance, but also act as mild vasodilators. When diuretics are prescribed for the treatment of fluid retention and oedema, three important principles have to be kept in mind. First, although a dramatic diuretic response may be required in pulmonary oedema and acute cardiac failure, a mild sustained diuresis is more appropriate in the majority of patients and will reduce any adverse effects. Second, plasma potassium concentration and hydration status must always be monitored. Third, diuretic therapy only treats the symptoms and does not influence the underlying cause or change the outcome of a patient with oedema.

Some diuretic drugs have other potentially beneficial effects, e.g. reduction of renal tubular oxygen consumption and theoretical improvements in renal blood flow. In acute kidney injury (AKI), they may increase flow of solute through injured renal tubules, theoretically help maintain tubular patency and decrease tubular back-leak. It has also been believed that the prognosis of oliguric AKI is worse than non-oliguric AKI. For these reasons, diuretics have been used in the management of the oliguria in surgical patients or the critically ill, but studies have shown no clinical benefit. There is also no clear evidence that polyuric renal dysfunction has a better outcome than oliguric renal failure. Furthermore, the use of diuretics in oliguric patients may have adverse effects. These include adverse effects on distribution of intrarenal blood flow and inhibition of important feedback mechanisms; reduced circulating volume and renal perfusion pressure, with subsequent activation of the RAAS; and by maintaining urine flow, the clinician may delay the correction of hypovolaemia or optimization of cardiac output.

Diuretics are classified according to their mechanism and site of action on the nephron (see Fig. 10.1):

- glomerulus and proximal renal tubule – e.g. osmotic diuretics, carbonic anhydrase inhibitors
- ascending limb of the loop of Henle – e.g. loop diuretics
- distal tubule – e.g. thiazides, potassium-sparing diuretics
- collecting ducts – e.g. aldosterone antagonists.

Carbonic Anhydrase Inhibitors

Acetazolamide

Acetazolamide is well absorbed, not metabolized, but excreted almost unchanged by the kidney within 24 h. Toxicity is very rare.

Acetazolamide is a carbonic anhydrase inhibitor. Under normal physiological conditions, the enzyme carbonic anhydrase is responsible for reabsorption of sodium and excretion of hydrogen ions in the proximal convoluted tubule of the nephron. Inhibition of carbonic anhydrase decreases hydrogen ion excretion and therefore sodium and bicarbonate ions stay in the renal tubule. This results in the production of alkaline urine with a high sodium bicarbonate content; the increased sodium excretion leads to a modest diuresis. Chloride ions are retained instead of bicarbonate to

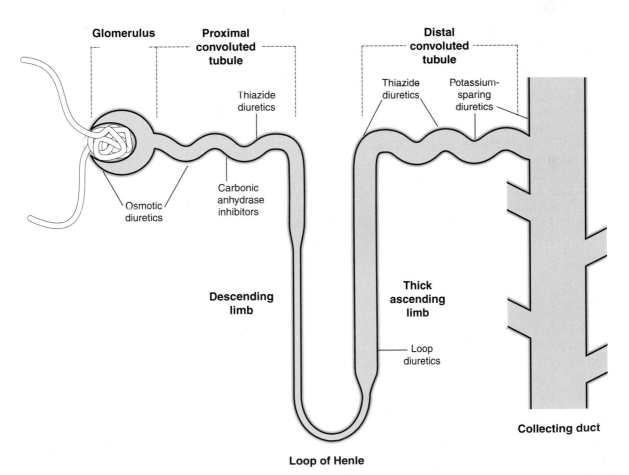

FIGURE 10.1 ■ Sites of action of diuretics.

maintain an ionic balance. All these changes result in a hyperchloraemic metabolic acidosis.

Carbonic anhydrase inhibitors are seldom used as primary diuretics because of their weak diuretic effect. They may be used in the management of salicylate overdose to produce an alkaline diuresis as this increases the urinary elimination of weak acids. The most common use of acetazolamide is to reduce the intraocular pressure of glaucoma patients. The inhibition of carbonic anhydrase results in a decreased formation of ocular aqueous humour and cerebrospinal fluid. It is also valuable in the prevention and management of acute mountain sickness. When used in patients with familial periodic paralysis, the metabolic acidosis increases the potassium concentration in the skeletal muscles and improves symptoms.

Osmotic Diuretics

Mannitol

Mannitol is an alcohol produced by the reduction of mannose. It is absorbed unreliably from the gastrointestinal tract and therefore has to be given by i.v. injection; doses of 0.25–1 g kg^{-1} are used. Initially it stays within the intravascular space but is then slowly redistributed into the extravascular compartment. Mannitol does not undergo metabolism and is excreted unchanged through the kidneys.

Mannitol expands the intravascular volume and then undergoes free glomerular filtration with almost no reabsorption in the proximal tubule. It also decreases the energy-consuming process of sodium and water reabsorption in the proximal tubule. This leads to an osmotic force that retains water and sodium in the tubule with a consequent osmotic diuresis, i.e. increased urinary excretion of sodium, water, bicarbonate and chloride. Mannitol does not alter urinary pH. The raised renal blood flow reduces the rate of renin secretion which decreases the urine-concentrating capacity of the kidney.

Mannitol has often been used prophylactically to protect the kidneys against an ischaemic incident (e.g. cardiopulmonary bypass, aortic cross-clamping or hypotensive episodes) and subsequent acute renal failure. Its theoretical effects include reduced proximal tubular oxygen demand, scavenging of oxygen free radicals, reduced tubular endothelial cell swelling and increased tubular flow which might maintain

tubular patency after ischaemic injury. However, there is no convincing evidence of a renal protective effect of mannitol in clinical practice. There is also little evidence that conversion from oliguric to non-oliguric renal failure decreases the mortality rate in critically ill patients. Nevertheless, mannitol is still used during renal transplantation to help 'preserve' the donor kidney.

Anaesthetists often administer mannitol to reduce intracranial pressure (Ch 32) and intraocular pressure.

Mannitol may precipitate pulmonary oedema in patients with compromised cardiac function. Occasionally, it may cause hypersensitivity reactions. If the blood–brain barrier is not intact after a head injury or neurosurgery, mannitol may enter the brain, draw water with it and cause rebound cerebral swelling.

Loop Diuretics

Loop diuretics act primarily on the medullary part of the ascending limb of the loop of Henle. After initial glomerular filtration and proximal tubular secretion, they inhibit the active reabsorption of chloride in the thick portion of the ascending limb. This leads to chloride, sodium, potassium and hydrogen ions remaining in the tubule to maintain electrical neutrality, and their increased excretion in the urine. The extent of the following diuresis is determined by the concentration of active drug in this part of the tubule. Because the ascending limb plays an important role in the reabsorption of sodium chloride in the kidney, these drugs produce a potent diuretic response. The decrease in sodium chloride reabsorption leads to a reduced urine-concentrating ability of the normally hypertonic medullary interstitium. Furosemide, bumetanide and torasemide are classified as loop diuretics because of their common site of action. Furosemide is the most commonly used.

Furosemide

Furosemide is usually administered intravenously (0.1–1 mg kg^{-1}) or orally (0.75–3 mg kg^{-1}). It is well absorbed orally and about 60% of the dose reaches the central circulation within a short period, with the peak effect after 1–1.5 h. Intravenous furosemide is usually started as a slow 20–40 mg injection in adults, but higher doses or even an infusion may be required in the case of elderly patients with renal failure or severe congestive cardiac failure. Typical doses in ICU patients are

2–5 mg per hour; i.v. infusions are associated with less toxicity than intermittent bolus doses. Approximately 90% of the drug is bound to plasma proteins and its volume of distribution is relatively low. Metabolism and excretion into the gastrointestinal tract contribute to about 30% of the elimination of a dose of furosemide. The remainder is excreted unchanged through glomerular filtration and tubular secretion. Impaired renal function affects the elimination process, but liver disease does not seem to influence this. The elimination half-life of furosemide is 1–1.5 h.

Furosemide increases renal artery blood flow if the intravascular fluid volume is maintained. It causes redistribution so that flow to the outer part of the cortex remains unchanged while inner cortex and medullary flow is increased. It leads to an improved renal tissue oxygen tension. This effect, together with the increased release of renin and the activation of the angiotensin–aldosterone axis, is mediated via prostaglandins. An advantage of loop diuretics is their high ceiling effect (i.e. increasing doses lead to increasing diuresis).

Furosemide is the diuretic of choice in acute pulmonary oedema or other states of fluid overload caused by cardiac, renal or liver failure. It reduces the intravascular fluid volume by promoting a rapid, powerful diuresis even in the presence of a low GFR. The pulmonary vascular bed and capacitance vessels are dilated by furosemide, and often a relief of dyspnoea and a reduction in pulmonary pressures may take place before the diuretic effect has occurred. In hypertensive patients, the vasodilatation and preload reduction lead to a decrease in arterial pressure.

Furosemide has been used widely in the management of the oliguric surgical or critically ill patient, but as with other diuretic drugs, studies have shown no clinical benefit. Furosemide should never be used to treat oliguria caused by a decreased intravascular fluid volume or dehydration, because the following diuresis could exaggerate hypovolaemia and renal ischaemic injury. It is important to restore the intravascular volume status first before any pharmacological intervention.

A raised intracranial pressure is often treated with furosemide. It mobilizes cerebral oedema fluid, decreases cerebrospinal fluid production and lowers intracranial pressure without changing plasma osmolarity. In contrast to mannitol, a disrupted blood–brain barrier does not influence the effect of furosemide on the intracranial pressure.

Excessive doses of furosemide often lead to fluid or electrolyte abnormalities. Severe hypokalaemia may precipitate dangerous cardiac arrhythmias, especially in the presence of high concentrations of digitalis. It may also enhance the effect of non-depolarizing neuromuscular blocking drugs. Hypovolaemia, dehydration and the consequent haemoconcentration may lead to changes in blood viscosity. Hyperuricaemia and prerenal uraemia may develop and may precipitate an acute gout attack in a patient with pre-existing gout.

Furosemide may cause high concentrations of aminoglycosides and cephalosporins in the kidneys and this may enhance their nephrotoxic effects. Prolonged high blood concentrations of furosemide may have a direct toxic action resulting in interstitial nephritis. It may also cause transient or permanent deafness because of changes in the endolymph electrolyte composition. Patients allergic to other sulphonamide drugs may have a cross-sensitivity, although idiosyncratic reactions are rare.

Bumetanide

The mechanism of action of bumetanide and its effects are similar to those of furosemide. The difference between these two drugs is the greater potency and bioavailability of bumetanide; smaller doses are needed. The normal adult dose is 0.5–3 mg i.v. over 1–2 min. The onset of diuresis is within 30 min and this usually lasts for about 4 h. The pharmacokinetics are similar to those of furosemide, with the exception that bumetanide is absorbed completely after oral administration and its rate of elimination is less dependent on renal function. Potassium loss is also a problem with bumetanide. Ototoxicity may be slightly less frequent than with furosemide, but renal toxicity is more of a problem. In clinical practice, there is no clear advantage or disadvantage over furosemide, providing equivalent doses are administered.

Thiazide Diuretics

Although thiazide diuretics are seldom used by anaesthetists, many patients scheduled for surgery are receiving these drugs for chronic hypertension or heart failure. There are a large number of thiazides available, all with a similar dose–response curve and diuretic effect.

Bendroflumethiazide, chlorothiazide, hydrochlorothiazide and chlorthalidone are a few examples of the better known thiazide diuretics. The majority have a duration of action of 6–12 h. In comparison with loop diuretics, thiazides have a longer duration of action, act at a different site, have a low 'ceiling' effect and are less effective in renal failure.

Thiazide diuretics are administered orally, absorbed rapidly from the gastrointestinal tract and initiate a diuresis within 1–2 h. The major distinction between the available thiazides is their difference in elimination rate. They are distributed in the extracellular space and eliminated in the proximal tubule of the nephron by active secretion.

Thiazides inhibit the active pump for sodium and chloride reabsorption in the cortical ascending part of the loop of Henle and the distal convoluted tubule. Therefore, the urine-concentrating ability of the kidney is not impaired, as normally this area is responsible for less than 5% of sodium reabsorption. The diuresis achieved by the thiazides is therefore never as effective as that of the loop diuretics. It is mild but sustained. In contrast with loop diuretics, the excretion of calcium is decreased and hypercalcaemia may become a problem. In the presence of aldosterone activity, the increase in sodium delivery to the distal renal tubules is associated with increased potassium loss, similar to that of the loop diuretics. The reduced clearance of uric acid by thiazides may cause hyperuricaemia.

Thiazides are used extensively in low doses, and often combined with a low-sodium diet, for the management of essential hypertension. A reduction in extracellular fluid volume and mild peripheral vasodilatation are responsible for the sustained antihypertensive effect. The full antihypertensive effect may take up to 12 weeks to become established. Higher doses of thiazides are used for the management of congestive cardiac failure and other oedematous conditions such as nephrotic syndrome and liver cirrhosis.

The most common side-effects of the thiazides are probably dehydration and hypovolaemia. This may present as orthostatic hypotension. When administered chronically, these drugs lead typically to a diuretic-induced hypokalaemic, hypochloraemic, metabolic alkalosis. In combination with magnesium depletion, the hypokalaemia may trigger serious cardiac arrhythmias, in addition to digitalis toxicity, muscle weakness and the potentiation of non-depolarizing muscle relaxants.

Thiazides decrease the tubular secretion of urate, which may lead to hyperuricaemia and gout. They are sulphonamide derivatives and may therefore cause inhibition of insulin release from the pancreas and blockade of peripheral glucose utilization. This may precipitate hyperglycaemia or an increase in insulin requirements in a patient with diabetes mellitus. They also lead to an increase in total blood cholesterol.

Potassium-Sparing Diuretics

Only a small part of sodium reabsorption into the renal cells takes place via the sodium–potassium exchange mechanism in the distal tubules. The potassium-retaining diuretics act on the distal convoluted tubules and the collecting ducts and therefore cause only a limited diuresis. There are two subgroups in this category: drugs acting independently of the aldosterone mechanism (e.g. triamterene and amiloride) and aldosterone antagonists (e.g. spironolactone).

These drugs increase the urinary excretion of sodium, chloride and bicarbonate and lead to an increase in urinary pH. They prevent excessive loss of potassium that occurs with the loop and thiazide diuretics by reducing the sodium–potassium exchange. Potassium-sparing drugs do, however, augment the diuretic response of these drugs when given in combination.

Amiloride and Triamterene

Amiloride acts directly on the distal tubule and collecting duct. It causes potassium retention and an increase in sodium loss. After oral intake, up to 25% is absorbed, onset of its peak effect is within 6 h and it is then excreted unchanged in the urine. Amiloride is almost always used in combination with thiazide or loop diuretics. It then has a synergistic action in terms of diuresis, although it opposes the potassium loss. Amiloride has few side-effects. Hyperkalaemia and acidosis may occur, and it is therefore contraindicated in patients with renal failure.

Triamterene has characteristics similar to those of amiloride.

Spironolactone

Aldosterone causes sodium reabsorption and potassium loss in the distal convoluted tubule. Spironolactone has a steroid molecular structure, acts as a competitive antagonist on the aldosterone receptors and inhibits sodium reabsorption and potassium loss. In the absence of aldosterone, it has no effect.

After oral absorption, spironolactone is immediately metabolized to a number of metabolites. Some of these are active and act for up to 15 h.

Spironolactone is the logical choice of diuretic in the management of liver cirrhosis, ascites and secondary hyperaldosteronism. Heart failure or hypertension in the presence of high mineralocorticoid levels (Conn's syndrome or prednisone therapy) is another indication. Spironolactone is often combined with thiazides to maximize the diuretic effect and prevent potassium loss.

Hyperkalaemia may develop if spironolactone is used in the presence of renal dysfunction. If used in high doses, it may cause gynaecomastia and impotence.

ACUTE RENAL FAILURE, SEPSIS AND THE INTENSIVE CARE UNIT

Acute renal failure is a common complication of sepsis and septic shock; the combination is associated with a mortality of over 50%. The arterial vasodilatation that accompanies sepsis is mediated in part by cytokines that upregulate inducible nitric oxide synthase with a subsequent increased release of nitric oxide. The potent vasodilatory effect of nitric oxide is partly responsible for the vascular resistance to the pressor response to noradrenaline and angiotensin II. Early in sepsis-related acute renal failure, cytokines such as tumour necrosis factor alpha (TNF-α) cause vasoconstriction of the renal vasculature, though trials of monoclonal antibodies against TNF-α have not shown any improvement in survival.

This early vasoconstrictor phase is potentially reversible and some clinical studies have suggested that measures to optimize haemodynamics with fluids and vasoactive drugs can reduce the incidence of established acute kidney injury though more data are needed. The administration of vasopressin (see above) in patients with septic shock may help maintain arterial pressure despite the relative ineffectiveness of other vasopressors such as noradrenaline and angiotensin II. It constricts the glomerular efferent arteriole and therefore increases the filtration pressure and glomerular filtration rate. There is early evidence in patients who have septic shock and are at risk of acute kidney injury that vasopressin may reduce progression to renal failure, and mortality.

ACUTE KIDNEY INJURY AFTER CARDIAC OR MAJOR VASCULAR SURGERY

The incidence of acute kidney injury (AKI) after cardiac surgery is approximately 10% and is associated with a high morbidity and mortality. Clinical evidence suggests that preoperative renal insufficiency, diabetes mellitus, prolonged cardiopulmonary bypass (CPB) time and postoperative hypotension are all independent risk factors for AKI in the cardiac patient. International consensus statements have recently been drawn up regarding the pathophysiology and treatment of AKI in cardiac surgical patients. Six pathophysiological processes were found to be most likely to contribute to this: exogenous and endogenous toxins, metabolic factors, ischaemia-reperfusion injury, neurohormonal activation, inflammation, and oxidative stress, which are probably all interrelated.

The most effective way to prevent AKI in this setting is by adequate hydration and perfusion pressure during CPB, and the maintenance of cardiac output throughout the perioperative period. Data for the effects of hypothermia during CPB, pulsatile CPB flow or avoiding CPB altogether through off-pump cardiac surgical techniques on the incidence of AKI are not conclusive. Many drugs have been studied for renal protection during CPB. Low-dose dopamine is ineffective and may even be harmful. Although mannitol is used in routine pump prime in many cardiac units and furosemide potentially reduces renal medullary oxygen consumption, neither prevents AKI after cardiac surgery. Recent therapeutic trials to reduce acute kidney injury in cardiac surgery patients fall broadly into reactive oxygen molecule scavengers, anti-inflammatory agents, and anti-apoptotic agents (tetracyclines, minocycline, human recombinant erythropoietin). However the results have been inconsistent and disappointing and there is currently no pharmacological strategy known to reliably reduce the incidence of AKI.

Aprotinin has been used to reduce transfusion requirements in high risk cardiac surgical patients.

Recent evidence has raised concerns that aprotinin is associated with an increased risk of AKI in cardiac surgery but the evidence is conflicting and the possibility of risk is not consistently supported by data from published, randomized, placebo-controlled clinical trials. Aprotinin is currently not recommended for routine use in cardiothoracic surgery.

DRUGS AND RENAL TRANSPLANTATION

The best treatment for end-stage renal failure is renal transplantation. Apart from optimizing the recipient's general health (e.g. correction of anaemia, preoperative dialysis, etc.), immunosuppression plays an extremely important role in graft survival.

Erythropoietin

Erythropoietin is a circulating hormone secreted by the kidneys. It stimulates the bone marrow to produce red blood cells. The ability of the kidney to secrete erythropoietin deteriorates as excretory function decreases. Patients with severe chronic renal failure are unable to produce adequate quantities of erythropoietin, which leads to diminished red blood cell production. The retention of toxic substances also contributes to bone marrow depression. In addition, red cell survival is reduced by 50% in advanced renal failure. Therefore these patients almost always develop a chronic anaemia.

Long-term administration of recombinant human erythropoietin (rHUEPO) in chronic renal failure patients results in global stimulation of the bone marrow, increasing red blood cell differentiation and maintaining cell viability, thereby improving anaemia. It also decreases bleeding by increasing platelet adhesion in haemodialysed uraemic patients. A side-effect of rHUEPO is the development of hypertension or exacerbation of existing hypertension.

Immunosuppression

Prednisolone and Azathioprine

Corticosteroids were the first drugs to be used as immunosuppressive agents. Initially, very high doses were used, producing the typical steroid side-effects, e.g. Cushingoid appearance, hypertension, hyperglycaemia and osteoporosis. Experience and research showed that large doses were not necessary and that better results and fewer side-effects were possible with lower doses.

The 'modern era' of immunosuppression started with the discovery of azathioprine. For a long period of time, the combination of azathioprine and corticosteroids was the 'gold standard' in transplant surgery. Azathioprine is a derivative of 6-mercaptopurine and is metabolized to its active form in the liver. It affects the synthesis of DNA and RNA and is broken down by the enzyme xanthine oxidase. Co-administration of allopurinol (xanthine oxidase inhibitor) is contraindicated because it may result in bone marrow suppression, agranulocytosis and leucopaenia. Patients receiving azathioprine are prone to develop viral warts or malignancies of the skin and hepatic dysfunction.

Ciclosporin A and Ciclosporin-Neoral

The next major advance in transplant surgery was the discovery of ciclosporin A. This fungal peptide prevents the proliferation and clonal expansion of T lymphocytes. The chance of acute rejection is reduced significantly by administration of this drug. In spite of the large number of side-effects of ciclosporin A, it has been accepted as the new standard against which all other immunosuppressants are judged. Ciclosporin A is lipophilic and incompletely absorbed in the small bowel. Serious side-effects such as gingival hypertrophy, hepatotoxicity and nephrotoxicity make this a less than perfect drug. For a long time, classic triple therapy consisted of prednisolone, azathioprine and ciclosporin A.

Recently, ciclosporin was released in a new form under the tradename Neoral. This form is a microemulsion that enhances the bioavailability of ciclosporin through improved absorption. Ciclosporin (Neoral) is equipotent to the parent drug and most renal transplant patients are presently receiving this agent.

Rapamycin

Rapamycin is a macrolide with antifungal and potent immunosuppressant effects. It prevents proliferation of T cells and antagonizes the action of interleukin-2 on its receptor. This agent is 100 times more potent than ciclosporin A. It has no adverse effects on liver or renal function, but has the potential to enhance the nephrotoxicity and hepatotoxicity of ciclosporin.

TABLE 10.2	
A Typical Perioperative Regimen for Renal Transplant	
Preoperative	Induction immunosuppression (ciclosporin-Neoral, FK506/tacrolimus, rapamycin, or sirolimus and mycophenolate mofetil (MMF) Heparin 5000 units subcutaneously Ranitidine 150 mg orally (stress ulcer prophylaxis) Nifedipine 20 mg orally (vasodilator, free radical scavenger)
At induction	Antibiotic prophylaxis – co-amoxiclav (augmentin) 1.2 g intravenously methylprednisolone 0.5 g i.v.
During vascular anastomosis	Mannitol $0.5\,g\,kg^{-1}$ intravenously $\pm$ dopamine $3{-}5\,\mu g\,kg^{-1}\,min^{-1}$
Postoperative	Antibiotic prophylaxis Heparin 5000 units subcutaneously, twice daily Aspirin 150 mg orally Ranitidine 150 mg orally, twice daily Co-trimoxazole 480 mg orally, daily (prophylaxis against *Pneumocystis carinii*) Immunosuppression ('triple therapy')

Tacrolimus

Tacrolimus is a macrolide antibiotic with a similar structure to rapamycin. It is a very potent immunosuppressant drug that inhibits the activation of T cells and interleukin-2 generation. The principal side-effects are nephrotoxicity and neurotoxicity.

Mycophenolate Mofetil

Mycophenolate mofetil (MMF) is a new immunosuppressant licensed for use in renal transplantation. It inhibits a key enzyme in the purine synthesis pathway and therefore has a specific effect on B and T lymphocytes. The synthesis of adhesion molecules is also inhibited by MMF. It seems as though MMF effectively prevents chronic rejection in renal transplant patients. MMF is neither nephrotoxic nor hepatotoxic.

There are a variety of substances with potent immunosuppressant properties which are usually used in combination with each other. Despite their powerful immunosuppressant effects, it is unlikely that any of the new or existing drugs may be used as monotherapy. The calcineurin inhibitors (CNIs), ciclosporin and tacrolimus, have revolutionized the overall success of renal transplantation through reduction in early immunological injury and acute rejection rates. However, the CNIs have a significant adverse effect on renal function and cardiovascular disease, and extended long-term graft survival has not been achieved.

CNI minimization using mycophenolate mofetil or sirolimus may be associated with a modest increase in creatinine clearance and a decrease in serum creatinine in the short term. A typical perioperative regimen for renal transplantation is shown in Table 10.2.

The role of drugs inhibiting antigen presentation and the use of monoclonal antibodies are still being defined.

FURTHER READING

Fischereder, M., Kretzler, M., 2004. New immunosuppressive strategies in renal transplant recipients. J. Nephrol. 17, 9–18.

Flechner, S.M., Kobashigawa, J., Klintmalm, G., 2008. Calcineurin inhibitor-sparing regimens in solid organ transplantation: focus on improving renal function and nephrotoxicity. Clin. Transplant. 22 (1), 1–15.

Garwood, S., 2010. Cardiac surgery-associated acute renal injury: new paradigms and innovative therapies. J. Cardiothorac. Vasc. Anesth. 24 (6), 990–1001.

Gordon, A.C., Russell, J.A., Whalley, K.R., et al., 2010. The effects of vasopressin on acute kidney injury in septic shock. Intensive Care Med. 36 (1), 83–91.

Gottlieb, S.S., 2008. Adenosine A1 antagonists and the cardiorenal syndrome. Curr. Heart Fail. Rep. 5 (2), 105–109.

Guyton, A.C., Hall, J.E., 2011. Diuretics, kidney diseases (Ch 31). In: Guyton, A.C., Hall, J.E. (Eds.), Textbook of Medical Physiology, eleventh ed. WB Saunders, Philadelphia, pp. 397–409.

Huang, D.T., Clermont, G., Dremsizov, T.T., et al., 2007. Implementation of early goal-directed therapy for severe sepsis and septic shock: a decision analysis. Crit. Care Med. 35 (9), 2090–2100.

Lindvall, G., Sartipy, U., Ivert, T., et al., 2008. Aprotinin is not associated with postoperative renal impairment after primary coronary surgery. Ann. Thorac. Surg. 86, 13–19.

Schrier, R.W., Wang, W., 2004. Acute renal failure and sepsis. N. Engl. J. Med. 351, 59–69.

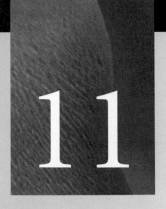

11

METABOLISM, THE STRESS RESPONSE TO SURGERY AND PERIOPERATIVE THERMOREGULATION

METABOLISM

Metabolism may be defined as the chemical processes which enable cells to function. Basal metabolic rate (BMR) is the minimum amount of energy required to maintain basic autonomic function and normal homeostasis. For example, energy is required by the myocardium to maintain heart rate and stroke volume and by nerve and muscle membranes to maintain membrane potentials. In a healthy resting adult, BMR is in the region of $2000\,\mathrm{kcal\,day^{-1}}$ (equivalent to $40\,\mathrm{kcal\,m^{-2}\,h^{-1}}$). One calorie is the energy required in joules to raise the temperature of $1\,\mathrm{g}$ of water from $15\,°C$ to $16\,°C$. Because this is a very small unit, a more practical measure in human physiology is the kcal or Calorie (C).

Adenosine triphosphate (ATP) is the 'energy currency' of the body. It contains two high-energy phosphate bonds and is present in all cells. Most physiological processes acquire energy from it. Oxidation of nutrients in cells releases energy, which is used to regenerate ATP. Conversion of one mole of ATP to adenosine diphosphate (ADP) releases 8 kcal of energy. Additional hydrolysis of the phosphate bond from ADP to AMP also releases 8 kcal (Fig. 11.1). Other high-energy compounds include creatine phosphate and acetyl CoA. The generation of energy through the oxidation of carbohydrate, protein and fat is termed catabolism, whereas the generation of stored energy as energy-rich phosphate bonds, carbohydrates, proteins or fats is termed anabolism (Fig. 11.2). The amount of energy released by carbohydrate, protein and fat metabolism is: carbohydrate $4.1\,\mathrm{kcal\,g^{-1}}$, protein $4.1\,\mathrm{kcal\,g^{-1}}$ and fat $9.3\,\mathrm{kcal\,g^{-1}}$.

CARBOHYDRATE METABOLISM

The final product of carbohydrate digestion is glucose, which is used to form ATP in cells. Because the cellular membrane is impermeable to glucose, it is transported by a carrier protein (GLUT4) across the membrane in a process termed *facilitated diffusion.* Activation of insulin receptors speeds translocation of GLUT4-containing endosomes into the cell membrane which then mediate glucose transport into the cell. Facilitated diffusion of glucose into cells is increased 10-fold in the presence of insulin, without which the rate of uptake would be inadequate. This is a passive process (i.e. it does not require energy expenditure by the cell). In contrast, glucose absorption in the gastrointestinal tract and reabsorption in the renal tubule are both active processes (i.e. are energy-consuming processes). They involve co-transport with sodium ions via sodium-dependent glucose transporters (SGLT).

Aerobic Glycolysis

After absorption into cells, glucose may be used immediately or stored in the form of glycogen, particularly in liver and muscle. The process of releasing glucose molecules from the glycogen molecule in times of high metabolic demand is termed *glycogenolysis.* This process is initiated by the enzyme *phosphorylase*, which is activated in the presence of adrenaline (epinephrine) and glucagon. Adrenaline is released by the sympathetic nervous system, while glucagon is released from the α cells of the pancreas in response to hypoglycaemia.

The mechanism of glucose catabolism involves an extensive series of enzyme-controlled steps, rather than a single reaction. This is because the oxidation of

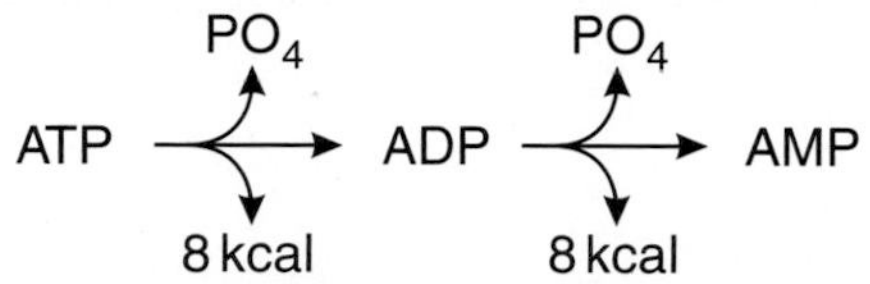

$$ATP \xrightarrow[8\,kcal]{PO_4} ADP \xrightarrow[8\,kcal]{PO_4} AMP$$

FIGURE 11.1 ■ Hydrolysis of adenosine triphosphate (ATP). ADP, adenosine diphosphate; AMP, adenosine monophosphate.

one mol of glucose (180 g) releases almost 686 kcal of energy, whereas only 8 kcal is required to form one molecule of ATP. Therefore, an elaborate series of reactions, termed the *glycolytic pathway,* releases small quantities of energy at a time, resulting in the synthesis of 38 mol of ATP from each mol of glucose (Fig. 11.3). As each molecule of ATP releases 8 kcal, a total of 304 kcal of energy in the form of ATP is synthesized. Hence, the efficiency of the glycolytic pathway is 44%, the remainder of the energy being released as heat.

The glycolytic pathway may be summarized as:

1. *Glycolysis,* i.e. splitting the glucose (6 carbon atoms) molecule into two molecules of pyruvic acid (3 carbon atoms each). This results in the net formation of two molecules of ATP anaerobically but also generates two pairs of H^+ for entry into the respiratory chain (see below) (Fig. 11.4).
2. *Oxidation* of each of the pyruvic acid (3 carbon atom) molecules in the Krebs citric acid cycle results in the generation of five pairs of H^+ per 3-carbon moiety, i.e. 10 pairs of H^+ per 6 carbon glucose molecule (Fig. 11.5).
3. *Oxidative phosphorylation,* i.e. the formation of ATP by the oxidation of hydrogen to water.

This process is also known as the respiratory chain. For each molecule of glucose, a total of 12 pairs of H^+ are fed into the respiratory chain, each pair generating three molecules of ATP. Thus, oxidative phosphorylation results in 36 molecules of ATP per molecule of glucose. A further two molecules of ATP are produced anaerobically. Therefore, one molecule of glucose generates 38 molecules of ATP. Uncoupling of oxidative phosphorylation allows ATP production to be sacrificed for heat production as part of thermoregulatory homeostasis.

Anaerobic Glycolysis

This is the process of ATP formation in the absence of oxygen and is possible because the first two steps of glycolysis do not require oxygen. In the absence of oxygen, pyruvic acid molecules and hydrogen ions accumulate, which would normally stop the reaction. However, pyruvic acid and hydrogen ions combine in the presence of the enzyme *lactic dehydrogenase* to form lactic acid, which diffuses easily out of cells, allowing anaerobic glycolysis to continue. Lactic acidosis is a feature of shock caused by, for example, severe sepsis. This is a highly inefficient use of the energy within glucose. When oxygen is again available to the cells, lactic acid is reconverted to glucose or used directly for energy.

The glycolytic pathway metabolizes 70% of glucose. A second mechanism, the phosphogluconate pathway (also known as the hexose monophosphate shunt) is responsible for metabolism of the remaining 30%. The importance of this pathway is that ATP is formed

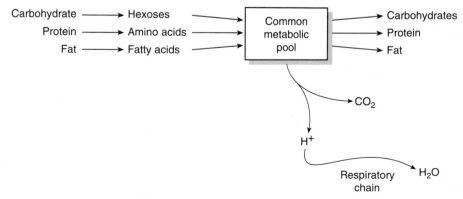

FIGURE 11.2 ■ Overview of metabolism.

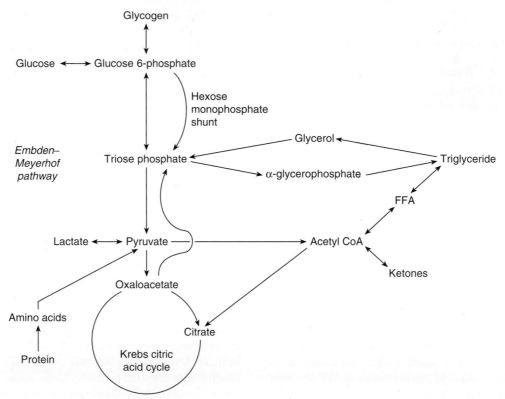

FIGURE 11.3 ■ Summary of the glycolytic pathway. Krebs citric acid cycle. FFA, free fatty acid. Note that two molecules of pyruvic acid are produced for each molecule of glucose metabolized. Each pyruvic acid molecule enters the Krebs citric acid cycle.

independently of the enzymes needed in the glycolytic pathway, and hence an enzymatic abnormality in the glycolytic pathway does not completely inhibit energy metabolism. It also provides for the production of pentoses, which are needed for nucleic acid production.

Gluconeogenesis

This is the formation of glucose from amino acids, which are usually used for protein formation. It occurs when stores of glycogen are depleted. Prolonged hypoglycaemia is the main trigger for this process, but ACTH, glucocorticoids and glucagon also have a role.

PROTEIN METABOLISM

Proteins are composed of amino acids, of which there are more than 20 different types in humans. All amino acids have a weak acid group (-COOH) and an amine group (-NH$_2$). They are joined by peptide linkages to form *peptide chains* (primary structure), a reaction which releases a molecule of water in the process. The blood concentration of amino acids is approximately 1–2 mmol L^{-1}. Entry into cells requires facilitated or active transport using carrier mechanisms. They are then conjugated into proteins by the formation of peptide linkages. Formation of the peptide link requires 0.5–4.0 kcal derived from ATP. Large proteins may be composed of several peptide chains wrapped around each other (secondary structure) and bound by weaker links, e.g. hydrogen bonds, electrostatic forces and sulfhydryl bonds (tertiary structure).

Some amino acids present in the body are not present in proteins to any appreciable extent including, for example, ornithine, 5-hydroxytryptophan, L-dopa and thyroxine. Catecholamines, histamine and serotonin are formed from specific amino acids. Sulphur-containing amino acids are the source of urinary sulphate and provide sulphur for incorporation into various proteins, e.g. Coenzyme A.

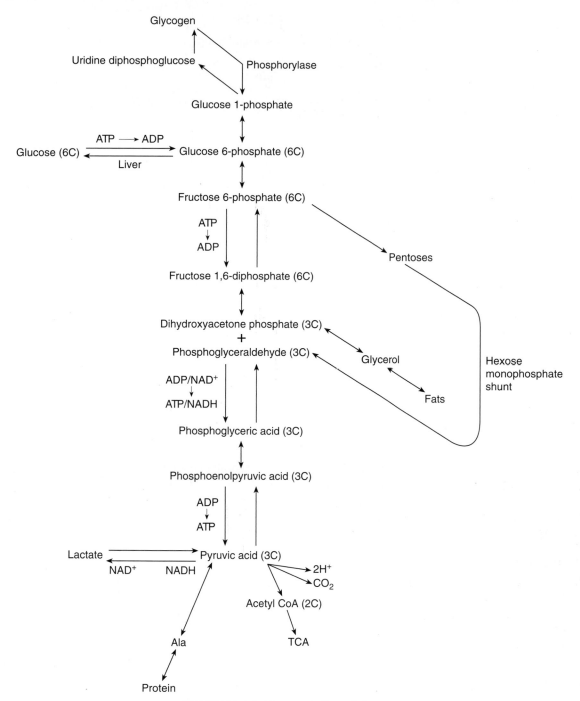

FIGURE 11.4 ■ The metabolism of glucose.

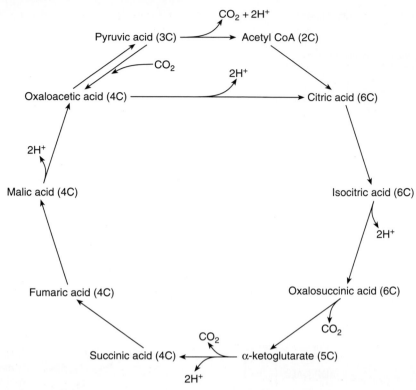

FIGURE 11.5 ■ The Krebs citric acid cycle. Note that five pairs of H^+ are generated by the oxidation of each pyruvate molecule. Each pair of H^+ generates three molecules of ATP in the respiratory chain in the mitochondria.

There is equilibrium between the amino acids in plasma, plasma proteins and tissue proteins. Proteins may be synthesized from amino acids in all cells of the body, the type of protein depending on the genetic material in the DNA, which determines the sequence of amino acids formed and hence controls the nature of the synthesized proteins. Essential amino acids must be ingested as they cannot be synthesized in the body. Table 11.1 lists the eight essential amino acids. If there is dietary deficiency of any of these, the subject develops a negative nitrogen balance. Others are *non-essential* (i.e. may be synthesized in the cells). Synthesis is by the process of *transamination*, whereby an amine radical (-NH_2) is transferred to the corresponding α-keto acid. Breakdown of excess amino acids into glucose (gluconeogenesis) generates energy or storage as fat, both of which occur in the liver. The breakdown of amino acids occurs by the process of *deamination*, which takes place in the liver. It involves the removal of the amine group with the formation of

TABLE 11.1
Essential Amino Acids
Leucine
Isoleucine
Lysine
Methionine
Phenylalanine
Threonine
Tryptophan
Valine

the corresponding ketoacid. The amine radical may be recycled to other molecules or released as ammonia. In the liver, two molecules of ammonia are combined to form urea (Fig. 11.6). Amino acids may also take up ammonia to form the corresponding amide.

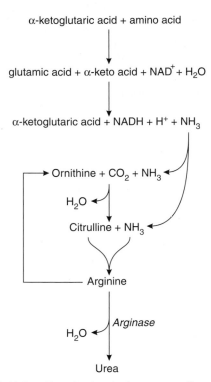

α-ketoglutaric acid + amino acid

↓

glutamic acid + α-keto acid + NAD^+ + H_2O

↓

α-ketoglutaric acid + NADH + H^+ + NH_3

Ornithine + CO_2 + NH_3

H_2O

Citrulline + NH_3

Arginine

H_2O — *Arginase*

Urea

FIGURE 11.6 ■ Deamination is the process of metabolizing amino acids. Ammonia is the end product. Two molecules of ammonia combine as shown to form urea. This occurs in the liver.

During starvation or when no protein is ingested (e.g. after major surgery), 20–30 g day^{-1} of protein is catabolized for energy purposes. This occurs despite the continuing availability of some stored carbohydrates and fats. When carbohydrate and fat stores are exhausted, the rate of protein catabolism is increased to >100 g day^{-1}, resulting in a rapid decline in tissue function. During the systemic inflammatory response syndrome (SIRS) or after major surgery, there is functional catabolism also. Several hormones influence protein metabolism. Growth hormone, insulin and testosterone are anabolic, i.e. they increase the rate of cellular protein synthesis. Other hormones, e.g. glucocorticoids, are catabolic, i.e. they decrease the amount of protein in most tissues, except the liver. Glucagon promotes gluconeogenesis and protein breakdown. Thyroxine indirectly affects protein metabolism by affecting metabolic rate. If insufficient energy sources are available to cells, thyroxine may contribute to excess protein breakdown. Conversely, if adequate amino acid and energy sources are available, thyroxine may increase the rate of protein synthesis.

LIPID METABOLISM

Lipids are a diverse group of compounds characterized by their insolubility in water and solubility in nonpolar solvents such as ether or benzene. They include fats, oils, steroids, waxes, etc. They serve as an immediate energy source but also provide storage energy. They include cholesterol, which is a precursor of steroids. They provide electrical insulation for nerve conduction and when combined with protein they are known as lipoproteins, an important component of cell membranes. Lipoproteins are also the predominant means for the transport of bloodstream lipids.

Lipids include triglycerides (TGs), phospholipids (PLs) and cholesterol. The basic structure of TGs and PLs is the *fatty acid*. Fatty acids are long-chain hydrocarbon organic acids. TGs are composed of three long-chain fatty acids bound with one molecule of glycerol (Fig. 11.7). Phospholipids have two long-chain fatty acids bound to glycerol with the third fatty acid replaced by attached compounds such as inositol, choline or ethanolamine. Although cholesterol does not contain fatty acid, its sterol nucleus is formed from fatty acid molecules.

Some polyunsaturated fatty acids are considered essential because they cannot be synthesized in humans and because they are precursors for eicosanoids. They must be acquired from plant sources. These essential fatty acids are linolenic acid and linoleic acid which together with their derivative arachidonic acid form prostaglandins, lipoxins and leukotrienes (collectively termed eicosanoids).

After absorption in the gastrointestinal tract, lipids are aggregated into droplets (diameter 90–1000 nm), termed chylomicrons, composed mainly of TGs. These molecules are too large to pass the endothelial cells of the portal system and so enter the circulation via

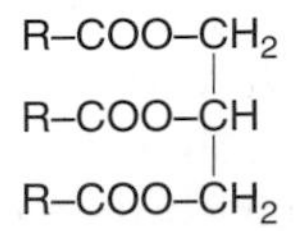

$R–COO–CH_2$

$R–COO–CH$

$R–COO–CH_2$

FIGURE 11.7 ■ Triglyceride structure. R represents a chain of carbon atoms.

the thoracic duct. Chylomicrons are metabolized by lipoprotein lipase adherent to the endothelium of many tissues throughout the body including adipose tissue but not adult liver. Chylomicrons carry cholesterol to the liver. The fatty acids and lipoproteins released from the liver into the circulation are derived from secondary products of chylomicron metabolism.

Transport of lipids from the liver or adipose cells to other tissues that need it as an energy source occurs by means of binding to plasma albumin. The fatty acids are then referred to as *free fatty acids* (FFAs), to distinguish them from other fatty acids in the plasma. After 12 h of fasting, all chylomicrons have been removed from the blood, and circulating lipids then occur in the form of *lipoproteins*. Lipoproteins are smaller particles than chylomicrons but are also composed of TGs, PLs and cholesterol. They may be classified as:

- very low-density lipoproteins (VLDLs), consisting mainly of TGs
- low-density lipoproteins (LDLs), consisting mainly of cholesterol
- high-density lipoproteins (HDLs), consisting mainly of protein.

Cholesterol

Cholesterol is a lipid with a sterol nucleus and is formed from acetyl CoA. It may be absorbed from food (animal sources only) but is also synthesized in the liver and to a lesser extent other tissue. Its function is predominantly the formation of bile salts in the liver, which promote the digestion and absorption of lipids. The remainder is used in the formation of adrenocortical and sex hormones and it is deposited also in the skin, where it resists the absorption of water-soluble chemicals.

The serum cholesterol concentration is correlated with the incidences of atherosclerosis and coronary artery disease. Prolonged elevations of VLDL, LDL and chylomicron remnants are associated with atherosclerosis. Conversely, HDL is protective. Factors affecting blood cholesterol concentration are outlined in Figure 11.8.

There is a feedback mechanism whereby increased cholesterol absorption from the diet results in inhibition of the enzyme *HMG-CoA reductase,* which regulates synthesis of cholesterol. There are many hormonal influences in cholesterol metabolism also,

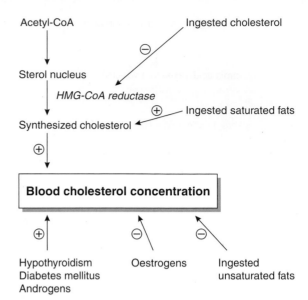

FIGURE 11.8 ■ Factors affecting blood cholesterol concentration.

including increased plasma concentrations in response to abnormally low concentrations of thyroid hormone, insulin and androgens. Oestrogen reduces cholesterol concentration by an unknown mechanism. The family of cholesterol-lowering drugs termed statins are inhibitors of the enzyme HMG-CoA reductase.

Lipids are ingested in similar proportions to carbohydrates and may be used as an energy source immediately or stored in the liver or adipose cells for later use as an energy source. The stages in the use of TGs as an energy source are as follows. TG is hydrolysed to its constituent glycerol and three fatty acids; glycerol is then conjugated to glycerol 3-phosphate and enters the glycolytic pathway, which generates ATP as described above. Fatty acids need *carnitine* as a carrier agent to enter mitochondria, where they undergo beta oxidation. The precise number of ATP molecules formed from a molecule of TG depends on the length of the fatty acid chain, longer chains providing more acetyl CoA and hence more molecules of ATP. Newborns have a special type of fat, termed brown fat, which on exposure to a cold stressor is stimulated to break down into free fatty acids and glycerol. In brown adipose tissue, oxidation and phosphorylation are not coupled and therefore the metabolism of brown fat is especially thermogenic.

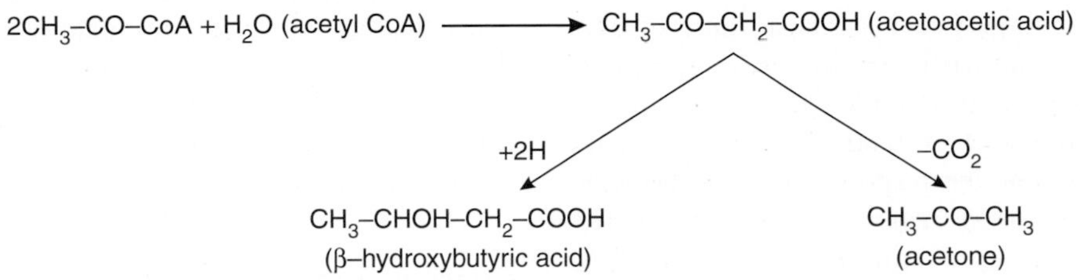

$$2CH_3-CO-CoA + H_2O \text{ (acetyl CoA)} \longrightarrow CH_3-CO-CH_2-COOH \text{ (acetoacetic acid)}$$

$$+2H \qquad\qquad\qquad -CO_2$$

$$CH_3-CHOH-CH_2-COOH \qquad\qquad CH_3-CO-CH_3$$
$$\text{(β–hydroxybutyric acid)} \qquad\qquad \text{(acetone)}$$

FIGURE 11.9 ■ Ketone formation.

Ketones

Initial degradation of fatty acids occurs in the liver, but the acetyl-CoA may not be used either immediately or completely. Ketones, or keto acids, are either *acetoacetic acid,* formed from two molecules of acetyl CoA, *β-hydroxybutyric acid,* formed from the reduction of acetoacetic acid, or *acetone,* formed when a smaller quantity of acetoacetic acid is decarboxylated (Fig. 11.9). These three substances are collectively termed ketones. They are organic acids formed in the liver, from which they diffuse into the circulation and are transported to the peripheral tissues where they may be used for energy. Their importance is that they accumulate in diabetes and starvation, such as may occur in the perioperative period. In both circumstances, no carbohydrates are being metabolized. In diabetes, decreased insulin results in a reduction in intracellular glucose, and in starvation, carbohydrates are lacking simply because they are not being ingested. The ensuing breakdown of fat as described above results in large quantities of ketones being released from the liver to the peripheral tissues. There is a limit to the rate at which ketones are used by the tissues, because depletion of essential carbohydrate intermediate metabolites slows the rate at which acetyl CoA can enter the Krebs cycle (see Fig. 11.5). Hence, blood ketone concentration may increase rapidly, causing metabolic acidosis and ketonuria. Acetone may be discharged on the breath to give a characteristic sweet odour.

Measuring Metabolic Rate

Basal metabolic rate (BMR) is determined at complete mental and physical rest 12–14h after food ingestion, if body temperature is within the normal range. Metabolic rate increases by approximately 8% for every 1 °C rise of body temperature. BMR may be measured by indirect calorimetry which involves the

TABLE 11.2
Factors Influencing Metabolic Rate
Malnutrition (20%)
Sleep (15%)
Exercise (up to 2000×BMR)
Protein ingestion
Age: <5 years has ×2 BMR of >70
Thyroid hormone imbalance (increase or decrease by 50%)
Sympathetic stimulation
Testosterone (by 15%)
Temperature
Anaesthesia (20% reduction) (regional anaesthesia – no effect)

measurement of water, CO_2 or protein breakdown products produced to enable the metabolic rate to be quantified. Alternatively, the O_2 consumption can be measured. A total of 4.82 kcal of energy is produced per litre of O_2 consumed although accurate assessment depends on information about the type of food ingested. Factors influencing BMR are listed in Table 11.2.

THE STRESS RESPONSE TO SURGERY

The stress response is a physiological response which has evolved to protect the body from injury and to enhance chances of survival. It involves cardiovascular, thermoregulatory and metabolic mechanisms and was first described by Cuthbertson in 1929.

Surgery or trauma consistently elicits a characteristic neuroendocrine and cytokine response in proportion to the extent of injury or metabolic insult. Minor surgery on a limb has a negligible stress response, in contrast to major surgery such as a laparotomy or thoracotomy. The characteristics of the stress response to surgery are summarized in Table 11.3. There are two principal components to the stress response to surgery: the *neuroendocrine* response and the *cytokine* response. The neuroendocrine response is stimulated by painful afferent neural stimuli reaching the CNS. It may be diminished and sometimes eliminated altogether by dense neural blockade from a regional anaesthetic technique.

The cytokine component of the stress response is stimulated by *local tissue damage* at the site of the surgery itself and is not inhibited by regional anaesthesia. It is diminished by minimally invasive surgery, especially laparoscopic techniques. Triggers are listed in Table 11.4.

There is growing evidence that the stress response is detrimental and is associated with postoperative morbidity. It has adverse effects on several key physiological systems, including the cardiovascular, respiratory and gastroenterological systems.

Consequences of the Neuroendocrine Element of the Stress Response

Protein Catabolism

Major surgery results in a net excretion of nitrogen-containing compounds, referred to as negative nitrogen balance, reflecting catabolism of protein into amino acids for gluconeogenesis. This is partly because of perioperative starvation, but mainly because of the stress response, which causes decreased total protein

---

TABLE 11.3
Components of the Stress Response to Surgery

Neuroendocrine Response	Consequence	Result
Hypothalamic–pituitary–adrenal	ACTH, GH, ADH, β-endorphin, prolactin all increased	Activation of adrenocortical hormones
		Mobilization of glucose reserves
		Water retention
		Protein catabolism and gluconeogenesis
Sympathetic nervous system stimulation	Catecholamines increased	Heart rate and cardiac output increased
		SVR and arterial pressure increased
	Hypothalamic–pituitary–adrenal	Activation of adrenocortical hormones; mobilization of glucose reserves; water retention; protein catabolism and gluconeogenesis
	Renin–angiotensin–aldosterone	Increased SVR, retention Na$^+$ and H$_2$O, secretion K$^+$
	Increased glucagon	Increased plasma glucose, lipolysis and insulin resistance
	Decreased insulin, testosterone	Hyperglycaemia, catabolic state
	Increased acute-phase proteins (liver)	Decreased liver synthesis of albumin
Cytokine Response		
Cytokine and inflammatory mediator release	IL-1, IL-6, TNF-α	Platelet adhesion
	Prostaglandins increased	Increased coagulation
		Increased hypothalamic–pituitary–adrenal activity
	Neutrophils increased	Local inflammation, pain
	Lymphocytes decreased	
Pyrexia (due to increased IL-1)	Increased metabolic rate	Increased demand on cardiovascular system

ACTH, adrenocorticotrophic hormone; GH, growth hormone; ADH, antidiuretic hormone; SVR, systemic vascular resistance; TNF-α, tumour necrosis factor alpha.

TABLE 11.4
Triggers of the Neuroendocrine and Cytokine Response in Patients After Surgery
Noxious afferent stimuli (especially pain)
Local inflammatory tissue factors, especially cytokines
Pain and anxiety
Starvation
Hypothermia and shivering
Haemorrhage
Acidosis
Hypoxaemia
Infection

synthesis, in addition to protein breakdown. Peripheral skeletal muscle is predominantly affected, but visceral protein may also be catabolized. Catecholamines, cortisol, glucagon and interleukins (IL-1 and IL-6) are involved in proteolysis and gluconeogenesis. Protein catabolism contributes to weight loss and impaired wound healing, and may delay overall postoperative recovery. Up to 0.5 kg day^{-1} of lean muscle mass may be lost postoperatively because of this aspect of the stress response.

Carbohydrate Mobilization

Hyperglycaemia and insulin intolerance are major features of the stress response and may persist for several days postoperatively. They result from increased blood concentrations of catecholamines, cortisol and glucagon and also from sympathetic nervous system stimulation (by further increasing catecholamine release from the adrenal medulla). These hormones also inhibit insulin and therefore glucose uptake into muscle, fat and liver. Moreover, there is decreased sensitivity of muscle and liver to circulating insulin during the stress response. Blood glucose concentrations may increase to over 11 mmol L^{-1}, leading to glycosuria and osmotic diuresis.

Fat Metabolism

The net effect of the hormonal alterations listed in Table 11.3 is lipolysis, stimulated by catecholamines acting at α_1-adrenoreceptors, with resultant increased concentrations of FFAs in the circulation. FFAs may be oxidized in the liver to form ketones (e.g. acetoacetate), which may be used as a source of energy by peripheral tissues.

Cardiovascular Effects

The stress response to surgery and postoperative pain activates the sympathetic nervous system (SNS), which may increase myocardial oxygen demand by increasing heart rate and arterial pressure. Activation of the SNS may also cause coronary artery vasoconstriction, reducing the supply of oxygen to the myocardium, which in turn can predispose to myocardial ischaemia. This effect may be aggravated by the fact that there is a hypercoagulable state postoperatively and the stress response is an important factor in causing this. The concentration of antidiuretic hormone (ADH) increases during the stress response, and this is known to contribute to increased platelet adhesiveness (Fig. 11.10).

Respiratory Effects

Postoperative pulmonary dysfunction may also result from pain and the stress response to major surgery. The most important alteration in respiratory function caused by the stress response is a reduction in functional residual capacity (FRC). This is the amount of air remaining in the lungs at the end of a normal expiration. The main cause of reduction in FRC is postoperative pain, which reduces the depth and rate of breathing. When FRC is reduced, it may become less than the closing capacity, the volume of air in the lungs required to prevent alveolar collapse. When FRC is less than closing capacity, airway closure occurs, with resultant ventilation-perfusion mismatch, shunting of blood and hypoxaemia.

Gastrointestinal Effects

The stress response to surgery stimulates both afferent nociceptive input and efferent SNS output, resulting in ileus and excessive SNS stimulation relative to parasympathetic nervous system (PNS) stimulation. Postoperative ileus is a temporary impairment of gastrointestinal motility after major surgery. It delays resumption of an enteral diet, and this starvation itself prolongs the stress response to surgery.

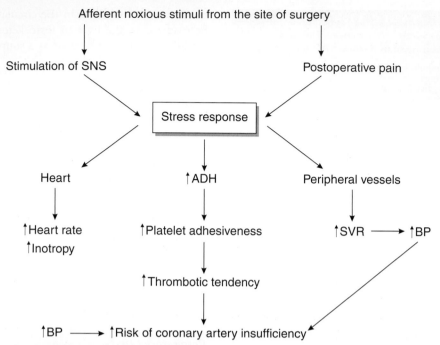

FIGURE 11.10 ■ Potential effect of the surgical stress response on coronary arterial blood flow. ADH, antidiuretic hormone; SVR, systemic vascular resistance; SNS, sympathetic nervous system.

Immunological System Effects

Many mediators of the stress response (cortisol, interleukins, prostaglandins, etc.) are cellular and humoral immunosuppressants. It is not known if stress response-mediated immunosuppression, which occurs for several days after surgery, influences patient outcome.

Afferent Neural Stimuli

Afferent noxious stimuli (such as pain, pressure, burning, distension) are transmitted by Aα and C nerve fibres. They enter the spinal cord via the dorsal root and synapse in the dorsal horn.

Local Factors and the Immunological (Cytokine) Response

Afferent neural stimuli are not the sole means of eliciting the stress response to surgery. Severe injury in a denervated limb also elicits the response, suggesting a non-neural stimulus. Cytokines and mediators of inflammation are released in response to local tissue destruction or trauma, increasing peripheral nociceptive activity. The magnitude of this response is proportional to the extent of tissue damage.

Effect of General Anaesthesia on the Stress Response

Intravenous (with the exception of etomidate) and inhalational anaesthetic agents have no appreciable effect on either the neuroendocrine or the cytokine elements of the stress response, irrespective of dose. Etomidate inhibits the 11β-hydoxylase enzyme involved in adrenal cortisol synthesis leading to reduced cortisol concentrations and is associated with increased mortality in the critically ill when infusions of etomidate are used for sedation. At much higher doses, adrenal 18β-hydroxylase and cholesterol side chain cleavage enzymes are inhibited, thus reducing aldosterone and other steroid hormone synthesis. There is some evidence that inhibition of 11β-hydroxylase occurs after a single induction dose of etomidate, reducing plasma cortisol concentrations for several hours, but the clinical significance of this is unclear. High-dose opioid analgesia (e.g. morphine $4\,mg\,kg^{-1}$ or fentanyl $50-100\,\mu g\,kg^{-1}$) may completely inhibit the neuroendocrine element (with the exception of that triggered by cardiopulmonary bypass). If the opioid is given *after* the surgical incision, it does not prevent the emergence of the stress response. These high doses of opioids are impractical for most operations.

Effect of Epidural Anaesthesia and Analgesia on the Stress Response

Neuroendocrine Element

While only very high-dose, opioid-based general anaesthesia completely inhibits the stress response to upper abdominal surgery epidural anaesthesia, commenced before the surgical incision and continued postoperatively, significantly reduces it. Epidural anaesthesia and analgesia for lower limb or pelvic surgery completely suppresses the response. Administration of local anaesthetic drugs into the epidural space is more effective in this respect than administration of opioids alone.

Cytokine Element

The systemic release of cytokines in response to local tissue damage is not influenced by any anaesthetic technique, including epidural anaesthesia and analgesia. However, the cytokine element of the stress response is reduced by limiting the extent of the surgical incision, in particular, by use of laparoscopic techniques.

Benefits of Modifying the Stress Response

It is generally agreed that it is beneficial to decrease the stress response in patients with cardiovascular disease. Neonates undergoing cardiac surgery show a decreased stress response when anaesthesia is supplemented with sufentanil and may suffer fewer postoperative complications.

There is actually no evidence that limiting the endocrine and metabolic responses to surgery is beneficial in all patients. However, regional anaesthesia may reduce complications in elderly high-risk patients (decreased cardiovascular and respiratory complications, reduced hospital stay) but further studies are needed to confirm this.

THERMOREGULATION AND ANAESTHESIA

Mammals are homeothermic, requiring a nearly constant internal body temperature; core temperature is one of the most closely guarded physiological parameters. Although core temperature varies daily with circadian rhythm and monthly in women, body temperature does not deviate more than a few tenths of a degree either side of normal. Anaesthesia and surgery have dramatic effects on temperature regulation, such that post-operative hypothermia is the rule rather than the exception. Hypothermia results in significant morbidity, including shivering, coagulopathy, prolonged duration of drug action and increased risk of surgical wound infection.

Physiology

It is useful to consider thermoregulatory physiology in terms of a two-compartment model. A central core compartment, comprising the major trunk organs and the brain (the main sources of heat production), accounts for two-thirds of body heat content. Core body temperature is maintained within a narrow range (36.8–37.2 °C), which facilitates optimal cellular enzyme function. This range is known as the 'interthreshold range', temperatures within this range result in little homeostatic regulation. The peripheral compartment consists of skin and subcutaneous tissues over the body surface, and the limbs. It amounts to about one-third of total body heat content. In contrast with the core, peripheral tissues have wide variation in temperature, ranging from 2–3 °C below to more than 20 °C below core temperature in extreme conditions. Peripheral tissue acts as a heat sink to absorb or give up heat in an attempt to maintain core temperature within its narrow range.

Heat Balance

Thermogenesis

Maintaining core temperature within a narrow range requires balancing heat production and loss. It is achieved by a control system consisting of afferent thermal receptors, central integrating systems and efferent control mechanisms (Fig. 11.11). It was formerly believed that the spinal cord and brainstem were passive conductors of afferent signals to the preoptic

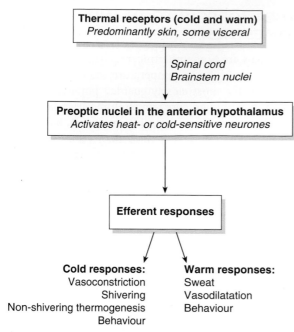

FIGURE 11.11 ■ Control of thermoregulation.

area of the hypothalamus, but it is now accepted that thermoregulation is a 'multi-level, multiple-input' system with the spinal cord, nucleus raphe magnus and locus subcoeruleus involved both in generating afferent thermal signals and modulating efferent thermoregulatory responses.

Body heat is produced by metabolism, shivering and exercise. Basal metabolic rate cannot be manipulated by thermoregulatory mechanisms. Vasoconstriction and shivering are the principal autonomic mechanisms of preserving body heat and increasing heat production.

Adjacent to the centre in the posterior hypothalamus on which the impulses from cold receptors impinge, there is a motor centre for shivering. It is normally inhibited by impulses from the heat-sensitive area in the anterior hypothalamus, but when cold impulses exceed a certain rate, the motor centre for shivering becomes activated by 'spillover' of signals and it sends impulses bilaterally into the spinal cord. Initially, this increases the tone of skeletal muscles throughout the body, but when this muscle tone increases above a specific level, shivering is observed. Shivering may increase heat production six-fold.

Non-shivering thermogenesis is also an important mechanism in increasing heat production, but is probably limited in its effectiveness to neonates. Its role in adult thermogenesis is thought to be minimal, increasing the rate of heat production by <10–15%, compared to the doubling seen in neonates. Non-shivering thermogenesis occurs mainly in brown adipose tissue (BAT). This subtype of adipose tissue contains large numbers of mitochondria in its cells, which are supplied by extensive SNS innervation. When sympathetic stimulation occurs, oxidative metabolism of the mitochondria is stimulated. However, it is *uncoupled* from phosphorylation, so that heat is produced instead of generating ATP. Exercise may increase heat production by as much as 20-fold for a short time at maximal intensity.

Heat Loss

Perioperative heat loss occurs predominantly by radiation (50–60%), convection (25–30%) evaporation (10–20%) and conduction (5%). Radiation is the major route of heat loss and is proportional to the difference in temperature between the patient and environment to the power of four. Conductive and convective heat losses are proportional to the difference between skin temperature and ambient temperature. Air flow accelerates cooling at a rate proportional to the square root of the air velocity. Evaporative heat loss from skin is usually minimal (<5% of overall heat loss) as is evaporation from the respiratory tract in a warm operating theatre, particularly when using a heat and moisture filter in the breathing system. Evaporative losses may become significant in surgery in which warm moist viscera are exposed to the air, e.g. laparotomy, and following the application of cleaning fluids (particularly alcoholic), when the latent heat of vaporization draws heat from the body to lower core temperature by as much as $0.2–0.4\,°C\,m^{-2}$.

Thermoregulation

Thermoregulation is achieved by a physiological control system consisting of peripheral and central thermoreceptors, an integrating control centre and efferent response systems (see Fig. 11.11).

Thermoreceptors. Afferent thermal input comes from anatomically distinct cold and heat receptors, located predominantly in the skin, but also centrally. The afferent thermal input comes from both core (80%) and peripheral (20%) compartments. The peripheral input is by thermally sensitive receptors located in the skin and mucous membranes, while core input occurs from thermoreceptors located in the hypothalamus itself (20%), brain (20%), spinal cord (20%), and thoracic and abdominal tissue (20%). Cold-specific receptors are innervated by Aδ fibres. Heat receptors are innervated by C fibres. Cold receptors in the skin outnumber heat receptors 10-fold and are the major mechanism by which the body protects itself against cold temperatures. Afferent input from these cold receptors in the skin is transmitted ultimately to the posterior hypothalamus.

Afferent thermal signals provide feedback to temperature-regulating centres in the hypothalamus. The preoptic area of the hypothalamus contains temperature-sensitive and temperature-insensitive neurones. The temperature-sensitive neurones, which predominate by 4:1, increase their discharge rate in response to increased local heat and this activates heat loss mechanisms. Conversely, cold-sensitive neurones increase their rate of discharge in response to cooling. Detection of cold differs from detection of heat, in that the principal mechanism of detection of cold is input from cutaneous cold receptors. At normothermia, most afferent input comes from cold receptors. Blockade of this afferent input by regional anaesthesia explains why the lower limbs are often perceived by the patient as feeling warm when epidural or spinal anaesthesia is established.

Central Control. The central control mechanism, situated in the hypothalamus, determines mean body temperature by integrating thermal signals from peripheral and core structures and comparing mean body temperature with a predetermined 'set point' temperature. The set point or physiological 'thermostat' of the thermoregulatory system is the temperature at which the system requires zero action to maintain that temperature (36.8–37.2 °C). The limits of this range represent the thresholds at which cold or heat responses are instigated, and hence it has been termed the 'interthreshold range'. Normally it is <1 °C, but this increases to 4 °C during general anaesthesia.

Effector Mechanisms. The most effective mechanisms for controlling body temperature are behavioural.

In extreme cold conditions, vasoconstriction and shivering are of limited effect compared to behavioural measures such as taking shelter and wearing protective clothing.

Physiological responses to heat result in vasodilatation and sweating which are the major autonomic mechanisms of increasing heat loss. Maximal sweating rates may reach over $1 L h^{-1}$ for a short time, resulting in heat loss of up to 15 times BMR.

Physiological responses to cold are generally of more relevance to anaesthesia because hypothermia is common during most procedures. In normal adults, the first response to a decrease in core temperature below the normal range (36.5–37.5 °C) is peripheral vasoconstriction. If core temperature continues to decrease, shivering commences. Vasoconstriction and shivering are characterized by *threshold onset, gain and maximal response intensity. Threshold* is the temperature at which the effector is activated. *Gain* is the rate of response to a given decrease in core temperature. Normally, the threshold core temperature for thermoregulatory vasoconstriction is 36.5 °C, with shivering commencing at 36.0–36.2 °C.

Measurement of Temperature

Core temperature may be evaluated reliably by an infrared thermometer at the tympanic membrane (provided that the external auditory meatus is free of ear wax) or by thermocouples positioned in the distal oesophagus, nasopharynx or pulmonary artery. Skin surface temperature varies with ambient temperature and induction of anaesthesia, and is usually also measured with a thermocouple. Rectal and bladder temperature may lag behind changes in core temperature because these organs are not perfused well enough to reflect rapid changes in body heat content.

Effect of General Anaesthesia on Thermoregulation

General anaesthesia has a number of effects on homeostatic mechanisms controlling thermoregulation which combine to cause hypothermia and impair the mechanisms which would normally limit the associated heat loss.

Widening of the Interthreshold Range

As discussed above, the interthreshold range is a narrow range of core temperature within which thermoregulatory mechanisms are relatively quiescent.

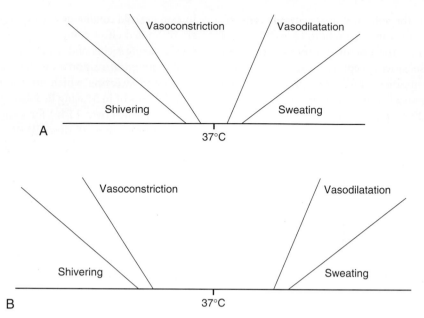

FIGURE 11.12 ■ Thresholds for thermoregulatory effectors. **(A)** Under normal conditions, the range of core temperatures within which no effector is active, i.e. normal temperature, is approximately 0.5 °C. **(B)** During general anaesthesia, the range of core temperatures within which no effector is active is increased to approximately 4.0 °C.

General anaesthesia causes a dose-dependent widening of this interthreshold range, with an increase in the temperature at which thermoregulatory responses to heat are activated and an even greater reduction in the temperature at which thermoregulatory responses to cold are activated. Typically, the interthreshold range widens by about 4 °C, with the body becoming poikilothermic within this temperature range (Fig. 11.12). However, once core temperature falls outside this range, the gain (the rate of response to a given decrease in core temperature) and maximal response intensity of homeostatic mechanisms are unaffected. All general anaesthetic agents, both volatile and intravenous, impair thermoregulatory responses to a similar, but not identical, extent.

Stages of Hypothermia

Mild hypothermia during general anaesthesia follows a distinctive pattern and occurs in three phases (Fig. 11.13):

Phase 1 (Redistribution Stage). Under normal conditions, the temperature gradient between core and peripheral compartments is maintained by tonic vasoconstriction. On induction of anaesthesia, normal vasoconstrictor tone is reduced, and vasodilatation occurs, allowing heat to flow down its concentration gradient from the warm core to the cooler periphery, resulting in a mild core hypothermia (core temperature about 35.5–36.0 °C). This core hypothermia occurs because of *redistribution* of body heat on induction of anaesthesia, and *overall* heat loss from the body is minimal. Redistribution hypothermia results in an initial rapid decrease in core temperature of approximately 1 °C over the first 30 min, but mean body temperature and body heat content remain constant during this 30 min (Fig. 11.14).

There are a number of factors which affect the magnitude of this initial phase 1 hypothermia.

- The greater the temperature gradient between the core and periphery, the greater is the decrease in core temperature. Patients who have been left in a cold reception room, for example, will have a relatively cold peripheral compartment and will suffer a greater degree of redistribution hypothermia.

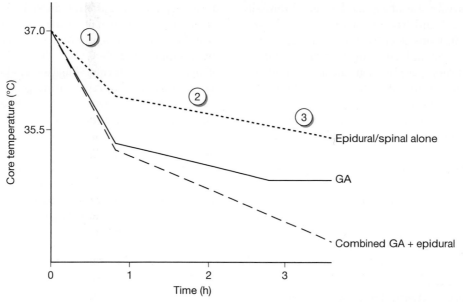

FIGURE 11.13 ■ Characteristic patterns of hypothermia during general anaesthesia (GA) alone, epidural or spinal anaesthesia alone and combined general and epidural anaesthesia. Patients in this last category are more likely to develop profound hypothermia than others (see text).

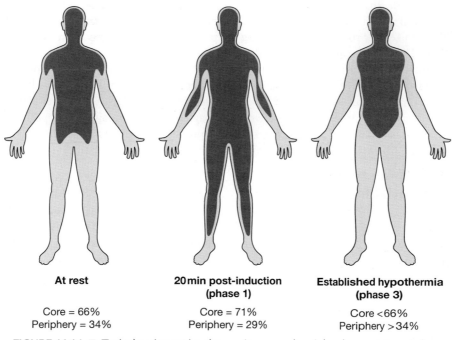

FIGURE 11.14 ■ Typical perioperative changes in core and peripheral compartment sizes.

- Patients who are obese tend to be chronically vasodilated and have a warm peripheral compartment. Consequently, they suffer less vasodilatation on induction of anaesthesia and the reduced core–peripheral gradient also limits the magnitude of the redistribution hypothermia.
- Neonates, and to a lesser extent children, have a much smaller peripheral compartment than adults and any decrease in core temperature on induction of anaesthesia is likely to be true heat loss rather than redistribution hypothermia.

Phase 2 (Heat Loss > Heat Production). Phase 2 is a slower linear decrease in core temperature to 34–35 °C over the next 2 h and occurs as a result of heat loss exceeding heat production. General anaesthesia reduces metabolic heat production by 15–40%, particularly through decreased brain metabolism and reduced respiratory muscle activity. Increased heat loss occurs through peripheral vasodilatation, evaporative heat loss from the body surface, and evaporative losses from exposed body cavities (some animal studies have shown that as much as 50% of total heat loss can come from exposed bowel).

Phase 3 (Plateau Phase). Phase 3 is a core temperature plateau (or thermal equilibrium), where heat loss equals heat production (either metabolic or warming devices) (Fig. 11.14). This core temperature plateau results largely from thermoregulatory vasoconstriction, triggered by a core temperature of 33–35 °C. Patients with impaired autonomic responses (e.g. elderly, diabetics, Parkinson's disease, Shy-Drager syndrome, etc.) are less able to establish effective vasoconstriction and in these patients, establishment of a plateau phase may be delayed or even absent.

Effect of Regional Anaesthesia on Thermoregulation

Regional anaesthesia has a similar effect to general anaesthesia on thermoregulation and hypothermia. Regional anaesthesia widens the interthreshold range. The reasons for this are not clear, but are probably related to a blockade of afferent input to the hypothalamus. As with general anaesthesia, redistribution of body heat during spinal or epidural anaesthesia is the main cause of hypothermia. Because redistribution

during spinal or epidural anaesthesia is confined usually to the lower half of the body, the initial core hypothermia is not as pronounced as in general anaesthesia (approximately 0.5 °C). Otherwise, the pattern of hypothermia during spinal or epidural anaesthesia is similar to that seen during general anaesthesia for the first two phases. The major difference for spinal or epidural anaesthesia is that the plateau phase does not emerge because vasoconstriction is blocked (see Fig. 11.13). Heat loss continues unabated during epidural anaesthesia despite the activation of effector mechanisms above the level of the block. Therefore, patients undergoing long procedures with combined general and epidural anaesthesia are at risk of a greater degree of hypothermia.

Consequences of Perioperative Hypothermia

In specific circumstances, hypothermia may have a protective effect in terms of reducing basal metabolic rate. The use of moderate hypothermia is routine practice in many centres during cardiopulmonary bypass. It is generally agreed, however, that, in most situations, the deleterious consequences of mild hypothermia outweigh the potential benefits, with evidence emerging that hypothermia *per se* is responsible for adverse postoperative outcomes. In particular, hypothermic patients are more likely than normothermic patients to have postoperative wound infections. The initial 3–4 h after bacterial contamination are thought to be crucial in determining whether clinical infection ensues. *In vitro* studies suggest that platelet function and coagulation are impaired by hypothermia, and mildly hypothermic patients lose >25% more blood in the perioperative period than do normothermic patients. In addition, perioperative thermal discomfort is often remembered by patients as the worst aspect of their perioperative experience (Table 11.5).

Physical, Active and Passive Strategies for Avoiding Perioperative Hypothermia

Preventing redistribution-induced hypothermia may be achieved by physical and pharmacological means (Table 11.6). Redistribution of heat results when anaesthetic-induced vasodilatation allows heat to flow from the core to the periphery down its concentration gradient. Pre-emptive skin surface warming does

TABLE 11.5
Consequences of Perioperative Hypothermia

Cardiac	CO↓, HR↓, BP↓ PR duration↑, QRS duration↑, QT prolongation, J waves Viscosity↑ Cardiac work↑ MI risk↑
Respiratory	Increased dead space Respiratory fatigue
Wound infection	Caused by vasoconstriction and hence low tissue oxygen tension (P_tO_2)
Prolonged drug action	
Negative nitrogen balance, metabolism↓, 8% per 1 °C below normal temperature	
Prolonged coagulation	
DVT/PE risk↑	
Oxyhaemoglobin dissociation curve shifted to right	
Stress response↑	
Patient discomfort/shivering	

TABLE 11.6
Strategies for Prevention of Perioperative Hypothermia

Intraoperative use of forced air convective warming device
Reflective space blankets
Heating and humidifying inspired gases
Increased ambient temperature to 23 °C
Warmed i.v. fluids

not increase core temperature but increases body heat content, particularly in the legs, and removes the gradient for heat loss via the skin. However, this approach is rarely used in clinical practice because it requires 1 h of prewarming. This is unfortunate because it is a far more effective method of minimizing peri-operative hypothermia than trying to rewarm patients who have become hypothermic.

Passive insulation with a single layer of any insulating material reduces cutaneous heat loss by 30–50%.

Because only 10% of metabolic heat production is lost in heating and humidifying inspired gases, this method is relatively ineffective. Heat and moisture exchange filters retain significant amounts of moisture and heat within the respiratory system, but are only 50% as effective as active mechanisms. Ambient temperature determines the rate of heat loss by radiation and convection and maintains normothermia if close to initial, preinduction, core temperature (36 °C). However, this is usually impractical, as operating room staff find this temperature uncomfortable. Water mattresses are demonstrably ineffective at preventing heat loss, possibly because relatively little heat is lost from the back. Moreover, decreased local tissue perfusion associated with local temperatures of 40 °C may lead to skin necrosis. Heat loss may be reduced if intravenous fluids are warmed before or during administration.

Forced air warming systems are undoubtedly the best way to maintain normothermia during long procedures and are particularly effective when used intra-operatively for vasodilated patients, allowing heat applied peripherally to be transferred rapidly to the core. Their use increases core temperature and reduces the incidence of postanaesthetic shivering (Table 11.6).

Postanaesthetic Shivering

Postanaesthetic shivering affects up to 65% of patients after general anaesthesia and 33% during epidural or regional anaesthesia. It is usually defined as readily detectable tremor of the face, jaw, head, trunk or extremities lasting longer than 15 s. Apart from the obvious discomfort, postanaesthetic shivering, in common with hypothermia, is associated with several potentially deleterious sequelae (see Table 11.5). Postanaesthetic shivering is usually preceded by core hypothermia and vasoconstriction. Two patterns of muscular activity, seen in electromyography studies, contribute to the phenomenon of postanaesthetic shivering; first, a tonic pattern (4–8 cycles min^{-1} characteristic of the response to hypothermia in awake patients) is observed, and then a phasic (6–7 Hz) pattern resembling clonus.

While hypothermia is one factor in the aetiology of postanaesthetic shivering, not all patients who shiver are hypothermic. Studies on postoperative patients have indicated that male gender, age (16–60 years) and anticholinergic premedication are risk factors for

TABLE 11.7
Treatment of Postanaesthetic Shivering
Pethidine 0.33 mg kg^{-1} (other opioids to a lesser extent)
Doxapram 1.5 mg kg^{-1}
Clonidine 2 μg kg^{-1}
Methylphenidate 0.1 mg kg^{-1}
Physostigmine 0.04 mg kg^{-1}
Ondansetron 0.1 mg kg^{-1}

postanaesthetic shivering, while the intraoperative use of pethidine virtually abolishes it. The use of propofol reduces the incidence of postoperative shivering compared with thiopental.

Postoperative shivering should not be treated in isolation from perioperative hypothermia. Not all patients who shiver are hypothermic, but most are, and successful treatment of shivering in these patients without concomitant management of hypothermia may result in deepening hypothermia. However, the mainstay of symptomatic treatment of postoperative shivering is radiant heating, forced air rewarming or pharmacological methods (Table 11.7).

A wide range of drugs is effective and it would be surprising if all worked on a single part of the thermoregulatory mechanism. Pethidine is remarkably effective in treating postoperative shivering, 25 mg being sufficient in the majority of adults. There is evidence that this may be the result of an action at the κ-opioid receptor.

One hypothesis for the mechanism of postanaesthetic shivering is that, because the brain recovers later than the spinal cord, uninhibited spinal clonic tremor occurs, resulting in shivering. Consistent with this hypothesis, doxapram (a cerebral stimulant) has also been shown to be an effective treatment, but it is not as effective as pethidine. Various drugs, the mechanisms of action of which are unclear, are also effective. Physostigmine prevents the onset of postanaesthetic shivering, implying that cholinergic pathways are involved in the thermoregulatory mechanisms which lead to shivering. Clonidine, an α_2-adrenergic agonist and ondansetron, a serotonergic antagonist, are also effective.

FURTHER READING

Buggy, D.J., Crossley, A.W.A., 2000. Thermoregulation, perioperative hypothermia and post-anaesthetic shivering. Br. J. Anaesth. 84, 615–628.

Desborough, J.P., 2000. The stress response to trauma and surgery. Br. J. Anaesth. 85, 107–117.

Guyton, A.C., Hall, J.E., 2005. Metabolism and temperature regulation. In: Guyton, A.C., Hall, J.E. (Eds.), Textbook of medical physiology, eleventh ed. WB Saunders, Philadelphia.

Hahnenkamp, K., Herroeder, S., Hollmann, M.W., 2004. Regional anaesthesia, local anaesthetics and the surgical stress response. Best Pract. Res. Clin. Anaesthesiol. 18, 509–527.

Inadvertent perioperative hypothermia. NICE clinical guideline. 2008. Available from www.nice.org.uk/CG065.

Kohl, B.A., Deutschman, C.S., 2006. The inflammatory response to surgery and trauma. Curr. Opin. Crit. Care 12, 325–332.

Reynolds, L., Beckmann, J., Kurz, A., 2008. Perioperative complications of hypothermia. Best Pract. Res. Clin. Anaesthesiol. 22, 645–657.

Sessler, D.I., 2008. Temperature monitoring and perioperative thermoregulation. Anesthesiology 109, 318–338.

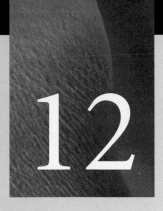

12

FLUID, ELECTROLYTE AND ACID–BASE BALANCE

■ ■ ■ ■ ■ ■ ■ ■ ■ ■ ■ ■

The realization that the enzyme systems and metabolic processes responsible for the maintenance of cellular function are dependent on an environment with stable electrolyte and hydrogen ion concentrations led Claude Bernard to describe the 'milieu interieur' over 100 years ago. Complex homeostatic mechanisms have evolved to maintain the constancy of this internal environment and thus prevent cellular dysfunction.

BASIC DEFINITIONS

Osmosis refers to the movement of *solvent* molecules across a membrane into a region in which there is a higher concentration of *solute*. This movement may be prevented by applying a pressure to the more concentrated solution – the effective osmotic pressure. This is a colligative property; the magnitude of effective osmotic pressure exerted by a solution depends on the number rather than the type of particles present.

The amounts of osmotically active particles present in solution are expressed in *osmoles*. One osmole of a substance is equal to its molecular weight in grams (1 mol) divided by the number of freely moving particles which each molecule liberates in solution. Thus, 180 g of glucose in 1 L of water represents a solution with a molar concentration of $1\,mol\,L^{-1}$ and an *osmolarity* of $1\,osmol\,L^{-1}$. Sodium chloride ionizes in solution and each ion represents an osmotically active particle. Assuming complete dissociation into Na^+ and Cl^-, 58.5 g of NaCl dissolved in 1 L of water has a molar concentration of $1\,mol\,L^{-1}$ and an osmolarity of $2\,osmol\,L^{-1}$. In body fluids, solute concentrations are much lower ($mmol\,L^{-1}$) and dissociation is incomplete.

Consequently, a solution of NaCl containing $1\,mmol\,L^{-1}$ contributes slightly less than $2\,mosmol\,L^{-1}$.

The term *osmolality* refers to the number of osmoles per unit of total weight of solvent, whereas *osmolarity* refers to the number of osmoles per litre of solvent. Osmolality (unlike osmolarity), is not affected by the volume of various solutes in solution. Confusion regarding the apparently interchangeable use of the terms osmolarity (measured in $osmol\,L^{-1}$) and osmolality (measured in $osmol\,kg^{-1}$) is caused by their numerical equivalence in body fluids; plasma osmolarity is 280–$310\,mosmol\,L^{-1}$ and plasma osmolality is 280–$310\,mosmol\,kg^{-1}$. This equivalence is explained by the almost negligible solute volume contained in biological fluids and the fact that most osmotically active particles are dissolved in water, which has a density of 1 (i.e. $osmol\,L^{-1}$=$osmol\,kg^{-1}$). As the number of osmoles in plasma is estimated by measurement of the magnitude of freezing point depression, the more accurate term in clinical practice is osmolality.

Cations (principally Na^+) and anions (Cl^- and HCO_3^-) are the major osmotically active particles in plasma. Glucose and urea make a smaller contribution. Plasma osmolality (P_{OSM}) may be estimated from the formula:

$$P_{OSM} = 2[Na^+]\,(mmol\,L^{-1}) + blood\,glucose\,(mmol\,L^{-1})$$
$$+ blood\,urea\,(mmol\,L^{-1}) = 290\,mosmol\,kg^{-1}$$

Osmolality is a chemical term and may be confused with the physiological term, *tonicity*. This term is used to describe the effective osmotic pressure of a solution relative to that of plasma. The critical difference between osmolality and tonicity is that *all* solutes contribute to osmolality, but only solutes that do not cross the cell membrane contribute to tonicity. Thus, tonicity expresses the osmolal activity of solutes restricted to the extracellular compartment, i.e. those which exert an osmotic force affecting the distribution of water between intracellular fluid (ICF) and extracellular fluid (ECF). As urea diffuses freely across cell membranes, it does not alter the distribution of water between these two body fluid compartments and does not contribute to tonicity. Other solutes that contribute to plasma osmolality but not tonicity include ethanol and methanol, both of which distribute rapidly throughout the total body water. In contrast, mannitol and sorbitol are restricted to the ECF and contribute to both osmolality and tonicity. The tonicity of plasma may be estimated from the formula:

$$\begin{aligned} \text{plasma tonicity} &= 2\left[Na^+\right]\left(mmol\,L^{-1}\right) \\ &\quad + \text{blood glucose}\ (mmol\,L^{-1}) \\ &= 285\,mosmol\,kg^{-1} \end{aligned}$$

COMPARTMENTAL DISTRIBUTION OF TOTAL BODY WATER

The volume of total body water (TBW) may be measured using radioactive dilution techniques involving either deuterium or tritium, both of which cross all membranes freely and equilibrate rapidly with hydrogen atoms in body water. Such measurements show

that approximately 60% of lean body mass (LBM) is water in the average 70 kg male adult. As fat contains little water, females have proportionately less TBW (55%) relative to LBM. TBW decreases with age, decreasing to 45–50% in later life.

The distribution of TBW between the main body compartments is illustrated in Figure 12.1. One-third of TBW is contained in the extracellular fluid volume (ECFV) and two-thirds in the intracellular fluid volume (ICFV). The ECFV is subdivided further into the interstitial and intravascular compartments. In addition to the absolute volumes of each compartment, Figure 12.1 shows the relative size of each compartment compared with body weight.

SOLUTE COMPOSITION OF BODY FLUID COMPARTMENTS

Extracellular Fluid

The capillary endothelium behaves as a freely permeable membrane to water, cations, anions and many soluble substances such as glucose and urea (but not protein). As a result, the solute compositions of interstitial fluid and plasma are similar. Each contains sodium as the principal cation and chloride as the principal anion. Protein behaves as a non-diffusible anion and is present in a higher concentration in

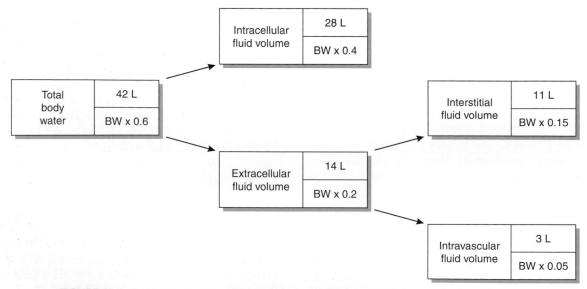

FIGURE 12.1 ■ Distribution of total body water in a 70 kg male, and related to body weight (BW).

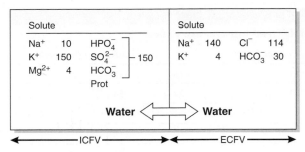

FIGURE 12.2 ■ Principal solute composition of body fluid compartments. All concentrations are expressed in mmol L⁻¹.

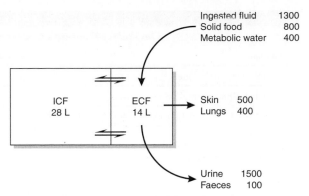

FIGURE 12.3 ■ Daily water balance. Input and output in millilitres.

plasma. The concentration of Cl⁻ is slightly higher in interstitial fluid in order to maintain electrical neutrality (Donnan equilibrium).

Intracellular Fluid

This differs from ECF in that the principal cation is potassium and the principal anion is phosphate. In addition, there is a high protein content. In contrast to the capillary endothelium, the cell membrane is permeable *selectively* to different ions and freely permeable to water. Thus, equalization of osmotic forces occurs continuously and is achieved by the movement of water across the cell membrane. The osmolalities of ICF and ECF at equilibrium must be equal. Water moves rapidly between ICF and ECF to eliminate any induced osmolal gradient. This principle is fundamental to an understanding of fluid and electrolyte physiology.

Figure 12.2 shows the solute composition of the main body fluid compartments. Although the total concentration of intracellular ions exceeds that of extracellular ions, the numbers of osmotically active particles (and thus the osmolalities) are the same on each side of the cell membrane (290 mosmol kg⁻¹ of solution).

WATER HOMEOSTASIS

Normal day-to-day fluctuations in TBW are small (<0.2%) because of a fine balance between input, controlled by the thirst mechanisms, and output, controlled mainly by the renal–ADH (antidiuretic hormone) system.

The principal sources of body water are ingested fluid, water present in solid food and water produced as an end-product of metabolism. Intravenous fluids are

another common source in hospital patients. Actual and potential outlets for water are classified conventionally as sensible and insensible losses. Insensible losses emanate from the skin and lungs; sensible losses occur mainly from the kidneys and gastrointestinal tract. Figure 12.3 depicts the daily water balance in a 70 kg adult in whom input and output balance. It should be noted that sources of potential loss are not evident in this diagram. For example, over 5 L of fluid are secreted daily into the gut in the form of saliva, bile, gastric juices and succus entericus, yet only 100 mL of fluid is present in faeces. This illustrates the potential that exists for significant fluid loss in the presence of disease.

PRACTICAL FLUID BALANCE

Calculation of the daily prescription of fluid is an arithmetic exercise to balance the input and output of water and electrolytes.

Table 12.1 shows the electrolyte contents of five intravenous solutions used commonly in the United Kingdom. These solutions are adequate for most clinical situations. Two self-evident but important generalizations may be made regarding solutions for intravenous infusion.

Rule 1. All infused Na⁺ remains in the ECF; Na⁺ cannot gain access to the ICF because of the sodium pump. Thus, if saline 0.9% is infused, all Na⁺ remains in the ECF. As this is an isotonic solution, there is no change in ECF osmolality and therefore no water exchange occurs across the cell membrane. Thus, saline 0.9%

TABLE 12.1
Electrolyte Contents of Commonly Used Intravenous Fluids

Solution		Electrolyte Content (mmol L^{-1})				Osmolality (mosmol kg^{-1})
Saline 0.9% ('normal saline')	Na$^+$	154	Cl$^-$		154	308
Saline 0.45% ('half-normal saline')	Na$^+$	77	Cl$^-$		77	154
Glucose 4%/saline 0.18% (glucose–saline)	Na$^+$	31	Cl$^-$		31	284
Glucose 5%		Nil				278
Compound sodium lactate (Hartmann's solution)	Na$^+$	131	Cl$^-$		112	281
	K$^+$	5	HCO$_3^-$ (as lactate)		29	
	Ca^{2+}	4				

expands ECFV only. However, if saline 0.45% is given, ECF osmolality decreases; this causes a shift of water from ECF to ICF. If saline 1.8% is administered, all Na$^+$ remains in the ECF, its osmolality increases and water moves from ICF to ECF to maintain osmotic equality.

Rule 2. Water without sodium expands the TBW. After infusion of a solution of glucose 5%, the glucose enters cells and is metabolized. The infused water enters both ICF and ECF in proportion to their initial volumes.

Table 12.2 illustrates the results of infusion of 1 L of saline 0.9%, saline 0.45% or glucose 5% in a 70 kg adult.

Assessment of daily fluid requirements may be allocated usefully into three processes:

- normal maintenance needs
- abnormal losses resulting from the underlying pathology
- correction of pre-existing deficits.

TABLE 12.2
Compartmental Expansion Resulting from Infusion of 1 L of Saline 0.9%, Saline 0.45% or Glucose 5%

Intravenous Infusion of 1000 mL	CHANGE IN VOLUME (ML)		Remarks
	ECF	ICF	
Saline 0.9%	+1000	0	Na$^+$ remains in ECF
Glucose 5%	+333	+666	66% of TBW is ICF
Saline 0.45%	+666	+333	33% of TBW is ECF

Normal Maintenance Needs

Water. Regardless of the disease process, water and electrolyte losses occur in urine and as evaporative losses from skin and lungs. It is evident from Figure 12.3 that a normothermic 70 kg patient with a normal metabolic rate may lose 2500 mL of water per day. Allowing for a gain of 400 mL from water of metabolism, this hypothetical patient needs about 2000 mL day^{-1} of water. As a rule of thumb, a volume of 30–35 mL kg^{-1} day^{-1} of water is a useful estimate for daily maintenance needs.

Sodium. The normal requirement is 1 mmol kg^{-1} day^{-1} (50–80 mmol day^{-1}) for adults.

Potassium. The normal requirement is 1 mmol kg^{-1} day^{-1} (50–80 mmol day^{-1}) for adults.

Thus, a 70 kg patient requires daily provision of 2000–2500 mL of water and approximately 70 mmol each of Na$^+$ and K$^+$. This could be administered as one of the following:

- 2000 mL of glucose 5% + 500 mL of saline 0.9%
- 2500 mL of glucose 4%/saline 0.18%; plus potassium as KCl, 1 g (13 mmol) added to each 500 mL of fluid.

Abnormal Losses

These are common in surgical patients. They may be sensible or insensible and either overt or covert.

Losses from the gut are common, e.g. nasogastric suction, diarrhoea and vomiting or sequestration of fluid within the gut lumen (e.g. intestinal obstruction). Although the composition of gastrointestinal secretions is variable, replacement should be with saline 0.9% with 13–26 mmol L^{-1} of potassium as KCl.

If losses are considerable ($>1000\,mL\,day^{-1}$), a sample of the appropriate fluid should be sent for biochemical analysis so that electrolyte replacement may be rationalized.

Increased insensible losses from the skin and lungs occur in the presence of fever or hyperventilation. The usual insensible loss of $0.5\,mL\,kg^{-1}\,h^{-1}$ increases by 12% for each °Celsius rise in body temperature.

Sequestration of fluid at the site of operative trauma is a form of fluid loss which is common in surgical patients. Plasma-like fluid is sequestered in any area of tissue injury; its volume is proportional to the extent of trauma. This fluid is frequently referred to as 'third-space' loss because it ceases to take part in normal metabolic processes. However, it is not contained in an anatomically separate compartment; it represents an expansion of ECFV. Third-space losses are not measured easily. Sequestered fluid is reabsorbed after 48–72 h.

Existing Deficits

These occur preoperatively and arise primarily from the gut. The difficulty in correcting these deficits relates to an inability to quantify their magnitude accurately. Fluid and electrolyte deficits occur directly from the ECF. If the fluid lost is isotonic, only ECFV is reduced; however, if water alone or hypotonic fluid is lost, redistribution of the remaining TBW occurs from ICF to ECF to equalize osmotic forces.

Dehydration with accompanying salt loss is a common disorder in the acutely ill surgical patient.

Assessment of Dehydration

This is a clinical assessment based upon the following.

History. How long has the patient had abnormal loss of fluid? How much has occurred, e.g. volume and frequency of vomiting?

Examination. Specific features are thirst, dryness of mucous membranes, loss of skin turgor, orthostatic hypotension or tachycardia, reduced jugular venous pressure (JVP) or central venous pressure (CVP) and decreased urine output. In the presence of normal renal function, dehydration is associated usually with a urine output of less than $0.5\,mL\,kg^{-1}\,h^{-1}$. The severity of dehydration may be described clinically as mild, moderate or severe and each category is associated with the following water loss relative to body weight:

- *mild:* loss of 4% body weight (approximately 3 L in a 70 kg patient) – reduced skin turgor, sunken eyes, dry mucous membranes
- *moderate:* loss of 5–8% body weight (approximately 4–6 L in a 70 kg patient) – oliguria, orthostatic hypotension and tachycardia in addition to the above
- *severe:* loss of 8–10% body weight (approximately 7 L in a 70 kg patient) – profound oliguria and compromised cardiovascular function.

Laboratory Assessment

The degree of haemoconcentration and increase in albumin concentration may be helpful in the absence of anaemia and hypoproteinaemia. Increased blood urea concentration and urine osmolality ($>650\,mosmol\,kg^{-1}$) confirm the clinical diagnosis.

Perioperative Fluid Therapy

In addition to normal maintenance requirements of water and electrolytes, patients may require fluid in the perioperative period to restore TBW after a period of fasting and to replace small blood losses, loss of ECF into the 'third space' and losses of water from the skin, gut and lungs.

Blood losses in excess of 15% of blood volume in the adult are usually replaced by infusion of stored blood. Smaller blood losses may be replaced by a crystalloid electrolyte solution such as compound sodium lactate; however, because these solutions are distributed throughout ECF, blood volume is maintained only if at least three times the volume of blood loss is infused. Alternatively, a colloid solution (human albumin solution or more usually a synthetic substitute) may be infused in a volume equal to that of the estimated loss.

Third-space losses are usually replaced as compound sodium lactate. In abdominal surgery (e.g. cholecystectomy), a volume of $5\,mL\,kg^{-1}\,h^{-1}$ during operation, in addition to normal maintenance requirements (approximately $1.5\,mL\,kg^{-1}\,h^{1}$) and blood loss replacement, is usually sufficient. Larger volumes may be required in more major procedures, but one should be guided by measurement of CVP or other measures of preload.

In the postoperative period, normal maintenance fluids should be administered (see above). Additional fluid (given as saline 0.9% or compound sodium lactate) may be required in the following circumstances:

- if blood or serum is lost from drains (colloid solutions should be used if losses exceed 500 mL)
- if gastrointestinal losses continue, e.g. from a nasogastric tube or a fistula
- after major surgery (e.g. oesophagectomy, total gastrectomy, aortic aneurysm repair), when additional water and electrolytes may be required for 24–48 h to replace continuing third-space losses
- during rewarming if the patient has become hypothermic during surgery.

Normally, potassium is not administered in the first 24 h after surgery as endogenous release of potassium from tissue trauma and catabolism warrants restriction. The postoperative patient differs from the 'normal' patient in that the stress reaction modifies homeostatic mechanisms; stress-induced release of ADH, aldosterone and cortisol causes retention of Na^+ and water and increased renal excretion of potassium. However, restriction of fluid and sodium in the postoperative period is inappropriate because of increased losses by evaporation and into the 'third space'.

This syndrome of inappropriate ADH secretion may persist for several days in elderly patients, who are at risk of symptomatic hyponatraemia if given hypotonic fluids in the postoperative period. Elderly, orthopaedic patients taking long-term thiazide diuretics are especially at risk if given 5% glucose postoperatively. Such patients may develop water intoxication and permanent brain damage as a result of relatively modest reductions in serum sodium concentration.

After major surgery, assessment of fluid and electrolyte requirements is achieved best by measurement of CVP and serum electrolyte concentrations. Fluid and electrolyte requirements in infants and small children differ from those in the adult (see Ch 36).

Patients with renal failure require fluid replacement for abnormal losses, although the total volume of fluid infused should be reduced to a degree determined by the urine output.

SODIUM AND POTASSIUM

Sodium Balance

Daily ingestion amounts to 50–300 mmol. Losses in sweat and faeces are minimal (approximately 10 mmol day^{-1}) and the kidney makes final adjustments. Urine sodium excretion may be as little as 2 mmol day^{-1} during salt restriction or may exceed 700 mmol day^{-1} after salt loading. Sodium balance is related intimately to ECFV and water balance.

Disorders of Sodium/Water Balance

Hypernatraemia

Hypernatraemia is defined as a plasma sodium concentration of more than 150 mmol L^{-1} and may result from pure water loss, hypotonic fluid loss or salt gain. In the first two conditions, ECFV is reduced, whereas salt gain is associated with an expanded ECFV. For this reason, the clinical assessment of volaemic status is important in the diagnosis and management of hypernatraemic states. The common causes of hypernatraemia are summarized in Table 12.3. The abnormality common to all hypernatraemic states is intracellular dehydration secondary to ECF hyperosmolality. Primary water loss resulting in

TABLE 12.3
Causes of Hypernatraemia

Pure Water Depletion	
Extrarenal loss	Failure of water intake (coma, elderly, postoperative) Mucocutaneous loss Fever, hyperventilation, thyrotoxicosis
Renal loss	Diabetes insipidus (cranial, nephrogenic) Chronic renal failure
Hypotonic Fluid Loss	
Extrarenal loss	Gastrointestinal (vomiting, diarrhoea) Skin (excessive sweating)
Renal loss	Osmotic diuresis (glucose, urea, mannitol)
Salt Gain	
	Iatrogenic ($NaHCO_3$, hypertonic saline) Salt ingestion Steroid excess

hypernatraemia may occur during prolonged fever, hyperventilation or severe exercise in hot, dry climates. However, a more common cause is the renal water loss that occurs when there is a defect in either the production or release of ADH (cranial diabetes insipidus) or an abnormality in response to ADH (nephrogenic diabetes insipidus).

The administration of osmotic diuretics results temporarily in plasma hyperosmolality. An osmotic diuresis may occur also in hyperglycaemia. During an osmotic diuresis, the solute causing the diuresis (e.g. glucose, mannitol) constitutes a significant fraction of urine solute, and the sodium content of the urine becomes hypotonic relative to plasma sodium. Thus, osmotic diuretics cause hypotonic urine losses which may result in hypernatraemic dehydration.

Hypertonic dehydration may occur also in paediatric patients. Diarrhoea, vomiting and anorexia lead to loss of water in excess of solute (hypotonic loss). Concomitant fever, hyperventilation and the use of high-solute feeds may combine to exaggerate the problem. ECFV is maintained by movement of water from ICF to ECF to equalize osmolality, and clinical evidence of dehydration may not be apparent until 10–15% of body weight has been lost. Rehydration must be undertaken gradually to prevent the development of cerebral oedema.

Measurement of urine and plasma osmolalities and assessment of urine output help in the diagnosis of hypernatraemic, volume-depleted states. If urine output is low and urine osmolality exceeds $800 \, \text{mosmol} \, \text{kg}^{-1}$, then both ADH secretion and the renal response to ADH are present. The most likely causes are extrarenal water loss (e.g. diarrhoea, vomiting or evaporation) or insufficient intake. High urine output and high urine osmolality suggest an osmotic diuresis. If urine osmolality is less than plasma osmolality, reduced ADH secretion or impairment of the renal response to ADH should be suspected; in both cases, urine output is high.

Usually, hypernatraemia caused by salt gain is iatrogenic in origin. It occurs when excessive amounts of hypertonic sodium bicarbonate are administered during resuscitation or when isotonic fluids are given to patients who have only insensible losses. Treatment comprises induction of a diuresis with a loop diuretic if renal function is normal; urine output is replaced in part with glucose 5%. Dialysis or haemofiltration is necessary in patients with renal dysfunction.

Consequences of Hypernatraemia. The major clinical manifestations of hypernatraemia involve the central nervous system. Severity depends on the rapidity with which hyperosmolality develops. Acute hypernatraemia is associated with a prompt osmotic shift of water from the intracellular compartment, causing a reduction in cell volume and water content of the brain. This results in increased permeability and even rupture of the capillaries in the brain and subarachnoid space. The patient may present with pyrexia (a manifestation of impaired thermoregulation), nausea, vomiting, convulsions, coma and virtually any type of focal neurological syndrome. The mortality and long-term morbidity of sustained hypernatraemia ($Na^+ > 160 \, \text{mmol} \, L^{-1}$ for over 48 h) is high, irrespective of the underlying aetiology. In many cases, the development of hypernatraemia can be anticipated and prevented, e.g. cranial diabetes insipidus associated with head injury, but in situations where preventative strategies have failed, treatment should be instituted without delay.

Treatment of Hypernatraemia. The magnitude of the water deficit can be estimated from the measured plasma sodium concentration and calculated total body water:

$$\text{water deficit} = (\text{measured} \, [Na^+]/140 \times TBW) - TBW$$

Thus, in a 75 kg patient with a serum sodium of $170 \, \text{mmol} \, L^{-1}$:

$$\begin{aligned} \text{water deficit} &= (170/140 \times 0.6 \times 75) - (0.6 \times 75) \\ &= 54.6 - 45 \\ &= 9.6L \end{aligned}$$

For hypernatraemic patients *without* volume depletion, 5% glucose is sufficient to correct the water deficit. However, the majority of hypernatraemic patients are frankly hypovolaemic and intravenous fluids should be prescribed to repair both the sodium and the water deficits. Regardless of the severity of the condition, isotonic saline is the initial treatment of choice in the volume-depleted, hypernatraemic patient, as even this fluid is *relatively* hypotonic in patients with severe hypernatraemia. When volume depletion has been corrected, further repair of any water deficit may be accomplished with hypotonic fluids. Fluid therapy should be prescribed with the intention of correcting hypernatraemia over a period of 48–72 h to prevent the onset of cerebral oedema.

Hyponatraemia

This is defined as a plasma sodium concentration of less than 135 mmol L^{-1}. Hyponatraemia is a common finding in hospital patients. It may occur as a result of water retention, sodium loss or both; consequently, it may be associated with an expanded, normal or contracted ECFV. As in hypernatraemia, the state of ECFV

is important in determining the cause of the electrolyte imbalance.

As plasma osmolality decreases, an osmolal gradient is created across the cell membrane and results in movement of water into the ICF. The resulting expansion of brain cells is responsible for the symptomatology of hyponatraemia or 'water intoxication': nausea, vomiting, lethargy, weakness and obtundation. In severe cases (plasma Na$^+$ <115 mmol L^{-1}), seizures and coma may result.

A scheme depicting the causes of hyponatraemia is shown in Figure 12.4. True hyponatraemia must be distinguished from pseudohyponatraemia. Sodium ions are present only in plasma water, which constitutes 93%

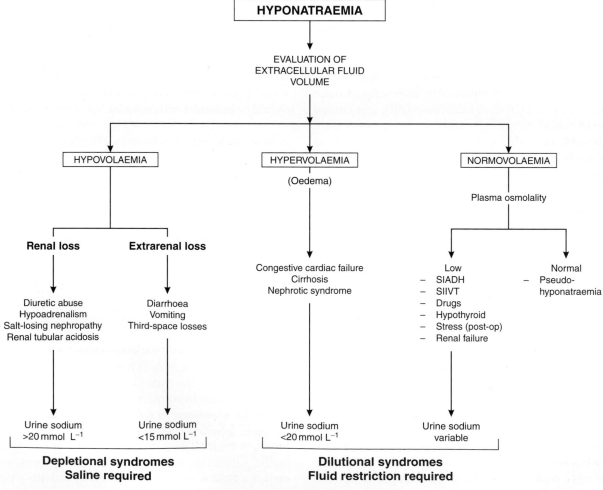

FIGURE 12.4 ■ Causes of hyponatraemia.

of normal plasma. In the laboratory, the concentration of sodium in plasma is measured in an aliquot of whole plasma and the concentration is expressed in terms of plasma volume (mmol L^{-1} of whole plasma). If the percentage of water present in plasma is decreased, as in hyperlipidaemia or hyperproteinaemia, the amount of Na$^+$ in each aliquot of plasma is also decreased, even if its concentration in plasma water is normal. A clue to this cause of hyponatraemia is the finding of a normal plasma osmolality. Pseudohyponatraemia is not encountered when plasma sodium concentration is measured by increasingly used ion-specific electrodes, because this method assesses directly the sodium concentration in the aqueous phase of plasma.

True hyponatraemic states may be classified conveniently into *depletional* and *dilutional* types. Depletional hyponatraemia occurs when a deficit in TBW is associated with an even greater deficit of total body sodium. Assessment of volaemic status reveals hypovolaemia. Losses may be *renal* or *extrarenal*. Excessive renal loss of sodium occurs in Addison's disease, diuretic administration, renal tubular acidosis and salt-losing nephropathies; usually, urine sodium concentration exceeds 20 mmol L^{-1}. Extrarenal losses occur usually from the gastrointestinal tract (e.g. diarrhoea, vomiting) or from sequestration into the 'third space' (e.g. peritonitis, surgery). Normal kidneys respond by conserving sodium and water to produce a urine that is hyperosmolal and low in sodium. In both situations, treatment should be directed at expanding the ECFV with saline 0.9%.

Dilutional hyponatraemic states may be associated with hypervolaemia and oedema or with normovolaemia. Again, assessment of volaemic status is important. If oedema is present, there is an excess of total body sodium with a proportionately greater excess of TBW. This is seen in congestive heart failure, cirrhosis and the nephrotic syndrome and is caused by secondary hyperaldosteronism. Treatment comprises salt and water restriction and spironolactone.

In normovolaemic hyponatraemia, there is a modest excess of TBW and a modest increase in ECFV associated with normal total body sodium. Pseudohyponatraemia is excluded by finding high protein or lipid levels and a normal plasma osmolality. True normovolaemic hyponatraemia is commonly iatrogenic in origin. The syndrome of inappropriate intravenous therapy (SIIVT) is caused usually by administration of intravenous fluids with a low sodium content to patients with isotonic losses.

A more chronic water overload may occur in patients with hypothyroidism and in conditions associated with an inappropriately elevated concentration of ADH. The syndrome of inappropriate ADH secretion (SIADH) is characterized by hyponatraemia, low plasma osmolality and an inappropriate antidiuresis, i.e. a urine osmolality higher than anticipated for the degree of hyponatraemia. It occurs in the presence of malignant tumours (e.g. lung, prostate, pancreas), which produce ADH-like substances, in neurological disorders (e.g. head injury, tumours, infections) and in some severe pneumonias. A number of drugs are associated with increased ADH secretion or potentiate the effects of ADH (Table 12.4). In patients with SIADH, the urine is concentrated in spite of hyponatraemia. Management comprises restriction of fluid intake to encourage a negative fluid balance. In severe or refractory cases, demeclocycline or lithium may result in improvement. Both drugs induce a state of functional diabetes insipidus and have been used effectively in SIADH if the primary disease cannot be treated.

Consequences of Hyponatraemia. Symptoms vary with the underlying aetiology, the magnitude of the reduction of plasma sodium and the rapidity with which the plasma sodium concentration decreases. Serious consequences involve the central nervous system and

TABLE 12.4
Drugs Associated with Antidiuresis and Hyponatraemia

Increased ADH Secretion
Hypnotics – barbiturates
Analgesics – opioids
Hypoglycaemics – chlorpropamide, tolbutamide
Anticonvulsants – carbamazepine
Miscellaneous – phenothiazines, tricyclics

Potentiation of ADH at Distal Tubule
Paracetamol
Indometacin
Chlorpropamide

result from intracellular overhydration, cerebral oedema and raised intracranial pressure. Nausea, vomiting, delirium, convulsions and coma result.

Treatment of Hyponatraemia. Acute symptomatic hyponatraemia is a medical emergency and requires prompt intervention using hypertonic saline. The rapidity with which hyponatraemia should be corrected is the subject of controversy because of observations that rapid correction may cause central pontine myelinolysis, a disorder characterized by paralysis, coma and death. As a causal relationship between this syndrome and the rate of increase of plasma sodium has not been established and it is clear that there is a prohibitive mortality associated with inadequately treated water intoxication, rapid correction of the symptomatic hyponatraemic state is warranted. Sufficient sodium should be given to return the plasma concentration to $125\,mmol\,L^{-1}$ only and this should be administered over a period of no less than 12 h. The amount of sodium needed to cause the desired correction in the plasma sodium can be calculated as follows:

$$Na^+ \, required(mmol) = TBW$$
$$\times (desired[Na^+] - measured[Na^+])$$

Hypertonic saline (3%) contains $514\,mmol\,L^{-1}$ of Na^+ and administration poses the risk of pulmonary oedema, especially in oedematous patients, in whom renal dialysis is preferable.

Potassium Balance

The normal daily intake of potassium is 50–200 mmol. Minimal amounts are lost via the skin and faeces; the kidney is the primary regulator. However, the mechanisms for the retention of potassium are less efficient than those for sodium. In periods of K^+ depletion, daily urinary excretion cannot decrease to less than 5–10 mmol. A considerable deficit of total body potassium occurs if intake is not restored. Hypokalaemia is a more common abnormality than hyperkalaemia.

Hypokalaemia

This is defined as a plasma potassium concentration of less than $3.5\,mmol\,L^{-1}$. Non-specific symptoms of hypokalaemia include anorexia and nausea, effects on skeletal and smooth muscle (muscle weakness,

TABLE 12.5
Causes of Hypokalaemia

Cause	Comments
Reduced intake	Usually only contributory
Tissue redistribution	Insulin therapy, alkalaemia, β_2-adrenergic agonists, familial periodic paralysis, vitamin B_{12} therapy
Increased Loss	
Gastrointestinal (urine K^+ <20 mmol L^{-1})	Diarrhoea, vomiting, fistulae, nasogastric suction, colonic villous adenoma
Renal	Diuretic therapy, primary or secondary hyperaldosteronism, malignant hypertension, renal artery stenosis (high renin), renal tubular acidosis, hypomagnesaemia, renal failure (diuretic phase)

paralytic ileus) and abnormal cardiac conduction (delayed repolarization with ST-segment depression, reduced height of the T wave, increased height of the U wave and a widened QRS complex).

The causes of hypokalaemia are summarized in Table 12.5. Management includes diagnosis and treatment of the underlying disorder in addition to repletion of total body potassium stores. As a general rule, a reduction in plasma K^+ concentration by $1\,mmol\,L^{-1}$ reflects a total body K^+ deficit of approximately 100 mmol. Potassium supplements may be given orally or intravenously. The maximum infusion rate should not exceed $0.5\,mmol\,kg^{-1}\,h^{-1}$ to allow equilibration with the intracellular compartment; much slower rates are generally used.

The potassium salt used for replacement therapy is important. In most situations, and especially in the presence of alkalosis, potassium should be replaced as the chloride salt. Supplements are available also as the bicarbonate and phosphate salts.

Hyperkalaemia

This is defined as a plasma potassium concentration exceeding $5\,mmol\,L^{-1}$. Vague muscle weakness progressing to flaccid paralysis may occur. However, the major clinical feature of an increasing plasma

TABLE 12.6
Causes of Hyperkalaemia

Factitious (Pseudohyperkalaemia)

In vitro haemolysis
Thrombocytosis
Leucocytosis
Tourniquet
Exercise

Impaired Excretion

Renal failure
Acute or chronic hyperaldosteronism
Addison's disease
K^+-sparing diuretics
Indometacin

Tissue Redistribution

Tissue damage (burns, trauma)
Rhabdomyolysis
Tumour necrosis
Hyperkalaemic periodic paralysis
Massive intravascular haemolysis
Succinylcholine

Excessive Intake

Blood transfusion
Excessive i.v. administration

TABLE 12.7
Treatment of Hyperkalaemia

Calcium gluconate 10% i.v. ($0.5\,ml\,kg^{-1}$ to maximum of 20 mL) given over 5 min. No change in plasma $[K^+]$. Effect immediate but transient

Glucose 50 g ($0.5–1.0\,g\,kg^{-1}$) plus insulin 20 units ($0.3\,unit\,kg^{-1}$) as single i.v. bolus dose. Then infusion of glucose 20%, plus insulin $6–20\,units\,h^{-1}$ (depending on blood glucose)

Sodium bicarbonate $1.5–2.0\,mmol\,kg^{-1}$ i.v. over 5–10 min

Calcium resonium 15 g p.o. or 30 g p.r. 8-hourly

Peritoneal or haemodialysis

potassium concentration is the characteristic sequence of ECG abnormalities. The earliest change is the development of tall, peaked T waves and a shortened QT interval, reflecting more rapid repolarization ($6–7\,mmol\,L^{-1}$). As plasma K^+ increases ($8–10\,mmol\,L^{-1}$), abnormalities in depolarization become manifest as widened QRS complexes and widening, and eventually loss, of the P wave; the widened QRS complexes merge finally into the T waves (*sine wave pattern*). Plasma concentrations in excess of $10\,mmol\,L^{-1}$ are associated with ventricular fibrillation. The cardiac toxicity of K^+ is enhanced by hypocalcaemia, hyponatraemia or acidaemia. The causes of hyperkalaemia are summarized in Table 12.6.

Immediate treatment is necessary if the plasma potassium concentration exceeds $7\,mmol\,L^{-1}$ or if there are any serious ECG abnormalities. Specific treatment may be achieved by four mechanisms:

- chemical antagonism of the membrane effects
- enhanced cellular uptake of K^+

- dilution of ECF
- removal of K^+ from the body.

Methods by which the plasma potassium concentration may be reduced are summarized in Table 12.7.

ACID–BASE BALANCE

Hydrogen ion homeostasis is a fundamental prerequisite to virtually all biochemical processes; hydrogen ion concentration $[H^+]$ significantly influences protein, including enzyme, structure and function and therefore nearly all biochemical pathways and many drug mechanisms. Unlike the majority of ions, $[H^+]$ is controlled at the nanomolar rather than millimolar level. Total body H^+ turnover per day is in the order of 150 mmol, although most of this is 'trapped' within metabolic pathways (particularly ATP hydrolysis). The resultant acids may be considered as volatile (from metabolic CO_2 production) and non-volatile (from carbohydrate, fat and protein metabolism). While the lungs and kidneys play a primary role in $[H^+]$ homeostasis, the liver and gastrointestinal tract are also important particularly in relation to ammonium metabolism.

Due to the very low concentration of hydrogen ions in body fluids the pH notation was adopted for the sake of practicality. This system expresses $[H^+]$ on a logarithmic scale:

$$pH = -\log_{10}\left[H^+\right]$$

A more logical arithmetic convention which expresses $[H^+]$ in $nmol\,L^{-1}$ is gaining popularity.

TABLE 12.8
Comparison of Logarithmic and Arithmetic Methods of Expressing Hydrogen Ion Concentration in the Range of Blood [H⁺] Compatible with Life

pH	[H⁺] (nmol L⁻¹)	
7.8	16	
7.7	20	
7.6	25	Alkalaemia
7.5	32	
7.4	**40**	Normal
7.3	50	
7.2	63	
7.1	80	
7.0	100	Acidaemia
6.9	125	
6.8	160	

Table 12.8 compares values of [H⁺] expressed as pH and nmol L⁻¹ and reveals several disadvantages of the pH notation. The most obvious disadvantage is that it moves in the opposite direction to [H⁺]; a decrease in pH is associated with increased [H⁺] and vice versa. It is also apparent that the logarithmic scale distorts the quantitative estimate of change in [H⁺]; for example, twice as many hydrogen ions are required to reduce pH from 7.1 to 7.0 as are needed to reduce it from 7.4 to 7.3. The pH scale gives the false impression that there is relatively little difference in the sensitivity of biological systems to an equivalent increase or decrease in [H⁺]. However, when [H⁺] is expressed in nmol L⁻¹, it becomes apparent that tolerance is limited to a reduction in [H⁺] of only 24 nmol L⁻¹ from normal, but to an increase of up to 120 nmol L⁻¹. Nevertheless, the pH notation remains the most widely used system and is used in the remainder of this chapter.

Basic Definitions

An *acid* is a substance that dissociates in water to produce H⁺; a *base* is a substance that can accept H⁺. Strong acids dissociate completely in aqueous solution, whereas weak acids (e.g. carbonic acid, H_2CO_3)

dissociate only partially. The *conjugate base* of an acid is its dissociated anionic product. For example, bicarbonate ion (HCO_3^-) is the conjugate base of carbonic acid:

$$H_2CO_3^- \rightarrow H^+ + HCO_3^-$$

A buffer is a combination of a weak acid and its conjugate base (usually as a salt) which acts to minimize any change in [H⁺] that would occur if a strong acid or base were added to it. Buffers in body fluids represent an important defence against [H⁺] change. The carbonic acid/bicarbonate system is an important buffer in blood and has historically been used as the principle determinant of physiological pH (this is in no small part due to the relationship this system has with the $PaCO_2$). However, it is important to appreciate the existence of other buffer systems such as plasma proteins, haemaglobin and phosphate. The pH of a buffer system may be determined from the Henderson–Hasselbalch equation, which, for the carbonic acid/bicarbonate system, relates pH, $[H_2CO_3]$ and $[HCO_3^-]$:

$$pH = pK + \log_{10}\left(\left[HCO_3^-\right]/\left[H_2CO_3\right]\right)$$

where K=dissociation constant and $pK = -\log_{10}K$.

This equation shows that [H⁺] in body fluids is a function of the *ratio* of base to acid. For the bicarbonate buffer system, pK is 6.1. As most of the carbonic acid pool exists as dissolved CO_2, the equation may be rewritten:

$$pH = 6.1 + \log_{10}\left\{\left[HCO_3^-\right]/\left(0.225 \times PCO_2\right)\right\}$$

The value 0.225 represents the solubility coefficient of CO_2 in blood (mL kPa⁻¹). Normally, $[HCO_3^-]$ is 24 mmol L⁻¹ and $PaCO_2$ is 5.3 kPa. Thus:

$$pH = 6.1 + \log_{10}\left[24/(0.225 \times 5.3)\right] = 7.4$$

Most acid–base disorders may be formulated in terms of the Henderson-Hasselbalch equation. The pH of plasma is kept remarkably constant at 7.36–7.44, i.e. a hydrogen ion concentration of 40±5 nmol L⁻¹. This is achieved by:

- regulation of H⁺ excretion and bicarbonate regeneration by the kidney
- regulation of CO_2 by the alveolar ventilation of the lungs.

Cellular metabolism poses a constant threat to buffer systems by the production of volatile and non-volatile acids. Thus, the acid–base status of body fluids reflects the metabolism of both H^+ and CO_2.

Acid–Base Disorders

The normal pH of body fluids is 7.36–7.44. Conventional acid–base nomenclature involves the following definitions:

- *acidosis* – a process that causes acid to accumulate
- *acidaemia* – this is present if pH <7.36
- *alkalosis* – a process that causes base to accumulate
- *alkalaemia* – this is present if pH >7.44.

Simple acid–base disorders are common in clinical practice and their successful management can usually be achieved by analysis of the carbonic acid/bicarbonate system as outlined above. In particular determination of pH, [HCO_3^-] and $PaCO_2$, along with calculation of *standard bicarbonate, base excess* and *anion gap* (see below) will enable meaningful diagnosis and treatment. The first step involves diagnosis of the primary disorder; this is followed by an assessment of the extent and appropriateness of any compensation.

Primary acid–base disorders are either *respiratory* or *metabolic*. The disorder is respiratory if the primary disturbance involves CO_2, and metabolic if it involves HCO_3^-. Thus, four potential primary disturbances exist (Table 12.9) and each may be identified by analysis of pH, [HCO_3^-] and $PaCO_2$. Both pH and $PaCO_2$ are measured directly by the blood gas machine. [HCO_3^-] is measured directly on the electrolyte profile but is derived in most blood gas machines. Other derived variables include *standard bicarbonate* and *base excess*. The standard bicarbonate is not the actual bicarbonate of the sample but an estimate of bicarbonate concentration after elimination of any abnormal respiratory contribution to [HCO_3^-], i.e. an estimate of [HCO_3^-] at a $PaCO_2$ of 5.3 kPa. The base excess (in alkalosis) or base deficit (in acidosis) is the amount of acid or base (in mmol) required to return the pH of 1 L of blood to normal at a $PaCO_2$ of 5.3 kPa; it is a measure of the magnitude of the metabolic component of the acid–base disorder.

After the primary disorder has been identified, it is necessary to consider if it is acute or chronic and if any compensation has occurred. The body defends itself against changes in pH by compensatory mechanisms, which *tend* to return pH towards normal. Primary respiratory disorders are compensated by a metabolic mechanism and vice versa. For example, a primary respiratory acidosis is compensated for by renal retention of HCO_3^-, whereas a primary metabolic acidosis is compensated for by hyperventilation and a decrease in $PaCO_2$. Thus, in each case, the *acidaemia* produced by the primary acidosis is reduced by a compensatory alkalosis. The response to a respiratory alkalosis is increased renal elimination of HCO_3^-, and metabolic alkalosis results in hypoventilation and increased $PaCO_2$, pH being restored towards normal by the compensatory respiratory acidosis. In each case, the efficiency of compensatory mechanisms is limited; compensation is usually only partial and rarely complete. Overcompensation does not occur.

TABLE 12.9				
Compensatory Mechanisms in Acid–Base Disturbances				
Primary Disorder	*pH*	*HCO_3^-*	*$PaCO_2$*	*Compensation*
Metabolic acidosis	↓	↓↓		Hyperventilation ↓ $PaCO_2$
Metabolic alkalosis	↑	↑↑		Hypoventilation ↑ $PaCO_2$
Respiratory acidosis	↓		↑↑	Renal retention of HCO_3^-
Respiratory alkalosis	↑		↓↓	Renal elimination of HCO_3^-

↓↓ or ↑↑ denotes the primary abnormality.
The final pH depends on the degree of compensation. Respiratory compensation for metabolic disorders is rapid; renal compensation for respiratory disorders is slow.

Metabolic Acidosis

The cardinal features of a metabolic acidosis are a decreased $[HCO_3^-]$, a low pH and an appropriately low $PaCO_2$. The extent of the acidaemia depends upon the nature, severity and duration of the initiating pathology in addition to the efficiency of compensatory mechanisms. The magnitude of the compensatory response is proportional to the decrease in $[HCO_3]$. The lower limit of the respiratory response is a $PaCO_2$ of 1.3 kPa. In a steady state:

$$predicted\ PaCO_2 = (0.2 \times observed\ bicarbonate) + 1.1\ (kPa)$$

If the observed $PaCO_2$ differs from the predicted value, then an independent respiratory disturbance is present.

In most instances, establishing the presence and the cause of a metabolic acidosis is straightforward. In difficult cases, an important clue to the nature of the abnormality is given by the measurement of the *anion gap* in plasma:

$$anion\ gap = \left(\left[Na^+\right] + \left[K^+\right]\right) - \left(\left[Cl^-\right] + \left[HCO_3^-\right]\right)$$

In reality, the numbers of cations and anions in plasma are the same and an anion gap exists because negatively charged proteins, together with phosphate, lactate and organic anions (which maintain electrical neutrality), are not measured. The normal anion gap is $12–18\ mmol\ L^{-1}$. In the critically ill population adjustments for hypoalbuminaemia (albumin itself being an anion) and hypophosphataemia should be made as follows:

$$corrected\ anion\ gap = \left(\left[Na^+\right] + \left[K^+\right]\right)$$
$$- \left(\left[Cl^-\right] + \left[HCO_3\right]\right)$$
$$- (0.2 \times [albumin]\,gdL^{-1} + 1.5$$
$$\times [phosphate]\,mmolL^{-1})$$

Clinically, it is useful to divide the metabolic acidoses into those associated with a normal anion gap and those with an increased anion gap. The former are caused by loss of HCO_3^- from the body and replacement with chloride. In acidoses associated with an increased anion gap, HCO_3^- has been titrated by either endogenous, e.g. lactic acidosis, diabetic ketoacidosis, or exogenous acids (e.g. poisons), thus increasing the number of unmeasured plasma anions

TABLE 12.10	
Types and Causes of Metabolic Acidosis	
High Anion Gap	
Overproduction of acid	Diabetic ketoacidosis
	Lactic acidosis: Type A - $\downarrow DO_2$ e.g. shock, hypoxaemia
	Type B – Normal DO_2 but impaired tissue O_2 utilization or lactate clearance e.g. metformin, hepatic failure
	Starvation
Exogenous acid	Salicylates
	Methanol
	Ethylene glycol
Reduced excretion	Renal failure
Normal Anion Gap	
Bicarbonate loss	*Extrarenal*
	Diarrhoea
	Biliary/pancreatic fistula
	Ileostomy
	Ureterosigmoidostomy
	Renal
	Renal tubular acidosis
	Carbonic anhydrase inhibitors
Addition of acid (with chloride)	HCl, NH_4Cl, arginine or lysine hydrochloride

without altering the plasma chloride concentration (Table 12.10). Another useful concept is the *osmolal/osmolar* (depending on units used) *gap*:

$$osmolal\ gap = measured\ osmolality - calculated\ osmolality$$

The concept is similar to the anion gap. A raised osmolal gap infers unrecognized/unmeasured osmotically active molecules within the plasma. A raised osmolal gap in conjunction with metabolic acidosis should immediately raise concern of methanol, ethylene glycol, paraldehyde or formaldehyde poisoning requiring urgent treatment. Other causes of raised osmolal gap in the absence of acidaemia include hyperglycaemia, hyperlipidaemias and paraproteinaemias.

Clinical Effects and Treatment. Metabolic acidosis results in widespread physiological disturbances, including reduced cardiac output, pulmonary hypertension, arrhythmias, Kussmaul respiration and hyperkalaemia; the severity of the disturbances is related to the extent of the *acidaemia*. Treatment should be directed initially at identifying and reversing the cause. If acidaemia is considered to be life-threatening (pH <7.2, [HCO_3^-] <10 mmol L^{-1}), measures may be required to restore blood pH to normal. Overzealous use of sodium bicarbonate may lead to rapid correction of blood pH, with the risks of tetany and convulsions in the short term and volume overload and hypernatraemia in the longer term. The required quantity of bicarbonate should be calculated:

$$\text{bicarbonate requirement (mmol)} = \text{body weight (kg)} \times \text{base deficit (mmol L}^{-1}) \times 0.3$$

Administration of sodium bicarbonate should be followed by repeated measurements of plasma [HCO_3^-] and pH. Sodium bicarbonate is available as isotonic (1.4%; 163 mmol L^{-1}) and hypertonic (8.4%; 1000 mmol L^{-1}) solutions. Slow infusion of the hypertonic solution is advisable to minimize adverse effects.

When considering the use of sodium bicarbonate in the context of metabolic acidaemia, it is important to realize that carbon dioxide is generated during the buffering process. This may result in a superimposed respiratory acidosis, especially in those patients with impaired ventilatory reserve or at the limit of compensation. It is also important to distinguish those acidoses associated with tissue hypoxia (e.g. cardiac arrest, septic shock) from those where tissue hypoxia is not a factor. It appears that therapy with sodium bicarbonate often exacerbates the acidosis if tissue hypoxia is present. For example, in patients with type A lactic acidosis, $NaHCO_3$ increases mixed venous $PaCO_2$, which rapidly crosses cell membranes resulting in an intracellular acidosis, particularly in cardiac and hepatic cells. Theoretically, this could result in decreased myocardial contractility and cardiac output and decreased lactate extraction by the liver, aggravating the lactic acidosis. Current guidelines for the management of cardiopulmonary arrest no longer recommend the routine use of sodium bicarbonate. However, if the acidosis is not associated with tissue hypoxaemia (e.g. uraemic acidosis) then the use of sodium bicarbonate results in a potentially beneficial increase in arterial pH.

Metabolic Alkalosis

The cardinal features of a metabolic alkalosis are an increased plasma [HCO_3^-], a high pH and an

TABLE 12.11
Types and Causes of Metabolic Alkalosis

Chloride-Responsive (urine chloride <20 mmol L^{-1})

Loss of acid
  Vomiting
  Nasogastric suction
  Gastrocolic fistula
Chloride depletion
  Diarrhoea
  Diuretic abuse
Excessive alkali
  $NaHCO_3$ administration
  Antacid abuse

Chloride-Resistant (urine chloride >20 mmol L^{-1})

Primary or secondary hyperaldosteronism
Cushing's syndrome
Severe hypokalaemia
Carbenoxolone

appropriately raised $PaCO_2$. The compensatory response of hypoventilation is limited and not very effective. For diagnostic and therapeutic reasons, it is usual to subdivide metabolic alkalosis into the chloride-responsive and chloride-resistant varieties (Table 12.11). The differential diagnosis of metabolic alkalosis, and in particular the classification of patients on the basis of the urinary chloride concentration, is important because of the differences in treatment of the two groups. In chloride-responsive alkalosis, the administration of saline causes volume expansion and results in the excretion of excess bicarbonate; if potassium is required, it should be given as the chloride salt. In patients in whom volume administration is contraindicated, the use of acetazolamide results in renal loss of HCO_3^- and an improvement in pH. H_2-receptor antagonists may be helpful if nasogastric suction is contributing to hydrogen ion loss.

Severe alkalaemia with compensatory hypoventilation may result in seizures or CNS depression. In life-threatening metabolic alkalosis, rapid correction is necessary and may be achieved by administration of hydrogen ions in the form of dilute hydrochloric acid. Acid administration requires central vein cannulation, as peripheral infusion causes sclerosis of veins. Acid is given as 0.1 normal HCl in glucose 5% at a rate no greater than 0.2 mmol kg^{-1} h^{-1}.

Respiratory Acidosis

The cardinal features of a respiratory acidosis are a primary increase in $PaCO_2$, a low pH and an appropriate increase in plasma bicarbonate concentration. The extent of the acidaemia is proportional to the degree of hypercapnia. Buffering processes are activated rapidly in acute hypercapnia and may remove enough H^+ from the extracellular fluid to result in a secondary increase in plasma $[HCO_3^-]$.

Usually, hypoxaemia and the manifestations of the underlying disease dominate the clinical picture, but hypercapnia *per se* may result in coma, raised intracranial pressure and a hyperdynamic cardiovascular system (tachycardia, vasodilatation, ventricular arrhythmias) resulting from release of catecholamines. There are many causes of respiratory acidosis, the most important of which are classified in Table 12.12. Treatment consists of reversing the underlying pathology if possible and mechanical ventilatory support if required.

Respiratory Alkalosis

The cardinal features of respiratory alkalosis are a primary decrease in $PaCO_2$ (alveolar ventilation in excess of metabolic needs), an increase in pH and an appropriate decrease in plasma bicarbonate concentration. Usually, hypocapnia indicates a disturbance of ventilatory control (in patients not receiving mechanical ventilation). As in respiratory acidosis, the manifestations of the underlying disease usually dominate the clinical picture. Acute hypocapnia results in cerebral vasoconstriction and reduced cerebral blood flow and may cause light-headedness, confusion and, in severe cases, seizures. Circumoral paraesthesia, hyperreflexia and tetany are common. Cardiovascular manifestations include tachycardia and ventricular arrhythmias secondary to the alkalaemia.

The causes of respiratory alkalosis are summarized in Table 12.13. Treatment comprises correction of the underlying cause and thus differential diagnosis is important.

TABLE 12.12
Causes of Respiratory Acidosis

Central Nervous System

Drug overdose
Trauma
Tumour
Degeneration or infection
Cerebrovascular accident
Cervical cord trauma

Peripheral Nervous System

Polyneuropathy
Myasthenia gravis
Poliomyelitis
Botulism
Tetanus
Organophosphorus poisoning

Primary Pulmonary Disease

Airway obstruction
  Asthma
  Laryngospasm
  Chronic obstructive airways disease
Parenchymal disease
  ARDS
  Pneumonia
  Severe pulmonary oedema
  Chronic obstructive airways disease
Loss of mechanical integrity
  Flail chest

TABLE 12.13
Causes of Respiratory Alkalosis

Supratentorial

Voluntary/hysterical hyperventilation
Pain, anxiety

Specific Conditions

CNS disease
  Meningitis/encephalitis
  Cerebrovascular accident
  Tumour
  Trauma
Respiratory disease
  Pneumonia
  Pulmonary embolism
  Early pulmonary oedema or ARDS
  High altitude
Shock
  Cardiogenic
  Hypovolaemic
  Septic
Miscellaneous
  Cirrhosis
  Gram-negative septicaemia
  Pregnancy
  IPPV
Drugs/hormones
  Salicylates
  Aminophylline
  Progesterone

Stewart's Physicochemical Theory of Acid–Base Balance

The 'traditional' model based on carbonic acid/bicarbonate chemistry with renal and pulmonary regulation of hydrogen ion concentration is relatively easy to understand and to apply in common clinical situations. However, it is at best a simplified model of a much more complex reality and as such has some limitations. It struggles to explain the phenomena of hyperchloraemic acidosis and the effect of other acids not buffered by the bicarbonate system, and the important role of plasma proteins. In the 1980s, Stewart, a Canadian physiologist, suggested that the bicarbonate system could not be viewed in isolation but rather the effect of fundamental physicochemical laws (mass action and electrochemical neutrality) on multiple biochemical reactions had to be considered, the bicarbonate system just being one of these, which in turn set $[H^+]$. He went on to theorize three independent variables which determine water dissociation, which is the major source of protons and therefore determinant of pH:

- *The strong ion difference* $(SID) = ([Na^+] + [K^+] + [Mg^{2+}] + [Ca^{2+}]) - ([Cl^-] - [lactate])$, i.e. the total concentration of fully dissociated cations minus the total concentration of fully dissociated anions
- *Total weak acid concentration* $(A_{TOT}) = 2.43 \times [total\ protein]$, i.e. this includes associated and dissociated ions (predominantly albumin)
- $\alpha \times PCO_2$, where α is the solubility coefficient for carbon dioxide

These three variables come together to form the Stewart equation:

$$pH = \frac{pKa + \log[SID] - Kb\ [A_{TOT}]/[Kb + 10 - pH]}{\alpha + PCO_2}$$

If albumin is removed from this equation it is remarkably similar to the Henderson–Hasselbach equation. In humans the strong ion difference equates to about 40 mmol/L, i.e. a net positive charge. This is the *apparent* SID (SIDa). However, we know plasma cannot be charged and SIDa is offset by the *effective* SID (SIDe) which is generated by poorly dissociated weak acids (albumin, phosphate and sulphate). The difference between SIDa and SIDe is the *strong ion gap* (SIG) which is analogous but superior to the anion gap as it accounts for total weak acid, and in particular albumin. Within this theory it is not just the function of the lungs (CO_2) and the kidneys (SID) being modelled but also the organs determining A_{TOT}, namely the gastrointestinal tract and liver. The Stewart equation also emphasizes the importance of $[Cl^-]$ as a key determinant of SID and therefore pH. An increasing $[Cl^-]$ in relation to $[Na^+]$, say after excessive normal saline administration, will decrease SID (with a normal SIG) and thereby decrease pH. This explains the common clinical phenomenon of hyperchloraemic acidosis. It is also worthy of note that Stewart's theory rejects HCO^- as an independent variable and therefore a determinant of pH, as in the classical model, being altered by both changes in $PaCO_2$ and SID.

This physicochemical approach does not fundamentally alter our clinical classification or management of acid base disturbance but may, in the view of some, improve our diagnostic resolution and understanding e.g. hyperchloraemic acidosis and hypoalbuminaemic alkalosis. It is, however, a relatively cumbersome equation and as such has not entered into common bedside usage. These different approaches to acid–base balance are not in themselves right or wrong but rather different viewing points of the same scene.

FURTHER READING

Arieff, A.I., 1991. Indications for the use of bicarbonate in patients with metabolic acidosis. Br. J. Anaesth. 67, 165–178.

Hubble, S.M.A., 2007. Acid–base and blood gas analysis. Anaesth. Int. Care Med. 8 (11), 471–473.

Kitching, J.K., Edge, C.J., 2002. Acid–base balance: a review of normal physiology. Br. J. Anaesth. CEPD reviews 2, 3–6.

Lane, N., Allen, K., 1999. Hyponatraemia after orthopaedic surgery. Br. Med. J. 318, 1363–1364.

Morris, C.G., 2008. Review: Metabolic acidosis in the critically ill: Part 1 Classification and pathophysiology. Anaesthesia 63, 294–301.

Sirker, A.A., Rhodes, A., Grounds, R.M., Bennett, E.D., 2002. Acid–base physiology: the 'traditional' and the 'modern' approaches. Anaesthesia 57, 348–356.

Swales, J.D., 1991. Management of hyponatraemia. Br. J. Anaesth. 67, 146–154.

Thomson, W.S.T., Adams, J.F., Cowan, R.A., 1997. Clinical acid–base balance. Oxford University Press, Oxford.

Wooten, E.W., 2004. Science review: quantitative acid–base physiology using the Stewart model. Crit. Care 8, 448–452.

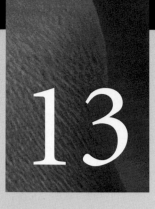

13 HAEMATOLOGICAL DISORDERS AND BLOOD TRANSFUSION

H aematological conditions can have a significant impact on the conduct of anaesthesia. Anaesthetists need to have an understanding of the pathophysiology associated with various haematological diseases which are known to increase the risk of thrombosis, infection, or haemorrhage. In addition, as one of the largest groups of clinicians responsible for the transfusion of various blood products, anaesthetists need to be familiar with the rationale for their safe use.

THE PHYSIOLOGY OF BLOOD

Blood Cells and Plasma

Red blood cells (RBCs, or erythrocytes) typically survive for about 120 days after their release into the circulation. They are created in bone marrow and are released as reticulocytes, which mature over two days into adult RBCs. In healthy adults, 1–2% of RBCs present in the circulation are reticulocytes. Reticulocytes and red blood cells do not have nuclei but residual RNA can still be found in reticulocytes as they mature into erythrocytes.

The classic shape of a red cell is a biconcave disk 8 μm in diameter, but because red cells deform easily they can pass through capillaries which are smaller than this.

At the end of their 120-day life-span, senescent red cells are destroyed by macrophages present in the liver, spleen and bone marrow. The iron present within the cells is made available for further red cell production, whilst the porphyrins are converted into unconjugated bilirubin.

The primary function of red cells is to carry oxygen, bound to haemoglobin, to the tissues of the body. In adults, the majority of haemoglobin present is HbA (which consists of two α and two β globin chains: $\alpha_2\beta_2$). A small amount of HbA_2 is also present ($\alpha_2\delta_2$), as is an even smaller amount of fetal haemoglobin, HbF ($\alpha_2\gamma_2$). HbF and HbA_2 typically represent less than 4% of the total amount of haemoglobin. Each globin chain contains a 'pocket' of haem in which iron is held in its ferrous state allowing it to bind reversibly with oxygen. As oxygen binds to each haem pocket in turn, the whole haemoglobin molecule changes shape, increasing its overall affinity for oxygen. When the haemoglobin molecule 'unloads' oxygen, the overall affinity for oxygen decreases because 2,3-diphosphoglycerate (2,3-DPG) displaces the two β chains. These changes account for the sigmoid shape of the oxygen–haemoglobin dissociation curve. Increased concentrations of carbon dioxide, hydrogen ions, 2,3-DPG, and sickle haemoglobin (HbS) shift the oxygen-haemoglobin dissociation curve to the right. Fetal haemoglobin does not bind with 2,3-DPG and so has a dissociation curve shifted to the left.

White blood cells (leukocytes) present in the circulation include granulocytes (neutrophils, eosinophils, basophils), lymphocytes and monocytes. The main purpose of white cells is to defend against infection from micro-organisms, and to do this they have to be able to travel across the endovascular wall and into the interstitial space. Once they are present in tissues, monocytes may differentiate into macrophages.

Neutrophils, monocytes and macrophages are the three major phagocytic cells responsible for the destruction of bacteria, fungi or damaged cells. Phagocytic

216

cells respond in three stages to foreign substances: chemotaxis, whereby phagocytes are attracted to sites of inflammation by chemical signals; phagocytosis, which is where the phagocyte ingests the material in question (often aided by a process called opsonization, in which particles are 'tagged' by immunoglobulins or complement); and destruction, which is achieved by the release of reactive oxygen species within the cell.

Eosinophils are involved in both allergic reactions and the response to parasitic infections. Lymphocytes are subdivided into B cell, T cell, and natural killer (NK) cells. B and T cells release immunoglobulins in response to antigens derived from bacteria, viruses and other foreign particles. Many of these antigens are processed and presented to the lymphocytes by specialist macrophages, termed antigen presenting cells. Lymphocytes which recognise specific antigens can proliferate and produce clones of themselves in response to a specific threat and this 'threat-response' is effectively memorized by the organism, resulting in an *adaptive immune response*. Natural killer lymphocytes do not need prior activation by antigens and are therefore part of an *innate immune response* which is responsible for identifying tumour cells or cells invaded by some viruses.

Platelets are produced by the natural breaking apart of megakaryocytes to form cell fragments with no nucleus. Their lifespan is approximately 5 days and they are chiefly involved in haemostasis, in which they are integral to the production of blood clots by adhering to the endothelium, aggregating, and catalysing procoagulant processes. They are also involved in the release of growth factors such as fibroblast growth factor.

All of the cells within the circulation are suspended in blood plasma, a mixture of water, electrolytes, proteins such as albumin and globulins, various nutrients such as glucose, and clotting factors.

Blood Coagulation

The physiology of haemostasis involves a complex interaction between the endothelium, clotting factors and platelets. Normally, the subendothelial matrix and tissue factor are separated from platelets and clotting factors by an intact endothelium. However, when a blood vessel is damaged, vasospasm occurs, which reduces initial bleeding and slows blood flow, increasing contact time between the blood and the area of injury. Initial haemostasis occurs through the action of platelets. Circulating platelets bind directly to exposed collagen with specific glycoprotein Ia/IIa receptors. Von Willebrand factor released from both endothelium and activated platelets strengthens this adhesion. Platelet activation results in a shape change, increasing platelet surface area, allowing the development of extensions which can connect to other platelets (pseudopods). Activated platelets secrete a variety of substances from storage granules, including calcium ions, ADP, platelet activating factor, von Willebrand factor, serotonin, factor V and protein S. Activated platelets also undergo a change in a surface receptor, glycoprotein GIIb/IIIa, which allows them to cross-link with fibrinogen. In parallel with all these changes, the coagulation pathway is activated and further platelets adhere and aggregate (Fig. 13.1).

The classical description of coagulation pathways includes an *intrinsic* pathway and an *extrinsic* pathway in which clotting factors are designated with Roman numerals (Fig. 13.1). Each pathway consists of a cascade in which a clotting factor is activated and in turn catalyses the activation of another pathway. The intrinsic pathway involves the sequential activation of factors XII, XI and IX. The extrinsic pathway involves the activation of factor VII by tissue factor, and is sometimes called the *tissue factor pathway*. Of the two pathways, the extrinsic pathway is considered to be the more important because abnormal expression of the intrinsic pathway does not necessarily result in abnormal clotting. The intrinsic pathway may have an additional role in the inflammatory response.

Both the intrinsic and extrinsic pathways result in a *final common pathway* which involves the activation of factor X. Activated factor X in turn converts prothrombin to thrombin (factor II to IIa), which allows the conversion of fibrinogen to fibrin (factor I to Ia). Fibrin then becomes cross-linked to form a clot.

It is important to note that this description of intrinsic and extrinsic pathways is essentially a description of what happens in laboratory *in vitro* conditions. The *in vivo* process is much more of an interplay between platelets, circulating factors and the endothelium.

The following steps can be conceptualized (Fig. 13.1):

Initiation. Damaged cells express tissue factor (TF) which, following activation by binding with circulating factor VIIa, initiates the coagulation process by

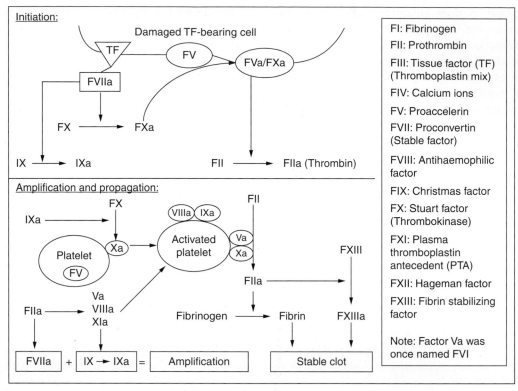

FIGURE 13.1 ■ Clotting processes. From Curry ANG, Pierce JMT. Continuing Education in Anaesthesia, Critical Care & Pain 2007; 2(2): 45–50.

activating factor IX to factor IXa and factor X to factor Xa. A rapid binding of factor Xa to factor II occurs, producing small amounts of thrombin (factor IIa).

Amplification. The amount of thrombin produced by these initiation reactions is insufficient to form adequate fibrin, so a series of amplification steps occurs. Activated factors IX, X and VII promote the activation of factor VII bound to tissue factor. Without this step, there are only very small amounts of activated factor VII present. In addition, thrombin generates activated factors V and VIII.

There is a parallel system of anticoagulation, involving antithrombins and proteins C and S, which help prevent an uncontrolled cascade of thrombosis. Thrombin binds to thrombomodulin on the endothelium. This prevents the procoagulant action of thrombin. In addition, the thrombin–thrombomodulin complex activates protein C. Along with its cofactor, protein S, activated protein C (APC) proteolyzes factor Va and factor VIIIa. Factor Va increases the rate of conversion of

prothrombin to thrombin and factor VIIIa is a cofactor in the generation of activated factor X. Inactivation of these two factors therefore leads to marked reduction in thrombin production. Activated protein C also has effects on endothelial cells and leukocytes, independent of its anticoagulant properties, including anti-inflammatory properties, reduction of leukocyte adhesion, and chemotaxis and inhibition of apoptosis.

Antithrombin is a serine protease inhibitor which is found in high concentrations in plasma. It inhibits the action of activated factors VII, X, XI, XII and thrombin. It is the site of action of heparin, which increases its rate of action several thousand-fold.

In addition, platelet adhesion and aggregation are normally inhibited in intact blood vessels by the negative charge present on the endothelium, which prevents platelet adhesion, and by substances which inhibit aggregation such as nitric oxide and prostacyclin.

Controlled fibrinolysis occurs naturally, involving the conversion of plasminogen to plasmin, which in turn degrades fibrin. Plasminogen can be activated by naturally occurring tissue plasminogen activator and urokinase.

Common laboratory tests used to investigate coagulation include:

- The activated prothrombin time (PT), which tests for factors involved in the extrinsic coagulation pathway (prothrombin, factors V, VII, X), normal range 12–14 s, but often expressed as a ratio (the international normalized ratio, INR)
- The activated partial thromboplastin time (APTT, also known as the kaolin cephalin clotting time, KCCT), which tests for factors present within the intrinsic pathway (including factors I, II, V, VIII, IX and X), normal range 26–33.5 s, often also expressed as a ratio (APTTR)
- Thromboplastin time (TT), which tests for the presence of fibrinogen and the function of platelets, normal range 14–16 s
- Fibrinogen assay, normal range 1.5–4 g L^{-1}

HAEMATOLOGICAL DISORDERS AND THEIR IMPACT ON ANAESTHESIA

Anaemia

Anaemia occurs as a result of decreased red cell production or increased loss due to bleeding or destruction. A number of congenital or acquired conditions can result in anaemia (Table 13.1). Anaemia is defined as a haemoglobin less than 13 g dL^{-1} (men) or 12 g dL^{-1} (women), but the level of anaemia at which physiological dysfunction occurs in everyday life, or under the stress of surgery, is unclear.

Symptoms associated with anaemia include dyspnoea, angina, vertigo and syncope, palpitations and limited exercise tolerance. These symptoms may be better tolerated in younger patients or in those in whom the onset is more gradual. Anaemia detected in the preoperative period should ideally be investigated and treated prior to surgery. This is true of even relatively mild anaemias because patients with a low haemoglobin concentration at the outset are more likely to receive blood transfusions as a result of their surgery, and there are occasions on which simple treatments, for example pre-operative iron supplementation, may prevent this. Anaemia is classically subdivided into three diagnostic categories:

- microcytic, hypochromic anaemia (anaemia with a low mean cell volume, MCV <78 fL, and low mean cell haemoglobin, MCH <27 pg); common causes include iron deficiency anaemia, chronic blood loss, anaemia of chronic disease, thalassaemia or sideroblastic anaemia.
- macrocytic anaemia (MCV <100 fL); common causes include vitamin B$_{12}$ or folate deficiency/malabsorption, alcoholism, liver disease, myelodysplasia or hypothyroidism. If the reticulocyte count is high (>2.5%), acute blood loss or haemolytic anaemia may be considered.
- normocytic normochromic anaemia (normal MCV and MCH); common causes include anaemia of chronic disease, aplastic anaemia, haematological malignancy, or bone marrow invasion or fibrosis. If the reticulocyte count is high, this may also represent acute blood loss or haemolysis.

Haemoglobinopathies

Causes of anaemia of particular interest to anaesthetists are the haemoglobinopathies, which include sickle-cell disease and thalassaemia. This is because both diseases may be associated with systemic complications, that in the case of sickle-cell disease may be triggered or exacerbated by anaesthetic techniques.

Sickle-Cell Disease

Sickle-cell disease is a genetic variation in the synthesis of haemoglobin which occurs most commonly in people with African or Mediterranean heritage. It involves a valine substitution in the β globin chain to make sickle haemoglobin (HbS), and because it is an autosomal recessive condition, individuals can either have HbA *and* HbS present (HbAS; sickle-cell trait), or just HbS (HbSS; sickle-cell anaemia). HbS becomes less soluble when deoxygenated, and aggregates, causing the red cell to deform into the classic sickle shape which can lodge in the microcirculation, becoming sequestrated and/or causing areas of ischaemia. Sickling is probably not the only cause of the pathology of sickle-cell disease. HbS is unstable as well as insoluble, resulting in cell breakdown, oxidative damage and endothelial damage. Surgical stress may therefore trigger vaso-occlusion through an inflammatory rather than sickling process. Sickle cell trait is relatively protected

TABLE 13.1
Causes of Anaemia

Decreased Production

Bone marrow failure	Aplastic anaemia
	Chemotherapy or bone marrow transplant conditioning
	Marrow infiltration or destruction
	■ Non-haematological cancers (e.g. breast, lung, kidney or thyroid cancers)
	■ Lymphoma
	■ Myelofibrosis
	■ Myeloma
	■ Tuberculosis
Decreased erythropoiesis	Alcoholism
	Chronic disease
	Hypothyroidism
	Infection
	Renal failure
	Sideroblastic anaemia
	Thalassaemia
Nutritional deficiencies	Iron
	Folic acid
	Vitamin B$_{12}$
	Vitamin C
	N.B. nutritional deficiencies may be caused or exacerbated by a number of conditions including:
	■ Alcoholism
	■ Drugs (e.g. methotrexate)
	■ Impaired absorption (e.g. Crohn's disease, pernicious anaemia, tropical sprue, Whipple's disease)
	■ Inherited disorders (e.g. homocystinuria)

Increased Loss

Bleeding	Acute haemorrhage
	Chronic bleeding (e.g. haematuria or occult gastrointestinal blood loss)
Haemolysis or sequestration	Acquired haemolytic disease
	■ Heart valve defects/mechanical heart valves
	■ Immune-mediated haemolysis (e.g. drug-related haemolysis, incompatible blood transfusion)
	■ Malaria
	■ Microangiopathic haemolytic anaemia (MAHA)*
	■ Paroxysmal nocturnal haematuria
	Inherited red cell disorders
	■ G6PD deficiency
	■ Pyruvate kinase deficiency
	■ Sickle-cell disease
	■ Spherocytosis
	■ Thalassaemia

Artefactual

	Hypervolaemic haemodilution
	Laboratory error

*Causes of MAHA include vasculitis, disseminated intravascular coagulation (DIC), HELLP syndrome (Haemolysis, Elevated Liver enzymes, Low Platelets) and thrombotic thrombocytopaenic purpura/haemolytic uraemic syndrome (TTP/HUS) (see Table 13.2).

from this effect because approximately 70% of red cells contain HbA, whereas up to 95% of red cells contain HbS in sickle-cell anaemia. HbS can be detected in a laboratory blood sample. However, it is extremely unlikely for adults to have unknown sickle-cell disease (as opposed to sickle-cell trait), particularly if they are not anaemic. Anaesthetic departments should have guidance about when sickle testing is required at routine preoperative anaesthetic assessment in susceptible patient populations.

As well as potentially being chronically anaemic, patients with sickle-cell disease are more likely to have preoperative renal or splenic disease (in which case splenectomy prophylaxis may be required, even in the absence of a surgical splenectomy). They are also more likely to have suffered from lung disease, or cardiovascular disease which may include previous cerebral infarctions or increased cardiac output at rest. Due to the recurrent painful episodes which these patients suffer, they are often not opioid-naïve, which may present problems with perioperative pain management.

During anaesthesia, and during the postoperative period, HbS is prone to sickling in the presence of hypoxaemia, dehydration, acidosis or mild hypothermia. In patients with HbSS, sickling may occur even at high oxygen saturations and become progressively worse, such that all red cells will be sickled at approximately 50% saturation. If sickling causes lung ischaemia, further hypoxaemia may develop. Patients with sickle-cell trait (HbAS) are less susceptible to ischaemic complications, but this does depend on the proportion of HbS present and there are case reports of thrombotic complications in this patient group. There is some evidence to suggest that patients with sickle trait are at increased risk of venous thromboembolism and pregnancy-related complications. In patients with sickle-cell disease, haematology input is required, and advice should be sought preoperatively, as an elective transfusion to lower the proportion of HbS may be indicated.

Intraoperative anaesthetic techniques should avoid hypoxaemia and acidosis, and this may involve general or regional anaesthesia. If general anaesthesia is required, intermittent positive pressure ventilation may be preferable as a means of optimizing oxygenation and avoiding respiratory acidosis (or potentially providing a respiratory alkalosis in high-risk patients).

Intravenous fluids (including in the preoperative period) and active warming of the patient are likely to be required to avoid dehydration and hypothermia. Vasopressors and limb tourniquets should be used with due consideration to risks and benefits. Intraoperative cell salvage is not currently recommended.

Continuation of monitoring and support with oxygen and intravenous fluids are likely to be required into the postoperative period, and the presence of a postoperative fever should alert clinicians to the possibility of an ischaemic crisis.

There are no specific guidelines as to which analgesic regimens should be used, although the presence of renal disease may be a relative contraindication to NSAIDs. Anaesthetists may also be called upon to provide analgesia, including patient-controlled morphine, to patients suffering from a non-surgical sickle-cell crisis. These are often extremely painful.

Thalassaemia

Thalassaemia is an abnormality of globin synthesis which occurs in patients of Mediterranean, Middle Eastern or Asian descent. There are two common forms, alpha and beta, and both forms are inherited in a recessive pattern and can thus be present in minor or major forms. The minor forms have few clinical implications except in states of increased haemodynamic stress such as pregnancy, when anaemia may occur. In the major forms, haemolytic anaemia occurs, which is often managed with regular blood transfusions in order to prevent anaemia and bony deformation caused by bone marrow hyperplasia. In untreated individuals, marrow hyperplasia can result in craniofacial abnormalities, which may directly affect anaesthetic techniques such as laryngoscopy. Iron overload can also occur, resulting in cardiac hypertrophy, pulmonary hypertension and liver disease; detailed cardiac history and preoperative assessment are required. In rare cases, the splenomegaly and/or folate deficiency associated with thalassaemia have resulted in thrombocytopaenia or neutropaenia being present, and this should be excluded preoperatively.

Various drugs are relatively contraindicated in thalassaemia because they may trigger haemolysis; these include prilocaine, nitroprusside, penicillin, aspirin and vitamin K. Advice should be sought before administering such agents.

Neutropaenia

Neutropaenia creates a significantly immunocompromised state, leaving patients at increased risk of infections, including those infections usually considered unusual or atypical. White cell counts of less than $1 \times 10^9 \, L^{-1}$ are considered significant and often require patients to be given medications for prophylaxis against fungal, viral or *Pneumocystis jirovecii* infections.

The commonest causes of neutropaenia are haematological malignancies and their treatments, as well as chemotherapy for other malignancies. When neutropaenic patients require surgery, the benefits must be weighed against the increased risk of postoperative infections. Strict asepsis is essential when dealing with neutropaenic patients, and it should be noted that they are at increased risk of ventilator-associated pneumonia, urinary catheter infections and infections associated with intravascular cannulation, particularly central venous catheters. If possible, these interventions should be avoided or limited to as short a time as possible.

Various antimicrobial regimens are recommended in patients with neutropaenic sepsis, which include broad spectrum agents with anti-pseudomonal and anti-fungal cover. Most hospitals have their own policies for management of suspected neutropaenic sepsis. If there is evidence of postoperative infection, specialist microbiological advice should be sought.

Inherited and Other Coagulopathies

Various conditions and drugs are known to be associated with increased blood loss during surgery (Tables 13.2 and 13.3). If a patient presents with a known condition or with a history of abnormal bleeding (e.g. menorrhagia or excessive bleeding after previous minor injuries), blood should be sent for a coagulation profile including a platelet count, prothrombin time (PT), thrombin time (TT) and activated partial thromboplastin time (APTT). A platelet count is often done as part of the full blood count, which is considered routine before major surgery. In contrast, coagulation screens should not be considered routine. They are designed for specific investigation of patients with bleeding disorders, not as screening tests. They have a low probability of detecting an abnormality in the absence of any relevant history.

Patients known to have inherited abnormalities of coagulation, such as haemophilias A and B, and von Willebrand disease, need specialist haematology input because they are likely to need supplementation of specific factor concentrates prior to surgery, guided by factor assays. This is particularly true of patients known to have antibodies (inhibitors) to the factor in question. Due to the incidence of spontaneous joint or muscle haemorrhage in patients with severe disease, it is rare for them to present for unrelated surgery with an occult diagnosis of haemophilia. Less severe disease (e.g. patients who are heterozygous for haemophilia and have abnormally low factor concentrations) or acquired disease (e.g. acquired von Willebrand disease) may occasionally present unexpectedly during surgery, and a suspicion of abnormal clotting during surgery should prompt the anaesthetist to send blood samples for assessment of the coagulation profile.

In the past, the use of factor concentrates from pooled donor units meant that many patients with haemophilia were infected with HIV or hepatitis viruses, and older patients may therefore be infected.

Depending on the type of haemophilia, tranexamic acid (an antifibrinolytic), desmopressin (DDAVP) or repeated factor infusions may need to be given intraoperatively. The use of desmopressin may be associated with water retention and, potentially, acute hyponatraemia.

Acquired coagulopathy can also occur as an acute event, for example: following major trauma, during major haemorrhage or in the presence of disseminated intravascular coagulopathy (DIC). In major haemorrhage, clotting factors can become depleted if not replaced promptly. The management of coagulopathy in major haemorrhage should be guided by clinical urgency and laboratory tests (Fig. 13.2).

Intramuscular injections are not recommended in coagulopathic patients because of the risk of intramuscular haemorrhage, and the use of NSAIDs may exacerbate the bleeding tendency.

Coagulopathy of Trauma. Patients who have suffered major trauma have a high incidence of coagulopathy. This is multifactorial and complex but certainly appears before administration of intravenous fluids or blood products, so is not solely an iatrogenic

TABLE 13.2		
Conditions Which are Known to Increase Blood Loss		
Conditions Which Cause Bleeding or Promote Blood Loss		
Coagulopathies	Anticoagulant drugs	See Table 13.3
	Auto-antibodies	Antibodies to individual factors, associated with haemophilia treatment
	Congenital diseases	Common disorders include: ■ Factor XI deficiency ■ Haemophilia A and Haemophilia B (Christmas disease) ■ von Willebrand disease
	Disseminated intravascular coagulation (DIC)	Common causes include: ■ Allergy ■ Embolism (e.g. pulmonary embolism, fat embolism) ■ Extracorporeal circulation ■ Infection ■ Malignancy ■ Pregnancy complications (e.g. abruption, amniotic fluid embolism, fetal death, pre-eclampsia) ■ Transfusion reactions ■ Trauma and burns
	Haemodilution	Massive transfusion
	Liver disease	As a result of thrombocytopaenia or reduced coagulation factor synthesis
	Vitamin K deficiency	Biliary tract or bowel disorders Inadequate diet
	Envenomation	Various snake venoms have the ability to cause hypofibrinogenaemia, DIC or platelet antagonism
Platelet disorders	Decreased production	Aplastic anaemia Congenital (e.g. Fanconi's) anaemia Folate deficiency Liver disease Malignancy with marrow infiltration Marrow fibrosis or myelodysplastic syndrome Radiation poisoning Toxins (drug or chemical reactions, including alcohol) Tuberculosis with marrow infiltration Vitamin B_{12} deficiency Viral infections (e.g. HIV)
	Increased consumption	Autoimmune thrombocytopaenic purpura DIC Drugs causing immune-mediated reactions (e.g. heparin/HIT*) HELLP syndrome (in pregnancy)** Hypersplenism Infections causing immune-mediated reactions (e.g. HIV, mononucleosis) Paroxysmal nocturnal haemoglobinuria Post-transfusion purpura Sepsis TTP/HUS[†]

Continued

	TABLE 13.2	
	Conditions Which are Known to Increase Blood Loss—Cont'd	
	Impaired function	Congenital (e.g. Glanzmann's thrombasthenia)
		Drugs (see Table 13.3)
		Hypergammaglobulinaemia
		Myeloproliferative diseases
		Uraemia
Vascular disorders	Acquired	Henoch-Schönlein purpura
		Vitamin C deficiency (scurvy)
	Congenital	Hereditary haemorrhagic telangiectasia
		Ehlers-Danlos syndrome

*Heparin-induced thrombocytopaenia (HIT)
**HELLP syndrome (Haemolysis, Elevated Liver enzymes, Low Platelets)
†Thrombotic thrombocytopaenic purpura/haemolytic uraemic syndrome (TTP/HUS)

	TABLE 13.3	
	Drugs which are Known to Increase or Reduce Blood Loss	
	Commonly Used Drugs Which Increase Blood Loss	
Antiplatelet agents	■ ADP receptor inhibitors	Clopidogrel, prasugrel, ticagrelor, ticlopidine
	■ cAMP inhibitors	Dipyridamole
	■ Cyclo-oxygenase inhibitors	Aspirin, non-steroidal anti-inflammatory drugs (NSAIDs)
	■ Glycoprotein IIb/IIIa antagonists	Abciximab, eptifibatide, tirofiban
	■ Phosphodiesterase inhibitors	Cilostazol
	■ Thromboxane inhibitors	Terutroban
	■ Thromboxane & PGDF inhibition	Prostacyclin (e.g. epoprostenol)
Anticoagulants	■ Factor X inhibitor	Rivaroxaban, fondaparinux
	■ Heparins (factors II, Xa)	Heparin (unfractionated), low molecular weight heparins (LMWH), heparinoids (e.g. danaparoid)
	■ Thrombin (factor II) inhibitors	Dabigatran, argatroban, hirudins (e.g. lepirudin, bivalirudin)
	■ Vitamin K antagonists (factors II, VII, IX, X)	Coumarins (e.g. warfarin), phenindione
Fibrinolytic drugs	■ Plasminogen activation	Alteplase, reteplase, streptokinase, tenecteplase, urokinase
Miscellaneous	■ Calcium (factor IV) antagonism	Citrate*
	■ Inhibition of factor conversion (V-Va; VIII-VIIIa)	Activated protein C**
		Drug-eluting stents***
	Drugs Which Reduce Blood Loss	
Aminocaproic acid	Plasminogen activation inhibitor	
Aprotinin	Inhibitor of plasmin, trypsin, chymotrypsin, kallikrein, thrombin and activated protein C	

Continued

TABLE 13.3	
Drugs which are Known to Increase or Reduce Blood Loss—Cont'd	
Conjugated oestrogens	Stimulate factors VII, XII and von Willebrand factor release
DDAVP (desmopressin)	Stimulates factor VIII and von Willebrand factor release
Etamsylate	Increased platelet aggregation, possible inhibition of prostacyclin metabolites
Protamine	Reverses the effects of heparin
Tranexamic acid	Plasminogen activation inhibitor (and plasmin inhibitor at high doses)
Vitamin K	Required for the production of factors II, VII, IX and X; therefore can reverse the effects of vitamin K antagonists
Miscellaneous	Topical haemostatic agents, e.g. oxidized cellulose, thrombin sealants, fibrin sealants, chitin dressings, platelet gels, cyanoacrylates Various blood components[†]

*Citrate may be used to anticoagulate some dialysis machines, and may be used to 'lock' central lines (i.e. keep them from becoming blocked with blood clot)

**Activated Protein C has been used in the treatment of severe sepsis

***Used in various angioplasty procedures; mechanism of action depends on drug being released by the stent

[†]See Table 13.8

Reproduced from Levi M, Toh CH, Thachil J, Watson HG. Guidelines for the diagnosis and management of disseminated intravascular coagulation. British Committee for Standards in Haematology. British Journal of Haematology 2009; 145(1): 24–33. © Blackwell Publishing.

haemodilution effect. The factors associated with co-agulopathy are listed in Table 13.4. These factors interact in particular in the 'lethal triad' of hypothermia, acidosis and coagulopathy. The effect of hypothermia is not seen in routine coagulation testing because these are performed at 37°C.

Most trauma centres now have well defined policies for managing major blood loss (see below). Following publication of the CRASH-2 study, tranexamic acid (1 g as soon as possible after injury, followed by 1 g given over 8 h) is recommended for patients presenting with major trauma.

Disseminated Intravascular Coagulation (DIC). In DIC, the microcirculation of different organs becomes damaged by fibrin clots generated by coagulation pathways which become hyperactive. The pathophysiological production of so many fibrin clots results in a consumptive coagulopathy rendering the patient susceptible to haemorrhage as a result of surgery or other invasive procedures. The causes of DIC are shown in Table 13.2. If DIC is suspected, the cause should be identified and corrected wherever possible. The diagnosis of DIC can be difficult to make and relies upon evaluating the results of several aspects of a coagulation profile. A scoring system exists to evaluate the likelihood of DIC (Table 13.5). Patients who develop DIC in the perioperative period, or who require surgery to treat the cause of DIC (e.g. patients with intra-abdominal sepsis), are at increased risk of major haemorrhage. They are likely to need replacement of consumed coagulation factors in the form of platelets, fresh frozen plasma and cryoprecipitate. Haematological advice should be sought whenever DIC is suspected.

Occasionally, DIC may present as a predominantly thrombotic condition, and in these cases, the use of heparin may be indicated.

Drug-Induced Coagulopathies. A list of drugs known to increase blood loss is shown in Table 13.3. If possible, provision should be made to discontinue these preoperatively, taking into account the amount of 'wash-out' time which may be required. For example, vitamin K inhibitors such as warfarin can take up to 5 or 6 days, and irreversible platelet inhibitors such as aspirin and clopidogrel may take up to 7 days (the time it takes to generate new platelets). In patients in whom continued anticoagulation is considered essential, for instance those at high risk of venous thromboembolic

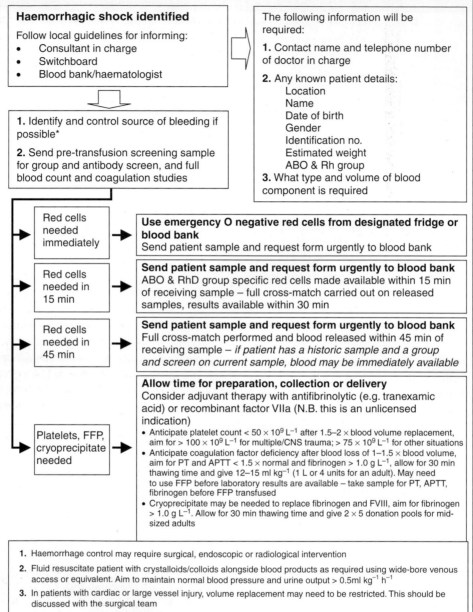

Haemorrhagic shock identified

Follow local guidelines for informing:
- Consultant in charge
- Switchboard
- Blood bank/haematologist

The following information will be required:

1. Contact name and telephone number of doctor in charge

2. Any known patient details:
    Location
    Name
    Date of birth
    Gender
    Identification no.
    Estimated weight
    ABO & Rh group
3. What type and volume of blood component is required

1. Identify and control source of bleeding if possible*

2. Send pre-transfusion screening sample for group and antibody screen, and full blood count and coagulation studies

Red cells needed immediately

Use emergency O negative red cells from designated fridge or blood bank
Send patient sample and request form urgently to blood bank

Red cells needed in 15 min

Send patient sample and request form urgently to blood bank
ABO & RhD group specific red cells made available within 15 min of receiving sample – full cross-match carried out on released samples, results available within 30 min

Red cells needed in 45 min

Send patient sample and request form urgently to blood bank
Full cross-match performed and blood released within 45 min of receiving sample – *if patient has a historic sample and a group and screen on current sample, blood may be immediately available*

Platelets, FFP, cryoprecipitate needed

Allow time for preparation, collection or delivery
Consider adjuvant therapy with antifibrinolytic (e.g. tranexamic acid) or recombinant factor VIIa (N.B. this is an unlicensed indication)
- Anticipate platelet count $< 50 \times 10^9$ L^{-1} after 1.5–2 × blood volume replacement, aim for $> 100 \times 10^9$ L^{-1} for multiple/CNS trauma; $> 75 \times 10^9$ L^{-1} for other situations
- Anticipate coagulation factor deficiency after blood loss of 1–1.5 × blood volume, aim for PT and APTT $< 1.5 \times$ normal and fibrinogen > 1.0 g L^{-1}, allow for 30 min thawing time and give 12–15 ml kg^{-1} (1 L or 4 units for an adult). May need to use FFP before laboratory results are available – take sample for PT, APTT, fibrinogen before FFP transfused
- Cryoprecipitate may be needed to replace fibrinogen and FVIII, aim for fibrinogen > 1.0 g L^{-1}. Allow for 30 min thawing time and give 2 × 5 donation pools for mid-sized adults

1. Haemorrhage control may require surgical, endoscopic or radiological intervention

2. Fluid resuscitate patient with crystalloids/colloids alongside blood products as required using wide-bore venous access or equivalent. Aim to maintain normal blood pressure and urine output > 0.5 ml kg^{-1} h^{-1}

3. In patients with cardiac or large vessel injury, volume replacement may need to be restricted. This should be discussed with the surgical team

4. Ensure the patient is kept warm, use blood warmers where possible

5. Consider cell salvage if possible

6. Use laboratory data to guide blood product requirements. Check FBC, PT, APTT, fibrinogen, biochemical profile, blood gases. Repeat FBC, PT, APTT, fibrinogen every 4h, or after 1/3 blood volume replacement, or after infusion of FFP

7. Treat any underlying causes of DIC where possible – shock, hypothermia, acidosis, sepsis

FIGURE 13.2 ■ Sample major haemorrhage protocol.

TABLE 13.4

Factors Associated with Coagulopathy in Trauma

Physiological dilution of clotting factors
Hypothermia
Acidosis
Red cell loss
Trauma-induced fibrinolysis
Injury-related inflammation
Hypoperfusion
Hypocalcaemia
Genetic predispositions
Iatrogenic – dilution by fluids, anticoagulant effects of intravenous fluids

TABLE 13.5

Diagnostic Scoring System for Disseminated Intravascular Coagulation (DIC)

If the patient has an underlying disorder known to be associated with overt DIC, score as below

Platelet count	
▪ >100 x 10^9 L^{-1}	0 points
▪ 50–100 x 10^9 L^{-1}	1
▪ <50 x 10^9 L^{-1}	2

Elevated fibrin marker (e.g. D-dimer or fibrin degradation products)	
▪ No increase	0
▪ Moderate increase	1
▪ Strong increase	2

Prolonged PT	
▪ <3 s more than normal	0
▪ 3–6 s more than normal	1
▪ >6 s more than normal	2

Fibrinogen level	
▪ >1 g L^{-1}	0
▪ <1 g L^{-1}	1

A calculated score ≥5 is compatible with overt DIC. The score should be repeated daily

A calculated score <5 may be suggestive of non-overt DIC. The score should be repeated every 1–2 days.

Adapted from the ISTH Diagnostic scoring system for DIC

disease, 'bridging' therapy during the wash-out period with shorter-acting anticoagulants such as an unfractionated heparin infusion or low molecular weight heparins (LMWHs) may be considered. These shorter acting agents can be stopped closer to the time of surgery in order to minimize the amount of time the patient is without anticoagulants. In the case of LMWHs, this should be 24 h before surgery, with the last dose being reduced to half normal. In the case of an unfractionated heparin infusion, this can be stopped 2–6 h prior to surgery and the level of anticoagulation monitored by measuring the APTT of the patient's blood.

For patients who have discontinued warfarin therapy, it is advised that the patient's INR is tested on the day of surgery. An INR of <1.5 is normally considered safe for most surgical procedures, although lower ratios may be preferred by surgeons working in highly sensitive areas, for example neurosurgery.

If surgery is required urgently, it may be necessary to reverse the effects of anticoagulant therapy acutely. This should be done under the guidance of a haematologist, but in the case of heparin may involve the use of protamine. Rapid reversal of vitamin K-dependent coagulopathy can be achieved safely with prothrombin complex concentrates (PCC). Vitamin K takes hours to work and should be given at the same time in order to reduce the risk of postoperative coagulopathy. In less urgent situations, vitamin K can be given alone, or the warfarin simply stopped for a few days. In acute circumstances where drugs are thought to be affecting platelet function, platelet transfusions may be considered.

Thrombocytopaenia. Thrombocytopenia is usually defined as a platelet count less than 100×10^9 L^{-1}, but the point at which thrombocytopaenia becomes clinically important depends upon the clinical scenario. Conditions which can result in thrombocytopaenia are shown in Table 13.2. In patients whose platelet count is low, or platelet function is thought to be impaired, a perioperative platelet transfusion may be required.

In the majority of patients with thrombocytopaenia, spontaneous bleeding is unlikely to occur if the platelet count is greater than 10×10^9 L^{-1}. There is no clear consensus as to what level of platelet count is acceptable for any given procedure, but the following guidance has been suggested:

- ▪ $\geq 20 \times 10^9$ L^{-1} – for a minor intervention (e.g. insertion of a urinary catheter or nasogastric tube)
- ▪ $\geq 30 \times 10^9$ L^{-1} – for the insertion of a central venous catheter under ultrasound guidance

- $\geq 60–80 \times 10^9\,L^{-1}$ – for epidural insertion or neuraxial blockade
- $\geq 80 \times 10^9\,L^{-1}$ – for uncomplicated surgery
- $\geq 100 \times 10^9\,L^{-1}$ – major haemorrhage, major trauma or CNS trauma

It should be noted that platelet transfusions are relatively contra-indicated in haemolytic uraemic syndrome/thrombotic thrombocytopaenic purpura (HUS/TTP) where their use may precipitate further thrombosis. In such cases, the risk of transfusion should be weighed against the risk of bleeding.

One cause of thrombocytopaenia of particular note in the perioperative setting is heparin-induced thrombocytopaenia (HIT). HIT is an antibody-mediated reaction which is thought to occur after exposure to heparin occurring concurrently with a physiological insult such as surgery. It is more strongly associated with unfractionated heparin than LMWHs, usually occurs 4–6 days after exposure and results in a falling platelet count, the nadir of which is 30–50% lower than the patient's 'normal' value. HIT rarely results in acute haemorrhage, but is thought to be associated with a pro-thrombotic tendency requiring the patient to be treated with an alternative anticoagulant such as danaparoid (warfarin is not suitable in this situation). Several scoring systems exist to evaluate the likelihood of HIT, and a laboratory ELISA can be used for confirmation.

INTERVENTIONAL PROCEDURES AND REGIONAL ANAESTHESIA IN COAGULOPATHIC PATIENTS

Interventional procedures such as the insertion of central venous catheters, epidural block or regional nerve blocks constitute a significant risk in coagulopathic patients in terms of haemorrhage or haematoma formation. Of particular note are the risks of airway obstruction from failed jugular venous catheter insertion, and paralysis caused by epidural haematoma formation.

It is likely that the routine use of ultrasound imaging has reduced the risks associated with many procedures, but in profoundly coagulopathic patients it may still be advisable to resort to alternative, 'safer' techniques; for example, central venous catheterization of the femoral vein may be preferable to the subclavian or internal jugular routes.

The level of coagulopathy at which various procedures can be considered 'safe' is far from clear. Regarding thrombocytopaenia, suggested platelet counts have been mentioned in the previous section, whilst INR and APTT ratios of ≤ 1.4 have been considered *relatively* safe for most procedures undertaken by anaesthetists.

Safe levels of clotting factors in patients with inherited disorders such as haemophilia are not known, and in these cases a risk/benefit analysis will be necessary.

Drugs causing coagulopathic problems which are difficult to measure present specific problems. A variety of consensus statements, based on evidence from case series, exist on the safety of neuraxial blockade in differing circumstances. Typical responses include:

- LMWH (*thromboprophylaxis* dose): needle insertion should be delayed until 12 h after last dose; epidural catheters should be removed at least 12 h after the last dose and at least 4 h before the next dose
- Subcutaneous unfractionated heparin thromboprophylaxis: needle insertion should be delayed until 4 h after the last dose; epidural catheters should be removed at least 1 h before the next dose
- NSAID therapy, including low-dose aspirin, can be continued and does not seem to represent an increased risk
- Ticlopidine: should be discontinued 14 days prior to neuraxial blockade
- Clopidogrel: should be discontinued 7 days prior to neuraxial blockade
- GIIb/IIIa inhibitors: should be discontinued 9–48 h prior to neuraxial blockade.

It should be noted that evidence in this area is sparse, and that these guidelines are incomplete, difficult to extrapolate into different settings (e.g. regional anaesthetic techniques with lower associated risk) and may not represent best practice. When in doubt, senior anaesthetic and/or specialist haematological advice should be sought.

THROMBOSIS AND ACUTE ISCHAEMIC EVENTS

All hospital patients should undergo an assessment of their risk of developing venous thromboembolism (VTE) in order to ensure that appropriate prophylactic measures are taken. Reassessment should be undertaken after 24h, and at any time that the patient's clinical condition changes. Any assessment should weigh the risk of developing VTE against the risk of bleeding which might occur when pharmacological prophylaxis is prescribed (Tables 13.6 and 13.7). Methods of pharmacological prophylaxis include subcutaneous low molecular weight heparins, subcutaneous unfractionated heparin and newer anticoagulants such as fondaparinux, dabigatran and rivaroxaban. Antiplatelet agents such as aspirin are not considered to provide adequate protection against VTE when used in isolation.

Mechanical methods of VTE prophylaxis are often also used, either as an adjunct to pharmacological methods, or as an alternative to them where the bleeding risk is considered high. Mechanical methods include anti-embolism stockings, and foot-impulse or pneumatic compression devices (both stockings and compression devices may be thigh or knee length). There is very little evidence to support the use of any one mechanical device rather than the alternatives. Mechanical methods may not be appropriate in patients with damaged skin, peripheral neuropathy,

oedema, peripheral arterial disease, or other conditions in which fitting the devices might be problematic or cause damage.

In patients who are at very high risk of both bleeding and thromboembolic events, the pre-emptive insertion of a vena cava filter may be required.

PATIENTS WITH HAEMATOLOGICAL MALIGNANCY

Unless the patient has an intercurrent coagulopathy or neutropaenia, the anaesthetic implications of haematological malignancies are relatively limited. If a patient has been treated previously with chemotherapeutic agents, special attention should be made to pre-operative cardiorespiratory assessment because some agents increase the risk of pulmonary fibrosis, pneumonitis, cardiomyopathy and hypertension. Patients who are likely to undergo haematopoietic stem cell transplants (bone marrow transplants), or who are treated with purine analogue, and who are needing blood product transfusions, are likely to need 'special measures' such as irradiated blood products or blood which is confirmed to be negative for cytomegalovirus (CMV negative). These patients should be discussed with a haematologist prior to transfusion.

BLOOD PRODUCTS AND BLOOD TRANSFUSION

The transfusion of whole blood is relatively uncommon and donated blood is usually separated into its constituent components, which are then available for transfusion. A wide range of blood products are available, the most common of which are listed in Table 13.8, along with their indications. Units of packed red cells are most commonly transfused during the resuscitation of acute haemorrhage, or as a treatment of symptomatic anaemia.

Red cell concentrates are commonly leukocyte depleted and resuspended to a haematocrit of 0.6. In the UK, the red cells are usually suspended in an additive solution: SAGM (*Saline* maintains isotonicity; *Adenine* as an ATP precursor to maintain red cell viability; *Glucose* for red cell metabolism; *Mannitol* to reduce red cell lysis). These additives are designed to extend the safe storage period and the packed red cells

TABLE 13.6

Conditions which are Known to Increase Thrombosis Risk

Acquired	Antiphospholipid syndrome
	Cardiac failure
	Diabetes
	Heparin-induced thrombocytopaenia
	Hyperlipidaemia
	Malignancy
	Myeloproliferative disorders
	Nephrotic syndrome
	Oral contraceptive pill (oestrogen therapies)
	Paroxysmal nocturnal haemoglobinuria
	Polycythaemia
	TTP/HUS*
Congenital	Antithrombin deficiency
	Dysfibrinogenaemia
	Factor V Leiden variant (activated protein C resistance)
	Hyperhomocysteinaemia
	Protein C deficiency
	Protein S deficiency
	Prothrombin genetic variant

*Thrombotic thrombocytopaenic purpura/haemolytic uraemic syndrome (TTP/HUS)

TABLE 13.7
Risk Assessment for Venous Thromboembolism (VTE)

Patients Who are at Risk of VTE

Medical patients

- Mobility significantly reduced for ≥3 days, OR
- Expected to have ongoing reduced mobility relative to normal state plus any VTE risk factor, OR
- If pregnant (or up to 6 weeks post partum) and expected to have significantly reduced mobility for ≥3 days or have one or more risk factor present

Surgical patients

- Total anaesthetic+surgical time >90 min OR
- Surgery involving pelvis or lower limbs and total anaesthetic+surgical time >60 min OR
- Acute surgical admission with inflammatory or intra-abdominal condition OR
- Expected to have significant reduction in mobility OR
- Any VTE risk factor present OR
- If pregnant (or up to 6 weeks post partum) and undergoing surgery

VTE risk factors

- Active cancer or cancer treatment
- Age >60 years (>35 years if pregnant, or up to 6 weeks post partum)
- Critical care admission
- Dehydration
- Known thrombophilias
- Obesity (body mass index > 30 kg m^{-2} – *if pregnant the BMI from pre- or early pregnancy should be used*)
- One or more significant medical comorbidities (e.g. heart disease; metabolic, endocrine, or respiratory pathologies; acute infectious diseases; inflammatory conditions)
- Personal history of, or first degree relative with, a history of VTE
- Use of hormone replacement therapy
- Use of oestrogen-containing contraceptive therapy
- Varicose veins or phlebitis
- Current, or recent, pregnancy-related risk factors (including: ovarian hyperstimulation, hyperemesis gravidarum, multiple pregnancy, pre-eclampsia, excess blood loss or blood transfusion)

Patients Who are at Risk of Bleeding

All patients who have the following:

- Active bleeding
- Acquired bleeding disorders (e.g. acute liver failure)
- Concurrent use of anticoagulants known to increase the risk of bleeding (e.g. warfarin with an INR >2)
- Lumbar puncture/epidural/spinal anaesthesia within the previous 4 h or expected within the next 12 h
- Acute stroke
- Thrombocytopaenia (platelets <70 x 10^9 L^{-1})
- Uncontrolled systolic hypertension (≥230 mmHg)
- Untreated inherited bleeding disorders (e.g. haemophilia or von Willebrand's disease)

Adapted from the NICE guidelines, Venous thromboembolism: reducing the risk, 2010

are kept refrigerated at 4 °C. Currently, red cells can be stored for up to 5–6 weeks. There is ongoing debate as to whether the 'storage lesion' which occurs during this time is clinically relevant, with some studies suggesting that outcomes are worse for patients who have had 'old' blood transfused.

Red Cell Storage Lesion

A variety of biochemical and immunological changes occur during red cell storage which may have clinical impact.

2,3-DPG concentrations fall rapidly (undetectable within 2 weeks). The clinical consequence is less clear,

TABLE 13.8		
Indications and Uses of Blood Products		
Blood Product	**Indication**	**Presentation and/or Dose**
Albumin (human albumin solution; HAS)	■ Fluid resuscitation/correction of hypovolaemia* ■ Therapeutic plasma exchange ■ Ascites and large volume paracentesis ■ Spontaneous bacterial peritonitis ■ Hepatorenal syndrome ■ Correction of hypoalbuminaemia**	Iso-oncotic (4.5%) Hyperoncotic (20%) Volume depends upon product.
Cryoprecipitate	*Correction of hypofibrinogenaemia* ■ Coagulopathy caused by major haemorrhage ■ Disseminated intravascular coagulopathy ■ Hereditary hypofibrinogenaemia	Typically issued as 10 x 20–40 ml bags or 1 x≈300 mL bag 300 ml contains 1.5–3 g fibrinogen In haemorrhage, maintain fibrinogen $>1\,g\,L^{-1}$
Fresh frozen plasma (FFP)	*Correction of coagulation factor deficiencies* ■ Coagulopathy caused by major haemorrhage ■ Liver disease ■ Inherited coagulation deficiencies if specific factor concentrates not available ■ Warfarin overdose if prothrombin complex concentrate not available ■ Therapeutic plasma exchange	Issued in bags of approximately 300 mL Dose is 12–15 ml kg^{-1} (typically 1000 mL for an adult) In haemorrhage, transfuse to maintain prothrombin time and activate partial thromboplastin time at <1.5 x normal ranges
Platelets	*Correction of thrombocytopaenia, or where there is evidence of platelet dysfunction* ■ Thrombocytopaenia caused by major haemorrhage ■ Haematological malignances and their treatment ■ Idiopathic or thrombotic thrombocytopaenic purpura ■ Disseminated intravascular coagulopathy	Issued in bags of 250–300 mL Each bag increases platelet count by approximately 20 x 10^9 L^{-1} In haemorrhage associated with multiple trauma or CNS trauma, maintain platelet count >100 x 10^9 L^{-1} In other situations, triggers may vary (see text)
Red cells (packed red cells; PRC)	■ Resuscitation of major haemorrhage ■ Correction of symptomatic anaemia ■ Treatment of sickle-cell crises	Packed red cells are issued in bags of approximately 300 mL which will raise the haemoglobin concentration in adults by approximately 1 g dL^{-1} Transfusion triggers vary according to context (see text) Suspended in SAGM (saline, adenine, glucose, mannitol).

*Albumin may be used safely for volume resuscitation, but there is little evidence to suggest that it is associated with improved outcomes when compared with other resuscitation fluids. It may be associated with worse outcomes when used in certain conditions such as traumatic brain injury.

**The use of human albumin solution to correct hypoalbuminaemia is contentious. Hypoalbuminaemia is associated with increased mortality in critically ill patients, but actively correcting it is not clearly associated with improved outcome. Hyperoncotic albumin has also been used in the management of adult respiratory distress syndrome (ARDS).

probably because 2,3-DPG concentrations are restored to normal very rapidly following transfusion.

ATP depletion occurs during storage, particularly beyond 5 weeks, and is associated with morphological changes. As with 2,3-DPG, ATP normalizes promptly following transfusion and the morphological changes reverse.

Haemoglobin has been shown to be an important part of the control of regional blood flow due to its interaction with nitric oxide. This ability is lost early (days) following blood storage, but the clinical impact of this is not yet clear.

Morphological changes during storage are complex, but in general, red cells become less deformable; these changes may be only partly reversible.

It has long been recognized that red cell transfusion can have systemic immunological effects including effects on organ transplants, infection and malignancy. The causes of these effects are not clear but may involve residual leukocytes and immunological mediators released by red cells.

In patients who are asymptomatic and not actively bleeding, current evidence suggests that there is no benefit in transfusion provided that the haemoglobin concentration is 7 g dL^{-1}, or greater. This 'trigger' of 7 g dL^{-1} is derived from the 'Transfusion requirements in critical care' trial (TRICC trial, Herbert P., et al, New England Journal of Medicine, 2009). Despite the publication of this study, there remains doubt as to what the 'safe' level of anaemia is for patients with some specific conditions, including ischaemic heart disease, head injury and acute burns. For patients who are symptomatic, or who are actively bleeding, a higher target haemoglobin concentration of 9–10 g dL^{-1} is often adopted.

Packed red cells must be checked before they are transfused to ensure that the donated blood is compatible with the recipient's blood, the most important aspect of which is ABO and Rhesus D (RhD) compatibility.

■ Patients of blood group O can receive only group O donated blood
■ Patients of blood group A can receive group O or group A donated blood
■ Patients of blood group B can receive group O or group B donated blood
■ Patients of blood group AB can receive groups O, A, B or AB donated blood

■ Patients with RhD positive blood can receive RhD positive or RhD negative blood
■ Patients with RhD negative blood will preferentially be given RhD negative blood, but occasionally may be transfused RhD positive blood unless they are an RhD negative female patient with child-bearing potential, in which case they should only ever receive RhD negative blood.

Other, less common, red blood cell antibody/antigen reactions may also occur, and if time allows, a full cross-match should be undertaken. In more urgent situations a more limited approach may be necessary (Fig. 13.2).

The transfusion of FFP also depends upon ABO grouping, but is more complex. Group O FFP may only be given to group O patients, whilst FFP of groups A, B and AB may given to any recipient, but only if it does not contain a 'high-titre' of anti-A or anti-B activity. If possible, the transfused unit of FFP should be of the same group as the recipient.

The transfusion of blood products is not without risk, and, if possible, should not be done without the informed consent of the recipient. A list of the most common complications of transfusion is shown in Table 13.9. Of particular note are the risks associated with the transfusion of incompatible blood products, which are considered to be 'Never Events' within the UK (the equivalent to 'No Pay' events within the US system). A 'zero-tolerance' approach to pre-transfusion sampling, and blood product checking and administration is recommended, which includes:

■ taking blood samples from one patient at a time
■ hand-writing all blood sample tubes and forms at the bedside after sampling, having positively identified the patient by full name, date of birth and hospital identification number
■ patient identification should involve checking any identification band which the patient is wearing as well as a verbal confirmation from the patient of full name and date of birth, if possible
■ all blood products should be prescribed on a record which also contains the above patient identification
■ all blood products should be checked prior to administration, and the patient's identity confirmed for a second time; all the patient details present on the prescribed unit of blood must match exactly the verbal response from the patient, the

TABLE 13.9

Errors and Complications of Blood Transfusion (as Classified and Defined by the SHOT Report 2009)

Acute transfusion reaction	Febrile, allergic or hypotensive reactions occurring within 24 h of a transfusion (excluding incorrect component transfusion, haemolytic reactions, TRALI, TACO, or bacterial contamination)
Anti-D related events	Failure to administer Anti-D when required, or incorrect dose Inappropriate administration of anti-D Expired or inappropriately stored medication
Autologous transfusion events	Incorrect use or assembly of cell-saving equipment Hypotension, bradycardia, pyrexia or rigors associated with the transfusion of autologous blood
Haemolytic transfusion reaction (HTR)	Can be acute (AHTR) or delayed (DHTR) More common in patients with sickle-cell disease Can involve antibodies not commonly associated with haemolytic transfusion reactions
Handling and storage errors	Failure to adhere to 'cold chain' Use of expired red cells Excessive unit transfusion time Technical error (e.g. leaking bag, wrong administration set)
Inappropriate and/or unnecessary transfusion	Erroneous, spurious or incorrectly documented laboratory results Unnecessary transfusions as a result of poor understanding and knowledge Delayed or inadequate transfusion
Incorrect blood component transfused (including ABO incompatible blood)	Phlebotomy or laboratory errors (e.g. mis-labelling of samples) Inadequate bedside transfusion checks Failure to meet patient's special requirements when necessary*
Post-transfusion purpura	Thrombocytopaenia 5–12 days after red cell transfusion caused by platelet antibody production
Transfusion-associated circulatory overload (TACO)	Circulatory overload as a result of transfusion resulting in tachycardia, hypertension, acute respiratory distress, or pulmonary oedema
Transfusion-associated dyspnoea (TAD)	Respiratory distress occurring within 24 h of transfusion, but not as a result of TACO, TRALI, allergy, or any co-existing medical condition
Transfusion-associated graft-versus-host disease (TA-GvHD)	The engraftment and clonal expansion of viable donor lymphocytes contained in blood components in a susceptible host characterized by fever, rash, liver dysfunction, diarrhoea, pancytopenia and bone marrow hypoplasia occurring less than 30 days following transfusion; generally fatal.
Transfusion-related acute lung injury (TRALI)	Acute dyspnoea with hypoxia and bilateral pulmonary infiltrates on chest X-ray; occurring within 6 h of transfusion and not associated with TACO. Thought to be more commonly associated with FFP and platelet transfusions from female donors.
Transfusion-transmitted infection	Potential contaminants include: ■ Bacterial contamination ■ Malaria ■ HIV ■ Hepatitis viruses ■ HTLV ■ New variant Creutzfeldt-Jakob disease

*Special requirements include irradiated blood, or blood where cytomegalovirus is absent (CMV negative blood) – for indications see text patient's identification band and the prescription record, and this should be confirmed by a second person performing an independent check

- if there are any discrepancies, the transfusion should not go ahead
- the details of the transfused product, including any serial numbers, should be recorded on the transfusion record

In Europe there is a legal obligation to keep a permanent record of all blood products that have been transfused.

MAJOR HAEMORRHAGE

When major haemorrhage occurs, it is often necessary to transfuse large volumes of both packed red cells and products which promote clotting, such as fresh frozen plasma (FFP), cryoprecipitate and platelets. Major haemorrhage protocols have been developed in order to aid this process, an example of which is shown in Figure 13.2. If possible, the transfusion of red cells and clotting products should be guided by laboratory results, or by near-patient testing (for example near-patient haemoglobinometers or thromboelastography – TEG). However, waiting for confirmation of coagulopathy before administering appropriate therapy is likely to lead to greater blood loss, use of more blood products and worse outcome. Major trauma is well recognized as causing early coagulopathy even before any fluids or blood products are given.

There is no universal agreement about the relative proportions of RBC:FFP:platelets:cryoprecipitate that should be given. However, there is reasonable evidence to suggest that early aggressive prevention/control of coagulopathy is beneficial in terms of overall blood product use and probably outcome.

Good communication among all members of the team and the haematology department are crucial to the management of major haemorrhage, whatever the setting. Prevention/correction of coagulopathy should always go hand in hand with control of the bleeding source.

Predictable Blood Loss

If large volumes of blood loss (>1000 mL or >20% of estimated total blood volume) are anticipated, for example during major elective surgery, it should be planned for in advance. In patients who are known to be anaemic, the cause of the anaemia should be investigated and, if possible, corrected before surgery. Some patients may require iron (either oral or intravenous) or vitamin supplementation in the weeks leading up to the operation. Some patients with pre-existing symptomatic anaemia, or requiring urgent surgery, may require preoperative blood transfusion. For patients who are not anaemic, autologous donation of blood is used occasionally. By donating blood in the preoperative period, patients can both regenerate their own red cell counts and have a supply of their own blood stored for later transfusion. The major drawback of this technique is that an established system needs to be in place within the hospital where surgery is planned, and multiple hospital visits are required in the weeks preceding surgery.

The management of patients with a known coagulopathy should be discussed with a haematologist before surgery because clotting factor replacement may be required. If patients are prescribed medication that is known to affect blood clotting, consideration should be given to stopping this prior to anaesthesia, if possible, as discussed above.

Blood conservation strategies should be employed whenever possible. These can involve the proactive or reactive use of pharmacological treatments, for example the administration of tranexamic acid, or topical fibrin sealants (Table 13.3). Alternatively, mechanical methods of blood conservation may be employed, for example the use of tourniquets for lower limb surgery.

Intraoperative cell salvage (ICS) is a method of blood conservation in which blood which is lost during surgery is collected by surgical suction, mixed with fluid containing an anticoagulant (usually citrate) and then centrifuged in order to create an autologous red cell concentrate which can be transfused back into the patient. The whole procedure is performed in the operating theatre, with an almost continuous circuit between surgical suction and transfusion. Cell salvage is particularly useful for patients in whom transfusion is complicated by a refusal to accept allogeneic blood, or by the lack of availability of a rare blood type. Cell salvage has been used successfully in a wide variety of surgical operations, including caesarean section and operations for malignancy. When used during obstetric haemorrhage, there is no evidence to suggest that the risk of amniotic fluid embolism is increased, despite the theoretical risk. The use of cell salvage during operations for malignancy remains controversial due to the potential risk of metastatic spread, which may be present even if salvaged blood is transfused through a leukocyte filter. At present, there is no evidence to support these concerns; and in the case of surgery for urological malignancy, there are case series which suggest no increased risk to survival if cell salvage is used in conjunction with a leukocyte filter. Cell salvage should not be used in procedures in which there is the potential for blood to become contaminated by faecal contents, pus, iodine, orthopaedic cement or topical clotting agents.

Jehovah's Witnesses

Blood transfusion is not acceptable to most patients who are Jehovah's Witnesses, even if refusal may increase their risk of death. In most cases, this principle also extends to blood products such as FFP and platelets, although this should be checked with each individual because each may interpret differently the definition of what constitutes a blood transfusion. If an adult Jehovah's Witness has clearly indicated that they will not accept a blood transfusion, and it is evident that they have the mental capacity to make such a decision, it is not ethical to proceed with a transfusion. This remains true even if, at some later point, the patient loses capacity, for example by becoming unconscious.

Many hospitals provide specific consent forms for Jehovah's Witnesses which cover the risks associated with transfusion refusal, and many hospitals also have a Jehovah's Witness liaison who may be able to advise on what alternative therapies are acceptable. For example, intraoperative cell-salvaged blood is often acceptable, as is the use of cardiopulmonary bypass technology where there has been no priming with autologous blood.

The general principles of blood conservation outlined above are the same in Jehovah's Witnesses as in other patients. However, when haemorrhage becomes extreme, it is likely that the patient will need extended postoperative critical care management, which may include elective mechanical ventilation, and measures to stimulate haemoglobin recovery such as iron supplementation and the administration of erythropoietin.

FURTHER READING

Association of Anaesthetists of Great Britain and Ireland, 1999. Management of anaesthesia for Jehovah's Witnesses. AAGBI.

Beed, M., Levitt, M., Bokhari, S.W., 2010. Intensive care management of patients with haematological malignancy. Continuing Education in Anaesthesia, Critical Care & Pain 10, 167–171.

Chee, Y.L., Crawford, J.C., Watson, H.G., et al., 2008. Guidelines on the assessment of bleeding risk prior to surgery or invasive procedures. Br. J. Haematol. 140, 496–504.

Curry, A.N.G., Pierce, J.M.T., 2007. Conventional and near-patient tests of coagulation. Continuing Education in Anaesthesia, Critical Care & Pain 2, 45–50.

Hoffbrand, A.V., Moss, P., 2010. Essential haematology. Wiley-Blackwell, Oxford.

Horlocker, T.T., Wedel, D.J., Benzon, H., et al., 2003. Regional anesthesia in the anticoagulated patient: defining the risks (The Second ASRA Consensus Conference on Neuraxial Anesthesia and Anticoagulation). Reg. Anesth. Pain Med. 28, 172–197.

Levi, M., Toh, C.H., Thachil, J., et al., 2009. Guidelines for the diagnosis and management of disseminated intravascular coagulation. Br. J. Haematol. 145, 24–33.

Mason, R., 2001. Anaesthesia databook, third ed. Greenwich Medical Media.

McClelland, D.B.L., 2007. Handbook of transfusion medicine, fourth ed. United Kingdom Blood Services.

National Institute for Health and Clinical Excellence (UK), 2010. Venous thromboembolism: reducing the risk. NICE.

Wilson, M., Forsyth, P., Whiteside, J., 2010. Haemoglobinopathy and sickle-cell disease. Continuing Education in Anaesthesia, Critical Care & Pain 10, 24–28.

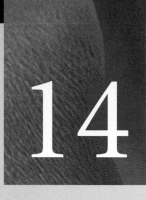

14 BASIC PHYSICS FOR THE ANAESTHETIST

K nowledge of some physics is required in order to understand the function of many items of apparatus for anaesthesia delivery and physiological monitoring. This chapter emphasizes the more elementary aspects of physical principles and it is hoped that the reader may be stimulated to study some of the books written specifically for anaesthetists and which examine this topic in greater detail (see 'Further reading'). Sophisticated measurement techniques may be required for more complex types of anaesthesia, in the intensive care unit and during anaesthesia for severely ill patients, and an understanding of the principles involved in performing such measurements is required in the later stages of the anaesthetist's training.

This chapter concentrates on the more common applications, including pressure and flow in gases and liquids, electricity and electrical safety. However, it is necessary first to consider some basic definitions.

BASIC DEFINITIONS

It is now customary in medical practice to employ the International System (Système Internationale; SI) of units. Common exceptions to the use of the SI system include measurement of arterial pressure and, to a lesser extent, gas pressure. The mercury column is used commonly to calibrate electronic arterial pressure measuring devices and so 'mmHg' is retained. Pressures in gas cylinders are also referred to frequently in terms of the 'normal' atmospheric pressure of 760 mmHg; this is equal to 1.013 bar (or approximately 1 bar). Low pressures are expressed usually in the SI unit of kilopascals (kPa) whilst higher pressures are referred to in bar (100 kPa = 1 bar). The basic and derived units of the SI system are shown in Table 14.1.

The fundamental quantities in physics are mass, length and time.

Mass (m) is defined as the amount of matter in a body. The unit of mass is the kilogram (kg), for which the standard is a block of platinum held in a Physics Reference Laboratory.

Length (l) is defined as the distance between two points. The SI unit is the metre (m), which is defined as the distance occupied by a specified number of wavelengths of light.

Time (t) is measured in seconds. The reference standard for time is based on the frequency of resonation of the caesium atom.

From these basic definitions, several units of measurement may be derived:

Volume has units of m^3.

Density is defined as mass per unit volume:

$$\text{density} \, (\rho) = \frac{\text{mass}}{\text{volume}} \, \text{kg m}^{-3}$$

Velocity is defined as the distance travelled per unit time:

$$\text{velocity} \, (v) = \frac{\text{distance}}{\text{time}} \, \text{ms}^{-1}$$

Acceleration is defined as the rate of change of velocity:

$$\text{acceleration} \, (a) = \frac{\text{velocity}}{\text{time}} \, \text{ms}^{-2}$$

TABLE 14.1
Physical Quantities

Quantity	Definition	Symbol	SI unit
Length	Unit of distance	l	metre (m)
Mass	Amount of matter	m	kilogram (kg)
Density	Mass per unit volume (m/V)	ρ	$kg\,m^{-3}$
Time		t	second (s)
Velocity	Distance per unit time (l/t)	v	$m\,s^{-1}$
Acceleration	Rate of change of velocity (v/t)	a	$m\,s^{-2}$
Force	Gives acceleration to a mass (ma)	F	newton (N) ($kg\,m\,s^{-2}$)
Weight	Force exerted by gravity on a mass (mg)	W	$kg\times9.81\,m\,s^{-2}$
Pressure	Force per unit area (F/A)	P	$N\,m^{-2}$
Temperature	Tendency to gain or lose heat	T	kelvin (K) or degree Celsius (°C)
Work	Performed when a force moves an object (force×distance)	U	joule (J) ($N\,m$)
Energy	Capacity for doing work (force×distance)	U	joule (J) ($N\,m$)
Power	Rate of performing work (joules per second)	P	watt (W) ($J\,s^{-1}$)

Force is that which is required to give a mass acceleration:

$$\text{force}(F) = \text{mass} \times \text{acceleration}$$
$$= ma$$

The SI unit of force is the newton (N). One newton is the force required to give a mass of 1 kg an acceleration of $1\,m\,s^{-1}$:

$$1\,N = 1\,kg\,m\,s^{-2}$$

Weight is the force of the earth's attraction for a body. When a body falls freely under the influence of gravity, it accelerates at a rate of $9.81\,m\,s^{-2}$ (g):

$$\text{weight }(W) = \text{mass} \times g$$
$$= m \times g$$
$$= m \times 9.81\,kg\,m\,s^{-2}$$

Momentum is defined as mass multiplied by velocity:

$$\text{momentum} = m \times v$$

Work is undertaken when a force moves an object:

$$\text{work} = \text{force} \times \text{distance}$$
$$= F \times l\,N\,m \text{ (or joules, J)}$$

Energy is the capacity for undertaking work. Thus it has the same units as those of work. Energy can exist in several forms, such as mechanical (kinetic energy [KE] or potential energy [PE]), thermal or electrical and all have the same units.

Power (P) is the rate of doing work. The SI unit of power is the watt, which is equal to $1\,J\,s^{-1}$:

$$\text{power} = \text{work per unit time}$$
$$= \text{joules per second}$$
$$= \text{watt (W)}$$

Pressure is defined as force per unit area:

$$\text{pressure}\,(p) = \frac{\text{force}}{\text{area}}$$
$$= N\,m^{-2}$$
$$= \text{pascal (Pa)}$$

As 1 Pa is a rather small unit, it is more common in medical practice to use the kilopascal (kPa): $1\,kPa \approx 7.5\,mmHg$.

FLUIDS

Substances may exist in solid, liquid or gaseous form. These forms or phases differ from each other according to the random movement of their constituent atoms or molecules. In solids, molecules oscillate about a fixed point, whereas in liquids the molecules possess higher velocities and therefore higher kinetic energy; they move more freely and thus do not bear a constant relationship in space to other molecules. The molecules of gases possess even higher kinetic energy and move freely to an even greater extent.

Both gases and liquids are termed fluids. Liquids are incompressible and at constant temperature occupy a fixed volume, conforming to the shape of a container; gases have no fixed volume but expand to occupy the total space of a container. Nevertheless the techniques for analysing the behaviour of liquids and gases (or fluids in general) in terms of their hydraulic and thermodynamic properties are very similar.

In the process of vaporization, random loss of liquid molecules with higher kinetic (thermal) energies from the liquid occurs while vapour molecules randomly lose thermal (kinetic) energy and return to the liquid state. Heating a liquid increases the kinetic energy of its molecules, permitting a higher proportion to escape from the surface into the vapour phase. The acquisition by these molecules of higher kinetic energy requires an energy source and this usually comes from the thermal energy of the liquid itself, which leads to a reduction in its thermal energy as vaporization occurs and hence the liquid cools.

Collision of randomly moving molecules in the gaseous phase with the walls of a container is responsible for the pressure exerted by a gas. The difference between a gas and a vapour will be discussed later.

Behaviour of Gases

The Gas Laws

There are three gas laws which determine the behaviour of gases and which are important to anaesthetists. These are derived from the kinetic theory of gases; they depend on the assumption that the substances concerned are perfect gases (rather than vapours), and they assume a fixed mass of gas.

Boyle's law states that, at constant temperature, the volume (V) of a given mass of gas varies inversely with its absolute pressure (P):

$$PV = k_1$$

Charles' law states that, at constant pressure, the volume of a given mass of gas varies directly with its absolute temperature (T):

$$V = k_2 T$$

The third gas law (sometimes known as Gay-Lussac's law) states that, at constant volume, the absolute pressure of a given mass of gas varies directly with its absolute temperature:

$$P = k_3 T$$

Combining these three gas laws:

$$PV = kT$$

or

$$\frac{P_1 V_1}{T_1} = \frac{P_2 V_2}{T_2}$$

where suffixes 1 and 2 represent two conditions different in P, V and T of the gas. Note that where a change of conditions occurs slowly enough for $T_1 = T_2$, conditions are said to be *isothermal*, and the combined gas law could be thought of as another form of Boyle's law.

The behaviour of a mixture of gases in a container is described by *Dalton's law of partial pressures*. This states that, in a mixture of gases, the pressure exerted by each gas is the same as that which it would exert if it alone occupied the container. Dalton's law can be used to compare volumetric fractions (concentrations) to calculate partial pressures, which are an important concept in anaesthesia. Thus, in a cylinder of compressed air at a pressure of 100 bar, the pressure exerted by nitrogen is equal to 79 bar, as the fractional concentration of nitrogen is 0.79.

Avogadro's Hypothesis

Avogadro's hypothesis, also deduced from the kinetic theory of gases, states that equal volumes of gases at the same temperature and pressure contain equal numbers of molecules.

Avogadro's number is the number of molecules in 1 gram-molecular weight of a substance and is equal to 6.022×10^{23}.

Under conditions of standard temperature and pressure (0 °C and 1.013 bar), 1 gram-molecular weight (i.e. 28 g of nitrogen or 44 g of carbon dioxide) of any gas occupies a volume of 22.4 litres (L).

These data are useful in calculating, for example, the quantity of gas produced from liquid nitrous oxide. The molecular weight of nitrous oxide is 44. Thus, 44 g of N_2O occupy a volume of 22.4 L at standard temperature and pressure (STP). If a full cylinder of N_2O contains 3.0 kg of liquid, then vaporization of all the liquid would yield:

$$\frac{22.4 \times 3.0 \times 1000 \text{ L}}{44}$$
$$= 1527 \text{ L at STP}$$

The gas laws can be applied to calculate its volume at, say, room temperature, bearing in mind that the Kelvin scale of temperature should be used for such calculations.

Critical Temperature

If the temperature of a vapour is low enough, then sufficient application of pressure to it will result in its liquefaction. If the vapour has a higher temperature, implying greater molecular kinetic energy, no amount of compression liquefies it. The critical temperature of such a substance is the temperature above which that substance cannot be liquefied by compression alone. A substance in such a state is considered a gas, whereas a substance below its critical temperature can be considered a vapour.

The critical temperature of oxygen is $-118\,°C$, that of nitrogen is $-147\,°C$, and that of air is $-141\,°C$. Thus, at room temperature, cylinders of these substances contain gases. In contrast, the critical temperature of carbon dioxide is $31\,°C$ and that of nitrous oxide is $36.4\,°C$. The critical pressures are 73.8 and 72.5 bar respectively; at higher pressures, cylinders of these substances at UK room temperature contain a mixture of gas and liquid.

Clinical Application of the Gas Laws

A 'full' cylinder of oxygen on an anaesthetic machine contains compressed gaseous oxygen at a pressure of 137 bar (2000 lb in^{-2}) gauge pressure. If the cylinder of oxygen empties and the temperature remains constant, the volume of gas contained is related linearly to its pressure (by Boyle's law). In practice, linearity is not followed because temperature falls as a result of adiabatic expansion of the compressed gas; the term adiabatic implies a change in the state of a gas without exchange of heat energy with its surroundings.

By contrast, a nitrous oxide cylinder contains liquid nitrous oxide in equilibrium with its vapour. The pressure in the cylinder remains relatively constant at the saturated vapour pressure for that temperature as the cylinder empties to the point at which liquid has totally vaporized. Subsequently, there is a linear decline in pressure proportional to the volume of gas remaining within the cylinder.

Filling Ratio. The degree of filling of a nitrous oxide cylinder is expressed as the mass of nitrous oxide in the cylinder divided by the mass of water that the cylinder could hold. Normally, a cylinder of nitrous oxide is filled to a ratio of 0.67. This should not be confused with the volume of liquid nitrous oxide in a cylinder. A 'full' cylinder of nitrous oxide at room temperature is filled to the point at which approximately 90% of the interior of the cylinder is occupied by liquid, the remaining 10% being occupied by nitrous oxide vapour. Incomplete filling of a cylinder is necessary because thermally induced expansion of the liquid in a totally full cylinder may cause cylinder rupture. Because vapour pressure increases with temperature, it is necessary to have a lower filling ratio in tropical climates than in temperate climates.

Entonox. Entonox is the trade name for a compressed gas mixture containing 50% oxygen and 50% nitrous oxide. The mixture is compressed into cylinders containing gas at a pressure of 137 bar (2000 lb in^{-2}) gauge pressure (see below). The nitrous oxide does not liquefy because the two gases in this mixture 'dissolve' in each other at high pressure. In other words, the presence of oxygen reduces the critical temperature of nitrous oxide. The critical temperature of the mixture is $-7\,°C$, which is called the 'pseudocritical temperature'. Cooling of a cylinder of Entonox to a temperature below $-7\,°C$ results in separation of liquid nitrous oxide. Use of such a cylinder results in oxygen-rich gas being released initially, followed by a hypoxic nitrous oxide-rich gas. Consequently, it is recommended that when an Entonox cylinder may have been exposed to low temperatures, it should be stored horizontally for a period of not less than 24 h at a temperature of $5\,°C$ or above. In addition, the cylinder should be inverted several times before use.

Pressure Notation in Anaesthesia

Although the use of SI units of measurement is generally accepted in medicine, a variety of ways of expressing pressure is still used, reflecting custom and practice. Arterial pressure is still referred to universally in terms of mmHg because a column of mercury is still used occasionally to measure arterial pressure and also to calibrate electronic devices.

Measurement of central venous pressure is sometimes referred to in cm H_2O because it can be measured using a manometer filled with saline, but it is more commonly described in mmHg when measured using an electronic transducer system. Note that, although we colloquially speak of 'cm H_2O' or 'mmHg', the actual expression for pressure measured by a column of fluid is $P = \rho.g.H$, where ρ is fluid density, g is acceleration due to gravity and H is the height of the column. Because mercury is 13.6 times more dense than water, a mercury manometer can measure a given pressure with a much shorter length of column of fluid. For

example atmospheric pressure (P_B) exerts a pressure sufficient to support a column of mercury of height 760 mm (Fig. 14.1).

$$
\begin{aligned}
1 \text{ atmospheric pressure} &= 760 \text{ mmHg} \\
&= 1.01325 \text{ bar} \\
&= 760 \text{ torr} \\
&= 1 \text{ atmosphere absolute (ata)} \\
&= 14.7 \text{ lb in}^{-2} \\
&= 101.325 \text{ kPa} \\
&= 10.33 \text{ metres of } H_2O
\end{aligned}
$$

In considering pressure, it is necessary to indicate whether or not atmospheric pressure is taken into account. Thus, a diver working 10 m below the surface of the sea may be described as compressed to a depth of 1 atmosphere or working at a pressure of 2 atmospheres absolute (2 ata).

In order to avoid confusion when discussing compressed cylinders of gases, the term *gauge pressure* is used. Gauge pressure describes the pressure of the

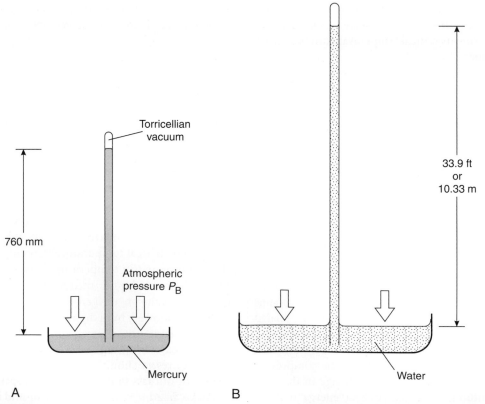

FIGURE 14.1 ■ The simple barometer described by Torricelli (not to scale). (**A**) Filled with mercury. (**B**) Filled with water.

contents above ambient pressure. Thus, a full cylinder of oxygen has a gauge pressure of 137 bar, but the contents are at a pressure of 138 bar absolute.

GAS REGULATORS

Pressure Relief Valves

The Heidbrink valve is a common component of many anaesthesia breathing systems. In the Magill breathing system, the anaesthetist may vary the force in the spring(s), thereby controlling the pressure within the breathing system (Fig. 14.2). At equilibrium, the force exerted by the spring is equal to the force exerted by gas within the system:

force (F) = gas pressure (P) × disc area (A)

Modern anaesthesia systems contain a variety of pressure relief valves, in each of which the force is fixed so as to provide a gas escape mechanism when pressure reaches a preset level. Thus, an anaesthetic machine may contain a pressure relief valve operating at 35 kPa, situated on the back bar of the machine between the vaporizers and the breathing system to protect the flowmeters and vaporizers from excessive pressures. Modern ventilators contain a pressure relief valve set at 7 kPa to protect the patient from barotrauma. A much lower pressure is set in relief valves which form part of

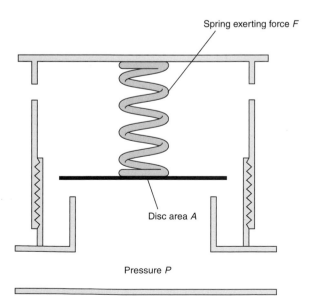

FIGURE 14.2 ■ A pressure relief valve.

anaesthetic scavenging systems and these may operate at pressures of 0.2–0.3 kPa to protect the patient from negative pressure applied to the lungs.

Pressure-Reducing Valves (Pressure Regulators)

Pressure regulators have two important functions in anaesthetic machines:

- They reduce high pressures of compressed gases to manageable levels (acting as pressure-reducing valves).
- They minimize fluctuations in the pressure within an anaesthetic machine, which would necessitate frequent manipulations of flowmeter controls.

Modern anaesthetic machines are designed to operate with an inlet gas supply at a pressure of 3–4 bar (usually 4 bar in the UK). Hospital pipeline supplies also operate at a pressure of 4 bar and therefore pressure regulators are not required between a hospital pipeline supply and an anaesthetic machine. In contrast, the contents of cylinders of all medical gases (i.e. oxygen, nitrous oxide, air and Entonox) are at much higher pressures. Thus, cylinders of these gases require a pressure-reducing valve between the cylinder and the flowmeter.

The principle on which the simplest type of pressure-reducing valve operates is shown in Figure 14.3. High-pressure gas enters through the valve and forces the flexible diaphragm upwards, tending to close the valve and prevent further ingress of gas from the high-pressure source.

If there is no tension in the spring, the relationship between the reduced pressure (p) and the high pressure (P) is very approximately equal to the ratio of the areas of the valve seating (a) and the diaphragm (A):

$$p.A = P.a$$

or

$$\frac{p}{P} = \frac{a}{A}$$

By tensing the spring, a force F is produced which offsets the closing effect of the valve. Thus, p may be increased by increasing the force in the spring.

Without the spring, the simple pressure regulator has the disadvantage that reduced pressure decreases

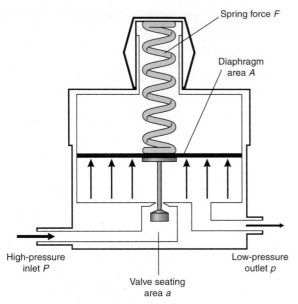

FIGURE 14.3 ■ A simple pressure-reducing valve.

proportionally with the decrease in cylinder pressure. The addition of a force from the spring considerably reduces but does not eliminate this problem, and in order to overcome it, newer pressure regulators contain an extra closing spring. During high flows, the input to the valve may not be able to keep pace with the output. This can cause the regulated pressure to fall. A two-stage regulator can be employed in order to overcome this. Simple one-stage regulators are often designed for use with a specific gas. A universal regulator, in which the body is used for all gases but has different seatings and springs fitted for each specific gas, is now available.

Pressure Demand Regulators

These are regulators in which gas flow occurs when an inspiratory effort is applied to the outlet port. The Entonox valve is a two-stage regulator and its mode of action is demonstrated in Figure 14.4. The first stage is identical to the reducing valve described above. The second-stage valve contains a diaphragm. Movement of this diaphragm tilts a rod, which controls the flow of gas from the first-stage valve. The second stage is adjusted so that gas flows only when pressure is below atmospheric.

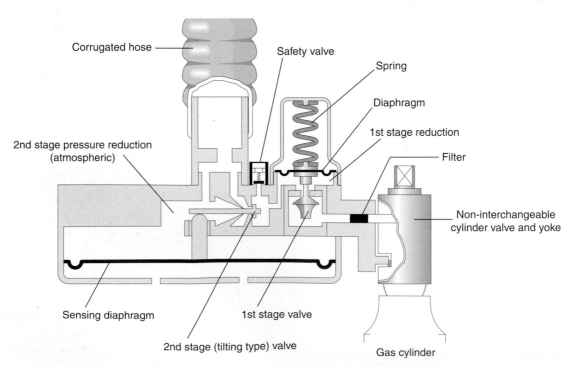

FIGURE 14.4 ■ The Entonox two-stage pressure demand regulator.

Flow of Fluids

Viscosity (η) is the constant of proportionality relating the stress (τ) between layers of flowing fluid (or between the fluid and the vessel wall), and the velocity gradient across the vessel, dv/dr.

Hence:

$$\tau = \eta \cdot \frac{dv}{dr}$$

or

$$\eta = \frac{\text{shear stress}}{\text{velocity gradient}}$$

In this context, velocity gradient is equal to the difference between velocities of different fluid layers divided by the distance between layers (Fig. 14.5B). The units of the coefficient of viscosity are Pascal seconds (Pa s).

Fluids for which η is constant are referred to as Newtonian fluids. However, some biological fluids are non-Newtonian, an example of which is blood; viscosity changes with the rate of flow of blood (as a result of change in distribution of cells) and, in stored blood, with time (blood thickens on storage).

Viscosity of liquids diminishes with increase in temperature, whereas viscosity of a gas increases with increase in temperature. An increase in temperature is due to an increase of kinetic energy of fluid molecules. This can be thought of as causing a freeing up of intermolecular bonds in liquids, and an increase in intermolecular collisions in gas.

Laminar Flow

Laminar flow through a tube is illustrated in Figure 14.5A. In this situation, there is a smooth, orderly flow of fluid such that molecules travel with the greatest velocity in the axial stream, whilst the velocity of those in contact with the wall of the tube may be virtually zero. The linear velocity of axial flow is twice the average linear velocity of flow.

In a tube in which laminar flow occurs, the relationship between flow and pressure is given by the Hagen–Poiseuille formula:

$$\dot{Q} = \frac{\pi \Delta P r^4}{8 \eta l}$$

where $\dot{Q}$ is the flow, ΔP is the pressure gradient along the tube, r is the radius of the tube, η is the viscosity of fluid and l is the length of the tube.

The Hagen–Poiseuille formula applies only to Newtonian fluids and to laminar flow. In non-Newtonian fluids such as blood, increase in velocity of flow may alter viscosity because of variation in the dispersion of cells within plasma.

Turbulent Flow: Flow of Fluids Through Orifices

In turbulent flow, fluid no longer moves in orderly planes but swirls and eddies around in a haphazard manner as illustrated in Figure 14.6. Essentially, turbulent flow is less efficient in the transport of fluids because energy is wasted in the eddies, in friction and in noise (bruits). Although viscosity is the important physical variable in relation to the behaviour of fluids in laminar flow, turbulent flow is more markedly affected by changes in fluid density.

It may be seen from Figure 14.7 that the relationship between pressure and flow is linear within certain limits. However, as velocity increases, a point is reached (the critical point or critical velocity) at which the characteristics of flow change from laminar to turbulent. The critical point is dependent upon several factors, which were investigated by the physicist Osborne Reynolds. These factors are related by the formula used for calculation of Reynolds' number:

$$\text{Reynolds' number} = v\rho r / \eta$$

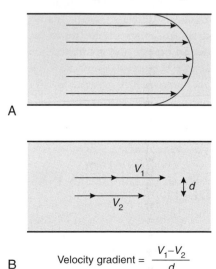

FIGURE 14.5 ■ (**A**) Diagrammatic illustration of laminar flow. (**B**) Velocity gradient.

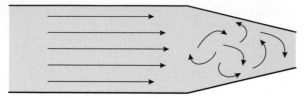

FIGURE 14.6 ■ Diagrammatic illustration of turbulent flow.

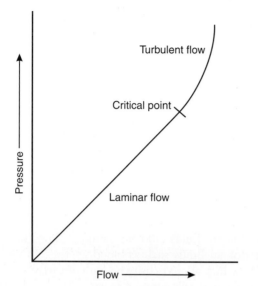

FIGURE 14.7 ■ The relationship between pressure and flow in a fluid is linear up to the critical point, above which flow becomes turbulent.

where v is the fluid linear velocity, r is the radius of the tube, ρ is the fluid density and η is its viscosity.

Studies with cylindrical tubes have shown that if Reynolds' number exceeds 2000, flow is likely to be turbulent, whereas a Reynolds' number of less than 2000 is usually associated with laminar flow. However, localized areas of turbulent flow can occur at lower Reynolds' numbers (i.e. at lower velocities) when there are changes in fluid direction, such as at bends, or changes in cross sectional area of the tube.

While the behaviour of fluids in laminar flow can be described by the Hagen–Poiseuille equation, the characteristics of turbulent flow are dependent on:

■ the square root of the pressure difference driving the flow
■ the square of the diameter of the vessel
■ the square root of density (ρ) of the fluid, i.e.:

$$Q = \alpha \cdot \frac{(\Delta P)^{\frac{1}{2}} \cdot R^2}{\rho^{\frac{1}{2}}}$$

A tube can be thought of as having a length many times its diameter. In an orifice by contrast, the diameter of the fluid pathway exceeds the length. The flow rate of a fluid through an orifice is much more likely to be turbulent and is described by the factors discussed above.

Applications of Turbulence in Anaesthetic Practice.
■ In upper respiratory tract obstruction of any severity, flow is inevitably turbulent downstream of the obstruction; thus for the same respiratory effort (driving pressure), a lower tidal volume is achieved than when flow is laminar. The extent of turbulent flow may be reduced by reducing gas density; clinically, it is common practice to administer oxygen-enriched helium rather than oxygen alone (the density of oxygen is $1360\,kg\,m^{-3}$ and that of helium is $160\,kg\,m^{-3}$). This reduces the likelihood of turbulent flow and reduces the respiratory effort required by the patient.
■ In anaesthetic breathing systems, a sudden change in diameter of tubing or irregularity of the wall may be responsible for a change from laminar to turbulent flow. Thus, tracheal and other breathing tubes should possess smooth internal surfaces, gradual bends and no constrictions.
■ Resistance to breathing is much greater when a tracheal tube of small diameter is used (Fig. 14.8). Tubes should be of as large a diameter and as short as possible.

In a variable orifice flowmeter, gas flow at low flow rates is predominantly laminar. Flow depends on viscosity. At higher flow rates, because the flowmeter behaves as an orifice, turbulent flow dominates and density is more important than viscosity.

THE VENTURI, THE INJECTOR AND BERNOULLI

A venturi is a tube with a section of smaller diameter than either the upstream or the downstream parts of the tube. The principles governing the behaviour of fluid flow through a venturi were formulated by Bernoulli in 1778, some 60 years earlier than Venturi himself. In any continuum, the energy of the fluid may be described by the Bernoulli equation, which

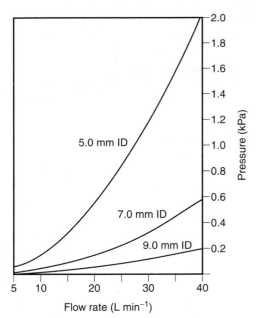

FIGURE 14.8 ■ Resistance to gas flow through tracheal tubes of different internal diameter (ID).

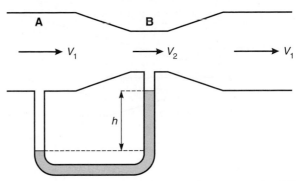

FIGURE 14.9 ■ The Bernoulli principle. See text for full details.

suggests that the sum of energies possessed by the fluid is constant, i.e.:

$$\frac{\rho v^2}{2}(KE) + P(PE) = constant,$$

assuming that the predominant fluid flow is horizontal such that gravitational potential energy can be ignored.

In a venturi, in order that the fluid flow be continuous, its velocity must increase through its narrowed throat ($v_2 > v_1$). This is associated with an increase in kinetic energy and Bernoulli's equation shows that where this occurs, there is an associated reduction in potential energy and therefore in pressure. Beyond the constriction, velocity decreases back to the initial value and the pressure rises again. The principle is illustrated in Figure 14.9. At point A, the energy in the fluid consists of potential (pressure) and kinetic (velocity), but at point B the amount of kinetic energy has increased because of the increased velocity. As the total energy state must remain constant, pressure is reduced at point B. A venturi has a number of uses, including that of a flow measurement device. For optimum performance of a venturi, it is desirable for fluid flow to remain laminar and this is achieved by gradual

opening of the tube beyond the constriction. In this way, if a U tube manometer is placed with one limb sampling the pressure at point A and the other at point B, then if the flow remains laminar, Hagen–Poiseuille's equation suggests a linear relationship between the pressure difference and the flow; this makes calibration of such a flowmeter relatively easy. This contrasts with an orifice, at the outflow of which the flow is usually turbulent. Although an orifice can be used as a flowmeter, the relationship between pressure difference and flow is non-linear. Another use of a venturi is as a device for entraining fluid from without. If a flow of oxygen is fed into a venturi through a nozzle, the low pressure induced at the throat may be used to entrain air, thus giving a metered supply of oxygen-enriched air, or acting as an injector by multiplying the amount of air flowing through the venturi towards the patient's lungs. If, instead, a hole is made in the side of the venturi at the throat, then the low pressure at that point may form the basis of a suction device (Fig. 14.10).

The injector principle may be seen in anaesthetic practice in the following situations:

■ *Oxygen therapy.* Several types of venturi oxygen masks are available which provide oxygen-enriched air. With an appropriate flow of oxygen (usually exceeding $4\,L\,min^{-1}$), there is a large degree of entrainment of air. This results in a total gas flow that exceeds the patient's peak inspiratory flow rate, thus ensuring that the inspired oxygen concentration remains constant, and it prevents an increase in apparatus dead space which always accompanies the use of low-flow oxygen devices.

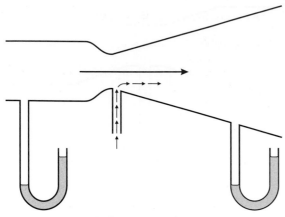

FIGURE 14.10 ■ Fluid entrainment by a venturi injector.

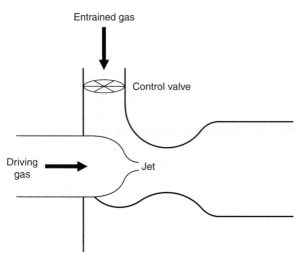

FIGURE 14.11 ■ A simple injector.

- *Nebulizers.* These are used to entrain water from a reservoir. If the water inlet is suitably positioned, the entrained water may be broken up into a fine mist by the high gas velocity.
- *Portable suction apparatus.*
- *Oxygen tents.*
- *As a driving gas in a ventilator* (Fig. 14.11).

The Coanda Effect

The Coanda effect describes a phenomenon whereby when gas flows through a tube and enters a Y-junction, gas tends to cling either to one side of the tube or to the other. This is because a Y-junction usually implies a reduction in downstream tube diameter, and thus an

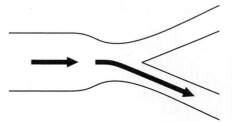

FIGURE 14.12 ■ The Coanda effect.

increase in velocity with a reduction in pressure adjacent to the wall. The gas is often not divided equally between the two outlets. The principle has been used in anaesthetic ventilators (termed fluidic ventilators), as the application of a small pressure distal to the restriction may enable gas flow to be switched (using an external cross flow of gas) from one side to another (Fig. 14.12).

HEAT

Heat is the energy which may be transferred from a body at a hotter temperature to one at a colder temperature. Its units are therefore Joules. As alluded to earlier, energy takes a number of forms and, if account is taken of energy losses, they are interchangeable. For example, if heat energy is applied to an engine, mechanical energy is the output. In a refrigeration cycle, mechanical energy is put in and heat is extracted from the cold compartment to the environment. Temperature is a measure of the tendency of an object to gain or lose heat.

Temperature and its Measurement

The Kelvin scale was adopted as an international temperature scale. The triple point of water is chosen as one reference point for the temperature scale; this is the point at which all three phases of water (ice, water, steam) are in equilibrium with each other, and although the pressure at which this occurs is very low (0.006 bar), the temperature at which this occurs is only fractionally greater than that of the ice point at atmospheric pressure (1.013 bar). The internationally agreed temperature 'number' of the triple point of water is 273.16, because it is this number of units above the recognized absolute zero of temperature, which was deduced from extrapolations of the relationships between pressure, volume and temperature of gases.

Hence the unit of thermodynamic temperature (the Kelvin; K) is the fraction 1/273.16 of the thermodynamic temperature of the triple point of water. The difference in temperature between the ice point for water and the steam point remains 100 units, which makes the range almost identical to the earlier, empirically derived, Celsius scale. It is not precisely the same, because this scale has its datum at 273.15 K, i.e. 0.01 K below the triple point. Although the unit on the thermodynamic Celsius scale is identical to that on the Kelvin scale, it is usual to denote 273.15 K as 0 °C.

Consequently, the intervals on the Celsius scale are identical to those on the Kelvin scale and the relationship between the two scales is as follows:

temperature (K) = temperature (°C) + 273.15

Temperature is measured in clinical practice by one of the following techniques:

- *Liquid expansion thermometer.* Mercury and alcohol are the more commonly used liquids.
- *Thermistor.* This is a semiconductor, which exhibits a reduction in electrical resistance with increase in temperature.
- *Thermocouple.* This relies on the Seebeck effect. When two metal conductors are joined together to form a circuit, a potential difference is produced which is proportional to the difference in the temperatures of the two junctions. In order to measure temperature, one junction has to be kept at a constant temperature.
- *Chemical thermometers.* These thermometers are described in more detail in Chapter 16.

Specific Heat Capacity

The specific heat capacity of a substance is the energy required to raise the temperature of 1 kg of the substance by 1 K, i.e.:

heat energy required = mass × specific heat capacity × temperature rise

Its units are $J\,kg^{-1}\,K^{-1}$. For gases, there are slight differences in specific heat capacities depending on whether the thermodynamic process being undergone is at constant pressure or at constant volume. The specific heat capacity of different substances is of interest because anaesthetists are frequently concerned with maintenance of body temperature in unconscious patients.

Heat is lost from patients by the processes of:

- conduction
- convection
- radiation, which is the most common mode of heat loss
- evaporation.

The specific heat capacity of gases is up to 1000 times smaller than that of liquids. Consequently, humidification of inspired gases is a more important method of conserving heat than warming dry gases; in addition, the use of humidified gases minimizes the very large energy loss produced by evaporation of fluid from the respiratory tract.

The skin acts as an almost perfect radiator; radiant losses in susceptible patients may be reduced by the use of reflective aluminium foil ('space blanket').

VAPORIZATION AND VAPORIZERS

In a liquid, molecules are in a state of continuous motion due to their kinetic energy, and are held in the liquid state because of intermolecular attraction by van der Waal's forces. Some molecules may develop velocities sufficient to escape from these forces, and if they are close to the surface of a liquid, these molecules may escape to enter the vapour phase. Increasing the temperature of a liquid increases its kinetic energy and a greater number of molecules escape. As the faster moving molecules escape into the vapour phase, the net velocity of the remaining molecules reduces; thus the energy state and therefore temperature of the liquid phase are reduced. The amount of heat required to convert a unit mass of liquid into a vapour without a change in temperature of the liquid is termed the 'latent heat of vaporization'.

In a closed vessel containing liquid and gas, a state of equilibrium is reached when the number of molecules escaping from the liquid is equal to the number of molecules re-entering the liquid phase. The vapour concentration is then said to be saturated at the specified temperature. Saturated vapour pressure of liquids is independent of the ambient pressure, but increases with increasing temperature.

The boiling point of a liquid is the temperature at which its saturated vapour pressure becomes equal to the ambient pressure. Thus, on the graph in

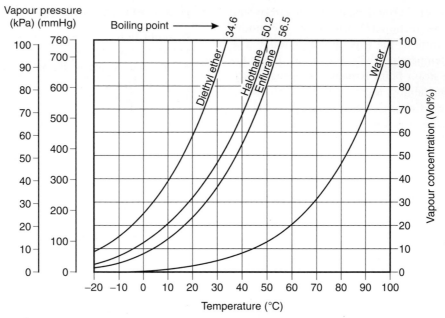

FIGURE 14.13 ■ Relationship between vapour pressure and temperature for different anaesthetic agents.

Figure 14.13, the boiling point of each liquid at 1 atmosphere is the temperature at which its saturated vapour pressure is 101.3 kPa.

Vaporizers

Vaporizers may be classified into two types:

- drawover vaporizers
- plenum vaporizers.

In the former type, gas is pulled through the vaporizer when the patient inspires, creating a subatmospheric pressure. In the latter type, gas is forced through the vaporizer by the pressure of the fresh gas supply. Consequently, the resistance to gas flow through a drawover vaporizer must be extremely small; the resistance of a plenum vaporizer may be high enough to prevent its use as a drawover vaporizer, although this is not necessarily so.

The principles of both devices are similar. If we consider the simplest form of vaporizer (Fig. 14.14), the concentration (C) of anaesthetic in the gas mixture emerging from the outlet port is dependent upon:

- *The saturated vapour pressure* of the anaesthetic liquid in the vaporizer. A highly volatile agent such as diethyl ether or desflurane is present in a much higher concentration than a less volatile

agent (i.e. with a lower saturated vapour pressure) such as halothane or isoflurane.
- *The temperature* of the liquid anaesthetic agent, as this determines its saturated vapour pressure.
- *The splitting ratio,* i.e. the flow rate of gas through the vaporizing chamber (F_v) in comparison with that through the bypass ($F - F_v$). Regulation of the splitting ratio is the usual mechanism whereby the anaesthetist controls the output concentration from a vaporizer.
- *The surface area* of the anaesthetic agent in the vaporizer. If the surface area is relatively small during use, the flow of gas through the vaporizing chamber may be too rapid to achieve complete saturation with anaesthetic molecules of the gas above the liquid.
- *Duration of use.* As the liquid in the vaporizing chamber evaporates, its temperature, and thus its saturated vapour pressure, decreases. This leads to a reduction in concentration of anaesthetic in the mixture leaving the exit port.
- *The flow characteristics* through the vaporizing chamber. In the simple vaporizer illustrated, gas passing through the vaporizing chamber may fail to mix completely with vapour as a result of

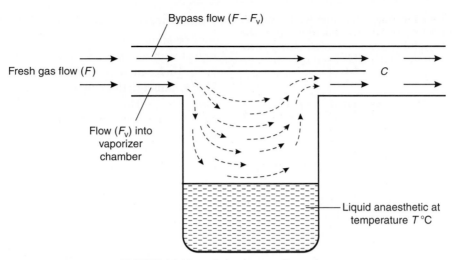

FIGURE 14.14 ■ A simple type of vaporizer.

streaming because of poor design. This lack of mixing is flow-dependent.

- Modern anaesthetic vaporizers overcome many of the problems described above. Maintenance of full saturation may be achieved by making available a large surface area for vaporization. In the TEC series of vaporizers, this is achieved by the use of wicks which draw up liquid anaesthetic by capillary pressure and provide a very large surface area. Efficient vaporization and prevention of streaming of gas through the vaporizing chamber are achieved by ensuring that gas travels through a concentric helix, which is bounded by the fabric wicks. Another method of ensuring full saturation is to bubble gas through liquid anaesthetic via a sintered disc; the final concentration is determined by mixing a known flow of fresh gas with a measured flow of fully saturated vapour.

Temperature Compensation

Temperature-compensated vaporizers possess a mechanism which produces an increase in flow through the vaporizing chamber (i.e. an increased splitting ratio) as the temperature of liquid anaesthetic decreases. In the TEC vaporizers, a bimetallic strip controls (by bending) a valve which alters flow through the exit port of the vaporizing chamber. In the EMO and Ohio vaporizers, a bellows mechanism is used to regulate the valve (by shortening with decreased temperature), whilst in the Drager Vapor 19 vaporizers, a metal rod acts in a similar fashion.

Back Pressure (Pumping Effect)

Some gas-driven mechanical ventilators (e.g. the Manley ventilator) produce a considerable increase in pressure in the outlet port and back bar of the anaesthetic machine. This pressure is highest during the inspiratory phase of ventilation. If the simple vaporizer shown in Figure 14.14 is attached to the back bar, the increased pressure during inspiration compresses the gas in the vaporizer; some gas in the region of the inlet port of the vaporizer is forced into the vaporizing chamber, where more vapour is added to it. Subsequently, there is a temporary surge in anaesthetic concentration when the pressure decreases at the end of the inspiratory cycle.

This effect is irrelevant with efficient vaporizers (i.e. those which saturate gas fully in the vaporization chamber) because gas in the outlet port is already saturated with vapour. However, when pressure reduces at the end of inspiration, some saturated gas passes retrogradely out of the inspiratory port and mixes with the bypass gas. Thus, a temporary increase in total vapour concentration may still occur in the gas supplied to the patient. Methods of overcoming this problem include:

- incorporation of a one-way valve in the outlet port
- construction of a bypass chamber and vaporizing chamber which are of equal volumes so that the gas in each is compressed or expanded equally

■ construction of a long inlet tube to the vaporizing chamber so that retrograde flow from the vaporizing chamber does not reach the bypass channel (as in the Mark 3 TEC vaporizers).

HUMIDITY AND HUMIDIFICATION

Absolute and Relative Humidity

Absolute humidity ($g\,m^{-3}$ or $mg\,L^{-1}$) is the mass of water vapour present in a given volume of gas. Relative humidity is the ratio of mass of water vapour in a given volume of gas to the mass required to saturate that volume of gas at the same temperature.

Since a mass of water vapour in a sample of air has an associated temperature-dependent vapour pressure, relative humidity (RH) may also be expressed as:

$$RH = \frac{actual\ vapour\ pressure}{saturated\ vapour\ pressure}$$

In normal practice, relative humidity may be measured using:

■ *The hair hygrometer.* This operates on the principle that a hair elongates if humidity increases; the hair length controls a pointer. This simple device may be mounted on a wall. It is reasonably accurate only in the range 15–85% relative humidity.
■ *The wet and dry bulb hygrometer.* The dry bulb measures the actual temperature, whereas the wet bulb measures a lower temperature as a result of the cooling effect of evaporation of water. The rate of vaporization is related to the humidity of the ambient gas and the difference between the two temperatures is a measure of ambient humidity; the relative humidity is obtained from a set of tables.
■ *Regnault's hygrometer.* This consists of a thin silver tube containing ether and a thermometer to show the temperature of the ether. Air is pumped through the ether to produce evaporation, thereby cooling the silver tube. When gas in contact with the tube is saturated with water vapour, it condenses as a mist on the bright silver. The temperature at which this takes place is known as the *dew point,* from which relative humidity is obtained from tables.

Humidification of the Respiratory Tract

Air drawn into the respiratory tract becomes fully saturated with water in the trachea at a temperature of 37 °C. Under these conditions, the SVP of water is 6.3 kPa (47 mmHg); this represents a fractional concentration of 6.2%. The concentration of water is $44\,mg\,L^{-1}$. At 21 °C, saturated water vapour contains 2.4% water vapour or $18\,mg\,L^{-1}$. Thus, there is a considerable capacity for patients to lose both water and heat when the lungs are ventilated with dry gases.

There are three means of humidifying inspired gas:

■ heated humidifier (water vaporizer)
■ nebulizer
■ condenser humidifier (also known as heat and moisture exchanging [HME] humidifier).

The hot water bath humidifier is a simple device for heating water to 45–60 °C. These devices have several potential problems, including infection if the water temperature decreases below 45 °C, scalding the patient if the temperature exceeds 60 °C (these high temperatures may be used to prevent growth of bacteria) and condensation of water in the inspiratory anaesthetic tubing. These devices are approximately 80% efficient.

Some nebulizers are based upon a Venturi system; a gas supply entrains water, which is broken up into a large number of droplets. The ultrasonic nebulizer operates by dropping water onto a surface, which is vibrated at a frequency of 2 MHz. This breaks up the water particles into extremely small droplets. The main problem with these nebulizers is the possibility that supersaturation of inspired gas may occur and the patient may be overloaded with water.

The condenser humidifier (or artificial nose) may consist of a simple wire mesh, which is inserted between the tracheal tube and the anaesthetic breathing system. More recently, humidifiers constructed of rolled corrugated paper have been introduced. These devices are approximately 70% efficient.

SOLUBILITY OF GASES

Henry's law states that, at a given temperature, the amount of a gas which dissolves in a liquid is directly proportional to the partial pressure of the gas in equilibrium with the liquid. If a liquid is heated and its temperature rises, the partial pressure of its saturated vapour increases. This will result in gas molecules coming out of solution, and a lesser amount of gas remaining dissolved in the liquid. This is exemplified by the carbon dioxide bubbles in a bottle of tonic water becoming more apparent as time elapses from its removal from the refrigerator.

It is customary to confine the term 'tension' to the partial pressure of a gas exerted by gas molecules in solution, but the terms are synonymous. The tension of the gas in solution is in equilibrium with the partial pressure of the gas above it. A relatively insoluble gas will reach equilibrium more quickly than a soluble one.

Solubility Coefficients

The Bunsen solubility coefficient is the volume of gas which dissolves in a unit volume of liquid at a given temperature when the gas in equilibrium with the liquid is at a pressure of 1 atmosphere.

The Ostwald solubility coefficient is the volume of gas which dissolves in a unit volume of liquid at a given temperature. Thus, the Ostwald solubility coefficient is independent of pressure.

The partition coefficient is the ratio of the amount of substance in one phase compared with a second phase, each phase being of equal volume and in equilibrium, e.g. the amount of carbon dioxide in the gas phase compared with the amount of carbon dioxide dissolved in blood. As with the Ostwald coefficient, it is necessary to define the temperature but not the pressure. The partition coefficient may be applied to two liquids, but the Ostwald coefficient applies to partition between gas and liquid. The blood/gas partition coefficient of an anaesthetic agent is an indicator of the speed with which the alveolar gas concentration equilibrates with the inspired concentration, a low coefficient (e.g. desflurane 0.42) leading to rapid equilibration. The oil/gas partition coefficient is a measure of its potency, a high coefficient (e.g. isoflurane 98.5) indicating an agent highly soluble in cerebral tissue, leading to high anaesthetic potency and low MAC. The Overton-Meyer hypothesis shows an inverse relationship between MAC and the logarithm of lipid potency.

Diffusion

If two different gases or liquids are separated in a container by an impermeable partition which is then removed, gradual mixing of the two different substances occurs as a result of the kinetic activity of each species

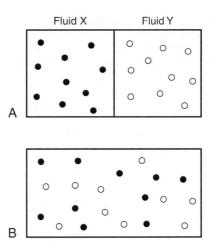

FIGURE 14.15 ■ Illustration of diffusion in fluids. (**A**) Fluids X and Y separated by partition. (**B**) Mixing of fluids after removal of partition.

of molecule. This is illustrated in Figure 14.15. The principle governing this process is described by Fick's law of diffusion, which states that the rate of diffusion of a substance across unit area is proportional to the concentration gradient. Graham's law (which applies to gases only) states that the rate of diffusion of a gas is inversely proportional to the square root of its molecular weight or density.

In the example shown in Figure 14.15B, the interface between fluids X and Y immediately after removal of the partition would be the interface between the two species of fluid. In biology, however, there is normally a membrane separating gases or separating gas and liquids.

The rate of diffusion of gases may be affected by the nature of the membrane. In the lungs, the alveolar membrane is moist and may be regarded as a water film. Thus, diffusion of gases through the alveolar membrane is dependent not only on the properties of diffusion described above but also on the solubility of gas in the water film. As carbon dioxide is more highly soluble in water than oxygen, it diffuses more rapidly across the alveolar membrane, despite the larger partial pressure gradient for oxygen.

Osmosis

In the examples given above, the membranes are permeable to all substances. However, in biology, membranes are frequently semipermeable, i.e. they allow the passage of some substances but are impermeable

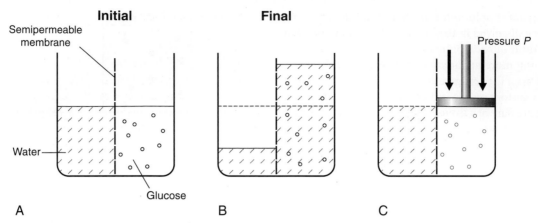

FIGURE 14.16 ■ Diagram to illustrate osmotic pressure. (**A**) Water and glucose placed into two compartments separated by a semipermeable membrane. (**B**) At equilibrium, water has passed into the glucose compartment to balance the pressure. (**C**) The magnitude of osmotic pressure of the glucose is denoted by a hydraulic pressure P applied to the glucose to prevent any movement of water into the glucose compartment.

to others. This is illustrated in Figure 14.16. In Figure 14.16A, initially equal volumes of water and glucose solution are separated by a semipermeable membrane. Water molecules pass freely through the membrane to dilute the glucose solution (Fig. 14.16B). This process continues until the volume of the diluted glucose solution supports a significantly greater head of fluid pressure than the water volume on the other side of the membrane. This hydrostatic pressure opposes the flow of water molecules through the membrane into the glucose solution, driven by the difference in solution constituents. This driving pressure is termed the osmotic pressure. Note that, depending on the membrane properties, the glucose molecules are probably too large to allow significant flow in the opposite direction. By application of a hydrostatic pressure on the glucose side (Fig. 14.16C), the process of further transfer of water molecules can be prevented or even reversed; this pressure (P) is equal to the osmotic pressure exerted by the glucose solution.

Substances in dilute solution behave in accordance with the gas laws. Thus, 1 gram-molecular weight of a dissolved substance occupying 22.4 L of solvent exerts an osmotic pressure of 1 bar at 273 K. Dalton's law also applies; the total osmotic pressure of a mixture of solutes is equal to the sum of osmotic pressures exerted independently by each substance.

The osmotic pressure of a solution depends on the number of dissolved particles per litre. Thus, a molar solution of a substance which ionizes into two particles (e.g. NaCl) exerts twice the osmotic pressure exerted by a molar solution of a non-ionizing substance (e.g. glucose). The osmotic pressure may be produced by all of a mixture of substances in a fluid. Thus, it is the sum of the individual molarities of each particle.

While osmolarity has units of osmoles per litre of solution the term osmolality refers to the number of osmoles per kilogram of water or other solvent. Thus, osmolarity may vary slightly from osmolality as a result of changes in density due to the effect of temperature on volume, although in biological terms the difference is extremely small.

In the circulation, water and the majority of ions are freely permeable across the endothelial membrane, but plasma proteins do not traverse into the interstitial fluid. The term oncotic pressure is used to describe the osmotic pressure exerted by the plasma proteins alone. Plasma oncotic pressure is relatively small (approximately 1 mosmol L^{-1} equivalent to 25 mmHg) in relation to total osmotic pressure exerted by plasma (approximately 300 mosmol L^{-1} equivalent to 6.5 bar).

ELECTRICITY

Basic Quantities and Units

An ampere (A) is the unit of electric current in the SI system. It represents the flow of 6.24×10^{18} electrons. The ampere is defined as the current which, if flowing in two parallel wires of infinite length, placed 1 m apart in a vacuum, produces a force of $2 \times 10^{-7}\,\mathrm{N\,m^{-1}}$ on each of the wires.

Electric charge is the measure of the amount of electricity and its SI unit is the coulomb (C). The coulomb is the quantity of electric charge that passes some point when a current of 1 ampere (A) flows for a period of 1 s:

$$\text{coulombs (C)} = \text{amperes (A)} \times \text{seconds (s)}$$

Electrical potential exists when one point in an electric circuit has more positive charge than another. Electrical potential is analogous to height in a gravitational field where a mass possesses potential energy due to its height; another analogy might be the pressure at the bottom of a water reservoir to drive a turbine. The electrical potential of the earth is regarded as the reference point for zero potential and is referred to as 'earth'. When a potential difference is applied across a conductor, it produces an electric current and current flows from an area of higher potential to one of lower potential.

The unit for potential difference is the volt. One volt is defined as the potential difference which produces a current of 1 ampere in a substance when the rate of energy dissipation is 1 watt, as demonstrated in the equation:

$$\text{potential difference (volts)} = \frac{\text{power (watts)}}{\text{current (amperes)}}$$

A volt can also be defined as a potential difference producing a change in energy of 1 J when 1 coulomb is moved across it. This definition is often used in connection with defibrillators.

Ohm's law states that the current flowing through a resistance is proportional to the potential difference across it. The unit for electrical resistance is the ohm (Ω). The ohm is that resistance which will allow 1 ampere of current to flow under the influence of a potential difference of 1 volt.

$$\text{resistance}\,(\Omega) = \frac{\text{potential}\,(V)}{\text{current}\,(I)}$$

The anaesthetist is in daily contact with a large amount of equipment which is powered by mains supply electricity; this includes monitoring equipment, many ventilators, suction apparatus, defibrillators and diathermy equipment.

Whilst a total understanding of this equipment and its mode of action may depend upon a detailed knowledge of electronics, the equipment can usually be used safely as a type of 'black box', i.e. the inside of the box may be a mystery, but the anaesthetist must be familiar with the operating controls and the ways in which the apparatus may malfunction or, if a recording instrument, give rise to artefacts.

It is not possible in this brief chapter to provide a full synopsis of the basic principles of electricity and electronics, but it is essential to stress some elements which have a bearing on the safety of both the patient and the anaesthetist in the operating theatre.

In the UK, the mains electricity is supplied at a voltage of 240 V with a frequency of 50 Hz, and in the USA at a voltage of 110 V and a frequency of 60 Hz. These voltages are potentially dangerous, although the danger is related predominantly to the current which flows through the patient as governed by Ohm's law.

When dealing with alternating current, it is necessary to use the term *impedance* in place of resistance, as impedance takes into account the frequency relationship between current and voltage, which is important in the presence of capacitors and inductors. The impedance offered to flowing current by a capacitor is inversely proportional to the current frequency. Hence a capacitor blocks direct current. If an increasing magnitude of electrical current at 50 Hz passes through the body, there is initially a tingling sensation at a current of 1 mA. An increase in the current produces increasing pain and muscle spasm until, at 80–100 mA, arrhythmias and ventricular fibrillation may occur. The electrical disturbance that current can cause to biological tissue is related to the current frequency, the greatest sensitivity occurring at mains frequencies of 50-60 Hz, with increasing resilience to such damage at lower and higher frequencies. The choice of 50-60 Hz for mains current is due to the lower energy losses which occur in transmission lines.

Electrical Safety

The damage to tissue by electrical current is related also to the current density; a current passing through a small area is more dangerous than the same current passing through a much larger area. Other factors relating to the likelihood of ventricular fibrillation are the duration of passage of the current and its frequency. Radiofrequencies in the megahertz range (such as those used in diathermy) have no potential for fibrillating the heart, but do cause burns.

It is clear from Ohm's law that the size of the current is dependent upon the size of the impedance to current flow. A common way of reducing the risk of a large current injuring the anaesthetist in the operating theatre is to wear antistatic shoes and to stand on the antistatic floor. This provides a high impedance (see below).

Mains electricity supplies may induce currents in other circuits or on cases of instruments. The resulting induced currents are termed leakage currents and may pass through either the patient or anaesthetist to earth. There are three classes of electrical insulation which are designed to minimize the risk of a patient or anaesthetist forming part of an electrical circuit between the live conductor of a piece of equipment and earth:

- *Class I equipment* (fully earthed). The main supply lead has three cores (live, neutral and earth). The earth is connected to all exposed conductive parts, and in the event of a fault developing which short-circuits current to the casing of the equipment, current flows from the case to earth. If small enough, the casing is rendered safe, if large enough the fuse on the live input to the device is blown and the equipment is rendered unusable, but safe.
- *Class II equipment* (double-insulated). This has no protective earth. The power cable has only live and neutral conductors and these are 'double-insulated'. The casing is normally made of non-conductive material.
- *Class III equipment* (low voltage). This relies on a power supply at a very low voltage produced from a secondary transformer situated some distance away from the device. Potentials do not exceed 24 V (AC) or 50 V (DC). Electric heating blankets, for example, are rendered safer in this way.

Isolation Circuits

All modern patient-monitoring equipment uses an isolation transformer so that the patient is connected only to the secondary circuit of the transformer, which is not earthed. Thus, even if the patient makes contact between the live circuit of the secondary transformer

and earth, no current is transmitted to earth. If the part of a circuit applied to the patient is not earthed, it is said to be 'floating', designated by 'F' in its safety classification (*vide infra*).

Microshock

Induced currents and leakage currents can also occur in electromedical equipment which has a component within the patient, such as a cardiac pacemaker or a saline-filled catheter connected to a transducer. With the skin breached as the first defence against shock, it only takes very small currents to cause manifestations of electrical shock, and this is termed *microshock*. 100 μA of current is enough to cause ventricular fibrillation under these circumstances.

Safety Testing

The International Electrotechnical Commission has produced recommendations (adopted by the British Standards Institute) defining the levels of permitted leakage currents and patient currents from different types of electromedical equipment. Whenever new equipment is bought for a hospital, it should be subjected to tests, which verify that the leakage currents and other electrical safety characteristics are within the allowed specifications. Equipment is labelled according to whether it is suitable for external (B, BF) or internal (CF) application to the patient, with testing to appropriate levels of leakage current. Regular servicing of equipment should be carried out by qualified engineers to ensure that these safe characteristics are maintained.

The Defibrillator

Capacitance is the ability to store electric charge. The defibrillator is an instrument in which electric charge is stored in a capacitor and then released in a controlled fashion. Direct current (DC) rather than alternating current (AC) energy is used. DC energy is more effective, causes less myocardial damage and is less arrhythmogenic than AC energy. However, biphasic defibrillators are now available, as they use a lower energy level, potentially resulting in less cardiac damage. Defibrillators are set according to the amount of energy stored and this depends on both the stored charge and the potential:

available energy (J) = stored charge (C) × potential (V)

To defibrillate a heart, two electrodes are placed on the patient's chest; one is placed just to one side of the sternum and the other over the apex of the heart. When it is discharged, the energy stored in the capacitor is released as a current pulse through the patient's chest and heart. This current pulse gives a synchronous contraction of the myocardium after which a refractory period and normal or near-normal beats may follow. The voltage may be up to 5000 V with a stored energy of up to 400 J. In practice, an inductor is included in the output circuit to ensure that the electric pulse has an optimum shape and duration. The inductor absorbs some of the energy which is discharged by the capacitor.

Diathermy

The effect of passing electric current through the body varies from slight physical sensation through muscle contraction to ventricular fibrillation. The severity of these effects depends on the amount and the frequency of the current. These effects become less as the frequency of the current increases, being small above 1 kHz and negligible above 1 MHz. However, the heating and burning effects of electric current can occur at all frequencies.

A diathermy machine is used to pass electric current of high frequency (about 1-2 MHz) through the body in order to cause cutting and/or coagulation by burning local tissue where the current density is high. In the electrical circuit involving diathermy equipment, there are two connections with the patient. In unipolar diathermy, these are the patient plate and the active electrode used by the surgeon (Fig. 14.17A). The current travels from the active electrode, through the patient and exits through the patient plate. The current density is high at the active end where burning or cutting occurs, but it is low at the plate end, where no injury occurs. If for any reason (e.g. a faulty plate) the current flows from the patient through a small area of contact between the patient and earth, then a burn may occur at the point of contact.

In bipolar diathermy, there is no patient plate, but the current travels down one side of the diathermy forceps and out through the other side (Fig. 14.17B). This type of diathermy uses low power and, because the current does not travel through the patient, it is advisable to use this in patients with a cardiac pacemaker.

ISOTOPES AND RADIATION

An atom consists of electrons which are negatively charged and these orbit around a nucleus which contains protons (positive charge) and neutrons (no charge) (Fig. 14.18). Isotopes are variations of similar atoms but with different numbers of neutrons. Isotopes with unstable nuclei are known as radioisotopes and are radioactive.

The process of change from one unstable isotope to another is known as radioactive decay. The rate of decay is measured by the half-life. The half-life of an isotope is the time required for half of the radioactive atoms present to disintegrate. When one atom changes from one unstable state to another, it emits energy in the form of gamma rays, or alpha or beta particles. Gamma rays, and alpha and beta particles all cause damage to or death of cells. Because of this, radioisotopes are used for the treatment of cancer (e.g. cobalt–60 and caesium–137) and for conditions such as thyrotoxicosis (iodine–131). They may also be used for diagnostic purposes. Technetium–99 m, krypton–81 m and xenon–133 are used in imaging techniques such as scanning. Chromium–51 is used in non-imaging techniques such as labelling of red blood cells in order to measure red cell volume.

Radiation may be detected using a scintillation counter. The SI unit for radioactivity is the becquerel.

X-Rays

X-rays are electromagnetic radiation produced when a beam of electrons is accelerated from a cathode to strike an anode (often made of tungsten). They are used for imaging purposes.

Radiation Safety

Exposure to radioisotopes and X-rays should be kept to a minimum because of the risks of tissue damage and chromosomal changes. Guidelines regarding the use of ionizing radiation were issued in the UK by the Department of Health in May 2000 in a document called Ionising Radiation (Medical Exposure) Regulations 2000 (IRMER 2000). The aims of this document are to protect patients against unnecessary exposure to radiation and to set standards for practitioners using ionizing radiation. The request of non-essential X-rays by clinicians is strongly discouraged. In the UK, a doctor requires a certificate of authorization

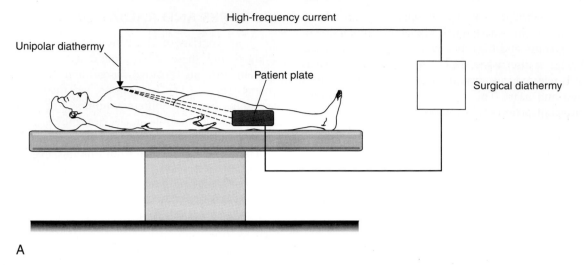

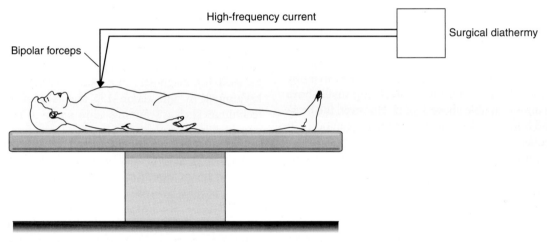

FIGURE 14.17 ■ Principle of the surgical diathermy system. (**A**) Unipolar diathermy. (**B**) Bipolar diathermy.

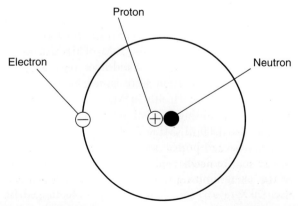

FIGURE 14.18 ■ Basic structure of an atom.

before he or she can administer radiation compounds to patients or use X-ray equipment. Lead absorbs X-rays and so it is incorporated into aprons worn by staff who are exposed to radiation. Staff who are exposed regularly to radiation should wear film badges. The film badge contains a piece of photographic film which permits estimation of the energy and dose of radiation received.

MAGNETIC RESONANCE IMAGING

Nuclear magnetic resonance (NMR) is a phenomenon that was first described by Bloch and Purcell in 1945 and has been used widely in chemistry and biochemistry. The more recent application of NMR to imaging came to be known as magnetic resonance imaging (MRI). The word nuclear was removed in order to emphasize that this technique was not associated with any radiation risk.

Physical Principles of MRI

Because of the presence of protons, all atomic nuclei possess a charge. In addition, the nuclei of some atoms spin. The combination of the spinning and the charge results in a local magnetic field. When some nuclei are placed in a powerful static magnetic field, they tend to align themselves longitudinally with the field. Approximately half of the nuclei are aligned parallel to the field and the other half antiparallel to it. However, there is an excess of nuclei which are parallel to the field and it is this population of nuclei which are of interest in the principles of MRI. When such a population of nuclei is subjected intermittently to a second magnetic field which is oscillating at the resonant frequency of the nucleus and at right angles to the static field, they tend to precess (i.e. they rotate about an axis different from the one about which they are spinning). The precession of the nuclei produces a rotating magnetic field and this is measured from the magnitude of the electrical signal induced in a set of coils within the MRI unit. The atoms then revert to their normal alignment. As they do so, images are made at different phases of relaxation known as T1, T2 and other sequences. These sequences are recorded. From the timings of these sequences, referred to as different weightings, the recorded images are compared with each other. The detected signals are then used to form an image of the body.

The hydrogen ion is used commonly for imaging because it is abundant in the body and has a strong response to an external magnetic field. Phosphorus may also be used.

The SI unit for magnetic flux density is the tesla (T) and magnets that are used in most MRI units have a magnetic flux density of 0.1–4 T. The powerful magnetic field may be created by either a permanent magnet (which cannot be switched on and off and tends to be heavy) or an electromagnet.

The presence of a strong magnetic field and restricted access to the patient imply that anaesthesia for patients undergoing an MRI scan presents unique problems which should be taken into account when planning MRI services. MRI-compatible anaesthetic equipment is essential. The hazards associated with using incorrect equipment include the projectile effect, burns and malfunction. Significant levels of acoustic noise are produced during MRI imaging because of vibrations within the scanner. Ear protectors should be provided to staff who may remain within the examination room during the scan and to the patients. The noise level may also make audible alarms inappropriate.

ULTRASOUND

Ultrasonic vibration is defined as between 20 kHz and the MHz range, outside hearing range. An ultrasound probe or transmitter consists of a piezo-electric crystal, which generates mechanical vibration, a vibrating pressure wave, in response to an electrical input (see Fig. 14.19A). Conversely it can also produce an electrical output in response to a mechanical pressure wave input. Hence the piezo-electric crystal can be used to transmit a pressure wave and to detect a reflected wave (see Fig. 14.19B).

The wavelength (λ) and the transmission frequency (f) are related to the propagation velocity c by the formula $c = f\lambda$.

The period T of such a wave is the time taken for one full cycle, and is given by $T = 1/f$.

Ultrasound velocity in a tissue and the attenuation of the wave varies depending on the tissue it is travelling through. In soft tissues the wave velocity is between 1460 and 1630 m s^{-1} whereas in bone it is 2700–4100 m s^{-1}. Bone attenuates the waveform about 10 times as quickly as soft tissue. The greatest penetration is achieved with the lowest frequency but with poor resolution, while the converse holds for high frequency waves. A compromise is to use the highest frequency that will give good resolution, and which will also ensure adequate penetration of the tissues being investigated. For example, a frequency of 3 MHz is normally used to visualize the kidneys, while 20 MHz is used to visualize intracorporeal devices inserted by the anaesthetist, such as needles and catheters. It is the reflection of the ultrasound wave at the interface between two tissues or at tissue-fluid (air) interfaces which provides a diagnostic image. The same piezo-electric crystal

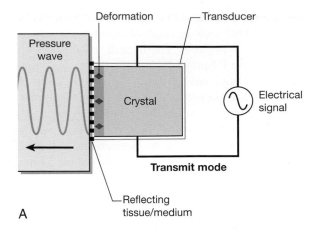

A

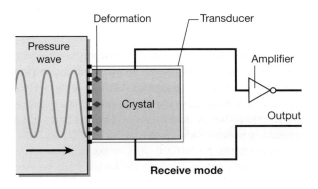

B

FIGURE 14.19 ■ Ultrasound generated from a piezo-electric crystal. An electrical signal input causes the crystal to deform (A), creating a pressure wave. Air conducts ultrasound poorly, so coupling between probe and surface requires gel. In (B) the reverse process occurs, and a reflected pressure wave induces an electrical signal, which can be used to create an image. *(Adapted from Fig: 10.1 'Ultrasound and Doppler' from Magee P, Tooley M (2011) Physics, Clinical Measurement and Equipment of Anaesthetic Practice for the FRCA by permission of Oxford University Press.)*

is usually used as the receiver, with the transmission mode switched off. The induced pressure changes coupled to the transducer induce electrical signals, which produce an image (see Fig. 14.19B). A real-time two dimensional image, using multiple probes, can be produced; this is known as a *B* scan.

Ultrasound can also be used in Doppler mode. When an ultrasonic wave reflects off a stationary object, the reflected wave has the same frequency as the transmitted wave. When the object (such as a collection of red blood cells) is moving towards the transmitter, however,

it encounters more oscillations per unit time than its stationary equivalent, so the frequency of the reflected wave is apparently increased. Conversely, when the object is moving away from the ultrasound wave, the frequency of the deflected wave is reduced. This property can be used as a non-invasive technique for measurement of blood velocity (not flow) within the body.

For a transmitted frequency f_t, of wavelength λ, and the velocity of sound in the medium c:

$$f_t = c/\lambda.$$

If the beam hits an object which is moving directly towards the transmitter at velocity v, the frequency of the waves arriving at the reflector (f_r) will now be:

$$f_r = (c+v)/\lambda.$$

The reflector will now act as a source which is moving towards the transmitter, and the actual frequency sensed by the transmitter (in receiver mode) will be $f_r = (c+2v)/\lambda$. The apparent increase in frequency is given by:

$$
\begin{aligned}
(f_r - f_t) &= (c+2v)/\lambda. - c/\lambda, \\
&= 2v/\lambda, \\
&= 2v f_t/c.
\end{aligned}
$$

The frequency difference can be transduced into an audible signal, or used to calculate the velocity of the blood cells. Normally the Doppler beam is applied non-invasively, not directly facing an oncoming flow of blood, but from outside the blood vessel, at an angle θ to it. The resulting frequency shift must be multiplied by $\cos\theta$.

Clearly the greatest accuracy in measuring blood velocity (e.g. to derive cardiac output) is achieved by having the probe aligned as far as is possible with the vessel (e.g. the aorta). Having measured mean velocity of the blood in a vessel in order to calculate blood flow, the mean diameter of the vessel must also be measured, and its cross sectional area calculated, using the formula: *flow = velocity × area*.

LASERS

A laser produces an intense beam of light which results from stimulation of atoms (the laser medium) by electrical or thermal energy. Laser light has three defining characteristics: coherence (all waves are in phase both in time and in space), collimation (all waves

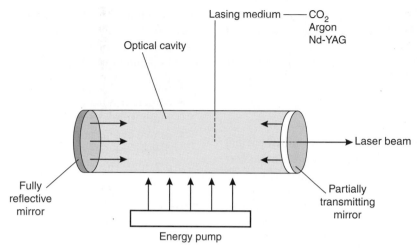

FIGURE 14.20 ■ Principle of a laser system.

travel in parallel directions) and monochromaticity (all waves have the same wavelength). The term *laser* is an acronym for Light Amplification by Stimulated Emission of Radiation.

Physical Principles of Lasers

When atoms of the lasing medium are excited from a normal ground state into a high-energy state by a 'pumping' source, this is known as the excited state. When the atoms return from the excited state to the normal state, the energy is often dissipated as light or radiation of a specific wavelength characteristic of the atom (spontaneous emission). In normal circumstances, when this change from higher to lower energy state occurs, the light emitted is likely to be absorbed by an atom in the lower energy state rather than meet an atom in a higher energy state and cause more light emission. In a laser, the number of excited atoms is raised significantly so that the light emitted strikes another high-energy atom and, as a result, two light particles with the same phase and frequency are emitted (stimulated emission). These stages are summarized below:

- *Excitation*: stable atom + energy → high-energy atom
- *Spontaneous emission*: high-energy atom → stable atom + a photon of light
- *Stimulated emission*: photon of light + high-energy atom → stable atom + 2 photons of light.

The light emitted is reflected back and forth many times between mirrored surfaces, giving rise to further stimulation. This amplification continues as long as there are more atoms in the excited state than in the normal state.

A laser system has four components (Fig. 14.20).

- *The laser medium* may be gas, liquid or solid. Common surgical lasers are CO_2, argon gas and neodymium-yttrium-aluminium-garnet (Nd-YAG) crystal. This determines the wavelength of the radiation emitted. The Nd-YAG and CO_2 lasers emit invisible infrared radiation and argon gives blue-green radiation.
- *The pumping source* supplies energy to the laser medium and this may be either an intense flash of light or electric discharge.
- *An optical cavity* is the container in which the laser medium is encased. It also contains mirrors used to reflect light in order to increase the energy of the stimulated emission. One of the mirrors is a partially transmitting mirror, which allows the laser beam to escape.
- *The light guide* directs the laser light to the surgical site. This may be in the form of a hollow tube or a flexible fibreoptic guide.

The longer the wavelength of the laser light, the more strongly it is absorbed, and the power of the light is converted to heat in shallower tissues, e.g. CO_2. The shorter the wavelength, the more scattered is the light, and the light energy is converted to heat in deeper tissues, e.g. Nd-YAG.

Lasers are categorized into four classes according to the degree of hazard they afford: class 1 is the least dangerous and class 4 the most dangerous. Surgical lasers which are specifically designed to damage tissue are class 4.

OPTICAL FIBRES

Optical fibres are used in the design of endoscopes and bronchoscopes in order to be able to see around corners. Optical fibres use the principle that when light passes from one medium to another, it is refracted (i.e. bent). If the direction of the light is altered, the light may be totally reflected instead and this allows transmission of the light along the optical fibres (Fig. 14.21). As a result, if light passes into one end of a fibre of glass or other transparent material, it may pass along the fibre by being continually reflected from the glass/air boundary. Endoscopes and bronchoscopes contain bundles of flexible transparent fibres.

FIRES AND EXPLOSIONS

Although the use of inflammable anaesthetic agents has declined greatly over the last two to three decades, ether is still used in some countries. In addition, other inflammable agents may be utilized in the operating theatre, e.g. alcohol for skin sterilization. Thus the anaesthetist should have some understanding of the problems and risks of fire occurring in the operating theatre.

Fires are produced when fuels undergo combustion. A conflagration differs from a fire in having a more rapid and more violent rate of combustion. A fire becomes an explosion if the combustion is sufficiently rapid to cause pressure waves that, in turn, cause sound waves. If these pressure waves possess sufficient energy to ignite adjacent fuels, the combustion is extremely violent and termed a detonation.

Fires require three ingredients:

- fuel
- oxygen or other substance capable of supporting combustion
- source of ignition, i.e. a source of heat sufficient to raise the fuel temperature to its ignition temperature. This quantity of heat is termed the activation energy.

Fuels

The modern volatile anaesthetic agents are non-flammable and non-explosive at room temperature in either air or oxygen.

Oils and greases are petroleum-based and form excellent fuels. In the presence of high pressures of oxygen, nitrous oxide or compressed air, these fuels may ignite spontaneously, an event termed dieseling (an analogy with the diesel engine). Thus oil or grease must not be used in compressed air, nitrous oxide or oxygen supplies.

Surgical spirit burns readily in air and the risk is increased in the presence of oxygen or nitrous oxide. Other non-anaesthetic inflammable substances include methane in the gut (which may be ignited by diathermy when the gut is opened), paper dressings and plastics found in the operating theatre suite.

Ether burns in air slowly with a blue flame, but mixtures of nitrous oxide, oxygen and ether are always explosive. It has been suggested that if administration of ether is discontinued 5 min before exposure to a source of ignition, the patient's expired gas is unlikely to burn provided that an open circuit has been used after discontinuation of ether.

The stoichiometric concentration of a fuel and oxidizing agent is the concentration at which all combustible vapour and agent are completely utilized. Thus the most violent reactions take place in stoichiometric mixtures, and as the concentration of the fuel moves away from the stoichiometric range, the reaction gradually declines until a point is reached (the flammability limit) at which ignition does not occur.

The inflammability range for ether is 2–82% in oxygen, 2–36% in air and 1.5–24% in nitrous oxide. The stoichiometric concentration of ether in oxygen

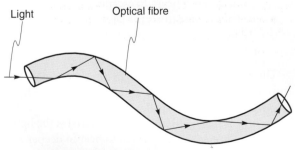

FIGURE 14.21 ■ Principle of the optical fibre.

Light   Optical fibre

is 14% and there is a risk of explosion with ether concentrations of approximately 12–40% in oxygen. In air, the stoichiometric concentration of ether is 3.4% and explosions do not occur.

Support of Combustion

It should always be remembered that as the concentration of oxygen increases, so does the likelihood of ignition of a fuel and the conversion of the reaction from fire to explosion.

Nitrous oxide supports combustion. During laparoscopy, there is a risk of perforation of the bowel and escape of methane or hydrogen into the peritoneal cavity. Consequently, the use of nitrous oxide to produce a pneumoperitoneum for this procedure is not recommended; carbon dioxide is to be preferred, as it does not support combustion (and, in addition, has a much greater solubility in blood than nitrous oxide, thereby diminishing the risk of gas embolism).

Sources of Ignition

The two main sources of ignition in the operating theatre are static electricity and diathermy.

Static Electricity

Electrostatic charge occurs when two substances are rubbed together and one of the substances has an excess of electrons while the other has a deficit. Electrostatic charges are produced on non-conductive material, such as rubber mattresses, plastic pillow cases and sheets, woollen blankets, nylon, terylene, hosiery garments, rubber tops of stools and nonconducting parts of anaesthetic machines and breathing systems. Static electricity may be a source of ignition.

Diathermy

Diathermy equipment has now become an essential element of most surgical practice. However, it should not be used in the presence of inflammable agents.

Other Sources of Ignition

- Faulty electrical equipment.
- Heat from endoscopes, thermocautery, lasers, etc.
- Electric sparks from switches, X-ray machines, etc.

Prevention of Static Charges

Where possible, antistatic conducting material should be used in place of non-conductors. The resistance of antistatic material should be between 50 kΩ cm^{-1} and 10 MΩ cm^{-1}.

All material should be allowed to leak static charges through the floor of the operating theatre. However, if the conductivity of the floor is too high, there is a risk of electrocution if an individual forms a contact between mains voltage and ground. Consequently, the floor of the operating theatre is designed to have a resistance of 25–50 kΩ when measured between two electrodes placed 1 m apart. This allows the gradual discharge of static electricity to earth. Personnel should wear conducting shoes, each with a resistance of between 0.1 and 1 Ω.

Moisture encourages the leakage of static charges along surfaces to the floor. The risk of sparks from accumulated static electricity charges is reduced if the relative humidity of the atmosphere is kept above 50%.

FURTHER READING

Association of Anaesthetists of Great Britain and Ireland, 2002. Provision of anaesthetic services in magnetic resonance units. The Association of Anaesthetists of Great Britain and Ireland http://www.aagbi.org/publications/guidelines/docs/mri02.pdf.

Association of Anaesthetists of Great Britain and Ireland, 2010. Safety in magnetic resonance units: an update. Anaesthesia 65, 766–770.

Davis, P.D., Kenny, G.N.C., 2003. Basic physics and measurement in anaesthesia, fifth ed. Heinemann, London.

Davey, A., Diba, A., 2005. Ward's anaesthetic equipment, fifth ed. WB Saunders, London.

Magee, P., Tooley, M., 2011. The physics, clinical measurement and equipment of anaesthetic practice, second ed. Oxford University Press, Oxford.

15

ANAESTHETIC APPARATUS

A naesthetists must have a sound understanding and firm knowledge of the functioning of all anaesthetic equipment in common use. Although primary malfunction of equipment has not featured highly in surveys of anaesthetic-related morbidity and mortality, failure to understand the use of equipment and failure to check equipment prior to use feature in these reports as a cause of morbidity and mortality. This is true especially of ventilators, where lack of knowledge regarding the function of equipment may result in a patient being subjected to the dangers of hypoxaemia and/or hypercapnia.

It is essential that anaesthetists check that all equipment is functioning correctly before they proceed to anaesthetize a patient (see Ch 21). In some respects, the routine of testing anaesthetic equipment resembles the airline pilot's checklist, which is an essential preliminary to aircraft flight.

The purpose of this chapter is to describe briefly apparatus which is used in delivery of gases, from the sources of supply to the patient's lungs. Clearly, it is not possible to describe in detail equivalent models produced by all manufacturers. Consequently, this chapter concentrates on principles and some equipment which is used commonly.

It is convenient to describe anaesthetic apparatus sequentially from the supply of gases to point of delivery to the patient. This sequence is shown in Table 15.1.

GAS SUPPLIES

Bulk Supply of Anaesthetic Gases

In the majority of modern hospitals, piped medical gases and vacuum (PMGV) systems have been installed. These obviate the necessity for holding large numbers of cylinders in the operating theatre suite. Normally, only a few cylinders are kept in reserve, attached usually to the anaesthetic machine.

The advantages of the PMGV system are reductions in cost, in the necessity to transport cylinders and in accidents caused by cylinders becoming exhausted. However, there have been several well-publicized incidents in which anaesthetic morbidity or mortality has resulted from incorrect connections in piped medical gas supplies.

The PMGV services comprise five sections:

- bulk store
- distribution pipelines in the hospital
- terminal outlets, situated usually on the walls or ceilings of the operating theatre suite and other sites
- flexible hoses connecting the terminal outlets to the anaesthetic machine
- connections between flexible hoses and anaesthetic machines.

Responsibility for the first three items lies with the engineering and pharmacy departments. Within the operating theatre, it is partly the anaesthetist's responsibility to check the correct functioning of the last two items.

Bulk Store

Oxygen

In small hospitals, oxygen may be supplied to the PMGV from a bank of several oxygen cylinders attached to a manifold.

Oxygen cylinder manifolds consist of two groups of large cylinders (size J). The two groups alternate in supplying oxygen to the pipelines. In both groups,

---

TABLE 15.1

Classification of Anaesthetic Equipment Described in this Chapter

Supply of gases:
  From outside the operating theatre
  From cylinders within the operating theatre, together with the connections involved

The anaesthetic machine:
  Unions
  Cylinders
  Reducing valves
  Flowmeters
  Vaporizers
Safety features of the anaesthetic machine
Anaesthetic breathing systems
Ventilators
Apparatus used in scavenging waste anaesthetic gases

Apparatus used in interfacing the patient to the anaesthetic breathing system:
  Laryngoscopes
  Tracheal tubes
  Catheter mounts and connectors

Accessory apparatus for the airway:
  Anaesthetic masks and airways
  Forceps
  Laryngeal sprays
  Bougies
  Mouth gags
  Stilettes
  Suction apparatus

---

all cylinder valves are open so that they empty simultaneously. All cylinders have non-return valves. The supply automatically changes from one group to the other when the first group of cylinders is nearly empty. The changeover also activates an electrical signalling system, which alerts staff to change the empty cylinders.

However, in larger hospitals, pipeline oxygen originates from a liquid oxygen store. Liquid oxygen is stored at a temperature of approximately $-165\,°C$ at 10.5 bar in what is in effect a giant Thermos flask – a vacuum insulated evaporator (VIE). Some heat passes from the environment through the insulating layer between the two shells of the flask, increasing the tendency to evaporation and pressure increase within the chamber. Pressure is maintained constant

by transfer of gaseous oxygen into the pipeline system (via a warming device). However, if the pressure increases above 17 bar (1700 kPa), a safety valve opens and oxygen runs to waste. When the supply of oxygen resulting from the slow evaporation from the surface in the VIE is inadequate, the pressure decreases and a valve opens to allow liquid oxygen to pass into an evaporator, from which gas passes into the pipeline system.

Liquid oxygen plants are housed some distance away from hospital buildings because of the risk of fire. Even when a hospital possesses a liquid oxygen plant, it is still necessary to hold reserve banks of oxygen cylinders in case of supply failure.

Oxygen Concentrators. Recently, oxygen concentrators have been used to supply hospitals and it is likely that the use of these devices will increase in future. The oxygen concentrator depends upon the ability of an artificial zeolite to entrap molecules of nitrogen. These devices cannot produce pure oxygen, but the concentration usually exceeds 90%; the remainder comprises nitrogen, argon and other inert gases. Small oxygen concentrators are provided for domiciliary use.

Nitrous Oxide

Nitrous oxide and Entonox may be supplied from banks of cylinders connected to manifolds similar to those used for oxygen.

Medical Compressed Air

Compressed air is supplied from a bank of cylinders into the PMGV system. Air of medical quality is required, as industrial compressed air may contain fine particles of oil.

Piped Medical Vacuum

Piped medical vacuum is provided by large vacuum pumps which discharge via a filter and silencer to a suitable point, usually at roof level, where gases are vented to atmosphere. Although concern has been expressed regarding the possibility of volatile anaesthetic agents dissolving in the lubricating oil of vacuum pumps and causing malfunction, this fear has not been realized.

Terminal Outlets

There has been standardization of terminal outlets in the UK since 1978, but there is no universal standard.

Six types of terminal outlet are found commonly in the operating theatre. The terminals are colour-coded and also have non-interchangeable connections specific to each gas:

- Vacuum (coloured yellow) – a vacuum of at least 53 kPa (400 mmHg) should be maintained at the outlet, which should be able to take a free flow of air of at least 40 L min^{-1}.
- Compressed air (coloured white/black) at 4 bar – this is used for anaesthetic breathing systems and ventilators.
- Air (coloured white/black) at 7 bar – this is to be used only for powering compressed air tools and is confined usually to the orthopaedic operating theatre.
- Nitrous oxide (coloured blue) at 4 bar.
- Oxygen (coloured white) at 4 bar.
- Scavenging – there is a variety of scavenging outlets from the operating theatre. The passive systems are designed to accept a standard 30-mm connection.

Whenever a new pipeline system has been installed or servicing of an existing pipeline system has been undertaken, a designated member of the pharmacy staff should test the gas obtained from the sockets, using an oxygen analyser. Malfunction of an oxygen/air mixing device may result in entry of compressed air into the oxygen pipeline, rendering an anaesthetic mixture hypoxic. Because of this and other potential mishaps, oxygen analysers should be used routinely during anaesthesia.

Gas Supplies

Gas supplies to the anaesthetic machine should be checked at the beginning of each session to ensure that the gas which issues from the pipeline or cylinder is the same as that which passes through the appropriate flowmeter. This ensures that pipelines are not connected incorrectly. Both the machine in the operating theatre and that in the anaesthetic room should be checked. Checking of anaesthetic machine and medical gas supplies is discussed fully in Chapter 20 ('The operating theatre environment').

CYLINDERS

Modern cylinders are constructed from molybdenum steel. They are checked at intervals by the manufacturer to ensure that they can withstand hydraulic pressures considerably in excess of those to which they are subjected in normal use. One cylinder in every 100 is cut into strips to test the metal for tensile strength, flattening impact and bend tests. Medical gas cylinders are tested hydraulically every 5 years and the tests recorded by a mark stamped on the neck of the cylinder and this includes test pressure, dates of test performed, chemical formula of the cylinder's content and the tare weight. Cylinders may also be inspected endoscopically or ultrasonically for cracks or defects on their inner surfaces. Light weight cylinders can be made from aluminium alloy with a fibreglass covering in an epoxy resin matrix.

The cylinders are provided in a variety of sizes (A to J), and colour-coded according to the gas supplied. Cylinders attached to the anaesthetic machine are usually size E. The cylinders comprise a body and a shoulder containing threads into which are fitted a pin index valve block, a bull-nosed valve or a hand-wheel valve.

The pin index system was devised to prevent interchangeability of cylinders of different gases. Pin index systems are provided for the smaller cylinders of oxygen and nitrous oxide (and also carbon dioxide) which may be attached to anaesthetic machines. The pegs on the inlet connection slot into corresponding holes on the cylinder valve.

Full cylinders are supplied usually with a plastic dust cover in order to prevent contamination by dirt. This cover should not be removed until immediately before the cylinder is fitted to the anaesthetic machine. When fitting the cylinder to a machine, the yoke is positioned and tightened with the handle of the yoke spindle. After fitting, the cylinder should be opened to make sure that it is full and that there are no leaks at the gland nut or the pin index valve junction, caused, for example, by absence of or damage to the washer. The washer used is normally a Bodok seal which has a metal periphery designed to keep the seal in good condition for a long period.

Cylinder valves should be opened slowly to prevent sudden surges of pressure and should be closed with no more force than is necessary, otherwise the valve seating may be damaged.

The sealing material between the valve and the neck of the cylinder may be constructed from a fusable material which melts in the event of fire and allows the contents of the cylinder to escape around the threads of the joint.

The colour codes used for medical gas cylinders in the United Kingdom are shown in Table 15.2.

Different colours are used for some gases in other countries. There is a proposal to harmonize cylinder colours throughout Europe. The body will be painted white and only the shoulders will be colour-coded. The shoulder colours for medical gases will correspond to the current UK colours but will be horizontal rings rather than quarters. Cylinder sizes and capacities are shown in Table 15.3.

Oxygen, air and helium are stored as gases in cylinders and the cylinder contents can be estimated from the cylinder pressure. The pressure gradually decreases as the cylinder empties. According to the universal gas law, the mass of the gas is directly proportional to the

TABLE 15.2
Medical Gas Cylinders Used Currently (2013) in the UK

| | COLOUR | | PRESSURE AT 15 °C | | |
	Body	Shoulder	lb in^{-2}	kPa	Bar
Oxygen	Black	White	1987	13700	137
Nitrous oxide	Blue	Blue	638	4400	44
CO_2	Grey	Grey	725	5000	50
Helium	Brown	Brown	1987	13700	137
Air	Grey	White/black quarters	1987	13700	137
O_2/helium	Black	White/brown quarters	1987	13700	137
N_2O/O_2 (Entonox)	Blue	White/blue quarters	1987	13700	137

TABLE 15.3
Medical Gas Cylinder Sizes and Capacities by Cylinder Size (A–J) and Height (inches)

| | CAPACITIES (L) | | | | | | | |
	A/10 in	B/10 in	C/14 in	D/18 in	E/31 in	F/34 in	G/49 in	J/57 in
Oxygen			170	340	680	1360	3400	6800
Nitrous oxide			450	900	1800	3600	9000	
CO_2			450	900	1800			
Helium				300		1200		
Air							3200	6400
O_2/helium					600	1200		
O_2/CO_2						1360	3400	
Entonox							3200	6400

pressure, and the volume of gas that would be available at atmospheric pressure can be calculated using Boyle's law.

Nitrous oxide and carbon dioxide cylinders contain liquid and vapour and the cylinders are filled to a known filling ratio (see Ch 14). The cylinder pressure cannot be used to estimate its contents because the pressure remains relatively constant until after all the liquid has evaporated and the cylinder is almost empty, though cylinder pressure may change slightly due to temperature changes during use. The contents of nitrous oxide and carbon dioxide cylinders can be estimated from the weight of the cylinder.

THE ANAESTHETIC MACHINE

The anaesthetic machine comprises:

- a means of supplying gases either from attached cylinders or from piped medical supplies via appropriate unions on the machine
- methods of measuring flow rate of gases
- apparatus for vaporizing volatile anaesthetic agents
- breathing systems and a ventilator for delivery of gases and vapours from the machine to the patient
- apparatus for scavenging anaesthetic gases in order to minimize environmental pollution.

Supply of Gases

In the UK, gases are supplied at a pipeline pressure of 4 bar (400 kPa, 60 lb in^{-2}) and this pressure is transferred directly to the bank of flowmeters and back bar of the anaesthetic machine. Flexible colour-coded hoses connect the pipeline outlets to the anaesthetic machine. The anaesthetic machine end of the hoses should be permanently fixed using a nut and liner union where the thread is gas-specific and non-interchangeable. The non-interchangeable screw thread (NIST) is the British Standard.

The gas issuing from medical gas cylinders is at a much higher pressure, necessitating the interposition of a pressure regulator between the cylinder and the bank of flowmeters. In some older anaesthetic machines (and in some other countries), the pressure in the pipelines of the anaesthetic machine may be 3 bar (300 kPa, 45 lb in^{-2}).

Pressure Gauges

Pressure gauges measure the pressure in the cylinders or pipeline. Anaesthetic machines have pressure gauges for oxygen, air and nitrous oxide. These are mounted usually on the front panel of the anaesthetic machine.

Pressure Regulators

Pressure regulators are used on anaesthetic machines for three purposes:

- to reduce the high pressure of gas in a cylinder to a safe working level
- to prevent damage to equipment on the anaesthetic machine, e.g. flow control valves
- as the contents of the cylinder are used, the pressure within the cylinder decreases and the regulating mechanism maintains a constant outlet pressure, obviating the necessity to make continuous adjustments to the flowmeter controls.

The principles underlying the operation of pressure regulators are described in detail in Chapter 14.

Flow Restrictors

Pressure regulators are omitted usually when anaesthetic machines are supplied directly from a pipeline at a pressure of 4 bar. Changes in pipeline pressure would cause changes in flow rate, necessitating adjustment of the flow control valves. This is prevented by the use of a flow restrictor upstream of the flowmeter (flow restrictors are simply constrictions in the low-pressure circuit).

A different type of flow restrictor may be fitted also to the downstream end of the vaporizers to prevent back-pressure effects (see Ch 14). The absence of such a flow restrictor may be detected if a gas-driven ventilator such as the Manley is used, as this leads to fluctuations in the positions of the flowmeter bobbins during the respiratory cycle.

Pressure Relief Valves on Regulators

Pressure relief valves are often fitted on the downstream side of regulators to allow escape of gas if the regulators were to fail (thereby causing a high output pressure). Relief valves are set usually at approximately 7 bar for regulators designed to give an output pressure of 4 bar.

Flowmeters

The principles of flowmeters are described in detail in Chapters 14 and 16.

Problems with Flowmeters

- *Non-vertical tube.* This causes a change in shape of the annulus and therefore variation in flow. If the bobbin touches the side of the tube, resulting friction causes an even more inaccurate reading.
- *Static electricity.* This may cause inaccuracy (by as much as 35%) and sticking of the bobbin, especially at low flows. This may be reduced by coating the inside of the tube with a transparent film of gold or tin.
- *Dirt* on the bobbin may cause sticking or alteration in size of the annulus and therefore inaccuracies.
- *Back-pressure.* Changes in accuracy may be produced by back-pressure. For example, the Manley ventilator may exert a back-pressure and depress the bobbin; there may be as much as 10% more gas flow than that indicated on the flowmeter. Similar problems may be produced by the insertion of any equipment which restricts flow downstream, e.g. Selectatec head, vaporizer.
- *Leakage.* This results usually from defects in the top sealing washer of a flowmeter.

It is unfortunate that, in the UK, the standard position of the oxygen flowmeters is on the left followed by either nitrous oxide or air (if all three gases are supplied). On several recorded occasions, patients have suffered damage from hypoxia because of leakage from a broken flowmeter tube in this type of arrangement, as oxygen, being at the upstream end, passes out to the atmosphere through any leak. This problem is reduced if the oxygen flowmeter is placed downstream (i.e. on the right-hand side of the bank of flowmeters) as is standard practice in the USA. In the UK, this problem is now avoided by designing the outlet from the oxygen flowmeter to enter the back bar downstream from the outlets of other flowmeters (Fig. 15.1). Most modern anaesthetic machines do not have a flowmeter for carbon dioxide. Some new anaesthetic machines such

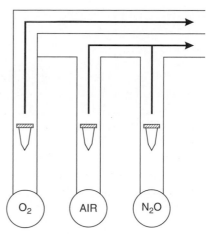

FIGURE 15.1 ■ Oxygen is the last gas to be added to the gas mixture being delivered to the back bar.

as Primus Dräger (Fig 15.2A) do not have traditional flowmeters; gas delivery is under electronic control and there is an integrated heater within a leak-tight breathing system. The gas flow is indicated electronically by a numerical display. In the event of an electrical failure, there is a pneumatic back-up which continues the delivery of fresh gas. These machines are particularly well suited to low and minimal flow anaesthesia and they use standard vaporizers.

The emergency oxygen flush is a non-locking button which, when pressed, delivers pure oxygen from the anaesthetic outlet. On modern anaesthetic machines, the emergency oxygen flush lever is situated downstream from the flowmeters and vaporizers. A flow of about 35–45 L min^{-1} at pipeline pressure is delivered. This may lead to dilution of the anaesthetic mixture with excess oxygen if the emergency oxygen tap is opened partially by mistake and may result in awareness. There is also a risk of barotrauma if the high pressure is accidentally delivered directly to the patient's lungs.

Quantiflex

The Quantiflex mixer flowmeter (Fig. 15.3) eliminates the possibility of reducing the oxygen supply inadvertently. One dial is set to the desired percentage of oxygen and the total flow rate is adjusted independently. The oxygen passes through a flowmeter to provide evidence of correct functioning of the linked valves. Both gases arrive via linked pressure-reducing regulators. The Quantiflex is useful in particular for varying the

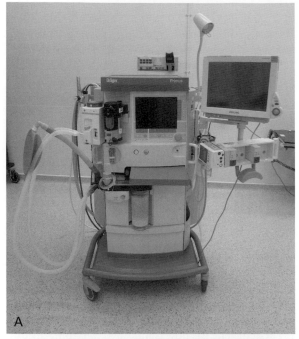

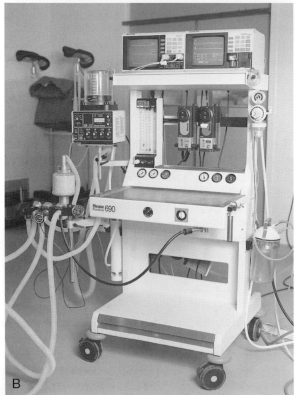

FIGURE 15.2 ■ (**A**) The Primus Dräger anaesthetic machine, which does not have conventional flowmeters. (**B**) A Blease Frontline anaesthetic machine.

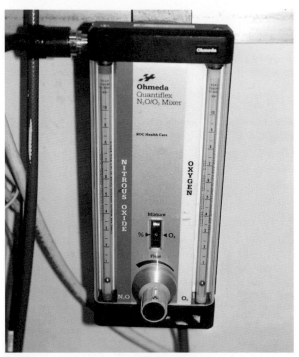

FIGURE 15.3 ■ A Quantiflex flowmeter. The required oxygen percentage is selected using the dial, and the total flow of the oxygen/nitrous oxide mixture is adjusted using the grey knob.

volume of fresh gas flow (FGF) from moment to moment whilst keeping the proportions constant. In addition, the oxygen flowmeter is situated downstream of the nitrous oxide flowmeter.

Linked Flowmeters

The majority of modern anaesthetic machines such as that shown in Figure 15.2B possess a mechanical linkage between the nitrous oxide and oxygen flowmeters. This causes the nitrous oxide flow to decrease if the oxygen flowmeter is adjusted to give less than 25–30% O_2 (Fig. 15.4).

Vaporizers

The principles of vaporizers are described in detail in Chapter 14.

Modern vaporizers may be classified as:

- *Drawover vaporizers.* These have a very low resistance to gas flow and may be used for emergency use in the field (e.g. Oxford miniature vaporizer; OMV) (Fig 15.5).

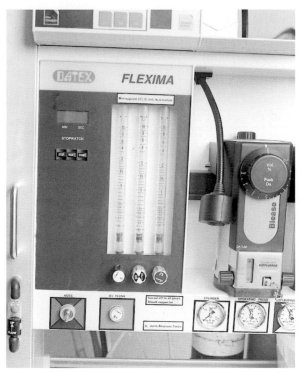

FIGURE 15.4 ■ Flowmeters with mechanical linkage between nitrous oxide and oxygen.

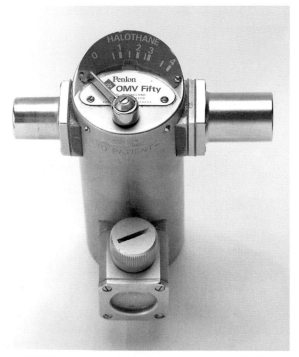

FIGURE 15.5 ■ Oxford miniature vaporizer (OMV).

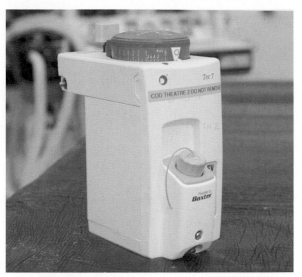

FIGURE 15.6 ■ Sevoflurane vaporizer.

- *Plenum vaporizers.* These are intended for unidirectional gas flow, have a relatively high resistance to flow and are unsuitable for use either as drawover vaporizers or in a circle system. Examples include the 'TEC' type in which there is a variable bypass flow. Commonly used plenum vaporizers are shown in Figures 15.6 and 15.7A.

Temperature regulation in the TEC vaporizers is achieved using a bimetallic strip.

There has been more than one model of the 'TEC' type of vaporizer. The TEC Mark 2 vaporizer is now obsolete. The TEC Mark 3 had characteristics which were an improvement on the Mark 2. These included improved vaporization as a result of increased area of the wicks, reduced pumping effect by having a long tube through which the vaporized gas leaves the vaporizing chamber, improved accuracy at low gas flows and a bimetallic strip which is situated in the bypass channel and not the vaporizing chamber. In the Mark 4, the improvements were as follows: no spillage into the bypass channel if the vaporizer was accidentally inverted, and the inability to turn two vaporizers on at the same time when on the back bar of the anaesthetic machine. The TEC Mark 5 vaporizer (Fig. 15.7A–C) has improved surface area for vaporization in the chamber, improved key-filling action and an easier mechanism for switching on the rotary

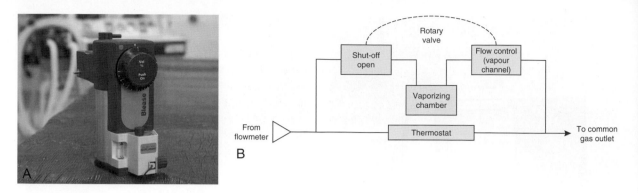

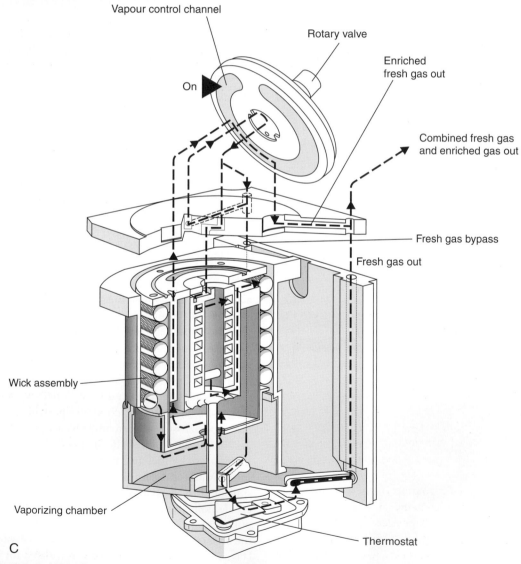

FIGURE 15.7 ■ (**A**) Isoflurane vaporizer. (**B**) Schematic diagram of the TEC mark 5 vaporizer. (**C**) Diagram of the TEC mark 5 vaporizer.

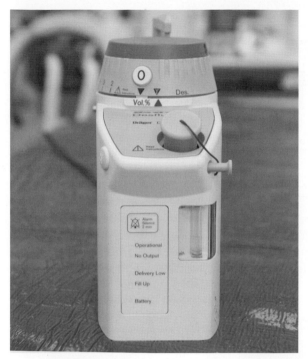

FIGURE 15.8 ■ Tec 6 desflurane vaporizer.

valve and lock with one hand. Desflurane presents a particular challenge because it has a saturated vapour pressure of 664 mmHg (89 kPa) at 20 °C and a boiling point of 23.5 °C. In order to combat this problem, a new vaporizer, the TEC 6, was developed (Fig. 15.8). It is heated electrically to 39 °C with a pressure of 1550 mmHg (approx. 2 bar). The vaporizer has electronic monitors of vaporizer function and alarms. The FGF does not enter the vaporization chamber. Instead, desflurane vapour enters into the path of the FGF. A percentage control dial regulates the flow of desflurane vapour into the FGF. The dial calibration is from 1% to 18%. The vaporizer has a back-up 9 volt battery in case of mains failure. The functioning of the vaporizer is shown diagrammatically in Figure 15.9.

Anaesthetic-specific connections are available to link the supply bottle (container of liquid anaesthetic agent) to the appropriate vaporizer (Fig. 15.10). These connections reduce the extent of spillage (and thus atmospheric pollution) and also the likelihood of filling the vaporizer with an inappropriate liquid. In addition

to being designed specifically for each liquid, the connections themselves may be colour-coded (e.g. purple for isoflurane, yellow for sevoflurane, orange for enflurane, red for halothane).

Halothane contains a non-volatile stabilizing agent (0.01% thymol) to prevent breakdown of the halothane by heat and ultraviolet light. Thymol is less volatile than halothane and its concentration in the vaporizer increases as halothane is vaporized. If the vaporizer is used and refilled regularly, the concentration of thymol may become sufficiently high to impair vaporization of halothane. In addition, very high concentrations may result in a significant degree of thymol vaporization, which may be harmful to the patient. Consequently, it is recommended that halothane vaporizers are drained once every 2 weeks. Sevoflurane and isoflurane vaporizers require to be emptied at much less frequent intervals.

SAFETY FEATURES OF MODERN ANAESTHETIC MACHINES

- Specificity of probes on flexible hoses between terminal outlets and connections with the anaesthetic machine. The flexible hoses are colour-coded and have non-interchangeable screw-threaded connectors to the anaesthetic machine.
- Pin index system to prevent incorrect attachment of gas cylinders to anaesthetic machine. Cylinders are colour-coded and they are labelled with the name of the gas that they contain.
- Pressure relief valves on the downstream side of pressure regulators.
- Flow restrictors on the upstream side of flowmeters.
- Arrangement of the bank of flowmeters such that the oxygen flowmeter is on the right (i.e. downstream side) or oxygen is the last gas to be added to the gas mixture being delivered to the back bar (Fig. 15.1).
- Non-return valves. Sometimes a single regulator and contents meter is used both for cylinders in use and for the reserve cylinder. When one cylinder runs out, the presence of a non-return valve prevents the empty cylinder from being refilled by the reserve cylinder and also enables the empty cylinder to be removed and

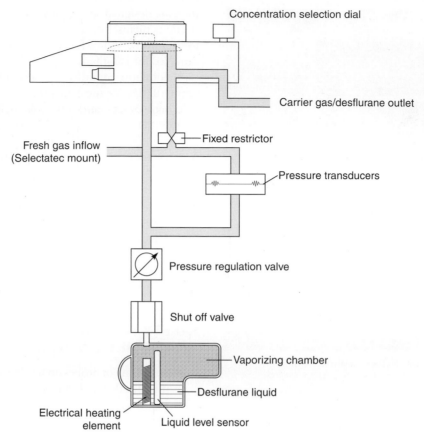

FIGURE 15.9 ■ The TEC 6 desflurane vaporizer. Liquid in the vaporizing chamber is heated and mixed with fresh gas; the pressure-regulating valve balances both fresh gas pressure and anaesthetic vapour pressure.

replaced without interrupting the supply of gas to the patient.

■ Pressure gauges indicate the pressures in the pipelines and the cylinders.

■ An oxygen bypass valve (emergency oxygen) delivers oxygen directly to a point downstream of the vaporizers. When operated, the oxygen bypass should give a flow rate of at least 35 L min^{-1}.

■ Mounting of vaporizers on the back bar. There is concern about contamination of vaporizers if two vaporizers are turned on at the same time. Temperature-compensated vaporizers contain wicks and these can absorb a considerable amount of anaesthetic agent. If two vaporizers are mounted in series, the downstream vaporizer could become contaminated to a dangerous degree with the agent from the upstream vaporizer. However, the newer TEC Mark 4 and 5 vaporizers have the interlocking Selectatec system (Fig. 15.11) which has locking rods to prevent more than one vaporizer being used at the same time. When a vaporizer is mounted on the back bar, the locking lever needs to be engaged (Mark 4 and 5). If this is not done, the control dial cannot be moved.

■ Modern anaesthetic machines have a mechanical linkage between the nitrous oxide and oxygen flowmeters which prevents the delivery of less than 25–30% oxygen.

■ A non-return valve situated downstream of the vaporizers prevents back-pressure (e.g. when using a Manley ventilator) which might otherwise cause output of high concentrations of vapour.

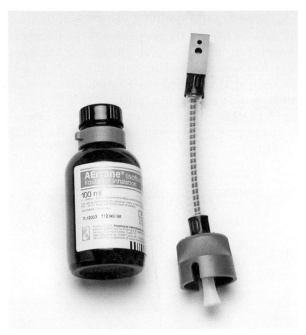

FIGURE 15.10 ■ An agent-specific connector for filling a vaporizer.

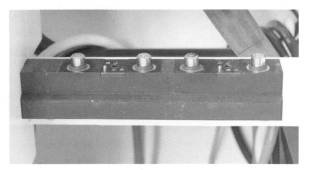

FIGURE 15.11 ■ A Selectatec block on the back bar of an anaesthetic machine. This permits the vaporizer to be changed rapidly without interrupting the flow of carrier gas to the patient.

- A pressure relief valve may be situated downstream of the vaporizer, opening at 34 kPa to prevent damage to the flowmeters or vaporizers if the gas outlet from the anaesthetic machine is obstructed.
- A pressure relief valve set to open at a low pressure of 5 kPa may be fitted to prevent the patient's lungs from being damaged by high pressure. The presence of such a valve prevents the use of

gas-driven minute volume divider ventilators, such as the Manley.

- Oxygen failure warning devices. Anaesthetic machines have a built in oxygen failure device. There are a variety of oxygen failure warning devices. The ideal warning device should have the following characteristics:
  - activation depends on the pressure of oxygen itself and does not depend on the pressure of any other gas
  - does not use a battery or mains power
  - gives a signal which is audible, of sufficient duration and of distinctive character
  - should give a warning of impending failure and a further warning that failure has occurred
  - should interrupt the flow of all other gases when it comes into operation.
  - The breathing system should open to the atmosphere, the inspired oxygen concentration should be at least equal to that of air, and accumulation of carbon dioxide should not occur. In addition, it should be impossible to resume anaesthesia until the oxygen supply has been restored.
- The reservoir bag in an anaesthetic breathing system is highly distensible and seldom reaches pressures exceeding 5 kPa.

MRI-compatible anaesthetic machines are available such as the Prima SP Anaesthetic machine (Penlon) which is made from non-ferrous metals and can be used up to the 1000 Gauss line.

BREATHING SYSTEMS

The delivery system which conducts anaesthetic gases from the machine to the patient is termed colloquially a 'circuit' but is described more accurately as a breathing system. Terms such as 'open circuits', 'semi-open circuits' or 'semi-closed circuits' should be avoided. The 'closed circuit' or circle system is the only true circuit, as anaesthetic gases are recycled.

Adjustable Pressure-Limiting Valve

Most breathing systems incorporate an adjustable pressure-limiting valve (APL valve, spill valve, 'popoff' valve, expiratory valve), which is designed to vent gas when there is a positive pressure within the system. During spontaneous ventilation, the valve opens when the patient generates a positive pressure within the system during expiration; during positive pressure ventilation, the valve is adjusted to produce a controlled leak during the inspiratory phase.

Several valves of this type are available. They comprise a lightweight disc (Fig. 15.12) which rests on a 'knife edge' seating to minimize the area of contact and reduce the risk of adhesion resulting from surface tension of condensed water. The disc has a stem which acts as a guide to position it correctly. A light spring is incorporated in the valve so that the pressure required to open it may be adjusted. During spontaneous breathing, the tension of the spring is low so that the resistance to expiration is minimized. During controlled ventilation, the valve top is screwed down to increase the tension in the spring so that gas leaves the system at a higher pressure than during spontaneous ventilation. Modern valves, even when screwed down fully, open at a pressure of 60 cm H_2O. Most valves are encased in a hood for scavenging.

Classification of Breathing Systems

In 1954, Mapleson classified anaesthetic breathing systems into five types (Fig. 15.13); the Mapleson E system was modified subsequently by Rees, but is classified as the Mapleson F system. The systems differ considerably in their 'efficiency', which is measured in terms of the fresh gas flow (FGF) rate required to prevent rebreathing of alveolar gas during ventilation.

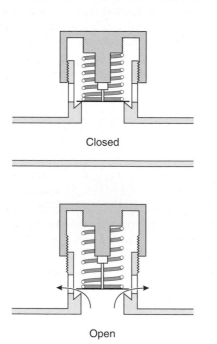

FIGURE 15.12 ■ Diagram of a spill valve. See text for details.

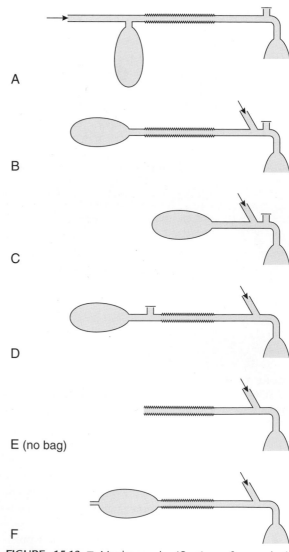

FIGURE 15.13 ■ Mapleson classification of anaesthetic breathing systems. The arrow indicates entry of fresh gas to the system.

Mapleson A Systems

The most commonly used version is the Magill attachment. The corrugated hose should be of adequate length (usually approximately 110 cm). It is the most efficient system during spontaneous ventilation, but one of the least efficient when ventilation is controlled.

During spontaneous ventilation (Fig. 15.14), there are three phases in the ventilatory cycle: inspiratory, expiratory and the expiratory pause. Gas is inhaled from

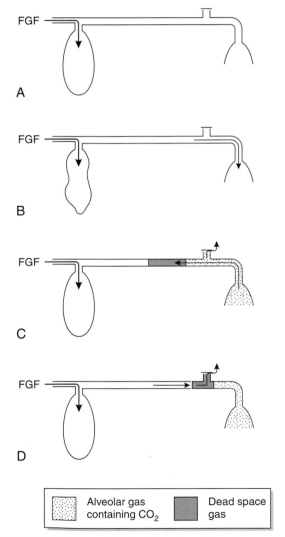

FGF

A

FGF

B

FGF

C

FGF

D

| Alveolar gas containing CO_2 | Dead space gas |

FIGURE 15.14 ■ Mode of action of Magill attachment during spontaneous ventilation. See text for details. FGF, fresh gas flow.

the system during inspiration (Fig. 15.14B). During the initial part of expiration, the reservoir bag is not full and thus the pressure in the system does not increase; exhaled gas (the initial portion of which is dead space gas) passes along the corrugated tubing towards the bag (Fig. 15.14C), which is filled also by fresh gas from the anaesthetic machine. During the latter part of expiration, the bag becomes full; the pressure in the system increases and the spill valve opens, venting all subsequent exhaled gas to atmosphere. During the expiratory pause, continued flow of fresh gas from the machine pushes exhaled gas distally along the corrugated tube to be vented through the spill valve (Fig. 15.14D). Provided that the FGF rate is sufficiently high to vent all *alveolar* gas before the next inspiration, no rebreathing takes place from the corrugated tube. If the system is functioning correctly and no leaks are present, an FGF rate equal to the patient's alveolar minute ventilation is sufficient to prevent rebreathing. In practice, a higher FGF is selected in order to compensate for leaks; the rate selected is usually equal to the patient's total minute volume (approximately $6\,L\,min^{-1}$ for a 70-kg adult).

The system increases dead space to the extent of the volume of the anaesthetic face mask and angle piece to the spill valve. The volume of this dead space may amount to 100 mL or more for an adult face mask. Paediatric face masks reduce the extent of dead space, but it remains too high to allow use of the system in infants or small children (<4 years old).

The characteristics of the Mapleson A system are different during controlled ventilation (Fig. 15.15). At the end of inspiration (produced by the anaesthetist squeezing the reservoir bag), the bag is usually less than half full (see below). During expiration, dead space and alveolar gas pass along the corrugated tube and are likely to reach the reservoir bag, which therefore contains some carbon dioxide (Fig. 15.15A). During inspiration, the valve does not open initially because its opening pressure has been increased by the anaesthetist in order to generate a sufficient pressure within the system to inflate the lungs. Thus, alveolar gas re-enters the patient's lungs and is followed by a mixture of fresh, dead space and alveolar gases (Fig. 15.15B). When the valve does open, it is this mixture which is vented (Fig. 15.15C). Consequently, the FGF rate must be very high

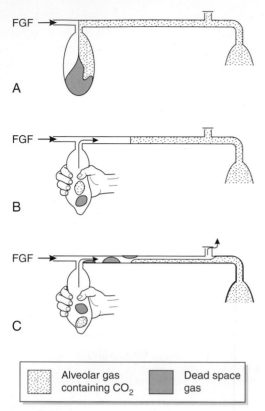

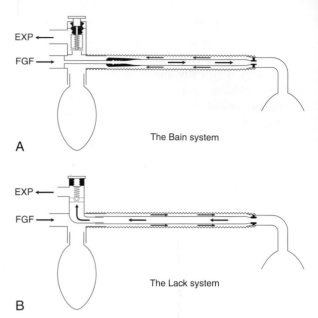

FIGURE 15.15 ■ Mode of action of Magill attachment during controlled ventilation. See text for details. FGF, fresh gas flow.

FIGURE 15.16 ■ Coaxial anaesthetic breathing systems. (**A**) Bain system (Mapleson D). (**B**) Lack system (Mapleson A). FGF, fresh gas flow; EXP, expired gas.

(at least three times alveolar minute volume) to prevent rebreathing. The volume of gas squeezed from the reservoir bag must be sufficient both to inflate the lungs and to vent gas from the system.

The major disadvantage of the Magill attachment during surgery is that the spill valve is attached close to the mask. This makes the system heavy, particularly when a scavenging system is used, and it is inconvenient if the valve is in this position during surgery of the head or neck. The Lack system (Fig. 15.16B) is a modification of the Mapleson A system with a co-axial arrangement of tubing. This permits positioning of the spill valve at the proximal end of the system. The inner tube must be of sufficiently wide bore to allow the patient to exhale with minimal resistance. The Lack system is not quite as efficient as the Magill attachment.

Mapleson B and C Systems

These systems cause mixing of alveolar and fresh gas during spontaneous or controlled ventilation. Very high FGF rates are required to prevent rebreathing. There is no clinical role for the Mapleson B system. The Mapleson C system is used in some hospitals to ventilate the lungs with oxygen during transport, but a self-inflating bag with a non-rebreathing valve is preferable.

Mapleson D System

The Mapleson D arrangement is inefficient during spontaneous breathing (Fig. 15.17). During expiration, exhaled gas and fresh gas mix in the corrugated tube and travel towards the reservoir bag (Fig. 15.17B). When the reservoir bag is full, the pressure in the system increases, the spill valve opens and a mixture of fresh and exhaled gas is vented; this includes the dead space gas, which reaches the reservoir bag first (Fig. 15.17C). Although fresh gas pushes alveolar gas towards the valve during the expiratory pause, a mixture of alveolar and fresh gases is inhaled from the corrugated tube unless the FGF rate is at least twice as great as the patient's minute volume

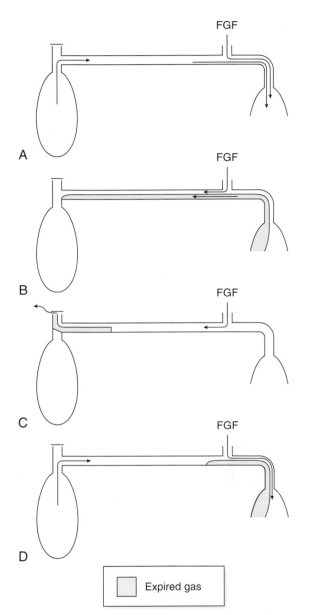

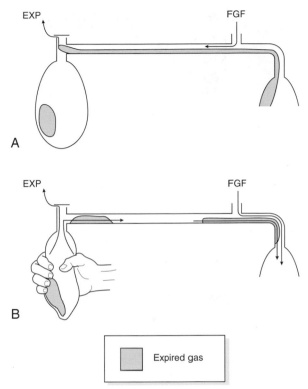

FIGURE 15.18 ■ Mode of action of Mapleson D breathing system during controlled ventilation. See text for details. FGF, fresh gas flow.

FIGURE 15.17 ■ Mode of action of Mapleson D breathing system during spontaneous ventilation. See text for details. FGF, fresh gas flow.

(i.e. at least $12\,L\,min^{-1}$ in the adult); in some patients, an FGF rate of $250\,mL\,kg^{-1}\,min^{-1}$ is required to prevent rebreathing.

However, the Mapleson D system is more efficient than the Mapleson A during controlled ventilation (Fig. 15.18), especially if an expiratory pause is incorporated into the ventilatory cycle. During expiration,

the corrugated tubing and reservoir bag fill with a mixture of fresh and alveolar gas (Fig. 15.18A). Fresh gas fills the distal part of the corrugated tube during the expiratory pause (Fig. 15.18B). When the reservoir bag is squeezed, this fresh gas enters the lungs, and when the spill valve opens a mixture of fresh and alveolar gas is vented. The degree of rebreathing may thus be controlled by adjustment of the FGF rate, but this should always exceed the patient's minute volume.

The Bain coaxial system (Fig. 15.16A) is the most commonly used version of the Mapleson D system. FGF is supplied through a narrow inner tube. This tube may become disconnected, resulting in hypoxaemia and hypercapnia. Before use, the system should be tested by occluding the distal end of the inner tube transiently with a finger or the plunger of a 2-mL syringe; there should be a reduction in the flowmeter bobbin reading during occlusion and an audible

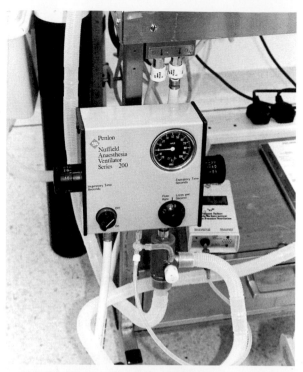

FIGURE 15.19 ■ The Penlon Nuffield 200 ventilator.

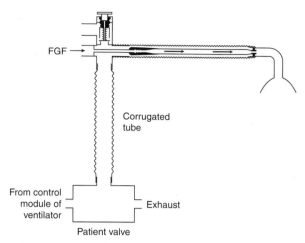

FIGURE 15.20 ■ The Bain system for controlled ventilation by a mechanical ventilator (e.g. Penlon Nuffield 200). A 1-m length of corrugated tubing with a capacity of at least 500 mL is required to prevent gas from the ventilator reaching the patient's lungs. $PaCO_2$ is controlled by varying the fresh gas flow (FGF) rate.

release of pressure when occlusion is discontinued. Movement of the reservoir bag during anaesthesia does not necessarily indicate that fresh gas is being delivered to the patient.

The Bain system may be used to ventilate the patient's lungs with some types of automatic ventilator (e.g. Penlon Nuffield 200; Fig. 15.19). A 1-m length of corrugated tubing is interposed between the patient valve of the ventilator and the reservoir bag mount (Fig. 15.20); the spill valve *must* be closed completely. An appropriate tidal volume and ventilatory rate are selected on the ventilator and anaesthetic gases are supplied to the Bain system. During inspiration, the gas from the ventilator pushes a mixture of anaesthetic and alveolar gas from the corrugated outer tube into the patient's lungs; during expiration, the ventilator gas and some of the alveolar gas are vented through the exhaust valve of the ventilator. The degree of rebreathing is regulated by the anaesthetic gas flow rate; a flow of 70–80 mL kg^{-1} min^{-1} should result in normocapnia and a flow of 100 mL kg^{-1} min^{-1} in moderate hypocapnia. A secure connection between the Bain system and

the anaesthetic machine must be assured. If this connection is loose, a leak of fresh gas occurs; this causes rebreathing of ventilator gas and results in awareness, hypoxaemia and hypercapnia.

Mapleson E and F Systems

The Mapleson E system, or Ayre's T-piece, has virtually no resistance to expiration and was used extensively in paediatric anaesthesia before the advantages of continuous positive airways pressure (CPAP) were recognized. It functions in a manner similar to the Mapleson D system in that the corrugated tube fills with a mixture of exhaled and fresh gas during expiration and with fresh gas during the expiratory pause. Rebreathing is prevented if the FGF rate is 2.5–3 times the patient's minute volume. If the volume of the corrugated tube is less than the patient's tidal volume, some air may be inhaled at the end of inspiration; consequently, an FGF rate of at least 4 L min^{-1} is recommended with a paediatric Mapleson E system.

During spontaneous ventilation, there is no indication of the presence, or the adequacy of ventilation. It is possible to attach a visual indicator, such as a piece of tissue paper or a feather, at the end of the corrugated tube, but this is not very satisfactory.

Intermittent positive pressure ventilation (IPPV) may be applied by occluding the end of the corrugated tube with a finger. However, there is no way of assessing the pressure in the system and there is a possibility of exposing the patient's lungs to excessive volumes and pressures.

The Mapleson F system, or Rees' modification of the Ayre's T-piece, includes an open-ended bag attached to the end of the corrugated tube. This confers several advantages:

- It provides visual evidence of breathing during spontaneous ventilation.
- By occluding the open end of the bag temporarily, it is possible to confirm that fresh gas is entering the system.
- It provides a degree of CPAP during spontaneous ventilation and positive end-expiratory pressure (PEEP) during IPPV.
- It provides a convenient method of assisting or controlling ventilation. The open end of the reservoir bag is occluded between the fourth and fifth fingers and the bag is squeezed between the thumb and index finger; the fourth and fifth fingers are relaxed during expiration to allow gas to escape from the bag. It is possible with experience to assess (approximately) the inflation pressure and to detect changes in lung and chest wall compliance.

However, one main disadvantage of the Mapleson F system is that efficient scavenging is unsatisfactory and is non-standard.

Mapleson ADE System

This system provides the advantages of the Mapleson A, D and E systems. It can be used efficiently for spontaneous and controlled ventilation in both children and adults.

It consists of two parallel lengths of 15-mm bore tubing; one delivers fresh gas and the other carries exhaled gas. One end of the tubing connects to the patient via a Y-connection and the other end contains the Humphrey block (Fig. 15.21). The Humphrey block (Fig. 15.22) consists of an APL valve, a lever to select spontaneous or controlled ventilation, a reservoir bag, a port to connect a ventilator and a safety pressure relief valve which opens at a pressure above 6 kPa.

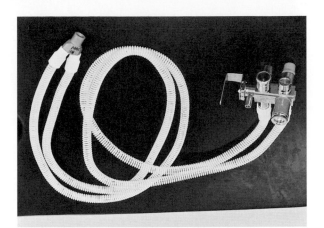

FIGURE 15.21 ■ The ADE system.

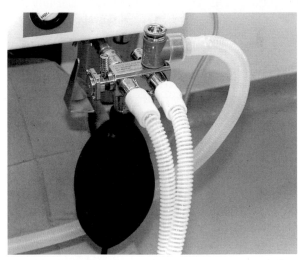

FIGURE 15.22 ■ The Humphrey block. This consists of an APL valve, a lever to select spontaneous or controlled ventilation, a reservoir bag, a port to connect to the ventilator and a safety pressure relief valve.

When the lever is in the A mode (up), the reservoir bag is connected to the breathing system as it would be in the Mapleson A system. The breathing hose connecting the bag to the patient is the inspiratory limb. The expired gases travel along the other tubing back to the APL valve, which is connected to the scavenging system.

With the lever in the D/E mode (down), the reservoir bag and the APL valve are isolated from the breathing system. What was the exspiratory limb in the A mode now delivers gas to the patient. The hose returning gas to the Humphrey block now functions as a reservoir to the T-piece. This hose would open to atmosphere via a port adjacent to the bag mount, but in practice this port is connected to a ventilator such as the Penlon Nuffield.

In adults, an appropriate FGF is 50–60 mL kg^{-1} min^{-1} in spontaneously breathing patients and 70 mL kg^{-1} min^{-1} in ventilated patients.

Drawover Systems

Occasionally, it is necessary to administer anaesthesia at the scene of a major accident. If inhalation anaesthesia is required, it is necessary to use simple, portable equipment. The Triservice apparatus has been designed by the British armed forces for use in battle conditions (Fig. 15.23). It comprises a self-inflating bag, a non-rebreathing valve (e.g. Ambu E, Rubens) which vents all expired gases to atmosphere, one or two Oxford miniature vaporizers (which have a low internal resistance), an oxygen supply and a length of corrugated tubing which serves as an oxygen reservoir. Either spontaneous or controlled ventilation may be employed using this apparatus.

Rebreathing Systems

Anaesthetic breathing systems in which some gas is rebreathed by the patient were designed originally to economize in the use of cyclopropane. In addition, they reduce the risk of atmospheric pollution and increase the humidity of inspired gases, thereby reducing heat loss from the patient. Rebreathing systems may be used as 'closed' systems, in which fresh gas is introduced only to replace oxygen and anaesthetic agents absorbed by the patient. More commonly, the system is used with a small leak through a spill valve, and the fresh gas supply exceeds basal oxygen requirements. Because rebreathing occurs, these systems must incorporate a means of absorbing carbon dioxide from exhaled alveolar gas.

Soda Lime

Soda lime is the substance used most commonly for absorption of carbon dioxide in rebreathing systems. The composition of soda lime is shown in Table 15.4. The major constituent is calcium hydroxide, but sodium and potassium hydroxides may also be present. Absorption of carbon dioxide occurs by the following chemical reactions:

$$CO_2 + 2NaOH \rightarrow Na_2CO_3 + H_2O + heat$$

$$Na_2CO_3 + Ca(OH)_2 \rightarrow 2NaOH + CaCO_3$$

Water is required for efficient absorption. There is some water in soda lime and more is added from the patient's expired gas and from the chemical reaction. The reaction generates heat and the temperature in the centre of a soda lime canister may exceed 60 °C. Sevoflurane has been shown to interact with soda lime to produce substances that are toxic in animals. However, this does not appear to impose any significant risk in humans (see Ch 2). There is new evidence suggesting that the presence of strong alkalis such as sodium and potassium hydroxides could be the trigger of the interaction between volatile agents and soda lime. New carbon dioxide absorbers are now being manufactured without these hydroxides in order to reduce this interaction.

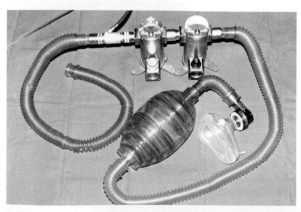

FIGURE 15.23 ■ The Triservice apparatus. *(Courtesy of Dr S. Kidd.)*

TABLE 15.4	
Composition of Soda Lime	
Ca(OH)$_2$	94%
NaOH	5%
KOH	<1% or nil
Silica	0.2%
Moisture content	14–19%

The size of soda lime granules is important. If granules are too large, the surface area for absorption is insufficient; if they are too small, the narrow space between granules results in a high resistance to breathing. Granule size is measured by a mesh number. Soda lime consists of granules in the range of 4–8 mesh. (A 4-mesh strainer has four openings per square inch and an 8-mesh strainer has eight openings.) Silica is added to soda lime to reduce the tendency of the granules to disintegrate into powder. In addition, soda lime contains an indicator which changes colour as the active constituents become exhausted. The rate at which soda lime becomes exhausted depends on the capacity of the canister, the FGF rate and the rate of carbon dioxide production. In a completely closed system, a standard 450-g canister becomes inefficient after approximately 2 h.

Baralyme

Baralyme is another carbon dioxide absorber. It is a mixture of approximately 20% barium hydroxide and 80% calcium hydroxide. It may also contain some potassium hydroxide, an indicator and moisture. Barium hydroxide contains eight molecules of water of crystallization, which help to fuse the mixture so that it retains the granular structure under various conditions of heat and moisture. The granules of Baralyme are similar to those of soda lime.

'To-and-Fro' (Waters') System

This breathing system comprises a Mapleson C breathing system with a canister of soda lime interposed between the spill valve and the reservoir bag (Fig. 15.24). The soda lime granules nearest the patient become exhausted first, increasing the dead space of the system;

in addition, the canister is positioned horizontally and gas may be channelled above the soda lime unless the canister is packed tightly. The system is cumbersome and there is a risk that patients may inhale soda lime dust from the canister.

Circle System

This system has replaced the 'to-and-fro' system. The soda lime canister is mounted on the anaesthetic machine, and inspiratory and expiratory corrugated tubing conducts gas to and from the patient (Fig. 15.25). The system incorporates a reservoir bag and spill valve and two low-resistance one-way valves to ensure unidirectional movement of gas (Fig. 15.26). These valves are normally mounted in glass domes so that they may be observed to be functioning correctly. The spill valve may be mounted close to the patient or beside the absorber; during surgery to the head or neck, it is more convenient to use a valve near the absorber. Fresh gas enters the system between the absorber and the inspiratory tubing.

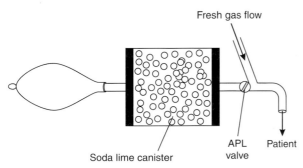

FIGURE 15.24 ■ Waters' anaesthetic breathing system, incorporating a canister of soda lime.

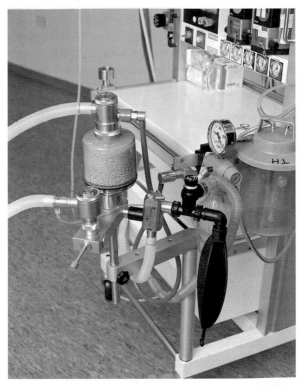

FIGURE 15.25 ■ The circle breathing system mounted on an anaesthetic machine.

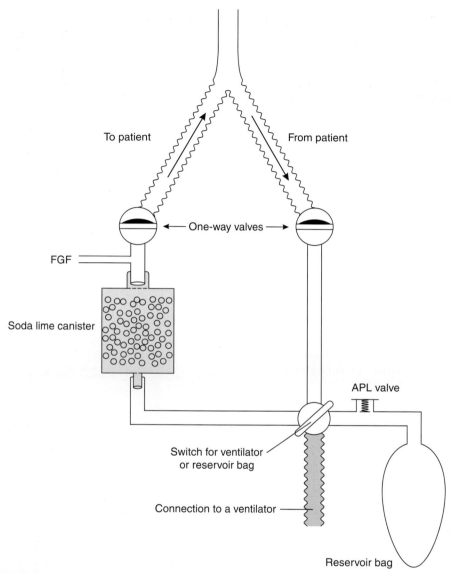

To patient

From patient

One-way valves

FGF

Soda lime canister

APL valve

Switch for ventilator
or reservoir bag

Connection to a ventilator

Reservoir bag

FIGURE 15.26 ■ Mechanism of the circle system. The direction of gas flow is controlled via the unidirectional valves. A lever allows the ventilation to be either spontaneous through the reservoir bag and APL valve, or controlled by a ventilator.

The soda lime canister is mounted vertically and thus channelling of gas through unfilled areas is not possible. The canister cannot contribute to dead space; consequently, a large canister may be used and the soda lime needs to be changed less often.

The major disadvantage of the circle system arises from its volume. If the system is filled with air initially, low flow rates of anaesthetic gases are diluted substantially and adequate concentrations cannot be achieved.

Even if the system is primed with a mixture of anaesthetic gases, the initial rapid uptake by the patient results in a marked decrease in concentrations of anaesthetic agents in the system, resulting in light anaesthesia. Consequently, it is necessary usually to provide a total FGF rate of 3–4 L min^{-1} to the system initially. This flow rate may be reduced subsequently, but it must be remembered that dilution of fresh gas continues at low flow rates and that rapid changes in depth of anaesthesia cannot be achieved.

Volatile anaesthetic agents may be delivered to a circle system in two ways:

- *Vaporizer outside the circle (VOC)* (Fig. 15.27A). If a standard vaporizer (e.g. TEC series) is used, it must be placed on the back bar of the anaesthetic

machine because of its high internal resistance. If low FGF rates ($<1\,L\,min^{-1}$) are used, the change in concentration of volatile anaesthetic agent achieved in the circle system is very small because of dilution, even if the vaporizer is set to deliver a high concentration (Fig. 15.28A). It may be

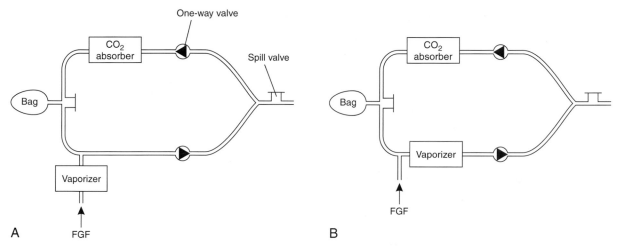

FIGURE 15.27 ■ Diagrammatic representation of the circle system. (**A**) Vaporizer outside the circle (VOC). (**B**) Vaporizer inside the circle (VIC).

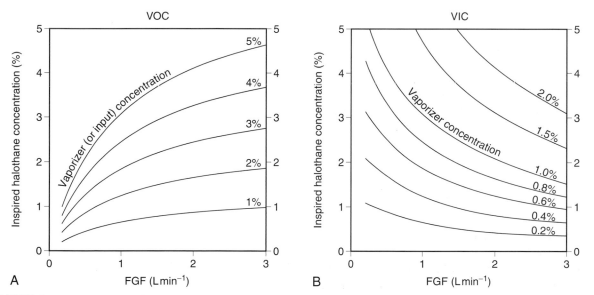

FIGURE 15.28 ■ Variation of inspired concentration of halothane with fresh gas flow (FGF) rate. Total minute ventilation is $5\,L\,min^{-1}$. (**A**) Vaporizer outside the circle (VOC); note that dilution of the fresh gas results in much lower concentrations in the circle system than the concentration set on the vaporizer unless FGF rate approaches $3\,L\,min^{-1}$. (**B**) Vaporizer inside the circle (VIC); at low flow rates, lack of dilution of expired halothane concentration, with additional halothane vaporized during each inspiration, results in inspired concentrations much higher than those set on the vaporizer. Even at an FGF rate of $3\,L\,min^{-1}$, inspired concentration is approximately 50% higher than the vaporizer setting.

necessary to change FGF rate rather than the vaporizer setting in order to achieve a rapid change in depth of anaesthesia. The concentration of volatile agent in the system depends on the patient's expired concentration (which is recycled), the rate of uptake by the patient (which decreases with time and is lower with agents of low blood/gas solubility coefficient), the concentration of agent supplied and the FGF rate.

- *Vaporizer inside the circle (VIC)* (Fig. 15.27B). Drawover vaporizers with a low internal resistance (e.g. Goldman) may be placed within the circle system. During each inspiration, vapour is added to the inspired gas mixture. In contrast to a VOC system, the inspired concentration is higher at low FGF rates because the expired concentration is diluted to a lesser extent (Fig. 15.28B) and the vaporizer *adds* to the concentration present in the expired gas. Very high concentrations of volatile agent may be inspired if minute volume is large; this risk is greatest if IPPV is employed.

If FGF rate is low, the use of the circle system by the inexperienced anaesthetist may result either in inadequate anaesthesia or in severe cardiovascular and respiratory depression. In addition, a hypoxic gas mixture may be delivered if low flow rates of a nitrous oxide/oxygen mixture are supplied, because after 10–15 min, oxygen is taken up in larger volumes than nitrous oxide. These difficulties can be overcome by monitoring the inspired concentrations of oxygen, carbon dioxide and volatile anaesthetic agent continuously (see Ch 16). The trainee anaesthetist *must* be aware that:

- It is inadvisable to use a VIC system unless inspired concentrations of anaesthetic agents are monitored continuously.
- IPPV must *never* be used with a VIC system unless inspired concentrations of anaesthetic agents are monitored continuously, because of the risk of generating very high concentrations of volatile agent.
- Nitrous oxide must *not* be used in any circle system if the total FGF rate is less than 1000 mL min^{-1}, unless inspired oxygen concentration is measured continuously.
- It is essential to monitor inspired concentrations of oxygen and inhalational anaesthetic agent and expired concentration of carbon dioxide when using the circle system.

- One-way valves may stick. These should be checked both at the pre-anaesthetic check of the machine and during anaesthesia.
- Because the circle system has many connections, the anaesthetist should be vigilant about checking for any leak or disconnection.

The advantages and disadvantages of the circle system are summarized in Table 15.5.

Manual Resuscitation Breathing Systems

Occasionally, a patient may require emergency ventilation support using a source which does not rely on pressurized gas or electricity. It is recommended that such a breathing system is readily available in all areas where anaesthetics are administered in case such an emergency arises.

There are many different types of manual resuscitation breathing systems but fundamentally they all have the following components:

- a self-inflating bag
- a non-rebreathing valve
- a fresh gas input with or without an oxygen reservoir bag.

The self-inflating bag has a volume of approximately 1500 mL, 500 mL and 250 mL for the adult, child and infant sizes, respectively. The non-rebreathing valve has several components which ensure that,

TABLE 15.5	
Disadvantages and Advantages of the Circle System	
Disadvantages	*Advantages*
Cumbersome equipment	Inspired gases are humidified and warmed
Risk of delivering hypoxic mixture	Economical
Increased resistance to breathing	Minimal pollution
Slow change in the depth of anaesthesia	
Risk of awareness	
Risk of a rise in end-tidal CO_2	
Risk of unidirectional valves sticking	
Not ideal for paediatric patients breathing spontaneously	
Some inhalational agents may interact with soda lime	

during the inspiratory phase, gas flows out of the bag into the patient and, during the expiratory phase, the valve ensures that exhaled gas escapes through the expiratory port without mixing with fresh gas. Three types of non-rebreathing systems are available, the Ruben, Ambu and Laerdal systems (Fig 15.29). Functionally, they are very similar but with some minor differences. The Ruben valve has a spring-loaded bobbin within the valve housing. The Ambu system has several series of valves which have either a single valve or double leaf valves to control unidirectional flow. The Laerdal system has three components: a duck-billed inspiratory/ expiratory valve, a valve body housing inspiratory and expiratory ports and a non-return flap valve in the expiratory port.

VENTILATORS

Mechanical ventilation of the lung may be achieved by several mechanisms, including the generation of a negative pressure around the whole of the patient's body except the head and neck (cabinet ventilator or 'iron lung'), a negative pressure over the thorax and abdomen (cuirass ventilators) or a positive pressure over the thorax and abdomen (inflatable cuirass ventilators). However, during anaesthesia, and in the majority of patients who require mechanical ventilation in the intensive care unit, ventilation is achieved by the application of positive pressure to the lungs through a laryngeal mask airway, tracheal tube or tracheostomy tube. Only this mode of ventilation is described here.

An enormous selection of ventilators exists and it is possible in this section to discuss only the principles involved in their use. Before using any ventilator, it is *essential* that the anaesthetist understands its functions fully; failure to do so may result in the delivery of a hypoxic gas mixture, rebreathing of carbon dioxide and/ or delivery of a mixture that contains no anaesthetic gases. If an unfamiliar ventilator is encountered, it may be helpful to use a 'dummy lung' (a small reservoir bag on the patient connection) and to discuss the capabilities and limitations of the machine with a senior colleague. In addition, the manufacturer's 'user handbook' may be consulted or details may be obtained from a specialist book.

Continuous clinical monitoring is essential when any ventilator is used, even those which incorporate sophisticated monitoring and warning devices. In addition to standard clinical monitoring systems attached to the patient (see Ch 16), the minimum acceptable monitoring of ventilator function includes measurement of expired tidal volume, airway pressure and inspired oxygen concentration; in addition, a ventilator disconnection alarm should be incorporated in the system. Continuous monitoring of end-tidal carbon dioxide, oxygen saturation and inspired anaesthetic gas concentrations is essential in the operating theatre.

The incorporation of a humidifier in the inspiratory limb, or of a condenser humidifier at the connection with the tracheal tube, is essential in long-term ventilation in the ICU. Bacterial filters (Fig. 15.30)

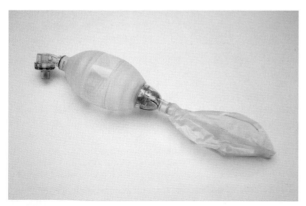

FIGURE 15.29 ■ The Laerdal manual resuscitation breathing system.

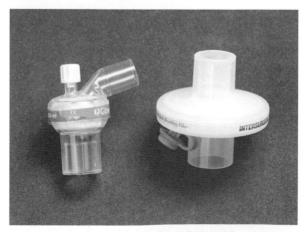

FIGURE 15.30 ■ Bacterial filters and humidifiers which are used in breathing systems: *left,* a paediatric filter incorporated into an angle piece; *right,* an adult filter.

are now recommended for all patients undergoing anaesthesia.

The principles of operation of ventilators are described best by considering each phase of the ventilatory cycle: inspiration; change from inspiration to expiration; expiration; and change from expiration to inspiration.

Inspiration

The pattern of volume change in the lung is determined by the characteristics of the ventilator. Ventilators may deliver a predetermined flow rate of gas (*constant flow generators*) or exert a predetermined pressure (*constant pressure generators*), although some machines produce a pattern which does not conform precisely to either category. Most flow generators produce a constant flow of gas during inspiration, although a few generate a sinusoidal flow pattern if the ventilator bellows is driven via a crank. The characteristics of constant flow and constant pressure generators are shown in Figure 15.31.

Constant Pressure Generator

The ventilator produces inspiration by generating a constant, predetermined pressure. However, if airway resistance increases or if compliance decreases, these

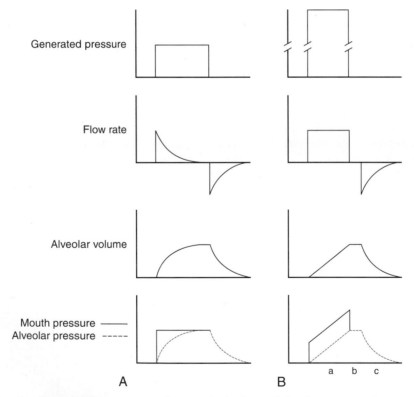

FIGURE 15.31 ■ Graphs of generated pressure, mouth (or tracheal tube) and alveolar pressures, flow rate and alveolar volume changes during inspiration and subsequent expiration produced by a constant pressure generator (**A**) and a constant flow generator (**B**). A constant pressure generator exerts a low pressure (e.g. 1.5 kPa, 15 cmH$_2$O). At the start of inspiration, the pressure in the alveoli is zero. Gas flows rapidly into the alveoli at a rate determined by airways resistance, resulting in rapid increases in alveolar volume and pressure. The mouth-alveolar pressure gradient decreases and flow rate, and consequently the rates of increase of alveolar volume and pressure, decrease also. When the alveolar pressure equals the ventilator pressure, flow ceases. A constant flow generator generates a very high internal pressure (e.g. 400 kPa) but has a high internal resistance to limit flow rate. The pressure gradient between machine and alveoli remains virtually constant throughout inspiration and thus flow rate is constant. The increases in alveolar volume and (assuming constant compliance) pressure are linear. Because flow rate is constant, the pressure gradient between mouth and alveoli is constant throughout inspiration. (a) Mouth pressure decreases to equal alveolar pressure during the inspiratory pause when flow ceases. (b) Gas flow out of the lung during expiration (c) is passive.

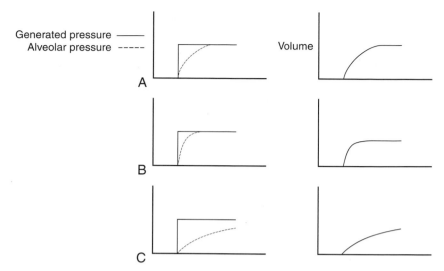

FIGURE 15.32 ■ Generated and alveolar pressures, and alveolar volume, during inspiration with a constant pressure generator. (A) Normal. (B) Decreased compliance. (C) Increased airway resistance. Note that both abnormalities reduce alveolar volume.

ventilators deliver a reduced tidal volume at the preset cycling pressure (Fig. 15.32). Consequently, their performance is variable.

Constant Flow Generator

These ventilators produce inspiration by delivering a predetermined constant flow rate of gas during inspiration. Changes in resistance or compliance make little difference to the volume delivered (unless the ventilator is pressure-cycled; see below), although airway and alveolar pressures may change (Fig. 15.33). For example, decreased compliance results in delivery of a normal tidal volume; however, the rate of increase of alveolar pressure is greater than normal (i.e. the slope is greater) and airway pressure is correspondingly higher to maintain an appropriate pressure gradient between the tracheal tube and the alveoli. If airway resistance increases, the pressure at the tracheal tube (and the gradient between tracheal tube and alveolar pressures) is higher than normal throughout inspiration, but alveolar pressure and the slopes of both pressure curves are normal. Constant flow generators do not compensate for leaks; the tidal volume delivered to the lungs decreases.

Some ventilators generate a pressure rather higher than that required to inflate the lungs but not high enough to maintain constant flow throughout

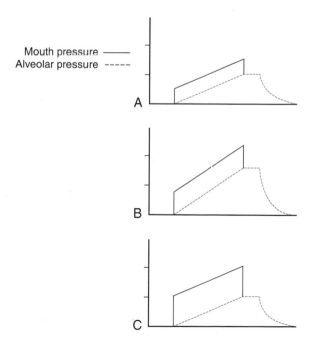

FIGURE 15.33 ■ Mouth and alveolar pressures during inspiration with a constant flow generator. (A) Normal. (B) Decreased compliance. (C) Increased airway resistance. Alveolar volume remains constant because flow rate is constant. Decreased compliance results in an increased rate of increase of alveolar pressure; mouth pressure also increases more steeply, but the gradient between mouth and alveolar pressures remains normal. Increased airway resistance increases the mouth-alveolar pressure gradient.

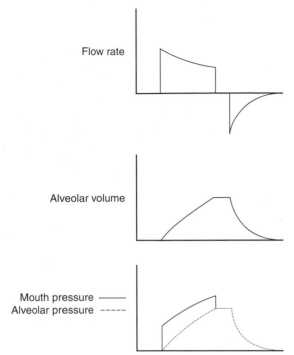

Flow rate

Alveolar volume

Mouth pressure ——
Alveolar pressure - - - -

FIGURE 15.34 ■ Pressure, flow and alveolar volume characteristics during inspiration with a ventilator with a moderately high internal pressure. At higher bellows pressures, and in a patient with normal compliance and airway resistance, the characteristics approximate to those of a constant flow generator (Fig. 15.33). At low bellows pressures, if compliance decreases or if airway resistance increases, the pattern is similar to that of a constant pressure generator.

inspiration. The flow, volume and pressure changes within the lung are shown in Figure 15.34.

Change from Inspiration to Expiration

This is termed 'cycling' and may be achieved in one of three ways:

Volume-cycling. The ventilator cycles into expiration whenever a predetermined tidal volume has been delivered. The duration of inspiration is determined by the inspiratory flow rate.

Pressure-cycling. The ventilator cycles into expiration when a preset airway pressure is achieved. This allows compensation for small leaks but, in common with a constant pressure generator, a pressure-cycled ventilator delivers a different tidal volume if compliance or resistance change. In addition, inspiratory time varies with changes in compliance and resistance.

Time-cycling. This is the method used most commonly by modern ventilators. The duration of inspiration is predetermined. With a constant flow generator, it may be desirable to preset a tidal volume; when this has been delivered, there is a short inspiratory pause (which improves gas distribution within the lung) before the inspiratory cycle ends. The use of this 'volume-preset' mechanism must be differentiated from volume-cycling, in which the ventilator cycles into expiration whenever the preset tidal volume has been delivered (and therefore the respiratory rate may be variable). When a constant pressure generator is time-cycled, the tidal volume delivered depends on the compliance and resistance of the lungs and on the pressure within the bellows.

Expiration

Usually, the patient is allowed to exhale to atmospheric pressure; flow rate decreases exponentially. Subatmospheric pressure should not be used during expiration as it induces closure of small airways and air trapping. PEEP may be applied in some circumstances (see Ch 45).

Change from Expiration to Inspiration

On most ventilators, this is achieved by time-cycling. However, it may be desirable occasionally to use pressure-cycling in response to a subatmospheric pressure generated by the patient's inspiratory effort.

Delivery of Anaesthetic Gas

Some ventilators deliver a minute volume determined by a preset tidal volume and rate. When used in anaesthesia, these machines must be supplied with a flow rate of anaesthetic gases which equals or exceeds the minute volume delivered, otherwise air, or gas used to drive the ventilator, is entrained and delivered to the patient. Ventilators such as the Bleen Manley ventilator (Fig. 15.35) are driven by the anaesthetic gas supply, can deliver only that gas, and divide it into predetermined tidal volumes (*minute volume dividers*).

Ventilators may be used to compress bellows in a separate system which contains anaesthetic gases ('bag-in-a-bottle'); it is possible to provide IPPV in a circle system in this way. The bag-in-a-bottle ventilator (Fig. 15.36) consists of a chamber with a tidal volume range of 0–1500 mL (adult mode) or

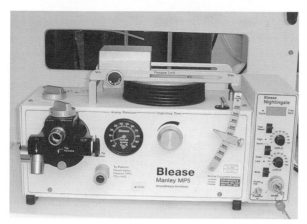

FIGURE 15.35 ■ The Blease Manley MP5 ventilator with ventilator alarm.

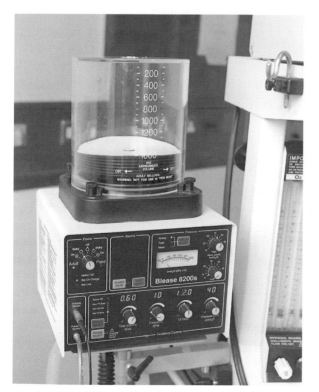

FIGURE 15.36 ■ Blease bag-in-a-bottle ventilator.

0–400 mL (paediatric mode) and ascending bellows which accommodate FGF. The control unit has controls, displays and alarms and these may include tidal volume, respiratory rate, inspiratory to expiratory (I:E) ratio, airway pressure and an on/off/standby switch. Compressed air or oxygen is used as the driving gas. On entering the chamber, the compressed gas forces the bellows down, delivering the FGF within the bellows to the patient. The driving gas in the chamber and the FGF in the bellows remain separate.

The Penlon Nuffield 200 ventilator (Fig. 15.19) is an intermittent blower. It is a very versatile ventilator, which may be used in different age groups and using different breathing systems. The control unit consists of an airway pressure gauge (cmH_2O), an on/off switch and controls to set inspiratory and expiratory time (seconds) and inspiratory flow rate (Ls^{-1}). Below the control unit, there is a connection for the driving gas (oxygen or air) and the valve block. A small tube connects the valve block to an airway pressure monitor and to a ventilator alarm. The valve block consists of a port for tubing to connect to the breathing system reservoir bag mount (Bain system) or the ventilator port (ADE system), an exhaust port which can be connected to the scavenging system and a pressure relief valve which opens at 6–7 kPa. With this standard valve, the ventilator is a time-cycled flow generator. The valve block can be changed to a paediatric Newton valve and this then converts the ventilator to a time-cycled pressure generator.

Older anaesthetic machine ventilators had a minimal number of controls, usually for minute volume, tidal volume, ventilator frequency and I:E ratio. The newer models resemble the critical care ventilators in the variable settings that are available. They perform self-tests which use dual processor technology when switched on, they have volume or pressure controlled ventilation modes, assisted spontaneous ventilation and electronically adjusted PEEP. They have sophisticated spirometry which compensates for factors such as leaks and patient compliance. They are suitable for a wider range of patients' weight, and can deliver tidal volumes as low as 20 mL. The ventilator in the Primus Dräger (Fig. 15.2A) anaesthetic machine is an electronically controlled piston ventilator, which provides several modes of ventilation including volume control, pressure control, pressure support and volume mode autoflow. All these modes can be synchronized with patient effort and can have additional pressure support.

Transport Ventilators

There are several types of ventilator available for use during the transport of critically ill patients, such as the Pneupac VR1 and the Oxylog. The Oxylog 3000 (Fig. 15.37) and 3000Plus ventilators offer sophisticated ventilation in emergency situations and during transport. They are time-cycled, constant volume and pressure-controlled ventilators and deliver tidal volumes of 50 mL or more. They incorporate various modes of ventilation suitable for critically ill patients including IPPV, synchronized intermittent mandatory ventilation (SIMV) with adjustable pressure assist during spontaneous breathing, continuous positive airways pressure (CPAP) and biphasic positive airway pressure (BIPAP), apnoea ventilation for switching over automatically to volume-controlled ventilation if breathing stops, and non-invasive ventilation (NIV). Other features include monitoring of airway pressure and expiratory minute volume, integrated capnography and enhanced data connectivity.

The characteristics of several common ventilators are summarized in Table 15.6.

High-Frequency Ventilation

High-frequency ventilation (HFV) may be defined as ventilation at a respiratory rate of greater than four times the resting respiratory rate of the subject. The different modes of HFV are shown in Table 15.7.

Of the three types of HFV, high-frequency jet ventilation (HFJV) is the most commonly used. The tidal volume used in HFJV is small compared with conventional ventilation. This is delivered at high pressure (up to 5 bar) through a cannula or catheter placed in the trachea. Inspiratory flow rates of up to 100 L min^{-1} may be required. The inspiratory time is adjustable from 20% to 50% of the cycle. The mechanism by which HFV is able to maintain gas exchange is not clear. Typical values for adult ventilation are:

- ventilation rate 100–150 cycles min^{-1}
- driving pressure 100–200 kPa
- inspiratory cycle of 20–40%.

HFJV is used during some operations on the larynx, trachea or lung and in a small number of patients in the ICU. Gases should be humidified when using HFJV. Gas exchange may be unpredictable and the technique should not be used by the trainee without supervision. Figure 15.38 illustrates a type of ventilator used for HFJV.

Venturi Injector Device

The Venturi injector consists of a high-pressure oxygen source (at about 400 kPa from either the anaesthetic

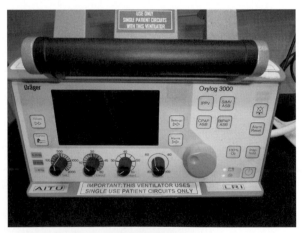

FIGURE 15.37 ■ Oxylog 3000 transport ventilator.

		TABLE 15.6				
		Classification of Some Common Ventilators Used During Anaesthesia				
Ventilator	Driven by	Cycling to Expiration	Cycling to Inspiration	Pressure/Flow Generator	Minute Volume Divider	Volume Preset
Manley MP3, MP5	Anaesthetic gases	Time/volume	Time	Pressure	Yes	Yes
Nuffield 200	Compressed air or oxygen	Time	Time	Flow	No	No
Bag-in-bottle	Compressed air or oxygen	Time	Time	Flow	No	Yes
Oxylog 3000 transport ventilator	Gas powered	Time	Time	Flow	No	Yes

TABLE 15.7	
Types of High-Frequency Ventilation	
Type of Ventilation	*Rate of Ventilation (Cycles min^{-1})*
High-frequency positive pressure ventilation (HFPPV)	60–100
High-frequency jet ventilation (HFJV)	100–400
High-frequency oscillation ventilation (HFOV)	400–2400

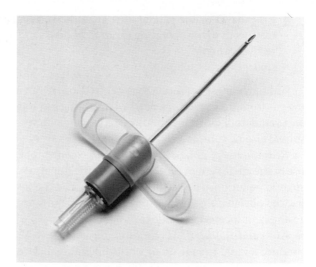

FIGURE 15.40 ■ Cricothyroid cannula to use with a Venturi injector device.

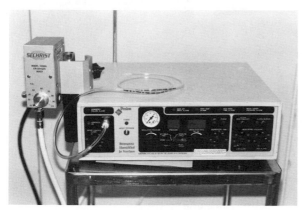

FIGURE 15.38 ■ Penlon Bromsgrove jet ventilator.

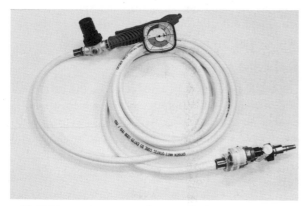

FIGURE 15.39 ■ Manually controlled Venturi injector.

machine or direct from a pipeline), on/off trigger and connection tubing that can withstand high pressure. The Manujet (Fig. 15.39) is a newer design of a Venturi injector device. It has a dial to alter the driving pressure to suit the size of patient from a neonate to an adult. This is connected to the side of a rigid bronchoscope, to a transtracheal catheter or to a cannula inserted through the cricothyroid membrane. The injector is controlled manually. A 14 gauge cannula or a specially designed cannula (Fig. 15.40) inserted through the cricothyroid membrane may be used to ventilate using the Venturi injector device. A Venturi effect is created which entrains atmospheric air and allows intermittent insufflation of the lungs with oxygen-enriched air at airway pressures of 2.5–3.0 kPa. It is used in operations on the larynx, trachea or lung. Possible complications include barotrauma, gastric distension and awareness if inadequate quantities of intravenous anaesthetic drugs are administered. When Venturi injector devices are employed, it is essential to ensure that gas is able to leave the lungs though the upper airway during expiration.

SCAVENGING

The possible adverse effects of pollution on staff in the operating theatre environment are discussed in Chapter 20. The principal sources of pollution by anaesthetic gases and vapours include:

- discharge of anaesthetic gases from ventilators
- expired gas vented from the spill valve of anaesthetic breathing systems
- leaks from equipment, e.g. from an ill-fitting face mask

■ gas exhaled by the patient after anaesthesia. This may occur in the operating theatre, corridors and recovery room

■ spillage during filling of vaporizers.

Although most attention has centred on removing gas from the expiratory ports of breathing systems and ventilators, other methods of reducing pollution should also be considered:

Reduced use of anaesthetic gases and vapours. The use of the circle system reduces the potential for atmospheric pollution. The use of inhalational anaesthetics may be obviated totally by using total intravenous anaesthesia or local anaesthetic techniques.

Air conditioning. Air conditioning units which produce a rapid change of air in the operating theatre reduce pollution substantially. However, some systems recycle air, and older operating theatres, dental surgeries and obstetric delivery suites may not be equipped with air conditioning.

Care in filling vaporizers. Great care should be taken not to spill volatile anaesthetic agent when a vaporizer is filled. The use of agent-specific connections (Fig. 15.10) reduces the risk of spillage. In some countries, vaporizers must be filled only in a portable fume cupboard.

Scavenging Apparatus

Anaesthetic gases vented from the breathing system are removed by a collecting system. A variety of purpose-built scavenging spill valves is available; an example of an adjustable pressure-limiting (APL) valve is shown in Figure 15.41. Waste gases from ventilators are collected by attaching the scavenging system to the expiratory port of the ventilator. Connectors on scavenging systems have a diameter of 30 mm to ensure that inappropriate connections with anaesthetic apparatus cannot be made.

Disposal systems may be active, semi-active or passive.

Active Systems

These employ apparatus to generate a negative pressure within the scavenging system to propel waste gases to the outside atmosphere. The system may be powered by a vacuum pump (Fig. 15.42) or a Venturi system (Fig. 15.43). The exhaust should be capable of accommodating 75 L min⁻¹ continuous flow with

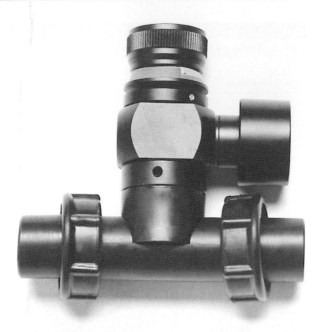

FIGURE 15.41 ■ An APL (adjustable pressure-limiting) valve with scavenging attachment.

a peak of 130 L min⁻¹. Usually, a reservoir system (Fig 15.42B) is used to permit high peak flow rates to be accommodated. In addition, there must be a pressure-limiting device within the system to prevent the application of negative pressure to the patient's lungs.

Semi-Active Systems

The waste gases may be conducted to the extraction side of the air-conditioning system, which generates a small negative pressure within the scavenging tubing. These systems have variable performance and efficiency.

Passive Systems

These systems vent the expired gas to the outside atmosphere (Fig. 15.44). Gas movement is generated by the patient. Consequently the total length of tubing must not be excessive or resistance to expiration is high. The pressure within the system may be altered by wind conditions at the external terminal; on occasions, these may generate a negative pressure, but may also generate high positive pressures. Each scavenging location should have a separate external

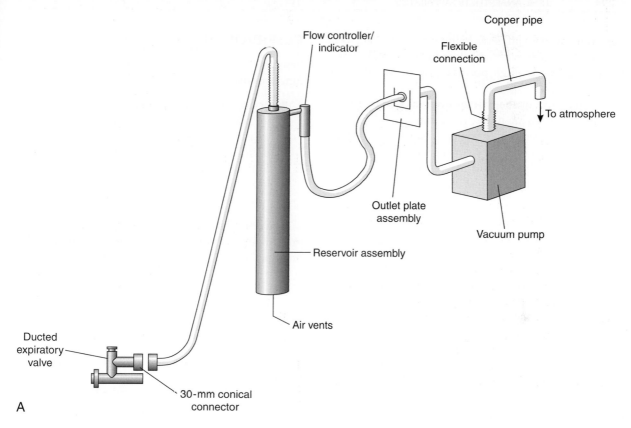

Flow controller/indicator

Copper pipe

Flexible connection

To atmosphere

Outlet plate assembly

Vacuum pump

Reservoir assembly

Air vents

Ducted expiratory valve

30-mm conical connector

A

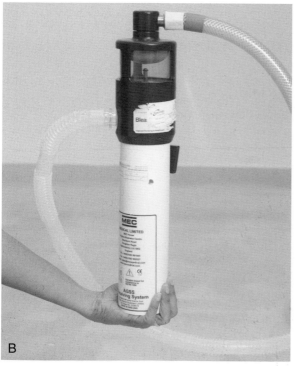

B

FIGURE 15.42 ■ An active scavenging system (**A**) and the reservoir assembly (**B**).

terminal to prevent gases being vented into adjacent locations. Relief valves must be incorporated to prevent negative or high positive pressures within the system.

Irrespective of the type of disposal system, tubing used for scavenging must not be allowed to lie on the floor of the operating theatre, as compression (e.g. by feet or by items of equipment) results in increased resistance to expiration and may generate dangerously high pressure within the patient's lungs.

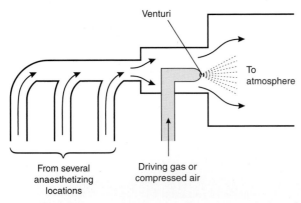

FIGURE 15.43 ■ A Venturi system for active scavenging of anaesthetic gases.

RESERVOIR BAGS

Reservoir bags are used in breathing systems. Their functions include:

- serving as a reservoir of inspired gases
- providing a means of manual ventilation of the lungs
- serving as a visual or tactile observation to monitor the patient's spontaneous respiration
- protecting the patient from excessive pressure in the breathing system.

The reservoir bag may accommodate an increase in pressure in the breathing system to a maximum of approximately 50 cmH$_2$O (5 kPa).

The standard adult size is 2 L and the paediatric size is 0.5 L. However, the size of reservoir bags may vary from 0.5 to 6 L.

LARYNGOSCOPES

A laryngoscope consists of a blade which elevates the lower jaw and tongue, a light source near the tip of the blade to illuminate the larynx, and a handle to apply leverage to the blade. There are many forms of blade and handle.

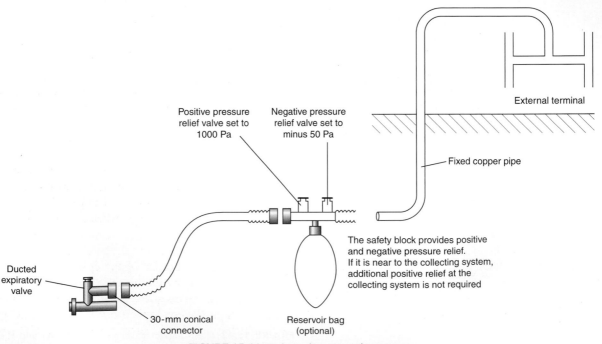

FIGURE 15.44 ■ A passive scavenging system.

Curved Blade

The most commonly used adult laryngoscope blade is the Macintosh curved blade, which is manufactured in several sizes (Figs 15.45, 15.46).

The tip of the laryngoscope blade is advanced carefully over the surface of the tongue until it reaches the vallecula (Ch 21, Fig. 21.3). The tip of the blade is rotated upwards and the laryngoscope lifted along the axis of the handle to lift the larynx; the incisor teeth must not be used as a fulcrum to lever the tip of the blade upwards. When the arytenoids and posterior part of the cords are seen, gentle pressure on the larynx using the right thumb, or provided by an assistant, may help to improve the view. Concerns have been raised about the possibility that multiple-use laryngoscopes may transfer between patients the prions thought to be responsible for causing variant Creutzfeldt–Jakob disease (vCJD), especially if used during surgery for tonsillectomy or adenoidectomy Therefore disposable laryngoscope blades are now used routinely. The quality of disposable laryngoscopes has improved enormously and is now indistinguishable from that of non-disposable devices.

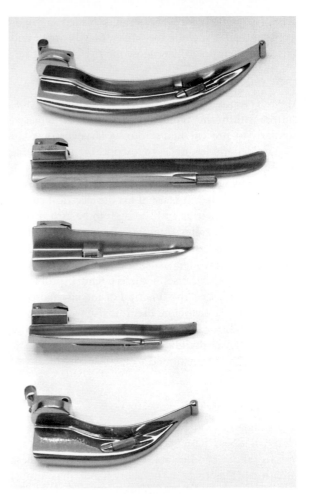

FIGURE 15.46 ■ A selection of laryngoscope blades. From the top downwards: Macintosh adult blade, Miller adult blade, Soper infant blade, Wisconsin infant blade and Macintosh infant blade.

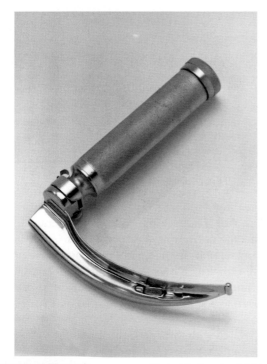

FIGURE 15.45 ■ A laryngoscope with the Macintosh adult blade.

Straight Blade

Straight-bladed laryngoscopes are useful adjuncts in safe airway management. However, they are not always as easy to use as curved blades. The technique of laryngoscopy is slightly different when a straight-bladed laryngoscope is used (see Fig. 21.3). Instead of placing the tip of the blade in the vallecula, it is advanced over the posterior border of the epiglottis, which is then lifted directly by the blade to provide a view of the larynx. This technique is useful particularly in babies, in whom the epiglottis is rather floppy and may obscure the view of the larynx if a curved blade is used. However, bruising of the epiglottis is more likely with a straight blade. The straight-bladed laryngo-scopes available include the Miller, Magill, Soper and Wisconsin (Fig 15.46) laryngoscopes.

Light Source

Most laryngoscopes are powered by batteries contained within the handle; these must be replaced regularly to prevent failure during laryngoscopy. On many older models of laryngoscope, the light source is a bulb which screws into a socket on the blade; a tight connection should be ensured before laryngo-scopy is attempted. It is usual for the electrical circuit between the batteries and the bulb to be closed by a switch which operates automatically when the blade is opened. However, the electrical contacts of the switch may become corroded, causing a reduction in power or total failure. Because of these potential problems, it is important that the function of the laryngoscope is checked carefully before use. It is also wise to have a spare functioning laryngoscope and a variety of blades available. Newer designs place the bulb in the handle and the light is transmitted to the blade by means of fibreoptics.

Laryngoscope Handle

The standard handle may result in difficult laryngoscopy in obese patients, and in women with large breasts. Short handles are available for use in these situations (Fig. 15.47). The short handle has almost replaced the use of the Polio blade (Fig. 15.48) in obstetric practice.

The McCoy laryngoscope (Fig. 15.49A) is based on the standard Macintosh blade but has a hinged tip. This is operated by a lever mechanism attached to the handle. When the lever is pressed (Fig. 15.49B), the tip of the blade bends forward and this improves the view of the larynx.

Video Laryngoscopes

Traditional direct laryngoscopy depends on achieving a straight line of vision to the patient's larynx. This requires alignment of the oral, pharyngeal and laryngeal axes. Videolaryngoscopes are a new class of laryngoscopes that have high resolution video cameras incorporated in the tip of a modified laryngoscope blade. The video image is relayed by either fibreoptic bundles, lenses or via cables to a dedicated LCD video

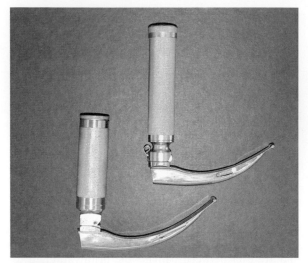

FIGURE 15.47 ■ Short and standard laryngoscope handles.

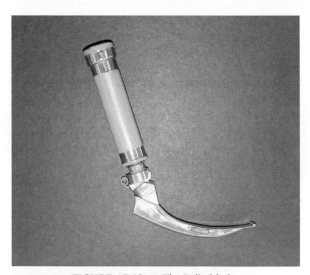

FIGURE 15.48 ■ The Polio blade.

display. Videolaryngoscopy allows the operator to see around the corners as the transmitted image is the view obtained from the tip of the laryngoscope blade. Aligning the three axes (oral, pharyngeal and laryngeal) and compression or distraction of tissues to achieve a line of sight are not required. With direct laryngoscopy, poor visualization of the glottic aperture is correlated with difficult intubation. The major difference with videolaryngoscopy when compared with conventional direct laryngoscopy is that it may be

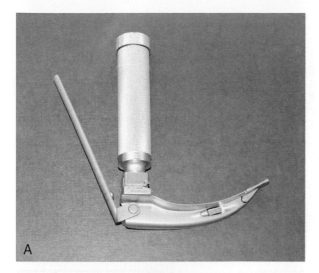

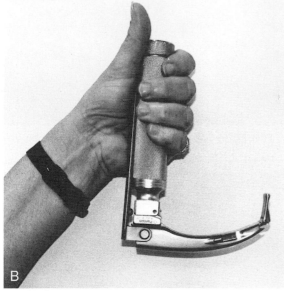

FIGURE 15.49 ■ (**A**) The McCoy laryngoscope. (**B**) The McCoy laryngoscope, demonstrating the hinged blade tip.

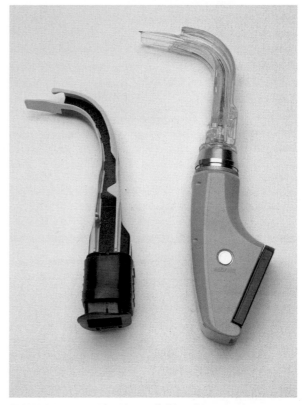

FIGURE 15.50 ■ The Airtraq (left) and Pentax Airway scope (right).

difficult to intubate the trachea despite a clear view of the glottis. Examples of videolaryngoscopes are those with a guiding channel such as the Pentax Airway scope and Airtraq (Fig. 15.50) and those without a guiding channel such as the Glidescope, McGrath and C-Mac (Fig. 15.51). The Venner AP Advance videolaryngoscope is a recent addition to the videolaryngoscope market (Fig. 15.52) in which the standard blade does not have a channel but the difficult airway blade does. The Airtraq is fully disposable whereas the other videolaryngoscopes have disposable blades but a reusable main unit. The C-Mac requires sterilization between uses.

Fibreoptic Laryngo/Bronchoscope

The fibreoptic scope (Fig. 15.53) is an endoscope which is used to view the upper and lower airway through either the nose or the mouth. The principle of the fibreoptic system is that light from a powerful external light source is transmitted through a flexible instrument and an image of the area is returned to an eyepiece or camera. The fibres which transmit the light have a diameter of approximately 20 μm and are made up of a central glass core coated with a thin layer of glass material with a lower refractive index. The light passing down the fibre is repeatedly reflected down the inner glass.

The fibreoptic scope consists of a light source, a universal cord and light guide connector, a control

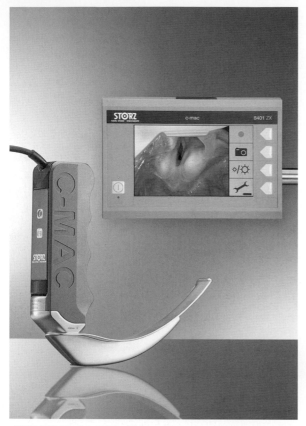

FIGURE 15. 51 ■ The C-Mac laryngoscope and monitor.

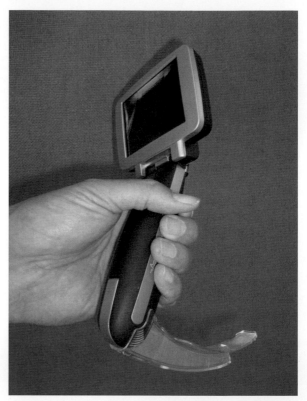

FIGURE 15.52 ■ Venner AP Advance laryngoscope.

unit, an eyepiece and an insertion tube. The light source (Fig. 15.54) is usually powered by mains electrical supply and contains either a xenon or a halogen lamp. The universal cord and light guide connector contain the light guide fibre bundle and transmits light from a light source to the fibreoptic bundle in the insertion tube. In some newer models, light is powered by a battery and this enables these scopes to be easily portable and be used in places outside the operating theatres, such as the emergency department.

The control unit consists of an angulation control lever, suction port and biopsy port. The angulation lever controls the deflection of the tip of the scope. The suction port is for connecting to a suction pump but it can also be used for insufflation of oxygen. The biopsy channel can be used for taking biopsy specimens but it can also be used to attach a syringe to instil local anaesthetic into the airway.

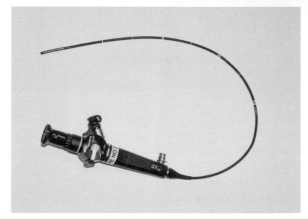

FIGURE 15.53 ■ The fibreoptic intubating laryngoscope which consists of a control unit, insertion cord and a connector for a light guide.

The eyepiece consists of the viewing lens and the dioptre adjustment ring. A camera can be attached to the eyepiece either to take photographs or to transmit the pictures to a television monitor (Figs 15.54 and

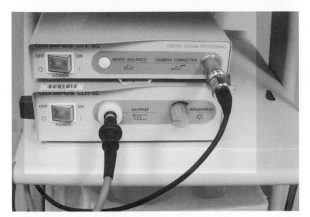

FIGURE 15.54 ■ The light source and a camera system for the fibreoptic intubating laryngoscope.

15.55A). A disposable fibreoptic scope (Ambuscope) is now available (Fig. 15.55B).

The insertion tube contains two optical fibre bundles: the light guide and the image guide. The fibres transmitting light (light guide) are arranged in a random fashion but those returning the image (image guide) are precisely located relative to each other. The insertion tube also contains the suction channel and the biopsy channel. At the distal end of each optical fibre, there is a lens. The size of the insertion tube varies from 1.8 to 6.4 mm to fit inside tracheal tubes of internal diameter 3.0–7.0 mm.

Most anaesthetists who use the fibreoptic scope now attach a camera to the eyepiece and view the airway on a television monitor. The use of a camera and TV monitor has been demonstrated to enhance the speed with which anaesthetists can be taught fibreoptic endoscopy skills.

TRACHEAL TUBES

Most tracheal tubes are constructed of red rubber, silicone rubber or plastic. Red rubber tubes are reusable, although they may start to show signs of deterioration after 2–3 years. Today, disposable plastic tubes are the preferred choice (Fig. 15.56) as they eliminate the need to collect, clean, sterilize and check tubes after use. Plastic tubes are presented in a sterile pack and should be cut to an appropriate length before use. The plastic disposable tubes have a cuff and a pilot balloon with a self-sealing valve. The cuff may be inflated with air, nitrous oxide or saline. The internal diameter of the tube is marked on the side of the tube in millimetres

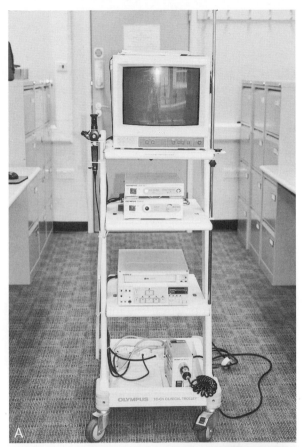

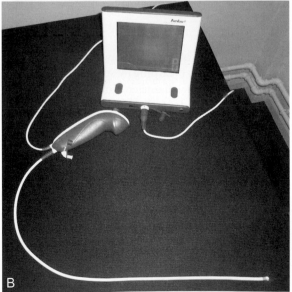

FIGURE 15.55 ■ (**A**) The television monitor, camera system and light source used with the intubating fibreoptic scope. (**B**) The Ambuscope – a disposable fibreoptic scope.

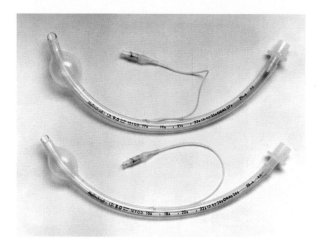

FIGURE 15.56 ■ 8- and 9-mm internal diameter plastic disposable tracheal tubes.

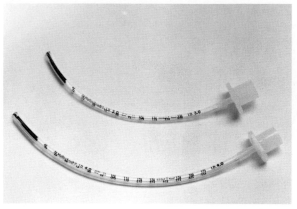

FIGURE 15.57 ■ Paediatric uncuffed plastic tracheal tubes.

and the length of the tube is marked along the length of the tube in centimetres. The tube also has a radio-opaque line running along its length. This enables the position of the tube to be determined on a chest X-ray.

Some tracheal tubes contain latex and must not be used in patients who have a history of latex allergy. Silicone rubber is increasingly being used in the manufacture of tracheal tubes. These are more expensive than the plastic tubes but they may be sterilized and re-used. They are softer than red rubber or plastic endotracheal tubes and they are non-irritant.

Tube Size

In adults, there is little to be gained in the way of reduced resistance to breathing by selecting a tube larger than 8.0 mm internal diameter. However, it is common to use a tube of 8.0–9.0 mm internal diameter for male and 7.0–8.0 mm for female adults. Tubes of wide diameter may exert pressure on the laryngeal cords after insertion. Appropriate sizes of tracheal tubes for children are shown in Appendix B (IX).

Plain Tubes

Uncuffed tubes are used in children (Fig. 15.57). A cuff is unnecessary to secure an airtight fit if the correct diameter of tube is selected, because the narrowest part of the airway is in the trachea at the level of the cricoid cartilage. However, the larynx is the narrowest part of the airway in the adult and a leak occurs if an uncuffed tube is used; in addition, there is a risk of aspiration of

fluid from the pharynx into the trachea. Nasotracheal intubation is less traumatic if an uncuffed tube is used. The incidence of sore throat is not influenced by the presence of a cuff on the tracheal tube.

Cuffed Tubes

It is usual to use a cuffed tube whenever tracheal intubation is required in the adult. It is mandatory if IPPV is to be used or if there is a risk of blood, pus or gastric fluid entering the pharynx. Tracheal tubes with a streamlined cuff are available and are suitable for nasotracheal intubation.

Cuff Volume

Tracheal tube cuffs may be either low-volume/high-pressure or high-volume/low-pressure. A tube with a low-volume cuff may require inflation to a high pressure to effect a seal within the trachea. The pressure within a low-volume cuff does not necessarily relate to the pressure exerted by the cuff on the tracheal mucosa. However, a high pressure may be exerted on the mucosa if the cuff is overinflated. This may occur inadvertently during anaesthesia because nitrous oxide diffuses through some types of plastic. Some anaesthetists inflate the cuff with an oxygen/nitrous oxide mixture to obviate this problem. Alternatively, the cuff volume may be readjusted after 10–15 min of anaesthesia.

High-volume/low-pressure ('floppy') cuffs cover a larger area of tracheal wall and may effect a seal with less pressure exerted on the mucosa. However, they may cause more trauma during insertion and may become puckered in a relatively small trachea.

Herniation of an overinflated cuff may occlude the distal end of the tracheal tube and cause partial or total airway obstruction.

Shape of Tube

In most centres, a curved tracheal tube is used. These should be cut to the correct length as there is a risk of accidental intubation of a bronchus (usually the right main bronchus) if the tip is inserted too far. Some plastic tracheal tubes are preformed in shapes which either fit the pharyngeal contour or carry the proximal end of the tube away from the mouth (Fig. 15.58); the latter design is useful when surgery on the face or head is planned. The RAE (Ring, Adair and Elwyn) tubes have preformed curves and they can be used either orally or nasally (Fig. 15.59). RAE tubes may be cuffed or uncuffed. Care should be taken not to insert these preformed tubes too far as there is a risk of bronchial intubation.

Specialized Tubes

An armoured latex tube is useful if there is a danger of the tube kinking during surgery; a nylon spiral is incorporated in the wall of the tube and prevents obliteration of the lumen. Alternatively, a reinforced flexometallic tube, with a metal spiral in the wall, may be used. These tubes are very floppy and a wire stilette is required for their insertion.

Reinforced flexometallic tubes are available in either uncuffed paediatric sizes or cuffed adult sizes (Fig. 15.60). These tracheal tubes are long and cannot be shortened because they have a fixed tracheal tube connector. Therefore, when inserting them into the trachea, care should be taken to avoid bronchial intubation. The adult cuffed tubes have two black rings and the paediatric uncuffed tubes have a black line at the distal end. These give guidance as to where the vocal cords should be, in order to avoid bronchial intubation.

A flexible metal tube (Fig. 15.61) may be used during procedures that require the use of lasers in the airway; plastic tubes may ignite if struck by the laser beam. Some designs have two cuffs. This ensures a tracheal seal if the upper cuff is damaged by laser. An air-filled cuff may ignite if it is hit by a laser beam. Therefore it is recommended that the cuffs are filled with saline instead of air.

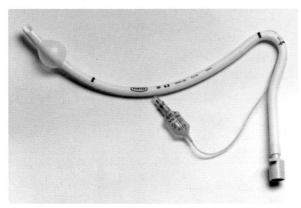

FIGURE 15.58 ■ Preformed north-facing nasotracheal tube.

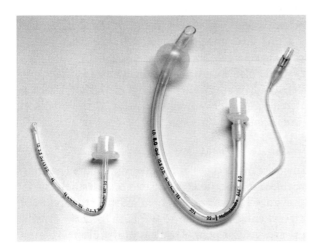

FIGURE 15.59 ■ Preformed RAE disposable plastic tracheal tubes: the uncuffed paediatric tube and the cuffed adult tube.

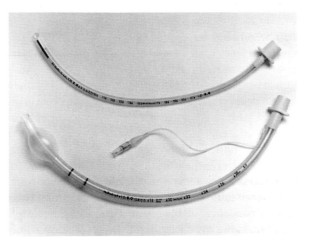

FIGURE 15.60 ■ The reinforced tracheal tube – the paediatric uncuffed and adult cuffed tubes.

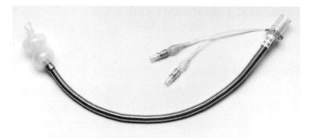

FIGURE 15.61 ■ Flexible metal tube suitable for use during laser surgery to the airway.

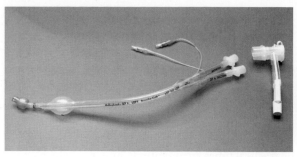

FIGURE 15.63 ■ Bronchocath double-lumen endobronchial tube with catheter mount.

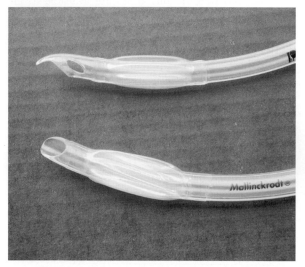

FIGURE 15.62 ■ The distal ends of a Parker (upper) and a conventional bevelled tracheal tube.

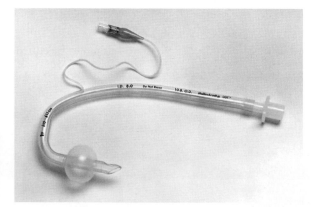

FIGURE 15.64 ■ Laryngectomy tube.

Laryngectomy tubes (Fig. 15.64) are designed to be inserted through a tracheostomy into the trachea to maintain the airway during surgery for laryngectomy. Because of its shape, the connection to the breathing system is some distance away from the surgical field and this gives the surgeon a relatively clear field in which to operate.

A microlaryngeal tube is a small tube (usually 5 mm internal diameter) with an adult-sized cuff which is used during surgery on the larynx. It allows better surgical access to the larynx.

Tracheostomy Tubes

There are many types of tracheostomy tube. They may be cuffed or uncuffed. The proximal end of a tracheostomy tube has a standard 15-mm connector and there are two wings with slots to which the securing tape is attached (Fig. 15.65). Tracheostomy tubes have a replaceable inner cannula which facilitates insertion and is removed once the tracheostomy tube is in place.

The Parker tube (Fig. 15.62) has a curved bevel on the inner curvature of the tube. The bevel therefore lies on the anterior aspect of the tube during insertion. The manufacturer claims that it is less likely than the conventional tube to cause trauma to the larynx or trachea, particularly during insertion over a bougie or fibreoptic laryngoscope.

Double-lumen endobronchial tubes are used during thoracic surgery when there is a need for one lung to be deflated. They allow selective deflation of one lung whilst maintaining ventilation of the other lung. The older Robertshaw double-lumen tubes are made of red rubber and are therefore reusable. The disposable Bronchocath double-lumen tubes (Fig. 15.63), which are made of plastic, are used more commonly now.

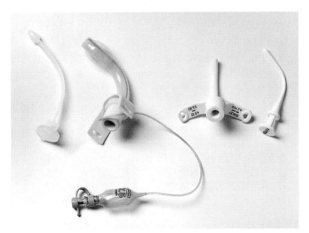

FIGURE 15.65 ■ Tracheostomy tubes. Adult cuffed (7.0 mm internal diameter) and paediatric Shiley uncuffed tubes with the replaceable inner cannulae.

The fenestrated tracheostomy tube has a hole (fenestration) along its greater curvature. This allows the patient to speak by directing some of the air past the vocal cords.

Silver tracheostomy tubes are used in many patients who require long-term intubation. They have an inner tube which may be removed for cleaning. Some designs have a one-way flap valve to allow the patient to speak. Silver is non-irritant and bactericidal.

Cricothyroidotomy Devices

Cricothyroidotomy is the creation of an opening in the cricothyroid membrane in order to gain access to the airway either as an elective prophylactic cricothyroidotomy in an anticipated difficult airway or in an emergency 'can't intubate and can't ventilate' (CICV) scenario (see Ch 22). Cricothyroidotomy can be carried out using either a small cannula (Fig. 15.40), large bore cannula (4 mm or larger internal diameter) or surgically using a tracheostomy tube (6 mm or greater). There are several types of large bore cannulae available. The cuffed or uncuffed Melker kit (Fig. 15.66) uses a Seldinger technique. The cuffed or uncuffed VBM Quicktrach (Fig. 15.67) is a rigid pre-assembled cannula-over-needle device that is inserted as a single step procedure. The cuffed Portex cricothyroidotomy kit is also a rigid cannula-over-needle device, which is packaged as a pre-assembled kit with

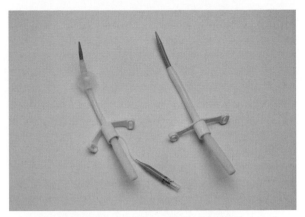

FIGURE 15.66 ■ Melker cricothyroidotomy set.

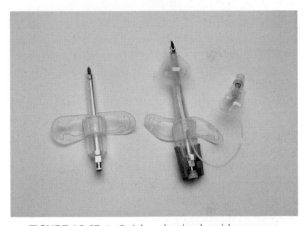

FIGURE 15.67 ■ Quicktrach cricothyroidotomy set.

a scalpel and syringe (Fig. 15.68). It has a spring-loaded Veress needle with a blunt stilette. The Portex Minitrach II is a wire-guided kit which provides an uncuffed 4-mm airway through the cricothyroid membrane. It is designed for tracheal suction and not for an emergency situation because it is not easy to insert quickly.

Connections

Catheter Mount

This is a flexible link between the breathing system and a tracheal tube, laryngeal mask airway, face mask or tracheostomy tube (Fig. 15.69). It may be made of rubber or plastic and some have a gas sampling port. The proximal end, which attaches to the breathing system, has a standard 22-mm connection and the distal end

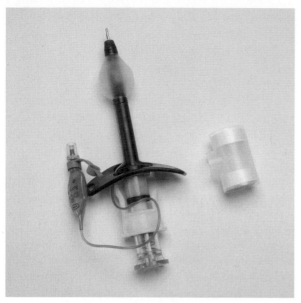

FIGURE 15.68 ■ Portex cricothyroidotomy kit.

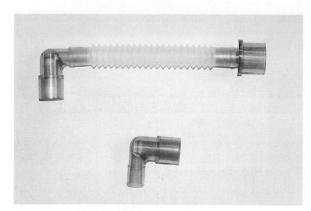

FIGURE 15.69 ■ A disposable catheter mount to connect the tracheal tube to the breathing system (top). A disposable angle piece to connect a face mask or tracheal tube to the breathing system (bottom).

is a 15-mm connector. The length of catheter mounts varies from 45 to 170 mm.

Tracheal Tube Connectors

Disposable 15-mm diameter connectors are provided with plastic disposable tubes; the diameter of the distal end is of an appropriate size to fit the

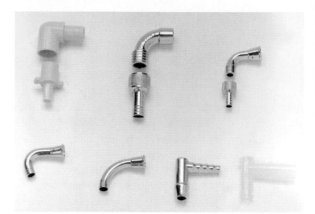

FIGURE 15.70 ■ A variety of new and old tracheal tube connectors. From top left in clockwise rotation: Portex with 15-mm tracheal tube connector, Nosworthy, Knight's paediatric connector, Cobbs, Rowbotham, Magill oral, Magill nasal.

internal diameter of the tube. Several older connections (Fig. 15.70) have been used with plastic or rubber tracheal tubes.

Angle Pieces

These are connectors which fit between the breathing system and the tracheal tube or mask (Fig. 15.69). They incorporate a 90° bend and have either 15- or 22-mm connectors at each end. Some angle pieces have a condenser humidifier, bacterial filter and a port for gas sampling incorporated into them (Fig. 15.30).

PROTECTING THE BREATHING SYSTEM IN ANAESTHESIA

Following recent fatal incidents in which anaesthetic tubing became blocked, the UK Department of Health has made recommendations to minimize the risk of recurrence. The recommendations include training and increasing awareness of the potential problem of anaesthetic tubing becoming blocked accidentally, and protecting vulnerable components of the breathing system by keeping the components individually wrapped until use. The Department of Health recommends the use of the Association of Anaesthetists of Great Britain and Ireland (AAGBI) document 'Checking anaesthetic equipment' and that all trainees should be trained in the correct procedure for checking anaesthetic equipment.

SUPRAGLOTTIC AIRWAY DEVICES (SADs)

Supraglottic airway devices (SADs) can be divided into two types. The first generation includes the classic laryngeal mask airway (LMA), flexible LMA and all the single-use LMAs. The second generation SADs include the I-gel, Pro-seal LMA and the Supreme LMA which are designed with a drainage tube to reduce aspiration, have an integral bite block and have increased airway seal to enable positive pressure ventilation to take place.

The Classic LMA (cLMA)

This device consists of a shortened conventional silicone tube with an elliptical cuff, inflated through a pilot tube, attached to the distal end (Fig. 15.71). The cuff, which resembles a miniature face mask, has been designed to form a relatively airtight seal around the posterior perimeter of the larynx (Fig. 15.72). A variety of sizes of cuff is available, ranging from size 1 which is used in the neonate to size 5 which is used in large adults. The mask is inserted and the cuff inflated until no air leak is detected. It is important to ensure that the maximum inflation volume is not exceeded (Table 15.8). The device is very effective in maintaining a patent airway in the spontaneously breathing patient. Positive pressure ventilation may be applied if necessary. The mask is not suitable for patients who are at risk from regurgitation of gastric contents (emergency

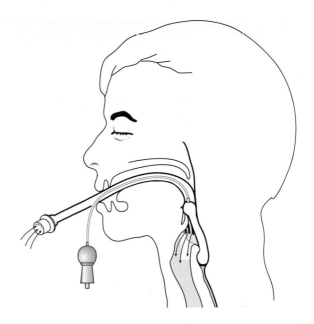

FIGURE 15.72 ■ A laryngeal mask airway *in situ*.

surgery, hiatus hernia or history of reflux, and obesity) and should be used with caution if pharyngeal soiling is anticipated.

The flexible LMA differs from the standard LMA in that it has a flexible, wire reinforced tube. The size of the cuff is similar to that of the standard LMA but the tube is longer and narrower and therefore offers more resistance to breathing (Fig. 15.71). Because of the wire in the tube, it is unsuitable for use in the MRI unit. The classic LMA is reusable up to 40 times. However, a large selection of disposable LMAs manufactured by different companies is available and these are now used more commonly.

Second Generation SADs

The Proseal LMA is a reusable LMA which has a drain tube, a posterior inflatable cuff, reinforced airway tube, integral bite block and an introducer (Fig.15. 73). The distal end must sit in the oesophageal inlet to ensure best performance. The drainage tube vents any gas leaking into the oesophagus as well as any fluid if regurgitation occurs and it can be used to insert an orogastric tube. The increased oesophageal and pharyngeal seal allows positive pressure ventilation to take place. The Pro-seal LMA is reusable up to

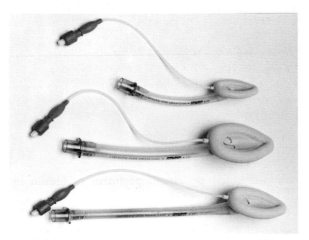

FIGURE 15.71 ■ Laryngeal mask airways (LMAs). A paediatric size 2 mask, an adult size 4 mask and a size 3 reinforced LMA.

TABLE 15.8
Characteristics of Laryngeal Mask Airways (LMAs)

Size of LMA	Length of LMA (cm)	Size of Patient	Volume of Cuff (mL)	Largest Size (mm) of Tracheal Tube that Fits into the LMA
1	8	Neonates and infants up to 6.5 kg	Up to 4	3.5
1.5	10	Infants 5–10 kg	Up to 7	4.0
2	11	Infants and children 10–20 kg	Up to 10	4.5
2.5	12.5	Children 20–30 kg	Up to 14	5.0
3	16	Children and small adults 30–50 kg	Up to 20	6.0
4	16	Normal adults 50–70 kg	Up to 30	6.0
5	18	Large adults >70 kg	Up to 40	7.0

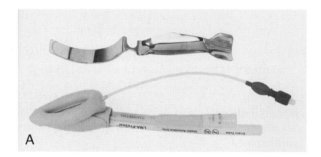 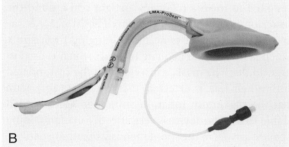

FIGURE 15.73 ■ (A) The LMA Pro-seal. (B) The LMA Pro-seal mounted on the LMA Pro-seal introducer.

40 times and all its components are latex-free. It can be mounted on an introducer (Fig. 15.73B) which facilitates the insertion of the LMA Pro-seal into the patient's mouth. The I-gel (Fig. 15.74) is a new single use SAD with a non-inflatable 'cuff' made of a soft thermoplastic elastomer. The 'cuff' is a preformed soft mould, which fits into the perilaryngeal structures. It has a narrow bore oesophageal drain tube, a short wide bore airway tube and an integral bite block. Both the Proseal and the I-gel come in adult and paediatric sizes. The Supreme LMA (SLMA) (Fig. 15.75) is the newest of the second generation SADs and it is sometimes described as a 'single use Pro-seal LMA'. However, in reality, it has features of the Pro-seal LMA and the intubating LMA (ILMA). Its features include a large inflatable plastic cuff but no posterior cuff found in the Pro-seal LMA, an oesophageal drain tube, a preformed semi-rigid tube, an integral bite block and fins in the mask bowl to

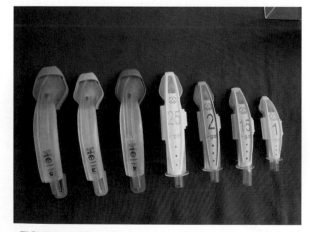

FIGURE 15.74 ■ The I-gel supraglottic device – sizes 1–5.

prevent epiglottic obstruction. It is made of PVC. Unlike a Pro-seal LMA, the SLMA does not require an introducer for insertion.

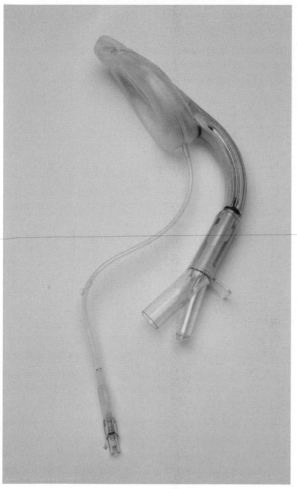

FIGURE 15.75 ■ Supreme LMA.

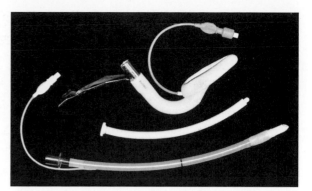

FIGURE 15.76 ■ An intubating laryngeal mask airway (ILMA) with the silicone tracheal tube and the introducer.

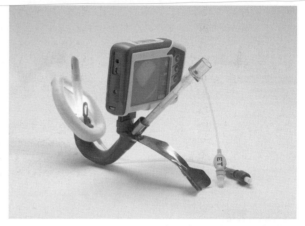

FIGURE 15.77 ■ LMA C-Trach with monitor attached.

The Intubating LMA

The intubating LMA (ILMA) is an advanced form of the standard LMA (Fig. 15.76). It has a shorter tube and a metal handle. The handle permits single-handed insertion without moving the head and neck and without placing fingers in the mouth. It may be passed through an interdental gap as narrow as 20 mm. The mask floor has an elevating bar which replaces the two bars in the standard LMA. The caudal end of the bar is not fixed to the mask floor and this allows a tracheal tube to be passed in order to intubate the trachea. The ILMA is available in sizes 3, 4 and 5. The recommended cuff volumes are similar to the corresponding sizes of the standard LMA. The rigid curved airway has a standard 15-mm connector at the proximal end.

The tube is wide enough to allow passage of a cuffed 8-mm tracheal tube. The ILMA is a reusable device which may be cleaned and sterilized up to 40 times but a single use version is now available.

The C-Trach LMA (Fig. 15.77) is a variant of the ILMA with fibreoptic components integrated into the device to allow direct vision at intubation. It has a digital screen with a light source and digital camera. The lens lies behind the epiglottis elevator bar (EEB) and captures the image from the front of the mask aperture. The image is transmitted to the viewing screen.

OTHER APPARATUS

Face Masks

These are designed to fit the face perfectly so that no leak of gas occurs, but without applying excessive pressure to the skin. An appropriate size of face mask must be selected to ensure a proper fit, but the smallest size possible should be used to minimize dead space. Disposable masks made of transparent material are available (Fig. 15.78). These allow the detection of vomitus or secretions.

A harness system (e.g. Clausen harness) is used by some anaesthetists to hold the mask on the face during surgery. However, airway obstruction may occur at any time and the excursion of the reservoir bag must be observed constantly. In many countries, the LMA is now used during maintenance of anaesthesia in almost all situations in which a face mask was formerly used.

Intubating Forceps

The most commonly used intubating forceps are those designed by Magill (Fig. 15.79A). The instrument is employed to manipulate a nasotracheal or nasogastric tube through the oropharynx and into the correct position. A laryngoscope is used to obtain a view of the oropharynx.

Laryngeal Spray

These are used to deposit a fine mist of local anaesthetic solution (usually lidocaine 4% or 10%) on the mucosa of the larynx and upper trachea (Fig. 15.80A and B). These sprays are particularly useful in applying local anaesthetic to the upper airway during awake fibreoptic intubation. The mucosal atomization device (MAD) is a single use atomizer which comes in two shapes, the oral and the nasal atomizer (Fig. 15.80B).

Mouth Gag

A mouth gag (Fig. 15.79B) may be used during dental anaesthesia and is required occasionally to open the mouth in patients with trismus, or if masseter spasm is present. It is positioned between the molar teeth and must be used with great care to avoid dental trauma.

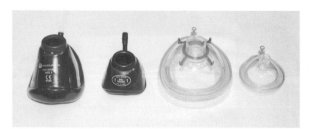

FIGURE 15.78 ■ Sizes 1 and 5 reusable (left) and disposable (right) face masks.

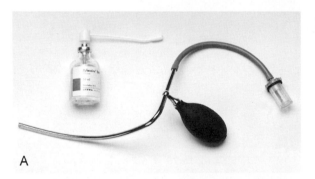

A

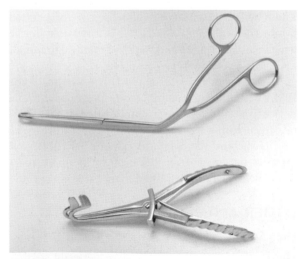

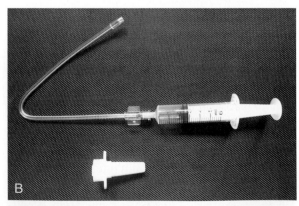

B

FIGURE 15.79 ■ Magill intubating forceps (above). The Ferguson mouth gag (below).

FIGURE 15.80 ■ Laryngeal sprays. (**A**) Forrester spray and the 10% lidocaine prefilled laryngeal spray. (**B**) The mucosal atomizing device (MAD).

Bougie

If the larynx cannot be seen adequately during laryngoscopy, or if the tracheal tube cannot be manoeuvred into the laryngeal inlet, a bougie may be used as an aid to tracheal intubation. The lubricated bougie is inserted into the trachea to act as a guide for the tracheal tube. The tube should be rotated so that the bevel does not become lodged against the aryepiglottic fold. In a difficult intubation scenario, the correct type of bougie should be used (Fig. 15.81). The bougie with a curved tip at the end is designed to assist in this situation whereas the straight-ended bougie is intended for endotracheal tube exchange only. Disposable bougies are now available but their efficacy over the reusable ones is yet to be demonstrated. The Eschmann (gum elastic) multiple-use bougie has the highest success rate, least likelihood of causing trauma and has reliable and clinically tested signs of confirmation of tracheal placement when compared with either the Frova single-use intubation introducer or the Portex single-use introducer.

Stilettes

A malleable metal stilette may be used to adjust the degree of curvature of a tracheal tube as an aid to its insertion. The stilette must not protrude from the distal end of the tube.

The Aintree Intubating Catheter (AIC)

This is a 56-cm hollow catheter with special adapters that connect to either a 15-mm connector for use with conventional anaesthetic circuits or a Luer lock for use with a jet ventilator (Fig. 15.82). The catheter has an internal diameter of 4.8 mm which allows it to be preloaded over a fibreoptic scope.

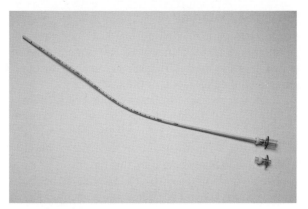

FIGURE 15.82 ■ Aintree Intubating Catheter (AIC).

The AIC is used for LMA-assisted orotracheal fibreoptic intubation. However, it should not be used without prior training as failure to follow the correct instructions can result in serious morbidity or mortality.

Airways

An oropharyngeal airway (Guedel airway, Fig. 15.83) may be required to prevent obstruction caused by the tongue or collapse of the pharynx in the patient without a tracheal tube. A nasopharyngeal airway (Fig. 15.83) is tolerated better during light anaesthesia and may also be used if it is difficult to insert an oropharyngeal airway, e.g. trismus. However, the use of nasopharyngeal airways may be associated with significant bleeding from the nose.

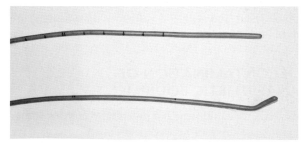

FIGURE 15.81 ■ The straight-ended multiple-use bougie (above) and the angled-end multiple-use bougie (below).

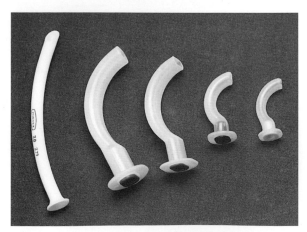

FIGURE 15.83 ■ A nasopharyngeal airway (left) and Guedel airways.

Suction Apparatus

Suction apparatus is vital during anaesthesia and re-suscitation to clear the airway of any mucus, blood or debris. It is also used during surgery to clear the operating field of either blood or fluid.

Suction apparatus consists of a source of vacuum, a suction unit and suction tubing. The source of vacuum can be either piped vacuum or electrically or manually operated units. Piped vacuum is the most commonly used source in many operating theatres.

The suction unit consists of a reservoir jar, bacterial filter, vacuum control regulator and a vacuum gauge (Fig. 15.84). The reservoir jar is graduated so that the volume of aspirate may be estimated. It contains a cut-off valve. The cut-off valve has a float that rises as the fluid level increases and shuts off the valve when the reservoir jar is full. This prevents liquid from the suction jar entering the suction system. There is a bacterial filter between the cut-off valve and the suction control unit to prevent air that has been contaminated during passage through the apparatus infecting the atmosphere when it is blown out. The filter also traps any particulate or nebulized matter. Filters should be changed at regular intervals.

The vacuum regulator adjusts the degree of vacuum. The vacuum is indicated on the pressure gauge. This is normally marked in mmHg or kPa. The needle on the gauge goes in an anticlockwise direction as the vacuum increases. Suction units can achieve flows of

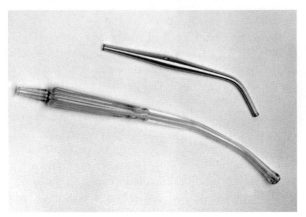

FIGURE 15.85 ■ Yankauer suction catheters. Paediatric (above) and adult apparatus.

greater than $25\,L\,min^{-1}$ and a vacuum of greater than $67\,kPa$. However, flows and vacuum as high as these are seldom necessary and can cause harm if used inappropriately, particularly in children.

The suction reservoir jar is connected to the patient via a suction tubing and either a Yankauer hand piece (Fig. 15.85) or suction catheters.

Head-Elevating Laryngoscopy Position Devices

Many studies have been conducted over the last ten years investigating the effect of a head-elevated position or ramping on laryngeal view. An imaginary line drawn between the patient's sternal notch should be in line with the auditory meatus in order to maximize the laryngeal view. Ramping or the head-elevated laryngoscopy position has been shown to improve the laryngeal view, particularly in obese patients. This has led to the development of devices such as the Oxford Head-Elevating Laryngoscopy Pillow (Oxford HELP) (Fig. 15.86). This device can be inserted and removed much faster and with less difficulty than using standard hospital pillows.

DECONTAMINATION OF ANAESTHETIC EQUIPMENT

Anaesthetic equipment is a potential vector for transmission of diseases between patients. Concerns have been raised about the possibility that multiple-use devices may transfer blood-borne infections between

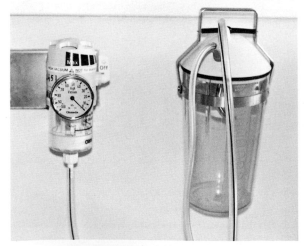

FIGURE 15.84 ■ Suction apparatus.

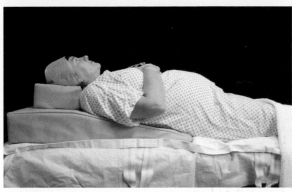

FIGURE 15.86 ■ The Oxford Head-Elevating Laryngoscopy Pillow (HELP).

patients and there is also the possibility of transfer of the prions thought to be responsible for causing variant Creutzfeldt-Jakob disease (vCJD). The guidelines of the AAGBI state that single-use, disposable anaesthetic equipment should always be used when possible. For reusable anaesthetic equipment, compliance with local hospital control policies and awareness of decontamination practices are important in minimizing the risk of cross-infection. Anaesthetic equipment such as breathing systems, laryngoscopes and fibreoptic endoscopes are classified as semi-critical items because they come in contact with mucous membranes and non-intact skin but do not ordinarily break the blood barrier. They present an intermediate risk of transmitting infection. It is therefore recommended that these should have a high level of disinfection. High concentrations of disinfectants such as glutaraldehyde, stabilized hydrogen peroxide, peracetic acid, chlorine and chlorine-releasing compounds should be used.

FURTHER READING

Al-Shaikh, B., Stacey, S., 2010. Essentials of anaesthetic equipment, third ed. Churchill Livingstone, London.

Association of Anaesthetists of Great Britain and Ireland, 2008. Infection control in anaesthesia 2. AAGBI, London.

Association of Anaesthetists of Great Britain and Ireland, 2012. Checking anaesthetic equipment. Anaesthesia 67, 660–668.

Davey, A., Diba, A., 2005. Anaesthetic equipment, fifth ed. WB Saunders, London.

Dorsch, J.A., Dorsch, S.E., 2008. Understanding anaesthetic equipment, fifth ed. Williams and Wilkins, London.

Gabbott, B.M., 2001. Recent advances in airway technology. BJA CEPD Reviews 1, 76–80.

Patel, B., Frerk, C., 2008. Large bore cricothyroidotomy devices. Continuing Education in Anaesthesia, Critical Care and Pain 8, 157–160.

Popat, M., 2009. Difficult airway management, first ed. Oxford University Press, Oxford.

Sabir, N., Ramachandra, V., 2004. Decontamination of anaesthetic equipment. Continuing Education in Anaesthesia, Critical Care and Pain 4, 103–106.

Sinclair, C., Thadsad, M.K., Barker, I., 2006. Modern anaesthetic machines. Continuing Education in Anaesthesia, Critical Care and Pain 6, 75–78.

16 CLINICAL MEASUREMENT AND MONITORING

■ ■ ■ ■ ■ ■ ■ ■ ■ ■ ■

The ability to measure and monitor the physiology of patients is fundamental to modern anaesthesia. The anaesthetist is responsible for the correct use of sophisticated instruments which extend clinical observations beyond the human senses and enhance patient care. This requires vigilance and awareness of the limitations of the processes of measurement and the many causes of error. Uncritical acceptance of the recordings of monitoring equipment in the face of contradictory evidence is a common mistake. Unreliable measurements that are taken at face value and used to change patient management compromise the safety and effectiveness of care. It is essential that those who use monitors understand their limitations and are able to justify their risks.

Clinical measurement is limited by four major constraints:

- *Feasibility of measurement.* The sensitivity and inherent variability of a clinical measurement depend on complex interactions and technical difficulties at the biological interface between the patient and the instrument.
- *Reliability* of measurements is determined by the properties of the measurement system. This is influenced by the calibration and correct use of the instrument. Simple examples include the correct placement of ECG electrodes, or the appropriate size of cuff for non-invasive measurement of arterial pressure. Delicate equipment, e.g. a blood gas analyser, requires regular maintenance and calibration.
- *Interpretation* depends on the critical faculties of the anaesthetist who interprets the significance of measurements in the context of complex physiological systems. Arterial pressure may be within the normal range despite severe hypovolaemia or derangement of cardiovascular function within the limits of physiological compensation. Global measurements of end-tidal carbon dioxide tension or oxygen saturation are influenced by many factors in a highly complex system. More information is required to deduce the cause of a change in the measurement.
- *Value* of clinical measurements in patient care is defined by the role of a measurement in improving patient care. This includes the ease, convenience, continuity and usefulness of a clinical measurement, and evidence of improvement in patient safety and clinical outcome.

Monitoring is the process by which clinical measurements are assessed and used to direct therapy. In general, monitors consist of four components (Table 16.1): (1) a device which connects to the patient – this may either be a direct attachment or via a tube or lead; (2) a measuring device, often a transducer which converts the properties of the patient into an electrical signal; (3) a computer which may amplify

TABLE 16.1
Four Components of a Monitor

Connection to patient
Measuring device
Electronic filter/amplifier
Display

the signal, filter it and integrate it with other variables to produce a variety of derived variables; (4) a display which may show the results as a wave, a number or a combination. It is important to appreciate that most monitors do not directly measure the displayed variable, and that the displayed variable may not reflect physiological function. For example, an electrocardiograph (ECG) does not measure cardiac function and therefore a normal ECG trace does not guarantee that the heart is pumping effectively. When interpreting measurements, the following questions should be asked:

- *What is being measured?* In the case of arterial pressure, there is an obvious answer. However, in some cases, for example 'depth of anaesthesia', it may not be clear what the monitor is measuring. In addition, many monitors use data from a variety of sources. For example, heart rate is usually derived from the ECG. However, if the ECG fails to provide the data required, the monitor often switches automatically to a rate from either a pulse oximeter or an arterial pressure waveform. Thus, the displayed value may change rapidly despite the patient remaining stable.
- *How is it measured?* Arterial pressure is often measured by either a transducer attached to an arterial cannula or an automated oscillometer. Although a transducer is often regarded as the more accurate, the readings must be compared with the preoperative values recorded on the ward, usually with an oscillometer. Therefore, where accurate control of arterial pressure is essential, it is advisable to start invasive pressure monitoring before anaesthesia to avoid any confusion with non-invasive measures.
- *Is the environment appropriate?* Many monitors have been designed for use in operating theatres and do not function correctly if exposed to the cold and vibration, for example in an ambulance or helicopter. Another example is the strong magnetic field produced by magnetic resonance imaging (MRI) scanners. The electrical currents induced may damage not only incompatible monitors but even produce burns to a patient's skin.
- *Is the patient appropriate?* Monitors designed for adult use often fail to produce reliable readings when used on small children. Particularly obese adults may require a large blood pressure cuff, and poor-quality ECG readings may be obtained.
- *Has the monitor been applied to the correct part of the patient?* For example, in aortic coarctation, arterial pressure may be markedly different in each arm. Pulse oximeters also fail to work reliably if placed on a limb distal to a blood pressure cuff.
- *Is the variable within the range of the monitor?* Most monitors are validated on healthy patients in laboratories. Whether such monitors continue to provide accurate results during the extreme physiological changes of, for example, anaphylaxis is uncertain. This does imply that the usefulness of monitors declines with the health of the patient: that is, they are least reliable when needed most. In most cases of acute perioperative patient deterioration, additional monitoring is needed.
- *Has the monitor been checked, serviced and calibrated at the correct intervals?* To reduce costs, departments may re-use single-use equipment and fail to ensure that service checks are carried out. All equipment should be tagged with a service sticker. This should identify the date serviced, when the next service is due and who to contact in case of malfunction. Equipment which has not been serviced or is past its service date should not be used.

Table 16.2 shows the checks which the anaesthetist should follow before using a patient monitor.

This chapter describes the feasibility and reliability of clinical measurements relevant to anaesthetic practice, and how such measurements are used to monitor the patient's physiology.

· TABLE 16.2
Premonitoring Checks
What is being measured?
What method is being used?
Has the monitor been serviced and calibrated?
Is the environment appropriate?
Is the patient appropriate?
Is it attached to the appropriate part of the patient?
Is the range appropriate?
Can the display be read?
Are the alarms on and have the limits been set?

PROCESS OF CLINICAL MEASUREMENT

Stages of Clinical Measurement

There are four stages of clinical measurement:

- detection of the biological signal, by a sensing device which responds to a characteristic signal in the form of electrical, mechanical, electromagnetic, chemical or thermal energy
- transduction, in which the output from the sensor is converted into another form of energy, usually to a continuous electrical signal
- amplification and signal processing to extract and magnify the relevant features of the signal and reduce unwanted noise
- display and storage – the output from the instrument is presented to the operator. Storage for future use may be achieved using mechanical markers, printed copy or computer memory.

Mechanical instruments use the signal energy to drive a display, with minimal intermediate processing. The height of a fluid-column manometer provides a visible index of pressure. The expansion of mercury within the confines of a thin glass column is a measure of temperature. Mechanical springs and gearing translate the rotation of a vane into the recording of expired volume on a dial. However, the overwhelming trend is for nonelectrical signals to be converted by a transducer to an electrical signal suitable for electronic processing by digital computers.

The Microprocessor Revolution

The development of digital microprocessors over the last 25 years has revolutionized anaesthetic practice. Beautifully engineered mechanical instruments, e.g. the von Recklinghausen oscillotonometer, are now obsolete in developed countries.

Advantages of digital signal processing include:

- continuous real-time detection, processing and recording of measurements
- increased range of measurements possible
- miniaturization of complicated and powerful instruments
- sophisticated artefact rejection and noise reduction algorithms
- complex on-line mathematical and statistical signal processing in upgradeable software, e.g. Fourier analysis of the EEG

- automated control of the apparatus and the timing and process of measurement, and integration of alarms
- storage in memory, permitting trend analysis, future display and further analysis
- user-friendly audio-visual display of recordings, integrating many simultaneous clinical measurements, and able to be customized by the user
- less maintenance than analogue instruments.

There are a few important disadvantages:

- dependence on electrically powered equipment
- degradation of clinical skills and alternative manual measurements through disuse
- impoverished understanding of the principles of complex measuring equipment and the requirements for correct use
- illusion of the unquestionable accuracy of measurements produced by expensive computer-controlled equipment and presented on an impressive display or typed copy.

Essential Requirements for Clinical Measurement

All clinical measurement systems detect a biological signal and reproduce this input signal in the form of a display or record which is presented to the operator. The degree to which a discrete measurement is a true reflection of the underlying signal is defined by its accuracy and precision.

Accuracy is the difference between the measurements and the real biological signal, or in practice, a different and superior 'gold standard' measurement. Calibration against predetermined signals is used to test and optimally adjust measuring instruments. For absolute measurements, e.g. arterial pressure, one point must be a fixed reference or 'zero'.

Precision describes the reproducibility of repeated measurements of the same biological signal. This dispersion is usually described by summary statistics, standard deviation for normally distributed measurements, or the range for non-normal distributions. A single recording is unreliable when the measurement is imprecise. This is especially true of tests which require patient cooperation, practised skill or effort, e.g. peak expiratory flow rate. Repeated measurements demonstrate the variability in response.

The Importance of Repeated Measurements

Differences in repeated clinical measurements arise from three causes:

- change in the clinical condition of the patient
- variability inherent in the biological signal or measuring instrument
- confounding errors – the recorded measurement does not reflect the signal.

The anaesthetist must be satisfied with the accuracy and precision of any clinical measurement used in patient management. Repeated measurements which are consistent ensure that the measurement is representative, i.e. precise, but do not ensure accuracy. For example, repeated recordings of invasive arterial pressure may be extremely consistent, but erroneous if the transducer is not calibrated against the correct zero point. Defences against the uncritical acceptance of inaccurate measurements include meticulous care in calibrating instruments and recording of clinical measurements, and reflection on clinical measurements which do not fit the clinical state of the patient or other related measurements. A discrepant result should be rechecked, using a different measurement technique if possible, before it is used to change patient management. This is especially true of complex, operator-dependent techniques such as measurement of cardiac output.

Measurement of Continuous Signals Over Time

Continuous signals, which include the majority of modern clinical measurements such as biological electrical signals and the electrical output of signal transducers, introduce the complication of the response of the measuring instrument to a changing signal over time. The reliability with which a continuous signal is reproduced is defined by the relationship between input and output of the measurement system over the clinical range of signal magnitude and frequency. The input–output function of an accurate clinical measurement system would demonstrate good zero and gain stability, minimal amplitude non-linearity and hysteresis, and an adequate frequency response. This cannot be taken for granted, particularly with older equipment or with variations in environmental temperature or humidity.

Zero Stability

The ability of a measurement to maintain a zero reading on the display or record when the input signal is zero defines the zero stability. The importance of zero instability depends on the magnitude relative to the signal, e.g. a zero drift of a few millimetres of mercury is much less important for the measurement of arterial pressure than it is for intracranial pressure.

Gain Stability

The majority of biological signals are amplified before reproduction. This 'gain' may be fixed or controlled by the user. When set, this should remain constant over the period of recording.

Amplitude Linearity

The degree of amplification of the signal should be constant over the whole range of signal amplitudes. Manufacturers usually specify the degree of linearity of electronic components over a certain amplitude range. The amplitude linearity of a complete clinical system may be confirmed easily in an electronics laboratory by comparing the output to known, standardized test signals.

Hysteresis

Some instruments, such as thermistors and humidity sensors, may display hysteresis. This is a special case of non-linearity, in which the output differs depending on whether the input signal is increasing or decreasing.

Frequency Response

Many biological signals vary in a complicated and rapidly changing pattern. Accurate reproduction of a complex waveform requires that all of the component frequencies which make up the waveform are processed in an identical manner. This requires more than simply equal amplification irrespective of frequency, i.e. no amplitude distortion. It also implies that the relative positions of the various frequency components of the waveform are not shifted, i.e. no phase distortion. In practice, accurate reproduction up to the 10th harmonic of the fundamental frequency is sufficient for clinical purposes, e.g. 30 Hz for an arterial pressure waveform associated with heart rates up to 180 beats min^{-1} (3 Hz).

Signal-to-Noise Ratio

Biological signals are obscured to a variable degree by unwanted or extraneous signals which have similar physical characteristics and are described as noise, e.g. heart sounds become difficult to detect in the presence of continuous, noisy breath sounds. The efficiency of isolation of the signal from unwanted biological signals and electronic noise sources in the equipment is defined by the signal-to-noise ratio. The variability of the amplitudes of signal and noise is enormous and the signal-to-noise ratio is described using a logarithmic scale of decibels. Microvolt EEG measurements are particularly susceptible to noise from many sources. Biological noise includes contaminating ECG and EMG potentials, particularly from the scalp muscles, and interference from electrochemical activity at the skin–electrode interface. Electrostatic and electromagnetic linkage between the recording wires and nearby sources of mains electricity generates noise which is predominantly 50 Hz frequency and harmonics. Radiofrequency noise from diathermy or transmitters may also be picked up at this stage. Physical disturbance of the recording wires causes tiny changes in capacitive potentials and may add low-frequency noise, called microphony. Thermal noise is added during amplification, particularly at the input stage when the signal is in the microvolt range. Good amplifier design, electronic filtering of unwanted frequencies and modern techniques of digital signal processing may extract small signals from considerable background noise, but this inevitably introduces some distortion of the signal. Prevention of contamination of the signal by minimizing sources of noise before the signal is amplified is always preferable. The operator is responsible for correctly using measuring instruments to optimize the signal and for applying knowledge of the physical principles of the measurement to minimize contamination by noise.

Analogue and Digital Processing

Following signal detection and appropriate transduction, the continuously variable analogue signal is amplified, processed and displayed for the attention of the clinician.

Mechanical Measuring Instruments

Measuring instruments based on mechanical principles lack the flexibility and automated control of computerized devices, but use ingenious methods for processing and displaying analogue measurements. For example, mechanical spirometers use precision-engineered gears to translate the movement of a piston or vane into the rotation of a calibrated dial.

Analogue Computers

Analogue computers use hardware comprising electronic circuits and operational amplifiers. Signals are processed in the form of continuously variable electric potentials. Analogue hardware components continuously perform a wide variety of mathematical functions on a rapidly changing input waveform. Integration and differentiation are formidable mathematical tasks for a digital computer, which can be solved simply and cheaply using analogue circuits comprising capacitors and resistors. Integration of the flow signal from a pneumotachograph produces a volume waveform.

Microcomputers and Digital Signal Processing

Digital signal processing offers a powerful alternative to mechanical processing and analogue computation. A fundamental step in this process is the conversion of a continuous analogue electrical signal into a discrete digital form. This analogue-to-digital conversion is achieved by measuring or 'sampling' the continuous input signal at regular intervals, to produce a series of discrete measurements over time which are in a suitable format for digital computation. The overwhelming advantage of digital processing is that the manipulation of the digitized signal is performed by a flexible and unlimited series of software calculations which range from mathematical functions to the analysis of statistical properties and trends.

Analogue-to-Digital Conversion

The core processing units of digital computers assume one of two stable states, i.e. a binary, rather than decimal, code. This imposes a limit on the resolving power of the digital processor, although with increasing processing power this limit has become negligible. Earlier 8-bit computing comprised a binary number of eight digits representing 2^8 integer decimal numbers, from binary 00000000=decimal 0 to binary 11111111=decimal 255. In short, an 8-bit converter can resolve an analogue signal with an accuracy of one part in 255, i.e. with an amplitude resolution of 0.4% of full scale. A 12-bit converter is more accurate, with a resolving power of one part in 4095 or 0.02% of full scale. More modern processors are capable of 32-bit computing corresponding to a range of 2^{32} integer decimal numbers (a resolving power of 0.00000002%), with 64-bit processors now commonly found in domestic computer equipment. Whilst highly accurate, the cost of this improvement in resolution is more expensive hardware to digitize, process and store considerably more digital information.

Amplitude resolution is not the only determinant of the accuracy of analogue-to-digital conversion. Resolution over time, determined by the sampling frequency, is also important. A relatively low sampling frequency may provide a representative sample of values for a slowly changing waveform but it may inadequately represent high-frequency components and introduce an aliasing error, in which different signals become indistinguishable. The Nyquist theorem suggests that the minimum sampling frequency to maintain the integrity of the waveform is at least twice the highest frequency component with significant amplitude in the input signal waveform, e.g. a sampling frequency of 100 Hz would adequately capture the fastest rate of change in a physiological pressure signal.

The immensely powerful and complicated hardware and software programming instructions responsible for performing the tasks of digitizing, processing, storing and displaying the input signal are hidden from view in the commercial 'black box'.

Data Display

Useful instruments communicate measurements in an appropriate and user-friendly manner.

Analogue Displays

A continuously variable signal, such as pressure or temperature, is represented by an analogue display in terms of the amplitude of a physical quantity on a calibrated scale, dial, electrical meter or printed record. The glass thermometer incorporates a wedge-shaped lens which magnifies the appearance of the mercury column against the calibrated background scale. The height of a water column manometer is a linear, visual scale of pressure. Simple mechanical displays are accurate and easily understood, but are inconvenient to read and most suitable for intermittent discrete measurements.

Mechanical spirometers and flowmeters record flow on a dial driven by gears. Electrical moving coil meters use a coil of wire suspended in a magnetic field which rotates in proportion to the applied current and moves a pointer on a calibrated dial. Alternatively, the amplified and filtered electrical signal could drive a chart recorder which produces a continuous printed record of the amplitude of measurements against time. Limitations common to these mechanical devices include fragile moving parts, and inertia which impairs the frequency response to rapidly changing signals.

The cathode ray oscilloscope is an effective screen-based display for continuous analogue electrical signals. A heated cathode generates a stream of electrons which are focused and accelerated onto a phosphorescent coating which lines the flat surface of the tube to generate a bright spot. The position of the electron beam in both x- and y-axes is controlled by electrostatic plates. The continuously varying input signal is applied to the y-plates so that deflection in the vertical y-axis is proportional to the amplitude of the signal. The absence of mechanical parts results in a high-frequency response. An electronic time-base circuit delivers a saw-tooth voltage to the x-plates which drives the electron beam across the x-axis at a constant rate and returns the beam to the left-hand side at the start of each sweep. This produces a dynamic image of signal amplitude against time. Alternatively, a second input signal may be applied to the x-plates to produce an x-y graphical plot, e.g. pressure–volume loop. Cathode ray oscilloscopes are widely used in electronic engineering and signal processing, but have been replaced in clinical practice by microprocessor-controlled displays.

Microprocessor-Controlled Displays

Digital signal processing has revolutionized clinical measurement. Modern monitors comprise a single system integrating various measurements of physiology, and display information as discrete measurements as well as continuous analogue waveforms (Fig. 16.1). This paradox, the conversion of analogue information into digital and then back to analogue, illustrates the real power of digital signal processing to manipulate and present information in a relevant and user-friendly manner. Data patterns (waveforms, trends, graphs) can be recreated or processed in other ways from the original digital signal to assist the anaesthetist, with

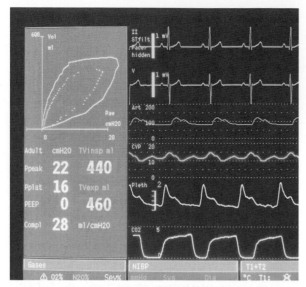

FIGURE 16.1 ■ Standard anaesthetic monitoring screen.

the original digital signal being stored in a computer record without degradation of the quality of the signal.

Most of the current monitoring systems follow good ergonomic principles, with different variables separated consistently by position on the screen and by colour. This allows the most important information to be placed centrally in large symbols or fonts and in bold colours, with less important data either relegated to small print, or placed in submenus. However, the flexibility of most monitors implies that it is still possible for individuals to change colours and priorities, often making the monitor much less effective. Whenever possible, departments should ensure that all monitors have identical default settings to reduce confusion (these are usually password protected). Unfortunately, the lack of international standards means that confusion may still occur if monitors from multiple sources are used in the same unit.

Despite many attempts to simplify patient data into geometric shapes or bar graphs, data continue to be displayed most often as simple numbers, supported by waveforms, e.g. invasive pressure, and a graphical display of trends over time. Trends are particularly useful when clinical problems may produce gradual change. For example, in neurosurgery, a gradual decrease in end-tidal carbon dioxide concentration is often associated with multiple air emboli.

BIOLOGICAL ELECTRICAL SIGNALS

The detection and recording of biological electrical potentials are important clinical measurements which incorporate many of the key principles of clinical measurement.

Depolarization of the cell membrane of excitable cells is fundamental to the action of these cells and generates a transient potential difference between the active cell and surrounding tissues. The summation of synchronous extracellular potentials from a large number of excitable cells generates a widespread electric field which can be detected by electrodes on the body surface. The electrocardiogram (ECG) and electroencephalogram (EEG) are two well-established measures of biological electrical activity.

Biological electrical signals are detected using electrodes constructed of silver and electrolytically coated with silver chloride. Low, stable impedances minimize mains interference. Symmetrical electrode impedance and insignificant polarization control drift. However, care is still required to achieve optimum results. The silver chloride layer is very thin, prone to deterioration and only suitable for single use. Movement artefacts which alter the electrode potential and impedance are greatly reduced if the electrode surface is separated from the skin by a foam pad impregnated with electrolyte gel. It is no longer necessary to abrade the skin to achieve ultra-low impedance, but de-greasing with alcohol before applying the electrode helps to reduce skin impedance and ensures satisfactory adhesion.

Amplification

The amplitude of tiny bioelectrical signals must be increased by amplification, and unwanted noise and interference minimized. Calibration voltages may be incorporated for correct adjustment of the gain of the amplifier.

Input Impedance and Common Mode Rejection

Amplifiers for biological signals require high common mode rejection and high input impedance. The input and electrode impedances act as a potential divider: high electrode impedance and low amplifier input impedance attenuate the electrical signal across the amplifier. The input impedance of modern amplifiers exceeds 5 MΩ to avoid problems, and careful attention must be paid to minimizing electrode impedance, particularly for EEG recordings.

Differential amplification is a powerful method of reducing unwanted noise. The potential difference between two input signals is amplified, but electrical signals common to both are attenuated. This feature is termed 'common mode rejection' and very effectively reduces mains interference in all biological signals and electrocardiographic contamination of much smaller electroencephalographic signals. The common mode rejection ratio (CMRR) for a typical differential amplifier exceeds 10000:1. In other words, a signal applied equally to both input terminals would need to be 10000 times larger than a signal applied between them for the same change in output.

Frequency Response

The bandwidth of the amplifier must cover the range of frequencies which are important in the signal. In practice, amplifiers require a flat frequency response for ECG from 0.14 to 50 Hz, for EEG from 0.5 to 100 Hz and for EMG from 20 Hz to at least 2 kHz.

Low-frequency interference, largely caused by slow fluctuating potentials generated in the electrodes, produces baseline instability and drift. This is removed by incorporating a network of resistors and capacitors which function as a simple high-pass filter allowing biological signals to pass, but attenuating low-frequency noise. This introduces a compromise in amplifier design between signal trace fidelity and stability of recording. For example, amplifiers designed for diagnostic electrocardiography have long time constants with optimal reproduction of the waveform at the expense of baseline instability, especially to movement. In comparison, continuity of recording is more important when the electrocardiogram is used for monitoring during anaesthesia; high-pass filtering produces a short time constant and good baseline stability at the expense of waveform reproduction. Low-frequency elements of the ECG, such as the T wave, may become differentiated by phase shift in the high-pass filter and appear distorted or biphasic.

Other filters can attenuate particular frequencies. Highly selective band reject filters attenuate 50 Hz interference from the signal. Low-pass filters are used to eliminate higher-frequency artefacts from an EEG

signal. The purpose of filtering is to reduce unwanted noise relative to the signal. When the frequency range of signal and noise overlap, some degree of signal degradation is inevitable.

Noise and Interference

Electrical noise arising from the patient, the patient-electrode interface or the surroundings may seriously interfere with accurate recording of biological potentials.

Noise Originating from the Patient. Millivolt ECG potentials on the body surface are hundreds of times larger than microvolt EEG signals on the scalp. EMG signals may be even larger, and muscular activity, especially shivering, causes severe interference. Two features of electronic amplifier design substantially improve the EEG signal-to-noise ratio. ECG potentials are essentially the same across the scalp and are ignored by amplifiers with a high common mode rejection. EMG activity has a higher frequency content than the EEG signal, and may be minimized by a low-pass filter which attenuates the higher-frequency response of the amplifier to a level which attenuates the EMG signals and does not interfere with the characteristics of the EEG.

Noise Originating from the Patient–Electrode Interface. Recording electrodes do not behave as passive conductors. All skin–metal electrode systems employ a metal surface in contact with an electrolyte solution. Polarization describes the interaction between metal and electrolyte which generates a small electrical gradient. Electrodes comprising metal plated with one of its own salts, e.g. silver—silver chloride, avoid this problem because current in each direction does not significantly change the electrolyte composition. Mechanical movement of recording electrodes may also cause significant potential gradients – alteration in the physical dimensions of the electrode changes the cell potential and skin–electrode impedance. Differences in potential between two electrodes connected to a differential amplifier are amplified and asymmetry of electrode impedance seriously impairs the common mode rejection ratio of the recording amplifier.

Noise Originating Outside the Patient. *Electrical interference.* Mains frequency interference with the recording of biological potentials may be troublesome, particularly in electromagnetically noisy clinical environments. Patients function physically as large unscreened conductors and interact with nearby electrical sources through the processes of capacitive coupling and electromagnetic induction.

Capacitance permits alternating current to pass across an air gap. A live mains conductor and nearby patient behave as the two plates of a capacitor. The very small mains frequency current which flows through the patient is of no clinical significance but confounds the detection and amplification of biological potentials, creating unwanted interference in the recording. Capacitive coupled interference is minimized by reducing the capacitance and the alternating potential difference. This is achieved by moving the patient away from the source of interference and by screening mains-powered equipment with a conductive surround which is maintained at earth potential by a low-resistance earth connection and by surrounding leads with a braided copper screen – stray capacitances couple with the screen instead of the lead.

Alternating currents in a conductor generate a magnetic flux. This induces voltages in any nearby conductors which lie in the changing magnetic flux, including the patient or signal leads to the amplifier, which function as inefficient secondary transformers. This source of interference is minimized by keeping patients as far as possible from powerful sources of electromagnetic flux, especially mains transformers. Electromagnetic inductance may be minimized by ensuring that all patient leads are the same length, closely bound or twisted together until very close to the electrodes. This ensures that the induced signals are identical in all leads and therefore susceptible to common mode rejection.

The importance of low electrode impedance. Low electrode impedance may exaggerate the effects of surrounding electrical interference. Capacitive and inductive coupling produce very small currents in the recording leads. If the electrode impedance is low, the potential at the amplifier input must remain close to the potential at the skin surface, so that minimal interference results. If electrode impedance is high, the small induced currents may create a significant potential difference across that impedance, leading to severe 50 Hz interference.

Radiofrequency interference from diathermy is a severe problem for the recording of biological potentials. ECG amplifiers may be provided with some protection by filtering the signal before it enters the isolated input circuit, filtering the power supply to block mains-borne radiofrequencies and enclosing the electronic components in a double screen, the outer earthed and the inner at amplifier potential.

BIOLOGICAL MECHANICAL SIGNALS

Pressure is a mechanical signal fundamental to measurement and monitoring in anaesthesia. Several physical principles and a wide range of instruments are used to measure pressure. Liquid column manometers display pressure according to the height of a column of fluid relative to a predefined zero-point, and the density of the fluid. Mechanical pressure gauges are used widely, particularly in high-pressure gas supplies; pressure-dependent mechanical movement is amplified by a gearing mechanism which drives a pointer across a scale.

For most physiological pressure measurements, diaphragm gauges are used – a flexible diaphragm moves according to the applied pressure. Mechanical display of diaphragm movement is limited by poor sensitivity to small pressures, inertia to changing pressure and a narrow range of linear response. In modern diaphragm gauges used for sensing dynamic pressures, movement of the diaphragm is sensed by a device which converts the mechanical energy imparted to the diaphragm into electrical energy.

Electromechanical Transducers

The first step in transduction is movement of the diaphragm caused by the relationship to applied pressure. This depends on the stiffness of the diaphragm and substantially determines the operating characteristics of the transducer. Linearity of amplitude and frequency response are improved by using small stiff diaphragms which require a more sensitive mechanism for sensing diaphragm movement.

Wire strain gauges are based on the principle that stretching or compression of a wire changes the electrical resistance. Changes in capacitance or inductance have also been coupled to movement of a diaphragm. Silicon strain gauges use the changes in resistance in a thin slice of silicon crystal which occur when it is compressed or expanded. They are very sensitive and suitable for incorporation into a small stiff diaphragm with excellent frequency response, but non-linearity and temperature dependence are difficult technical problems.

Optical transduction senses movement of the diaphragm by reflecting light from the silvered back of the convex diaphragm on to a photocell. Applied pressure causes the silvered surface to become more convex. This causes the reflected light beam to diverge, reducing the intensity of reflected light sensed by the photoelectric cell. This design is used in a fibreoptic cardiac catheter for intravascular pressure measurement. These miniature pressure transducers are expensive but have a high-frequency response and fibreoptic light sources eliminate the risk of microshock.

THE CARDIOVASCULAR SYSTEM

The principal aim of an anaesthetist is to ensure the delivery of oxygen to the patient's tissues. In physiological terms, oxygen delivery is the product of the cardiac output, the concentration of haemoglobin and its oxygen saturation. Clinically, if the patient is pink, with a normal volume pulse and has warm extremities, then these aims are being met. When combined with a urine output of greater than 0.5 mL h^{-1} it is unlikely that the patient has any cardiovascular problems. A further confirmatory test, especially useful in children, is the capillary refill time. When an extremity is compressed for 5 s, if capillary refill occurs in less than 1.5 s, cardiac output is adequate. If the refill time is greater than 5 s, then shock is likely to be present.

The need for direct patient observation cannot be overestimated. Literally having a 'finger on the pulse' and being able to see the patient are the most important safety factors. While factors such as drapes and dimmed theatre lights may make direct observation difficult, there should not be complete reliance on electronic monitoring.

Electrocardiography

The electrocardiogram (ECG) is a well-established measure of myocardial electrical activity. The synchronous depolarization and prolonged action potentials in cardiac muscle summate to generate a potential field of high amplitude. This potential difference is detected between two electrodes placed on the body surface. In the three-lead system commonly in use, the third lead is used as a reference electrode. The voltage changes are very small (1 mV in amplitude with a frequency response of 0.05–100 Hz) and require amplification before being displayed as the familiar waveform.

Different lead positions detect electrical activity from different parts of the myocardium. The commonest position of the electrodes used in the operating theatre is the CM5 arrangement, as this is the best position to detect ischaemia of the left ventricle (Fig. 16.2).

The ECG is a standard monitor used on all anaesthetized patients. The visible waveform allows the cardiac rhythm to be identified and may often be printed for further analysis. Alarms may be set to identify arrhythmias and brady/tachycardias. Many monitors are able to display a numerical value of the heart rate in addition to a measure of any ST segment depression/elevation produced by cardiac ischaemia/infarction. This may be displayed as a trend over time and the success of treatment observed.

Unfortunately, the relatively small voltages measured are easily swamped by skeletal muscle activity or surgical diathermy, often leading to false alarms. The signal may also be severely degraded if the gel of the electrodes has been allowed to dry out or if the weight of the leads is allowed to pull on the electrodes.

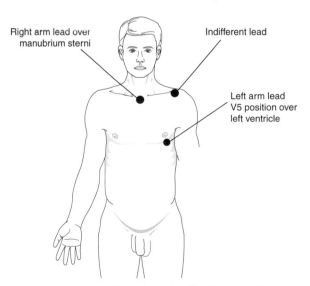

Right arm lead over manubrium sterni

Indifferent lead

Left arm lead V5 position over left ventricle

FIGURE 16.2 ■ CM5 configuration for electrocardiograph monitoring.

In addition, the monitor only identifies ischaemia in a single area; multiple lead systems are required to monitor the whole myocardium. While the ECG has become a standard monitor, it adds little to the information provided by palpating the pulse. It must be remembered that electrical activity does not always produce a cardiac output. Complications are rare, although the electrode adhesive may produce skin damage in susceptible patients.

Arterial Pressure

Indirect Methods

An adequate arterial pressure is essential for tissue perfusion; even when perfusion is adequate, hypotension may lead to renal failure. Indirect methods of measuring arterial pressure do not depend on contact between arterial blood and the system for signal recognition and transduction. Arterial pressure may be most rapidly estimated by palpating a pulse, although this method is too unreliable as a single technique. The majority depend on signals generated by the occlusion of a major artery using a cuff, known as the Riva-Rocci method. Systolic pressure can be estimated by the return of a palpable distal pulse; auscultation of the Korotkoff sounds can determine systolic and diastolic pressures. These methods, however, are too time-consuming during anaesthesia and often impossible because of poor access to the patient's arm.

Oscillometric Measurement of Arterial Pressure

The oscillometric measurement of arterial pressure estimates arterial pressure by analysis of the pressure oscillations which are produced in an occluding cuff by pulsatile blood flow in the underlying artery during deflation of the cuff (Fig. 16.3). The original automatic oscillometers used two cuffs. The upper cuff was inflated to occlude the arterial flow and then gradually deflated. As the blood flow began to pass under the upper cuff, the small changes in volume were detected by the lower cuff with an electromechanical pressure transducer. Modern machines use a single cuff with two tubes for inflation/measurement. During slow deflation, each pulse wave produces a pressure transient in the cuff which may be distinguished from the slowly decreasing ambient pressure in the cuff. Above systolic pressure, the transients are small, but suddenly increase in magnitude when the cuff pressure reaches the systolic point. As the cuff pressure decreases further, the amplitude reaches a peak and then starts to diminish. The mean arterial pressure correlates closely with the lowest cuff pressure

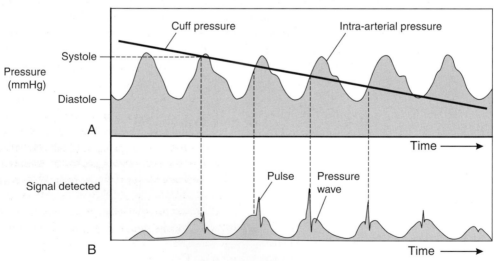

FIGURE 16.3 ■ Diagram showing: (**A**) Relationship between cuff pressure and intra-arterial pressure as cuff pressure decreases during oscillometry; (**B**) the signal created by the relative pressure changes in A. The sharp spikes of pressure in B are created by the walls of the artery opening and closing. These spikes are detected by a transducer first when the cuff pressure is just below systolic arterial pressure; their amplitude reaches a peak at mean arterial pressure and they cease when the cuff pressure is below diastolic pressure.

at which the maximum amplitude is maintained. As the cuff pressure reaches diastolic pressure, the transients abruptly diminish in amplitude. To avoid high cuff pressures and long deflation times, monitors inflate the cuff to just above a normal systolic pressure and then slowly decrease the pressure until a pulse is detected. Consequently, estimates of diastolic pressure can be unreliable. If a pulse is not detected, the cuff is then inflated to a higher pressure. This process may be repeated several times before a measurement is made.

Commercial instruments incorporate mechanisms for improving the reliability of the measurement. For example, at each successive plateau pressure during the controlled deflation, successive pressure fluctuations are compared and accepted only if they are similar. All automatic oscillometric instruments require a regular cardiac cycle with no great differences between successive pulses. Accurate and consistent readings may be impossible in patients with an irregular rhythm, particularly atrial fibrillation.

Clinical studies comparing automatic oscillometric instruments with direct arterial pressure have demonstrated good correlation for systolic pressure with a tendency to overestimate at low pressures and underestimate at high pressures. Mean and diastolic pressures were less reliable. The 95% confidence interval for all three indices exceeded 15 mmHg. The disadvantages of automated oscillometry are shown in Table 16.3.

Other Techniques. Measuring devices depend on the detection of movement of the arterial wall using changes in pressure or sound below audible frequencies

TABLE 16.3
Disadvantages of Automated Oscillometry

Delayed measurement with arrhythmias or patient movement

Inaccuracy with systolic pressure <60 mmHg

Inaccurate if the wrong size cuff used

May be inaccurate in obese patients

Discomfort in awake patients

Skin and nerve damage in prolonged use

Delay in injected drugs reaching the circulation

Backflow of blood into i.v. cannulae

Pulse oximeter malfunction as cuff is inflated

and detection of blood flow using the Doppler shift of an ultrasound signal, or plethysmography. Several other techniques have been used to measure arterial pressure, but have failed to find widespread usage. These include the Penaz technique, which measures the effect of external pressure on the blood flow through a finger, and other devices relying on pressure measurements over an artery, Doppler probes or detection of Korotkoff sounds with a microphone.

Direct Measurement

To measure arterial pressure directly, a cannula (usually 20–22G parallel-sided Teflon) must first be inserted into an artery (usually the radial because occlusion of the artery may be compensated for by flow through the ulnar artery). As fluids are incompressible, the pressure in the artery is transmitted directly to a transducer, which converts pressure into an electrical signal which is displayed by the monitor. The cost and complexity of pressure transducers are compensated by convenience, accuracy, continuity of measurement and an electrical output which may be processed, stored and displayed according to the requirements. The transducer should be at the level of the left ventricle and the transducer opened to the atmosphere to provide a zero reading before use. Monitors usually display systolic and diastolic pressures as well as the mean pressure, calculated automatically by integrating the area under the pressure waveform. The waveform provides useful additional information: a rapidly appreciated estimate of pressure, a qualitative assessment of the adequacy of the frequency response and damping, and an assessment of relative hypovolaemia during positive pressure as identified by the variability or 'swing' in the waveform.

The advantage of direct measurements is a real-time measure of arterial pressure, which is essential when administering drugs such as vasopressors to critically ill patients (Table 16.4). Such measurement systems also provide a means for obtaining samples for arterial blood gas analysis and other blood tests. The use of arterial cannulae has therefore become standard practice for severely ill patients, both in the operating theatre and in the intensive care unit.

However, errors are common as a result of malpositioning of the transducers and failure to zero the transducer before use. For example, if the operating

TABLE 16.4
Advantages of Direct Arterial Pressure Measurement

Accuracy of pressure measurement

Beat-by-beat observation of changes when blood pressure is variable or when vasoactive drugs are used

Accuracy at low pressures

Ability to obtain frequent blood samples

table is moved upwards while the transducer remains static, the difference in height artificially increases the pressure reading. Further, while modern disposable sets are usually reliable and accurate, they may occasionally malfunction. Unusual readings should therefore be checked against a reading from a non-invasive monitor. Complications relating to arterial cannulae are shown in Table 16.5.

Resonant Frequency and Damping. Fourier showed that all complex waveforms may be described as a mixture of simple sine waves of varying amplitude, frequency and phase. These consist of a fundamental wave, in this case at the pulse frequency, and a series of harmonics. The lower harmonics tend to have the greatest amplitude and a reasonable approximation to the arterial pressure waveform may be obtained by accurate reproduction of the fundamental and first 10 harmonics. In other words, to reproduce an arterial waveform at 120 beats min^{-1} accurately would require

TABLE 16.5
Complications Relating to Arterial Cannulae

Requires skill to insert

Bleeding

Pain on insertion

Arterial damage and thrombosis

Embolization of thrombus or air

Ischaemia to tissues distal to puncture site

Sepsis

Inadvertent injection of drugs

Late development of fistula or aneurysm

transduction with a linear frequency response up to a frequency of at least $(120{\times}10)/60{=}20\,Hz$. Accurate reproduction of a waveform requires that both the amplitude and phase difference of each harmonic are faithfully reproduced. This requires a transduction system with a natural frequency higher than the significant frequency components of the system, and the correct amount of damping.

The fluid and diaphragm of the transducer constitute a mechanical system which oscillates in simple harmonic motion at the natural resonant frequency. This determines the frequency response of the measurement system (Fig. 16.4). The resonant frequency of a catheter-transducer measuring system is highest, and the frictional resistance to fluid flow which dampens the frequency response is lowest, when the velocity of movement of fluid in the catheter is minimized. This is achieved with a stiff, low-volume displacement diaphragm and a short, wide, rigid catheter.

Determination of the Resonant Frequency and Damping. The resonant frequency and the effects of damping may be estimated by applying a step change in pressure to the catheter-transducer system and recording the response (Fig. 16.5). The underdamped system responds rapidly but overshoots and oscillates close to the natural resonant frequency of the system; frequency components of the pressure wave close to the resonant frequency are exaggerated. By contrast,

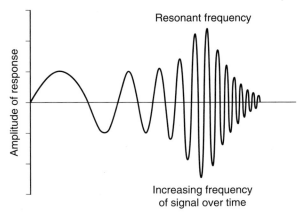

FIGURE 16.4 ■ Stimulation of the output of a catheter-transducer system with increasing frequency of a constant amplitude input signal. The linearity of response is lost as the frequency approaches the resonant frequency of the system.

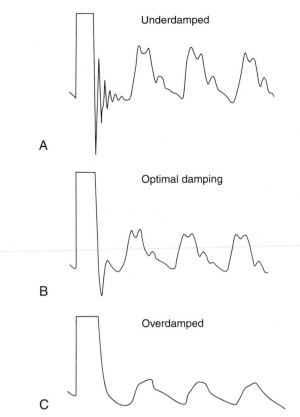

A — Underdamped

B — Optimal damping

C — Overdamped

FIGURE 16.5 ■ Damping of arterial pressure waves and the response to a square wave signal from the fast flush device.

minimum of constrictions or connections, approximate to this ideal. The system also includes a pressurized bag of saline which produces a flow of 1–3 mL h^{-1} through a restrictor to prevent clot formation, as well as the facility to allow a higher flow rate to flush the system, for example after a blood sample has been taken. Air bubbles in the system, clotting or kinking in the vascular catheter, and arterial spasm lower the natural resonant frequency and increase the damping.

In clinical practice, the resonant frequency of the whole system is uncomfortably close to the frequency content of the signal, and accurate measurements require optimal damping. However, damping is difficult to measure and control, and is poor compensation for an inadequate frequency response in the pressure recording system. Adjustment of damping is difficult to achieve and mechanical methods which include inserting constrictions or a compliant tube into the system to increase damping further reduce the resonant frequency. Electronic damping of the electrical output from the transducer cannot correct for non-linear amplification and attenuation of frequencies in the pressure wave before transduction.

Accuracy of Arterial Pressure Measurements

The accuracy of pressure measurements, particularly using indirect methods, needs to be considered. Invasive direct measurement of arterial pressure is the usual standard for comparison. However, the catheter-transducer system must be carefully set up and tested for optimal performance and this is hard to achieve in clinical practice. Arterial pressure varies throughout the arterial tree and the measured pressure depends on the site of measurement. As the pulse wave travels from the ventricle to peripheral arteries, changes in vessel diameter and elasticity affect the pressure waveform, which becomes narrower with increased amplitude. Differences in arterial pressure between limbs are common, particularly in patients with arterial disease.

Indirect methods using an occluding cuff make intermittent measurements, with the systolic and diastolic readings reflecting the conditions in the artery at two instants at which the end-points are detected. By contrast, direct pressure measurements are the average of a number of cycles, more precisely reflecting mean pressures. Indirect measurements may be

the overdamped system responds slowly and the recorded signal decreases slowly to reach the baseline, with no overshoot. High-frequency oscillations are damped, underestimating the true pressure changes. These extremes are undesirable.

Optimal Damping. Optimal damping maximizes the frequency response of the system, minimizes resonance and represents the best compromise between speed of response and accuracy of transduction. A small overshoot represents approximately 7% of the step change in pressure, with the pressure then following the arterial waveform (Fig. 16.5).

Damping is relatively unimportant when the frequencies being recorded are less than two-thirds of the natural frequency of the catheter-transducer system. Modern transducer systems using small compliance transducers connected to a short, stiff catheter, with a compromised by taking a small number of infrequent samples from a variable signal.

Central Venous Pressure

Central venous pressure is often considered a measure of the amount of blood within the venous system; a pressure less than normal (2–3 mmHg) indicates hypovolaemia and a higher pressure indicates volume overload. While such a view is reliable for healthy patients with acute blood loss, it is not so simple in other circumstances. For example, patients with damage to the right side of the heart may have raised central venous pressure even when the filling pressure of the left side of the heart is low. Single measurements rarely provide an accurate reflection of the fluid status of the patient. However, repeated measurements taken while a fluid challenge is given can be informative.

There are four common routes for central venous catheterization.

- Long catheters inserted via the antecubital fossa are relatively easy and safe to insert but are of small diameter. Catheters inserted via the basilic or cephalic vein are sometimes difficult to advance past the shoulder. It is also difficult to determine if the tip of the catheter is within a central vein without X-ray imaging. Thrombosis of the veins is common if the catheter is left *in situ* for more than 24 h.
- Femoral venous catheters are inserted just below the inguinal ligament. They are also relatively easy to insert and may be of large gauge to allow rapid transfusion of fluids. This route is often chosen in children. However, the site of insertion is often within a skin fold, making skin sepsis more likely.
- Internal jugular catheters are used most commonly because the vein is superficial, of larger diameter, and easily managed. This is the route which is often most appropriate for use in an emergency. However, the insertion point is adjacent to several vital structures, including the carotid artery, lung, brachial plexus and cervical spine, with the result that direct needle trauma to these structures can occur. Current guidelines recommend the use of an ultrasound probe for insertion of a catheter via the internal jugular route to improve the accuracy of insertion and to minimize complications.
- Subclavian catheters suffer the same problems as those in the internal jugular vein, although the point of insertion under the clavicle may make it easier to anchor the catheter to the skin. However, if accidental arterial puncture occurs, the overlying clavicle obscures bleeding and makes direct compression of the artery impossible. The proximity of the pleura is associated with a risk of accidental lung puncture. The subclavian route should therefore be used only when the internal jugular approach is contraindicated.

As the central venous pressure is relatively low, it may be measured using a simple manometer. However, a central venous catheter is usually connected to the same type of transducer and flush system described for arterial cannulae. This provides a continuous readout of pressure, allowing the effect of infusions of fluids to be assessed in real time. However, because the central venous pressure is low, great care is required to ensure that the pressure is measured relative to the correct zero point (the right atrium) on the patient (Fig. 16.6). Although a single reading of central venous pressure is of little diagnostic use, a change in response to fluid challenge is more useful. In general, if a fluid challenge has little effect on the central venous pressure, the patient is likely to be hypovolaemic. In contrast, a marked increase in pressure indicates fluid overload. However, in unwell patients, the correlation between the CVP response to a fluid challenge and circulating volume is poor. Caution is required in using this principle to guide fluid therapy in hospitalized patients.

Complications are infrequent but potentially serious, and are shown in Table 16.6.

Pulmonary Artery Pressure

Although a central venous cannula may be used to estimate venous volume, it measures the filling of the right side of the heart. However, cardiac output and systemic arterial pressure are determined primarily by the filling pressure of the left side of the heart. When introduced, the pulmonary artery flotation catheter (PAFC), with its ability to measure cardiac output and left atrial pressure, appeared to be a major advance. Recently, however, frequent complications, a lack of

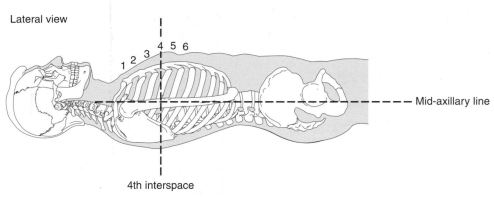

Lateral view

4 5 6

1 2 3

Mid-axillary line

4th interspace

FIGURE 16.6 ■ Surface markings used to identify the position of the right atrium.

TABLE 16.6
Complications of Central Venous Catheterization

Acute
Arrhythmias
Bleeding
Air embolus
Pneumothorax
Damage to thoracic duct, oesophagus, carotid artery, stellate ganglion
Cardiac puncture
Catheter embolization
Delayed
Sepsis
Thrombosis
Cardiac rupture

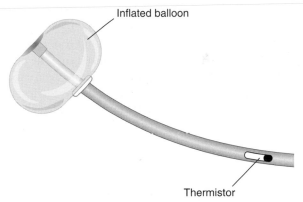

Inflated balloon

Thermistor

FIGURE 16.7 ■ Distal end of a pulmonary artery catheter showing inflated balloon and thermistor.

evidence of improved survival and the introduction of non-invasive techniques to estimate cardiac output have led to a decline in its use. The PAFC is also known as a Swan-Ganz or balloon tip catheter (Fig. 16.7).

A PAFC is a long catheter with three or four lumens, and a thermistor near the tip. It is inserted into a neck vein through a large cannula. A flexible plastic sheath allows the catheter to be inserted, withdrawn and rotated after insertion without desterilizing it. After insertion into the superior vena cava, saline is injected to inflate a balloon at the tip. The pressure at the tip is measured via a transducer and displayed on a monitor. The catheter is then advanced slowly so that the blood

flow directs the catheter toward the pulmonary artery. As the catheter is advanced, a series of changes in pressure is observed, marking the progression through the right atrium and right ventricle into the pulmonary artery (Fig. 16.8). Eventually, the balloon 'wedges' into a pulmonary artery. At this point, the tip is isolated from the pulmonary artery and measures the pressure in the pulmonary capillaries, which is taken to reflect left atrial pressure. Although the ability to estimate left atrial pressure is useful, the interpretation of measurements is as problematic as for central venous pressure (see above). For the same reasons, measuring the changes after a fluid challenge is more useful than a single reading.

The ability to measure the filling pressure of the left ventricle as well as the cardiac output was a major advance, and has led to many advances in

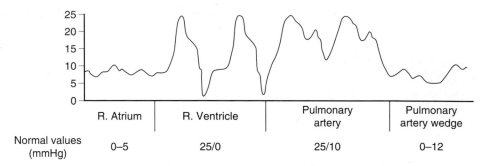

FIGURE 16.8 ■ Diagrammatic representation of pressure waveforms.

our understanding of cardiac physiology and the mechanisms and treatments of diseases such as sepsis. However, the process of insertion described above is not always straightforward and prolonged manipulation may be needed to direct the catheter into the pulmonary artery. Arrhythmias are extremely common with catheter insertion and the technique carries all the risks of central venous catheterization noted above in addition to the risks shown in Table 16.7.

Cardiac Output

Cardiac output is closely linked to oxygen delivery; in addition, studies have shown that low cardiac output is linked to increased mortality. However, it must be remembered that cardiac output is intermittent and not continuous and that factors such as the pressure changes caused by ventilation (especially positive pressure ventilation), changes in heart rate and arrhythmias produce complex changes. Therefore, monitors do not produce consistent results even when synchronized with the heartbeat and respiratory cycle.

TABLE 16.7
Risks of Pulmonary Artery Catheterization (in Addition to those Shown in Table 16.6)
Arrhythmias with catheter manipulation
Damage to tricuspid and pulmonary valves
Knotting of catheter
Pulmonary infarction if balloon left inflated
Pulmonary artery rupture with balloon inflation
Cardiac rupture

Dilution techniques have been regarded as the 'gold standard' against which other methods are compared.

The Fick Principle. The Fick principle defines flow by the ratio of the uptake or clearance of a tracer within an organ to measurements of the arteriovenous difference in concentration. It may be used to measure cardiac output, notably when applied to oxygen uptake or indicator dilution, and also regional blood flow, e.g. cerebral blood flow using the uptake of nitrous oxide, and renal blood flow from the excretion of compounds cleared totally by the kidney, such as *para*-aminohippuric acid.

In subjects with minimal cardiac shunt and reasonable pulmonary function, pulmonary blood flow may be calculated from the ratio of the oxygen consumption and the difference in oxygen content between arterial and mixed venous blood, as follows:

$$\frac{\text{Pulmonary}}{\text{blood flow}} = \frac{\text{oxygen consumption}}{\text{arteriovenous oxygen content difference}}$$

Oxygen consumption from a reservoir is measured using an accurate spirometer, and oxygen content of blood requires a co-oximeter. The patient should be at steady state when the measurements are made, with constant inspired oxygen concentration and blood samples obtained slowly whilst the oxygen consumption is being determined. True mixed venous blood samples must be obtained from a pulmonary artery catheter, and alternative indicator dilution techniques described below are less demanding. The effects of ventilation and beat-to-beat variation in cardiac output are averaged over the long period of measurement of oxygen consumption. Errors in measurement of oxygen consumption limit the accuracy of this technique (± 10%).

Indicator Dilution. An indicator is injected as a bolus into the right heart and the concentration reaching the systemic side of the circulation is plotted against time (Fig. 16.9). The average concentration is calculated from the area under the concentration–time curve divided by the duration of the curve. The cardiac output during the period of this measurement is the ratio of the dose of indicator to the average concentration.

The general formula is:

$$\frac{\text{Cardiac}}{\text{output}} = \frac{\text{indicator dose (units)} \times 60}{\text{average concentration (units L}^{-1}) \times \text{time(s)}}$$

The main problem with this technique is that when the dye has been measured at the artery it passes back to the heart and then back to the arteries (known as recirculation), making the calculations more complex. This may be circumvented by extrapolation of the early exponential downslope to define the tail of the curve which would have been recorded if recirculation had not occurred (Fig. 16.9). The area under the curve is calculated by integration.

Chemical Indicator Dilution. Original studies used indocyanine green as the chemical indicator. It is non-toxic and has a relatively short half-life so that repeated measurements may be made. It also has a peak spectral absorption at 800 nm, which is the wavelength at which absorption of oxygenated haemoglobin is identical to that of reduced haemoglobin. The measurement is therefore not affected by arterial saturation. However, because the dye is cleared from the circulation only slowly, recirculation makes repeated measurements impossible. More recent monitors use an injection of lithium as a marker which is detected with a modified arterial catheter.

Thermal Indicator Dilution. This technique requires a PAFC to be in the pulmonary artery. The principle of the method is similar to other indicator dilution methods, but the injection and sampling are performed on the right side of the heart. A bolus of 10 mL of saline at room temperature is injected into the right atrium and the temperature change is recorded by a thermistor at the tip of the PAFC in the pulmonary artery. The smaller the temperature drop, the larger is the cardiac output. The recorded temperatures generate an exponential dilution curve with no recirculation. The 'heat dose' is the product of the difference in temperature

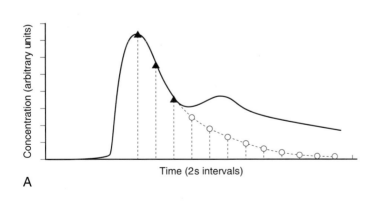

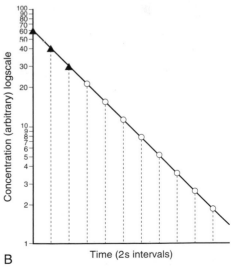

FIGURE 16.9 ■ (**A**) Single injection indicator dilution curve showing distortion of downslope produced by recirculation. (**B**) Re-plot on semi-logarithmic paper. ▲ = points taken from the downslope in **A** to establish the slope of the re-plot in **B**; ○ = points taken from **B** to plot tail of curve in **A**. *(Reproduced with permisssion from Sykes, M.K., Vickers, M.D., Hull, C.J., 1991. Principles of clinimeasurement, third ed. Blackwell Scientific Publications, Oxford.)*

between the injectate and blood multiplied by the density, specific heat and volume of the injectate. The average change in heat content is the area under the temperature–time graph multiplied by the density and specific heat of blood.

Thermal dilution techniques offer many advantages:

- the indicator is cheap and non-toxic
- repeated measurements may be made without accumulation of the indicator
- arterial puncture and blood sampling are not required
- absence of recirculation greatly facilitates measurement of the area under the curve, particularly in low output states.

Disadvantages of thermal dilution include the following:

- invasive and expensive pulmonary artery catheterization is required: the mortality associated with PAFC use may outweigh improvements in care
- the thermistor probe must be matched to the cardiac output processor
- mixing of the large bolus with venous blood may be incomplete
- pulmonary artery flow varies more with ventilation than does systemic flow
- corrections are required, e.g. for changes in injectate temperature during injection through the catheter
- time-consuming: three separate readings are required to produce a reliable mean result, and the procedure needs to be repeated after each change of therapy.

The measurement of cardiac output using both dye and thermodilution is now automated with computer-controlled sampling, calculation of indicator dilution curves, rejection algorithms for artefacts or curves which are not exponential, and on-line calculation of cardiac output.

'Continuous' cardiac output monitors have also been introduced. These use a similar principle, but instead of using a bolus of cold saline, the catheter has an electrical coil which is heated at intervals, creating a bolus of warm blood which passes into the pulmonary artery. This eliminates much of the operator error

and produces frequently updated measurements of cardiac output, allowing the effect of interventions to be observed.

Monitors have also been developed which do not require a pulmonary artery catheter, but use a bolus of iced saline injected into a modified central venous catheter and a peripheral arterial catheter with a built-in thermistor (e.g. the PiCCO monitor).

Most of the current monitors allow cardiac output data to be integrated with other measurements such as arterial pressure to provide calculated values of, for example, systemic vascular resistance and stroke volume. This aids the choice and administration of drugs such as vasoconstrictors.

Pulse Contour Analysis. The shape of the arterial pulse (the pulse contour) is a product of the rate of ejection of blood into the aorta and the elasticity of the arterial tree. Therefore, if some assumptions are made about the arterial tree, the volume ejected at each heartbeat (stroke volume) may be calculated from the shape of the arterial pulse contour. Multiplying this by the heart rate provides an estimate of cardiac output. This system has the advantage of being able to calculate the cardiac output in near real-time using an arterial cannula alone.

However, the technique relies on assumptions on arterial tree elasticity which may not always be correct in every patient. Therefore, these systems often require calibration by another method such as thermodilution every 8–12 h to ensure accuracy. The costs of the computer and consumables are also considerable.

Doppler Ultrasonography. Ultrasound techniques can detect the shape, size and movement of tissue interfaces, especially soft tissues and blood, including the echocardiographic measurement of blood flow and the structure and function of the heart. Sound waves are transmitted by the oscillation of particles in the direction of wave transmission and are defined by the amplitude of oscillation (the difference between ambient and peak pressures) and the wavelength (distance between successive peaks) or frequency (inversely proportional to wavelength, the number of cycles per second). These characteristics are measured by a pressure transducer placed in the path of an oncoming wave. The human ear detects frequencies within the range of

20–20 000 Hz. Diagnostic ultrasound uses frequencies in the range of 1–10 MHz. Short-term diagnostic use of ultrasound appears to be free from hazard.

Generation and Detection of Ultrasound. Generation and sensing of ultrasound are performed by transducers which are manufactured from ceramic materials containing lead zirconate and lead titanate which display the piezoelectric effect: the generation of an electrical charge in response to mechanical pressure. These substances are cheap, easily shaped and very efficiently transform mechanical to electrical energy and *vice versa*. Pressure on the surface of these materials generates a related and measurable electric charge. Conversely, applying a high-frequency alternating potential difference across the transducer changes the thickness and generates pressure waves in the form of ultrasound of the same frequency as the applied voltage.

Properties of Ultrasound. Shorter wavelengths and higher frequencies improve the resolution of distance, but tissue penetration is simultaneously reduced. Amplitude determines the intensity of the ultrasound beam, the number and size of echoes recorded and therefore the sensitivity of the instrument. Ultrasound is absorbed by tissues and reflected at tissue interfaces. The intensity of the beam decreases exponentially as it passes through tissue. Attenuation depends on the nature and temperature of the tissue, and is related linearly to the frequency of the ultrasound.

The reflection of the ultrasound beam from the junction between two tissues or from tissue–fluid or tissue–air interfaces forms the basis of the majority of diagnostic techniques. Reflections at most soft-tissue interfaces are therefore weak, but bone–fat and tissue–air interfaces reflect the majority of incident energy. Structures lying behind a bone or air interface cannot be studied using ultrasound.

Ultrasound scanning techniques have been developed which are suited to different applications and which have extremely sophisticated two-dimensional, real-time, brightness- and colour-modulated displays under microprocessor control.

Detection of Motion by the Doppler Effect: Cardiac Output. When ultrasound waves reflect off an object moving towards the transmitter, there is an apparent increase in frequency as the object encounters more oscillations in a given time. This physical phenomenon is termed the Doppler effect. The change in frequency is proportional to the velocity of the object and two constants: the frequency of the transmitted ultrasound and the velocity of ultrasound in the medium. The velocity of the object can be calculated using the Doppler equation:

$$\text{Velocity} = \frac{(Fd \times C)}{(2Ft \times \cos\theta)}$$

(Fd = change in Doppler frequency; C = speed of sound in medium; Ft = transmitted frequency; θ = angle of probe relative to the flow of blood)

In practice, a beam of ultrasonic waves is focused on the descending aorta and reflections from red cells are measured by a transducer in the same probe. Probes may be transthoracic (usually placed in the sternal notch) or placed in the oesophagus. The speed–time curve of the red cells (Fig. 16.10) is integrated to calculate the average velocity over each cardiac cycle. The stroke volume can be calculated by multiplying the average velocity per cycle with an estimation of the cross-sectional area of the aorta (using pre-determined values based on population data, or estimated echocardiographically).

Current Oesophageal Doppler Monitors derive the total cardiac output utilising a nomogram created by 'calibration' of total left ventriculated Stroke Volume as measured by the pulmonary artery catheter against

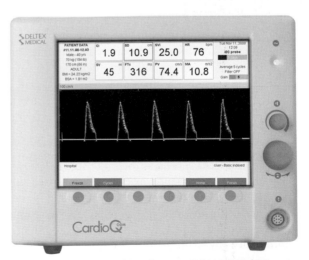

FIGURE 16.10 ■ Display of an oesophageal Doppler cardiac output monitor showing the pulse waveform from which a variety of haemodynamic variables are derived.

descending aortic blood flow velocity and Stroke Distance as measured by the ODM.

The advantage of these systems is that they produce an almost real-time reading of cardiac output so that changes in output in response to drugs or fluids are seen almost immediately, and so are a useful guide to further therapy, particularly fluid responsiveness.

However, there are a number of problems with this technology. These systems are reliant on the ultrasound beam being directed at the centre of the aorta and the aorta being a smooth tube. In practice, even small movements of the sensor may lead to marked changes in readings because the speed of red cells near the aortic wall is measured. Furthermore, the aorta is not completely circular, may also contain atheroma, and the diameter (usually an estimate) can change by as much as 12% during systole. The Doppler shift also depends on the direction of the ultrasound beam relative to the axis. Provided that the angle is less than 20°, the error in cardiac output is only about 6%. Conscious patients do not always tolerate the more accurate oesophageal probes, and certain surgical procedures preclude their use (e.g. oesophagectomy surgery). Most machines now provide a visual (and audible) measure of signal strength to allow the user to identify when the probe has moved.

Despite these limitations, these probes are very useful in high-risk patients who require relatively minor surgery because they may be used to monitor cardiac output during anaesthesia without the risks associated with the insertion of multiple intravascular catheters. They are also useful in patients undergoing surgery requiring precise control of intravascular volume and cardiac output. However, although they may be used to determine whether a change in therapy has had a positive or negative effect, they are unable to provide reliable estimates of cardiac output in absolute terms. Complications are rare.

Transoesophageal Echocardiography. Transoesophageal echocardiography uses a miniaturized ultrasonic probe inserted into the oesophagus under anaesthesia. It provides a real-time picture of all four cardiac chambers and valves. Its advantage is that it can identify any malfunctioning valves in addition to any wall-motion abnormalities related to myocardial ischaemia. It can also identify if therapy has successfully treated the ischaemia.

However, these probes are expensive to purchase and require an operator who is trained both to use the equipment and to interpret the results. They are useful as patients come off bypass after cardiac surgery to ensure that both the myocardium and valves are functioning correctly. Through use of Doppler, they can also measure cardiac output. However, they remain suitable only for anaesthetized or sedated patients, and cannot provide prolonged continuous measurements. They are rarely used in non-cardiac surgery.

Thoracic Electrical Bioimpedance. Tissue impedance depends on blood volume. Measurement of thoracic impedance provides an index of stroke volume. Two circumferential electrodes are placed around the neck and two around the upper abdomen. A small (<1 mA) constant, high-frequency (>1 kHz) alternating current is passed between the outer electrodes and the resulting potential difference is detected by the inner pair. This potential is rectified, smoothed and filtered to record voltage fluctuations which reflect changes in impedance due to ventilation and cardiac activity. The cardiac activity is extracted by signal-averaging relative to the ECG R wave. This represents changes in thoracic blood volume and clearly resembles the pulse waveform.

Modern instruments show a modest agreement with invasive measurements of cardiac output, although trends and rapid changes in cardiac output are reliably demonstrated. This method is inaccurate when there are intracardiac shunts or arrhythmias, and underestimates cardiac output in a vasodilated circulation.

THE RESPIRATORY SYSTEM

Clinical

Continuous visual monitoring of the colour and the pattern of ventilation of the patient are essential for safe anaesthesia. When the patient is breathing spontaneously, observation should detect signs of airway obstruction, e.g. tracheal tug, paradoxical movement and failure of the anaesthetic reservoir bag to move.

Maintenance of the airway in an anaesthetized patient is a skilled task. Although the introduction of supraglottic airways has led to a reduction in the frequency of need for airway skills, airway maintenance still remains one of the most basic tasks for the anaesthetist. Auscultation of the chest with a stethoscope may confirm the presence of normal breath sounds and also detect additional sounds caused by secretions, oedema or bronchospasm. Although useful, clinical signs cannot reliably disprove oesophageal placement of a tracheal tube.

Oesophageal Stethoscope

This consists of a balloon-tipped catheter which may also carry a temperature probe. It is connected to either an earpiece or stethoscope and inserted into the patient's oesophagus. The catheter is advanced until the heart sounds are maximal and then taped at the nose. It provides a constant monitor of both heart rate and ventilation and is said to be able to identify the characteristic 'millwheel murmur' of an air embolus. It is most often used in children. In addition to being inexpensive, it carries little morbidity and has the great advantage of forcing the anaesthetist to remain beside the patient.

Respiratory Rate

The rate may be timed clinically or more often derived from the capnograph. Many ECG monitors use the leads to pass a very small high-frequency alternating current across the chest; the increase in electrical impedance (resistance to an alternating current) produced by inhalation is measured and the respiratory rate calculated.

Airway Pressure

The lungs are damaged easily and although anaesthetic machines incorporate pressure relief valves, these are designed to protect the machine rather than the patient. Although electronic ventilators usually allow a maximum airway pressure to be set to protect the patient, excessive pressure may still be exerted by manual compression of the reservoir bag. The self-inflating bags used for resuscitation are often capable of exerting extremely high pressures. As even transient peaks of pressure may lead to lung trauma or pneumothorax, a pressure monitor should be used whenever positive-pressure ventilation is used.

As all ventilators now incorporate pressure monitors, separate airway pressure monitors are rarely used. Most ventilators include a pressure transducer in the form of a piezoelectric crystal that converts pressure to an electrical potential, which is then measured by the monitor and displayed.

Although such monitors are both accurate and reliable, it must be remembered that they measure the pressure within the monitor and not the airway pressure. Therefore, the measured pressure may not be reliable if a narrow tracheal tube, long breathing circuit or high-frequency ventilation are used. High lung pressures may be a particular problem in obese patients, those positioned head down and those with bronchospasm.

In devices without electronic components, such as ventilators used for transport, pressure is measured by devices in which the air pressure deforms a bellows or a metal tube. The deformation is linked to a needle with the pressure read from a scale. These are simple devices and are usually reliable, but are susceptible to damage by excess pressure.

Measurement of Gas Flow and Volume

The relationships between volume, flow and velocity are central to understanding gas flow and volume. Flow rate is defined as the volume passing a fixed point in unit time, i.e. volume per second. Integration of a continuous flow signal is the volume which has flowed over a defined period. Velocity is the distance moved by gas molecules in unit time. These are related directly and depend upon the cross-sectional area of flow:

$$Velocity = flow\ rate/area$$

The concept of velocity is important in flow measurement because several instruments measure the velocity of flow and not the flow rate. The velocities of all molecules in a gas or liquid are not the same. Axial streaming is characteristic of laminar flow (Fig. 16.11).

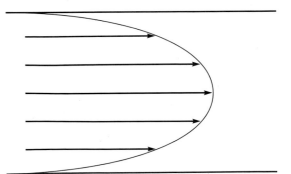

FIGURE 16.11 ■ Velocity profile during laminar flow. Velocity is zero at the walls of the containing tube and maximal in the axial stream.

Measuring Volume

Measurements of gas volume depend on collecting the gases in a calibrated spirometer, or passing the gases through some type of gas meter. However, volume can also be derived from measuring gas flow. Gas flow when integrated over time produces a calculated volume.

Spirometers

Wet spirometers consist of a rigid cylinder suspended over an underwater seal and counterbalanced. Gas entering the bell causes it to rise. This linear displacement is proportional to the volume of gas. Wet spirometers are accurate at steady state and have been used to calibrate other volume-measuring devices. However, they are bulky and inconvenient to use, and the frequency response is damped by friction between the moving parts, causing the instrument to under-read with rapidly changing rates of flow.

Dry spirometers are more convenient for clinical work. Gas displaces a rolling diaphragm or bellows and the expansion is recorded and related to gas volume. The 'Vitalograph' is a specialized type of bellows spirometer used for lung function testing. The patient makes a maximal forced exhalation into the spirometer through a wide-bore tube. The expansion of the wedge-shaped bellows is recorded by a stylus on a pressure-sensitive chart. The stylus moves across the x-axis (time) at a constant rate. The resultant plot represents the volume–time plot of the patient's expiration (Fig. 16.12). The FVC is the maximal volume expired.

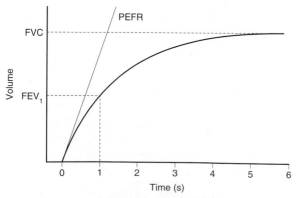

FIGURE 16.12 ▪ Forced vital capacity (FVC), forced expiratory volume in 1 second (FEV1) and peak expiratory flow rate (PEFR) can all be derived from the volume–time plot of the Vitalograph (Sykes et al 1991).

Understanding of technique and active cooperation of the patient are essential for accurate and precise recordings. The patient must make an airtight seal with the mouthpiece and the nose is occluded with a nose clip. Expiration should be as forcible and rapid as possible. Several attempts are recorded. The highest value measured is recorded because the technique is dependent on voluntary effort, which usually improves with practice.

Gas Meters

Dry gas meters are widely used in the gas industry and are used also in medicine, e.g. in some mechanical ventilators, to measure large volumes of gas. Displacement of bellows controls valves which alternately direct gas flow to fill and empty the bellows, and also drives the pointer on a calibrated recording dial. Irregularities within each cycle disappear when the meter has returned to the same position in the cycle; hence, accuracy of measurements improves with increasing multiples of meter volume.

The Dräger Volumeter

The volume of gas which flows through the Dräger volumeter is related to the rotation of two light, interlocking, dumbbell-shaped rotors. It is a simple meter and accurate when dry, but is affected by moisture.

The Wright Respirometer

This device contains a light mica vane which rotates within a small cylinder (Fig. 16.13). Inflowing air is directed on to the vane by tangential slits. Rotation of the vane drives a gear chain and pointer on a dial. This mechanism is described as inferential because it does not measure either the volume or the flow of all of the gas flowing through the device. It is calibrated for normal tidal volumes and breathing rates by a sine wave pump. However, the meter seriously over-reads at high tidal volumes and under-reads at low tidal volumes because of the inertia of the moving parts.

Integration of the Flow Signal

The flow signal from a rapidly responding flowmeter may be integrated electronically over time to calculate volume. However, the process of integration exaggerates the effect of baseline drift; a small and insignificant change in the baseline of the flow signal may produce substantial and increasing error in the volume signal

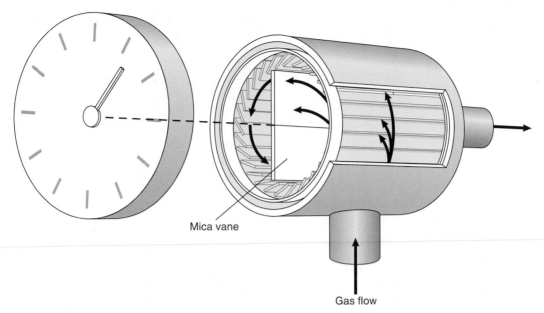

Mica vane

Gas flow

FIGURE 16.13 ■ Diagrammatic representation of the mechanism of the Wright respirometer.

over time. This effect is minimized by limiting the duration of integration, e.g. to a single tidal volume by resetting the integrator to zero at the end of each inspiration.

Indirect Methods of Measuring Tidal Volume

Methods which depend on measuring inspired or expired gases require a leak-free connection. This is feasible with tracheal intubation. A physiological mouthpiece and connection to the measuring apparatus may change the pattern of breathing and is suitable only for short-term use. Several indirect methods have been developed which enable tidal volume to be derived from measurements of chest wall movement.

Pneumography. Pneumographs sense changes in chest and abdominal circumference. Non-elastic tapes are placed around the chest and abdomen and the ends are connected to a displacement sensor. The output may be calibrated to provide a tidal volume signal. However, these devices are sensitive to position and require frequent calibration.

Respiratory Inductance Plethysmography. Respiratory inductance plethysmography uses a wire coil sewn into an elasticated strap. Expansion of the chest or abdomen increases the space between the coils and so alters the inductance generated by a high-frequency alternating (AC) current. The change in inductance depends on the cross-sectional area enclosed by the coil, which is closely related to change in volume. Inductance plethysmography has been used in various physiological studies to monitor postoperative respiratory depression and to detect apnoea.

Measuring Gas Flow

Volume–Time Methods

Flow rate may be calculated from spirometric measurements of volume of gas per unit time. These methods are accurate when corrected for temperature and pressure and are used widely to calibrate other flowmeters, but are slow, cumbersome and have limited clinical application.

Most clinical methods are based on the relationship between pressure decrease and flow across a resistance – either a fixed pressure decrease across a variable orifice or a variable pressure change across a fixed orifice.

Variable Orifice (Constant Pressure Change) Flowmeters

The orifice through which gas flows enlarges with the flow rate so that the pressure difference across the orifice remains constant. This is the physical principle of the Rotameter.

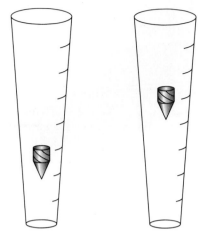

FIGURE 16.14 ■ Physical principle of the Rotameter flow-meter. The weight of the bobbin is exactly opposed by the pressure drop across the cross-sectional area of the annular space around the bobbin.

Rotameter. The Rotameter consists of a vertical glass tube inside which rotates a light metal alloy bobbin (Fig. 16.14). The flow of gas is controlled by the fine-adjustment flow control valve at the bottom of the Rotameter, and when this is opened, the pressure of the gas forces the bobbin up the tube. The inside of the tube is shaped like an inverted cone, so that the cross-sectional area of the annular space exactly opposes the downward pressure resulting from the weight of the bobbin. The pressure decrease remains constant throughout the range of flows for which the tube is calibrated and the bobbin rotates freely in the steady stream of gas. Each Rotameter must be calibrated for a specific gas. Laminar flow predominates at low flow rates and depends on the viscosity of gas. Turbulent flow increases at higher flow rates and the density of the gas becomes an important factor. Both density and viscosity of a gas vary with temperature and pressure, and each Rotameter must be calibrated for one specific gas in appropriate conditions.

The Peak Flowmeter. This useful clinical instrument is capable of measuring flow rates up to $1000 \, L \, min^{-1}$. Air flow causes a vane to rotate or a piston to move against the constant force of a light spring. This opens orifices which permit air to escape. The position adopted by the vane or piston depends primarily on the flow rate and on the area of the orifice which must be exposed to the air flow to maintain a constant pressure. The light moving vane or piston rapidly attains a maximum position in response to the peak expiratory flow. It is held in this position by a ratchet. The reading is obtained from a mechanical pointer which is attached to the vane or piston.

Accurate results demand good technique. These devices must be held horizontally to minimize the effects of gravity on the position of the moving parts. The patient must be encouraged to exhale as rapidly as possible. Consistency of repeated recordings suggests maximal effort and the peak expiratory flow rate is the maximum reading recorded.

Variable Pressure Change (Fixed Orifice) Flowmeters

The resistance is maintained constant so that changes of flow are accompanied by changes in pressure across the resistance element.

Bourdon Gauge Flowmeter. A Bourdon gauge is used to sense the pressure change across an orifice and is calibrated to the gas flow rate. These rugged meters are not affected by changes in position and are useful for metering the flow from gas cylinders at high ambient pressure. Back-pressure causes over-reading of the actual flow rate.

Pneumotachograph. The pneumotachograph measures flow rate by sensing the pressure change across a small but laminar resistance. Careful design ensures that the differential manometer senses the true lateral pressure exerted by the gas on each side of the resistance element (Fig. 16.15). The differential manometer needs to be very sensitive to record the tiny changes in pressure across the resistance and transduce them to a continuous electrical output. This signal may be integrated to give volume and the manometer must have good zero and gain stability.

Pneumotachographs are sensitive instruments with a rapid response to changing gas flow and are used widely for clinical measurement of gas flows in respiratory and anaesthetic practice. However, practical application requires frequent calibration and correction or compensation for differences in temperature, humidity, gas composition and pressure

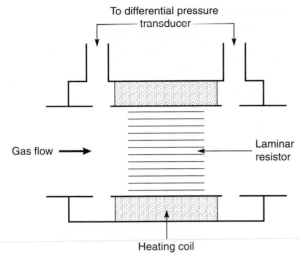

To differential pressure
transducer

Gas flow →

Laminar
resistor

Heating coil

FIGURE 16.15 ■ The Fleisch pneumotachograph.

changes during mechanical ventilation. They are also susceptible to particle blockage, particularly by water condensation.

Other Devices for Measuring Gas Flow

Measurements other than pressure change across an orifice have been used to measure flow.

Hot-Wire Flowmeters. These employ the rate of cooling of a heated wire, which depends on the gas flow rate and is measured by sensing the change in temperature. It also depends on the thermal conductivity of the gas, which is affected by changes in the gas composition and the presence of water vapour. This method is inexpensive, robust, reliable and works over a wide range of flows. However, it is not able to determine the direction of gas flow.

Ultrasonic Flowmeters. These flowmeters use the vortex-shedding technique. Gas is passed through a tube containing a rod 1–2 mm in diameter, mounted at right angles to the direction of gas flow. Vortices form downstream of the rod, the number of vortices formed being directly related to the flow rate. The vortices are detected using ultrasound and integrated to give a volume signal. Measurement is not affected greatly by temperature, humidity or changes in gas composition. A critical flow rate is required for the formation

of vortices and the flowmeter is most accurate when the tidal volume is large.

GAS AND VAPOUR ANALYSIS

Measurement of the concentration of gases and vapours in anaesthetic breathing systems is vital to prevent hypoxaemia and ensure the delivery of anaesthetic agents.

Chemical Methods

Chemical methods are important historically for measurement of oxygen and carbon dioxide concentrations. They involve the removal of fractional volumes from the gas phase by chemical reactions to nongaseous compounds, the fractional concentration being determined by the reduction in volume which occurs:

$$\text{Fractional concentration} = \frac{\text{reduction in gas volume}}{\text{original volume}}$$

Several types of apparatus have been described, e.g. the Haldane. Carbon dioxide is absorbed in a strongly alkaline potassium hydroxide solution. Subsequently oxygen is absorbed in alkaline pyrogallol or sodium anthraquinone.

Physical Methods

In contrast with chemical methods, instruments based on the physical properties of a gas or vapour are convenient, responsive and more suitable for continuous operation.

Speed of response of the system is determined by two components:

- *Transit time* required for the sample to flow along the sampling catheter usually accounts for the greater part of the total delay. It is minimized by using a narrow and short sampling catheter with a rapid sampling flow rate.
- *Response time* required for the instrument to react to the change in gas concentration. It consists of the time required to wash out the analysis cell and delays imposed by the sensing mechanism.

Zero drift and variations in gain are common problems and most gas analysers have to be calibrated frequently, ideally against gas mixtures of known composition.

Non-Specific Methods

Non-specific methods use a property of the gas which is common to all gases, but which is possessed by each gas to a differing degree.

Thermal Conductivity

A gas with a high thermal conductivity conducts heat more readily than one with a low conductivity. In the katharometer, gas is passed over a heated wire and the degree of cooling of the wire depends on the temperature of the gas, the rate of gas flow and the thermal conductivity of the gas. The reduction in temperature of the wire reduces its resistance and produces an electrical signal related to the gas concentration. In clinical practice, katharometers are usually used for the measurement of CO_2 and He, and as detectors in gas chromatography systems.

Refractive Index: Interference Refractometers

The speed of light slows through transparent materials to a degree determined by the refractive index of that substance. The delay caused by the passage of light through the gas depends on the number of gas molecules present; hence the refractive index also depends on the pressure and temperature of the gas. This extremely small delay is measured using the phase lag by the principle of interference. When light waves from a common source are passed through two linear slits in an opaque sheet and focused on to a screen, an interference pattern is produced. Bright areas where light from the two sources in phase is reinforced alternate with dark bands where the light paths differ in length by half a wavelength, i.e. they are out of phase and attenuating each other. When a gas is introduced into one light path, it delays transmission of the light waves with a reduction in wavelength and an alteration in the position of the dark bands. If the refractive index of the gas is known, the change in position can be related to the number of gas molecules in the light path and hence to the partial pressure of the gas. Interference refractometers are calibrated using known concentrations of gas or vapour. The response is essentially linear and remains stable after calibration.

This method of analysis is used to calibrate flowmeters and vaporizers accurately. Portable devices are useful for monitoring pollution by anaesthetic gases and vapours.

Specific Methods

Specific methods identify and measure a gas using some unique property and are particularly suitable for complex mixtures of gases. These methods include:

- Magnetic susceptibility
- Absorption of radiation
- Mass spectrometry
- Gas–liquid chromatography.

Their principles may be explored further by reference to specific gases relevant to the practice of anaesthesia.

Oxygen

Oxygen concentration in a breathing system is measured using either a fuel cell or a paramagnetic analyser.

The fuel cell is the more common device. It contains a lead anode within a small container of electrode gel. When exposed to oxygen, the lead is converted to lead oxide, producing a small voltage which may be measured and amplified. Fuel cells are small, robust and reliable, although they require calibration at regular intervals. After a period of around 6 months, they require replacement because the lead becomes oxidized. Accuracy is better than $\pm$ 1% with a response time of $<10\,s$.

The principle of the paramagnetic analyser is that oxygen molecules are attracted weakly to a magnetic field (paramagnetic). Most other anaesthetic gases are repelled by a magnetic field (diamagnetic). In the original analysers, a powerful magnetic field was passed across a chamber which contained two nitrogen-containing spheres suspended on a wire. When oxygen was introduced into the chamber, it tended to displace the spheres, causing them to rotate. The degree of rotation was measured to estimate the oxygen concentration.

A fast differential paramagnetic oxygen sensor has been designed on the pneumatic bridge principle. The sample and reference gas are drawn by a common pump through two tubes surrounded by an electromagnet alternating at 110 Hz. Pressure differences between the two tubes are related to the paramagnetic properties of the sample and reference gases. The phasic changes in pressure are extremely small and measured with a miniature microphone. The output of the device is linear, very stable and has a fast response time of less than 150 ms.

These monitors are accurate, reliable and do not need frequent maintenance. The monitors measure the partial pressure of oxygen, but display oxygen as a percentage. If the pressure within the circuit is increased, for example when a gas-driven ventilator is employed, they can overestimate the oxygen concentration.

Carbon Dioxide and Anaesthetic Gases

Absorption of Radiation. Infrared radiation (1–15 µm) is absorbed by all gases with two or more dissimilar atoms in the molecule. Carbon dioxide, nitrous oxide and anaesthetic vapours absorb light at different wavelengths. Therefore, a cell is arranged with light sources on one side of a chamber and photoelectric cells on the other. Infrared light is dispersed through a prism or diffraction grating into a spectrum of different wavelengths. The test gas is then passed through the chamber and the amount of light absorbed is measured. The absorption spectrum is specific to each gas, and according to Beer–Lambert laws (see 'Oximetry'), the amount of light absorbed is proportional to the concentration of the gas. In practice, the chambers have mirrors on each side so the light passes across the chamber many times to amplify the absorption. The chamber is also heated to avoid condensation. Accuracy is around 0.5% with a response time of <0.5 s.

There are several sources of error with infrared analysis:

- The absorption wavebands of different gases may be coincident. For instance, the peak absorption bands for carbon dioxide, nitrous oxide and carbon monoxide are at 4.3, 4.5 and 4.7 µm respectively, and the absorption spectra inevitably overlap. Error is minimized by narrowing the band of infrared light
- The phenomenon of 'collision broadening' describes the apparent widening of the absorption spectrum of CO_2 by the physical presence of certain other gases, notably N_2 and N_2O. Correction factors have been described, but the error may be minimized by calibrating the instrument with similar background gas mixtures as the gas to be analysed
- Absorption is related to the number of molecules in the absorbent gas in the cuvette, i.e. partial pressure. The reading is affected by changes in atmospheric pressure, pressurization of a breathing system or variation in the resistance of the sampling flow line
- Unexpected vapours, such as ethanol from an intoxicated patient, may introduce errors.

Modern gas analysers for clinical use are very stable but require regular calibration of the zero point and scale. Accuracy at normal breathing frequencies also requires a satisfactory response time, typically a 90% or 95% rise time less than 150 ms. Slow response is usually caused by blockage of the sampling line with condensation or sputum, or failure of the suction pump.

Most analysers pump a small flow of gas out of the breathing system to be analysed in the main monitoring box, a 'side stream' system. This involves some delay while the gas is pumped to the monitor. The movement of gas may also reduce accuracy if mixing of inspiratory and expiratory gas occurs. In most cases, the sampled gas is passed into the scavenging system, but when low flows are required it may be returned to the breathing system. This arrangement allows the sensing chamber to be housed within a monitor, making it more robust.

The alternative 'main stream' system places the sensing chamber in a connector within the patient breathing system and so reduces any delay in measurement. However, it also makes the sensor more prone to accidental damage.

The carbon dioxide concentration in respired gases is displayed most often as a graph of concentration against time (capnogram). This provides visual confirmation that the airway is patent and that ventilation is occurring. It also provides the only reliable guarantee after tracheal intubation that the tube is not in the oesophagus.

At the start of expiration, the carbon dioxide concentration is zero (dead space gas). The concentration then increases to a plateau level (alveolar gas). The end-tidal value of carbon dioxide concentration is used usually as a measure of the adequacy of ventilation because it approximates to alveolar and therefore arterial carbon dioxide partial pressure. However, when the respiratory rate is high, if tidal volume is low, if the sampling point is distant from the airway or if the gases tend to mix in the circuit, the 'end-tidal' value tends to be artificially low. This may give the impression that the lungs are being hyperventilated. For these reasons, it is difficult to measure end-tidal carbon dioxide meaningfully in small children. This is also true in patients, often smokers, who have marked ventilation/perfusion mismatch; there is often a prolonged upstroke on the capnograph trace and the relationship between end-tidal and arterial carbon dioxide tensions becomes less reliable (Fig. 16.16). If the capnograph trace does not appear to resemble a square wave, problems should be suspected and the arterial carbon dioxide partial pressure should be checked by blood gas analysis.

If lung perfusion is compromised, either by a low cardiac output or by pulmonary emboli or an air embolus, the end-tidal carbon dioxide tension decreases because carbon dioxide delivery to the lungs decreases. Paradoxically, arterial carbon dioxide partial pressure increases. Therefore, in situations where air emboli are likely, for example in neurosurgery, any alteration in end-tidal carbon dioxide should be investigated by blood gas analysis.

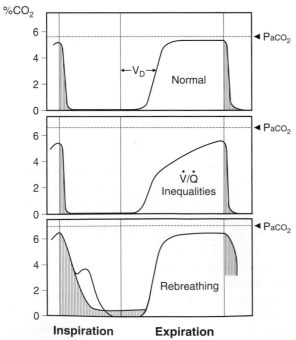

FIGURE 16.16 ■ Carbon dioxide traces recorded from the connector of the tracheal tube. $\dot{V}/\dot{Q}$, ventilation/perfusion.

Although infrared analysers are used usually for measuring the concentration of anaesthetic agents, other methods are used occasionally either for calibration or for complex analyses.

Mass Spectrometry. Mass spectrometers are capable of separating the components of complex gas mixtures according to their mass and charge by deflecting the charged ions in a magnetic field. When a sample is introduced into a mass spectrometer, it passes into a vacuum where it is bombarded with high-energy electrons. These break up larger molecules and strip off their outer electrons. The resulting positively charged ions are then accelerated by a negatively-charged plate into a magnetic field. The magnetic field causes the moving particles to curve depending on how heavy they are (their mass:charge ratio). A row of sensors then measures the number of molecules and their sizes, in proportion to the partial pressure of the sampled gas. A mass spectrum is produced by relating the detector output on the y-axis (calibrated to concentration of gas) to the accelerating voltage on the x-axis (calibrated to molecular weight).

Some molecules may lose two electrons and become doubly charged – they behave like ions with half the mass. Some fragmentation of molecules also occurs in the ionization process, resulting in the production of a mass spectrum rather than a single peak for each molecule. These secondary peaks may be used to advantage, e.g. in the identification and quantification of CO_2 and N_2O, both of which share a parent peak at 44 Da, but produce secondary peaks at 12 and 30 Da, respectively.

Mass spectrometers are expensive to purchase and maintain, but are extremely accurate, have a very short response time, use very small sample flow rates (approx. 20 mL min^{-1}) and can identify a wide range of compounds. They may be sited centrally within large theatre complexes as part of a calibration and quality control system.

Gas–Liquid Chromatography. A gas chromatograph consists of two components: a column packed with inert beads covered in a thin film of oil ('the stationary phase'), and a constant stream of inert gas which passes through the column. When a sample of gas is introduced at one end, the mixture passes into the column and past the oil. Insoluble gases tend to stay in the carrier gas and move through the column quickly, while soluble gases tend to dissolve in the oil, slowing their progress. At the other end of the column is a non-specific detector unit which yields an electronic signal proportional to the quantity of each substance present. Commonly used detectors include katharometers, flame ionization and electron capture detectors. Thus, any gas may be identified by the time it takes to pass through the column and its quantity measured by the detector unit. Their chief advantage is the ability to identify the components in a mixture of unknown compounds.

In addition to gas analysis, the gas–liquid chromatograph may be used to analyse blood samples containing volatile or local anaesthetic agents, anticonvulsants and intravenous anaesthetic drugs.

Raman Scattering. Passing a high-powered laser through a sample of gas causes a scattering of light of different wavelengths in a process known as the 'Raman effect'. The change in wavelength is characteristic of the molecule under study. Thus, sensors placed at the side of the chamber may detect this radiation and identify the gases present. The size and complexity of this technique have restricted its use.

BLOOD GAS ANALYSIS

The Glass pH Electrode

A potential difference is generated across hydrogen ion-sensitive glass depending on the gradient of hydrogen ions. The hydrogen ion concentration within the pH electrode is fixed by a buffer solution, so that the potential across the glass is dependent on the hydrogen ion concentration in the sample (Fig. 16.17).

Measurement of this potential gradient is complicated by the difficulty in making stable electrical contact with the sample and buffer solutions. Two silver:silver chloride electrodes generate an electrode potential, but this is constant at a fixed temperature and provides a stable electrical connection with the buffer solution in the pH electrode, and with a potassium chloride solution in the reference electrode separated from the test sample by a semi-permeable membrane. The potential difference between the electrodes is determined by the pH of the test solution and the temperature, and is calibrated using two phosphate buffers of known and fixed pH. Careful daily

The pH electrode

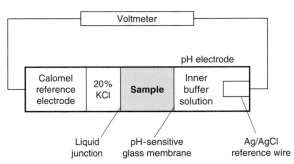

FIGURE 16.17 ■ Component parts of the pH electrode. *(Reproduced from the Radiometer Reference Manual. Permission from Radiometer A/S, Åkandevej 21, DK-2700 Brønshøj, Denmark.)*

calibration is required to maintain accuracy and the electrodes must be regularly cleaned of protein deposits. Reliable measurement of blood pH also depends on the quality of the blood sample, which must be free from air bubbles, heparinized and analysed promptly.

Dissociation of acids and bases is temperature-dependent and the electrodes and blood sampling channel are maintained at 37°C. The measured pH is then corrected to indicate the pH at the temperature of the patient.

The CO_2 Electrode

The main methods of measuring CO_2 tension in liquids are based on pH measurement: CO_2 equilibrates in solution with hydrogen and bicarbonate ions. A glass pH electrode is in contact with a thin layer of bicarbonate buffer. The buffer is trapped in a nylon mesh spacer and separated by a thin Teflon or silicone membrane which is permeable to CO_2 but not to blood cells, plasma or charged ions.

The whole unit is maintained at 37°C. Carbon dioxide diffuses from the blood into the buffer, and so changes the hydrogen ion concentration. The electrode is calibrated by equilibrating the buffer with two known CO_2 concentrations to establish the relationship between pH and PCO_2.

Oxygenation

Oxygenation may be assessed by measuring the tension, saturation or content of oxygen, the relationship between these three measurements being determined by the shape and position of the oxyhaemoglobin dissociation curve. There are many causes of variations in both the shape and position of the curve and it is usually necessary to measure the oxygen tension or saturation directly. Tension measurements are required for most respiratory problems, although saturation or content may be required for calculation of the percentage shunt.

Oxygen tension is usually measured using an oxygen electrode. Content is measured by vacuum extraction and chemical absorption, by driving the O_2 into solution and measuring the increase in PO_2 or by a galvanic cell analyser. Saturation is determined by photometric techniques, involving the transmission or reflection of light at certain wavelengths.

Oxygen Tension

Oxygen Electrode: the Polarographic Method. The oxygen electrode (Clark) consists of a platinum wire, nominally 2nm in diameter, embedded in a rough-surfaced glass rod. This is immersed in a phosphate buffer which is stabilized with KCl and contained in an outer jacket which incorporates an oxygen-permeable polyethylene or polypropylene membrane (Fig. 16.18). A polarizing voltage of between 600 and 800 mV is applied to the platinum wire and as oxygen diffuses through the membrane electro-oxidoreduction occurs at the cathode:

$$O_2 + 2H_2O + 2e^- = H_2O_2 + 2OH^-$$

Corresponding oxidation occurs at the Ag:AgCl anode:

$$4Ag \rightarrow 4Ag^+ + 4e^-$$

$$4Ag^+ + 4Cl \rightarrow 4AgCl$$

Thus a half cell is set up and a tiny current is generated dependent on the oxygen tension at the platinum cathode. The change in current is measured as a change in voltage using the same potentiometric circuit as the pH and PCO_2 measurement systems. The oxygen electrode may be used with gas mixtures or blood. Two-point calibration includes zero with an oxygen-free reference gas or an electronic zero with no electrode output, and the second point with 12% O_2. Temperature control is important and the electrode is maintained at 37°C. Accuracy is compromised by

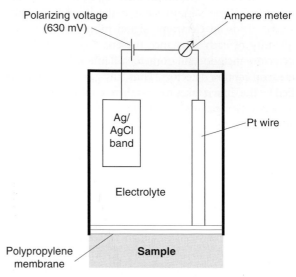

The pO₂ electrode

FIGURE 16.18 ■ The oxygen electrode. *(Reproduced from the Radiometer Reference Manual. Permission from Radiometer A/S, Åkandevej 21, DK-2700 Brønshøj, Denmark.)*

protein deposits or perforation of the delicate plastic membrane, which must be inspected regularly. Oxygen continues to be consumed in blood samples, which should be taken anaerobically, heparinized and analysed promptly.

Galvanic or Fuel Cell. Galvanic cells convert energy from an oxidation-reduction chemical process into electrical energy. The potential generated is dependent on the oxygen concentration.

A gold mesh cathode catalyses the reduction of oxygen by reaction with water to hydroxyl ions, while lead is oxidized at the anode. Unlike the oxygen electrode, no battery is required. The reaction in the fuel cell generates a potential gradient. The chemical reaction uses up the components of the cell, so that its life depends on the concentration of oxygen to which it is exposed and on the duration of exposure: in practice, 6–12 months. Fuel cells are widely used in reliable and portable oxygen analysers which incorporate a digital readout and audible alarms. These are cheap and require little maintenance. Inaccurate responses to calibration with oxygen and air suggest that the fuel cell is exhausted and should be replaced.

Transcutaneous Electrodes. Transcutaneous electrodes are non-invasive and used extensively for monitoring neonatal blood gas tensions. The electrodes are based on principles similar to those used in blood gas analysers but also incorporate a heating element. The electrode is attached to the skin to form an airtight seal using a contact liquid and the area is heated to 43°C. At this temperature, the blood flow to the skin increases and the capillary oxygen diffuses through the skin, allowing measurement of the diffused gases by the attached electrode. The values obtained from the transcutaneous electrode are lower than those from a simultaneous arterial specimen. Many factors affect the transcutaneous measurement of oxygen tension, including the skin site and thickness. Most importantly, the electrode depends on local capillary blood flow and under-reads in the presence of hypotension and microcirculatory perfusion failure. Problems occur with surgical diathermy; the heating current circuit provides a return path for the cutting current which may cause the transcutaneous electrode to overheat.

Other methods of measuring oxygen tension in blood include mass spectrometry and optodes, which employ the quenching of fluorescence from illuminated dye.

Oxygen Content

The total amount of oxygen in blood may be measured directly, but this is technically demanding and rarely used. The van Slyke technique uses a chemical and volumetric or manometric analysis of oxygen content. Oxygen is driven from a small sample by denaturing the haemoglobin with acid. The volume of gas at atmospheric pressure, or the pressure at constant volume, is recorded before and after the chemical absorption of oxygen. The change is related directly to the oxygen content of the fixed volume of blood. Alternative detectors have been used to measure oxygen displaced from haemoglobin, e.g. a galvanic cell.

These time-consuming and operator-dependent laboratory techniques have been replaced by calculation of oxygen content from measurements of the oxygen saturation of haemoglobin, haemoglobin concentration and the tension of oxygen in blood:

$$\begin{aligned}\text{Oxygen content} \\ \text{of blood}\left(\text{mL dL}^{-1}\right)\end{aligned} = \begin{aligned}&\left[So_2(\%) \times Hb\left(g\,dL^{-1}\right) \times 1.34\right] \\ &+ \left[0.0225 \times Po_2(\text{kPa})\right]\end{aligned}$$

Accurate estimates require that the oxygen saturation of haemoglobin is measured directly, and not calculated from oxygen tension and an arbitrary but unmeasured oxyhaemoglobin dissociation curve.

Oximetry: Measurement of Oxygen Saturation

In Vitro Oximetry. Oximetry relies on the differing absorption of light at different wavelengths by the various states of haemoglobin. The absorption of radiation passing through a sample is measured. The degree of absorption of light, defined by the ratio of incident to emergent light intensities on a logarithmic scale, is proportional to the concentration of the molecules absorbing light (Beer's law) and the thickness of the absorbing layer (Lambert's law).

Oxyhaemoglobin and deoxyhaemoglobin differ at both the red and infrared portions of the absorption spectrum (Fig. 16.19). The differential absorption of two wavelengths of red and infrared light permits the calculation of the ratio of the concentrations of oxygenated and reduced haemoglobins. Additional wavelengths are added in co-oximeters for the calculation of the proportions of other species of haemoglobin, such as carboxyhaemoglobin and methaemoglobin, and the absolute absorbance is used to estimate total haemoglobin concentration from the sum of the various haemoglobins. This is important in measurements of oxyhaemoglobin for use in the calculation of oxygen content.

Commercial co-oximeters draw a small blood sample which is haemolysed before entering a cuvette. Light is filtered to produce monochromatic beams, shone through the cuvette and detected by a photocell. The absorption by the sample is the difference in the intensity of incident and transmitted light and both must be measured. Spectrophotometers apply a double-beam technique which improves the accuracy and precision. Light from the monochromator is split into two beams, which pass through the test sample or a reference sample. Photocells generate two signals corresponding to the sample and the reference light intensities. Electronic processing compares the two signals and generates an output proportional to the difference. This greatly improves the signal-to-noise ratio because any variation which affects both the sample and reference beams equally is ignored and the difference remains constant.

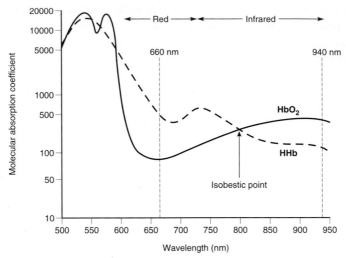

FIGURE 16.19 ■ Absorption spectra of reduced (HHb) and oxygenated (HbO$_2$) haemoglobin.

The saturation of mixed venous blood may be measured using an oximeter incorporated into a pulmonary artery catheter. Fibreoptic cables transmit incident light of at least two wavelengths, and carry reflected light from red blood cells back to a detector.

The same spectrophotometric principles used by co-oximeters in vitro on haemolysed blood samples have been applied to patients in vivo.

Pulse Oximetry. Light transmitted through tissues is absorbed not only by arterial blood but also by other tissue pigments and venous blood. However, the variation in light absorption with each pulse beat results almost entirely from pulsatile arterial blood flow. Two light-emitting diodes – red (660 nm) and infrared (940 nm) – shine light through a finger or earlobe and a photocell detects the transmitted light. The output of the sensor is processed to display a pulse waveform and the arterial oxygen saturation.

The pulse oximeter progresses through the following steps.

1. The sensor first measures the ambient light and subtracts this value from all other measurements. This implies that sudden changes in ambient light levels, e.g. after drapes are moved, may cause transient errors.

2. An LED is turned on and off rapidly. The absorption of transmitted light is then measured and the variations with time are recorded. The result is a waveform with a trough as blood flows into the finger (more absorption) during systole and a peak as blood flows into the veins in diastole. The monitor requires around eight heartbeats to make a calculation and then assumes the frequency of this waveform is the heart rate. Frequent ectopic beats or atrial fibrillation may lead to a delay in calculation or unreliable results.

3. The monitor then analyses the measurements and splits the absorption into two components. The fixed or unchanging absorption is assumed to result from tissues such as skin, muscle and bone (Fig. 16.20). The varying absorption is then assumed to be caused by arterial blood moving into the tissue. In situations such as hypotension, hypovolaemia or hypothermia, pulsation may be reduced to a point at which the monitor is not able to make any calculations and it fails to read. When a patient is on cardiac bypass the tissues are perfused, but if the flow is non-pulsatile, pulse oximeters cannot provide a reading.

4. Steps 1–3 are repeated sequentially using light of at least two different wavelengths at around 120 Hz. When the absorptions of each different wavelength are known, the proportion of oxygenated and deoxygenated haemoglobin may be calculated. The measurements are processed and

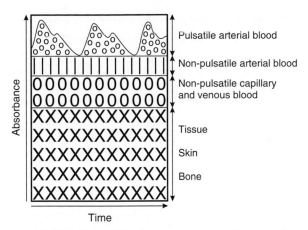

FIGURE 16.20 ■ Schematic representation of the contribution of pulsatile arterial blood, non-pulsatile blood and tissues to the absorbance of light.

| Pulsatile arterial blood |
| Non-pulsatile arterial blood |
| Non-pulsatile capillary and venous blood |
| Tissue |
| Skin |
| Bone |

| TABLE 16.8 |
Disadvantages of Pulse Oximetry
Damage to skin caused by pressure from probe
Failure to detect hypoxaemia in carbon monoxide poisoning
Failure to detect hypoventilation
Slow response times: instrument and circulatory delay
Signal quality adversely affected by hypoperfusion
Inter-instrument variability

a new value displayed around every 8 s. Whilst improving reliability, this averaging introduces delay. Another source of delay is circulatory, dependent on the distribution of blood from the lungs to the tissues. The response time can exceed 1 min in normal subjects, and is exaggerated by low cardiac output or vasoconstriction.

Pulse oximeter calculations are based on the assumption that the blood contains only normal haemoglobin and that no abnormal light-absorbing substances (dyes) are present. For example, if the patient has breathed carbon monoxide, the monoxycarboxyhaemoglobin (as it has a similar absorption spectrum) is measured as oxyhaemoglobin. The result is that the pulse oximeter reading in patients suffering from carbon monoxide poisoning is usually close to 100%, even though they have severe hypoxaemia. The use of intravascular dyes as markers, or even nail varnish, may produce unpredictable results. Lastly, if the probe slips partially off the patient, some light passes directly from the LEDs to the light sensor and also through the sensor. This also causes unreliable readings.

Pulse oximeters provide rapid, non-invasive measurement of pulse rate and an estimate of oxygen saturation. The pulse oximeter has become one of the most widely used monitors and is particularly useful in situations in which it is difficult to identify cyanosis, e.g. if light levels are low, in pigmented patients and in areas where access is difficult such as CT/MRI

scanners. Pulse oximeters are also used to measure the oxygen saturation in patients with intermittent respiratory problems, e.g. postoperative patients and those with sleep apnoea. Advances in technology have resulted in several small battery-powered devices becoming available for out-of-hospital use. Calibration points between 80% and 100% are derived from volunteer studies, and accuracy of pulse oximeters is around ± 2% above an oxygen saturation of 70%. Accuracy below 70% is not known precisely, because it is not ethical to conduct trials at these levels. It is important to note that, especially when oxygen therapy is used, normal oxygen saturation does not equate to normal ventilation. For example, in opioid overdose, hypoventilation may lead to potentially fatal hypercapnia without any decrease in oxygen saturation if the patient is breathing a high concentration of oxygen. Complications are rare. The major drawbacks and source of error of pulse oximetry are summarized in Table 16.8.

THE NERVOUS SYSTEM

The best monitor of cerebral function is the patient, who is able to report symptoms such as numbness, loss of function or pain. During general anaesthesia, this monitoring function is lost and it is possible for patients to develop major neurological deficits during anaesthesia which become evident only during the recovery phase. For example, patients who have suffered head trauma may develop undiagnosed cerebral oedema under anaesthesia if appropriate monitoring, such as intracranial pressure measurement, is not used. During procedures which carry a high risk of ischaemia or seizure activity, such as carotid endarterectomy, this problem may be avoided by performing the procedure under local anaesthesia; however, this may not always be acceptable to patients or possible because of unrelated medical problems. In general, therefore, patients at risk of cerebral malfunction should be given general anaesthesia only if there is no alternative.

When general anaesthesia is used, estimating the 'depth of anaesthesia' has traditionally been a function of the anaesthetist using clinical signs such as heart rate, blood pressure, sweating and pupillary dilatation. Unfortunately, especially in the presence of autonomic neuropathy, such clinical signs are not reliable enough to avoid the risk of awareness during surgery.

It should be noted that there is no widely accepted definition of what 'anaesthesia' represents. Although it may be characterized in terms of lack of perception, lack of responsiveness and inability to recall, these are all poorly defined concepts. Therefore, no monitor can measure 'depth of anaesthesia' in the same way as is possible, for example, with arterial pressure. Further, what is required is not a monitor which can detect awareness, but a monitor which can predict the onset of awareness and allow the anaesthetist to act before awareness occurs. Another reason to measure depth of anaesthesia is the ability to ensure that each patient receives only the minimum amount of anaesthetic required to maintain unconsciousness. This may have the potential to greatly reduce the side-effects of anaesthesia and improve recovery time.

Depth of Anaesthesia

The Isolated Forearm Technique

In this method, a patient is anaesthetized, and then a tourniquet is applied to the upper arm and inflated to above systolic arterial pressure. A muscle relaxant is then administered (if required as part of the appropriate anaesthetic technique). Because the tourniquet prevents the muscle relaxant passing to the arm, the forearm muscles still function and are supplied by nerves passing under the tourniquet. If awareness occurs, the patient is able to signal by moving the forearm. Unfortunately, the technique signals only that the patient is already awake and its duration is limited by the ischaemia caused by the tourniquet.

The electroencephalogram and evoked potentials

The electroencephalogram (EEG) is a small, complex signal which is recorded usually from at least four electrodes fixed to specially prepared sites around the head. It has an amplitude of 50–200 µV and a frequency content which is classified conventionally into four categories:

- delta waves: 0–4 Hz
- theta waves: 4–8 Hz
- alpha waves: 8–13 Hz
- beta waves: 13 Hz and above.

The spiking, transient depolarization, then repolarization, of action potentials in neurones in the brain is sufficiently asynchronous and transient to be unrecordable from the scalp or surface of the brain. It is believed that the EEG is generated by the summation of synchronous postsynaptic potentials on the dendrites of sheets of large and symmetrically arranged pyramidal cells in cortical layers III and IV. Recording of these microvolt signals with acceptable levels of artefact and interference is difficult. Visual analysis of EEG recordings is subjective and requires experience.

The complexity of the raw EEG signals makes its use in the operating theatre impractical. Cerebral function monitors using fewer electrodes have been developed which average the EEG signal, but have been shown to be unreliable in monitoring depth of anaesthesia. However, the Cerebral Function Analysing Monitor (CFAM) has found a role in neurosurgery, and in other specialities in which monitoring cerebral function is crucial. For example, sedated and paralysed patients are unable to display classical tonic-clonic activity during generalized seizures. CFAM enables clinicians to detect seizure activity in neurosurgical intensive care patients and titrate sedation against burst-suppression of the EEG. Two symmetrical pairs of EEG electrodes are placed on either side of the patient's head. The monitor then analyses the EEG amplitude and the frequency of the waveforms into delta, theta, alpha and beta waves as well as displaying wave suppression information.

Two further methods make the EEG signal easier to interpret, based on spectral analysis. The principle is that any complex wave may be broken down into a series of sine waves. Fast Fourier analysis produces an output in terms of the proportion of each frequency which contributes to the total signal. Bispectral analysis uses relationships between the phase and power of different frequencies within the original signal.

Initial attempts using spectral analysis showed that general anaesthesia produces a reduction in the mean frequency and spectral edge (frequency below which 95% of activity occurs). Ultimately, increasing doses of anaesthetic drugs produce a suppressed or isoelectric EEG. Unfortunately, these changes have not proved to be reliable as a measure of depth of anaesthesia.

The bispectral index (BIS monitor) is a number from 100 (awake) to 0 (deeply anaesthetized) produced by a commercially available monitor. Although the exact methods used have not been published, it identifies patterns within 30-s periods of EEG recording by first excluding episodes likely to be produced by diathermy or muscle activity, and periods of burst suppression. The remaining activity is subjected to bispectral analysis with the final result adjusted to take account of the proportion of suppressed EEG. It appears to provide reliable measurements in clinical use. However, it is not clear how factors such as different anaesthetic agents, hypoxaemia or epileptic activity affect the results.

Auditory Evoked Potentials

Auditory evoked potential monitors measure the slowing of auditory information processing produced by anaesthetic agents. The patient wears headphones which repeatedly play soft 'clicks'. Each click produces neuronal activity in the auditory cortex. While the signal from a single click is masked by other brain activity, the signal from repeated clicks can be averaged to isolate the auditory signal. The activity in the auditory cortex may therefore be displayed as the auditory evoked potential, which has a characteristic waveform (Fig. 16.21). The time delay for some waves can then be measured and the result converted into a value typically from zero to 100, reflecting depth of anaesthesia. The equipment cannot be used in patients who have impaired hearing and may require several seconds to generate enough data to process. Monitors using this principle are commercially available, but have yet to be used widely. Equipment using either visual or somatosensory stimulation has also been developed.

Other Techniques

Respiratory sinus arrhythmia is the normal variation in heart rate related to the respiratory cycle. This variability is reduced by anaesthesia and has formed the basis of a commercially available monitor. However, it has not achieved widespread use.

Monitors based on physiological measures such as frontalis muscle myography and lower oesophageal contractility have not proved reliable enough for clinical use.

Intracranial Pressure

Intracranial pressure (ICP) is frequently measured in neurointensive care units, and forms the basis of neuroprotective treatment strategies in brain injuries. The principle is similar to measurement of vascular pressure: an invasive device is connected via a rigid fluid-filled column to an electromechanical transducer which enables display of the waveform on a monitor. Classically, this is achieved using a catheter inserted into the lateral ventricle - the 'gold standard' for ICP measurement. Alternatively, the subdural space can be used, although this provides a less accurate monitor of ICP. More modern systems are less invasive and use either a catheter-tip miniature transducer or a microchip sensor which sits within the parenchyma of the brain. These systems do not require a fluid-filled column or an external transducer, so avoid errors of positioning. However, they cannot be re-calibrated once inserted and do not necessarily reflect global ICP.

Brain Oxygenation

The crucial need to ensure brain oxygenation and the inability to monitor consciousness during anaesthesia imply that an electronic monitor would be very valuable, especially during neurosurgery and in head-injured patients. Unfortunately, none of the currently available techniques has proved suitable for general use in the theatre environment. Their role is essentially limited to the neurosurgical Intensive Care Unit.

Near-infrared spectroscopy (NIRS) uses a pulse oximeter probe attached to the patient's head to detect light reflected from the brain. While the technique may be used in small children, whose skulls are thin, doubts remain in adults as to whether this technique reflects brain oxygenation or merely scalp blood flow.

Transcranial Doppler involves a trained operator using a Doppler probe to measure the speed of red cells in cerebral arteries. It may detect vasospasm after

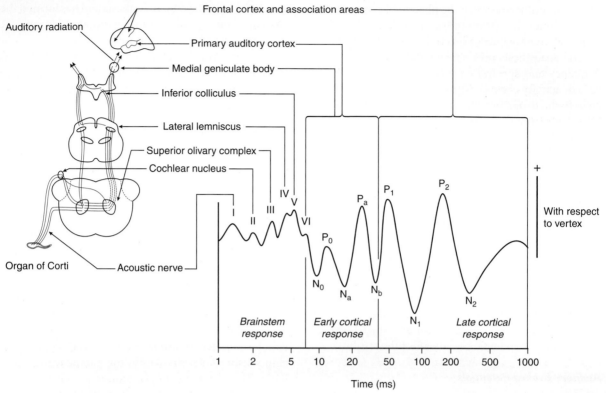

FIGURE 16.21 ■ The auditory evoked response consists of a series of waves generated from specific anatomical sites in the auditory pathway as indicated. Activity passes from the cochlea through the brainstem to the cortex.

subarachnoid haemorrhage, but has little use in routine anaesthesia apart from during carotid endarterectomy when it may be used to demonstrate adequacy of blood flow in the circle of Willis during contralateral carotid artery clamping.

Jugular venous oxygen saturation monitoring involves passing a catheter retrogradely up the internal jugular vein into the jugular venous sinus. A saturation of less than 55% indicates increased oxygen extraction and therefore relative ischaemia. It is a useful technique in the Intensive Care Unit but only measures global perfusion and fails to detect small areas of ischaemia. It also does not inform the clinician as to whether a low saturation is due to inadequate oxygen supply or increased cerebral demand.

Cerebral oxygenation can also be measured directly through the use of specialized intracerebral sensors. The Licox® PMO is a combined brain tissue oxygen and brain temperature monitor which detects regional changes

in oxygenation. It is in essence a Clark polarographic electrode with a thermistor and sits within the brain parenchyma, ideally within the damaged but salvageable region of tissue (the penumbra). Assuming the monitor is sited in the correct area, it is able to measure regional oxygen tension accurately, although with a slight tendency to under-read.

More recently, microdialysis catheters have been introduced. These comprise a catheter with a surface dialysis membrane, and a perfusion system which slowly circulates dialysis fluid within the catheter. The returning fluid is analysed, either remotely or continuously, for cerebral metabolites such as lactate, pyruvate and other indicators of cerebral stress such as glutamate and glycerol. The lactate/pyruvate ratio is useful as a marker of cerebral ischaemia. As with intraparenchymal ICP monitors and the Licox system, the measurements are necessarily regional and dependent on accurate positioning of the catheter.

TEMPERATURE

The body is considered to have an inner core temperature and an outer peripheral temperature. In reality, the temperature decreases with distance down limbs and proximity to the skin. The difference between core and peripheral temperatures is related strongly to the cardiac output and degree of vasoconstriction. In practice, a core-periphery difference of >2°C indicates a low cardiac output state and has been used as a marker of hypovolaemia.

Commercial thermometers make use of several temperature-dependent phenomena.

Direct Reading Non-Electrical Thermometers

Liquid Expansion Thermometers

Liquid expansion thermometers are simple, reliable instruments. A glass bulb is filled with a liquid (generally alcohol or mercury) and connected to an evacuated, closed capillary tube. The temperature is recorded by the position of the meniscus in the capillary tube against a calibrated scale. If the cross-sectional area of the capillary tube is constant, movement of the meniscus with changing temperature is linear.

Several simple and elegant design features improve usability. A large bulb and very narrow capillary increase the sensitivity. Visibility of the narrow capillary is improved by shaping the thermometer so that the glass forms a lens and by incorporating a strip of white glass behind the capillary. A constriction in the capillary tube permits the mercury to expand but hinders its return to the bulb so that the reading is preserved until the mercury is shaken down. However, glass thermometers are fragile. A large thermal capacity results in a slow response. The instrument is handheld, awkward to read and reset, and cannot be used for remote measurement or recording. Traditional mercury-in-glass thermometers are no longer used because of the risk of breakage and mercury contamination.

Chemical Thermometers

Thermometers based on temperature-dependent changes in chemical mixtures have been marketed. Reversible chemical thermometers contain several cells filled with liquid crystals, each of slightly different composition. At a critical temperature, the optical properties change because of realignment of the molecules, causing reflection instead of absorption of the incident light. An alternative technique consists of rows of cells filled with chemical mixtures which melt at specific temperatures releasing a dye; this single-use, disposable design prevents cross-infection but is relatively expensive.

Infrared Thermometers

The amount of infrared radiation emitted by the tympanic membrane depends on its temperature, emissivity compared to a black body at the same temperature and the Stefan-Boltzmann constant. Infrared tympanic membrane thermometers based on this principle are in common clinical use. They are inserted into the external ear with the tip protected by a disposable sheath. They measure the infrared radiation produced from the eardrum and produce a digital readout in less than 3 s. Unfortunately, because of factors such as earwax and variations in the angle of insertion, results are less reliable than fixed probes and they cannot produce continuous readings. They are therefore used principally in recovery and ward areas.

Remote Reading Instruments

Temperature-dependent electrical properties may be incorporated into thermometers suitable for automation (e.g. targeted temperature management systems for therapeutic cooling of patients), and are also commonly used for monitoring peripheral and core temperature.

Resistance-Wire Thermometers

Resistance-wire thermometers are based on the principle that the resistance of some metal wires increases as their temperature increases. Platinum resistance thermometers have a large temperature coefficient of resistance and are very sensitive to small changes in temperature, but are fragile and slow to respond. Single-use probes which incorporate a tiny copper element have been marketed with an acceptable clinical accuracy and response time.

Thermistor Thermometers

Thermistors are semiconductors made from the fused oxides of heavy metals such as cobalt, manganese and nickel. They demonstrate marked and non-linear variation in resistance with temperature, which is usually compensated by electronic processing. Disadvantages include inconsistent variation between individual thermistors, change in resistance over time, and hysteresis during rapid heating and cooling. However, the large temperature coefficient permits the detection of small temperature changes and the tiny 'pin-head' size results in a rapid response. They are used widely in invasive temperature monitoring, e.g. in pulmonary artery catheters.

Thermocouple Thermometers

If two dissimilar metals are joined to create an electrical circuit and the junctions are at different temperatures, current flows from one metal to the other. The potential difference which is generated is a function of the temperature difference between the two junctions. All junctions made from the same metals have identical properties. The reference junction must be kept at a constant temperature, or incorporate temperature compensation into the measurement. Common combinations of metals include copper-constantan or platinum-rhodium. The output is small (about 40 mV per °C temperature difference between the junctions), but this is sufficient to be sensed by a galvanometer.

Temperature probes using these properties can continuously measure peripheral and core temperatures. Peripheral temperature is measured by attaching a probe to either a finger or toe. Core temperature probes may be inserted into the nasopharynx, oesophagus or rectum, and although complications are rare, it is possible to cause mucosal trauma, bleeding and even penetration of the pharynx or rectum. When used for prolonged periods, mucosal damage is possible as a result of pressure-related ischaemia. Core temperature probes may also form part of an intravascular catheter, for example within a PAFC. Many monitors accept two probes and automatically display the temperature difference. Care must be taken to avoid the peripheral probe being exposed to warmth from heating blankets.

Equipment Temperature

The performance of some anaesthetic equipment is temperature dependent (e.g. vaporizers) and alternative thermometric principles may be used.

Dial Thermometers

Dial thermometers exploit the increase in pressure caused by the temperature-dependent expansion of a liquid or gas in an enclosed cavity. This is sensed by a Bourdon pressure gauge and recorded on a dial. Although cheap and robust, they are relatively inaccurate, slow to respond and are only suitable for large temperature changes in heated equipment, e.g. autoclaves.

Bimetallic Strip Thermometers

If strips of two metals with different coefficients of expansion are fastened together throughout their length, the combined strip will bend when heated. Sensitivity is improved by using a long strip which is usually bent in a spiral or coil, with one end fixed and the other connected to a recording pointer. This technique is used for temperature compensation in some anaesthetic vaporizers, and in cheap mechanical thermometers for measuring air temperature.

BLOOD LOSS AND TRANSFUSION

During surgery, blood loss is common but it may be difficult to measure accurately because blood may soak into surgical drapes and swabs, find its way into suction bottles or fall on to the floor. Although it is usually impossible to measure the blood loss accurately, an attempt should be made to estimate blood loss in all cases. This is particularly important in paediatric cases, where, for example, in a 2-kg child, a major haemorrhage equates to a blood loss of more than 20 mL.

Red Cell Loss

This may be estimated by weighing the swabs after use, but is notoriously inaccurate. Measuring the haemoglobin concentration of a known volume of solution after all the swabs have been washed in it provides a more accurate result, but usually too late to be of immediate clinical use. Regular estimation of blood haemoglobin concentration is the only reliable method of determining the effect of blood loss.

Blood Clotting

Clotting efficacy is assessed by measuring the platelet count, prothrombin time (intrinsic system), activated partial thromboplastin time (extrinsic system) and fibrinogen concentration. Although these are traditional laboratory-based tests, there are increasing numbers of methods of analysing blood clotting in the operating theatre. These require the user to add a sample of blood to a reagent in a chamber, which is then inserted into a measuring device. The Sonoclot™ device uses a probe which is moved up and down in the sample. As the clot forms, the increasing resistance is measured and plotted as a graph against time. In thromboelastography, a pin is lowered into the sample and rotated intermittently. As a clot forms, there is increasing resistance to rotation.

Laboratory-based tests of clotting should be used whenever there is a risk of a clotting defect and after a significant blood transfusion. The main advantage of these tests is that they can be interpreted by haematologists, who provide advice on suitable treatments. Bedside monitors are used increasingly to measure clotting in procedures such as coronary artery surgery, where anticoagulants are usually used and significant blood loss is common.

Near-Patient Testing

During long operations, or when there is a need for infusion of large volumes of fluid, it may be necessary to measure physiological variables such as pH, haemoglobin and electrolyte concentrations and carboxyhaemoglobin. These have traditionally been performed on samples sent to laboratories and analysed by trained staff. The machines used are often complex and subject to regular servicing and quality control. More recently, it has become possible to use a variety of devices for 'bedside' analysis.

These devices usually comprise a small disposable cartridge which contains a combination of reagents and often some electronic circuitry. A sample is placed in the cartridge, which is then inserted into a larger analyser. Serum glucose concentration may be measured by a reagent strip which is compared with a colour chart or by insertion into a reader. These machines provide rapid results at the bedside and avoid the delays of transporting samples to the laboratory. However, the accuracy of the results produced by such devices is usually dependent on the skill of the operator and they may be affected by poor storage of the reagent or monitor. They also usually lack the organized quality control checks used in laboratories. Results are therefore less reliable and should be confirmed by laboratory analysis where possible.

MONITORING STANDARDS

The presence of an appropriately trained and experienced anaesthetist is the most essential patient monitor. However, human error is inevitable and there is substantial evidence that many incidents are attributable, at least in part, to error by anaesthetists.

Appropriate monitoring will not prevent all adverse incidents in the perioperative period. However, there is substantial evidence that it reduces the amount of harm to patients, not only by detecting problems as they occur but also by alerting the anaesthetist that an error has occurred. In one study, the introduction of modern standards of monitoring halved the number of cardiac arrests, principally because of the reduction in arrests caused by preventable respiratory causes. In the Australian Incident Monitoring Study, 52% of incidents were detected first by a monitor and in more than half of these cases, it was the pulse oximeter or capnograph which detected the problem.

There has never been a study comparing outcomes from anaesthesia with and without monitoring, and now that there are mandatory standards of monitoring in most countries, it will be impossible to prove that monitors make a difference.

The current recommendations from the Association of Anaesthetists of Great Britain and Ireland are shown in Table 16.9. However, it is not sufficient that the monitors are available. Departmental heads are responsible for ensuring not only that equipment is available but also that it works correctly, that it is maintained to appropriate standards, that staff are trained in its use and that it is used appropriately.

All anaesthetists must ensure that they are familiar with the equipment used in their hospital and that all equipment has been checked before use. The need for training and practice cannot be overemphasized because the increasing complexity of modern monitoring devices implies that they can behave in unexpected ways at inopportune moments.

ALARMS

All electronic monitors now include alarms which sound (and illuminate) when a variable moves outside a preset range. These limits are usually set by the manufacturer as part of the monitoring system's basic functions and may be changed by the user (although the default values are often protected by a password). Failure to reset the

TABLE 16.9

Summary of Recommendations for Standards of Monitoring During Anaesthesia and Recovery

The anaesthetist must be present and care for the patient throughout the conduct of an anaesthetic.*

Monitoring devices must be attached before induction of anaesthesia and their use continued until the patient has recovered from the effects of anaesthesia.

The same standards of monitoring apply when the anaesthetist is responsible for a local/regional anaesthetic or sedative technique for an operative procedure.

A summary of information provided by monitoring devices should be recorded on the anaesthetic record. Electronic record keeping systems are now recommended.

The anaesthetist must ensure that all equipment has been checked before use. Alarm limits for all equipment must be set appropriately before use. Audible alarms must be enabled during anaesthesia.

Table 16.10 indicates the monitoring devices which are essential and those which must be immediately available during anaesthesia. If it is necessary to continue anaesthesia without a device categorized as 'essential', the anaesthetist must clearly note the reasons for this in the anaesthetic record.

Additional monitoring may be necessary as deemed appropriate by the anaesthetist.

A brief interruption of monitoring is only acceptable if the recovery area is immediately adjacent to the operating theatre. Otherwise monitoring should be continued during transfer to the same degree as any other intra- or inter-hospital transfer.

Provision, maintenance, calibration and renewal of equipment is an institutional responsibility.

*In hospitals employing Anaesthetic Practitioners (APs), this responsibility may be delegated to an AP supervised by a consultant anaesthetist in accordance with guidelines published by the Royal College of Anaesthetists (www.rcoa.ac.uk).
Reproduced with permission from the Association of Anaesthetists of Great Britain and Ireland 2007.

alarm limits to appropriate values before starting anaesthesia is a common cause of false alarm signals. This often results in the anaesthetist cancelling a series of false alarms, with the risk that an alarm for a real problem is also cancelled without any action being taken.

Alarms alert the anaesthetist to a developing physiological change and allow it to be corrected. However, alarms may not respond to a serious problem. For example, marked hypotension in an elderly hypertensive patient may still fall within the range of a 'normal' arterial pressure as set for the monitor. Alarms must therefore be set to appropriate levels before induction so that they are triggered only by real abnormalities. This is particularly true during procedures involving children, when values for respiratory rate, for example, are not within the 'normal' adult range.

More commonly, alarms are triggered by artefacts: for example, the electrical interference produced by diathermy often triggers an alarm for arrhythmia from the ECG. Also common is the production of alarms by spurious problems such as an apparently low endtidal carbon dioxide concentration during induction of anaesthesia, produced by the gas leak around a face mask. The frequency of such false alarms implies that many alarms are ignored, or may lead the anaesthetist

to concentrate on the monitoring equipment and ignore the patient.

Further, because of the lack of standardization of alarm signals and the uniformity of alarms, in a genuine crisis, the cacophony of multiple alarms and series of flashing lights may cause staff to concentrate on a relatively unimportant complication, such as bradycardia, with the cause, such as a disconnection in the breathing system, going unnoticed.

Oxygen Supply

The use of an oxygen analyser with an audible alarm is mandatory for all patients breathing anaesthetic gases. The sampling port must be placed such that the gas mixture delivered to the patient is monitored continuously. The analyser should provide a clearly visible readout of the concentration of oxygen in the inspired gas and sound an audible alarm if a hypoxic mixture is delivered.

Breathing Systems

The principal problems are of disconnection, leak or excessive pressure. During spontaneous ventilation, the movement of a reservoir bag usually provides evidence of continuing ventilation. However, a capnograph is required to ensure that ventilation is adequate. When positive-pressure ventilation is used, a measure of airway pressure and appropriate alarms are also required.

Monitors do not always detect every abnormality. For example, if a capnograph is attached to an airway filter in a spontaneously breathing patient, the breathing system may become disconnected from the filter, leading to a risk of awareness. However, because the patient continues to breathe room air through the filter, the capnograph trace is unchanged and no alarm is triggered.

Vapour Analyser

A vapour analyser is essential whenever anaesthetic vapours are used, both to prevent accidental overdose and also to prevent awareness. A particular problem with many commonly used vaporizers is that they are not able to detect when the vaporizer is empty (the Tec 6 Desflurane vaporizer is one exception). During a long procedure, it is possible for a vaporizer to become empty without warning unless an agent monitor is in place.

Cardiovascular

Non-invasive arterial pressure and ECG are always required as monitors of the cardiovascular system. Although these provide useful information, clinical measures such as capillary refill and urine output are more reliable monitors.

Infusion Devices

Increasingly, anaesthetic drugs are being delivered by infusion devices. As with most equipment, individual devices are becoming more complex. For example, rather than using simple infusion pumps, anaesthesia may be delivered using devices containing computers, allowing the infusion to maintain a constant plasma concentration, e.g. the Diprifusor™ infusion pump.

These devices contain sophisticated alarm systems and usually need to be programmed with a variety of patient data to function effectively. Anaesthetists also need to be trained in their use and must understand how these devices work before attaching them to a patient. In particular, it must be emphasized that although many infusion devices display information about the amount of drug administered and/or plasma concentration, these are dependent on absence of leaks and on assumptions about the patient. A common problem is disconnection of the infusion line under surgical drapes, leading to underdosage. A further

problem is that, in sick patients, factors such as the size of fluid compartments or rate of drug transport may differ greatly from those assumed by the pump, leading to over- or underdosage.

GENERAL GUIDELINES FOR MONITORING DURING ANAESTHESIA

Table 16.10 summarizes the required monitors for different components of anaesthesia. Monitors should be applied to the awake patient and readings taken to ensure that they are functioning correctly before induction of anaesthesia. If uncooperative patients make

---

TABLE 16.10
Essential Monitoring

A. Induction and Maintenance of Anaesthesia
  i. Pulse oximeter
  ii. Non-invasive blood pressure monitor
  iii. Electrocardiograph
  iv. Airway gases: oxygen, carbon dioxide and vapour
  v. Airway pressure

The following must also be available:
- A nerve stimulator whenever a muscle relaxant is used
- A means of measuring the patient's temperature

B. Recovery from Anaesthesia
  i. Pulse oximeter
  ii. Non-invasive blood pressure monitor

The following must also be immediately available:
- Electrocardiograph
- Nerve stimulator
- Means of measuring temperature
- Capnograph

C. Additional Monitoring
- Some patients will require additional, mainly invasive monitoring.
- The AAGBI endorses the views of the American Society of Anesthesiologists (ASA): "Brain function monitoring is not routinely indicated for patients undergoing general anaesthesia, either to reduce the frequency of intra-operative awareness or to monitor depth of anaesthesia"

D. Regional Techniques & Sedation for Operative Procedures
  i. Pulse oximeter
  ii. Non-invasive blood pressure monitor
  iii. Electrocardiograph

Reproduced with permission from the Association of Anaesthetists of Great Britain and Ireland 2007.

application of monitoring impossible before induction, the monitors should be applied as soon as possible after induction and the reason recorded on the anaesthetic chart.

For short procedures such as electroconvulsive therapy (ECT) or orthopaedic manipulations, the standards for induction of anaesthesia are appropriate. However, if the procedure is prolonged then the standards for maintenance of anaesthesia should be applied. A high standard of monitoring should be applied continuously until the patient has recovered fully from anaesthesia. If the recovery room is not immediately adjacent to the operating theatre, or if the patient's condition is poor, equipment should be available so that the above standards are applied during transfer of the patient.

Additional Monitoring

The standards in Table 16.10 are the minimum acceptable levels and apply to healthy patients undergoing minor surgery. If the patient is unwell before surgery or major surgery is planned, additional monitoring should be applied. It is difficult to give strict guidelines on what conditions or surgery should prompt the use of each monitor. Suggestions are given in Table 16.11.

Monitoring During Transfer

It is essential that the standard of care and monitoring during transfer is as high as that applied in the operating theatre and that staff with appropriate training and experience accompany the patient.

During transfer, vibrations may make devices which rely on pressure change, such as non-invasive arterial pressure monitors, inaccurate or non-functional. Vibration may also cause connections to work loose and equipment may suffer physical damage. Movement may make an ECG trace useless for diagnosis of arrhythmias. Noise and poor lighting make the displays of many monitors difficult to read and make audible alarms inaudible. Adequate supplies must be taken for the entire journey, together with additional supplies

---

TABLE 16.11
Variables that it may be Appropriate to Monitor During Anaesthesia in some Patients in Addition to the Essential Monitoring for all Anaesthetized Patients

Indications	Monitors
Operative duration >3 h	Direct arterial pressure measurement
Blood loss >10% blood volume	Central venous pressure
Operations on: 　Chest 　Central nervous system 　Cardiovascular system	Pulmonary capillary wedge pressure Cardiac output Transoesophageal echocardiography Blood loss measurement
Clinically significant coexisting disease	Urine output Temperature: 　Patient 　Blood warmer, mattress 　Inspired gas Blood gas analysis Serum electrolyte concentrations Haemoglobin concentration Coagulation status

to anticipate any unforeseen delays. This includes oxygen cylinders, batteries (the internal batteries of a monitor may have short lives) and anaesthetic drugs.

Before transfer, the patient should be in a stable physiological state. The patient should be moved on to the transport trolley, all of the transport monitors should be applied to the patient and their functions should be checked. All equipment should then be fastened securely and all catheters and leads taped into position. A check should be made that, from a single position, the anaesthetist is able to attend to the airway, see all the monitors and be able to administer drugs and fluids. The process is made much easier and safer with a dedicated transport trolley, so that all the equipment is fixed permanently in place.

ANAESTHETIC RECORD-KEEPING

It is the professional responsibility of every doctor to maintain accurate records of the treatment which patients receive, and their response to it. The anaesthetic record forms a part of a patient's medical record. The principal purpose of the anaesthetic chart is to provide details of the anaesthetic technique used, of the physiological changes which were associated with the technique and with surgery, and of complications or problems which were encountered during the procedure. This information may assist other doctors if complications ensue, or if anaesthesia is required in the future. In addition, the anaesthetic record may be a valuable source of information if a subsequent complication results in litigation; the absence of a full record makes it difficult for an anaesthetist to demonstrate, for example, that postoperative renal failure was not attributable to untreated intraoperative hypotension.

The design of anaesthetic records varies widely, and is probably unimportant provided that it facilitates recording and display of all the relevant data. Suggestions for the reasonable content of an anaesthetic record data set are shown in Table 16.12.

In addition to the data described above, the record should include details of the techniques discussed with the patient, together with any risks or benefits outlined and the management plan agreed. If the patient has any specific requests or concerns, such as a desire to avoid blood transfusion, it is also best to record them in writing.

Automated Records

It has been estimated that up to 20% of the anaesthetist's time is taken up with documentation. While the anaesthetic record is usually completed as the anaesthetic proceeds, there are times, such as during induction or a crisis, when it is not possible to complete the chart contemporaneously. This delay leads to inaccuracies. In addition, studies have shown that anaesthetists tend to record 'normalized' data, i.e. the record tends to minimize any physiological changes which occur.

To counteract these problems, most anaesthetic monitors and anaesthetic machines may be connected to automatic data recording systems. These log all the monitoring data and have the facility for the anaesthetist to add data such as drugs used and comments on events, such as the start of surgery. The data may be stored electronically for later study and printed out in a variety of formats. They have the potential to interact with other sources of information so that patient details, laboratory results, scans and outpatient letters can all be accessed. These systems have the potential to make audits and quality control much easier to perform. The AAGBI recommends that departments consider their procurement.

However, these systems are expensive and it must be recognized that all monitors have numerous sources of error; while most anaesthetists tend to ignore erroneous readings, they are recorded and printed by an automated system. Printouts should therefore be checked and errors marked before being included in the patient's medical record.

TABLE 16.12

Suggested Data for Inclusion on Anaesthetic Records

PREOPERATIVE INFORMATION

Patient identity
Name/ID number/gender
Date of birth

Assessment and risk factors
Date of assessment
Assessor, where assessed
Weight (kg) [height (m) optional]
Base vital signs (BP, HR)
Medication, incl. contraceptive drugs
Allergies
Addiction (alcohol, tobacco, drugs)
Previous GAs, family history
Potential airway problems
Prostheses, teeth, crowns
Investigations
Cardiorespiratory fitness
Other problems
ASA grade±comment

Urgency
Scheduled – listed on a routine list
Urgent – resuscitated, not on a routine list
Emergency – not fully resuscitated

PERIOPERATIVE INFORMATION

Checks
Nil by mouth
Consent
Premedication, type and effect

Regional anaesthesia
Consent
Block performed
Entry site
Needle used, aid to location
Catheter: y/n

Patient position and attachments
Thrombosis prophylaxis
Temperature control
Limb position

Postoperative instructions
Drugs, fluids and doses
Analgesic techniques

Place and time
Place
Date, start and end times

Personnel
All anaesthetists named
Check performed, anaesthetic room, theatre

Operation planned/performed

Apparatus
Check performed, anaesthetic room, theatre

Vital signs recording/charting
Monitors used and vital signs recorded not less frequently
than every 5 min

Drugs and fluids
Dose, concentration, volume
Cannulation
Injection site(s), time & route
Warmer used
Blood loss, urine output

Airway and breathing system
Route, system used
Ventilation: type & mode
Airway type, size, cuff, shape
Special procedures, humidifier, filter
Throat pack
Difficulty

Special airway instructions, incl. oxygen
Monitoring

Untoward events
Abnormalities
Critical incidents
Preoperative, perioperative, postoperative
Context, cause, effect

Hazard flags
Warnings for future care

Based on recommendations of the Royal College of Anaesthetists and the Association of Anaesthetists of Great Britain and Ireland

FURTHER READING

Association of Anaesthetists of Great Britain and Ireland, 2012. Checklist for anaesthetic equipment. AAGBI, London.

Association of Anaesthetists of Great Britain and Ireland, 1998. Risk management 1998. AAGBI, London.

Association of Anaesthetists of Great Britain and Ireland, 2007. Recommendations for standards of monitoring during anaesthesia and recovery, fourth ed. AAGBI, London.

Cruikshank, S., 1998. Mathematics and statistics in anaesthesia. Oxford Medical Publications, Oxford.

Davis, P.D., Kenny, G., 2003. Basic physics and measurement in anaesthesia, fifth ed. Butterworth-Heinemann, Oxford.

Sykes, M.K., Vickers, M.D., Hull, C.J., 1991. Principles of clinical measurement, third ed. Blackwell Scientific Publications, Oxford.

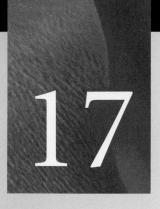

17

PREOPERATIVE ASSESSMENT AND PREMEDICATION

All patients scheduled to undergo surgery should be assessed in advance with a view to planning optimal preparation and perioperative management. This is a standard of care of the Association of Anaesthetists of Great Britain and Ireland, and similar bodies worldwide. It is one mechanism by which the standard and quality of care provided by an individual anaesthetist or an anaesthetic department may be measured. Failure to undertake this activity places the patient at increased risk of perioperative morbidity or mortality.

The overall aims of preoperative assessment should include the following:

- To enable the most appropriate treatment for the patient, taking into consideration the patient's current health, the nature of the proposed surgery and anaesthetic technique, and the skills and expertise of the anaesthetist.
- To confirm that the surgery proposed is realistic and allow assessment of the likely benefit to the patient and the possible risks involved.
- To anticipate potential problems and ensure that adequate facilities and appropriately trained staff are available to provide satisfactory perioperative care.
- To ensure that the patient is prepared correctly for the operation and allow time for further investigations and specialist referral to improve any existing factors which may increase the risk of an adverse outcome.
- To provide appropriate information to the patient, and obtain informed consent for surgery and the planned anaesthetic technique.

- To prescribe premedication and/or other specific prophylactic measures if required.
- To ensure that proper documentation is made of the assessment process.

It is implicit that the anaesthetist has sufficient knowledge and experience of both the proposed surgery and necessary anaesthetic management to predict the potential progress of an individual patient during the perioperative period. Appropriate skills must be achieved and maintained by an ongoing commitment to education, both individually and within the profession overall. There are organizational issues to be considered within any hospital in order that preoperative assessment and preparation of patients can be accomplished successfully. Increasingly, this makes use of a nurse-led assessment process combined with gaining an anaesthetic opinion when appropriate, guided and supported by the use of evidence-based protocols.

THE PROCESS OF PREOPERATIVE ASSESSMENT

Who, When and Where?

The decision regarding the need for an operation is normally made by an experienced surgeon on the basis of the patient's presenting pathology. The patient subsequently undergoes a more extensive assessment of general health closer to the time of admission for surgery. This is undertaken usually by the least experienced member of the surgical team, and in some circumstances is delegated (in part) to an experienced

357

nurse practitioner. Identification of potential problems by these individuals relies upon their application of general medical knowledge and common sense, often assisted by the use of screening protocols developed either nationally, or locally by the anaesthetic department. When a patient is recognized to be at special risk, referral to an appropriate anaesthetist should be made. This need not be the anaesthetist ultimately responsible for the patient's care if surgery is not urgent, provided that decisions made regarding preoperative preparation are communicated and recorded clearly in the medical notes. If surgery is more imminent, it is preferable to involve the anaesthetist who will be responsible for the patient's perioperative care.

The need to improve efficiency of hospital bed occupancy has led to the increasing use of pre-admission clerking appointments, arranged to allow completion of the majority of the necessary administrative details. This is an ideal opportunity for anaesthetic assessment to take place, but in reality it is often not feasible to guarantee the availability of an experienced anaesthetist for these sessions. One direct consequence of this change is that patients are subsequently admitted on to the ward close to the time of surgery, allowing significantly less time for the anaesthetist to organize perioperative management. In order to optimize preparation for surgery within this system, many hospitals now use preoperative questionnaires which are completed by the patient in advance of clerking and are designed specifically to identify key features in the medical history which need further clarification. In addition, guidelines may be provided by the anaesthetic department for the surgical team or nurse practitioner to ensure that appropriate investigations are undertaken and that suitable action is taken if problems are identified.

Regardless of the timing and the individual personnel involved in clerking patients before surgery, the fundamental process of taking a detailed history and performing a systematic clinical examination remains the foundation on which preoperative assessment relies, backed up by ordering appropriate investigations where indicated. This allows the anaesthetist to concentrate on areas of particular relevance to perioperative care.

History

Direct questions should be asked about the following items of specific relevance to anaesthesia.

Presenting Condition and Concurrent Medical History

The indication for surgery determines its urgency and thus influences aspects of anaesthetic management. There are many surgical conditions which have systemic effects and these must be sought and quantified, e.g. bowel cancer may be associated with malnourishment, anaemia and electrolyte imbalance. The presence of coexisting medical disease must also be identified, together with an assessment of the extent of any associated limitations to normal activity. The most relevant tend to be related to cardiovascular and respiratory diseases because of their potential effect on perioperative management. Specific questioning should ascertain the degree of exertional dyspnoea, paroxysmal nocturnal dyspnoea, orthopnoea, angina of effort, etc. Functional capacity is frequently defined in terms of the ability to exercise to a certain degree of metabolic equivalents (METs) where 1 MET is equivalent to basal oxygen consumption at rest (i.e. $3.5\,mL\,min^{-1}\,kg^{-1}$). The Duke Activity Status Index approximates certain physical activities with multiples of the MET and so may be used to quantify patients' ability to exercise. The inability to climb two flights of stairs (which approximates to 4 METs) is associated with an increased risk of cardiac complications after major surgery. Limitations to exercise because of other factors should be identified, e.g. intermittent claudication, arthritis, etc., so that effort-related symptoms such as dyspnoea and angina may be interpreted correctly.

Anaesthetic History

Details of the administration and outcome of previous anaesthetic episodes should be documented, especially if problems were encountered. Some sequelae such as sore throat, headache or postoperative nausea may not seem of great significance to the anaesthetist but may form the basis of considerable preoperative anxiety for the patient. The patient may be unaware of anaesthetic problems in the past if managed uneventfully and hence the anaesthetic records should be examined if they are available. More serious problems such as difficulty maintaining a patent airway, performing tracheal intubation or some other specific procedure (e.g. insertion of an epidural catheter) should have been documented. Other serious problems such as unexpected admission to the intensive care unit following surgery should be explored carefully in order to identify contributing factors which might be encountered once again.

Family History

There are several hereditary conditions which influence planned anaesthetic management, such as malignant hyperthermia, cholinesterase abnormalities, porphyria, some haemoglobinopathies and dystrophia myotonica. Some of these disorders may not limit the patient's normal activities, but their presence is usually confirmed by asking about details of anaesthetic problems encountered by immediate family members and any subsequent investigations required; the family history is particularly important in patients who have not undergone surgery and anaesthesia previously.

It is important to remember that a negative family history does not imply that there are no familial issues. A positive history is relatively specific, but a negative history is very insensitive.

Drug History

A complete history of concurrent medication must be documented carefully. Many drugs interact with agents or techniques used during anaesthesia but problems may occur if drugs are withdrawn suddenly during the perioperative period (Table 17.1). Knowledge of pharmacology is essential to permit the anaesthetist to

TABLE 17.1
Drugs with Potential Anaesthetic Interaction During Anaesthesia

Drug Group	Comments
Cardiovascular	
Angiotensin-converting enzyme inhibitors Captopril Enalapril Lisinopril	Hypotensive effects may be potentiated by anaesthetic agents. Sudden withdrawal tends not to produce haemodynamic effects, perhaps because of relatively long duration of action
Angiotensin II receptor blockers Losartan Valsartan	May be associated with severe hypotension at induction or during maintenance of anaesthesia; consideration should be given to stopping treatment 24 h preoperatively
Antihypertensives Clonidine Guanethidine Methyldopa Reserpine	Hypotension with all anaesthetic agents, requiring extreme care with dosage and administration. *Clonidine* (or *dexmedetomidine*) allows reduction in dosage of anaesthetic agents and opioids. Acute withdrawal of long-term treatment may result in a hypertensive crisis. *Guanethidine* potentiates effect of sympathomimetics. *Reserpine* depletes noradrenaline (norepinephrine) stores, so attenuating the action of pressor agents acting via noradrenaline release
β-Blockers	Negative inotropic effects additive with anaesthetic agents to cause exaggerated hypotension. Mask compensatory tachycardia. Caution with concomitant use of any cardiovascular depressant drugs. Acute withdrawal may result in angina, ventricular extrasystoles, or even precipitate myocardial infarction
Ca^{2+} channel blockers Verapamil	Depresses AV conduction and excitability. Interacts with volatile anaesthetic agents leading to bradyarrhythmias and decreased cardiac output
Diltiazem Nifedipine	Negative inotropic effect and vasodilatation. Interact with volatile anaesthetic agents to cause hypotension. May augment action of competitive muscle relaxants. Acute withdrawal may exacerbate angina
Others Digoxin	Arrhythmias enhanced by calcium. Toxicity is enhanced by hypokalaemia, which must be corrected preoperatively. Succinylcholine enhances toxicity and should therefore be used with caution. Beware of bradyarrhythmias

Continued

TABLE 17.1	
Drugs with Potential Anaesthetic Interaction During Anaesthesia—Cont'd	
Drug Group	**Comments**
Diuretics	Can cause hypokalaemia, which may potentiate the effect of competitive muscle relaxants
Magnesium	Potentiates action of muscle relaxants, the dosage of which may need to be reduced
Quinidine	Intravenous administration can produce neuromuscular blockade, notable particularly following succinylcholine
Central nervous system	
Anticonvulsants	Cause liver enzyme induction. May increase requirements for sedative or anaesthetic agents. Sudden withdrawal may produce rebound convulsive activity
Benzodiazepines	Additive effect with many CNS-depressant drugs. Caution with dosage of intravenous anaesthetic agents and opioids. Additive effect with competitive muscle relaxants, causing potentiation of their action. Action of succinylcholine may be antagonized
Monoamine oxidase inhibitors (MAOIs)	React with opioids causing coma or CNS excitement. Severe hypertensive response to pressor agents. Treatment of regional anaesthetic-induced hypotension may be difficult, especially as indirect sympathomimetics (e.g. ephedrine) are contraindicated due to unpredictable and exaggerated release of noradrenaline (norepinephrine). Adverse effects do not always occur, but recommended to withdraw drugs 2–3 weeks before surgery and use alternative medication
Tricyclic antidepressants	Inhibit the metabolism of catecholamines, increasing the likelihood of arrhythmias. Imipramine potentiates the cardiovascular effects of adrenaline (adrenaline). Delay gastric emptying
Phenothiazines	Interact with other hypotensive agents, necessitating care with administration of all agents
Butyrophenones	with potential cardiovascular effect
Others	
Lithium	Potentiates non-depolarizing muscle relaxants. Consider changing to alternative treatment 48–72 h prior to anaesthesia
L-Dopa	Risks of tachycardia and arrhythmias with halothane. Actions antagonized by droperidol. Augments hyperglycaemia in diabetes. Some suggest discontinuing on day of surgery, but this must be balanced against possible detrimental effects as a result
Antibiotics	
Aminoglycosides	Potentiation of neuromuscular block. Caution with the use of neuromuscular blockers. Effect may be partially antagonized with Ca^{2+}
Sulphonamides	Potentiation of thiopental
Non-steroidal anti-inflammatory drugs	Interfere with platelet function to varying degrees by inhibition of platelet cyclo-oxygenase.
Steroids	Potential adrenocortical suppression. Additional steroid cover may be required for the perioperative period. Risk of hyperglycaemia
Anticoagulants	Problems with minor trauma resulting from cannulation, laryngoscopy and intubation (especially nasotracheal), intramuscular injections and the use of local anaesthetic blocks. Full anticoagulation is an absolute contraindication to the use of regional anaesthetic techniques. Surgical haemorrhage more likely. Preoperative management of anticoagulant therapy is discussed elsewhere
Anticholinesterases	
Organophosphorus insecticides	Caution should be exercised with the use of succinylcholine
Oral contraceptive pill	Increased risk of thromboembolic complications with oestrogen-containing formulations. Recommended that OCP is stopped 4 weeks before elective surgery or that some form of prophylactic therapy is provided
Antimitotic agents	Inhibition of plasma cholinesterase. Caution should be exercised with the use of succinylcholine

adjust the doses of anaesthetic agents appropriately and to avoid possibly dangerous interactions. In addition, the anaesthetist must maintain up-to-date knowledge of pharmacological advances as new drugs continue to emerge on the market. Any potential interactions observed with new drugs must always be reported to the Medicines and Healthcare products Regulator Agency (MHRA), or comparable body outside the UK.

In general terms, administration of most drugs should be continued up to and including the morning of the operation, although some adjustment in dose may be required (e.g. antihypertensives, insulin). Consideration must also be given to possible perioperative events which influence subsequent drug administration (e.g. postoperative ileus) and appropriate plans made to use an alternative route or an alternative product with similar action. It is advised that some drugs should be discontinued several weeks before surgery if feasible (e.g. oestrogen-containing oral contraceptive pill, long-acting monoamine oxidase inhibitors), because of the potential severity of perioperative complications with which they are associated. Consideration must be given to the potential consequences of stopping drugs preoperatively and appropriate advice or alternative treatment provided to the patient.

There are occasions when patients with an illicit drug habit present for surgery. The patterns of abuse geographically are prone to frequent change, as are the specific drugs taken. Abuse of opioids and cocaine is not uncommon and there is significant information available about potential perioperative problems related to acute or chronic toxicity; however, the same is not true for the increasing number of 'designer drugs' available.

There are significant potential interactions between 'herbal' remedies and drugs used during the perioperative period. Garlic, ginseng and gingko are associated with increased bleeding; St John's Wort induces cytochrome P4503A4 and cytochrome 2C9; valerian modulates GABA pathways; and traditional Chinese herbal medicines have a variety of potential adverse effects including hypertension and delayed emergence. The clinical importance of these interactions is not clear. Current guidance is that the anaesthetist should ask explicitly about their use and if possible discontinue use 2 weeks before surgery (tapering if necessary). There is no evidence to postpone surgery purely because patients are taking herbal remedies.

History of Allergy

A history of allergy to specific substances must be sought, whether it is a drug, foods or adhesives, and the exact nature of the symptoms and signs should be elicited in order to distinguish true allergy from some other predictable adverse reaction. Latex allergy is becoming an increasing problem and requires specific equipment to be used perioperatively. Atopic individuals do not have an increased risk of anaphylaxis but may demonstrate increased cardiovascular or respiratory reactivity to any vasoactive mediators (e.g. histamine) released following administration of some drugs.

A small number of patients describe an allergic reaction to previous anaesthetic exposure. A careful history and examination of the relevant medical notes should clarify the details of the problem, together with the documentation of any postoperative investigations.

Reported allergy to local anaesthetics is usually a manifestation of anxiety or a response to peak concentrations of local anaesthetic or adrenaline. There are a small number of individuals who are allergic to sulphites which are commonly found in local anaesthetic preparations (and other drugs).

Smoking

Long-term deleterious effects of smoking include vascular disease of the peripheral, coronary and cerebral circulations, carcinoma of the lung and chronic bronchitis. It has been suggested that there are good theoretical reasons for advising all patients to cease cigarette smoking for at least 12 h prior to surgery, although there is little evidence to suggest that this influences patients' behaviour in this period.

There are several potential mechanisms by which cigarette smoking can contribute to an adverse perioperative outcome. The cardiovascular effects of smoking are caused by the action of nicotine on the sympathetic nervous system, producing tachycardia and hypertension. Furthermore, smoking causes an increase in coronary vascular resistance; cessation of smoking improves the symptoms of angina. Cigarette smoke contains carbon monoxide, which converts haemoglobin to carboxyhaemoglobin. In heavy smokers, this may result in a reduction in available oxygen by as much as 25%. The half-life of carboxyhaemoglobin is short and therefore abstinence for 12 h leads to an increase in arterial oxygen content. Finally, the effect of smoking on the respiratory tract leads to a six-fold increase in postoperative respiratory morbidity. It has been suggested that abstinence for 6 weeks results in reduced bronchoconstriction and mucus secretion in the tracheobronchial tree.

There is some evidence to suggest that the preoperative period is an effective moment to introduce smoking cessation interventions in those patients who are motivated to stop.

Alcohol

Patients may present with acute intoxication from alcohol or sequelae of chronic consumption. The latter are mainly non-specific features of secondary organ damage such as cardiomyopathy, pancreatitis and gastritis. Establishing the diagnosis may be far from straightforward and needs to be complemented by a decision about whether to allow continued alcohol consumption during the hospital admission or risk the development of a withdrawal syndrome.

Obstructive Sleep Apnoea

Patients with obstructive sleep apnoea have a higher incidence of difficult airway management and current recommendations are that they should have careful observation in the postoperative period. The gold standard for diagnosis is polysomnography. However, this is not always available and current guidance supports the use of screening tools such as the Berlin or STOP–BANG questionnaires (Tables 17.2a and 17.2b).

Physical Examination

A physical examination should be performed on every patient admitted for surgery and the findings documented in the medical notes. It might be argued that this is unnecessary in young healthy patients undergoing short or minor procedures. However, the exercise is a simple and safe method for confirming good health or otherwise, and provides important information in case unexpected morbidity arises postoperatively, e.g. foot drop as a result of incorrect positioning on the operating theatre table, prolonged sensory anaesthesia following local anaesthetic techniques, etc. The information obtained from clinical examination should complement the patient's history and

TABLE 17.2a	
Berlin Questionnaire	
Positive Response	
Category 1	
Do you snore?	Yes
How loud is your snoring?	My snoring is louder than talking My snoring is very loud
How frequently do you snore?	Almost every day 3–4 times per week
Does your snoring bother other people?	Yes
How often have your breathing pauses been noticed?	Almost every day 3–4 times per week
Category 2	
Are you tired after sleeping?	Almost every day 3–4 times per week
Are you tired during daytime?	Almost every day 3–4 times per week
How often do you nod off or fall asleep while driving?	Almost every day 3–4 times per week
Category 3	
Do you have high blood pressure?	Yes
BMI	$>30\,kg\,m^{-2}$

High likelihood of obstructive sleep apnoea is indicated by 2 or more positive categories.
Category 1 is positive with ≥2 positive responses.
Category 2 is positive with ≥2 positive responses.
Category 3 is positive with ≥1 positive responses.

allows the anaesthetist to focus further on features of relevance (Table 17.3).

In addition, the anaesthetist must assess the patient for any potential difficulty in maintaining the airway during general anaesthesia. The teeth should be inspected closely for the presence of caries, caps, loose teeth and particularly protruding upper incisors. The extent of mouth opening is assessed, together with the degree of flexion of the cervical spine and extension of the atlanto-occipital joint. The thyromental distance should also be documented. Specific features associated with difficulty in performing tracheal intubation are described elsewhere (Ch 22).

TABLE 17.2b
STOP–BANG Questionnaire

S: Do you **s**nore loudly (louder than talking or loud enough to be heard through closed doors)?

T: Do you often feel **t**ired, fatigued, or sleepy during daytime?

O: Has anyone **o**bserved you stop breathing during your sleep?

P: Do you have or are you being treated for high blood **p**ressure?

STOP (alone): High risk of OSA: Yes to ≥2 questions out of 4.

BMI: >35 kg m^{-2}

Age: >50 years

Neck circumference: >40 cm

Gender: Male

STOP–BANG: High risk of OSA: Yes to ≥3 questions from 8 questions of STOP–BANG

TABLE 17.3
Features of the Clinical Examination Relevant to the Anaesthetist

System	Features of Interest
General	Nutritional state, fluid balance Condition of the skin and mucous membranes (anaemia, perfusion, jaundice) Temperature
Cardiovascular	Peripheral pulse (rate, rhythm, volume) Arterial pressure Heart sounds Carotid bruits Dependent oedema
Respiratory	Central vs. peripheral cyanosis Observation of dyspnoea Auscultation of lung fields
Airway	Mouth opening Neck movements Thyromental distance Dentition
Nervous	Any dysfunction of the special senses, other cranial nerves, or peripheral motor and sensory nerves

Special Investigations

In general, the results of many investigations may be predicted if a detailed history and examination have been performed. Routine laboratory tests in patients who are apparently healthy on the basis of the history and clinical examination are invariably of little use and a waste of resources. Before ordering extensive investigations, the following questions should be considered:

- Will this investigation yield information not revealed by clinical assessment?
- Will the results of the investigation give additional information on diagnosis or prognosis relevant to planned surgery?
- Will the results of the investigation alter the management of the patient?

In order to reduce the volume of routine preoperative investigations, the following suggestions are made. It should be noted that these are guidelines only and should be modified according to the assessment obtained from the history and clinical examination (Table 17.4). Attention should be paid to ensuring that the results of any investigations requested are seen by the surgical team and properly documented, and that this process is undertaken in a timely manner to allow any necessary intervention with the patient's management to be considered and implemented. The National Institute for Health and Clinical Excellence in the UK has produced a comprehensive summary of suggested testing approaches based on the patient and nature of surgery. The European Society of Anaesthesiology has also adopted these recommendations.

Urine Analysis

This should be performed in every patient. It is inexpensive and may reveal undiagnosed diabetes mellitus or the presence of urinary tract infection. Positive results should be confirmed by seeking further evidence of pathology.

All women of childbearing age should have pregnancy excluded before surgery. For many, this will involve a urine test on the day of surgery.

Full Blood Count

This provides information about the haemoglobin concentration, white blood cell count and platelet count, together with details of red cell morphology. Haemoglobin concentration tends to be of greatest interest to the anaesthetist. Patients whose ethnic origin or family history suggests that a haemoglobinopathy may be present should have their haemoglobin

TABLE 17.4	
Guidelines for Preoperative Investigations	
Urinalysis	All patients
Full blood count	All female adults Before surgery which is likely to result in significant blood loss When indicated clinically, e.g. history of blood loss, previous anaemia or haemopoietic disease, cardiovascular disease, malnutrition, etc.
Urea, creatinine and electrolytes	All patients over 65 years (increased likelihood of CVS disease), or with a positive urinalysis result Any patient with cardiopulmonary disease, or taking cardiovascular active medication, diuretics or corticosteroids Patients with renal or liver disease, diabetes or abnormal nutritional status Patients with a history of diarrhoea, vomiting or metabolic disorder Patients receiving intravenous fluid therapy for greater than 24 h
Blood glucose	Patients with diabetes mellitus, vascular disease or taking corticosteroids
Liver function tests	Any history of liver disease, alcoholism, previous hepatitis or an abnormal nutritional state
Coagulation screen	Any history of a coagulation disorder, drug abuse, significant chronic alcohol abuse, acute or chronic liver disease or anticoagulant medication
ECG	Male smokers older than 45 years; all others older than 50 years Any history (actual or suspected) of heart disease or hypertension Any patient taking medication active on the cardiovascular system or a diuretic Patients with chronic or acute-on-chronic pulmonary disease
Chest X-ray	Rarely indicated unless active cardiac or respiratory disease or possible pulmonary metastases. Previously abnormal chest X-ray is not an indication in its own right to repeat a chest X-ray

concentration measured and haemoglobin electrophoresis undertaken if it has not been performed previously or if the result is not available. If such patients are scheduled for emergency surgery, a Sickledex test may be requested and, if positive, haemoglobin electrophoresis should be undertaken as soon as possible. However, this should not delay emergency surgery because, in practice, in teenagers and adults without a personal history of sickle disease, the result is unlikely to change management.

Moderate degrees of anaemia increase the risk of requiring blood transfusion. Preoperative assessment clinics should have agreed processes for investigation and/or treatment to avoid either missing important pathology such as bowel malignancy or undertaking unnecessary investigations.

Blood Chemistry

The measurements available include the serum concentrations of urea, creatinine and electrolytes, blood glucose concentration and liver function tests. There are specific conditions in which knowledge of preoperative values is important (e.g. diuretic therapy, impaired renal function, chronic alcohol abuse). Beyond these situations, the value of preoperative screening is less clear and detection of an unexpected abnormality seldom alters anaesthetic management. Blood sugar measurement is informative in patients receiving corticosteroid drugs and in those who have diabetes mellitus or vascular disease; a fasting sample is usually required.

Coagulation Tests

These should be ordered solely if the patient has a high likelihood of a bleeding disorder. This is based on the history (alcohol, liver disease, bleeding/bruising tendency, family history, drug history, etc.). They have no value as a screening test. They do not detect abnormalities of platelet function so have no role in patients taking antiplatelet drugs.

Chest X-Ray

This investigation should be reserved for patients with a clear indication and if the clinician believes that the result will change management significantly. There is little evidence that chest X-rays change management even in a higher risk population. It has little value as a preoperative baseline because postoperative abnormalities are treated predominantly on the basis of their clinical relevance.

Other X-rays

Cervical spine X-rays should be considered in any patient in whom there is a possibility of vertebral instability, e.g. in the presence of rheumatoid arthritis. Thoracic inlet X-rays may be required in patients with thyroid enlargement.

Cardiac Investigation

The extent of cardiac investigation should be based on the urgency of surgery, the presence of active cardiac conditions which require treatment, the risk of complications from surgery and the patient's physical fitness. A schematic of an approach to patients at risk of cardiac events is shown in Figure 17.1.

ECG

A 12-lead electrocardiogram can demonstrate many acute or longstanding pathological conditions affecting the heart, particularly changes in rhythm or the occurrence of myocardial ischaemia or infarction. It has little value as a preoperative baseline in patients with known or potential cardiovascular disease; in the resting state, the trace may appear normal despite the presence of clinically significant coronary artery disease. More extensive investigations are available in many departments to supplement the 12-lead ECG and these are discussed elsewhere (see Chs 18 and 34).

Echocardiography

Echocardiography is indicated in patients with undiagnosed heart murmurs. It should be noted that systolic murmurs are common and, in the absence of cardiac symptoms, they are unlikely to represent significant valve disease. Static (i.e. non-exercise/non-dobutamine) transthoracic echocardiography gives some information about the presence of left ventricular hypertrophy and function but is not a good investigation for patients with suspected ischaemic heart disease. As with all investigations, echocardiography should be requested only if the result is likely to change management. Formal protocols detailing which patients

should be referred for echocardiography should be agreed between the anaesthesia and cardiology departments.

Dobutamine stress echocardiography (DSE) utilizes an infusion of dobutamine to increase heart rate and work whilst monitoring cardiac function using transthoracic echocardiography, usually to a maximum heart rate of 120 beats min^{-1} in patients aged over 65 years. It is used to assess left ventricular wall motion abnormalities, which occur in heart failure or ischaemic cardiomyopathy. The test is considered positive if symptoms of angina, headaches, vomiting, ST depression or elevation, or hypotension occur. DSE has a low (25–30%) positive predictive value but a high (95%) negative predictive value for perioperative cardiovascular complications after major surgery. A patient who has a positive DSE test should be referred to a cardiologist for consideration of coronary angiography and revascularisation.

Pulmonary Function Tests

Pulmonary function tests (peak expiratory flow rate (PEFR), forced vital capacity (FVC) and forced expiratory volume in 1 s (FEV_1)) have a poor predictive value for postoperative problems apart from possibly some specific situations such as thoracic surgery and correction of spinal deformity.

Patients with stable asthma do not require PFTs, but note should be made of home recorded PEFR if patients are poorly controlled.

Patients with significant dyspnoea on mild or moderate exertion may require PFTs as part of a diagnostic work-up to elucidate the cause. Reversibility with bronchodilators is an important question to be answered as this may have an impact on perioperative management. Arterial blood gas analysis is prudent in patients with dyspnoea at rest and in patients scheduled for elective thoracotomy; the information is a useful supplement to spirometry values. In patients with progressive disease, these investigations may serve as a useful reference for future admissions.

Cardiopulmonary Exercise Testing

Cardiopulmonary exercise (CPEX) testing has been used in respiratory and sports medicine for some time, but has more recently been applied to the assessment of physical fitness in patients scheduled for major

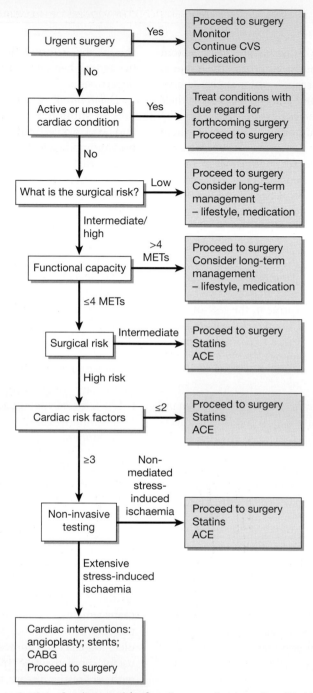

FIGURE 17.1 ■ Approach to investigation of patients at risk of cardiac complications. Simplified from European and American Guidelines.

METs: metabolic equivalents – inability to climb two flights of stairs or run a short distance equates to <4 METs.

Cardiac risk factors:

➢ Angina pectoris
➢ Prior MI
➢ Heart failure
➢ Stroke/transient ischaemic attack
➢ Renal dysfunction (serum creatinine >170 mmol L^{-1} or 2 mg dL^{-1} or a creatinine clearance of <60 mL min^{-1})
➢ Diabetes mellitus requiring insulin therapy

surgery. The usual protocol for CPEX testing is that patients exercise on a bicycle against progressively increasing resistance while ECG, oxygen consumption, carbon dioxide production and other variables are measured. These variables include anaerobic threshold (AT, the oxygen consumption at the point where anaerobic metabolism starts to occur) and ventilatory equivalents for CO_2 and O_2 (V_E/Vco_2 and V_E/Vo_2, expired volume required for adequate CO_2 exchange or oxygen intake). All of these reflect physical fitness, cardiac and pulmonary function. Peak oxygen consumption, V_E/Vco_2 and AT have been related to outcome and long-term survival after major surgery.

Alternatively, simple measures of exercise tolerance such as the Incremental Shuttle walk test may be used to quantify aerobic fitness.

PREDICTION OF PERIOPERATIVE MORBIDITY OR MORTALITY

After the patient's history, examination and relevant investigations have been collated the anaesthetist must answer two questions:

- Is the patient in optimum physical condition for anaesthesia and surgery?
- Are the anticipated benefits of surgery greater than the combined risks of undergoing anaesthesia and surgery, taking into account any concurrent disease?

In principle, if there is any medical condition which may be improved (e.g. pulmonary disease, hypertension, cardiac failure, chronic bronchitis, renal disease), surgery should be postponed and appropriate therapy instituted. The reasoning behind such a decision must be recorded clearly in the patient's medical notes, with the anticipated time required to achieve reasonable improvement. At this stage, the patient should be reassessed and the decision about when or whether to proceed with surgery reviewed.

There is continued interest in quantifying factors preoperatively which correlate with the occurrence of postoperative morbidity and mortality. Some accuracy is possible for populations of patients, but precision does not extend to accurate prediction of risk for an individual patient. Frequently, the decision to proceed may be made only by discussion between surgeon and anaesthetist.

Scoring systems for determining the likelihood of adverse outcome may be divided into two main groups:

- general scoring systems designed to predict non-specific undesirable events
- systems which focus on prediction of specific morbidity or technical difficulty, e.g. adverse cardiac events, difficulty with tracheal intubation.

Prediction of Non-Specific Adverse Outcome

Over a broad range of operations and age, the overall mortality rate within 7 days of surgery is approximately 4% across Europe as a whole. This is many times greater than the incidence of deaths to which anaesthesia has made a significant contribution or has been the sole cause (approximately 1 in 10 000). In many large studies of mortality, e.g. NCEPOD reports, common factors which have emerged as contributing to anaesthetic mortality include inadequate assessment of patients in the preoperative period, inadequate supervision and monitoring in the intraoperative

FIGURE 17.1 ■ Cont'd
Surgical risk of MI and cardiac death within 30 days after surgery

Low risk (<1%)	Intermediate risk (1–5%)	High risk (>5%)
Breast	Abdominal	Aortic/major vascular
Dental	Carotid surgery	Peripheral vascular
Endocrine	Peripheral angioplasty	
Eye	Endovascular aneurysm repair	
Gynaecology	Head and neck	
Reconstructive	Neurological	
Orthopaedic – minor	Orthopaedic – major	
Urology – minor	Transplant	
	Urology – major	

period and inadequate postoperative supervision and management. It remains difficult to evaluate formally whether the patient's characteristics, the surgical features or the anaesthetic technique are the most influential in terms of final outcome. This is primarily a result of the high standards of practice which exist, the relative infrequency with which significant perioperative morbidity or mortality occurs and the multifactorial background for many adverse events.

However, there is an increasing body of evidence to suggest that postoperative complications are not benign. Patients who have postoperative complications and who survive the postoperative period have an increased mortality several months and even years after their operation compared to those without. Some data indicate that reducing complications improves outcome, suggesting that this link is not solely identifying patients with poor reserve.

Any prospective studies intended to evaluate predictive factors of perioperative risk rely upon the incorporation of large numbers of patients and scrupulous design. Those that have been published tend to agree on several factors identified from physiological, demographic and laboratory data which can combine to indicate the likelihood of adverse outcome (Table 17.5).

In an effort to better manage patients with increased risk of postoperative morbidity and mortality, clinicians have been encouraged to document the predicted risk of complications both before and after surgery. There is reasonable evidence that clinical judgement alone is not a particularly good predictor of the need for critical care in the postoperative period.

ASA (American Society of Anesthesiologists) Grading

The ASA grading system (Table 17.6) was introduced in the 1960s as a simple description of the physical state of a patient, along with an indication of whether surgery is elective or emergency. Despite its apparent simplicity, it remains one of the few prospective descriptions of the patient which correlates with the risks of anaesthesia and surgery. However, it does not embrace all aspects of anaesthetic risk, as there is no allowance for inclusion of many criteria such as age or difficulty in intubation. In addition, it does not take into account the severity of either the presenting disease or the surgery proposed, nor does it identify factors which can be improved preoperatively in order to influence outcome. Nevertheless, it is extremely useful and should be applied to all patients who present for anaesthesia.

More recently, the combination of ASA with age of patient, urgency and extent of surgery has been shown to be a reliable predictor of outcome at a population level and uses information readily available preoperatively.

TABLE 17.5
Typical Preoperative Features which may Increase the Likelihood of Significant Perioperative Complications or Mortality

Demographic/Surgical	Pathophysiological	Laboratory
Age >70 years	Dyspnoea at rest or on minimal exertion	Serum urea >20 mmol L^{-1}
Major thoracic, abdominal or cardiovascular surgery	MI within 30 days or unstable angina, untreated heart failure or high grade arrhythmias	Serum albumin <30 g L^{-1}
Perforated viscus (excluding appendix), pancreatitis or intraperitoneal abscess	Cardiac symptoms requiring medical treatment	Haemoglobin <10 g dL^{-1}
Intestinal obstruction	Confusional state	
Palliative surgery	Clinical jaundice	
Smoking	Significant weight loss (>10%) in 1 month	
Cytotoxic or corticosteroid treatment	Productive cough with sputum, especially if persistent	
Controlled diabetes	Haemorrhage or anaemia requiring transfusion	

TABLE 17.6

ASA Classification of Physical Status and the Associated Mortality Rates (for Elective and Emergency Cases)

ASA Rating	Description of Patient	Mortality Rate (%)
Class I	A normally healthy individual	0.1
Class II	A patient with mild systemic disease	0.2
Class III	A patient with severe systemic disease that is not incapacitating	1.8
Class IV	A patient with incapacitating systemic disease that is a constant threat to life	7.8
Class V	A moribund patient who is not expected to survive 24 h with or without operation	9.4
Class E	Added as a suffix for emergency operation	

TABLE 17.7

Factors Contributing to the POSSUM Score for Risk of Perioperative Mortality and Morbidity. A Higher Score is Awarded for Increasing Deviation from the 'Normal' Value or Range

Physiological Factors	Operative Factors
Age (years)	Operative complexity
Cardiac status	Single vs. multiple procedures
Respiratory status	Expected blood loss
Systolic blood pressure	Peritoneal contamination (blood, pus, bowel content)
Pulse rate	Extent of any malignant spread
Glasgow Coma Score	Urgency of surgery
Haemoglobin concentration	
White cell count	
Serum urea concentration	
Serum sodium concentration	
Serum potassium concentration	
ECG rhythm	

POSSUM

This stands for 'Physiological and Operative Severity Score for the enUmeration of Mortality and morbidity'. First reported in 1991, this tool was developed to compare mortality and morbidity over a wide range of general surgical procedures, and takes into account 12 physiological and six operative factors which are either readily available or predictable in the immediate preoperative period (Table 17.7). These factors are weighted according to their value, and a logistic regression formula applied to calculate 'risk' of mortality or morbidity. Some groups have modified the formula (P-POSSUM) after suggestions that the original system overestimated the risk of death in low-risk patient groups, and others have produced speciality-specific variants (e.g. V-POSSUM for elective vascular surgery). It should be emphasized that the POSSUM scoring system was designed to compare observed with expected death rates among populations rather than to predict mortality for an individual, and should be applied only in this way.

Prediction of Specific Adverse Events

The Difficult Airway

There are specific medical or surgical conditions which are associated with potential airway problems during anaesthesia, such as obesity, the later stages of pregnancy, a large neck, mediastinal tumours and some faciomaxillary deformities. Apart from these, it requires an experienced anaesthetist to collate various physical features which can predict likely difficulty. Several classifications or scoring systems have been designed for this purpose, although none is entirely reliable; they are discussed elsewhere (see Chs 21 and 22).

Adverse Cardiac Events

Over 25 years ago, Goldman and colleagues published a retrospective analysis of preoperative risk factors which were associated with an adverse cardiac event following non-cardiac surgery. This topic has been re-evaluated extensively in the intervening years, with many studies agreeing broadly with Goldman's conclusions. However, conflicting opinions exist regarding identification of the most accurate predictors, probably as a result of the diversity of methods used in these studies together with the significant and continued advances made in the understanding and management of cardiovascular pathophysiology. The most widely used risk index currently is Lee's Revised Cardiac Risk Index (Table 17.8).

It should be noted that many aspects of perioperative care have changed since the production of these cardiac risk indices.

Respiratory Complications

Patients at risk of developing postoperative pulmonary complications include smokers, those with pre-existing lung disease, the obese and those undergoing thoracic or abdominal surgery. Unfortunately, predicting the likelihood and severity of such adverse events remains difficult. Sophisticated tests of pulmonary function (e.g. functional residual capacity, closing capacity, pulmonary

---

TABLE 17.8
Lee's Revised Cardiac Risk Index

	Indicators
High risk surgical procedures	Intraperitoneal Intrathoracic Suprainguinal vascular
History of ischaemic heart disease	History of myocardial infarction History of positive exercise test Current ischaemic chest pain Use of nitrate therapy ECG with pathological Q waves
Congestive heart failure	History of congestive heart failure, pulmonary oedema or paroxysmal nocturnal dyspnoea Physical examination showing bilateral rales or S3 gallop Chest X-ray showing pulmonary vascular redistribution
Cerebrovascular disease	History of transient ischaemic attack or stroke

Risk for Major Cardiac Event (Myocardial Infarction, Pulmonary Oedema, Ventricular Fibrillation, Primary Cardiac Arrest, and Complete Heart Block): Complication Rates in Patients with 0, 1, 2, or More than 2 of these Variables were Reported as 0.4%, 1.0%, 7% and 11%. Reprinted from Thomas H. Lee, Edward R. Marcantonio, Carol M. Mangione et al. Derivation and Prospective Validation of a Simple Index for Prediction of Cardiac Risk of Major Noncardiac Surgery. Circulation. 1999;100:1043–1049.

---

diffusing capacity, etc.) are no more valuable in assessment of lung disease than simple spirometric tests, particularly vital capacity, FVC and FEV_1. Blood gas analysis should be performed preoperatively if there is concern about postoperative lung function; the presence of a preoperative arterial oxygen tension of less than 9 kPa, together with the presence of dyspnoea at rest, is the most sensitive method of predicting the need for mechanical ventilation in the postoperative period.

There are scoring tools available for prediction of postoperative respiratory complications such as pneumonia and respiratory failure.

PREOPERATIVE PREPARATION

Having taken a full clinical history, performed a physical examination and reviewed the relevant investigations, the anaesthetist should decide whether further measures are required to prepare the patient satisfactorily before proceeding to anaesthesia and surgery. This is the time to address any factors which place the patient at increased risk of adverse outcome and which could be improved to the patient's benefit before surgery. It is also appropriate to consider factors such as preoperative fasting; providing information to the patient and obtaining consent to proceed; ensuring blood products are available during the perioperative period if this is thought necessary; and organizing appropriate staff and equipment within the operating theatre suite.

Postponing Surgery for Clinical Reasons

There are several common reasons for postponing surgery, some of which are mentioned below. One key issue relates to communication; the reason(s) for the decision to postpone surgery must be clear to the patient, the surgical team and any other staff who have been contacted to review the patient (e.g. cardiologists, physiotherapists). This helps to ensure that the time course for any improvement remains realistic and apparent to everyone involved, and that it can be balanced against the possible detriment of delaying surgery.

Acute Upper Respiratory Tract Infection

Although many patients may admit to the presence of a cold, clarification of such an admission should be made. In general, the presence of nasal secretions, pyrexia or the unexpected presence of physical signs on clinical examination of the chest indicate that non-urgent surgery should be postponed for a few weeks until the patient has recovered.

Coexisting Medical Disease and Drug Therapy

If the patient has coexisting medical disease which may affect outcome adversely if not under optimum control, there is a strong argument to postpone non-urgent surgery until further specialized advice has been sought. Examples include thyroid disease, and acute exacerbations of inflammatory diseases such as multiple sclerosis, inflammatory bowel disease and autoimmune diseases.

Emergency Surgery for Which the Patient has not been Resuscitated Adequately

In some emergency patients, it may be necessary to delay surgery to optimize the patient's physiology, but this should be balanced against the risks of deterioration due to the underlying disease process. Acutely unwell patients with surgical pathology are unlikely to make significant improvements if the underlying condition is not addressed, unless they are grossly hypovolaemic. In practice, resuscitation should proceed at the same time that preparations for surgery are made.

Surgery for haemorrhage control in trauma is discussed elsewhere (see Ch 37).

Recent Ingestion of Food

In general, anaesthesia for elective surgery should not be undertaken within 6 h of ingestion of food, although clear fluids may be taken up to 2 h before surgery (see below).

Failure to Obtain Consent

Consent for surgery should be obtained from all adult patients unless the patient is incapable of providing consent and the treatment proposed is clearly in his or her best interests (see below). If there is any doubt regarding the validity of the consent, surgery should be postponed where feasible until appropriate advice has been obtained.

Preoperative Fasting

The time of last oral intake of solid and fluid must be established. One of the commonest causes of anaesthetic-related mortality and morbidity is aspiration of gastric contents.

Many anaesthetic departments have re-evaluated their standing orders on the issue of preoperative fasting for clear fluids in light of clinical studies which have demonstrated the speed of gastric emptying in healthy adults. Several important points need to be emphasized on this topic:

- There are many factors which can increase the likelihood of significant gastric content regardless of the period of starvation (e.g. pain, anxiety, some drugs and premedication including opioid analgesics, paralytic ileus, later stages of pregnancy, etc.).
- The normal daily secretion of gastric fluid can approach 2000 mL in adults; consequently, the stomach is never truly 'empty'.
- Clinical studies which encourage changes in practice should be scrutinized carefully to ensure that the results are not extrapolated beyond the sample of the population upon which they were based.

Providing Information to the Patient and Obtaining Consent

Consent for anaesthesia is a vital part of preoperative preparation. It is discussed more fully in Chapter 19. It must be obtained by an individual with sufficient knowledge of the procedure and the risks involved. In order for consent to be valid, it must encompass three elements:

- The patient must have the capacity to consent to the treatment offered.
- The patient must have sufficient information to enable him/her to make a balanced decision to consent.
- The consent must be voluntary.

Capacity to consent refers to the patient's ability to comprehend the information provided, come to a decision on what is involved and communicate that decision. There is no fixed age limit below which a minor cannot consent to treatment, although caution should be exercised when dealing with patients aged less than 16 years; if in doubt, consent should also be sought from a person with parental responsibility. Capacity may also be invalidated by a patient's confusion, pain, shock or fatigue, and administration of some drugs such as opioid analgesics or benzodiazepine premedication. Appropriate advice should be sought if there is any concern.

Patients are confronted by a barrage of information on arrival in hospital, in addition to having to comply with an often alien environment with its own routines and practices. It is common for surgical consent forms to include consent to anaesthesia, despite the fact that the surgical team rarely has the knowledge to inform the patient fully on this subject. During the preoperative visit, the anaesthetist must ensure that the patient has been given an adequate amount of information about the proposed anaesthetic technique, and in particular its nature and consequences. The amount of information provided should be determined by an assessment of the needs of the patient to receive detailed information and the likelihood of adverse events.

- All patients should be told of common complications associated with the proposed anaesthetic technique (e.g. succinylcholine pains, postdural puncture headache).
- All patients should be told what they may experience in the perioperative period, including temporary numbness and weakness in the postoperative period if a local or regional technique is to be used.
- If a technique of a sensitive nature (e.g. insertion of an analgesic suppository) is to be used during anaesthesia, the patient should be informed.
- Patients should be informed of any increased risk related to their preoperative condition (e.g. damage to loose or crowned teeth, or cardiac complications in the presence of severe coronary artery disease).
- All patients should be given the opportunity to ask questions, and specific questions relating to anaesthesia must be answered honestly; if the questions relate to surgery, then the anaesthetist should ensure that a surgeon speaks to the patient before anaesthesia is induced.

- A summary of the matters discussed, the risks explained and the techniques agreed should be documented on the anaesthetic record.

In many hospitals, patients receive information leaflets which describe anaesthesia and its associated risks.

Blood Transfusion Requests

Blood products are an expensive commodity and blood transfusion carries small but finite risks of incompatibility reactions and transmission of infection. In addition, there is the potential for supplies to be short, and the need for transfusion should be considered very carefully. The object of transfusion is to ensure that adequate oxygen delivery to the tissues can be maintained throughout the perioperative period. The amount of blood ordered from the blood transfusion service depends on both the patient's preoperative haemoglobin concentration and the anticipated extent of surgery. Consideration should also be given to the use of anaesthetic techniques which reduce intraoperative blood loss, the use of cell salvage techniques perioperatively if available, preoperative red cell donation immediately before surgery or acute normovolaemic haemodilution.

Common operations should have agreed policies in place regarding transfusion requests. With the advent of electronic issue of blood in many hospitals, formal cross-matching before surgery is less commonly needed than previously.

Preoperative Organization of the Operating Theatre and the Postoperative Period

The process of preoperative assessment provides the anaesthetist with a wealth of information about the patient and the proposed surgery. This allows the anaesthetist to plan various aspects of perioperative management. Some aspects must be conveyed to staff in the operating theatre suite in advance. Examples include the planned use of invasive monitoring, issues related to patient positioning and any special needs the patient might have, such as an interpreter. If senior anaesthetic assistance is needed, this should be arranged in advance, and organization of appropriate postoperative care should also be initiated.

This information should be discussed, as a minimum, at the preoperative briefing. Clearly, many of these issues need addressing before this time.

PREMEDICATION AND OTHER PROPHYLACTIC MEASURES

Premedication refers to the administration of drugs in the period 1–2 h before induction of anaesthesia. The traditional intramuscular opioid premedication is no longer a routine part of preoperative preparation, but the need for premedication must be considered after all of the relevant factors have been identified. The objectives of premedication are to:

- allay anxiety and fear
- reduce postoperative nausea and vomiting
- assist with intra- and postoperative analgesia
- reduce secretions
- reduce the volume and increase the pH of gastric contents
- attenuate vagal reflexes
- attenuate sympathoadrenal responses.

Relief from Anxiety

Surgical patients have a high incidence of anxiety and there is a significant inverse relationship between anxiety and smoothness of induction of anaesthesia. Relief from anxiety is accomplished most effectively by non-pharmacological means, which may be termed psychotherapy. This is effected at the preoperative visit by establishment of rapport, explanation of events which occur in the perioperative period and reassurance regarding the patient's anxieties and fears. There is good evidence that this approach has a significant calming effect.

In some patients, reassurance and explanation may be insufficient to allay anxiety. In these patients, it is appropriate to offer anxiolytic medication; benzodiazepine drugs are the most effective for this purpose.

Sedation

Sedation is not synonymous with anxiolysis. Some drugs, e.g. barbiturates and to a lesser extent opioids, provide sedation but have no anxiolytic properties. In general, it is unnecessary to use a sedative preoperatively. An exception to this may be in paediatric practice. It is unwise to administer any sedative medication if the patient is in a critical condition, particularly if the airway and/or respiratory function are at risk of compromise.

Postoperative Antiemesis

Nausea and vomiting are extremely common after anaesthesia. Opioid drugs administered during and after operation are often responsible. Antiemetics may be given usefully as an oral premedication, particularly in day-case surgery.

Analgesia

Paracetamol. Paracetamol is a cheap and effective analgesic when given as an oral premedication. Many day-case and children's surgery units do this as routine. Logistical reasons prevent many main theatre units from doing this, but the anaesthetist should always consider prescribing paracetamol at the preoperative visit.

Non-Steroidal Anti-Inflammatory Drugs (NSAIDs). Similarly to paracetamol, NSAIDs can be given safely and effectively as premedication, with due consideration to contraindications and ensuring that a second dose is not given inadvertently in theatre or the recovery room.

Opioid Analgesics. The main indication for preoperative opioid therapy is treatment of pain but, otherwise, premedication with opioids is rarely used now. Opioids should always be used in combination with an antiemetic agent.

Reduction in Secretions

Ether stimulates the production of secretions from pharyngeal and bronchial glands and premedication with an anticholinergic agent was common before ether anaesthesia. This problem occurs rarely with modern anaesthetic agents and anticholinergic premedication is no longer used as a routine. However, premedication with an anticholinergic drug is advisable for patients in whom an awake fibreoptic intubation is planned (when excessive salivation can create extra difficulty), or before using ketamine.

Reduction in Gastric Volume and Elevation of Gastric pH

In patients who are at risk of vomiting or regurgitation (e.g. emergency patients with a full stomach or elective patients with hiatus hernia), it may be desirable to promote gastric emptying and elevate the pH of residual gastric contents. Gastric emptying may be enhanced by the administration of metoclopramide, which also possesses some antiemetic properties, while elevation of the pH of gastric contents may be produced by administration of sodium citrate. This topic is described in greater detail in Chapter 37.

Reduction in Vagal Reflexes

Premedication with an anticholinergic drug may be considered in specific situations in which vagal bradycardia may occur.

- Traction of the eye muscles, particularly the rectus medialis, during squint surgery may result in bradycardia and/or arrhythmias (the oculocardiac reflex). Premedication with atropine protects against this but it is not as effective as the intravenous administration of atropine at induction of anaesthesia or in anticipation of traction of the muscles.
- Repeated administration of succinylcholine often results in bradycardia, which sometimes proceeds to asystole. Administration of atropine should always precede the administration of a second dose of succinylcholine.
- Surgical stimulation during a balanced anaesthetic technique may be associated with bradycardia – particularly during laparoscopy.
- The administration of propofol to patients with a slow heart rate may result in dangerous degrees of bradycardia.

Limitation of Sympathoadrenal Responses

Induction of anaesthesia and tracheal intubation may be associated with marked sympathoadrenal activity, manifest by tachycardia, hypertension and elevation of plasma catecholamine concentrations. These responses are undesirable in the healthy individual and may be harmful in patients with hypertension or ischaemic heart disease. A β-blocker drug or clonidine may be given as premedication in order to attenuate these responses.

Drugs Used for Premedication

Some of the objectives listed above may be achieved by administration of drugs at induction or during maintenance of anaesthesia. The ability to achieve all objectives by administration of a variety of drugs either preoperatively or at induction is responsible for the wide variation in prescribing habits among anaesthetists.

Benzodiazepines

Benzodiazepines possess several properties which are useful for premedication, including anxiolysis, sedation and amnesia. The extent of each of these effects differs among individual drugs. Diazepam was the first drug of this group to be used commonly, although temazepam (10–30 mg) is now often preferred because of its shorter duration of action. Lorazepam (1–5 mg) produces a greater degree of amnesia than the other drugs in this group. Benzodiazepines produce anxiolysis in doses which do not produce excessive sedation and this is advantageous if respiratory function is compromised; however, great caution should be exercised in these patients because depression of ventilation may be precipitated even by small doses. Some benzodiazepines may be administered by intramuscular injection but evidence suggests that oral administration gives better results. There is a very wide variation in response to benzodiazepines and effects may be unpredictable. A specific antagonist (flumazenil) is available.

Anticholinergic Agents

The three anticholinergic agents used commonly in anaesthesia are atropine, hyoscine and glycopyrronium. Atropine and hyoscine are tertiary amines which cross the blood–brain barrier; glycopyrronium is a quaternary amine which does not cross the blood–brain barrier and which is not absorbed from the gastrointestinal tract. Although atropine is absorbed from the gastrointestinal tract, this occurs in an unpredictable manner and is dependent on gastric content, pH and motility.

These three drugs differ in respect of their dose-response effects at various cholinergic receptors. In standard clinical doses, hyoscine 0.4 mg produces a greater antisialagogue effect than atropine 0.6 mg and has little action on cardiac vagal receptors. Hyoscine possesses sedative and amnesic actions and, in contrast to atropine, does not cause stimulation of higher centres. Hyoscine should be avoided in the elderly (over 60 years of age) as it can produce dysphoria and restlessness. Glycopyrronium has no central effects, a much longer duration of action and, in a standard clinical dose of 0.4 mg, causes less change in heart rate than atropine 0.6 mg.

Anticholinergic drugs are used clinically to produce the following effects:

- *Antisialagogue effects.* Glycopyrronium and hyoscine are more potent than atropine in this respect. These drugs block secretions when irritant anaesthetic gases are used and reduce excessive secretions and bradycardia associated with succinylcholine when it is given either repeatedly or as an infusion.
- *Sedative and amnesic effects.* In combination with morphine, hyoscine produces powerful sedative and amnesic effects.
- *Prevention of reflex bradycardia.* Anticholinergics are given for both prophylaxis and treatment of bradycardia. Atropine is used commonly as premedication in ophthalmic surgery to block the oculocardiac reflex in patients undergoing squint surgery and has been used also in small children to reduce the bradycardia which may occur in association with halothane anaesthesia.

Side-effects of anticholinergic drugs include the following:

- *CNS toxicity.* The central anticholinergic syndrome is produced by stimulation of the CNS (usually by atropine). Symptoms include restlessness, agitation and somnolence and, in extreme cases, convulsions and coma. With hyoscine, there is more commonly prolonged somnolence. Physostigmine 1–2 mg i.v. has been recommended to reverse the central anticholinergic syndrome, but is no longer available in the UK. Diazepam has been reported to have a beneficial effect but the patient must be observed closely and steps taken if necessary to deal with depression of ventilation or upper airway obstruction.
- *Reduction in lower oesophageal sphincter tone.* Theoretically, a reduction in tone may lead to an increased risk of gastro-oesophageal reflux, although in clinical practice there is no suggestion that the use of anticholinergics for premedication is associated with an increased incidence of regurgitation and aspiration.
- *Tachycardia,* which should be avoided in patients with cardiac disease (e.g. obstructive cardiomyopathy, valvular stenosis or ischaemic heart disease) or when a hypotensive anaesthetic technique is planned.
- *Mydriasis and cycloplegia,* which lead to visual impairment. This may be troublesome, but is not a serious side-effect. Theoretically, mydriasis may be associated with reduced drainage of aqueous humour from the anterior chamber of the eye, thereby increasing intraocular pressure in patients with glaucoma. However, this effect is not important in practice and atropine may be prescribed safely to patients with glaucoma provided that appropriate therapy is maintained.
- *Pyrexia.* By suppressing secretion of sweat, anticholinergics predispose to an increase in body temperature. These drugs should therefore be avoided in the presence of pyrexia, particularly in children.
- *Excessive drying.* Although anticholinergics are given for the specific purpose of producing antisialagogue effects, this may be most unpleasant for the patient.
- *Increased physiological dead space.* Atropine and hyoscine increase physiological dead space by 20–25%, but this is compensated for by an increase in ventilation.

β-Blockers

The use of β-blockers (e.g. atenolol) during the perioperative period limits the haemodynamic response to nociceptive stimuli, such as tracheal intubation and surgical stimulation, and inhibits the neuroendocrine stress response. Recent studies concerning the use of β-blockers in patients at risk of coronary artery disease are still controversial. Current advice is not to prescribe prophylactic β-blockers indiscriminately in the perioperative period, but withdrawal of β-blockers in patients receiving chronic treatment may be harmful; such patients should continue their β-blocker therapy.

TABLE 17.9
Prophylactic Measures Against Specific Complications

Complication	Methods of Prophylaxis
Deep vein thrombosis	Early postoperative mobilization Leg exercises (active/passive) Pneumatic compression of limbs Electrical stimulation of calf muscles Graduated stockings Low-dose subcutaneous heparin Warfarin anticoagulation (Regional anaesthetic techniques, especially for orthopaedic lower-limb procedures)
Aspiration of gastric contents	Nil by mouth Antacids: sodium citrate H_2-antagonists Omeprazole Metoclopramide

Infection
    Surgical procedure
    Infective endocarditis
	
	Directed by local or national practice with advice of microbiologists
	Follow guidelines of the Endocarditis Working Party

Adrenocortical suppression – suggested for patients who have received exogenous systemic steroids (>10 mg prednisolone/day) during the 2 months preceding surgery	Hydrocortisone 25 mg 6-hourly, or continue usual steroids if this is in excess of the current requirements (i.e. >300 mg hydrocortisone equivalent, which is the maximum daily production in response to stress). Consult local guidance.

Clonidine and Dexmedetomidine

These are α_2-agonists which potentiate anaesthetics by decreasing central noradrenergic activity. Dexmedetomidine is more specific for the α_2-receptor and probably has greater potential as a premedicant. Administration results in decreased intraoperative requirements for inhaled anaesthetic agents or propofol, although recovery times may be prolonged. These agents may also have a role in attenuating sympathoadrenal responses at induction of anaesthesia.

Other Prophylactic Measures

Thought should be given to the value of giving prophylactic treatment for the specific situations summarized in Table 17.9.

FURTHER READING

American Heart Association Task Force on Practice Guidelines, 2007. (Writing Committee to revise the 2002 guidelines on perioperative cardiovascular evaluation for noncardiac surgery) Developed in collaboration with the American Society of Echocardiography, American Society of Nuclear Cardiology, Heart Rhythm Society, Society of Cardiovascular Anesthesiologists, Society for Cardiovascular Angiography and Interventions, Society for Vascular Medicine and Biology, and Society for Vascular Surgery. Circulation 116, 1971–1996.

Association of Anaesthetists of Great Britain and Ireland, 2001. Preoperative assessment: the role of the anaesthetist. www.aagbi.org.

De Hert, S., Imberger, G., Carlisle, J., et al., 2011. Preoperative evaluation of the adult patient undergoing non-cardiac surgery: guidelines from the European Society of Anaesthesiology. Eur. J. Anaesthesiol. 28, 684–722.

Donati, A., Ruzzi, M., Adrario, E., et al., 2004. A new and feasible model for predicting operative risk. Br. J. Anaesth. 93, 393–399.

Janke, E., Chalk, V., Kinley, H., 2002. Pre-operative assessment: setting a standard through learning. University of Southampton.

National Institute for Clinical Excellence, 2003. CG3 – pre-operative testing, the use of routine pre-operative tests for elective surgery. www.nice.org.uk.

Pearse, R.M., Moreno, R.P., Bauer, P., et al., 2012. Mortality after surgery in Europe: a 7 day cohort study. Lancet 380, 1059–1065.

Poldermans, D., Bax, J.J., Boersma, E., et al., 2009. Guidelines for preoperative cardiac risk assessment and perioperative cardiac management in noncardiac surgery: the Task Force for Preoperative Cardiac Risk Assessment and Perioperative Cardiac Management in Noncardiac Surgery of the European Society of Cardiology (ESC) and endorsed by the European Society of Anaesthesiology (ESA). Eur. Heart J. 30, 2769–2812.

Stoelting, R.K., Diedrorf, S.F., 2002. Handbook of anesthesia and co-existing disease, fourth ed. Elsevier Health Sciences, Edinburgh.

18

INTERCURRENT DISEASE AND ANAESTHESIA

■ ■ ■ ■ ■ ■ ■ ■ ■ ■ ■ ■ ■

Many patients presenting for anaesthesia and surgery suffer from intercurrent disease and are often receiving a variety of medications. Many are elderly with limited physiological reserve, and may also be suffering from more advanced intercurrent disease. All these factors influence the conduct of anaesthesia and surgery and must be considered when assessing and managing a patient perioperatively.

Intercurrent diseases may have a variety of effects on anaesthesia and surgery:

- the course of the disease may be modified by anaesthesia and surgery
- the disease may influence the effects of anaesthesia
- concurrent drug therapy may influence the effects of anaesthesia
- the choice of anaesthetic technique may be affected
- normal compensatory responses may be affected.

In severe cases, the patient's condition may preclude a successful outcome from the proposed anaesthesia and surgery. In assessing the patient with co-existing disease, it is important to consider:

- the patient's physiological reserve or functional capacity
- the extent of surgery
- the disease processes involved and whether they can be improved before surgery.

Physiological Reserve

It is increasingly recognized that physiological reserve is an important predictor of outcome from major surgery. Cardiopulmonary exercise (CPEX)

testing is a useful tool to allow preoperative assessment of cardiovascular and respiratory reserve and the ability to withstand the stresses of major surgery. More simply, or where CPEX testing is unavailable, the capacity of the cardiorespiratory system to respond adequately to perioperative stress can be estimated in terms of metabolic equivalents (METs). If a patient has no major cardiac risk factors (see below) and can achieve more than 4 METs of activity without significant cardiorespiratory symptoms then the perioperative risk of an adverse cardiac event is low (Table 18.1). It may be possible to improve cardiorespiratory reserve before surgery in some patients. Knowledge of physiological reserve will guide the choice of anaesthetic technique, the level of monitoring used and the requirement for Level 2 or Level 3 care postoperatively.

Extent of Surgery

This determines the level of physiological stress which the patient will experience. High-risk operations (cardiac morbidity >5%) include aortic and other major vascular procedures; intermediate risk procedures include intraperitoneal, intrathoracic, major orthopaedic or urological surgeries, and also procedures anticipated to be prolonged and to involve significant fluid shifts and blood loss (Table 18.2). Following discussion with the patient and surgeon, it may be appropriate in some cases to consider alternatives to surgery or a less major operation if the patient is considered at too high a risk. In some cases the appropriate decision is not to undergo surgery.

TABLE 18.1
Metabolic Equivalent (MET) Levels for Readily Assessed Activity Levels

MET Score	Approximate Level of Activity
1	Dress, walk indoors
2	Light housework, slow walk
4	Climb one flight of stairs, run a short distance
6	Moderate sport, e.g. golf, doubles tennis or dancing
10	Strenuous sports or exercise

One MET is approximately equivalent to an oxygen consumption of 3.5 mL kg^{-1} min^{-1}.
Adapted from Fleisher LA, Beckman JA, Brown KA et al 2007 ACC/AHA guidelines on perioperative cardiovascular evaluation and care for noncardiac surgery: executive summary: a report of the American College of Cardiology/American Heart Association Task Force on Practice Guidelines. J Am Coll Cardiol 50:1707–1732.

TABLE 18.2
Cardiac Risk* Stratification for Non-Cardiac Surgical Procedures ·

Risk Stratification	Procedure Examples
Vascular (reported cardiac risk often more than 5%)	Aortic and other major vascular surgery Peripheral vascular surgery
Intermediate (reported cardiac risk generally 1% to 5%)	Intraperitoneal and intrathoracic surgery Carotid endarterectomy Head and neck surgery Orthopaedic surgery Prostate surgery
Low[†] (reported cardiac risk generally less than 1%)	Endoscopic procedures Superficial procedures Cataract surgery Breast surgery Ambulatory surgery

*Combined incidence of cardiac death and non-fatal myocardial infarction.
[†]These procedures do not generally require non-invasive testing.
Adapted from Fleisher LA, Beckman JA, Brown KA et al 2007 ACC/AHA guidelines on perioperative cardiovascular evaluation and care for noncardiac surgery: a report of the American College of Cardiology/American Heart Association Task Force on Practice Guidelines. J Am Coll Cardiol 50:1707–1732.

Specific Disease Processes

All patients presenting for surgery should have a full clinical history and examination. Past medical history, including previous anaesthesia, regular medications and allergies (including food) are important. Previous anaesthetic records should be reviewed where available. Appropriate targeted investigations may then be planned.

CARDIOVASCULAR DISEASE

Ischaemic Heart Disease

The presence of coronary, cerebral or peripheral vascular disease defines a group of patients at increased risk from anaesthesia and surgery, manifesting as postoperative cardiovascular events such as myocardial ischaemia and infarction, arrhythmias, cardiac failure and in some cases death. Major surgery causes physiological stress leading to increased sympathetic activity, cardiac work and oxygen demand. Activation of coagulation and associated reduction in fibrinolysis leads to a prothrombotic state which predisposes to coronary thrombosis in some at-risk patients.

The presence of uncompensated left ventricular failure and a low left ventricular ejection fraction are also defined as active cardiac conditions. This is a result partly of the close association with coronary vascular disease and is also due to the resultant reduction in cardiac reserve. These should be assessed and treated before any non-emergency surgery.

Diabetes mellitus, a history of stroke, previous or treated heart failure and impaired renal function (creatinine >177 µmol L^{-1}) are independent risk factors associated with perioperative myocardial ischaemia and infarction. The extent of preoperative testing required is dictated by the patient's functional status and the type of intended surgery.

Hypertension alone is now considered to be a relatively low risk factor. However, it is often a marker of significant underlying vascular disease.

Preoperative Assessment

The aims of preoperative assessment in this group are to:

■ define the fitness of the patient for the proposed anaesthetic and surgery
■ delineate the level of risk of the procedure

- decide on the most appropriate anaesthetic technique
- assess the requirement for preoperative therapy to be initiated, for example β-blockade or blood transfusion
- assess the level of perioperative monitoring required
- decide on the patient's postoperative management, including where this should take place.

The Lee revised cardiac risk index for patients undergoing non-cardiac surgery identifies several intermediate risk factors (Table 18.3). The presence of two or more of these factors has been shown to identify patients with moderate (7%) and high (10%) risk of cardiac complications. There is evidence that this increased risk may continue for 6 months following surgery.

- high-risk surgery (defined as intraperitoneal, intrathoracic or suprainguinal vascular surgery)
- ischaemic heart disease diagnosed either from the history or investigation
- congestive heart failure
- cerebrovascular disease
- insulin-dependent diabetes mellitus
- renal impairment (creatinine $>177\mu$mol L^{-1}).

TABLE 18.3

Stratification of Risk Factors for Patients Undergoing Non-Cardiac Surgery

Active cardiac condition:
Unstable coronary syndrome (MI within 30 days, PCI within last 6 weeks)
Decompensated heart failure
Significant arrhythmias
Severe valvular disease

Intermediate Factors according to the Revised Cardiac Risk Index:
History of heart disease
History of compensated or prior heart failure
History of cerebrovascular disease
Diabetes mellitus*
Renal impairment

---

*The original Lee Revised Cardiac Risk Index included only diabetes treated with insulin, though it is now thought that Type II diabetes is also an intermediate risk factor.
Adapted from Fleisher LA, Beckman JA, Brown KA et al 2007 ACC/AHA guidelines on perioperative cardiovascular evaluation and care for noncardiac surgery: a report of the American College of Cardiology/American Heart Association Task Force on Practice Guidelines. J Am Coll Cardiol 50:1707–1732.
MI, myocardial infarction; PCI, percutaneous coronary intervention.

History. Symptoms of cardiovascular disease include chest pain, dyspnoea, palpitations, ankle swelling and intermittent claudication. Past medical history and medical records usually reveal the nature and severity of disease, as many patients with cardiovascular symptoms will already have undergone relevant investigations.

Examination. Preoperative cardiovascular examination should include measurement of heart rate, arterial pressure and assessment of peripheral pulses and perfusion. Signs of heart failure should be sought, including a third heart sound, elevated jugular venous pressure and fine basal crepitations on auscultation of the lung fields. The heart should be auscultated for murmurs indicative of valvular disease. In particular, it is vital to make the diagnosis of aortic stenosis pre-operatively.

Testing the patient's exercise capacity in the ward or on a flight of stairs is a simple, but useful, assessment of functional reserve. The inability to climb two flights of stairs indicates a very high risk of cardiopulmonary complications after major high-risk surgery.

Risk Stratification. Assessment of the patient's risk of a perioperative cardiac event provides prognostic information. These issues may be discussed with the patient and appropriate written information provided. Adequate provision of information and the opportunity to ask questions has been shown to allay preoperative anxiety. Assessment also guides perioperative investigation and management.

In patients with an active cardiac condition defined as unstable coronary syndrome, decompensated heart failure, significant arrhythmias or severe valvular disease (Table 18.3), only emergency procedures should be considered. Elective procedures should be postponed for evaluation, testing and optimization of the patient's active cardiac condition to minimize perioperative risk. The need for evaluation and further testing depends on the risks associated with a particular surgical procedure, the patient's physiological reserve or functional capacity, and whether testing would change management. Patients undergoing low-risk surgery, or those with proven good functional capacity undergoing intermediate or higher risk surgery, can usually proceed to surgery. They will only require further invasive cardiac investigations if it would change management (i.e. they would require medical optimization or be a candidate for coronary revascularization) (Fig. 18.1).

For example, patients who have sustained a myocardial infarction (MI) within the 30 days before proposed surgery are a high-risk group. As a result of increased sympathetic stimulation and the coagulation activation secondary to surgery, such patients have a very high risk (up to 28%) of perioperative MI, which carries a high (10–15%) mortality. A history of uncomplicated MI more than 30 days before surgery is no longer considered an absolute contraindication to elective surgery, provided that the patient is symptom-free and has a good exercise capacity (see Table 18.1).

If there is no urgency for surgery however, it is best to wait until 3 months after MI when, if patients are asymptomatic with a good exercise capacity, they rejoin the low-risk group.

Asymptomatic patients who have undergone successful coronary artery bypass grafting more than 6 weeks before surgery constitute a low-risk group. Indeed, the mortality in this group is less than in a matched group with well-controlled angina on medical therapy. However, the risk of coronary artery surgery itself negates this benefit. It is therefore recognized that major cardiac interventions such as bypass grafting are indicated before non-cardiac surgery only if the patient's underlying cardiac condition merits intervention for its own sake. This is the case for patients with severe triple vessel disease or significant left main stem stenosis.

Increasing numbers of patients now present for non-cardiac surgery having undergone percutaneous coronary interventions (PCI), particularly intracoronary stenting (ICS). Guidelines for the optimal perioperative management of these patients have been produced (Fig. 18.2). There are a number of important points. Firstly, it is beneficial to discuss the patient's management with an experienced cardiologist. The risk of non-cardiac surgery in patients with intracoronary stents depends on the timing of surgery related to insertion of the stent and the type of stent used. Bare metal stents have been largely superseded by drug-eluting stents, which contain a cytotoxic agent. This is slowly released from the ICS to limit endothelialization, which reduces the incidence of thrombosis

and stenosis within the stent itself. However, more prolonged and intensive antiplatelet therapy is required for drug-eluting stents because they are at increased risk of thrombosis until re-endothelialization has occurred. Following insertion of any ICS, there is an initial requirement for dual antiplatelet therapy (e.g. aspirin and clopidogrel). Non-cardiac surgery should be avoided during this time if possible. If antiplatelet therapy is stopped, the risk of stent thrombosis (which carries a 7% mortality) is high, while continuing therapy increases the risk of perioperative bleeding. The duration of dual antiplatelet therapy should be a minimum of one month after bare metal stents and up to 12 months for drug-eluting stents. It is recommended that even urgent surgery should be postponed for at least 4–6 weeks after ICS insertion, and elective surgery deferred for 3 months after bare metal stent, and for 12 months after drug-eluting stent insertion. If possible, even beyond these times, aspirin should be continued throughout the perioperative period, particularly because abrupt cessation of aspirin increases thrombogenicity. In the future, the possibility of bridging therapy with short-acting glycoprotein IIb/IIa inhibitors such as tirofiban may be considered.

As with coronary revascularization procedures, and due to the risks outlined, there is no place for prophylactic coronary stenting before surgery unless this is independently indicated for the cardiac condition.

Investigations. Standard investigations including haematology, biochemistry, an ECG and chest X-ray are necessary in all patients with proven or suspected cardiovascular disease. A coagulation screen may be indicated.

Subsequent investigations depend on the assessed risk for the patient and the clinical findings.

All patients found to have a murmur should have preoperative echocardiography. Significant aortic stenosis, for example, is associated with an increased risk of perioperative cardiovascular events and may be difficult to confirm and grade on clinical grounds alone. Echocardiography also provides useful information on left ventricular function.

Additional cardiovascular investigations are indicated only if they influence management. The

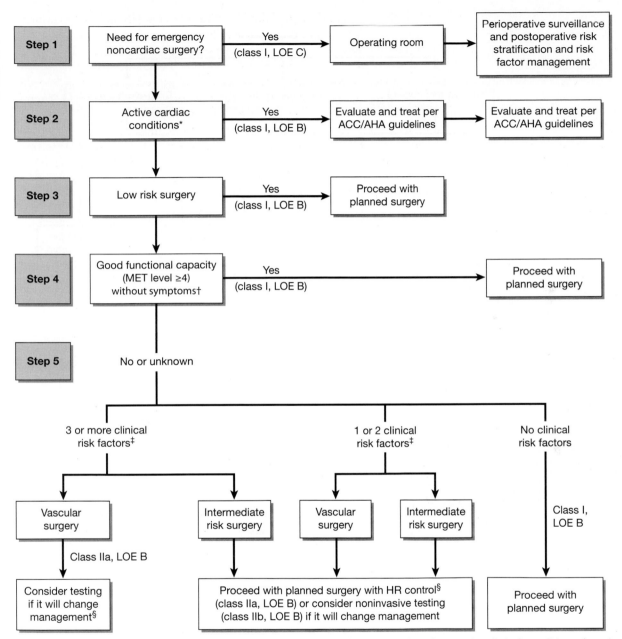

FIGURE 18.1 ■ Cardiac evaluation and care algorithm for noncardiac surgery based on active clinical conditions, known cardiovascular disease, or cardiac risk factors for patients 50 years of age or greater. *See Table 18.3 for active cardiac conditions. †See Table 18.1 for estimated MET level equivalent. ‡Clinical risk factors include ischaemic heart disease, compensated or prior heart failure, diabetes mellitus, renal insufficiency, and cerebrovascular disease (Table 18.3). §Consider perioperative beta blockade for populations in which this has been shown to reduce cardiac morbidity/mortality. ACC/AHA indicates American College of Cardiology/American Heart Association. HR, heart rate; LOE, level of evidence; and MET, metabolic equivalent. *(Adapted from Fleisher LA, Beckman JA, Brown KA et al 2007 ACC/AHA guidelines on perioperative cardiovascular evaluation and care for noncardiac surgery: a report of the American College of Cardiology/American Heart Association Task Force on Practice Guidelines. J Am Coll Cardiol 50:1707–1732.)*

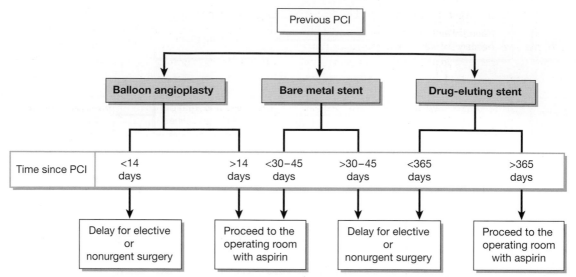

FIGURE 18.2 ■ Recommended timing of noncardiac surgery following percutaneous coronary intervention (PCI) depends on whether a stent was placed and the type of stent used. *(Adapted from Fleisher LA, Beckman JA, Brown KA et al 2007 ACC/AHA guidelines on perioperative cardiovascular evaluation and care for noncardiac surgery. J Am Coll Cardiol 50:1707–1732.)*

incidence of asymptomatic coronary artery disease in the population is approximately 4%, and screening tests are unlikely to be helpful in patients with no cardiac symptoms. Patients with active cardiac conditions, in whom specific management of cardiovascular disease is indicated independent of the need for noncardiac surgery, should undergo non-invasive cardiac testing, with or without coronary angiography and further treatment as indicated.

Between these two extremes lies a group of patients at increased risk of perioperative cardiovascular events in whom further assessment is indicated because perioperative care is influenced by the results. Moreover, accurate determination of risk to the patient may help decision-making with regard to the need for surgery and/or the type of operation and anaesthetic (Fig. 18.1).

Patients who should be considered for further preoperative testing include:

- patients with poor or unknown functional capacity
- patients with clinical risk factors undergoing intermediate or high-risk surgery
- patients with diabetes mellitus
- patients with poor left ventricular function

The choice of preoperative test is dictated by local and patient factors, but commonly it includes exercise stress testing, dobutamine stress echocardiography and dipyridamole thallium scanning. Cardiological advice should be sought for both the test required and interpretation of the results with regard to predicting the perioperative risk of a serious cardiovascular event.

Preoperative Therapy

There are two main areas to be addressed. Pre-existing cardiovascular disease should be treated and management optimized where necessary. In addition, there may be interventions which, appropriately initiated in patients at risk, may improve outcome.

Pre-Existing Cardiovascular Disease. Ischaemic heart disease. Medical therapy should be reviewed and optimized if symptoms are poorly controlled.

Hypertension. Raised arterial pressure is a major cause of morbidity and mortality in the general population because of the detrimental effects on the myocardial, cerebrovascular and renal circulations. It is now recognized that both hypertension and isolated systolic hypertension should be treated because effective control of arterial pressure reduces the incidence of complications from target organ damage. The British Hypertension Society guidelines recommend starting antihypertensive therapy for sustained pressures above 140/90 mmHg. However, in the perioperative setting, there is little evidence that patients with isolated hypertension of less than 180/110 mmHg have a significantly increased risk of cardiovascular complications and isolated hypertension below this level is classified as a low-risk factor. If hypertension is identified preoperatively, evidence of target organ damage should be sought. If target organ damage is found, then the risks of anaesthesia and surgery are dependent on this. Subsequent investigation and management should be based on target organ function rather than on the hypertension *per se*. Postoperative follow-up and treatment are indicated.

For non-urgent surgery, patients with severe hypertension, i.e. >180/110 mmHg, should be treated to lower the arterial pressure in a controlled manner before embarking on surgery. In the case of urgent surgery, more rapid control may be achieved. In light of their beneficial effects in high-risk cardiovascular patients, β-blockers are probably the agents of choice. Care must be taken, however, because rapid decreases in arterial pressure may be detrimental.

Antihypertensive therapy should be continued as far as possible throughout the perioperative period.

Many patients seen at preadmission clinic or admitted to hospital have hypertension which subsequently settles or which is not in keeping with the recordings made by their general practitioner. There is no evidence that so called 'white coat hypertension' carries an increased perioperative risk. Often, these patients benefit from a benzodiazepine premedication.

Heart failure. A history of treated heart failure and low left ventricular ejection fraction are intermediate clinical risk factors. Treatment should be optimized as far as possible pre-operatively and investigation of underlying coronary artery disease undertaken as appropriate, as outlined above.

Treatment and Additional Interventions. *β-Blockers.* Established β-blocker therapy should be maintained throughout the perioperative period either orally or intravenously if necessary. Sudden preoperative cessation may be associated with rebound effects such as

angina, myocardial infarction, arrhythmias and hypertension. The dose of β-blocker may be reduced if there is undue bradycardia preoperatively (<50 beat min^{-1}). Intraoperative bradycardia usually responds to intravenous atropine or glycopyrrolate. Some studies have shown that institution of perioperative β-blockade reduces short and long term cardiovascular morbidity and mortality in patients with *definite evidence of ischaemic heart disease undergoing high-risk surgery.*

These advantages are not seen in patients receiving chronic therapy and do not appear to be restricted to any particular β-blocker. Beta blockade should therefore be considered for these patients but the optimal time to begin therapy and the optimal duration of β-blockade are uncertain. In a non-urgent situation, it may be preferable to introduce β-blockade cautiously over several weeks, particularly if there is evidence of left ventricular dysfunction. It should be noted that several studies in lower risk patients (e.g. those with risk factors for ischaemic heart disease but no symptoms) have shown no overall benefit from perioperative β-blockade. In the POISE study, perioperative β-blockade actually increased the overall mortality and the incidences of stroke, bradycardia and hypotension.

Angiotensin-converting enzyme inhibitors and angiotensin II receptor blockers. These agents have disease-modifying effects in patients with vascular disease, cardiac failure and diabetes, with a reduction in cardiac morbidity and mortality. They may predispose to renal failure and hyperkalaemia and may be associated with intractable intraoperative hypotension. There is currently no consensus as to whether or not these agents should be continued intraoperatively.

Antiplatelet agents. Aspirin and clopidogrel are used increasingly in combination to maintain vessel patency following percutaneous coronary intervention (PCI) and to reduce thrombosis in patients with unstable angina or recent MI. Both agents have irreversible effects on platelet action and their effect therefore continues for the life of the platelet. Aspirin inhibits cyclo-oxygenase-mediated production of thromboxane. Clopidogrel is a non-competitive antagonist of platelet ADP receptors. They have a synergistic effect in inhibiting platelet aggregation. Both agents need to be stopped for at least 7 days to see these effects reversed by new platelet production. Whether or not these agents are continued perioperatively depends on the perceived risk of bleeding against the increased risk of cardiovascular events. If the drugs are continued, both the surgeon and anaesthetist must be aware of the increased risk of haemorrhage and take appropriate anticipatory measures. Platelet transfusion is the only effective therapy for uncontrolled haemorrhage secondary to these agents.

In general, if a patient is anticoagulated (see below) or receiving clopidogrel, neuraxial blockade is contraindicated because of the increased risk of haematoma and neurological damage. Aspirin alone is not considered a significant risk factor.

Anticoagulants. Where long-term therapy is indicated, perioperative control must be monitored closely. Warfarin should be stopped at least 48 h preoperatively and the prothrombin time monitored daily. The prothrombin time should be less than 1.5 times control at the time of surgery. If prolonged, the use of vitamin K may be considered; however, this takes 6–12 h to act and may compromise subsequent anticoagulation, so its use depends on the reasons for anticoagulation. In an emergency or where excessive haemorrhage occurs, fresh frozen plasma should be given to supply coagulation factors. For patients at high risk from thrombosis, e.g. with a prosthetic heart valve, an intravenous heparin infusion should be started when the prothrombin time decreases and continued until 2 h preoperatively. After minor surgery with low risk of haemorrhage, warfarin may be restarted postoperatively. After major surgery, an infusion of unfractionated heparin should be used to maintain anticoagulation until warfarin therapy is reinstituted safely. The heparin infusion may be titrated to activated partial thromboplastin time (aPTT) to maintain good control and if necessary may be reversed rapidly with intravenous protamine. Protamine should be given slowly to avoid hypotension and if given in excessive dose is itself an anticoagulant.

Statins. Statins reduce morbidity and mortality in patients with vascular disease even in the presence of a normal cholesterol concentration. This is thought to result from stabilization of atheromatous plaques. There is also increasing evidence in patients undergoing high-risk vascular surgery that initiating statin therapy may reduce cardiovascular complications. The introduction of a statin preoperatively should therefore be considered in this group. Again, the optimal timing of this intervention is unknown but it has been suggested that therapy should be started 1 month before surgery.

α_2-Agonists. Drugs such as clonidine reduce sympathetic activity, reduce arterial pressure and heart rate and have analgesic properties. There is some evidence to suggest they may be of benefit in patients at high risk of perioperative cardiovascular events, but this is insufficient to recommend their routine use.

Continued administration mandates a greater degree of cardiovascular monitoring, particularly with regard to maintenance of intravascular volume. Vasoactive agents may be required to maintain an adequate arterial pressure.

Preoptimization. Measures to improve cardiac output and oxygen delivery have been shown to improve outcome in some high-risk patients with limited physiological reserve undergoing major surgery. These measures include monitored fluid therapy, vasoactive support, blood transfusion and mechanical ventilation, and are aimed at improving tissue oxygen delivery and hence oxygen delivery/consumption balance. The level of monitoring required, patient selection and the risk/benefit balance of increasing myocardial oxygen demand in the face of ischaemic heart disease, versus improving cardiac output and hence oxygen delivery, need to be considered on an individual basis.

This management strategy may be undertaken in a critical care area or in the anaesthetic room and requires close cooperation between relevant medical staff.

It is not known yet if combining preoptimization with preoperative therapy with agents such as β-blockers is helpful. However, the two approaches are not necessarily mutually exclusive.

Premedication. Anxiety is a cause of sympathetic nervous system activation which may be detrimental in patients with cardiovascular disease. While not all patients require anxiolytic premedication, there should be a low threshold for use in these patients. A benzodiazepine such as temazepam is usually satisfactory. In patients with low or fixed cardiac output states, e.g. mitral or aortic stenosis, constrictive pericarditis or congestive cardiac failure, and other high-risk patients, it is important to avoid hypotension or excessive sedation, respiratory depression and hypoxaemia which could result from premedication, and in these situations it may be preferable to omit sedative premedication.

The patient's usual cardiac medications and any additional therapy started preoperatively should be continued and included in the premedication.

High-risk patients benefit from oxygen therapy before transfer to the anaesthetic room, especially if sedative premedication has been given.

Anaesthesia: General Principles

- Anaesthesia should comprise a balanced technique aimed at maintaining cardiovascular stability. A variety of options may be suitable, including both general and regional anaesthesia or a combination.
- Tachycardia should be avoided and an adequate arterial pressure maintained (there should not be a sustained reduction in arterial pressure of more than 20% of the patient's normal pressure). Coronary perfusion and myocardial oxygen delivery are thus maintained without increasing myocardial work and oxygen requirements.
- For patients identified as high risk, consideration should be given to stress reduction. Measures to achieve this are dictated by the patient and operative factors. These include the following:
  - *Use of neuraxial blockade.* This has been associated with reduced perioperative myocardial ischaemia and infarction. However, this must be balanced against the sympathetic block and associated hypotension. This may be pronounced, particularly with a high spinal block. Early judicious use of vasopressors coupled with maintenance of intravascular volume should limit this problem. However, neuraxial blockade, particularly spinal block, is relatively contraindicated if there is severely limited cardiovascular reserve and if maintenance of adequate arterial pressure is critical, e.g. severe aortic stenosis (see below).
  - Perioperative β-blockade.
  - High-dose opioids, e.g. fentanyl or remifentanil.
- The level of intraoperative monitoring should be dictated by risk assessment. The following should be considered in addition to standard monitoring.
  - *Five-lead ECG.* The usual ECG configuration for anaesthetic monitoring is standard limb lead II. Whilst this is useful for identifying arrhythmias, myocardial ischaemia occurs most commonly in the left ventricle and is detected more sensitively with a CM5 configuration (see Fig. 16.2).
  - *Direct arterial pressure recording.*
  - *CVP monitoring* with or without central venous oxygen saturations.
  - *Oesophageal Doppler*, providing a measurement of cardiac output and intravascular filling.
  - Other minimally invasive cardiac output monitors are now available and may prove useful as intraoperative monitors. Examples include devices which derive cardiac output and other variables from the arterial pressure waveform using internal algorithms. Some devices (*FloTrac/Vigileo* or *LiDCO*) use a standard arterial catheter whereas others (*PiCCO*) require a dedicated thermistor tipped catheter in a proximal (femoral or axillary artery).
  - *Pulmonary artery flotation catheter* with continuous cardiac output and mixed venous oxygen saturation monitoring.
- Patients should be well oxygenated and normocapnic.
- Close attention to fluid balance is mandatory. This begins preoperatively when fluid depletion secondary to factors such as excessive fasting times and bowel preparation should be corrected. As far as possible, normovolaemia should be maintained. Intravascular volume depletion is known to compromise organ perfusion and oxygen delivery but there is increasing evidence that postoperative recovery is also compromised by excessive volume and sodium loading in the immediate perioperative period.
- Patients at high risk from cardiovascular disease do not tolerate anaemia. The optimal level of haemoglobin is the subject of much discussion but is probably around $10\,g\,L^{-1}$.
- Patients should be actively warmed to avoid hypothermia, which activates the stress response, predisposes to arrhythmias and increases oxygen consumption postoperatively as a result of shivering.

- Effective perioperative analgesia is essential. Pain is a potent stimulator of the stress response and uncontrolled sympathetic activation increases myocardial work and oxygen demand, predisposing to myocardial ischaemia or infarction.
- Before embarking on anaesthesia and surgery, consideration needs to be given to the patient's management and destination postoperatively, e.g. would benefit be derived from a period of artificial ventilation or continued close monitoring in a high dependency or intensive care area postoperatively?
- Good communication between all of the relevant carers, including cardiology, critical care and the surgical team, is important.

Anaesthetic Agents. Most intravenous anaesthetic induction agents are cardiovascular depressants, causing both vasodilatation and myocardial depression. This is exaggerated in patients with low fixed cardiac output states and by concurrent hypovolaemia. Of the agents in regular use, etomidate is the least cardiac depressant. Care with dosing and rate of administration limits the hypotension caused by drugs such as propofol or thiopental. Co-induction with more than one agent may be beneficial in reducing the dose requirements of each and limiting hypotension. Concurrent administration of midazolam and a short-acting opioid (alfentanil or fentanyl) is often used. Remifentanil may be useful in these patients, in a low-dose infusion of $0.1–0.2\,\mu g\;kg^{-1}\;min^{-1}$. It limits the dose of induction agent required and blunts the cardiovascular response to laryngoscopy and tracheal intubation. However, used in high doses, it may induce respiratory muscle stiffness and make bag and mask ventilation difficult before the onset of neuromuscular blockade.

For patients naive to β-blockers, esmolol (a short-acting i.v. β-blocker) may be used to obtund the cardiovascular response to airway manoeuvres.

Of the neuromuscular blocking agents, rocuronium and vecuronium are the most cardiostable.

Brief periods of cardiac ischaemia provide protection against the damaging effects of subsequent more prolonged episodes; this is known as ischaemic preconditioning. Much is now known about the physiology of this in experimental situations, including the fact that volatile anaesthetic agents and opioids help to induce ischaemic preconditioning, while other agents, e.g. the sulphonylureas, inhibit it.

There is clinical evidence of its relevance, e.g. patients with pre-infarct angina generally have a better prognosis than those who are asymptomatic, and this may be a result of preconditioning. The clinical application of these findings is as yet unknown, but may favour the use of volatile agents in this high-risk group.

Arrhythmias

Preoperative arrhythmias should be treated before surgery. The patient should be screened for predisposing factors such as ischaemic or valvular heart disease and electrolyte and endocrine abnormalities. In atrial fibrillation, the ventricular rate should be controlled preoperatively if possible.

Antiarrhythmic therapy should continue throughout the perioperative period.

The indications for antiarrhythmic therapy and pacing are identical to those applicable in the absence of surgery and anaesthesia.

Indications for preoperative temporary pacing include:

- bradyarrhythmia unresponsive to atropine if associated with syncope, hypotension or ventricular arrhythmias
- risk of asystole
- complete heart block
- second-degree heart block (Mobitz 2)
- first-degree heart block associated with bifascicular block
- sick sinus syndrome.

Intraoperative Arrhythmias. Arrhythmias are common in the perioperative period and are often self-limiting and require no specific treatment. However, precipitants of these arrhythmias should be sought and corrected if possible as they are more likely to occur and cause cardiovascular compromise in patients with underlying heart disease.

Factors predisposing to intraoperative arrhythmias include the following.

Patient factors:

- hypoxaemia
- hypo- and hypercapnia

- acidosis
- hypo- and hyperthermia
- electrolyte abnormalities, particularly of potassium and magnesium
- hypovolaemia.

Autonomic effects:

- surgical stimulation and pain
- vagal stimulation, e.g. anal or cervical dilatation, traction on mesentery, traction on extraocular muscles
- laryngoscopy and tracheal intubation
- laparascope insertion or intra-abdominal insufflation of gas with peritoneal stretching during laparascopic procedures.

Direct stimulation:

- CVP catheter and guide wire insertion
- PA catheter insertion.

Drugs:

- adrenaline
- local anaesthetic toxicity (bupivacaine)
- halothane.

Management. This depends on the nature of the arrhythmia, likely causes and the degree of haemodynamic compromise.

- The precipitant should be removed if possible. Reflex arrhythmias tend to occur more commonly during light anaesthesia and may often be prevented by deepening anaesthesia.
- Physiological abnormalities should be corrected, as specific antiarrhythmic therapy may be ineffective in the presence of uncorrected hypoxaemia, hypovolaemia or electrolyte abnormalities. Treatment of these should be concurrent with specific management of the arrhythmia.

Intraoperative Bradyarrhythmias. Bradyarrhythmias may often be prevented and may be treated using an intravenous anticholinergic, e.g. atropine or glycopyrrolate.

External pacing defibrillators are now widely available and can be used for temporary cardiac pacing for patients unresponsive to anticholinergics pending insertion of a transvenous pacemaker.

Intraoperative Tachyarrhythmias. These are either supraventricular or ventricular in origin. Generally, but not exclusively, supraventricular arrhythmias are narrow-complex, in distinction to broad-complex ventricular arrhythmias.

Supraventricular tachycardia. If there is haemodynamic compromise, the treatment of choice is synchronized DC cardioversion, particularly as the patient is already anaesthetized. This applies to all supraventricular tachyarrhythmias. If cardioversion fails, amiodarone 300 mg be given i.v. over 10–20 min and electrical cardioversion re-attempted.

If the patient is not severely compromised, management depends on the individual arrhythmia:

- *Atrial fibrillation.* This is the commonest supraventricular arrhythmia seen intraoperatively. Often, a return to sinus rhythm cannot be achieved until the underlying precipitants are resolved. Improvements in oxygenation, volume status and analgesia may all improve the situation. However, ventricular rate control may also require treatment with either amiodarone or digoxin. Beta blockers or verapamil may also be used to slow ventricular rate. When surgery is complete, anticoagulation should be considered to avoid the embolic complications of atrial fibrillation.
- *Atrial flutter.* This should be managed in the same way as atrial fibrillation if it occurs intraoperatively.
- *AV node/AV re-entry tachycardia and atrial tachycardia.* Vagal manoeuvres, e.g. carotid sinus massage, may be tried, as can intravenous adenosine. Adenosine transiently slows AV conduction and may convert supraventricular tachycardia (SVT) to sinus rhythm. Alternatively, it may aid diagnosis by revealing flutter or fibrillation waves. A rapid i.v. bolus of 6 mg is given, followed by 12 mg a maximum of three times at 2-min intervals. Adenosine is contraindicated in patients with asthma, second- or third-degree heart block, patients receiving carbamazepine or dipyridamole and patients with a denervated heart, e.g. after cardiac transplant. Care must be taken with its use if the patient has Wolff-Parkinson-White syndrome. Verapamil,

β-blockers and amiodarone may control the ventricular rate. Intravenous verapamil should never be given to a β-blocked patient.

■ *Ventricular tachycardia.* Synchronized DC cardioversion is the treatment of choice. Alternatively, amiodarone (300 mg i.v. over 20-60 min, followed by an infusion of 900 mg over 24 h) may be given if the arrhythmia is well tolerated. Lidocaine 1 mg kg^{-1} may be used as an alternative if amiodarone is not available, but should not be given if amiodarone has been given already.

Permanent Pacemakers. Many patients with these devices have underlying heart disease which should be managed accordingly.

Permanent pacemakers are inserted in an increasing number of patients and are becoming increasingly complex. Pacemakers are classified by a series of 5 letters relating to the functions they possess (Table 18.4).

Specific Issues in Anaesthetic Management

■ Preoperative assessment: the pacemaker clinic should be contacted to find out the indication for pacemaker insertion, its history and mode of action noted, and any evidence of malfunction sought. The underlying rhythm and rate should be determined and the consequences in case of pacemaker malfunction failure known to determine the need for backup support.

■ The main intraoperative hazards are electromagnetic interference, which may reprogramme the pacemaker, cause inappropriate inhibition or trigger a defibrillator discharge, or damage the pacemaker circuitry.

■ Routine investigations should include ECG, chest X-ray and electrolytes.

■ The pacemaker should have been checked within 3 months of elective surgery. The battery life should be known; consider replacing any device near its elective replacement time.

■ Due to the complexity of programming available, it is no longer acceptable practice to use a magnet to return the pacemaker to a fixed rate mode. Magnets should not be used, as they have an unpredictable effect on programming.

■ Some pacemakers have a rate modulation facility. This implies that they can vary the rate of pacing with the patient's activity detected usually by muscle activity or respiratory activity so that heart rate may be increased with exercise. In general, rate modulation features should be inactivated before anaesthesia and surgery as shivering and muscle fasciculation may be misinterpreted and lead to inappropriate increases in heart rate.

■ Central venous or pulmonary artery catheters may dislodge pacing leads, particularly if the pacemaker has only recently been inserted. Consideration should be given to use of the femoral vein for central venous access and to alternative monitors of cardiac output.

■ Alternative pacing should be available in the event of pacemaker failure; external pacing is a rapid and effective back-up.

TABLE 18.4		
Pacemaker Classification		
Letter Position	*Function*	*Chamber/Function*
1st	Chamber paced	Atrium/ventricle/both
2nd	Chamber sensed	Atrium/ventricle/both
3rd	Response to sensing	None/triggered/inhibited/both
4th	Programmable? Rate modulation?	Simple/multiple/communicating Yes/no
5th	Anti-tachyarrhythmia functions	None/pacing/shock/both

For example: a VVI pacemaker both paces and senses with a ventricular wire and is inhibited by the patient's own heart beat.

- Pacemakers should be routinely checked postoperatively either before discharge or via an early appointment at the pacemaker clinic. Electromagnetic interference may unpredictably reprogramme the pacemaker or cause damage to it.
- Diathermy: bipolar diathermy should be used if possible. If unipolar diathermy is used, the diathermy and ground plate should be as far from the pacemaker as possible and the current pathway should be placed at right angles to the pacing wire(s).
- Lithotripsy: the lithotriptor should be at least 12 cm away from the pacemaker and rate modulation should be deactivated.
- Peripheral nerve stimulators and transcutaneous electrical nerve stimulators (TENS) should be kept at least 12 cm from the pacemaker.
- Defibrillator paddles should be 12 cm away from the pacemaker.
- MRI is contraindicated.

Implantable Cardioverter Defibrillators (ICDs).
Increasingly, these devices are used for the management of patients with recurrent life-threatening episodes of VF and VT. ICDs may also have a pacemaker function. As with permanent pacemakers, they may be subject to electromagnetic interference and the same precautions apply.

The antitachycardia and defibrillator actions should be switched off before surgery involving diathermy. Diathermy could be interpreted as VF and a shock delivered unnecessarily. An external defibrillator must be available and the patient should be in a high-dependency area postoperatively until the ICD is checked and reactivated.

Valvular Heart Disease

In both aortic and mitral stenosis, there is a low fixed cardiac output which leaves no reserve to compensate for changes in heart rate or vascular resistance. Regurgitant lesions are usually better tolerated.

As with ischaemic heart disease, specific intervention such as valve replacement or valvuloplasty is indicated before non-cardiac surgery only if the valvular lesion merits intervention anyway. Clearly, in an emergency situation, this is not an option.

General Principles

- The patient's functional reserve is a good indicator of the severity of a valve lesion
- Routine antibiotic prophylaxis is no longer recommended for all patients with valvular heart disease
- Patients with valvular heart disease may be receiving anticoagulants; perioperative heparinization is necessary
- No specific anaesthetic technique is preferred for valvular heart disease. The aim is to maintain cardiovascular stability. In severe disease, this is often best achieved using a general anaesthetic technique with opioids and controlled ventilation
- Invasive monitoring is often required in these patients.

Aortic Stenosis

Isolated aortic stenosis is associated most commonly with calcification, often on a congenitally bicuspid valve. In rheumatic heart disease, aortic stenosis occurs rarely in the absence of mitral disease and is combined usually with regurgitation. The diagnosis is suggested by the findings of an ejection systolic murmur, low pulse pressure and clinical and ECG evidence of left ventricular hypertrophy. It is important to distinguish between aortic stenosis and the murmur of aortic sclerosis found in some elderly patients. Clinical signs provide a guide; a slow-rising, low-volume pulse with reduced pulse pressure, reduced intensity of the second heart sound and the presence of a click are suggestive of stenosis, as is evidence of left ventricular hypertrophy on ECG. However, echocardiography with Doppler flow monitoring is essential for confirmation and assessment of severity. The heart size on chest X-ray is normal until late in the disease, while symptoms of angina, effort syncope and left ventricular failure indicate advanced disease.

Perioperative mortality is increased in patients with aortic stenosis.

Left ventricular systolic function is usually good but the hypertrophied ventricle has reduced compliance. Tachycardia and arrhythmias which compromise ventricular filling are poorly tolerated and should be avoided. Normally, 30% of ventricular filling results from atrial systole; therefore, maintenance of sinus rhythm is important. Tachycardia also reduces the duration of coronary perfusion, compromising blood supply to the hypertrophied ventricle, particularly if there is concomitant coronary artery disease. The resulting myocardial ischaemia causes further cardiovascular deterioration, which may be catastrophic. Excessive bradycardia also compromises cardiac output. Adequate venous return must be maintained to ensure ventricular filling and hypotension, which compromises coronary flow, must be avoided.

Mitral Stenosis

This is usually a manifestation of rheumatic heart disease. Characteristic features include atrial fibrillation, arterial embolism, pulmonary oedema, pulmonary hypertension and right heart failure. Acute pulmonary oedema may be precipitated by the onset of atrial fibrillation.

Patients with mitral stenosis who present for surgery are frequently receiving digoxin, diuretics and anticoagulants. Preoperative control of atrial fibrillation, treatment of pulmonary oedema and management of anticoagulant therapy (see Ch 13) are necessary. During anaesthesia, control of heart rate is important. Tachycardia reduces diastolic ventricular filling and thus cardiac output, while bradycardia also results in decreased cardiac output because stroke output is limited. As with aortic stenosis, drugs which produce vasodilatation may cause severe hypotension. As a result of pre-existing pulmonary hypertension, patients are particularly vulnerable to hypoxaemia. Both hypoxaemia and acidosis are potent pulmonary vasoconstrictors and may produce acute right ventricular failure. Thus, opioid analgesics should be prescribed cautiously, and airway obstruction avoided.

Aortic Regurgitation

Acute aortic regurgitation, e.g. resulting from infective endocarditis, causes rapid left ventricular failure and may require emergency valve replacement, even in the presence of unresolved infection.

Chronic aortic regurgitation is asymptomatic for many years. Left ventricular dilatation occurs, with eventual left ventricular failure.

Patients with mild or moderate aortic regurgitation without left ventricular failure or major ventricular dilatation tolerate anaesthesia well. A slightly increased heart rate of approximately 100 beat min^{-1} is desirable because this reduces left ventricular dilatation. Bradycardia causes ventricular distension and should be avoided. Vasodilator therapy increases net forward flow by decreasing afterload and is useful in severe aortic regurgitation; isoflurane anaesthesia may be beneficial. Vasopressors should be avoided. Careful monitoring is required, and in severe cases a pulmonary artery catheter may be useful to aid management.

Mitral Regurgitation

Acute mitral regurgitation usually results from infective endocarditis, or myocardial infarction with papillary muscle dysfunction or ruptured chordae tendineae. Acute pulmonary oedema results, and urgent valve replacement is required. Left ventricular failure with ventricular dilatation may cause functional mitral regurgitation.

Chronic mitral regurgitation is commonly associated with mitral stenosis. In pure mitral regurgitation, left atrial dilatation occurs with a minimal increase in pressure. The degree of regurgitation may be limited by reducing the size of the left ventricle and the impedance to left ventricular ejection. Thus, inotropic agents and vasodilators may be useful, while vasopressors should be avoided. A slight increase in heart rate is desirable unless there is concomitant stenosis.

Infective Endocarditis

This is caused predominantly by the viridans group of streptococci, occasionally by Gram-negative organisms or enterococci and also by staphylococci, especially after cardiac surgery or in intravenous drug abusers. Coxiella burnetii also accounts for some cases. Patients with rheumatic or congenital heart disease, including asymptomatic lesions, e.g. bicuspid aortic valve, are at risk.

Hypertrophic Cardiomyopathy

Hypertrophic cardiomyopathy (HOCM) is a genetic cardiac disorder affecting 1 in 500 adults. There is a variable degree of ventricular muscle hypertrophy affecting mainly the interventricular septum. Patients may remain asymptomatic, or they may suffer dyspnoea, angina and syncope as a result of muscle hypertrophy and subsequent left ventricular outflow obstruction. HOCM is also a cause of sudden cardiac death caused by arrhythmias.

Diagnosis is confirmed by echocardiography.

Anaesthetic issues include:

- Acute changes in volume status cause severe haemodynamic consequences and hypovolaemia should be avoided
- Outflow obstruction is exacerbated by catecholamines so that inotropic agents should be avoided
- Patients are usually receiving a β-blocker which should be continued perioperatively
- Patients with previous malignant ventricular arrhythmias are likely to have an ICD *in situ*.

RESPIRATORY DISEASE

Successful anaesthetic management of the patient with respiratory disease is dependent on accurate assessment of the nature and extent of functional impairment and an appreciation of the effects of surgery and anaesthesia on pulmonary function.

Assessment

History

Of the six cardinal symptoms of respiratory disease (cough, sputum, haemoptysis, dyspnoea, wheeze and chest pain), dyspnoea provides the best indication of functional impairment. Specific questioning is required to elicit the extent to which activity is limited by dyspnoea. Dyspnoea at rest or on minor exertion clearly indicates severe disease. A cough productive of purulent sputum indicates active infection. Chronic copious sputum production may indicate bronchiectasis. A history of heavy smoking or occupational exposure to dust may suggest pulmonary pathology.

A detailed drug history is important. Long-term steroid therapy within 3 months of the date of surgery necessitates augmented cover for the perioperative period and may cause hypokalaemia and hyperglycaemia. Bronchodilators should be continued during the perioperative period. Patients with cor pulmonale may be receiving digoxin and diuretics.

Examination

A full physical examination is required, with emphasis on detecting signs of airway obstruction, increased work of breathing, active infection which may be treated preoperatively, and evidence of right heart failure. The presence of obesity, cyanosis or dyspnoea should be noted. In addition, a simple forced expiratory manoeuvre may reveal prolonged expiration, and a simple test of exercise tolerance may be useful, e.g. a supervised walk up stairs.

Measurement of oxygen saturation provides a quick and useful indication of oxygenation; an SpO_2 >95% on air excludes significant hypoxaemia and, by inference, hypercapnia.

Investigations

Chest X-ray. The preoperative chest X-ray is a poor indicator of functional impairment but may be indicated in certain situations:

- when history and/or examination suggest acute disease, e.g. infection, effusion, neoplasm
- in patients with chronic lung disease
- in patients from countries where tuberculosis is endemic.

ECG. This may indicate right atrial enlargement or right ventricular hypertrophy (P pulmonale in II; dominant R wave in III, V_{1-3}). Associated ischaemic heart disease is common, and ECG abnormalities may confirm this (Fig. 18.1).

Haematology. Polycythaemia occurs secondary to chronic hypoxaemia, while anaemia aggravates tissue hypoxia. Leucocytosis may indicate active infection.

Sputum Culture. Sputum culture is essential in patients with chronic lung disease or suspected acute infection.

Pulmonary Function Tests. Peak expiratory flow rate, forced expiratory volume in 1 s (FEV_1) and forced vital capacity (FVC) can be measured easily at the bedside. The FEV_1:FVC ratio is decreased in obstructive lung disease and normal in restrictive disease. In the presence of obstructive disease, the test should be repeated 5–10 min after administration of a bronchodilator aerosol to provide an indication of reversibility. An FVC <1–1.5 L is indicative of limited ability to take large sigh breaths, expand lung bases and clear secretions by coughing.

Fuller investigation involves measurement of functional residual capacity (FRC), residual volume and total lung capacity, but these are rarely of value in determining clinical management.

Blood Gas Measurement. Arterial blood gas measurement is indicated in patients with chronic respiratory disease scheduled to undergo significant surgery and also if there is suspected acute hypoxaemia. It is also advisable when pulmonary function tests are markedly abnormal, e.g. in obstructive disease where the FEV_1 is less than 1.5 L. A raised $PaCO_2$ with normal pH indicates chronic hypercapnia with renal compensation; a combined raised $PaCO_2$ and acidosis indicates an acute event. Hypercapnia, particularly if acute, associated with acidosis, is likely to be associated with postoperative pulmonary complications. With a $PaCO_2$ of 6.7 kPa (50 mmHg) or greater, elective controlled ventilation may be required after major surgery. The combination of a low preoperative arterial oxygen tension (PaO_2) and dyspnoea at rest is also associated with a high likelihood of the need for planned ventilation after abdominal surgery.

Effects of Anaesthesia and Surgery

The effects of anaesthesia alone on respiratory function are generally minor and short-lived, but may tip the balance towards respiratory failure in patients with severe disease. These effects include:

- mucosal irritation by anaesthetic agents
- ciliary paralysis
- introduction of infection by aspiration or tracheal intubation
- respiratory depression by muscle relaxants, opioid analgesics or volatile anaesthetic agents.

In addition, anaesthesia is associated with a decrease in FRC, especially in the elderly and in obese patients, which leads to closure of basal airways and shunting of blood through underventilated areas of lung, an effect which is magnified by inhibition of the hypoxic pulmonary vasoconstrictor reflex.

Following recovery from anaesthesia, residual concentrations of anaesthetic agents and the presence of opioids inhibit the hyperventilatory responses to both hypercapnia and hypoxaemia, so that without close monitoring with pulse oximetry and appropriate blood gas analysis, serious hypoxaemia and hypercapnia may occur. Following thoracic and upper abdominal surgery, the decrease in FRC is more profound and persists for 5–10 days after surgery, with a parallel increase in alveolar–arterial oxygen tension difference ($P_{A-a}O_2$). Complications including atelectasis and pneumonia occur in approximately 20% of these patients.

Regional Anaesthesia. The use of appropriate regional anaesthetic techniques, where possible, confers several advantages in patients with respiratory disease both intra- and post-operatively, including:

- possible avoidance of tracheal intubation and controlled ventilation
- reduced or absent requirement for respiratory depressant agents such as volatile agents and opioids
- epidural analgesia may reduce postoperative hypoxaemia by diminishing the decrease in FRC associated with anaesthesia and abdominal surgery
- effective analgesia, allowing the patient to undergo chest physiotherapy, to mobilize early and to avoid prolonged bed rest.

The effects of surgery are dependent on its type and magnitude. Clearly, patients with pre-existing respiratory disease are at much greater risk following upper abdominal and thoracic surgery than after limb, head and neck or lower abdominal surgery.

Laparoscopic Surgery. The use of laparoscopic techniques for cholecystectomy, fundoplication and other abdominal procedures has markedly reduced postoperative pulmonary morbidity with the result that patients with severe pulmonary disease can usually undergo these procedures without the need for postoperative ventilatory support. The reasons for reduced morbidity include the relative lack of postoperative pain and the preservation of lung volumes postoperatively. These techniques should be encouraged in patients with chronic pulmonary disease. Nevertheless, cardiopulmonary function may be considerably compromised intraoperatively by raised intra-abdominal pressure, and judicious use of invasive haemodynamic monitoring has been recommended in patients with severe cardiorespiratory disease.

Obstructive Pulmonary Disease

This includes both chronic obstructive pulmonary disease and bronchial asthma. Patients with bronchiectasis and cystic fibrosis may also demonstrate marked airways obstruction, and justify a similar approach to management.

Chronic Obstructive Pulmonary Disease

Chronic obstructive pulmonary disease (COPD) is characterized by the presence of productive cough for at least 3 months in 2 successive years. Airways obstruction is caused by bronchoconstriction which has minimal or no reversibility, bronchial oedema and hypersecretion of mucus. In the postoperative period, pulmonary atelectasis and pneumonia result if sputum is not cleared. Severe disease may be accompanied by the signs and symptoms of right heart failure.

ASTHMA

Asthma may affect all age groups; it is characterized by recurrent generalized reversible airways obstruction, caused by bronchial smooth muscle spasm, mucus plugs and bronchial oedema. Asthma may be classified into two types: *extrinsic,* where an external allergen is demonstrable, and *intrinsic.* Intrinsic asthma tends to occur in adults, is more chronic and continuous and often requires long-term steroid therapy. There is an overlap between intrinsic asthma and COPD.

Preoperative Management

The current state of the patient's disease is assessed by:

- History – frequency and severity of attacks, factors provoking attacks, recent episodes of infection, drug history.
- Examination – presence or absence of wheeze, prolonged expiratory phase, overdistension, evidence of infection (cough, sputum, temperature, WBC).

- Pulmonary function tests – peak expiratory flow rate or FEV_1/FVC before and after inhalation of bronchodilator.
- Blood gas analysis including changes in $PaCO_2$ to varying inspired oxygen concentrations.

Treatment of Airways Obstruction

Elective surgery should not be undertaken unless or until airways obstruction is well controlled. Existing bronchodilator therapy should be continued perioperatively. Asthmatic patients are more likely to respond to inhaled β_2-adrenoceptor agonists, e.g. salbutamol, either by metered dose inhaler or nebulizer. Chronic asthmatics and patients with COPD may benefit from an inhaled anticholinergic agent (ipratropium bromide). The role of the phosphodiesterase inhibitor aminophylline is still controversial; it remains useful in the treatment of acute bronchospasm. If patients are receiving long-term theophyllines, the plasma concentration should be checked. Magnesium i.v. may be beneficial in acute asthma.

Corticosteroids are also important in the prevention and treatment of bronchospasm in asthmatics as they modify the underlying inflammatory process. Patients prescribed long-term inhaled or systemic steroid therapy who are suboptimally controlled may require a course of augmented steroid therapy, e.g. prednisolone 40–60 mg daily or hydrocortisone 100 mg four times daily, to cover the anaesthetic and postoperative periods. Equivalent doses of steroid preparations are shown in Table 18.5. The steroid dose should be gradually reduced postoperatively, titrated against the severity of the asthma.

TABLE 18.5
Equivalent doses of Glucocorticoids

Glucocorticoid	Dose (mg)
Betamethasone	3
Cortisone acetate	100
Dexamethasone	3
Hydrocortisone	80
Methylprednisolone	16
Prednisolone	20
Triamcinolone	16

Treatment of Active Infection

Amoxicillin or co-amoxiclav are appropriate, the common infecting organisms being *Streptococcus pneumoniae* and *Haemophilus influenzae*. Clarithromycin may be used if the patient is allergic to penicillin. Sputum for culture and sensitivities should be obtained to allow an appropriate choice of antibiotic. Chest physiotherapy and humidification of inspired gases aid expectoration.

Treatment of Cardiac Failure

Biventricular failure resulting from concurrent ischaemic heart disease and cor pulmonale frequently complicates COPD. Diuretics are indicated, while nitrates or digoxin may have a role.

Weight Reduction

This should be encouraged before elective surgery in obese patients with respiratory disease.

Smoking

Patients should be strongly encouraged to stop smoking for at least 6 weeks before elective surgery.

Premedication

A benzodiazepine to allay anxiety is appropriate for asthmatic patients, plus a dose of bronchodilator 30 min before induction of anaesthesia.

Anaesthesia

The anaesthetic technique in obstructive airways disease should be guided by the nature of the surgery, and also the severity of the disease.

An Approach with Minimal Intervention. Spontaneous ventilation with the option of local or regional anaesthesia is indicated for minor body surface operations. The use of a laryngeal mask airway (LMA) avoids tracheal intubation with its attendant risk of provoking bronchoconstriction, and if undue respiratory depression occurs, manifested by an increased $PaCO_2$, ventilation may be readily assisted via the LMA. Volatile anaesthetic agents, being bronchodilators, are well tolerated in asthmatics. Plexus blocks and low subarachnoid or epidural anaesthesia enable limb, lower abdominal or pelvic surgery in patients with severe respiratory impairment. Sedation should be administered carefully to avoid respiratory compromise.

Elective Mechanical Ventilation. A decision may be made to undertake intermittent positive-pressure ventilation (IPPV) during anaesthesia and for a variable period after operation, at least until elimination of neuromuscular blockers and anaesthetic agents has occurred. This also permits optimal provision of analgesia without fear of opioid-induced depression of ventilation. This technique is usually preferred if the preoperative $PaCO_2$ is greater than 6.7 kPa (50 mmHg) or if major thoracic or abdominal surgery is planned. Care should be taken with ventilator settings. A sufficiently long expiratory phase should be allowed to enable lung deflation and prevent gas trapping, while the inspiratory time should be adequate to avoid unduly high inflation pressures, with the attendant risk of pneumothorax.

Regional Anaesthesia. A combined general/epidural anaesthetic technique is often useful for major abdominal or thoracic surgery, as there is good evidence of a reduction in postoperative pulmonary complications with effective epidural analgesia. This approach may avoid a need for postoperative IPPV in some patients or may be usefully combined with noninvasive ventilation.

Anaesthetic Agents. Drugs which are associated with histamine release, e.g. atracurium and morphine, are perhaps best avoided, whilst rocuronium and fentanyl are preferred. β-Blocking drugs should also be avoided. If bronchospasm occurs during anaesthesia, it may result from easily remedied causes such as light anaesthesia or tracheal tube irritation and these should be corrected. If bronchospasm persists, nebulized salbutamol 2.5–5 mg should be administered into the anaesthetic breathing system and if this is not immediately beneficial, salbutamol 125–250 μg or aminophylline 250 mg should be administered by slow i.v. injection over at least 20 minutes, under ECG monitoring. The aminophylline dose should be modified if the patient is receiving oral theophylline. Thereafter, an infusion of aminophylline, up to 0.5–0.8 mg kg^{-1} h^{-1}, or salbutamol, possibly in combination with nebulized salbutamol by positive-pressure ventilation (solution of 50–100 µg mL^{-1} of water, run at 3–20 µg min^{-1}), should be maintained until improvement occurs. Hydrocortisone 200 mg i.v. should be given simultaneously, although it has no immediate effect. Inhaled volatile anaesthetic agents, e.g. sevoflurane, and intravenous ketamine have also been used with success when other agents have failed to relieve acute bronchospasm. Intravenous magnesium should also be considered in refractory cases.

Postoperative Care

Postoperative care of the patient with severe COPD or asthma should be conducted in an HDU or an ICU to allow close respiratory monitoring and ventilatory support if required.

Elective postoperative controlled ventilation allows adequate oxygenation, analgesia without respiratory depression, clearance of secretions by physiotherapy, tracheal suction and, if necessary, therapeutic fibreoptic bronchoscopy. Cardiac output and peripheral perfusion should be optimized before restoration of spontaneous ventilation. Unless there is pre-existing pulmonary infection, a period of 24 h of elective controlled ventilation is usually adequate and many patients may be weaned to spontaneous breathing much sooner. Analgesia produced by regional, e.g. epidural, blockade often allows earlier return to spontaneous ventilation, and permits pain-free coughing and clearing of secretions.

Oxygen and Respiratory Care.

Asthmatic patients rarely lose carbon dioxide responsiveness, and therefore high inspired oxygen concentrations are well tolerated and should be given. In patients with COPD, a controlled concentration of oxygen is generally required during spontaneous ventilation, using a 24% or 28% Venturi mask. Arterial blood gases should be checked frequently to ensure an adequate PaO_2 (>8 kPa) without excessive carbon dioxide retention ($PaCO_2$ <7.5–8 kPa). Using a pulse oximeter, the FiO_2 may be titrated to achieve an SpO_2 of around 90%. Hypoxaemia may seriously aggravate existing pulmonary hypertension and precipitate right ventricular failure.

Percutaneous cricothyroid puncture and insertion of a minitracheostomy permits aspiration of secretions while preserving the ability of the patient to cough and speak. This may be indicated postoperatively if sputum retention is a major problem.

The use of non-invasive respiratory support via a face-mask may be beneficial in the postoperative period. Non-invasive ventilation with a bilevel ventilator may aid carbon dioxide clearance and avoid postoperative invasive ventilation, or bridge the gap from invasive ventilation to spontaneous breathing. Face mask CPAP increases lung volumes and may prevent or treat lung atelectasis, with consequent improvement in oxygenation but without any significant effect on CO_2 clearance.

Techniques such as intermittent positive-pressure breathing (IPPB) supervised by a physiotherapist after surgery, can be used to expand the lungs and aid clearance of secretions. These techniques may also be effective if used and taught preoperatively in patients with large volumes of pulmonary secretions.

Analgesia.

Simple, non-opioid analgesics and/or local and regional techniques should be used where possible. Non-steroidal anti-inflammatory drugs (NSAIDs) such as diclofenac or ibuprofen are useful in reducing the opioid requirements following major surgery and may be adequate on their own after minor surgery. However, NSAIDs may aggravate bronchospasm in some asthmatics as a result of increased leukotriene production. These agents should not be given to patients with a history of aspirin hypersensitivity or to asthmatics who have never taken NSAIDs previously. Opioid analgesics are best administered, where necessary, in small i.v. doses, under direct supervision, or using patient-controlled analgesia. Physiotherapy, bronchodilators and antibiotics should be continued postoperatively.

Bronchiectasis

The patient should receive intensive physiotherapy with postural drainage for several days before surgery. Appropriate antibiotics, based on sputum culture, should be prescribed. Severe disease localized in one lung should be isolated during anaesthesia using a double-lumen tube.

Restrictive Lung Disease

This category includes a wide range of conditions which affect the lung and chest wall. Lung diseases include sarcoidosis and fibrosing alveolitis, while lesions of the chest wall include kyphoscoliosis and ankylosing spondylitis. Pulmonary function tests reveal a decrease in both FEV_1 and FVC, with a normal FEV_1/FVC ratio and decreased FRC and total lung capacity (TLC). Small airways closure occurs during tidal ventilation, with resultant shunting and hypoxaemia. Lung or chest wall compliance is decreased; thus, the work of breathing is increased and the ability to cough and clear secretions is impaired. There is an increased risk of postoperative pulmonary infection.

Anaesthesia causes little additional decrease in lung volumes and is tolerated well, provided that hypoxaemia is avoided. However, postoperatively, inadequate basal ventilation and retention of secretions may occur, partly as a result of pain, opioid analgesics and the residual effects of anaesthetic agents. High concentrations of oxygen may be used without risk of respiratory depression. A short period of mechanical ventilation may be necessary in patients with severe disease to allow adequate analgesia and clearing of secretions. Minitracheostomy may aid sputum clearance in the postoperative period, while non-invasive ventilation may avert the need for prolonged intubation and IPPV. Effective epidural analgesia helps to reduce postoperative respiratory complications.

Bronchial Carcinoma

Patients with bronchial carcinoma frequently suffer from coexisting COPD. In addition, there may be infection and collapse of the lung distal to the tumour. Patients with bronchial carcinoma may have myasthenic syndrome (see p. 413), while oat-cell tumours may secrete a variety of hormones, among the commonest being adrenocorticotrophic hormone (ACTH), (producing Cushing's syndrome), and antidiuretic hormone (ADH) (producing dilutional hyponatraemia, the syndrome of inappropriate ADH secretion).

Tuberculosis

Tuberculosis should be considered in patients with persistent pulmonary infection, especially if associated with haemoptysis or weight loss. It is becoming commoner in the UK. If active disease is present, all anaesthetic equipment should be changed after use to avoid cross-infection.

GASTROINTESTINAL DISEASE

Gastrointestinal disease presents several problems for the anaesthetist:

- malnutrition
- anaemia
- fluid and electrolyte depletion
- gastro-oesophageal reflux.

Malnutrition cannot usually be corrected fully before surgery but fluid and electrolyte depletion may be remedied, and appropriate measures may be taken to minimize the risk of regurgitation and aspiration.

Malnutrition

This may be caused by decreased nutritional intake, malabsorption or gut losses. Patients are at increased risk of perioperative morbidity and mortality, with infections, poor wound healing and thromboembolic complications being prominent. If patients are undergoing major surgery, consideration should be given to commencing preoperative nutritional support with enteral or total parenteral nutrition (TPN) before surgery. Vitamin supplementation is essential. Anaemia should be corrected.

Fluid and Electrolyte Depletion

This may result from decreased fluid intake caused by dysphagia or vomiting, or diarrhoea, for example. Significant fluid depletion may be caused by preoperative bowel preparation with hypertonic solutions and fluid may be given i.v. before surgery to maintain hydration.

Clinical assessment of volume depletion (poor perfusion, decreased tissue turgor, postural hypotension) should be supplemented by measurement of serum urea and electrolyte concentrations, and fluid and electrolyte deficits replaced. Patients with intestinal obstruction may have extreme fluid and electrolyte depletion, with a consequent risk of cardiovascular collapse, if vigorous fluid resuscitation is not provided before induction of anaesthesia. These patients require invasive cardiovascular monitoring throughout the perioperative period.

Gastrointestinal Reflux

Patients at risk include those with symptoms such as heartburn and regurgitation, and those with proven hiatus hernia. Patients with intestinal obstruction, ileus secondary to peritonitis from any cause and those presenting with vomiting may have a full stomach and be prone to regurgitation.

Other factors associated with reflux include raised intra-abdominal pressure, with obesity, pregnancy and the lithotomy position being particular risk factors.

The risk of aspiration of gastric acid and subsequent pneumonitis is reduced by administration of a histamine H_2-receptor antagonist, e.g. ranitidine, on the night before and morning of surgery, or a proton pump inhibitor, e.g. omeprazole. Sodium citrate 30 mL 5 min before induction neutralizes residual gastric acid. Metoclopramide is sometimes given to promote gastric emptying.

In patients with intestinal obstruction, emptying the stomach before induction of anaesthesia, using a large bore nasogastric tube, may be attempted. However, this may precipitate vomiting and, even if apparently effective, an empty stomach cannot be assumed.

Prevention of regurgitation and aspiration of gastric contents is based on early securing of the airway; preoxygenation, followed by rapid-sequence induction of anaesthesia with cricoid pressure to prevent regurgitation, is mandatory.

LIVER DISEASE

By far the commonest cause of liver disease in patients presenting for anaesthesia and surgery is alcoholic cirrhosis. This ranges in severity from asymptomatic to hepatic failure. Anaesthesia and surgery may affect liver function adversely, e.g. by decreasing liver blood flow, while pre-existing liver dysfunction may affect the conduct of anaesthesia because of impaired drug metabolism.

Preoperative Assessment

Preoperative assessment should be directed both to the degree of liver dysfunction and to the complications of liver disease.

Clinical features of liver disease include jaundice, ascites, oedema and impaired conscious level (encephalopathy).

Preoperative investigations should include full blood count, a coagulation screen, serum urea and electrolytes, bilirubin, alkaline phosphatase and transaminases, protein, albumin and blood sugar concentrations. Hypoglycaemia and hyperlactataemia may indicate hepatic metabolic dysfunction and a prolonged PT ratio impaired synthetic function. The patient should be screened for viral hepatitis. Universal precautions should be taken to protect staff and patients from transmission of viral hepatitis.

As far back as 1963, Child identified an increased mortality in patients with liver disease and classified surgical risk in patients with liver disease on the basis of:

- bilirubin and albumin concentrations
- nutritional state
- presence of ascites
- neurological disturbance
- surgical risk.

Particular problems relevant to the anaesthetist include the following:

Cardiovascular function. Patients with liver disease tend to be vasodilated and hypotensive. This may be aggravated by loss of fluid from the circulation as a result of hypoalbuminaemia and hence low oncotic pressure. Hypotension may also be aggravated by alcoholic cardiomyopathy.

Respiratory function. There may be respiratory compromise caused by diaphragmatic splinting by ascites and by pleural effusions. In severe disease, intrapulmonary shunting may cause disproportionate hypoxaemia.

Acid–base and fluid balance. Many patients are overloaded with salt and water. Hypoalbuminaemia results in oedema and ascites and predisposes to pulmonary oedema. Secondary hyperaldosteronism produces sodium retention (even though the plasma sodium concentration may be low) and also hypokalaemia. Diuretic therapy, often including spironolactone, may also affect the serum potassium concentration. In hepatic failure, a combined respiratory and metabolic alkalosis may occur, which shifts the oxygen dissociation curve to the left, potentially impairing tissue oxygenation.

Hepatorenal syndrome. This is defined as acute renal failure developing in patients with pre-existing chronic liver failure. Jaundiced patients are at risk of developing postoperative renal failure. This may be precipitated by hypovolaemia. Prevention involves adequate preoperative hydration, with i.v. fluids for at least 12 h before surgery and close monitoring of urine output, intra- and postoperatively. Intravenous 20% mannitol 100 mL may be given preoperatively and postoperatively if the hourly urine output decreases below 50 mL, though there is limited evidence for its efficacy. Close cardiovascular monitoring is essential and measurement of cardiac output should be considered.

Bleeding problems. Production of clotting factors II, VII, IX and X is reduced as a result of decreased vitamin K absorption. Production of factor V and fibrinogen is also reduced. Thrombocytopenia occurs if portal hypertension is present. Gastrointestinal haemorrhage from gastro-oesophageal varices may cause major management problems. Vitamin K should be administered preoperatively and fresh frozen plasma given to provide clotting factors during surgery, with regular checks made on coagulation. Infusion of platelet concentrate is indicated to cover surgery in cases of severe thrombocytopenia (platelet count $<50\times10^9$ L^{-1}) or if there is overt bleeding in a thrombocytopenic patient. Close liaison with the haematology service is essential and local protocols should be in place for the management of major haemorrhage.

Infection. Impairment of the filtering function of the liver's Kupffer cells leads to a higher incidence of endotoxaemia and infection. Bacterial peritonitis is a potential problem in patients with ascites.

Drug metabolism. Impairment of liver function slows elimination of drugs, including anaesthetic induction agents, opioid analgesics, benzodiazepines, succinylcholine, local anaesthetic agents and many others. Because the duration of action of many of these drugs is determined initially by redistribution, prolongation of action may not become apparent until a subsequent dose has been given.

In addition, many drugs have toxic effects on the liver. Halothane was previously well recognized as a cause of postoperative hepatitis, or even fulminant hepatic failure. Modern volatile anaesthetic agents, e.g. isoflurane, sevoflurane, are minimally metabolized and this complication is now rare.

Hepatic failure. The management of hepatic failure is beyond the scope of this chapter. The main issues are recognition, assessment and initial resuscitation and transfer to a specialist centre.

Initial Management Issues

- The airway and breathing may be compromised by impaired conscious level, diaphragmatic splinting by ascites or both. Intubation of the trachea and IPPV may be required, especially for transport.
- Direct monitoring of arterial and central venous pressures is required. Hypotension requires correction, generally with a vasopressor, e.g. noradrenaline (noradrenaline). Intravascular hypovolaemia and poor cardiac output need to be considered as possible additional factors.
- Conscious level: airway protection and IPPV may be required. Blood glucose concentration must be checked and hypoglycaemia corrected with intravenous glucose infusion. The presence of blood in the gastrointestinal tract following variceal or other haemorrhage is commonly a precipitating factor for encephalopathy; it is treated with lactulose by nasogastric tube.
- Electrolyte problems such as hypokalaemia should be corrected.
- Active bleeding should, if possible, be controlled before transfer to a specialist centre, e.g. by banding of gastro-oesophageal varices, or insertion of a Linton or Sengstaken-Blakemore tube.

Conduct of Anaesthesia

Anaesthesia with tracheal intubation and IPPV is commonly required to enable procedures to control gastrointestinal bleeding, e.g. upper GI endoscopy with injection or banding of oesophageal varices, to be undertaken safely.

The liver is particularly vulnerable to hypoxia, hypovolaemia and hypotension. During anaesthesia, cardiovascular stability should be maintained as far as possible. Lost blood should be replaced promptly, and overall fluid balance maintained. Careful arterial and central venous pressure monitoring is required. Drugs which depress cardiac output or arterial pressure, including volatile anaesthetic agents and β-blockers, should be used with caution to avoid reduction in hepatic blood flow.

The neuromuscular blockers of choice are those with cardiovascular stability and a short duration of action; atracurium may be preferable because its elimination is independent of hepatic and renal function. Opioids should be administered with caution unless ventilatory support is planned postoperatively. Short-acting agents such as remifentanil should be infused intraoperatively and fentanyl PCA may be suitable for postoperative analgesia. NSAIDs should be avoided.

Controlled ventilation to a normal $PaCO_2$ is important, as hypocapnia is associated with decreased hepatic blood flow. Hypoxaemia should be avoided throughout the perioperative period. In the adequately volume-expanded patient, hypotension may be reversed by infusion of noradrenaline (noradrenaline). However, in the unstable patient, expert help should be sought and monitoring should include measurement of cardiac output. In the presence of oesophageal varices, oesophageal doppler monitoring is contraindicated and other cardiac output monitors should be used.

RENAL DISEASE

Renal dysfunction has several important implications for anaesthesia, and therefore full assessment is required before even minor surgical procedures are contemplated.

Measurement of blood urea and electrolyte concentrations should be undertaken before all major surgery and in all elderly or potentially unwell patients; a raised blood urea concentration demonstrated preoperatively may be the first indication of renal disease. Severity of renal dysfunction may be assessed further by measurement of serum creatinine concentration and creatinine clearance, urinary:plasma osmolality ratio and urinary urea and electrolyte excretion (Table 18.6).

TABLE 18.6
Urinary Measurements in Prerenal and Renal Failure

Variable	Prerenal	Renal
Specific gravity	High >1.020	1.010–1.012
Sodium (mmol L^{-1})	Low <20	High >40
U:P urea ratio	High >20	Low <10
U:P creatinine ratio	High >40	Low <10
U:P osmolality ratio	High >2.1	Low <1.2
U, urine; P, plasma		

Chronic kidney disease (CKD) is currently classified according to estimated glomerular filtration rate (eGFR). It should be noted that, while eGFR can be a useful estimate of renal function, it requires a steady-state creatinine concentration for calculation and is therefore inaccurate in acute renal failure, and it should not be used in the acutely ill or unstable patient. It is also inaccurate where muscle mass or creatinine intake are at extremes, e.g. in cachectic patients or those on a vegetarian diet.

CKD 1&2: eGFR>60 but with other evidence of kidney disease such as haematuria or proteinuria.

- CKD 3: eGFR 30–59
- CKD 4: eGFR 15–29
- CKD 5: eGFR <15

Pre-Anaesthetic Assessment

Pre-anaesthetic assessment of the patient should be directed to several specific problems which require correction before anaesthesia.

Fluid Balance

In acute renal failure (acute kidney injury), fluid overload may develop suddenly and is uncompensated. In chronic renal failure, overload may be controlled with diuretic therapy or dialysis. Pulmonary oedema and hypertension may result from fluid overload and must be treated before induction of anaesthesia. This may require fluid removal using dialysis or haemofiltration.

In patients with nephrotic syndrome, hypoalbuminaemia results in oedema and ascites. Circulating blood volume in these patients is often decreased, and care should be taken at induction of anaesthesia to avoid hypotension. Invasive monitoring and measurement of cardiac output should be considered in these patients.

Electrolyte Disturbances

Sodium. Sodium retention occurs in renal failure, and through increased secretion of ADH, is associated with water retention, oedema and hypertension.

Hyponatraemia is also common in renal disease. It is the result either of sodium losses through the kidney or gastrointestinal tract, or of water overload causing dilutional hyponatraemia. The renal tubules may have a reduced ability to conserve sodium, e.g. in pyelonephritis, analgesic nephropathy or recovering acute renal failure, or sodium may be lost through diuretic therapy, vomiting or diarrhoea. Dilutional hyponatraemia is caused by either inappropriate fluid administration (glucose 5%), inappropriate ADH secretion, or both. Following transurethral prostatectomy, hyponatraemia may result from absorption of glycine irrigation fluid. Diagnosis of the cause of hyponatraemia involves measurement of urinary and plasma osmolality and urinary sodium concentration.

Potassium. Hyperkalaemia occurs typically in renal failure, frequently in association with metabolic acidosis. It causes delayed myocardial conduction and, if untreated, leads to cardiac arrest in asystole or ventricular fibrillation.

Hyperkalaemia should be treated promptly when the serum potassium concentration exceeds 6 mmol L^{-1} or when ECG changes are evident:

- calcium chloride 10% titrated up to 20 mL i.v. to antagonize the cardiac effects of hyperkalaemia, under ECG guidance
- glucose 50%, 50 mL with 5–15 units of soluble insulin followed by an infusion of 20% glucose with insulin as required, depending on BM-test blood sugar estimation
- nebulized salbutamol 5 mg repeated regularly
- sodium bicarbonate 1.26% to improve the metabolic acidosis
- an ion exchange resin, e.g. calcium polystyrene sulphonate, orally, provides longer-term control in chronic renal failure
- haemodialysis or haemofiltration. The former is more effective in lowering serum potassium concentration rapidly, but haemofiltration may be more easily set up as an emergency in a general intensive care unit.

Hypokalaemia occurs commonly in patients receiving diuretic therapy. These patients require preoperative measurement of serum potassium concentration and replacement if necessary. Hypokalaemia is associated with ventricular irritability, notably in patients taking digoxin.

Calcium. Retention of phosphate and vitamin D depletion (1,25-dihydroxycholecalciferol) in chronic renal failure lead to hyperparathyroidism. The development of a parathyroid adenoma leads to hypercalcaemia (tertiary hyperparathyroidism).

Cardiovascular Effects

Hypertension may occur for several reasons:

- a raised plasma renin concentration secondary to decreased perfusion of the juxtaglomerular apparatus results in hypertension through increased secretion of angiotensin and aldosterone
- fluid retention also causes hypertension by increasing the circulating blood volume.

Conversely, hypertension from other causes results in renal impairment. The precise cause of hypertension in these patients should be sought and the hypertension treated.

Both pulmonary and peripheral oedema may occur from a combination of fluid overload, hypertensive cardiac disease and hypoproteinaemia. Heart failure should be treated preoperatively. Uraemia may cause pericarditis and a haemorrhagic pericardial effusion, which may embarrass cardiac output and require aspiration. Good control of blood urea concentration with haemodialysis or haemofiltration usually prevents this complication and is essential for its resolution.

Neurological Effects

Severe uraemia causes drowsiness and eventually coma. Electrolyte disturbances and rapid fluid shifts, e.g. during dialysis, may also affect conscious level by causing cerebral oedema. Sedative drugs, including opioids, should be used with care in these patients. Morphine may be a particular problem because renally excreted metabolites, in particular morphine-6-glucuronide, accumulate. In addition, a combined motor and sensory peripheral neuropathy may occur in uraemic patients.

Haematological Effects

Patients with chronic kidney disease suffer from normochromic anaemia, which results from marrow depression, partly as a result of erythropoietin deficiency. They also have an increased incidence of gastrointestinal bleeding, and so iron deficiency may also be present. These patients are usually well compensated, with an increased cardiac output, so that excessive preoperative blood transfusion should be avoided. Increasingly, such patients are treated with long-term erythropoietin. There is often a bleeding tendency, in part caused by platelet dysfunction. Conventional tests of coagulation (platelet count, PTT, APPT) are normal but bleeding time is prolonged and correlates with the degree of bleeding tendency. Platelet dysfunction may be improved with cryoprecipitate 10 iu i.v. over 30 min or desmopressin (DDAVP) $0.3\,\mu g\,kg^{-1}$ i.v. or s.c.

Other Factors

Patients with chronic kidney disease are frequently undernourished and tend to be vulnerable to infection. Patients who have received a renal transplant and are immunosuppressed are particularly vulnerable to opportunistic pathogens, e.g. *Pneumocystis jirovecii.*

Drug Treatment

This is important for several reasons:

- patients are frequently receiving concurrent medication for attendant problems, e.g. antihypertensive therapy
- many drugs are renally excreted; dosages require modification and plasma concentrations may require monitoring, e.g. aminoglycosides, digoxin
- some drugs have active metabolites which are renally excreted, e.g. morphine, midazolam. Dosage requires careful titration, or use of alternative agents should be considered, e.g. fentanyl, oxycodone
- some drugs adversely affect renal function, even in normal dosage. NSAIDs and the newer specific cyclo-oxygenase 2 inhibitors inhibit vasodilator prostaglandin production in the kidney and thus reduce glomerular blood flow and sodium excretion. This may be critical in septic or shocked patients, those with pre-existing renal dysfunction or those undergoing surgery associated with major blood loss. Their use should be avoided in such high-risk patients.

ACE inhibitors dilate the postglomerular arterioles in the kidney and thus reduce glomerular filtration pressure. They may therefore precipitate renal failure in hypotensive patients. Patients receiving these agents should be monitored carefully and fluid should be replaced adequately to avoid hypotension. It may be prudent to omit the immediate preanaesthetic dose in the high-risk patient. ACE inhibitors may also cause hyperkalaemia, particularly in patients with renal dysfunction.

Anaesthesia

Minor procedures, such as the establishment of vascular access for dialysis, may be carried out satisfactorily under regional anaesthesia. The potential benefits of neuraxial blockade need to be weighed against the risks associated with impaired coagulation for individual patients.

Patients who suffer from acute renal failure, and those receiving long-term dialysis for chronic renal failure, may require dialysis before surgery to correct fluid overload, acid-base disturbances and hyperkalaemia. Ideally, there should be some delay before surgery to allow correction of anticoagulation.

The i.v. cannula for induction and fluid infusion should be sited in the contralateral limb from the arteriovenous shunt or fistula in patients undergoing dialysis and care should be taken to protect the fistula during the operation. Careful monitoring of arterial pressure and ECG is required and CVP measurement may be indicated in patients who are clinically fluid overloaded. Intravenous fluid administration should be cautious and in some instances titrated against CVP measurements. Excessive sodium administration and potassium-containing solutions should be avoided in renal failure. If the patient is anaemic preoperatively, intraoperative blood loss should be replaced promptly.

Succinylcholine should be avoided in hyperkalaemic patients in view of its effect of releasing potassium from muscle cells. An increase of up to $0.6\,mmol\,L^{-1}$ may be expected in normal dosage.

Drugs excreted primarily via the kidneys should be used with caution in renal failure. In anaesthetic practice, the principal drugs involved are the neuromuscular blockers. Atracurium, elimination of which is independent of kidney and liver function, and which has minimal cardiovascular effects, is the drug of choice. All other neuromuscular blockers depend to some extent on renal elimination and should be avoided, particularly in repeated doses. In addition, many drugs, including morphine, are conjugated in the liver before excretion in the urine. Depending on the activity of the conjugated metabolite, these drugs may have adverse effects following repeated doses. Morphine-6-glucuronide, an active metabolite of morphine, accumulates in renal failure and may result in prolongation of clinical effects after administration of morphine.

Modern volatile anaesthetic agents avoid metabolism to fluoride ions to any great extent, and are free of any deleterious effects on renal function.

Postoperative Renal Failure

In the absence of severe sepsis or pre-existing renal dysfunction, this is now relatively uncommon. In high-risk patients, such as those undergoing major surgery which involves large blood loss, surgery following trauma, and septic patients, avoidance of renal failure involves close monitoring of the cardiovascular state, including CVP and urinary output, avoidance of hypoxaemia and hypotension, and adequate fluid and blood replacement. In many instances, e.g. in patients with pre-existing renal dysfunction, shock, sepsis or liver disease, a pulmonary artery catheter may be required to optimize cardiac output and oxygen delivery, and to guide vasoactive drug therapy. Low-dose ($2–5\,\mu g$ $kg^{-1}\,min^{-1}$) dopamine was formerly recommended to prevent renal failure in such situations, but it has been demonstrated by randomized controlled trial to be ineffective. The only proven therapy in the prevention and early treatment of acute renal failure is adequate fluid resuscitation titrated against CVP and maintenance of an adequate cardiac output and mean arterial pressure ($>80\,mmHg$). This may involve use of a vasoactive agents such as dobutamine (mainly inotropic) and/or noradrenaline (mainly vasoconstrictor).

Other measures, such as use of an osmotic diuretic (mannitol 100 mL of 20% solution over 15 min) or loop diuretic (furosemide by bolus or infusion), are also of doubtful value. Mannitol continues to be recommended in jaundiced patients at risk of developing the hepatorenal syndrome and in patients with rhabdomyolysis. In some cases of oliguric acute renal failure, where adequate resuscitation has failed to achieve diuresis, furosemide i.v. does appear to 'kick-start' a urine output which is then maintained.

Postoperative oliguria may also be the result of postrenal causes. Patients with prostatic enlargement are particularly liable to develop acute urinary retention. Examination to exclude a full bladder and catheterization should always be carried out in the anuric postoperative patient. Abdominal ultrasound is mandatory in all cases of acute renal failure to exclude obstruction as a causative or contributory factor. It also allows assessment of the size and presence of two kidneys which provides prognostic information.

DIABETES MELLITUS

Diabetes mellitus is common. Approximately 10% of patients admitted to hospital have diabetes either as a cause of admission or coincidentally. Fifty per cent of all diabetic patients present for surgery during their lifetime, most commonly for ophthalmic or vascular disease or for drainage of an abscess. Perioperative morbidity and mortality are greater in diabetic than in non-diabetic patients, for several reasons:

- hyperglycaemia leading to increased risk of infectious complications and impaired healing (including anastomotic failure)
- hypoglycaemia, the clinical signs of which may be masked completely by anaesthesia
- complications of diabetes:
  - ischaemic heart disease
  - autonomic neuropathy
  - infection
  - renal impairment.

There are two main types of diabetes: type 1, pancreatic β-cell destruction (insulin dependent); type 2, defective insulin secretion and insulin resistance (non-insulin-dependent diabetes mellitus). Both groups suffer from hyperglycaemia. However, the complete lack of insulin in the former group allows unrestrained glycogenolysis, gluconeogenesis, and protein and fat catabolism with subsequent production of keto acids if insulin treatment is interrupted. These effects are limited by residual insulin production in type 2 diabetics. However, additional significant stress such as major surgery or sepsis may be sufficient to precipitate ketoacidosis in this group too.

The specific problems of managing diabetic patients who undergo surgery are a result of the attendant period of starvation and the stress response to surgery with catabolic hormone release. The aim is to minimize the metabolic disturbance by ensuring an adequate intake of glucose and insulin, thus controlling hyperglycaemia and reducing proteolysis, lipolysis and production of lactate and ketones. Adequate control of blood glucose concentration must be established preoperatively and maintained until oral feeding is resumed after operation.

The availability of accurate near-patient monitoring of blood glucose has allowed close glycaemic control to be achieved perioperatively and there is now strong evidence that good glycaemic control improves outcome following major surgery.

Precise diabetic management depends upon:

- the nature of the diabetes and its treatment (insulin-dependent or non-insulin-dependent)
- the magnitude of the surgery contemplated, in particular duration of fasting
- the time available for improving control of the diabetes preoperatively if necessary.

Preoperative Assessment

Preoperative assessment is aimed at evaluating blood glucose control, the treatment regimen used and the presence of complications.

Control of Blood Glucose

This is assessed by inspection of the patient's urine-testing or BM-testing records, by random blood glucose measurements and by measurement of glycosylated haemoglobin (HbA_{1c}). Whenever possible, blood glucose concentration should be maintained between 6 and 10 mmol L^{-1}. HbA_{1c} should be 48–59 mmol mol^{-1} or 6.5–7.5% in a well-controlled diabetic patient; higher values indicate poor control. In an elective situation, a patient with poor preoperative glycaemic control should benefit from review and optimization of treatment before surgery.

Treatment Regimens. *Oral hypoglycaemic agents*:

- the sulphonylureas, e.g. glipizide and gliclazide, stimulate release of insulin from the pancreatic islets. Hypoglycaemia may be induced by these agents.
- biguanides, e.g. metformin, which increase peripheral uptake of glucose and decrease gluconeogenesis, are used either alone or in combination with sulphonylureas. These agents may cause

lactic acidosis, usually, but not exclusively, in patients with a degree of renal or hepatic impairment. Guidelines for the administration of i.v. contrast media include the instructions to withhold metformin for 24 h before and 48 h after the investigation. Lactic acidosis carries a very high mortality. Metformin, the only biguanide now available, should usually be discontinued on the morning of surgery. Newer guidelines however suggest that it may be safely continued provided the patient does not have renal impairment and hypovolaemia is avoided.

- acarbose inhibits intestinal glucosidases, delaying carbohydrate digestion and reducing post-prandial glucose surges.

Insulins:

Insulin therapy is required by all type 1 diabetics and some type 2 patients. Most insulins in clinical use are now human insulins produced via recombinant DNA technology. The durations of action of insulin preparations vary:

- Short-acting insulins. Soluble insulins, e.g. Humulin S and Actrapid, have an onset time of 30 min, peak effect 2–4 h and duration 8 h when given subcutaneously. Given intravenously, their effect is much shorter, with a half-life of around 2.5 min and a duration of action of 30 min. Insulin aspart (NovoRapid) and insulin lispro (Humalog) are human insulin analogues and have an even faster onset and shorter duration of action.
- Intermediate, e.g. isophane insulin, insulin zinc suspension and the human insulin analogues: insulin detemir (levemir) and insulin glargine (lantus) have a more prolonged duration of action up to 16–35 hours. Onset time is 1–2 hours with peak effect at 4–12 hours. The longest acting agents, detemir and glargine, are often given once daily.
- Biphasic fixed mixtures, e.g. Mixtard (soluble and isophane insulin), Humalog (insulin lispro and insulin lispro protamine), NovoMix (insulin aspart and insulin aspart protamine). These are a combination of soluble and longer-acting insulins available in a variety of different proportions.

Insulin is given by subcutaneous injection and the patient's specific regimen is tailored to provide optimal glycaemic control. Often this is a twice-daily biphasic insulin injection. However, with the increasing requirement to achieve near normoglycaemia, more complex regimens are increasingly seen, e.g. a single 'background' injection of long-acting insulin with soluble insulin given before meals.

In well-controlled diabetic patients it is not usually necessary to change the insulin regimen on the day before surgery. Often, a change of regimen results in poorer control.

Complications of Diabetes Mellitus

- *Cardiovascular disorders* (coronary artery, cerebrovascular and peripheral vascular) are common in diabetic patients and there is an increased risk of perioperative myocardial infarction. There may be significant ischaemic heart disease in the absence of warning symptoms and, as discussed earlier, this is a group which may merit further cardiovascular investigation before major surgery.
- *Renal disease.* Microvascular damage produces glomerulosclerosis with proteinuria, oedema and eventually chronic renal failure. Anaesthetic implications of renal disease are discussed on page 401, and in Chapter 10.
- *Ocular problems.* Cataracts, exudative or proliferative retinopathy, vitreous haemorrhage and retinal detachment may occur. In the long term, good blood glucose control has been shown to reduce the frequency of such complications.
- *Infection.* Diabetic patients are prone to infection and an increased risk of septicaemia, abscess formation and wound infection. Infection is associated with increased insulin requirements, which return to normal on its eradication.
- *Neuropathy.* Chronic sensory peripheral neuropathies are common; mononeuropathies and acute motor neuropathies (amyotrophy) are associated with poor control of blood glucose. Loss of sensation together with peripheral vascular disease may lead to ulceration after trivial trauma. Consequently, care in positioning patients in the operating theatre is important. Local anaesthetic nerve or plexus blocks should be avoided in patients with an acute neuropathy, as neurological deficits may be attributed to the local anaesthetic solution.
- *Autonomic neuropathy* may cause postoperative urinary retention or vasomotor instability, e.g. postural hypotension or hypotension during anaesthesia. IPPV or subarachnoid or epidural block may be associated with significant hypotension; preoperative intravascular volume status should be assessed and fluids given to achieve normovolaemia before performing a block. Precise cardiovascular monitoring, use of vasopressors and careful anaesthetic management are essential.

Concurrent Drug Therapy

Thiazide diuretics, adrenergic agents, e.g. salbutamol, and corticosteroids tend to increase the blood glucose concentration. β-Adrenergic blockers tend to potentiate hypoglycaemia and may mask its clinical signs. Blood glucose concentration should be monitored if any of these drugs is administered, and insulin dosage altered accordingly.

Some drugs, including phenylbutazone, displace sulphonylureas from protein-binding sites and potentiate their hypoglycaemic effect.

Perioperative Diabetic Management

There are national guidelines in the UK for the perioperative management of diabetes but advice regarding perioperative management of diabetes should be sought from the metabolic team; local guidelines should be followed where available.

Type 2 non-insulin-dependent diabetics undergoing minor surgery and able to recommence oral intake immediately postoperatively do not require perioperative insulin therapy. These patients should be scheduled early on the operating list. They should omit the usual morning hypoglycaemic agents. Blood glucose monitoring should continue throughout the fasting period. If hyperglycaemia occurs (blood glucose $>12\,mmol\,L^{-1}$) or if there is any delay in recommencing normal diet and therapy, insulin treatment should be started.

In type I diabetes, a combination of glucose and insulin is the most satisfactory method of overcoming the deleterious metabolic consequences of starvation and surgical stress in the diabetic patient. A no glucose/no insulin regimen results in ketosis and is not advocated.

Minor procedures, e.g. cystoscopy or examination under anaesthesia, may be carried out at the start of an operating list by delaying the morning dose of insulin until a late breakfast is taken after recovery from anaesthesia. Attention must be paid to avoiding postoperative nausea and vomiting, with adequate hydration, limitation of opioids if possible and with prophylactic antiemetic administration. This may be facilitated by the use of regional anaesthesia with or without sedation, which allows the patient to resume normal oral intake earlier than is usually possible following general anaesthesia.

Individual units have local protocols for the perioperative management of diabetes.

A variable rate insulin infusion should be instituted for patients with type 1 diabetes anticipating a longer fasting period. A solution of soluble insulin (1 unit mL^{-1}) is co-administered with 5% or 10% glucose (with appropriate potassium replacement), or a combined saline/dextrose solution. Hourly blood glucose monitoring is undertaken and the insulin infusion rate varied to maintain glucose levels between 6 and 12 mmol L^{-1}.

This regimen is also used for type 2 diabetic patients who have poor diabetic control or where a prolonged fasting time is expected. The choice of intravenous fluids should be made to match the patients fluid and electrolyte requirements in addition to supplying glucose.

A variable rate insulin infusion should be continued until the patient is able to eat and drink. A dose of subcutaneous insulin should be given with a meal and the insulin infusion stopped 30–60 minutes later. It should be noted that patients who normally receive oral hypoglycaemics may be very sensitive to insulin therapy.

Blood transfusion may increase insulin requirements as citrate stimulates gluconeogenesis.

Emergency Surgery and Diabetic Ketoacidosis

Diabetic ketoacidosis results from inadequate insulin dosage or increased insulin requirements, often precipitated by infection, trauma or surgical stress. Diabetic patients who require emergency surgery often have a grossly increased blood glucose concentration and occasionally overt ketoacidosis. Such patients require i.v. volume resuscitation, correction of sodium depletion, correction of potassium depletion and i.v. soluble insulin by infusion at an initial rate of 4–8 unit h^{-1}, aiming to reduce glucose levels by approximately 5 mmol L^{-1} per hour.

Initial fluid replacement should consist of isotonic (0.9%) saline: 1 L in the first 30 min, 1 L in the next hour and an additional 1 L over the next 2 h, guided by clinical reassessment, cardiovascular monitoring and local protocols.

Progress is monitored by regular measurements of blood glucose, sodium and potassium concentrations, and arterial pH and blood gas tensions. Correction of acidosis with bicarbonate is very rarely, if ever, required. Cellular potassium depletion is present from the outset, but hyperkalaemia or normokalaemia may be found initially because potassium shifts out of the cells in the presence of acidosis. Potassium replacement is required as the plasma concentration begins to decrease with correction of the acidosis. Phosphate and magnesium are also usually required. An infusion of glucose 5% should be given, in conjunction with continued insulin therapy, when the blood glucose concentration decreases to approximately 15 mmol L^{-1}. When volume resuscitation is underway, and some reversal of acidosis and hyperglycaemia has been achieved, surgery may be carried out while management of the diabetes is continued intra- and postoperatively.

OTHER ENDOCRINE DISORDERS

Pituitary Disease

The clinical features of pituitary disease depend on the local effects of the lesion and its effects on the secretion of pituitary hormones. Local effects include headache and visual field disturbances. The effects on hormone secretion depend on the cells involved in the pathological process.

Acromegaly. Acromegaly is caused by increased secretion of growth hormone from eosinophil cell tumours of the anterior pituitary gland. If this occurs before fusion of the epiphyses, gigantism results. Problems for the anaesthetist include the following:

- upper airway obstruction may result from an enlarged mandible, tongue and epiglottis, thickened pharyngeal mucosa and laryngeal narrowing. Maintenance of a clear airway and tracheal intubation may be difficult, and postoperative care of the airway must be meticulous. Consideration may be given to awake fibreoptic tracheal intubation.
- cardiac enlargement, hypertension and congestive cardiac failure occur commonly and require preoperative treatment.
- growth hormone increases blood sugar concentration. Hyperglycaemia should be controlled perioperatively.
- thyroid and adrenal function may be impaired because of decreased release of thyroid-stimulating hormone (TSH) and ACTH. Thyroxine and steroid replacement may be required.

Treatment involves hypophysectomy which requires steroid cover preoperatively and steroid, thyroxine and possibly ADH replacement thereafter.

Cushing's Disease. Cushing's disease results from basophil adenomas, which secrete ACTH (see below).

Hypopituitarism (Simmonds' Disease). Causes include chromophobe adenoma, tumours of surrounding tissues, e.g. craniopharyngioma, skull fractures, infarction following postpartum haemorrhage and infection. Clinical features include loss of axillary and pubic hair, amenorrhoea, features of hypothyroidism and adrenal insufficiency, including hypotension, but with a striking pallor, in contrast to the pigmentation of Addison's disease (see p. 408).

The fluid and electrolyte disturbances are not as marked as in primary adrenal failure as a result of intact aldosterone production, but may be unmasked by surgery, trauma or infection. Anaesthesia in these patients requires steroid cover (pp. 408–409), cautious administration of induction agent and volatile anaesthetic agents, and careful cardiovascular monitoring.

Diabetes Insipidus. This is caused by disease or damage affecting the hypothalamic posterior pituitary axis.

Common causes are pituitary tumour, craniopharyngioma, basal skull fracture and infection, or it may occur as a sequel to pituitary surgery. In 10% of cases, diabetes insipidus is renal in origin.

Dehydration with hypernatraemia follows excretion of large volumes of dilute urine. Patients require fluid replacement and treatment with parenteral vasopressin, or desmopressin, which can be also be given orally or intranasally.

Thyroid Disease

Goitre. Thyroid swelling may result from iodine deficiency (simple goitre), autoimmune (Hashimoto's) thyroiditis, adenoma, carcinoma or thyrotoxicosis. Nodules of the thyroid gland may be 'hot' (secreting thyroxine) or 'cold'.

The goitre may occasionally cause respiratory obstruction. Retrosternal goitre may also cause superior vena caval obstruction. The presence of a goitre should alert the anaesthetist to the possibility of tracheal compression or displacement. A preoperative X-ray of neck and thoracic inlet may be useful, and a selection of small-diameter, armoured tracheal tubes should be available. Preoperative assessment of thyroid function is essential.

Thyrotoxicosis. This is characterized by excitability, tremor, tachycardia and arrhythmias (commonly atrial fibrillation), weight loss, heat intolerance and exophthalmos. Diagnosis is confirmed by measurement of total serum thyroxine, tri-iodothyronine (T_3) and TSH concentrations.

Elective surgery should not be carried out in hyperthyroid patients; they should first be rendered euthyroid with carbimazole or radioactive iodine. However, urgent surgery and elective subtotal thyroidectomy may be carried out safely in hyperthyroid patients using β-adrenergic blockade alone or in combination with potassium iodide to control thyrotoxic symptoms and signs. Emergency surgery carries a significant risk of thyrotoxic crisis. Control is best achieved in these circumstances by i.v. potassium iodide and a nonselective β-blocker (e.g. propranolol). If patients are unable to absorb oral medication, i.v. infusion is indicated (for propranolol, the daily i.v. dose is approximately one-tenth of the oral dose).

The doses of sedative drugs for premedication, and of anaesthetic agents, should be increased to compensate for faster distribution and elimination. Larger doses of sedative drugs than normal are required to avoid anxiety when procedures are carried out under regional anaesthesia.

Preparation for Thyroidectomy

Conventional management involves at least 6–8 weeks administration of carbimazole to render the patient euthyroid, followed by potassium iodide 60 mg 8-hourly for 10 days to decrease the vascularity of the gland. However, if a hyperthyroid patient is presented for urgent surgery, a β-blocker can be used. Propranolol 160 mg daily for 2 weeks preoperatively and a further 7–10 days postoperatively provides adequate control in most patients. However, control with β-blockers depends on maintaining an adequate plasma concentration of the drug. Because β-blockers, in common with other drugs, are cleared more rapidly than normal in thyrotoxic patients, propranolol should be prescribed more frequently than usual, e.g. four times daily. Alternatively, a long-acting β-blocker, e.g. atenolol once daily, continued on the morning of surgery, provides satisfactory control and avoids the problem of impaired drug absorption immediately after operation. A combination of β-blocker and potassium iodide 60 mg 8-hourly provides control in even the most severely thyrotoxic patient. Postoperatively, laryngoscopy should be carried out to check vocal cord function, and to exclude recurrent laryngeal nerve injury.

Hypothyroidism.

This may result from primary thyroid failure, Hashimoto's thyroiditis, as a consequence of thyroid surgery, or secondary to pituitary failure. The diagnosis is suggested by tiredness, cold intolerance, loss of appetite, dry skin and hair loss. It may be confirmed by the finding of a low serum thyroxine concentration associated, in primary thyroid failure, with a raised serum TSH concentration.

Basal metabolic rate is decreased. Cardiac output is decreased, with little myocardial reserve, and hypothermia may be present. Treatment is with thyroxine, which should be started in a small dose of 25–50 µg daily. Rapid correction of hypothyroidism may be achieved using i.v. T_3, but this is inadvisable in elderly patients and those with ischaemic heart disease, which is common in hypothyroidism, as

the sudden increase in myocardial oxygen demand may provoke ischaemia or infarction. ECG monitoring is advisable during treatment. Elective surgery should be avoided in myxoedematous patients, but if emergency surgery is necessary, close cardiovascular, ECG and blood gas monitoring is essential. Drug distribution and metabolism are slowed, and thus all anaesthetic agents must be administered in reduced doses.

Disease of the Adrenal Cortex

Clinical symptoms are associated with increased or decreased secretion of cortisol or aldosterone.

Hypersecretion of Cortisol (Cushing's Syndrome).

Most instances are caused by pituitary adenomas which secrete ACTH and thus cause bilateral adrenocortical hyperplasia (Cushing's disease). In 20–30% of patients, an adrenocortical adenoma or carcinoma is present. Rarely, an oat-cell carcinoma of bronchus, secreting ACTH, is the cause. ACTH and corticosteroid therapy present similar pictures. Clinical features include obesity, hypertension, proximal myopathy and diabetes mellitus. Biochemically, there is a metabolic alkalosis with hypokalaemia. Depending on the cause, treatment may involve hypophysectomy or adrenalectomy.

Anaesthetic management of these patients involves preoperative treatment of hypertension and congestive cardiac failure, and correction of hypokalaemia. Intraoperative management is directed towards careful monitoring of arterial pressure and maintenance of cardiovascular stability, with careful choice and administration of anaesthetic agents and muscle relaxants. Etomidate and atracurium or rocuronium would be an appropriate choice of induction agent and neuromuscular blocker, respectively. Postoperative steroid therapy is required for hypophysectomy and adrenalectomy (see below). Fludrocortisone 0.1–0.3 mg daily is required after bilateral adrenalectomy.

Primary Hypersecretion of Aldosterone (Conn's Syndrome).

Conn's syndrome is caused by an adenoma of the zona glomerulosa of the adrenal cortex and presents with hypertension, hypernatraemia, hypokalaemia and oliguria. Anaesthetic management involves preoperative treatment of hypertension, administration of spironolactone and potassium replacement; meticulous intra- and postoperative monitoring of arterial pressure is essential.

Adrenocortical Hypofunction. Primary adrenocortical insufficiency (*Addison's disease*) may be caused by an autoimmune process, tuberculosis, HIV infection, amyloid, metastatic carcinoma, or bilateral adrenalectomy. Haemorrhage into the glands during meningococcal septicaemia may cause acute adrenal failure in association with septic shock. Secondary failure results from hypopituitarism or prolonged corticosteroid therapy. In secondary failure resulting from pituitary insufficiency, aldosterone secretion is maintained, and fluid and electrolyte disturbances are less marked.

Clinical features include weakness, weight loss, hyperpigmentation, hypotension, vomiting, diarrhoea and volume depletion. Hypoglycaemia, hyponatraemia, hyperkalaemia and metabolic acidosis are characteristic but late biochemical findings. The stress of infection, trauma or surgery provokes profound hypotension. Diagnosis is made by measurement of plasma cortisol concentration and the response to ACTH stimulation.

All surgical procedures in these patients must be covered by increased steroid administration (see below). Patients with acute adrenal insufficiency require urgent fluid and sodium replacement with arterial pressure and CVP monitoring, glucose infusion to combat hypoglycaemia and hydrocortisone 100 mg 6-hourly i.v. They should be cared for in a high dependency or critical care area. Antibiotics are advisable to cover the possibility that infection has provoked the crisis. In cases of primary adrenal failure, mineralocorticoid replacement with fludrocortisone is required. If emergency surgery is required in acute adrenal failure, all precautions necessary for anaesthetizing the shocked patient should be taken (see Ch 37).

Congenital Adrenal Hyperplasia (Adrenogenital Syndrome). This is associated with overproduction of androgens as a result of deficiency of the hydroxylase enzyme required for production of cortisol. Hydrocortisone treatment overcomes adrenal insufficiency and, by suppressing ACTH production, decreases androgen accumulation. Augmented steroid cover is required for surgery in these patients.

Steroid Therapy

Replacement therapy in cases of primary adrenocortical failure and hypopituitarism is given as oral hydrocortisone 20 mg in the morning and 10 mg in the evening. Fludrocortisone 0.05–0.1 mg daily is given additionally to replace aldosterone in primary adrenocortical failure. Equivalent doses of other steroid preparations are shown in Table 18.5. Prednisolone and prednisone have less mineralocorticoid effect, while betamethasone and dexamethasone have none. Requirements increase following infection, trauma or surgery.

Corticosteroids are also prescribed for a wide range of medical conditions, including asthma and collagen diseases. Prolonged therapy suppresses adrenocortical function.

Steroid Cover for Anaesthesia and Surgery

Indications for augmented perioperative steroid cover and the dosage required are the subject of ongoing debate. Suggested indications:

- patients with pituitary adrenal insufficiency, receiving steroid replacement therapy
- patients undergoing pituitary or adrenal surgery
- patients receiving systemic steroid therapy for more than 2 weeks before surgery
- patients no longer receiving systemic steroid therapy, but who received steroids within the three months before surgery.

Topical fluorinated steroid preparations applied widely to the skin and high-dose inhaled steroids may be absorbed sufficiently to produce adrenal suppression. An ACTH stimulation (short Synacthen) test can be carried out to assess adrenal function. Preoperative assessment should identify fluid and electrolyte abnormalities, which should be corrected. Evidence of infection should be sought in patients receiving long-term steroid therapy.

The following corticosteroid cover is recommended for patients taking more than 10 mg prednisolone daily (or equivalent) within 3 months of operation. In all cases the usual morning dose of steroid should also be given:

- minor diagnostic procedures – usual morning dose of steroid OR i.v. hydrocortisone 25–50 mg at induction; recommence patient's usual dose after surgery

- intermediate operations, e.g. inguinal herniorrhaphy – usual morning dose of steroid AND i.v. hydrocortisone 25–50 mg at induction, then 25–50 mg 8-hourly for 24 h
- major surgery – usual morning dose of steroid AND i.v. hydrocortisone 25–50 mg at induction, then 8-hourly for 48–72 h.

The requirements may need to be increased if infection is present, or be continued beyond 3 days if infection or the effects of major trauma persist. Oral steroid preparations should be resumed as soon as oral intake allows and i.v. supplementation stopped.

If steroids are prescribed for asthma or other medical conditions, the perioperative dosage may require modification according to the activity of the disease.

Disease of the Adrenal Medulla

Phaeochromocytoma. This is discussed in Chapter 31.

NEUROLOGICAL DISEASE

General Considerations

Neurological disease embraces a wide range of differing conditions, the effects of which may influence the conduct of perioperative care in a number of ways:

- a depressed level of consciousness may prejudice airway protection and result in depressed respiratory drive
- peripheral neuromuscular disease may lead to impaired ventilatory function and reduced ability to clear secretions
- autonomic dysfunction may result in blood pressure instability, cardiac arrhythmias and dysfunction of gastrointestinal motility
- there may also be significant adverse effects from specific drug treatment, and there are several important drug interactions which need to be recognized.

Assessment

In addition to standard history and examination, a detailed drug history should be obtained. Many patients with neurological disease should have their medication continued up to the time of surgery and reinstated as soon as possible thereafter, e.g. epilepsy, Parkinsonism, myasthenia gravis. Respiratory function should be assessed by the use of pulmonary function tests including vital capacity and measurement of arterial blood gas tensions. Erect and supine arterial pressure should be measured when appropriate and a 12-lead ECG performed to assess QT interval and possible heart block.

Respiratory Impairment

Inadequate ventilatory function may result from:

- reduced central drive, e.g. because of an impaired conscious level
- motor neuropathy, e.g. Guillain–Barré syndrome, motor neurone disease
- neuromuscular dysfunction, e.g. myasthenia gravis
- muscle weakness, e.g. muscular dystrophies
- rigidity, e.g. Parkinson's disease.

These patients are sensitive to anaesthetic agents, opioids and neuromuscular blockers. If intraoperative artificial ventilation is undertaken, a period of elective postoperative ventilation may be needed until full recovery from the effects of anaesthesia has occurred. If appropriate, procedures may be carried out under a regional anaesthetic technique.

Bulbar muscle involvement may lead to inadequate protection of the airway such that regurgitation and aspiration can occur. Chest infection should be effectively treated preoperatively, and in the elective situation this may necessitate postponing surgery.

Altered Innervation of Muscle and Hyperkalaemia

Succinylcholine my cause life-threatening hyperkalaemia in some neurological conditions. An altered ratio of intracellular to extracellular potassium tends to produce sensitivity to nondepolarizing, and resistance to depolarizing, muscle relaxants. Consideration should be given to the use of short-acting anaesthetic agents such as propofol, sevoflurane and remifentanil. If there is widespread denervation of muscle with lower motor neurone damage, e.g. in Guillain–Barré syndrome, disorganization of the motor end-plate occurs, resulting in hypersensitivity to acetylcholine and succinylcholine, with increased permeability of muscle cells to potassium. A similar potassium efflux occurs in the presence of direct muscle damage, widespread burns involving muscle, upper motor neurone lesions, spinal cord lesions with paraplegia, and tetanus. In upper motor neurone and spinal cord lesions, the reason for this shift is less clear. Patients undergoing mechanical ventilation in the ICU who are suffering from sepsis and multiple organ failure may develop a critical illness polyneuropathy, with a similar hyperkalaemic response to succinylcholine.

The resulting increase in serum potassium concentration after succinylcholine may be 3 mmol L^{-1} (in comparison with 0.5 mmol L^{-1} in the normal patient) and may occur from 24 h after acute muscle denervation or damage. In such patients, succinylcholine is clearly contraindicated.

Autonomic Disturbances

These may occur as part of a polyneuropathy e.g. diabetes mellitus, Guillain-Barré syndrome and porphyria, or from central nervous system involvement, e.g. in Parkinsonism. Sympathetic stimulation, e.g. during light anaesthesia, tracheal intubation or following administration of pancuronium or catecholamines, may produce severe hypertension and arrhythmias. More commonly, blood loss, head-up posture, IPPV or neuraxial regional blocks may be associated with severe hypotension. Cardiac arrhythmias may also occur.

Conscious Level

Patients with pre-existing marked reduction in conscious level for whatever reason require tracheal intubation and artificial ventilation of the lungs for airway protection and control of carbon dioxide and oxygen partial pressures.

Increased Intracranial Pressure

Elective surgery should be postponed if raised intracranial pressure is suspected, until investigation by CT scan and treatment have been undertaken. Anaesthetic agents which cause an increase in cerebral blood flow must be avoided. Hypercapnia must also be avoided, and controlled ventilation to a $PaCO_2$ of approximately 4 kPa (30 mmHg) is indicated. This is discussed fully in Chapter 32.

Medicolegal

Perioperative alteration in neurological deficit may be attributed to anaesthesia. This may render subarachnoid or epidural anaesthesia inadvisable in some patients.

Epilepsy

Epilepsy may be associated with birth injury, hypoglycaemia, hypocalcaemia, drug overdose or withdrawal, fever, head injury, cerebrovascular disease and cerebral tumour, the most likely cause depending on the age of onset. In most patients with epilepsy, no identifiable cause is found. Epilepsy developing after the age of 20 years usually indicates organic brain disease.

Anaesthesia

Patients should receive maintenance anticonvulsant therapy throughout the perioperative period. Some anaesthetic agents, e.g. enflurane, have cerebral excitatory effects and should be avoided. Sevoflurane and isoflurane do not cause cerebral excitation. Convulsions and abnormalities of muscle posture have been reported after operation in patients who have received propofol and it is currently recommended that this drug should not be used in patients known to have epilepsy. Interestingly, it is an effective anticonvulsant agent in some patients with status epilepticus. Thiopental is a potent anticonvulsant and is the i.v. induction agent of choice, while isoflurane is currently the volatile agent of choice. Local anaesthetic agents may cause convulsions at lower than normal concentrations and the safe maximum dose should be reduced. The anticonvulsants phenobarbital and phenytoin induce hepatic enzymes and accelerate elimination of drugs metabolized by the liver.

In cases of late-onset epilepsy, where increased intracranial pressure may be present as a result of tumour, controlled ventilation is advisable to avoid any further increase in intracranial pressure.

Status Epilepticus

Management is aimed at cessation of the fits while maintaining tissue oxygenation. Initial treatment should be Diazemuls, titrated intravenously in a dose of up to 10–20 mg or until fitting ceases. An alternative is lorazepam 2–4 mg i.v. slowly. A loading dose of phenytoin 10–15 mg kg^{-1} should be administered i.v. under ECG monitoring over 30–60 min. High-concentration oxygen should be administered, and a clear airway maintained throughout. If the convulsions persist or conscious level diminishes to the extent of compromising the airway and ventilation, the patient should be anaesthetized, the trachea intubated and mechanical ventilation commenced. While propofol has been associated with convulsive episodes when used for standard general anaesthesia, it is also highly effective in the treatment of status epilepticus and indeed may be the anaesthetic agent of choice in this condition. Propofol may be used in seizures refractory to benzodiazepines and phenytoin, both as the anaesthetic induction agent and as maintenance by infusion.

The conventional anaesthetic induction agent used is thiopental. Thereafter, an infusion of propofol may be used to control the fits. This has the advantage over thiopental of being short acting, allowing the patient's conscious level to be assessed more readily.

With status epilepticus, patients undergoing mechanical ventilation should not be paralysed, but if they are, a cerebral function monitor/electroencephalogram monitor must be used so that continued fitting is noted and treated.

Parkinson's Disease

The clinical signs of resting tremor, muscle rigidity and bradykinesia characterize Parkinson's disease. This illness affects around 3% of individuals over 66 years of age. It is caused by cell death in areas of the basal ganglia, with loss of dopaminergic neurones. Similar symptoms and signs occur with loss of dopaminergic function secondary to drugs such as antipsychotic agents and following encephalitis in some patients.

Patients commonly present for urological, ophthalmic or orthopaedic surgery. There are various considerations for the anaesthetist.

Respiratory. The airway may be difficult because of fixed flexion of the neck. Upper airway muscle dysfunction may lead to aspiration. Excessive salivation may necessitate administration of a preoperative antisialagogue. An obstructive ventilatory pattern is present in around 35% of patients and muscle rigidity and tremor may also impair ventilation.

Cardiovascular. Postural hypotension may be present and there is an increased risk of cardiac arrhythmias. Autonomic failure may cause or exacerbate these problems.

Gastrointestinal. There is an increased risk of reflux.

Medications. These may have cardiovascular side-effects and there are several potential interactions with anaesthetic agents, analgesics and neuromuscular blocking drugs. These are detailed in Table 18.7.

Anaesthetic Management

Preoperatively. Medication should be continued up to the time of surgery and reinstated as soon as possible thereafter. Regional techniques offer several advantages such as the avoidance of opioid drugs and less effect on respiratory function.

General anaesthesia. A technique which avoids pulmonary aspiration should be used when appropriate. Isoflurane and sevoflurane are the inhalational agents of choice although hypotension

TABLE 18.7	
Potential Drug Interactions in Patients with Parkinson's Disease	
Drug	**Comments**
Induction Agents	
Propofol	Avoid for stereotactic procedures (dyskinetic, may abolish tremor)
Etomidate	Probably safe
Thiopental	Probably safe
Analgesics	
Fentanyl	Possible muscle rigidity
Morphine	Possible muscle rigidity
Volatile Agents	
Isoflurane	Probably safe
Sevoflurane	Probably safe
Neuromuscular Blocking Agents	
Succinylcholine	Possible hyperkalaemia
Nondepolarizing agents	Probably safe
Antiemetics	
Metoclopramide	Precipitates or exacerbates Parkinsonism

Reproduced from Nicholson et al 2002 Parkinson's disease and anaesthesia. British Journal of Anaesthesia 89(6):904–916. Copyright The Board of Management and Trustees of the British Journal of Anaesthesia. Reproduced by permission of Oxford University Press/British Journal of Anaesthesia.

may be a problem, particularly in the presence of autonomic neuropathy and when bromocriptine or selegiline have been administered. In the patient requiring general anaesthesia, nasogastric L-dopa can be administered during prolonged operations. If the enteral route is not possible, parenteral apomorphine can be used. This should be preceded by administration of domperidone for 72 h. Parkinsonian patients have an increased risk of postoperative confusion and hallucinations and may exhibit abnormal neurological signs such as decerebrate posturing, upgoing plantars and hyperreflexia following general anaesthesia.

Drugs. Phenothiazines, haloperidol and metoclopramide are contraindicated. Opioids must be used with caution but paracetamol and NSAIDs can be used as normal.

Multiple Sclerosis

Deterioration of symptoms tends to occur after surgery, but no specific anaesthetic technique has been implicated. It may be advisable to avoid epidural and subarachnoid anaesthesia, but only for medicolegal reasons, as there is no evidence that these techniques affect the disease adversely. They may be used if indicated strongly, e.g. in obstetrics, provided that a full explanation has been given to the patient.

If a large motor deficit is present, there may be increased potassium release from muscle following administration of succinylcholine, which should be avoided.

Peripheral Neuropathies

These may exhibit axonal 'dying back' degeneration or segmental demyelination. They are classified by anatomical distribution, the commonest being a symmetrical peripheral polyneuropathy.

Motor, sensory and autonomic fibres are involved. Causes include:

- metabolic disorders (diabetes, porphyria)
- nutritional deficiency
- toxicity (heavy metals, drugs)
- collagen disease
- carcinoma
- infection
- inflammation
- critical illness polyneuropathy.

Problems for the anaesthetist include the effects of autonomic neuropathy, respiratory impairment and bulbar involvement.

Acute Demyelinating Polyneuropathy (Guillain–Barré Syndrome)

This autoimmune polyneuropathy appears some days after a respiratory or gastrointestinal infection. Progression is variable, ranging from nearly total paralysis in 24 h to development over several weeks. Respiratory and bulbar muscles may be affected and, if so, tracheal intubation and IPPV are necessary. Several techniques may be used for induction of anaesthesia and tracheal intubation. We recommend either the combination of an i.v. induction agent with rocuronium or the combination of propofol and alfentanil. The patient's general state, particularly the presence of cardiovascular instability, dictates which agents should be used. Autonomic neuropathy may result in hypotension after commencing IPPV. This may be minimized by adequate fluid preloading and gradual increases in minute volume. Succinylcholine should be avoided. There is evidence that either high-dose immunoglobulin therapy or plasmapheresis beneficially modifies the course of the disease, although mortality is not affected. Severe pain in a girdle distribution and peripheral neuropathic pain are particular problems in many patients and require a multimodal approach to analgesia.

Motor Neurone Disease (Progressive Muscular Atrophy, Amyotrophic Lateral Sclerosis, Progressive Bulbar Palsy)

Motor neurone disease is characterized by slow-onset and progressive deterioration in motor function. Several patterns of motor loss occur, with both upper and lower motor neurone loss. Problems for the anaesthetist include sensitivity to all anaesthetic agents and muscle relaxants, respiratory inadequacy and laryngeal incompetence. Regional techniques may be useful. Long-term IPPV should generally be avoided, but non-invasive ventilation has a definite role in palliation of dyspnoea.

Hereditary Ataxias

Friedreich's ataxia is the most common of these. Spinocerebellar, corticospinal and posterior columns are involved, and the course of the disease is slowly progressive. Problems for the anaesthetist include scoliosis, respiratory failure and cardiomyopathy with cardiac failure and arrhythmias.

Spinal Cord Lesions with Paraplegia

Release of potassium from muscle cells by succinylcholine precludes its use within 6–12 months of cord injury. Assessment of ventilatory function is important, as impaired cough and poor inspiration may indicate a need for postoperative controlled ventilation.

In cervical spine lesions, patients are dependent on the diaphragm for breathing. In the acute situation, the loss of intercostal muscle function, to which patients may take some time to adjust, coupled with general anaesthesia, may lead to postoperative respiratory failure necessitating controlled ventilation.

Regional anaesthetic techniques may be useful in these patients, reducing the autonomic reflexes stimulated by surgery and avoiding compromise of ventilatory function.

Huntington's Chorea

It has been reported that thiopental may cause prolonged apnoea, and decreased serum cholinesterase activity may prolong the action of succinylcholine.

Myasthenia Gravis

This disease usually presents in young adults and is characterized by episodes of increased muscle fatigue caused by decreased numbers of acetylcholine receptors at the neuromuscular junction. Treatment comprises an anticholinesterase (pyridostigmine 60 mg 6-hourly or neostigmine 15 mg 6-hourly) with a vagolytic agent (atropine or propantheline) to block the muscarinic side-effects. Steroid therapy is useful in some cases and thymectomy may benefit many patients considerably.

The principal problems concern adequacy of ventilation, ability to cough and clear secretions, and the increased secretions resulting from anticholinesterase therapy. If there is evidence of respiratory infection, surgery should be postponed. Serum potassium concentration should be kept within the normal range because hypokalaemia potentiates myasthenia. Local and regional anaesthesia, including subarachnoid or epidural block, may be suitable alternatives to general anaesthesia, although the maximum dose of local anaesthetic agents should be reduced because of their neuromuscular blocking action. The minimum possible dose of induction agent should be used and neuromuscular blockers should be avoided if possible. For major procedures requiring relaxation, the anticholinesterase may be omitted for 4 h preoperatively, and a small dose of muscle relaxant may be given if necessary. Atracurium is the relaxant of choice because of its short duration of action, and should be administered in a reduced dose. Succinylcholine has a variable effect in myasthenia and is best avoided.

After major surgery, the patient's lungs should be ventilated electively, usually for a few hours, but in some cases for significantly longer. Frequent chest physiotherapy and tracheal suction are required. Steroid cover is given if appropriate. If extreme muscle weakness occurs, i.v. neostigmine 1–2 mg and atropine 0.6–1.2 mg may be given. Care must be taken to titrate the doses of anticholinesterase, or a cholinergic crisis may occur, characterized by a depolarizing neuromuscular block, with sweating, salivation and pupillary constriction. An infusion of neostigmine is required if resumption of oral intake is delayed after surgery; 0.5 mg i.v. is equivalent to 15 mg neostigmine or 60 mg pyridostigmine orally, and should be combined with an anticholinergic agent. Edrophonium may be used to test the end-plate response to acetylcholine.

A myasthenic state may also be associated with carcinoma, thyrotoxicosis, Cushing's syndrome, hypokalaemia and hypocalcaemia. In these patients, nondepolarizing relaxants should be avoided or used in reduced dosage.

Familial Periodic Paralysis

This is also associated with prolonged paralysis after administration of nondepolarizing muscle relaxants.

Progressive Muscular Dystrophy

Several types of muscular dystrophy exist, of varying patterns of heredity and described according to their anatomical distribution. Muscle weakness occurs and must be distinguished from myasthenia and lower motor neurone disease. The anaesthetic complications comprise sensitivity to muscle relaxants, opioids and other sedative and anaesthetic drugs, and liability to respiratory infection. Myocardial involvement may occur. These patients may be treated long-term with domiciliary ventilation.

Dystrophia Myotonica

This is a disease of autosomal dominant inheritance characterized by muscle weakness and muscle contraction persisting after the termination of voluntary effort. Other features may include frontal baldness, cataract, sternomastoid wasting, gonadal atrophy and thyroid adenoma. Problems which affect anaesthetic management include the following:

- *Respiratory muscle weakness.* Respiratory function should be assessed fully before operation. Respiratory depressant drugs, e.g. thiopental or opioids, should be used with care; there is sensitivity also to nondepolarizing neuromuscular blockers. Planned IPPV may be required after surgery. Postoperative care of the airway must be meticulous. Chest infections are common.
- *Cardiovascular effects.* There may be a cardiomyopathy and conduction defects, including complete heart block. Patients may have a cardiac pacemaker *in situ*. Arrhythmias are common, particularly during anaesthesia, and may result in cardiac failure. Careful monitoring is essential.
- *Muscle spasm.* This may be provoked by administration of depolarizing neuromuscular blockers or anticholinesterases; succinylcholine and neostigmine should thus be avoided. The spasm is not abolished by nondepolarizing relaxants.
- *Gastrointestinal.* Oesophageal dysmotility may predispose to regurgitation and aspiration.

PSYCHIATRIC DISEASE

There are several considerations in the anaesthetic management of patients with psychiatric disease.

- Psychiatric patients are frequently depressed, with little understanding of, or interest in, anaesthesia.
- Patients are receiving a variety of medications with potential for serious drug interactions with anaesthetic agents.
- Patients may have associated pathology as a result of drug and/or alcohol abuse.

- Repeated anaesthetics are required for electroconvulsive therapy.

Electroconvulsive Therapy

Electroconvulsive therapy (ECT) involves application of an electrical stimulus to the patient's head with the intention of inducing seizure activity. It is a successful treatment for severe depression and some other psychiatric conditions. Anaesthesia is given to render the procedure safe and acceptable. However, it is important that seizure induction and duration are not compromised by the anaesthetic agents so that ECT is ineffective.

Seizure activity dramatically increases cerebral oxygen consumption, associated with an increase in intracranial pressure. Autonomic activation, with an initial parasympathetic followed by sympathetic stimulation, occurs. This results in an initial bradycardia followed by tachycardia and hypertension. Myocardial ischaemia may result in susceptible individuals.

Anaesthesia
Preoperative assessment
- Cardiorespiratory function must be assessed in the light of the autonomic effects described.
- Previous anaesthetic records – common in this group of patients.
- Antidepressants with anticholinergic effects slow gastric emptying so that an adequate fasting time (8 h) is important. However, patient reports of fasting time may be unreliable.

Anaesthetic Management
- Premedication is not usually given because it may influence seizure activity and prolong recovery time unnecessarily.
- Anaesthesia is induced usually with either etomidate or propofol. The use of propofol is uncertain because, although it provides suitable anaesthesia, it may impair seizure activity.
- A short-acting muscle relaxant is used to prevent trauma caused by seizure activity, and succinylcholine is the most frequently used agent.
- Hyperventilation by bag and mask before seizure induction lowers the seizure threshold and prolongs duration, whilst ventilation continued in the post-ictal phase avoids desaturation.

ECT is frequently undertaken in isolated units. However, the availability of monitoring, anaesthetic assistance and recovery facilities should be of an equivalent standard to those required for surgical patients.

Drug Interactions

In general, it is usually more likely that a patient may be harmed by discontinuing long-term medications than by continuing them with the risk of drug-related complications, provided that potential complications are recognized and the anaesthetic technique is tailored to avoid detrimental interactions. Traditionally, it has been recommended that monoamine oxidase inhibitors (MAOIs) are discontinued 2 weeks before surgery. However, it is recognized that, because this group of drugs is reserved for patients who have failed on other therapy or have particularly severe symptoms, it may be preferable to continue treatment. Stopping MAOIs early is not an option in the emergency situation. There is also a risk of precipitating unpleasant withdrawal symptoms if antidepressants are discontinued acutely.

Tricyclic Antidepressants.
Tricyclic antidepressants, e.g. amitriptyline and dothiepin, inhibit reuptake of noradrenaline into the presynaptic nerve terminals. These drugs have the following side-effects:

- anticholinergic – dry mouth, constipation, delayed gastric emptying, urinary retention
- arrhythmias and heart block, postural hypotension, which may occur during anaesthesia
- sedation
- the hypertensive response to direct-acting sympathomimetics is increased
- increased risk of CNS toxicity with tramadol.

Monoamine Oxidase Inhibitors

- MAOIs, e.g. phenelzine and tranylcypromine, inhibit intraneuronal metabolism of sympathomimetic amines.
- Tyramine (noradrenaline precursor) precipitates hypertensive crises ('cheese reaction').
- They inhibit metabolism of indirect-acting sympathomimetic amines, e.g. ephedrine, resulting in severe hypertension if these drugs are given concurrently. There may also be an exaggerated sympathomimetic response if directly acting sympathomimetics are given concurrently.
- CNS excitation occurs with pethidine, manifest as agitation, hypertension, convulsions and hyperthermia. Other opioids appear to be safe although excessive sedation has been described. Note the antibacterial agent Linezolid is a reversible nonselective MAO inhibitor.

Selective Serotonin Reuptake Inhibitors.
These selectively inhibit serotonin reuptake, e.g. fluoxetine, sertraline. They have fewer cardiac and anticholinergic effects than tricyclic antidepressants and may cause CNS toxicity in conjunction with tramadol.

Phenothiazines.
This is a broad group of drugs and their therapeutic actions and side-effects vary considerably, e.g. chlorpromazine, thioridazine, prochlorperazine:

- antipsychotic, antiemetic
- sedation, extrapyramidal effects, antimuscarinic effects, antihistamine, α-adrenoceptor blockade, inhibition of normal temperature regulation
- drug interactions are generally related to enhanced effects such as excess sedation, hypotension and anticholinergic actions.

Lithium.
Lithium inhibits release and increases reuptake of noradrenaline:

- lithium is used to treat manic states
- lithium acts as a sodium ion, and may potentiate muscle relaxants
- it is renally excreted, and toxicity is enhanced by hyponatraemia because lithium is conserved along with sodium
- its toxic effects include tremor, ataxia, nystagmus, renal impairment and convulsions
- it is recommended that lithium is discontinued 24 h before major surgery if possible.

CONNECTIVE TISSUE DISORDERS

These are multisystem diseases which can therefore present with a variety of problems relevant to anaesthesia and surgery and which show a wide degree of overlap, well illustrated by rheumatoid arthritis.

Rheumatoid Arthritis

Rheumatoid arthritis is by far the most common connective tissue disorder; it is a multisystem disease, with several implications for anaesthesia which must be considered at the time of preoperative assessment.

Airway Problems

The arthritic process may involve the temporomandibular joints, rendering laryngoscopy and intubation difficult. The cervical spine may be fixed or subluxed, and thus unstable, especially when the patient is anaesthetized and paralysed. Cricoarytenoid involvement should be suspected if hoarseness or stridor is present.

Respiratory Function

Costochondral involvement causes a restrictive defect with reduced vital capacity. Pulmonary involvement with interstitial fibrosis produces ventilation/perfusion abnormalities, a diffusion defect and thus hypoxaemia.

Cardiovascular System

Endocardial and myocardial involvement may occur. Coronary arteritis, conduction defects and peripheral arteritis are other, uncommon, features. Immobility caused by arthritis may make assessment of cardiorespiratory function difficult.

Anaemia

A chronic anaemia, hypo- or normochromic, but refractory to iron, occurs. Preoperative transfusion to a haemoglobin concentration of approximately $100\,g\,L^{-1}$ is advisable before major surgery. Treatment with salicylates or other NSAIDs may cause gastrointestinal blood loss.

Renal Function

Renal impairment, or nephrotic syndrome, may occur as a result of amyloidosis or drug treatment. NSAIDs should be used with caution in the perioperative period.

Steroid Therapy and Immunosuppression

Many patients are receiving long-term steroid therapy and require augmented steroid cover for the perioperative period (see pp. 408–409). They are more vulnerable to postoperative infection due both to the disease and concurrent therapy.

Routine Preoperative Investigation

This should include full blood count, serum urea and electrolyte concentrations, chest X-ray, cervical spine X-ray and ECG. Other investigations, e.g. pulmonary function tests, may be required in some instances.

Conduct of Anaesthesia

Specific anaesthetic considerations include:

- consideration of general versus regional anaesthesia
- how to secure and maintain the patient's airway if a general anaesthetic is required
- vascular access
- steroid replacement where indicated
- positioning for surgery
- analgesia for a group of patients who may have significant preoperative pain and may be on regular opioids and other analgesics.

Particular care should be taken with venepuncture and insertion of i.v. cannulae because of atrophy of skin and subcutaneous tissues, and fragility of veins. Careful positioning of the patient on the operating table is required because these patients may have multiple joint involvement. Padding may be required to prevent pressure sores.

The anaesthetist should be prepared for a difficult tracheal intubation. If intubation is essential, an awake fibreoptic-assisted intubation is often the technique of choice. When intubation is not essential, a laryngeal mask airway is often satisfactory, but a back-up plan should be made in case of difficulties. Alternatively, the use of regional anaesthesia may pre-empt the need for complex airway management.

Other Connective Tissue Diseases

Implications for the anaesthetist are similar to those associated with rheumatoid arthritis. However, some specific features may be more prominent, e.g. vasculitis (including cerebral vasculitis), glomerulonephritis, pulmonary fibrosis, or peri- or myocarditis. Steroid and immunosuppressive therapy are other potential problems.

Scleroderma

Scleroderma (systemic sclerosis) is particularly associated with restricted mouth opening, lower oesophageal involvement with increased risk of regurgitation, pulmonary involvement, renal failure, steroid therapy and peripheral vascular disease.

Systemic Lupus Erythematosus

Anaemia, renal and respiratory involvement may be severe. Cardiac involvement may include mitral valve disease. Cerebral vasculitis may occur. Steroid therapy is usual.

Ankylosing Spondylitis

The rigid spine makes intubation difficult, and spinal and epidural anaesthesia may be technically impossible. Awake fibreoptic-assisted intubation is often required for airway control and may be difficult. Costovertebral joint involvement restricts chest expansion. Postoperative ventilatory support may be required.

Marfan's Syndrome

This is a disorder of connective tissue of autosomal dominant inheritance, which is characterized by long, thin extremities, a high arched palate, lens subluxation and aortic and mitral regurgitation. Regurgitation may be severe, and the valve lesions may be complicated by infective endocarditis. Antibiotic cover is necessary for dental and other surgical procedures.

NUTRITIONAL PROBLEMS

Obesity

Obesity poses several problems to the anaesthetist and surgeon.

Cardiovascular Function

Obesity is associated with increased blood volume, increased cardiac work, hypertension and cardiomegaly. Atherosclerosis and coronary artery disease are common. Diabetes mellitus may coexist.

Respiratory Function

Vital capacity and FRC are decreased. Closing volume is increased. As a result, increased shunting occurs through underventilated, dependent lung regions, with consequent hypoxaemia. These changes, brought about by abdominal splinting of the diaphragm, are accentuated in the supine, Trendelenburg and lithotomy positions. Total thoracic compliance is decreased, the work of breathing increased, and increased oxygen consumption and carbon dioxide production cause hyperventilation.

Other Factors

There may be difficulty in cannulating a vein, and arterial pressure measurement may be inaccurate unless the appropriate size of cuff is used. Direct arterial measurement is often preferable. Assessment of volume state is generally more difficult than in the normal patient. Surgery is technically more difficult, with a risk of heavy blood loss and increased incidences of wound infection and wound dehiscence. Hiatus hernia with the risk of regurgitation is more common, and maintenance of the airway and tracheal intubation may be more difficult.

Obese patients require careful preoperative respiratory and cardiovascular assessment (see Ch 17). The inspired oxygen fraction should be increased and positive end-expiratory pressure (PEEP) applied to maintain a satisfactory SpO_2. Fluid balance should be monitored carefully. Elective postoperative artificial ventilation should be considered, especially after abdominal surgery. Pulmonary, thromboembolic and wound complications are more common, and appropriate prophylactic measures and/or early recognition and treatment are important.

Pickwickian Syndrome

Pickwickian syndrome is characterized by a combination of obesity, episodic somnolence and hypoventilation with cyanosis, polycythaemia, pulmonary hypertension and right ventricular failure. Avoidance of hypoxaemia is important, and elective postoperative ventilation may be necessary, especially after abdominal surgery.

Malnutrition

As a result of persistent anorexia, dysphagia or vomiting, malnourished patients may have severe depletion of fluid and electrolytes. Anaemia and hypoproteinaemia are common. The anaemia may result from iron, vitamin B_{12} or folate deficiency, and if megaloblastic in nature, it may be associated with thrombocytopenia.

Preoperative correction of fluid and electrolyte deficits is required, with CVP monitoring in severe cases. Infusion of albumin may be advisable in some instances to raise the colloid osmotic pressure. A parenteral multivitamin preparation should be administered in view of probable thiamine deficiency.

Induction agents should be administered carefully to avoid hypotension, while smaller doses of relaxants than normal are required.

ANAESTHETIC CONSIDERATIONS IN THE ELDERLY

With a steady increase in life expectancy, there is an associated increase in the need for surgery and anaesthesia in elderly people.

The normal ageing process is associated with progressive loss of functional reserve in several vital organ systems, so that an elderly patient may be unable to increase functional capacity adequately to cope with the stress of major surgery. Several other factors increase the risk for elderly patients undergoing anaesthesia and surgery:

- associated comorbidity
- concomitant drug therapy
- increased sensitivity to many drugs
- impaired drug metabolism
- nutritional impairment.

Organ System Changes

Central Nervous System

- Autonomic dysfunction, leading to attenuated baroreceptor reflexes and susceptibility to hypotension, impaired temperature regulation and impaired gut motility.
- Cognitive impairment, resulting in a reduced capacity to cope with new situations and increased likelihood of confusional states. This effect may be compounded by sensory deprivation associated with impaired hearing and vision.

Cardiovascular

- There is a loss of atrial pacemaker cells, resulting in an increasing tendency to develop atrial fibrillation.
- Maximum heart rate decreases and the elderly are increasingly dependent on increased stroke volume to increase cardiac output. This renders them more sensitive to hypovolaemia and reduced preload.
- Peripheral vascular resistance is increased as a result of loss of blood vessel compliance, and compensatory left ventricular hypertrophy is common.

- Catecholamine receptors are downregulated, resulting in a less predictable response to adrenergic agents used therapeutically.

Respiratory System

- Closing volume increases and encroaches on tidal volume such that, when supine, significant shunting, hypoxaemia and later atelectasis may occur.
- Obstructive sleep apnoea is more common with associated episodes of desaturation and these episodes may be potentiated by opioid analgesia.
- Silent regurgitation and aspiration of gastric contents occurs more commonly.

Renal

- There is a progressive loss of functioning glomeruli and a resultant reduction in the ability to excrete or conserve sodium and water.

ANAESTHETIC CONSIDERATIONS

There is no preferred anaesthetic technique for elderly patients and their management must be tailored to the individual patient in the context of the surgery required.

Conditions limiting mobility such as arthritis and Parkinson's disease make assessment of cardiorespiratory function more difficult. In high-risk situations, dobutamine stress testing may be appropriate for cardiovascular assessment.

Cognitive impairment is associated with reduced cholinergic function and, generally, centrally active anticholinergics should be avoided in the elderly. This includes antiemetics such as cyclizine. The elderly are generally more sensitive to sedative agents, which should be given slowly and titrated to effect. Opioid sensitivity increases with age, so that bolus doses of these agents should be reduced in the elderly and titrated to effect.

The elderly are at increased risk from drug side-effects, e.g. renal dysfunction and gastrointestinal bleeding with NSAIDs. They are also at increased risk of adverse drug interactions because of multiple concurrent therapies. Particular care is required when prescribing. Drug doses must be adjusted where appropriate.

The elderly are less resilient in the face of profound changes in volume status and may require a greater degree of monitoring to guide fluid replacement effectively.

The elderly are also at increased risk of complications such as chest infections and thromboembolic events secondary to prolonged immobilization. Anaesthetic techniques should be used which allow prompt mobilization after surgery, e.g. effective epidural analgesia.

HUMAN IMMUNODEFICIENCY VIRUS

With a steady increase in the prevalence of human immunodeficiency virus (HIV) carriage, there is a commensurate increase in patients who are HIV positive and require anaesthesia and surgery. This raises issues both for patients and for their carers.

Initial infection with HIV is associated with a high viral load which stimulates an immune reaction which is initially effective in reducing the viral load. HIV replicates in T-helper (CD4) cells. Ten per cent of patients who seroconvert develop acquired immunodeficiency syndrome (AIDS) in the first 2–3 years. The remainder develop it over a median duration of 10 years. Development of AIDS is associated with a reduction of CD4 cells and an increase in viral load.

Transmission of HIV requires a large infecting dose. HIV is present in body fluids and may be transmitted by contamination with body fluids. Of particular relevance to anaesthesia is the risk of transmission via needle stick injury. Wearing gloves reduces the size of the inoculum of virus, and double gloving improves on this further. It is imperative that universal precautions are used in the theatre environment to reduce the risk of blood-borne infection transmission, including HIV. Sharps safety is particularly important.

Patient-to-patient transmission via contaminated equipment is also possible and appropriate precautions must be taken to avoid exposure of patients to this risk. Increasingly, a move to single-use equipment is being introduced where direct patient contact occurs to avoid the possibility of transmission of infection, including HIV.

In the event of significant exposure to infected body fluids, postexposure prophylaxis should be given. The local occupational health department and/or the local infectious diseases unit should be contacted for advice urgently, because treatment should commence within 1–2 h.

With regard to anaesthesia, there is little specific information available.

- General anaesthesia is known to be immunosuppressant so that, theoretically, a regional technique, e.g. epidural anaesthesia, might be preferable. However, this must be balanced against the risk of pre-existing immunosuppression leading to epidural abscess and the potential to exacerbate pre-existing neuropathy. At present, individual decisions should be made at the discretion of the anaesthetist and the patient involved.
- Pain is a common symptom of late HIV infection and AIDS, and pain should be assessed and treated as part of the patient's perioperative management.
- Drug interactions may occur with antiretroviral agents. For example, the protease inhibitors inhibit cytochrome P450, resulting in reduced metabolism of many drugs, including fentanyl and benzodiazepines. Conversely, non-nucleoside reverse transcriptase inhibitors induce cytochrome P450. Patients with HIV infection are usually receiving a combination of three agents so that interactions may be complex.

MYELOMA

This neoplastic condition affects plasma cells and has several features of significance to the anaesthetist.

- Widespread skeletal destruction occurs and careful handling of the patient on the operating table is essential. Pathological fractures are common.
- Bone pain may be severe and often requires large doses of analgesics.
- Hypercalcaemia occurs as a result of bone destruction and may precipitate renal failure.
- Chronic renal failure may also result from direct nephrotoxicity.
- Anaemia is almost invariable, and preoperative blood transfusion is often necessary.
- Thrombocytopenia is common during cytotoxic therapy.
- Patients are susceptible to infection, including chest infection, especially during chemotherapy.

TABLE 18.8

Safety of Drugs Commonly used in Clinical Anaesthesia for Patients with Acute Porphyrias

Drug Group

Intravenous induction agents	Propofol Midazolam	PS PS	Ketamine	C	Barbiturates Etomidate	U PU
Inhalation agents	Nitrous oxide	S	Isoflurane	ND	Enflurane	PU
Muscle relaxants	Succinylcholine Vecuronium	S PS	Atracurium Pancuronium	ND C		
Neuromuscular blockade reversal	Atropine Neostigmine	S S	Glycopyrronium	ND		
Local anaesthetics			Lidocaine Prilocaine Bupivacaine	C C C		
Analgesics	Morphine Fentanyl Buprenorphine Naloxone Paracetamol	S S S PS S	Alfentanil	ND		
Anxiolytics	Temazepam Lorazepam Phenothiazines	S PS S	Diazepam	C	All other benzodiazepines	U
Antiarrhythmics	β-Blockers	S			Verapamil Nifedipine Diltiazem	U U U
Other cardiovascular drugs	Adrenaline Phentolamine	S S	Beta-agonists Alpha-agonists	ND ND		
Bronchodilators	Corticosteroids Salbutamol	PS S			Aminophylline	U
Premedication for caesarean section	Metoclopramide Domperidone	PS S	Ranitidine	C	Cimetidine	PU

PS, possibly safe; S, safe; C, contentious; ND, no data; U, unsafe; PU, probably unsafe.
An up-to-date list of drugs considered safe in acute porphyria can be found at www.wmic.wales.nhs.uk/porphyria_info.php.

■ Increased plasma immunoglobulin concentrations may increase blood viscosity, predisposing to arterial and venous thrombosis. Drug binding may be affected.

■ Neurological manifestations include spinal cord and nerve root compression.

PORPHYRIA

The porphyrias are an inherited group of disorders of porphyrin metabolism characterized by increased activity of D-aminolaevulinic acid synthetase with excessive production of porphyrins or their precursors. In the UK, acute intermittent porphyria is the most common type. It is characterized by acute attacks which may arise spontaneously or be precipitated by infection, starvation, pregnancy or administration of some drugs. Inheritance is Mendelian dominant and thus patients with a family history of porphyria require further investigation. Clinical features include the following:

■ Gastrointestinal – abdominal pain and tenderness, vomiting, constipation and occasionally diarrhoea.

- Neurological – a motor and sensory peripheral neuropathy is common. It may involve bulbar and respiratory muscles. Epileptic fits and psychological disturbance may occur.
- Cardiovascular – hypertension and tachycardia often occur during the attacks. Hypotension has also been reported.
- Fever and leucocytosis occur in 25–30% of patients.

Drugs which can provoke the attack include alcohol, barbiturates, chlordiazepoxide, steroid hormones, chlorpropamide, pentazocine, phenytoin and sulphonamides.

Anaesthesia in such patients is directed to avoiding drugs which may provoke attacks. Induction with propofol, followed by muscle relaxation with succinylcholine or vecuronium, ventilation with nitrous oxide, and oxygen, and analgesic supplementation with morphine or fentanyl is satisfactory (Table 18.8). If fits occur, diazepam is a suitable anticonvulsant, while chlorpromazine, promethazine or promazine are suitable sedatives.

FURTHER READING

Avidan, M.S., Jones, N., Pozniak, A.L., 2000. The implications of HIV for the anaesthetist and the intensivist. Anaesthesia 55, 344–354.

Benumof, J.L. (Ed.), 1998. Anesthesia and uncommon diseases, fourth ed. WB Saunders, Philadelphia.

British Journal of Anaesthesia, 2004. Postgraduate educational issue, cardiovascular disease in anaesthesia and critical care. Oxford University Press, Oxford.

British National Formulary, sixty third ed, 2012. British Medical Association and Royal Pharmaceutical Society of Great Britain, London.

Chassot, P.G., Delabays, A., Spahn, D.R., 2002. Preoperative evaluation of patients with, or at risk of, coronary artery disease undergoing non-cardiac surgery. Br. J. Anaesth. 89, 747–759.

Fleisher, L.A., Beckman, J.A., Brown, K.A., et al., 2007. ACC/AHA guidelines on perioperative cardiovascular evaluation and care for noncardiac surgery: executive summary. J. Am. Coll. Cardiol. 50, 1707–1732.

Management of adults with diabetes undergoing surgery and elective procedures. Available from: http://www.diabetes.nhs.uk/areas_of_care/emergency_and_inpatient/perioperative_management/.

McAnulty, G.R., Robertshaw, H.J., Hall, M., 2000. Anaesthetic management of patients with diabetes mellitus. Br. J. Anaesth. 85, 80–90.

Nicholson, G., Pereira, A.C., Hall, G.M., 2002. Parkinson's disease and anaesthesia. Br. J. Anaesth. 89, 904–916.

Priebe, H.J., 2000. The aged cardiovascular risk patient. Br. J. Anaesth. 85, 763–778.

Riddell, J.W., Chiche, L., Plaud, B., et al., 2007. Coronary stents and non cardiac surgery. Circulation 116, e378–e382.

Stoelting, R.K., Dierdorf, S.R., 1993. Anaesthesia and co-existing disease, third ed. Churchill Livingstone, London.

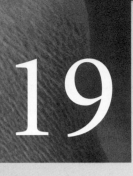

19 CONSENT AND INFORMATION FOR PATIENTS

C ompetent adults have a fundamental right to give or withhold their consent to medical examination, investigation or treatment. Other than in specific or exceptional circumstances, anaesthetists must therefore at all times have been given the **valid** consent of their patients. Several important points must be borne in mind when considering consent. Is it given freely? Does the patient have the requisite information to make a decision? Do they have the capacity to make this decision?

TYPES OF CONSENT

In clinical anaesthetic practice, the vast majority of consent is *implied* consent. The person's consent is inferred from his or her actions (or inactions). If an anaesthetist asks to check a patient's pulse and he or she offers his/her wrist, then consent is implied. The same principle of *implied* consent applies to documenting the patient's history in the medical notes, attaching monitoring, insertion of a venous cannula or positioning a patient for a local anaesthetic block. Conversely, refusal to participate in these acts would imply that the patient did not give his or her consent at that time.

Verbal consent may be simply an extension of implied consent. The anaesthetist may ask the patient if it is all right to insert a venous cannula and the patient says yes. At the other extreme, verbal consent may be a very thorough process in which the anaesthetist has explained specific risks and benefits of a proposed procedure in great detail and, following some deliberation, the patient agrees verbally.

Written consent involves the patient agreeing to the proposed procedure and confirming this in writing. This is most commonly facilitated by a pre-printed consent form for operative procedures, but there may be occasions on which the medical notes are used for this purpose. It is important to understand that the written form simply documents that the patient has given their consent. It does not necessarily provide any information about the quality of that consent. Written consent is no more 'valid' than verbal consent but the documentation may provide some evidence of the process in the event of problems.

At present, anaesthetists use a combination of all these types of consent in their daily practice: the patient implies consent to blood pressure monitoring by holding his or her arm in position; he or she may have agreed verbally to general anaesthesia and its attendant risks and benefits with the anaesthetist; he or she will almost certainly have signed a consent form for the proposed surgical procedure. Currently, the Association of Anaesthetists of Great Britain and Ireland (AAGBI) is of the view that a formal signed consent form is not necessary for anaesthesia and anaesthesia-related procedures, since it is the process of consent itself that is important, and a signed form does not increase the validity of the consent. However, it is recommended, particularly for procedures which are invasive or which carry significant risks, that both a patient's agreement to the intervention and the discussions which led up to that agreement are documented. This can be done on a standard consent form, on the anaesthetic record or separately in the patient's notes.

CONSENT AS AN ACTIVE PROCESS

Gaining consent should be considered a process, not an event. For most patients, the process starts long before they meet the anaesthetist when they are seen by their family doctor and then the surgeon. At each step in this process, they are being given information and consenting, however informally, to the next stage in the process. Healthcare professionals, family, friends and other sources will all be providing information which will help them to come to a decision. The anaesthetist adds to this process with information about planned anaesthetic techniques, risks and benefits. The final consent from the patient should reflect this whole process – and documentation should support this.

Voluntariness

A fundamental principle of valid consent is that it should be voluntary. Consent is always **given** or withheld by the patient. It is not something done **to** a patient. Anaesthetists, along with other healthcare professionals, should avoid references to 'consenting the patient.' The anaesthetist should take appropriate steps to satisfy him/herself that the patient is not being coerced by other people, however well meaning, or by the situation. In normal practice, this involves nothing more than straightforward discussion with the patient. Anaesthetists should be aware that the context of consent must be considered, not just whether there is undue pressure from family or friends. An elective patient who is in the anaesthetic room and given new, significant information about the anaesthetic technique may be viewed as being in a coercive context because it would be difficult to refuse the interventions offered.

The anaesthetist has a professional duty to offer his or her opinion about what he or she believes the best course of action might be, but this should not cross the line into coercion. Patients have the right to refuse offered treatments. However, this does not mean that anaesthetists have to provide a treatment which they feel is unsafe just because a patient requests it. In the unusual event that this problem arises, clear documentation and discussion with senior colleagues are vital.

Information

In broad terms, the anaesthetist should provide the individual patient with sufficient information to make a reasonable decision. The patient should have some understanding of what he or she is consenting to. The anaesthetist must consider the individual patient – as suggested by the AAGBI: 'What would *this* patient regard as relevant when coming to a decision about which, if any, of the available options to accept?'. Conversely, information should not be withheld solely because the anaesthetist feels it may deter a patient from undergoing a particular intervention or therapy.

There is no statute which clearly defines what information should be given to patients about anaesthesia, and different countries' legal systems have taken slightly divergent views. The AAGBI guidance is shown in Table 19.1. It must be emphasized that the anaesthetist should adapt this to the individual patient and surgery. For instance, visual loss after prone surgery is a rare but significant procedure-related complication which is relevant to specific patients.

Patients may sometimes state that they do not wish to know anything at all. The anaesthetist has a responsibility to ensure that the patient has sufficient information to provide valid consent. When handled with sensitivity, it is usually possible to provide an appropriate degree of information without unnecessary distress.

Quantity

It is impossible to provide patients with complete information about every anaesthetic and to attempt to do so would be counterproductive. The anaesthetist is responsible for providing the patient with sufficient information – professional training and communication skills should allow the anaesthetist to provide adequate information in a form that the patient can understand without overburdening the patient.

Most studies have demonstrated that patients wish to know more than healthcare professionals think, although conversely, they are usually satisfied with the information they are given. Most patients would like to receive written information, but only a minority read it when it is given. In general, women wish to know more than men, and parents wish to know more on their children's behalf than they might wish to know for themselves. Although clearly every patient is different, in general, anxious patients have the same desire for information as non-anxious patients.

TABLE 19.1
AAGBI Guidance on Information Which Should be Provided to Patients Relating to Anaesthesia

- Generally what may be expected as part of the proposed anaesthetic technique. For example, fasting, the administration and effects of premedication, transfer from the ward to the anaesthetic room, cannula insertion, noninvasive monitoring, induction of general and/or local anaesthesia, monitoring throughout surgery by the anaesthetist, transfer to a recovery area, and return to the ward. Intraoperative and postoperative analgesia, fluids and antiemetic therapy should also be described.
- Postoperative recovery in a critical care environment (and what this might entail), where appropriate.
- Alternative anaesthetic techniques, where appropriate.
- Commonly occurring, 'expected' side-effects, such as nausea and vomiting, numbness after local anaesthetic techniques, succinylcholine pains and post-dural puncture headache.
- Rare but serious complications such as awareness (with and without pain), nerve injury (for all forms of anaesthesia), disability (stroke, deafness and blindness) should be provided in written information, as should the very small risk of death.
- It is good practice to include an estimate of the incidence of the risk. Anaesthetists must be prepared to discuss these risks at the preoperative visit if the patient asks about them.
- Specific risks or complications that may be of increased significance to the patient, for example, the risk of vocal cord damage if the patient is a professional singer.
- The increased risk from anaesthesia and surgery in relation to the patient's medical history, nature of the surgery and urgency of the procedure. If possible, an estimate of the additional risk should be provided.
- The risks and benefits of local and regional anaesthesia in comparison to other analgesic techniques.
- The risk of intra-operative pain, and the need to convert to general anaesthesia, should a proposed local or regional technique be inadequate or ineffective. The risks and benefits of adjunctive sedation or general anaesthesia should be discussed.
- The benefits and risks of associated procedures such as central venous catheterization, where appropriate.
- Techniques of a sensitive nature, such as the insertion of an analgesic suppository.

Methods of Information Provision

There are numerous ways of conveying information to patients. Traditionally, the face-to-face preoperative consultation was the only method used by anaesthetists. This is clearly still very valuable, partly to help establish rapport between patient and anaesthetist, but also to allow the anaesthetist to discover any specific issues of concern to the patient. However, numerous studies have shown that understanding and information retention following simple verbal consultation are poor. As the AAGBI states:

'It is neither practical nor desirable for all information to be provided to patients at the preoperative meeting with the anaesthetist.'

Written information is a complement to the preoperative consultation, not a replacement. It provides an opportunity to give more extensive information about the process of anaesthesia, and about benefit and risks, which the patient can read at leisure and discuss with friends, family and other healthcare professionals. Producing good written information is a time-consuming process which requires consultation with patients, colleagues and experts in clear writing. Ideally, such information should be supported by published evidence and updated regularly to ensure that new information is included. Individual clinicians are unlikely to have the time or skill-sets to achieve this to a high standard; nor are most anaesthetic departments. There are various sources of high quality information available from national bodies and commercial organizations which meet these requirements.

Multimedia/video information is an attractive alternative approach. As with written information, it is not a straightforward task to produce high quality information. The studies that have been published generally demonstrate that it aids understanding and information retention, at least in the short term. However, there are practical issues to be resolved, including how to make it available to all patients, and cost.

Whatever approach used, it is the anaesthetist's final responsibility to ensure that the patient has had sufficient information to provide valid consent.

Communicating Risk

Humans are not very good at assessing risk. A variety of factors influence people's acceptance and interpretation of risk. Self-inflicted risk is generally better accepted than externally imposed risk – as evidenced by smokers concerned about relatively small risks from anaesthesia. Immediate and high impact risks (e.g. hypoxic brain damage) are rated more strongly than short-term or distant risks even though they may be far less likely to occur. There is also a natural tendency to overestimate rare risks and underestimate common ones.

The context of risk is relevant. In general, when given identical data concerning themselves and other people, individuals tend to rate the risk of 'bad things' happening to other people as greater than the risk to themselves; the converse is true for 'good things.' Even if they understand the risks, people are subject to the myth of invulnerability – the risk is real, but applies only to other people.

Taking all the above into account, how should an anaesthetist give information about risks and benefits? It is important to remember that the information is for the benefit of the patient, not solely as a defence against possible legal action. However, there are legal consequences of failure to obtain consent or failure to provide sufficient information. If a Court finds that consent was invalid, there may be a finding that provision of treatment amounted to battery or assault. Alternatively, the patient may argue that, by refusing to undergo the procedure if appropriate warnings had been given, the complication would have been avoided. If this argument is successful, then the patient is entitled to compensation for the consequences of the injury, even if the injury occurred despite all reasonable care in undertaking the procedure.

Patients prefer to be given numerical estimates of risk; doctors prefer to provide less precise qualitative estimates. Given the current state of evidence, neither is more accurate. The risk to the individual patient is usually unknown with sufficient precision. There is reasonable evidence that patients (and doctors) do not have sufficient understanding of probabilities for these to be used alone. Verbal likelihood scales are therefore most commonly used. The problem lies in the interpretation by anaesthetist and patient of the scale. 'Never' and 'always' are straightforward, but 'common', 'rare' and 'unusual' are subjective terms. Even within anaesthesia information systems, these are used differently. Drug information uses the 'Calman' scale; the Royal College of Anaesthetists (RCOA) uses a different scale. In order to provide more personal context, the population scale is sometimes used, comparing the risk to the number of people on a street, village, town, etc. (Table 19.2).

The framing of risk changes perception of risk. A 90% success rate is better received than a 10% failure rate. Relative risks and benefits may have a greater influence on an individual than is necessarily warranted. The absolute risk of dying due to anaesthesia-related complications is very small, regardless of technique. However, the relative risk (e.g. regional versus general anaesthesia for Caesarean section) may be quite large.

TABLE 19.2
Commonly Used Methods of Expressing the Risk of Medical Treatments

Level of Risk	Calman Scale	RCOA Leaflets	Population Comparison: One Person in
1 in 1 to 1 in 9		Very common	A family
1 in 10 to 1 in 99	High	Common	
1 in 100 to 1 in 999	Moderate	Uncommon	A street
1 in 1000 to 1 in 9999	Low	Rare	A village
1 in 10,000 to 1 in 1,000,000	Minimal	Very rare	A small town
1 in 1,000,000 to 1 in 9,999,999	Negligible		A city
1 in 10,000,000 to 1 in 99,999,999			A province or country
1 in 100,000,000 to 1 in 999,999,999			A large country

Capacity

The vast majority of patients clearly have capacity to make their own decisions. However, there are a number of patients who may be unable to give valid consent, either temporarily or permanently. The largest group is children (see below). In adults, the Mental Capacity Act (2005) in the UK, and similar legislation in other countries, provides a legal framework for patients unable to provide their own consent.

1. Adult patients are assumed to have capacity unless it is established that they lack capacity. Capacity is the ability to (a) understand and remember the information and (b) use it to arrive at a decision.
2. Patients must be given a reasonable chance to demonstrate their capacity. A person's lack of capacity cannot be assumed solely because they have taken drugs, alcohol or premedication, nor because they are making seemingly 'wrong' choices. In particular, the inability to communicate verbally does not imply a lack of capacity. Doctors (including anaesthetists) must make reasonable attempts to provide information for the patient so that they can decide on treatment options for themselves.
3. The treatment of adults without capacity must be in their best interests. This is a wider definition of best interests than solely medical best interests. Although generally more relevant to critical care than anaesthesia, the Act is clear that the treatment must be necessary, the least restrictive and in the patient's wider best interests.
4. Patients may appoint proxy decision-makers with Lasting Power of Attorney (LPA). These individuals have the legal right to give or receive consent on behalf of a patient without capacity for carrying out or continuation of treatment. The exception is for life-sustaining treatment or treatment considered inappropriate by the doctor.

Advance directives have varying legal standing across the world. Within the UK, an advance directive is held to be legally valid if:

■ at the time of the directive, the patient makes the decision voluntarily, with adequate information, and they have capacity

■ the specific refusal is clear, e.g. blood transfusion
■ the circumstances of when the refusal should apply are clear, e.g. resuscitation may be accepted after witnessed cardiac arrest, but not following a disabling stroke.

Advance directives should be honoured provided that the treating doctor believes the above conditions are met. Although most advance directives are written, oral directives are acceptable. Only decisions regarding refusal of life-sustaining treatment **must** be in writing; these should be witnessed and countersigned.

In emergency situations, doctors should not unreasonably delay treatment but should make reasonable efforts to ascertain whether a valid advance directive exists.

Consent in Special Circumstances

Emergency

Most emergency patients have capacity and the same considerations about consent and information apply. However, the urgency of a situation may necessitate a shortened time-frame for consideration. This does not preclude the requirement to clearly document any discussions held.

For patients who lack capacity (e.g. loss of consciousness due to head injury), the stipulations of the Mental Capacity Act (or similar) apply. The doctor should act in the patient's best interests in the least restrictive way possible.

Children

Although legal definitions vary, consent, or refusal of consent, is usually given on behalf of the child by a parent. Up-to-date guidance should be referred to, because professional and legal frameworks change. In general, an adult with legal parental responsibility can give or refuse consent. Teachers may be acting *in loco parentis*, although in practice for truly emergency care, the provisions of the Mental Capacity Act apply. Older children who have capacity are able to consent for themselves, though under the age of 18 years, they may not legally be allowed to refuse consent.

Occasionally, anaesthetists become involved in complex issues around refusal of consent on religious grounds by parents on behalf of the child. This almost invariably should be discussed with experts such as hospital solicitors and medical defence societies.

When taking parental consent, the anaesthetist should be very clear about the limits of that consent, particularly if it is anticipated that the child may become distressed at induction of anaesthesia.

Pregnancy

The pregnant woman has exactly the same rights to give or withhold consent as any other person. She does not have to justify her decisions and the fetus has no legal rights until it is born. This raises two main issues for the anaesthetist.

The first is the provision of information for regional analgesia in the labour suite. A significant number of women are extremely anxious and in severe pain by the time that the anaesthetist is asked to insert an epidural catheter. They may therefore not wish to hear (and almost certainly will not retain) a long list of potential complications. However, the anaesthetist has a responsibility to provide at least a minimum amount of information about risks and benefits of the procedure. This **must** be documented at the time because there is good evidence that the mother's recollection of the discussion may not be complete, even the next day.

The second is the refusal of regional anaesthesia for emergency Caesarean section. The anaesthetist may believe that general anaesthesia is the riskier option for the mother. However, due to the emergency nature of Caesarean section, the option of refusing to provide general anaesthesia may be the most risky for the fetus.

SUMMARY

Patients have a fundamental right to give or withhold consent for anaesthesia. Anaesthetists must respect that and assist the patient in coming to a decision by providing sufficient information, in a way that the patient can understand.

FURTHER READING

Consent for Anaesthesia 2. 2006. Association of Anaesthetists of Great Britain and Ireland. http://www.aagbi.org/sites/default/files/consent06.pdf.

Hardman, J.G., Moppett, I.K., Aitkenhead, A.R. (Eds.), 2009. Consent, benefit, and risk in anaesthetic practice. Oxford University Press, Oxford.

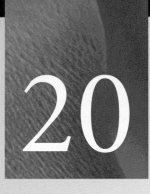

20 THE OPERATING THEATRE ENVIRONMENT

▪ ▪ ▪ ▪ ▪ ▪ ▪ ▪ ▪ ▪ ▪

Until the middle of the nineteenth century, surgery was carried out in any convenient room, frequently one which was used for other purposes. Although the introduction of antisepsis resulted in the washing of instruments and the operating table, the operating room itself was ignored as a source of infection. Operating rooms were designed with tiers of wooden benches around the operating table for spectators; thus the term operating *theatre* was introduced. During the early part of the twentieth century, large windows were incorporated, as artificial light was relatively ineffective, and high ceilings were introduced to improve ventilation. Additional facilities became necessary for preparing and anaesthetizing the patient, for sterilization of instruments and for the surgeon and other theatre staff to change clothes and scrub up. In addition, the design of operating theatres changed, and smaller theatres were introduced to facilitate frequent cleaning.

A modern operating theatre incorporates the following design features:

- environmental controls of varying degrees of complexity, to reduce the risk of airborne infection
- services for surgical and anaesthetic equipment
- an operating table on which the patient may be placed in the position required for surgery
- artificial lighting appropriate for the requirements of both surgeon and anaesthetist
- measures to ensure the safety of patient and staff.

In addition, provision should be made immediately adjacent to the operating theatre for preparing instruments, cleaning dirty instruments and for the surgeon to scrub up. Traditional practice in the UK has been to have

428

a separate room for anaesthetizing the patient. Many countries around the world do not use separate anaesthetic rooms and some operating theatres are now designed with shared or no anaesthetic rooms. Procedure rooms are becoming more common where aspects of perioperative care can be carried out such as regional anaesthesia and insertion of central venous catheters. There should also be separate areas for reception and recovery of patients. It is the usual practice for each hospital to have a suite of theatres, rather than operating theatres close to each of the surgical wards, which was formerly a common feature. The use of theatre suites permits more flexible and efficient use of staff and resources.

THE OPERATING THEATRE SUITE

The number of operating theatres required is difficult to calculate, but approximates in most British cities to one for every 40 000 of the population served. Ideally, the operating theatre suite should be close to the surgical wards, and adjacent to, and on the same floor as, the accident and emergency department, intensive care unit, X-ray department, day-case ward and sterile supplies unit. It is logical for the anaesthetic department to be immediately adjacent to, or an integral part of, the operating theatre suite, although this seldom occurs in practice.

The main purpose of the operating theatre environment is to provide a safe environment for patients and staff. A key component of this is to minimize the risk of transmission of infection to the patient from the air, the building or the staff. The operating theatre suite contains four zones of increasing degree of cleanliness (Table 20.1).

TABLE 20.1
Zones of Cleanliness in the Operating Theatre Suite

Outer zone – hospital areas up to and including the reception area

Clean zone – the circulation area used by staff after they have changed, and the route taken by patients from the transfer bay to the anaesthetic room

Aseptic zone – scrub-up and gowning area, anaesthetic room, theatre preparation room, operation room, exit bay

Disposal zone – disposal area for waste products and soiled or used equipment and supplies

Transfer of Patient

There is some evidence that anxiety in the surgical patient peaks as transfer from the ward to the operating theatre begins, and it is important that facilities for transfer minimize stress. A member of staff from the ward usually accompanies the patient, but it is customary for the ward staff to leave adult patients before anaesthesia has been induced. In paediatric practice, it is the normal routine that a ward nurse or play therapist and parent remain with the child during induction of anaesthesia.

On arrival at the reception area, the patient's identity and surgical procedure are checked. In a theatre suite, it may be necessary for patients to wait for some time in the reception area to prevent delays in the operating schedules. Consequently, adequate space should be provided for several beds, and there should be screens for patients who wish privacy. The staff in the reception area should include nurses. The décor should be cheerful, and the lighting subdued.

Transport should involve the minimum number of changes of trolley. A trolley is used frequently to transfer the patient to the operating theatre suite, and changes of trolley may be required to enter the clean area and also for transfer to the operating table after anaesthesia has been induced. Because sedative premedication is now unusual, patients not infrequently walk to the operating theatre suite and climb on to a trolley on arrival.

Alternatively, the patient's own bed may be taken to the operating theatre suite. If the patient is infirm or in severe pain, the bed may be taken to the anaesthetic room and transfer delayed until after induction of anaesthesia, but this is appropriate only if the bed has the facility to be tipped head-down if necessary. In some hospitals, a single transfer is effected by transporting the patient to the theatre suite in bed, where the patient is moved on to the operating theatre table-top, which is mounted on a wheeled frame. After induction of anaesthesia, the table-top is wheeled into the theatre and the top attached to a fixed base, which allows it to be positioned for surgery.

There is increasing awareness of the risk of injury to operating theatre personnel as a result of lifting patients, and thus an increasing tendency to install transfer systems which do not require great physical effort. There are also risks to patients arising from transfer to and from trolleys, operating tables and beds, including physical injury, disconnection of intravenous infusions or intravascular catheters, displacement of a tracheal tube and disconnection of monitoring apparatus. The anaesthetist is responsible for ensuring the safety of the patient and of themselves during transfer. There is no universal method of transferring patients from one trolley to another. All hospitals should provide training on safe transfer techniques.

All trolleys in the operating theatre suite should be equipped with oxygen, and this should be administered routinely to patients during transfer from theatre to the recovery room at the end of the procedure if general anaesthesia has been used or if there is any other clinical indication.

Anaesthetic Room

In several countries, the anaesthetic room has developed from a small annexe to the theatre to an integral part of the operating theatre suite. However, this is not universal, and in many parts of the world anaesthesia is induced in the operating theatre after the patient has been transferred onto the operating table. The following are the main advantages of the anaesthetic room.

- The patient's anxiety may be reduced by avoiding the sights and sounds of the operating theatre. This is of special importance in children.
- The equipment which may be necessary during induction of anaesthesia can be stored in an uncluttered manner, with each item readily available and its location obvious, in contrast to the cramped 'cart' which is usually employed to provide equipment and drugs when anaesthesia is induced in the operating theatre.
- Time is saved by inducing anaesthesia while surgery is being completed on another patient. This

is useful particularly if preparation is prolonged, e.g. performance of local anaesthetic blocks or establishment of invasive cardiovascular monitoring, but is safe only if at least two anaesthetists and two trained assistants are present.

However, there are several disadvantages.

- Anaesthetic and monitoring equipment must be duplicated, or moved to the operating theatre with the patient; this usually necessitates temporary disconnection from electrical or gas supplies.
- Hazards are involved in transferring an unconscious patient from a trolley to the operating table.
- Construction and maintenance of anaesthetic rooms are expensive.

Even in countries where anaesthetic rooms are used, it is customary to induce anaesthesia in the high-risk patient on the operating table, as the delay between onset of unconsciousness and the start of surgery must be kept to a minimum, e.g. for emergency caesarean section or severe haemorrhage.

The design of the anaesthetic room should allow easy access all round the patient's trolley, and should provide space for anaesthetic and monitoring equipment, and storage cupboards and shelves. The minimum floor area recommended by the Department of Health in the UK is $17\,m^2$, but this is inadequate. A floor area of $21\,m^2$ is more appropriate. Piped gases and suction, and electrical sockets, are required near the head of the trolley. An anaesthetic machine, mechanical ventilator and monitoring system are also necessary. Cupboards must be available to store equipment and drugs, and worktops must be of sufficient size to allow syringes, needles, cannulae and drugs to be prepared. There should be a clock with a second hand.

The layout of the anaesthetic room has an impact on both safety and efficiency of operating lists. Clear labelling, prioritization of commonly used items and avoidance of overstocking are important factors. Anaesthetists commonly work in several different theatres and a consistent layout between anaesthetic rooms may facilitate safe and smooth working.

Operating Room

The operating room is designed around its centrally situated operating table with overhead lighting and ventilation systems. The ideal shape for the operating room is circular, but this is inefficient and most operating rooms are square or nearly square. The Royal College of Surgeons of England has suggested that the floor should be $625\,ft^2$ (approximately $58\,m^2$) in area, and no smaller than $484\,ft^2$ (approximately $45\,m^2$). Theatres for specialized surgery may require a larger area to accommodate bulky equipment.

Outlets for piped gases and electrical sockets must be positioned close to the head of the operating table; they are provided most conveniently by a boom or stalactite system. Electrical cables should not lie across the floor. The operating room should be of sufficient size to allow all types of surgery without moving the position of the head of the table; this location should be reached easily and without complex manoeuvres as the patient enters the theatre from the anaesthetic room.

Temperature, Humidity and Ventilation

The temperature in the operating theatre and anaesthetic room should be sufficiently high to minimize the risk of inducing hypothermia in the patient, but must be comfortable for theatre staff. The patient may develop hypothermia at an ambient temperature of less than 21 °C. Temperatures of 22–24 °C are usually acceptable in the operating room, with a relative humidity of 50–60%; a higher environmental temperature is required during surgery in the neonate or infant. Slightly lower temperature and humidity are acceptable in other parts of the theatre suite. Controls for temperature and humidity should be located within the operating theatre so that adjustments can be made by theatre staff. The theatre temperature is less of a concern when patient warming devices are used, but anaesthetists should be aware that there are often significant periods when the patient is exposed without warming. A cold theatre will put the patient at greater risk of inadvertent hypothermia.

Heating and humidity are controlled usually by an air-conditioning and ventilation system, which provides an ambient pressure inside the operating room slightly higher than atmospheric. In general, air is introduced directly over the operating table, and leaves at the periphery through ducts positioned near floor level. In the area of the table, 400 air changes per hour are required to minimize the risk of airborne transmission of infection. More effective systems of ventilation, involving radial exponential air flow away from the operating table, or laminar flow, are used in some centres for some types of surgery, e.g. joint replacement, in which infection is especially undesirable. High-flow systems may accelerate cooling of the patient (and staff).

Light

Daylight is not necessary in the operating theatre, although it is more pleasant for staff if there are windows in the theatre suite, e.g. in corridors and common rooms. A high level of illumination is required over the operating table, and ceiling-mounted lamps are standard; it is preferable if they can be positioned directly by the surgeon.

The intensity and colour temperature of general lighting are very important to the anaesthetist, as appreciation of skin colour is affected by the spectrum of the source of illumination. The spectrum provided by lighting tubes should be similar to that of daylight, with an emission temperature of 4000–5000 K. The colour of the décor should be neutral and uniform. The intensity of general illumination should be up to 325 lm m^{-2} in the operating theatre, and it should be diffuse to avoid glare. In the anaesthetic room and recovery area, a light intensity of approximately 220 lm m^{-2} is acceptable, but a spotlight should be available if increased illumination is required for specific procedures.

Safety in the Operating Theatre

Trailing electrical wires, gas supply hoses, ventilator tubing, intravenous tubing and monitoring cables represent a hazard to both staff and patients in the operating theatre. Staff may trip and suffer injury, and it is easy to disconnect the electrical supply to vital equipment. If the power to modern anaesthetic machines is disconnected, monitoring, ventilation and gas supplies may fail simultaneously. In addition, there may be a risk to staff from pollution of the atmosphere with anaesthetic gases and vapours, and of contracting infection, particularly human immunodeficiency virus (HIV) or hepatitis, from infected patients. Potential hazards in the operating theatre are shown in Table 20.2.

Electrical Safety

Although some mention is made of electrical hazards in the operating theatre in Chapter 14, a detailed description is beyond the scope of this book, and the

TABLE 20.2
Potential Hazards in the Operating Theatre
Electricity
Liquids
Gases and vapours
Temperature
Humidity
Fire
Cables and tubes

reader is referred to the article by Boumphrey and Langton (2003) in the further reading list. The electrical supply to the operating theatre and all electrical equipment connected to the patient incorporate design features which minimize the risk of electrical currents being transmitted through the patient to earth.

However the theatre is designed, there will always be some electrical connection between the anaesthetic machine and the wall or ceiling sockets. Anaesthetists should develop a system which minimizes the risk of disconnection and trip hazard from these cables. Stopping staff from walking behind the anaesthetic machine is a simple but effective approach.

Explosions

Explosive anaesthetic gases and vapours (diethyl ether, cyclopropane, ethyl chloride) are no longer used in developed countries. However, diethyl ether is still used occasionally in some countries. Ether burns in air, but forms an explosive mixture with oxygen. An explosion may be initiated by a spark of very low energy ($<1\,\mu J$) or by contact with a temperature of 300 °C or higher. The risk of explosion is highest within and close to the anaesthetic breathing system because of the presence of a high oxygen concentration. Beyond a distance of 10 cm from the breathing system, the oxygen concentration diminishes and the risk is reduced. Ethyl chloride is used in some centres to generate a cold stimulus when testing the extent of regional or local anaesthetic blocks, and the risk of fire or explosion should not be forgotten.

The construction of anaesthetic apparatus is designed to minimize explosion hazards from generation of sparks caused by accumulation of static electricity.

All rubber is conductive, so that electrical charges leak to earth, and non-conductive substances are treated with antistatic material. In most operating theatres more than 15–20 years old, the floor has a high but finite resistance, so that static charges leak to earth but electrocution risks are minimized. Until recently, theatre footwear was also designed to earth static charges. Sparks may be generated by clothing made of synthetic materials such as nylon. The risk of accumulation of static electricity on walls and equipment is reduced if the environment humidity exceeds 70%.

Diathermy must not be used if flammable or explosive anaesthetics are employed. However, because the use of these agents has ceased in developed countries, many of the precautions against generation of sparks, and the use of expensive antistatic flooring, have become unnecessary.

Fire is still a hazard if alcohol-based solutions are used by the surgeon to sterilize the skin; the usual ignition source is a spark from the diathermy probe, and paper drapes provide a fuel.

Atmospheric Pollution

There has been considerable controversy regarding the risk to theatre staff from atmospheric pollution by anaesthetic gases and vapours. Earlier investigations suggested that theatre staff are more likely than other hospital personnel to suffer from hepatic and renal disease, to have non-specific neurological symptoms and for their children to have an increased risk of congenital abnormality. However, none of these problems has been substantiated.

There was more convincing evidence from some studies that female staff who worked in the operating theatre during the early months of pregnancy suffered an increased incidence of spontaneous abortion, and there is experimental evidence to suggest that constant exposure of rats to a concentration of more than 1000 ppm of nitrous oxide produces adverse results on their reproduction. However, the most recent, comprehensive and only randomized prospective investigation of operating theatre staff failed to demonstrate any increased health risk.

Trace concentrations of anaesthetic gases have been implicated in another area of concern – impairment of professional performance. Motor and intellectual performance were shown in an early laboratory study in volunteers to deteriorate in the presence of concentrations of nitrous oxide of 500 ppm, with or without halothane 15 ppm. However, subsequent studies failed to confirm these findings, and the consensus of several studies is that concentrations of 8–12% nitrous oxide are required before significant impairment of performance occurs. Such concentrations might be inhaled if the anaesthetist is close to an unscavenged expiratory valve, or during inhalation induction of anaesthesia, but exceed those present in other areas of an adequately ventilated operating theatre.

Nevertheless, it is sensible to minimize atmospheric pollution in the operating theatre, and hospital regulations in both western Europe and North America require the installation of anaesthetic gas-scavenging systems in all areas where anaesthesia is administered. In the USA, the National Institute of Occupational Safety and Hygiene (a federal regulatory body) dictates that environmental concentrations of anaesthetic gases should not exceed a value of 25 ppm of nitrous oxide and 2 ppm of volatile agent. In the UK, the Health and Safety Executive introduced maximum limits of exposure to anaesthetic agents in January 1996; these are shown in Table 20.3. Scavenging systems are described in Chapter 15.

Anaesthetic gases are not the only source of environmental pollution in the operating theatre; volatile skin-cleaning fluids and aerosol sprays, e.g. iodine or plastic skin dressing, should be used sensibly, and inhalation of vapours should be avoided.

TABLE 20.3
Maximum Levels of Exposure to Anaesthetic Agents in the Operating Theatre Suite Over an 8-h Time-Weighted Average Reference Period, as Laid Down in the UK by the Health and Safety Executive

Agent	Maximum Concentration (ppm)
Nitrous oxide	100
Halothane	10
Enflurane	50
Isoflurane	50
Sevoflurane	20*

*Manufacturer's recommendation.

Infection

The most serious types of acquired infection in operating theatre staff are HIV and hepatitis, which may be contracted by contact with blood or body fluids from an infected patient. Several healthcare workers have been infected in this way, either by a needlestick injury or through cuts and abrasions. The risk of percutaneous transmission of HIV is believed to be low; the risk of acquiring HIV following needlestick injury is estimated to be around 1 in 300 needlestick injuries. The annual risk of HIV infection for anaesthetists is estimated at between 1 in 3100 and 1 in 80000 in the US (depending upon the local HIV rate). High-risk fluids for HIV transmission include: CSF, pleural, peritoneal, synovial fluid and breast milk; vomit, urine, faeces and saliva are considered low-risk.

Two thousand cases of hepatitis B are reported each year in the UK, although the true incidence is probably very much higher. The prevalence of evidence of previous or current infection (antibodies to hepatitis B core antigen – anti-HBc) is around 1–2% in the UK; it is about 96% in parts of China and South Korea. Hepatitis B surface antigen persists for at least 6 months in 5–10% of infected individuals. Up to 20% of the population may have chronic hepatitis in South Asia, East Asia and sub-Saharan Africa. The virus is highly infectious, and minute amounts of blood may transmit the disease. The Association of Anaesthetists of Great Britain and Ireland (AAGBI) recommends that all anaesthetists should receive active immunization against hepatitis B and most hospitals in the UK insist that evidence of immunity to the virus is present in an anaesthetist's serum before allowing employment to start. A single dose of hepatitis B immunoglobulin combined with active immunization is required immediately if an unprotected individual is inoculated with infected material.

Hepatitis C and D viruses are also blood-borne. Up to 50% of people infected with the hepatitis C virus develop chronic liver disease. Occupational transmission of this virus has been reported.

The prevalence of HIV infection in the community is increasing. Thus, anaesthetists are likely to be exposed to an increasing number of patients who may transmit HIV. Compulsory screening of hospital patients for HIV is regarded as unacceptable and impractical. Anaesthetists should therefore assume that all patients potentially carry blood-borne diseases and precautions should be taken with all patients.

The following precautions are recommended to reduce the risks of transmission of HIV and other blood-borne diseases. These precautions are largely the same as those for reducing the risk of hospital-acquired infections for the patient.

- Gloves must be worn during induction of anaesthesia, performance of venepuncture or insertion of any intravascular cannula, and during insertion or removal of airways and tracheal tubes; this should be a routine when dealing with any patient. A plastic apron, mask and eye protection should be worn if substantial spillage of blood is anticipated, e.g. during insertion of an arterial cannula. Gloves should normally be discarded on taking the patient into the operating theatre and a fresh pair donned when any of these procedures is carried out during or at the end of anaesthesia.
- Equipment, notes and other articles must not be handled with contaminated gloves.
- Needles which have been in contact with the patient must not be resheathed or handed from one person to another.
- Cuts or abrasions on the anaesthetist's hands should be covered with a waterproof dressing. An anaesthetist with considerable skin lesions, such as eczema, chapping or several scratches, is particularly at risk of being infected.
- If a needlestick injury or contamination of a cut or abrasion occurs, bleeding should be encouraged and the skin washed thoroughly with soap and water.
- Advice should be obtained immediately from the hospital's occupational health department if there is reason to believe that contamination has occurred. Post-exposure prophylaxis following potential HIV exposure should be started within one hour of injury.
- Disposable equipment should be used where possible. Non-disposable equipment should be decontaminated with 2% glutaraldehyde, washed with soap and water and left in glutaraldehyde for a further 3 h. Contaminated floors and surfaces should be washed with 1% hypochlorite solution. Gloves must be worn.

There have been a number of instances in which items of disposable equipment, e.g. angle-pieces and catheter mounts, have been re-used, but in which the lumen has become obstructed, probably accidentally, by other items of equipment kept in the anaesthetic room. Equipment intended for single use must be discarded after use; re-usable equipment should be checked carefully to ensure that it is functioning correctly.

It is standard practice that a bacterial filter should be placed between the tracheal tube or airway and the anaesthetic breathing system in all patients to prevent cross-infection from a patient with undiagnosed infection.

In some countries, and particularly the UK, there has been increasing concern in recent years about the possibility of transmission of the prion responsible for the development of variant Creutzfeldt-Jakob disease (vCJD), attributed to infection from cows affected by bovine spongiform encephalitis (BSE). In infected patients, the prion is believed to be present in high concentrations in the tonsils. It is resistant to conventional methods of cleaning or sterilizing equipment. Consequently, hospitals in the UK have taken steps to stop the use of non-disposable items of equipment which could come in contact with structures in the pharynx. These items include laryngoscopes, bougies and laryngeal mask airways, and single-use devices have been introduced.

Prevention of Hospital-Acquired Infection

Anaesthetists are responsible for patients when they are at significant risk of hospital-acquired infection both at the operative site and through invasive procedures. There is some evidence linking better outcomes for patients with improved hand hygiene practice amongst anaesthetists.

Effective hand hygiene is the single most important measure to reduce the risk of infection of patients. All anaesthetic rooms and operating theatres should have ready access to hand-washing sinks, antiseptic hand-rubs and clean gloves. The anaesthetist has a responsibility to comply with hand hygiene policies in their work place. Typically these include the following:

- Washing hands with soap and water at the start of the day, after eating or drinking, visiting the toilet or if hands are visibly soiled.
- Frequent hand hygiene with an appropriate agent (often antiseptic hand-gel) whenever there is the possibility of cross-contamination. Of particular relevance to the anaesthetist is the risk of transfer

of organisms around the airway to intravascular devices.
- Washing/cleaning hands between patients – particularly after handover in recovery.

A good handwashing technique is a key component. The six-stage technique is recommended due to the frequency with which areas are missed with less rigorous handwashing.

- Wet hands with water (if using soap and water)
- Apply enough soap and handwash or hand-gel to cover all hand surfaces
  1. Rub hands palm to palm
  2. Right palm over the other hand with interlaced fingers and vice versa (back of hands)
  3. Palm to palm with fingers interlaced (between the fingers)
  4. Backs of fingers to opposing palms with fingers interlocked (backs of fingers)
  5. Rotational rubbing of left thumb clasped in right palm and vice versa (thumbs)
  6. Rotational rubbing, backwards and forwards with clasped fingers of right hand in left palm and vice versa (finger tips).
- Rinse hands with water (if relevant)
- Dry thoroughly with towel (if using water)/allow to air-dry
- Duration of procedure: at least 15 seconds.

The anaesthetist should also wear clean, disposable gloves for all procedures where he/she is exposed to body fluids (e.g. cannulation, airway management). This is mainly for the protection of the anaesthetist. It is important that these gloves are removed promptly to avoid cross-contamination.

There is some evidence that drugs drawn up and administered by anaesthetists may not be sterile by the time they reach the patient. This break in sterility may occur at any point in the preparation, storage and administration process. Anaesthetists must therefore ensure that they have a process which actively avoids inadvertent contamination of syringes and their contents.

Noise

Noise in the operating theatre should be kept to a minimum. Patients in the anaesthetic room before induction of anaesthesia may be made more anxious by boisterous laughter or loud conversation coming from the operating theatre. Similarly, as patients recover consciousness after the operation, undue noise is undesirable.

Surgeons and operating theatre staff may enjoy listening to music during surgery, and it is not uncommon for sound systems to be installed in operating theatres. The anaesthetist must ensure that sounds from the monitoring system, e.g. the tone indicating arterial oxygen saturation and the sounds of alarms, can be heard, either by turning up the volume of tones from the monitoring system or turning down the volume of the sound system.

The evidence regarding beneficial or detrimental effects of music in theatre is mixed. There are clearly times when it may hinder the ability of staff to concentrate or monitor the patient. Conversely, there may be times when it is an aid to concentration.

Equipment Checks

Anaesthetic equipment should be up to date, maintained regularly and the instruction manuals should be available and accessible. Monitoring apparatus should be in accordance with contemporary guidelines. Appropriate alarm limits must be set, and alarms must not be permanently disabled. An equipment check must be performed before an operating theatre session begins because a frequent cause of misadventure is the use of a machine which has not been checked properly, and which malfunctions. An adequate check of anaesthetic apparatus is an integral part of good practice; failure to check the anaesthetic equipment properly may amount to malpractice.

Operating theatre staff usually carry out checks when setting up an operating theatre for use, or after apparatus has been serviced or repaired, but the ultimate responsibility for ensuring that the apparatus is safe for its intended use rests with the anaesthetist. Sophisticated tests may have been performed after major servicing, but key control settings may have been altered and it is essential that the anaesthetist checks that the equipment is in proper working order and ready for clinical use. The final pre-use check is the sole responsibility of the anaesthetist who is to use the machine. It cannot be delegated to any other person.

There is no justification for proceeding with an anaesthetic when faults have been identified in the equipment. If there is no record of an adequate preoperative check of equipment and a problem occurs as a result of equipment failure, it is very difficult to defend an allegation of negligence.

At its most basic, the function of an anaesthetic machine is to enable the anaesthetist to administer to a patient oxygen under pressure without leaks. If all else fails, this allows the anaesthetist to preserve life.

Anaesthetic apparatus should be checked before the start of each operating session in a logical sequence as recommended in the AAGBI checklist shown in Tables 20.4 and 20.5. Further checks shown in Table 20.6 should be undertaken between cases. The primary intention of the check of the anaesthetic machine is to ensure that it is safe to use and to deliver gases under pressure without leaks. These checklists are available as laminated cards, intended to be attached to all anaesthetic machines in the UK and Ireland.

In most industries in which complex equipment is used, full training is provided for users. It is not acceptable for anaesthetists to assume that they intuitively understand an anaesthetic machine which they have not used before. Those new to the speciality require detailed instruction and training in the use of anaesthetic equipment, but even experienced anaesthetists need tuition in the use of new equipment.

Alternative Means of Ventilation

The early use of an alternative means of ventilation (a self-inflating bag which does not rely on a source of oxygen to function) may be life-saving. A self-inflating bag must be immediately available in any location where anaesthesia might be given. An alternative source of oxygen should also be readily available.

Perform Manufacturer's Machine Check

Modern anaesthesia workstations may perform many of the following checks automatically during start-up. Anaesthetists must know which are included and ensure that the automated check has been performed.

Power Supply

The anaesthetic workstation and relevant ancillary equipment must be connected to the mains electrical supply (where appropriate) and switched on. The anaesthetic workstation should be connected directly to the mains electrical supply, and only correctly

TABLE 20.4		
The Association of Anaesthetists of Great Britain and Ireland Checklist for Pre-Session Checking of Anaesthetic Equipment		
Checklist for Anaesthetic Equipment 2012 AAGBI Safety Guideline		
Checks at the start of every operating session Do not use this equipment unless you have been trained		
Check self-inflating bag available		
Perform manufacturer's (automatic) machine check		
Power supply	■ Plugged in ■ Switched on ■ Back-up battery charged	
Gas supplies and suction	■ Gas and vacuum pipelines – 'tug test' ■ Cylinders filled and turned off ■ Flowmeters working (if applicable) ■ Hypoxic guard working ■ Oxygen flush working ■ Suction clean and working	
Breathing system	■ Whole system patent and leak-free using 'two-bag' test ■ Vaporizers – fitted correctly, filled, leak-free, plugged in (if necessary) ■ Soda lime – colour checked ■ Alternative systems (e.g. Bain, T-piece) – checked ■ Correct gas outlet selected	
Ventilator	■ Working and configured correctly	
Scavenging	■ Working and configured correctly	
Monitors	■ Working and configured correctly ■ Alarms limits and volume set	
Airway equipment	■ Full range required working, with spares	
RECORD THIS CHECK IN THE PATIENT RECORD		
Don't Forget!	■ Self-inflating bag ■ Common gas outlet ■ Difficult airway equipment ■ Resuscitation equipment ■ TIVA and/or other infusion equipment	

This guideline is not a standard of care. The ultimate judgement with regard to a particular clinical procedure or treatment plan must be made by the clinician in the light of the clinical data presented and the diagnostic and treatment options available.
© The Association of Anaesthetists of Great Britain and Ireland 2012.
Adapted from *Checking Anaesthetic Equipment 2012*, with permission.

rated equipment connected to its electrical outlets. Multisocket extension leads must not be plugged into the anaesthetic machine outlets or used to connect the anaesthetic machine to the mains supply.

Hospitals should have back-up generators and many operating theatres have their own back-up system. Anaesthetists should know what is available where they are working. Back-up batteries for anaesthetic machines and other equipment should be charged.

Switch on the gas supply master switch (if one is fitted).

Check that the system clock (if fitted) is set correctly.

TABLE 20.5
The Association of Anaesthetists of Great Britain and Ireland 'Two-Bag' Test

THE TWO-BAG TEST

A two-bag test should be performed after the breathing system, vaporizers and ventilator have been checked individually

1. Attach the patient end of the breathing system (including angle piece and filter) to a test lung or bag.

2. Set the fresh gas flow rate to 5 L min^{-1} and ventilate manually. Check that the whole breathing system is patent and that the unidirectional valves are moving. Check the function of the APL valve by squeezing both bags.

3. Turn on the ventilator to ventilate the test lung. Turn off the fresh gas flow, or reduce to a minimum. Open and close each vaporizer in turn. There should be no loss of volume in the system.

Adapted from *Checking Anaesthetic Equipment 2012*, with permission.

TABLE 20.6
The Association of Anaesthetists of Great Britain and Ireland Checklist for Checking Anaesthetic Equipment between Cases

CHECKS BEFORE EACH CASE

Breathing system	▪ Whole system patent and leak-free using 'two-bag' test
	▪ Vaporizers – fitted correctly, filled, leak-free, plugged in (if necessary)
	▪ Alternative systems (e.g. Bain, T-piece) – checked
	▪ Correct gas outlet selected
Ventilator	▪ Working and configured correctly
Airway equipment	▪ Full range required working, with spares
Suction	▪ Clean and working

Adapted from *Checking Anaesthetic Equipment 2012*, with permission.

Gas Supplies and Suction

On some workstations, it is necessary to disconnect the oxygen pipeline in order to check the correct function of the oxygen failure alarm, although on machines with a gas supply master switch, the alarm may be operated by turning the master switch off. Repeated disconnection of gas hoses may lead to premature failure of the

Schrader socket and probe, and current guidelines recommend that the regular pre-session check of equipment includes a 'tug test' to confirm correct insertion of each pipeline into the appropriate socket. It is also recommended that the oxygen failure alarm is checked once a week by disconnecting the oxygen pipeline with the oxygen flowmeter turned on. The alarm must sound for at least 7 s. Oxygen failure warning devices are also linked to a gas shut-off device. Anaesthetists must be aware of both the tone of the alarm and also which gases will continue to flow on the anaesthetic machine in use.

Suction

The suction apparatus should be checked to ensure that it is clean, functioning, that all connections are secure and that an adequate negative pressure is generated.

Medical Gas Supplies

Identify the gases which are being supplied by pipeline, confirming with a 'tug test' that each pipeline is correctly inserted into the appropriate gas supply terminal. Only gentle force is required; excessive force during a 'tug test' may damage the pipeline or gas supply terminal.

It is essential to check that the anaesthetic machine is connected to a supply of oxygen and that an adequate reserve supply of oxygen is available from a spare cylinder. It is also necessary to check that adequate supplies of any other gases intended for use are available and connected. All cylinders should be securely seated and turned off after checking their contents.

Carbon dioxide cylinders should not be present on the anaesthetic machine. If a blanking plug is supplied, it should be fitted to any empty cylinder yoke.

All pressure gauges for pipelines connected to the anaesthetic machine should indicate a pressure of 400–500 kPa.

If flowmeters are present, their function should be checked, ensuring that each control valve operates smoothly and that the bobbin moves freely throughout its range without sticking. If nitrous oxide is to be used, the anti-hypoxia device should be tested by first turning on the nitrous oxide flow and ensuring that at least 25% oxygen also flows. The oxygen flow should then be turned off to check that the nitrous oxide flow also stops. The oxygen flow should be turned back on, the nitrous oxide flow should be turned off and a check should be made that the oxygen analyser display approaches 100%. Turn off all flow control valves. Machines fitted with a gas supply master switch will continue to deliver a basal flow of oxygen.

The emergency oxygen bypass control should be operated to ensure that flow occurs from the gas outlet without a significant decrease in the pipeline supply pressure. It is important to ensure that the emergency oxygen bypass control ceases to operate when released; there is a risk of awareness if it continues to operate.

Breathing System and Vaporizers

All breathing systems which are to be used must be checked and a 'two-bag test' performed before use (Table 20.5). Breathing systems should be inspected visually for correct configuration and assembly. All connections within the system and to the anaesthetic machine should be checked to ensure that they are secured by 'push and twist'. Ensure that there are no leaks or obstructions in the reservoir bags or breathing system and that they are not obstructed by foreign material. A pressure leak test (between 20 and 60 cmH$_2$O) should be performed on the breathing system by occluding the patient end and compressing the reservoir bag.

Manual leak testing of vaporizers was previously recommended routinely. It should only be performed on basic 'Boyle' machines because it may be harmful to modern anaesthetic workstations. **Refer to the manufacturer's recommendation before performing a manual test**.

Check that vaporizers for the required volatile agents are fitted correctly to the anaesthetic machine, that any locking mechanism is fully engaged and that the control knobs rotate fully through the full ranges. Check that the vaporizers are adequately filled but not overfilled, and that the filling port is tightly closed. Vaporizers must always be kept upright. Tilting a vaporizer can result in delivery of dangerously high concentrations of vapour.

All vaporizers must be turned off after they have been checked.

Manual Leak Test of Vaporizer. A flow rate of oxygen of 5 L min^{-1} should be set and, with the vaporizer turned off, the common gas outlet should be temporarily occluded. There should be no leak from any part of the vaporizer, and the flowmeter bobbin (if present) should dip.

If more than one vaporizer is present, turn each one on in turn and repeat this test. After the tests, ensure that the vaporizers and flowmeters are turned off.

It may be necessary to change a vaporizer during use although this should be avoided if at all possible. If a change is necessary, repeat the leak test because failure to do so is a common cause of critical incidents. Some anaesthetic workstations automatically test the integrity of vaporizers.

It is only necessary to remove a vaporizer from a machine to refill it if the manufacturer recommends this.

Carbon Dioxide Absorber

The contents and connections should be checked to ensure that there is an adequate supply of carbon dioxide absorbent and that it is of an appropriate colour.

Alternative Breathing Systems

If a co-axial system is in use, an occlusion test should be performed on the inner tube and a check should be made that the adjustable pressure limiting (APL) valve, where fitted, can be fully opened and closed.

Correct Gas Outlet

Special care must be exercised if the anaesthetic machine incorporates an auxiliary common gas outlet (ACGO). Incidents of patient harm have resulted from misconnection of a breathing system to an ACGO or mis-selection of the ACGO.

Whenever a breathing system is changed, either during a case or a list, its integrity and correct configuration must be confirmed. This is particularly important for paediatric lists when breathing systems may be changed frequently during an operating list.

Ventilator

It is important to check that the ventilator is configured correctly for its intended use and that the ventilator tubing is attached securely. The controls should be set according to the intended use of the ventilator and the system should be checked to ensure that adequate pressure is generated during the inspiratory phase. Ventilator alarms should be checked to ensure that they are working and correctly configured. The pressure relief valve should be checked to ensure that it functions correctly at the set pressure.

Two-Bag Test

A two-bag test should be performed after the breathing system, vaporizers and ventilator have been checked individually (see Table 20.5). Breathing systems should be protected with a test lung or bag when not in use to prevent intrusion of foreign bodies.

Scavenging

The anaesthetic gas scavenging system should be checked to ensure that it is switched on and functioning, and that the tubing is attached to the appropriate exhaust port of the breathing system, ventilator or anaesthetic workstation.

Monitoring Equipment

Before using the anaesthetic machine, all monitoring devices must be checked to ensure that they are functioning and that appropriate parameters and alarms have been set. This includes the cycling times, or frequency of recordings, of automatic non-invasive blood pressure monitors. Gas sampling tubing must be properly attached and free from obstruction or kinks. It is particularly important to check that the oxygen analyser, pulse oximeter and capnograph are functioning correctly and that appropriate alarm limits are set.

Airway Equipment

This includes bacterial filters, catheter mounts, connectors and tracheal tubes, laryngeal mask airways, etc. These should all be available in the appropriate sizes for patients on the operating list and **must** be checked for patency.

A new, single-use bacterial filter and angle piece/catheter mount must be used for each patient. It is important that these are checked for patency and flow, both visually and by ensuring that gas flows through the whole assembly when connected to the breathing system. This check must occur whenever new airway equipment is provided, and is a standard part of the WHO checklist for every patient.

Appropriate laryngoscopes must be available and checked to ensure that they function reliably. Equipment for the management of the anticipated or unexpected difficult airway must be available and checked regularly in accordance with departmental policies. The anaesthetist and anaesthetic assistant should both be aware of the location of the nearest 'difficult airway' trolley.

Single-Use Devices

Any part of the breathing system, ancillary equipment or other apparatus that is designated 'single-use' must be used for one patient only, and not reused. Packaging should not be removed until the point of use, for infection control, identification and safety.

Total Intravenous Anaesthesia (TIVA)

When TIVA is used, there must be a continuous intravenous infusion of anaesthetic agent or agents; interruption from whatever cause may result in awareness. A thorough equipment check is therefore the most important step in minimizing the incidence of awareness. Anaesthetists using TIVA must be familiar with the drugs, the technique and all equipment and disposables being used.

The following recommendations have been made to minimize the risks of awareness during TIVA.

1. An anti-reflux/non-return valve should always be used on the intravenous fluid infusion line when administering TIVA to prevent accumulation of drug in the fluid infusion tubing.
2. Sites of intravenous infusions should be visible so that they can be monitored for disconnection, leaks or subcutaneous leakage.
3. The anaesthetist must know how to use, and to check, the equipment before use.
4. Hospitals should give preference to purchasing intravenous connectors and valves which are clearly labelled.

Ancillary and Resuscitation Equipment

The patient's trolley, bed or operating table must be capable of being placed rapidly into a head-down position; as with all equipment, the anaesthetist must be familiar with the operating mechanism before anaesthesia starts.

A resuscitation trolley and defibrillator must be available in all locations where anaesthesia is given and checked regularly in accordance with local policies. Equipment and drugs for rarely encountered emergencies, such as malignant hyperthermia and local anaesthetic toxicity, must be available and checked regularly in accordance with local policies. The location of these must be clearly signed.

Machine Failure

In the event of failure, some modern anaesthetic workstations may default to little or no flow, or oxygen only with no vapour. The anaesthetist must know the default setting for the machine in use. Alternative means of oxygenation, ventilation and anaesthesia must be available.

'Shared Responsibility' Equipment

As a member of the theatre team, the anaesthetist has shared responsibility for the safe use of other equipment, e.g. diathermy, intermittent compression stockings, warming devices, cell salvage and tourniquets, and should have received appropriate training. Involvement with this equipment, especially 'troubleshooting' problems which arise intraoperatively, must not be allowed to distract anaesthetists from their primary role.

Recording and Audit

A clear note must be made in the patient's anaesthetic record that the anaesthetic machine check has been performed, that appropriate monitoring is in place and functional, and that the integrity, patency and safety of the whole breathing system has been assured. A logbook should also be kept with each anaesthetic machine to record the daily pre-session check and weekly check of the oxygen failure alarm. Modern anaesthesia workstations may record electronic self-tests internally. Such records should be retained for an appropriate time. Documentation of the routine checking and regular servicing of anaesthetic machines and patient breathing systems should be sufficient to permit audit on a regular basis.

Recovery

There must be clear departmental procedures for the daily and other checks of equipment which is used in recovery. This may also include pre-use checks of patient-controlled analgesia and epidural pumps, etc.

Emergencies

Some eventualities are unpredictable. There are many action plans available to guide anaesthetists during emergency situations, and these protocols, guidelines and action plans should be displayed prominently in the operating theatre suite.

Recovery Room/Post-Anaesthesia Care Unit

A recovery room or ward is an essential requirement in the operating theatre. All patients require close surveillance in the immediate postoperative period and, after major surgery or in vulnerable patients, for up to 24 h.

The recovery room should be an integral part of the operating theatre suite and should be located within the clean area. Department of Health guidelines suggest that there should be 1.5 places in the recovery area for each operating theatre, although a greater number may be required for surgery with a high turnover, e.g. gynaecology or day-case surgery. Each place requires a minimum floor area of approximately $10\,m^2$, and there must be sufficient space to move a patient without disturbing the others in the room.

It is appropriate for many patients to lie on a trolley in the recovery room, but beds should be available for those who are likely to stay for more than 30–45 min, e.g. patients who have undergone major surgery, or ASA (American Society of Anesthesiologists) grade III or IV patients who may require prolonged observation even after minor surgery. Each place should have piped oxygen and suction outlets on the wall, with an oxygen flowmeter and suction apparatus attached to a wall rail. Lighting should conform to the same standards as apply to the operating theatre, and additional spotlights should be provided. It is not common practice in the UK to monitor the electrocardiogram in all patients in the recovery ward, but oxygen saturation and blood pressure should be monitored routinely and the facility to monitor ECG and invasive arterial blood pressure should be available. Most large recovery areas have two or three places which are fully equipped with piped nitrous oxide, a mechanical ventilator and complete cardiovascular monitoring facilities.

An anaesthetic machine, a defibrillator, and equipment and drugs for resuscitation must be available in the recovery room. Oxygen is usually administered by disposable face mask, but each place should have a self-inflating resuscitation bag and anaesthetic mask.

Drug cupboards and storage space for equipment should be provided as well as dedicated telephones. Nursing staff spend most of their time with the patient, but require a nursing station at which notes may be written and from which wards can be contacted by telephone. At least one nurse is required for each three bed spaces. At present, specific training in the UK for recovery room nurses is somewhat haphazard. Student nurses may receive as little as 1 week of training in this area.

In many hospitals, it is possible to provide supervision of patients in the recovery ward for up to 24 h after major surgery, although it is now usual for patients who require close supervision for more than a few hours to be transferred to a high-dependency unit.

Clinical aspects of recovery room care are discussed in Chapter 40.

High-Dependency Unit

A high-dependency unit is an area for patients who require more invasive observation, treatment and nursing care than can be provided on a general ward. It would not normally accept patients requiring mechanical ventilation, but could manage those who require invasive monitoring. A survey conducted by the AAGBI in the 1990s indicated that many intensive care units admitted patients who could have been managed appropriately in a high-dependency unit. An unknown number of patients return from the recovery area to a general ward requiring monitoring or an intensity of nursing or medical care which cannot be provided safely in that location.

The facilities required to provide high-dependency care vary. Essential features are a high nurse-to-patient ratio, provision of piped oxygen and suction at every bed, and appropriate monitoring equipment. Protocols must be in place for admission and discharge criteria, and medical staffing must be clearly defined. In large hospitals, several units may be desirable, each dedicated to the care of specific groups of patients; in smaller hospitals, a single, multi-user unit may be more appropriate.

Procedure Rooms

With an increasing use of regional blocks as the sole mode of anaesthesia, many theatre suites now have dedicated 'block rooms.' These should be of the same standard as an anaesthetic room, with appropriate gas supplies, monitoring equipment and access to resuscitation facilities. Due consideration should be given to providing privacy in these rooms as more than one patient may be present at a time. Appropriate assistance for the anaesthetist must be present at all times.

Other Accommodation

Storage space is required for large items of equipment. In most modern operating theatre suites, instruments are sterilized in a separate department, which is not always on-site.

Near-patient testing of a variety of blood tests is now available and most theatre suites provide these in a single location. Arterial blood gas analysis and measurement of serum electrolyte concentrations is essential, especially if major surgery is to be undertaken, and if the equipment is not available in theatre then it should be readily available in an adjacent ITU.

The theatre coordinator needs adequate facilities for the smooth administration of theatres which should be accessible to non-theatre staff for the booking of cases and discussion of requirements.

Staff accommodation includes changing rooms and rest rooms. There should be facilities for staff to take their breaks. Theatre team leaders need office accommodation for their non-clinical time. Ideally, there should be a tutorial or seminar room for staff training. Some theatre suites incorporate offices for the anaesthetic department.

Other Anaesthetizing Locations

The anaesthetist is often required to work in areas outside the operating theatre suite. Many hospitals have peripheral theatres for some types of surgery, e.g. a self-contained day-case unit or treatment centre. In addition, patients may require anaesthesia in the emergency department, the radiology and radiotherapy departments or, in some instances (e.g. paediatric oncology), the side room of a ward. In these circumstances, where conditions are frequently not ideal, it is essential that the same precautions are taken as in the operating theatre suite to ensure that the identity of the patient and the nature of the proposed procedure are checked, that equipment is functioning correctly, that skilled help for the anaesthetist is available and that recovery facilities and staff are satisfactory. It is wise to avoid sending junior and inexperienced anaesthetists to these remote locations without direct senior supervision.

Ancillary Staff

Skilled and dedicated help should be available to the anaesthetist at all times. In the majority of hospitals in the UK, this is provided by operating department practitioners (ODPs), who undergo a 2-year training programme in recognized institutions and are required to sit examinations. In some hospitals, anaesthetic nurses assist the anaesthetist. It is important to differentiate between anaesthetic nurses and the nurse anaesthetists who are trained to deliver anaesthesia in some countries (e.g. CRNAs in the USA). The anaesthetic nurse performs essentially the same functions as the ODP. These include the following:

- Preparation and preliminary checking of equipment. It should be stressed that this does not absolve the anaesthetist from the responsibility of checking the equipment fully before an operating list is started.
- Alleviation of anxiety by reassurance and constant communication with the patient while awaiting anaesthesia.
- Checking the correct identity of the patient and participating in the WHO checklist procedures. It is the responsibility of the surgeon to ensure that the appropriate procedure is undertaken on the correct patient, but the anaesthetist must also confirm the identity of the patient and, as far as is possible, confirm that the surgeon is performing the correct operation. This is one of the many reasons why the anaesthetist must see every patient preoperatively.
- Preparation of intravenous infusions, cardiovascular monitoring transducers, etc.
- Assistance during anaesthesia, particularly during induction, when special manoeuvres such as cricoid pressure may be required, and after transfer to the operating theatre to assist in re-establishment of monitoring.
- Assistance in positioning the patient for local or regional blocks.
- Assistance in obtaining drugs or equipment if complications arise during anaesthesia.
- Assistance in the immediate postoperative period before the patient is transferred to the recovery room.

The ODP or anaesthetic nurse should never be left alone with an anaesthetized patient unless a dire emergency requires the anaesthetist's presence elsewhere.

Physicians' Assistants (Anaesthesia)

Physicians' assistants (anaesthesia) (PA(A)s) are fully trained professionals who have completed a specific postgraduate diploma. They work under the direction and supervision of a consultant anaesthetist at all times, often in a 2:1 model where one consultant supervises two theatres with a trainee and a PA(A) or two PA(A)s. They are allowed to provide anaesthesia without an anaesthetist present but overall responsibility for the care of the patient remains with the supervising consultant anaesthetist. Their role is to improve theatre utilization through reductions in theatre downtime, assisting with preoperative assessment and regional anaesthesia. However, for every case, the supervising consultant anaesthetist must:

- be present in the theatre suite, must be easily contactable and must be available to attend within 2 min of being requested to attend by the PA(A)
- be present in the anaesthetic room/operating theatre during induction of anaesthesia
- regularly review the intraoperative anaesthetic management
- be present during emergence from anaesthesia until the patient has been handed over safely to the recovery room staff
- remain in the theatre suite until control of airway reflexes has returned and artificial airway devices have been removed, or the ongoing care of the patient has been handed on to other appropriately qualified staff, e.g. in the intensive care unit.

Individual departments of anaesthesia are responsible for precise details of the scope of practice for PA(A)s. At present, they are not allowed to prescribe drugs but may administer drugs using locally developed patient-specific tools. At qualification, PA(A)s are not qualified to undertake regional anaesthesia, obstetric or paediatric practice or initial airway assessment/management of the acutely unwell or injured patient unless they are the first team members to arrive. Following extended training, PA(A)s have taken on some of these roles safely.

FURTHER READING

Association of Anaesthetists of Great Britain and Ireland, 2013. Immediate postanaesthetic recovery. AAGBI, London.

Association of Anaesthetists of Great Britain and Ireland, 2008. Infection control and anaesthesia 2. AAGBI, London.

Association of Anaesthetists of Great Britain and Ireland, 2012. Checking anaesthetic equipment 2012. AAGBI, London.

Boumphrey, S., Langton, J.A., 2003. Electrical safety in the operating theatre. BJA CEPD Reviews 3, 10.

Johnston, I.D.A., Hunter, A.R. (Eds.), 1984. The design and utilization of operating theatres. Edward Arnold, London.

Royal College of Anaesthetists, 2011. PA(A) supervision and limitation of scope of practice (May 2011 revision). http://www.rcoa.ac.uk/node/1927.

Spence, A.A., 1987. Environmental pollution by inhalation of anaesthetics. Br. J. Anaesth. 59, 96.

Taylor, T.H., Major, E. (Eds.), 1994. Hazards and complications of anaesthesia, second ed. Churchill Livingstone, Edinburgh.

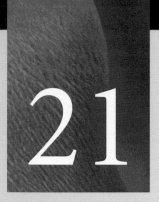

21

THE PRACTICAL CONDUCT OF ANAESTHESIA

T he conduct of anaesthesia is planned after details concerning the surgical procedure and the medical condition of the patient have been obtained at the preoperative visit. Preoperative assessment and selection of appropriate premedication are discussed in Chapter 17.

PREPARATION FOR ANAESTHESIA

Before starting, consideration should be given to induction and maintenance of anaesthesia, the position of the patient on the operating table, the equipment necessary for monitoring, the use of intravenous (i.v.) fluids or blood for infusion and the postoperative care and recovery facilities that will be required.

The anaesthetic machine must be tested before use for leaks, misconnections and proper function. A checklist, e.g. that published by the Association of Anaesthetists of Great Britain and Ireland (AAGBI 2004), is recommended. This is discussed in Chapter 20. The breathing system to be used should be new for each patient, or a new filter of appropriate size for each patient should be placed between the patient and the system, according to the AAGBI recommendations (2008).

The availability and function of all anaesthetic equipment should be checked before starting (see Table 21.1). The anaesthetist should be satisfied that the correct operation is being performed upon the correct patient and that consent has been given. Surgical Safety checklists are available for all the theatre team. The patient must be on a tilting bed or trolley and the anaesthetist should have a competent, trained assistant.

INDUCTION OF ANAESTHESIA

Anaesthesia is induced using one of the following techniques:

Inhalational Induction

The most common indications for inhalational induction of anaesthesia are listed in Table 21.2.

The proposed procedure should be explained to the patient before starting. A technique using a cupped hand around the fresh gas delivery tube may be preferred for young children, otherwise a face mask is used. The mask or hand is introduced *gradually* to the face from the side; the use of a transparent perfumed mask can render the procedure less unpleasant. While talking to the patient and encouraging normal breathing, the anaesthetist adjusts the mixture of the fresh gas flow and observes the patient's reactions. Initially, nitrous oxide 70% in oxygen is used and anaesthesia is deepened by the gradual introduction of increments of a volatile agent, e.g. sevoflurane which can can be increased up to an inspired concentration of 6%. Maintenance concentrations of isoflurane (1–2%) or sevoflurane (2–3%) are used when anaesthesia has been established.

A single-breath technique of inhalational induction has been advocated for patients who are able to cooperate. One vital capacity breath from a prefilled 4 L reservoir bag containing a high concentration of volatile agent (e.g. sevoflurane 8%) in oxygen (or nitrous oxide 50% in oxygen) results in smooth induction of anaesthesia within 20–30 s.

Observation of the colour of the patient's skin and pattern of ventilation, palpation of the peripheral

TABLE 21.1
Equipment Required for Tracheal Intubation

Correct size of laryngoscope and spare (in case of light failure)

Tracheal tube of correct size + an alternative smaller size

Tracheal tube connector

Wire stilette

Gum elastic bougies

Magill forceps

Cuff-inflating syringe

Artery forceps

Securing tape or bandage

Catheter mount(s)

Local anaesthetic spray – 4% lidocaine

Cocaine spray/gel for nasal intubation

Tracheal tube lubricant

Throat packs

Anaesthetic breathing system and face masks – tested with O_2 to ensure no leaks present

TABLE 21.2
Indications for Inhalational Induction

Young children

Upper airway obstruction, e.g. epiglottitis

Lower airway obstruction with foreign body

Bronchopleural fistula or empyema

No accessible veins

pulse, ECG and SpO_2 monitoring, and measurement of arterial pressure are important accompaniments to the technique of inhalational induction.

If spontaneous ventilation is to be maintained during the procedure, airway patency is ensured by use of an oropharyngeal airway, a laryngeal mask airway or a tracheal tube once anaesthesia has been established.

Complications and Difficulties

- Slower induction of anaesthesia
- Problems particularly during stage 2 of anaesthesia (see below)
- Airway obstruction, bronchospasm
- Laryngeal spasm, hiccups
- Environmental pollution.

Intravenous Induction

Induction of anaesthesia with an i.v. agent is suitable for most routine purposes and avoids many of the complications associated with the inhalational technique. It is the most appropriate method for rapid induction of the patient undergoing emergency surgery, in whom there is a risk of regurgitation of gastric contents. All drugs which may be required at induction should be prepared, and a cannula inserted into a suitable vein. The anaesthetist should wear rubber gloves for this and for other procedures such as airway manipulations and insertion of an airway or tracheal tube.

If an existing i.v. cannula is to be used, its function must be checked. Cannulae with a side injection port ('Venflon' type) are useful; large cannulae (e.g. 16G, 14G) are necessary for transfusion of fluids or blood. A vein in the forearm or on the back of the hand is preferable; veins in the antecubital fossa should be avoided because of the risks of intra-arterial injection and problems with elbow flexion. After selection of a suitable vein and skin preparation with 2% chlorhexidine in alcohol, subcutaneous local anaesthetic can be used . Alternatively, local anaesthetic cream ('EMLA' or 'Ametop') may have been applied preoperatively. Intravenous entry is confirmed and the cannula is secured firmly with tape. 'Opsite' or other specific cannula dressings may be used when long-term use is anticipated.

Patient monitors, including SpO_2, ECG and arterial pressure should be attached before induction of anaesthesia. Preoxygenation of the lungs may begin, using a close-fitting face mask and 100% oxygen delivered by a suitable breathing system for 5 min. Alternatively, three to four large (vital capacity) breaths may be used. Preoxygenation before routine elective induction of anaesthesia avoids transient hypoxaemia before establishment of effective lung ventilation.

Doses of the common i.v. agents are shown in Table 21.3. The induction dose varies with the patient's weight, age, state of nutrition, circulatory status, premedication and any concurrent medication. A small test dose is commonly administered and its effects are observed. Slow injection is recommended in the aged and in those with a slow circulation time (e.g. shock, hypovolaemia, cardiovascular disease) while the effects

TABLE 21.3
Intravenous Induction Agents

Agent	Induction Dose (mg kg^{-1})
Thiopental	3–5
Etomidate	0.3
Propofol	1.5–2.5
Ketamine	2

of the drug on the cardiovascular and respiratory systems are assessed.

A rapid-sequence induction technique is indicated for patients undergoing emergency surgery and for those with potential for vomiting or regurgitation. After i.v. induction, a rapid transition to stage 3 anaesthesia (see below) is achieved; this is maintained by the introduction of an inhalational agent or by repeated bolus injections or a continuous infusion of an i.v. anaesthetic agent. Emergency anaesthesia is discussed fully in Chapter 37.

Complications and Difficulties

Regurgitation and vomiting. If pharyngeal regurgitation occurs, the patient should be placed immediately into the Trendelenburg position and material aspirated with suction apparatus. Should inhalation of gastric contents occur, treatment is with 100% oxygen, bronchodilators and tracheal suction. Steroids and antibiotics are not routinely administered but may be considered. Continued IPPV may be required if the resultant pneumonitis is severe.

Intra-arterial injection of thiopental. This rare complication should nowadays be avoided by the appropriate choice of venous site and by checking the 'flashback' of blood on cannulation before injection. Pain and blanching in the hand and fingers occurs as a result of crystal formation in the capillaries. The cannula should be left in the artery and 40 mg papaverine injected with local anaesthetic (e.g. lidocaine 1% 5 mL). Further treatment includes stellate ganglion block, brachial plexus block or sympathetic block with i.v. guanethidine.

Perivenous injection. This causes blanching and pain and may result in a small degree of tissue necrosis. Propofol produces less tissue damage than thiopental. Hyaluronidase may be used to speed dispersal of the drug.

Cardiovascular depression. This is likely to occur particularly in the elderly, the hypovolaemic or the untreated hypertensive patient. Reducing the dose and speed of injection is essential in these patients. Infusion of i.v. fluid (e.g. 500 mL colloid or 1000 mL crystalloid solution) is usually successful in restoring arterial pressure but other agents e.g. ephedrine 3–12 mg i.v. may be required.

Respiratory depression. Slow injection of an induction agent can reduce the extent of respiratory depression. Respiratory adequacy must be assessed carefully and the anaesthetist should be ready to assist ventilation of the lungs if necessary.

Histamine release. Thiopental in particular may cause release of histamine with subsequent formation of typical wheals. Severe reactions may occur to individual agents, and appropriate drugs and fluids should be available in the anaesthetic room for treatment. Guidelines for emergency management of acute major anaphylaxis are available (AAGBI) and may be displayed in the anaesthetic room. This is discussed further in Chapter 43.

Porphyria. An acute porphyric episode may be precipitated by barbiturates in susceptible individuals.

Other complications. Pain on injection (especially with etomidate or propofol), hiccup or dystonic muscular movements may occur. The use of lidocaine 10–40 mg per 20 mL propofol 1% reduces the incidence of pain on injection.

POSITION OF PATIENT FOR SURGERY

After induction of anaesthesia, the patient is placed on the operating table in a position appropriate for the proposed surgery. When positioning the patient, the anaesthetist should take into account surgical access, patient safety, anaesthetic technique, monitoring and position of i.v. cannulae, etc.

Some commonly used positions are shown in Figure 21.1. Each may have adverse effects in terms of skeletal, neurological, ventilatory and circulatory effects.

The lithotomy position may result in nerve damage on the medial or lateral side of the leg from pressure exerted by the stirrups, which must be well padded. Care must be taken to elevate both legs simultaneously

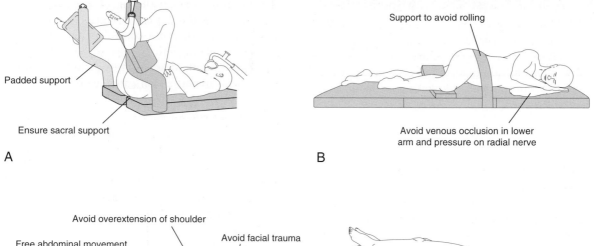

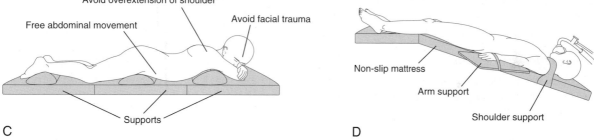

FIGURE 21.1 ■ Positions on the operating table. **(A)** Lithotomy position. **(B)** Lateral position. **(C)** Prone position. **(D)** Trendelenburg position.

so that pelvic asymmetry and resultant backache are avoided. The sacrum should be supported and not allowed to slip off the end of the operating table.

The lateral position may result in asymmetrical lung ventilation. Care is required with arm position and i.v. infusions. The pelvis and shoulders must be supported to prevent the patient from rolling either backwards (with a risk of falling from the table) or forwards into the recovery position.

The prone position may cause abdominal compression which may result in ventilatory and circulatory embarrassment. To prevent this, support must be provided beneath the shoulders and iliac crests. Excessive extension of the shoulders should be avoided. The face, and particularly the eyes, must be protected from external pressure or trauma. The tracheal tube must be secured firmly in place as it is almost impossible to reinsert it with the patient in this position.

The Trendelenburg position may produce upward pressure on the diaphragm because of the weight of the abdominal contents. Damage to the brachial plexus may occur as a result of pressure from shoulder supports, especially if the arms are abducted.

The sitting position requires careful support of the head. In addition, venous pooling and resultant cardiovascular instability may occur.

The supine position carries the risk of the supine hypotensive syndrome during pregnancy (see Ch 35) or in patients with a large abdominal mass.

Positioning during anaesthesia is discussed extensively by Martin & Warner (1997).

MAINTENANCE OF ANAESTHESIA

Anaesthesia may be continued using inhalational agents, i.v. anaesthetic agents or i.v. opioids either alone or in combination. Tracheal intubation with or without muscle relaxants may be used. Regional anaesthesia may be used to supplement any of these techniques to achieve the components of the familiar anaesthetic triad of sleep, neuromuscular relaxation and analgesia.

Inhalational Anaesthesia with Spontaneous Ventilation

This is an appropriate form of maintenance for superficial body surgery, minor procedures which produce little reflex or painful stimulation and operations for which profound neuromuscular blockade is not required.

Conduct

After induction of anaesthesia, nitrous oxide 67% in oxygen and a volatile agent is used in the patient breathing spontaneously. Depending on the nature of surgery, the use of analgesia in premedication (if used), and the patient's response (assessed by observation of ventilation, circulation and heart rate and rhythm), the volatile agent is used in an inspired concentration of isoflurane 1–2%, sevoflurane 2–3%, or desflurane 3–6%.

Minimum Alveolar Concentration

Minimum alveolar concentration (MAC) is the minimum alveolar concentration of an inhaled anaesthetic agent which prevents reflex movement in response to surgical incision in 50% of subjects. MAC values of commonly used inhalational agents are shown in Appendix C. MAC varies little with metabolic factors but is reduced by opioid medication and in the presence of hypothermia. MAC is higher in neonates and is reduced in the elderly (see Ch 2). The effects of inhalational anaesthetics are additive: thus 1 MAC-equivalent could be achieved by producing an alveolar concentration of 70% nitrous oxide (0.67 MAC) and 0.4% isoflurane (0.33 MAC).

The rate at which MAC is attained may be increased by raising the inspired concentration and by avoidance of airway obstruction. Increasing ventilation at a constant inspired concentration produces more rapid equilibration between inspired and alveolar concentrations. The time taken for equilibration increases with the blood/gas solubility coefficient of the agent; those with a high blood/gas solubility coefficient (e.g. halothane) do not reach equilibrium for several hours (see Ch 2). It follows, therefore, that the inspired concentration must be considerably higher than MAC to produce an adequate alveolar concentration when such agents are used.

Control of the depth of anaesthesia to achieve adequacy without overdose by varying the inspired concentration of volatile agent requires constant assessment of the patient's reaction to anaesthesia and surgery. This rapid control is one of the main advantages of inhalational anaesthesia. The signs of inadequate depth of anaesthesia include tachypnoea, tachycardia, hypertension and sweating.

Signs of Anaesthesia

Guedel's classic signs of anaesthesia are those seen in patients premedicated with morphine and atropine and breathing ether in air. The clinical signs associated with anaesthesia produced by other inhalational agents follow a similar course, but the divisions between the stages and planes are less precise (Fig. 21.2).

Stage 1: the stage of analgesia. This is the stage attained when using nitrous oxide 50% in oxygen, as used in the technique of relative analgesia (see Ch 29).

Stage 2: stage of excitement. This is seen with inhalational induction, but is passed rapidly during i.v. induction. Respiration is erratic, breath-holding may occur, laryngeal and pharyngeal reflexes are active and stimulation of pharynx or larynx, e.g. by insertion of a Guedel or laryngeal mask airway, may produce laryngeal spasm. The eyelash reflex (used as a sign of unconsciousness with i.v. induction) is abolished in stage 2, but the eyelid reflex (resistance to elevation of eyelid) remains present.

Stage 3: surgical anaesthesia. This deepens through four planes (in practice, three – light, medium, deep) with increasing concentration of anaesthetic drug. Respiration assumes a rhythmic pattern and the thoracic component diminishes with depth of anaesthesia. Respiratory reflexes become suppressed but the carinal reflex is abolished only at plane IV (therefore, a tracheal tube which is too long may produce carinal stimulation at an otherwise adequate depth). The pupils are central and gradually enlarge with depth of anaesthesia. Lacrimation is active in light planes but absent in planes III and IV – a useful sign in a patient not premedicated with an anticholinergic.

Stage 4: stage of impending respiratory and circulatory failure. Brainstem reflexes are depressed by the high anaesthetic concentration. Pupils are enlarged and unreactive. The patient should not be permitted to reach this stage. Withdrawal of the anaesthetic agents and administration of 100% oxygen lightens anaesthesia.

STAGE	RESPIRATION	PUPILS	EYE REFLEXES	URT & RESPIRATORY REFLEXES
1 Analgesia	Regular Small volume	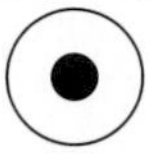		
2 Excitement	Irregular	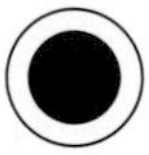	Eyelash absent	
3 Anaesthesia Plane I	Regular Large volume	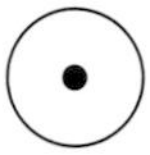	Eyelid absent Conjunctival depressed	Pharyngeal & vomiting depressed
Plane II	Regular Large volume	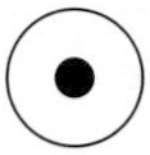	Corneal depressed	
Plane III	Regular Becoming diaphragmatic Small volume	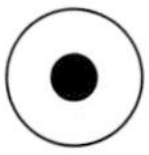		Laryngeal depressed
Plane IV	Irregular Diaphragmatic Small volume	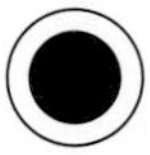		Carinal depressed
4 Overdose	Apnoea	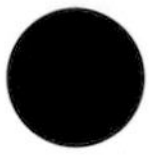		

FIGURE 21.2 ■ Stages of anaesthesia (modified from Guedel).

Observation of other reflexes provides a guide to depth of anaesthesia. Swallowing occurs in the light plane of stage 3. The gag reflex is abolished in upper stage 3. Stretching of the anal sphincter produces reflex laryngospasm even at plane III of stage 3.

Complications and Difficulties

Airway obstruction. This is relieved by appropriate positioning and the use of airway equipment (see below).

Laryngeal spasm. This may occur above light-medium planes of stage 3 as a result of stimulation. Treatment is to stop the stimulation and gently deepen anaesthesia. If spasm is severe, 100% oxygen is applied with the face mask held tightly, while the airway is maintained by hand and pressure is applied to the reservoir bag. Attempts to ventilate the patient's lungs usually result only in gastric inflation. However, as the larynx partially opens, 100% oxygen flows

through under pressure. Further gentle deepening of anaesthesia may then take place. In severe laryngeal spasm, i.v. succinylcholine may be required, and after the lungs have been inflated with oxygen it is advisable to intubate the trachea.

Bronchospasm. This may occur if volatile anaesthetic agents are introduced rapidly, particularly in smokers or those with excessive bronchial secretions. Humidification and warming of gases may minimize the problem. Bronchospasm may accompany laryngospasm. Administration of bronchodilators may be required. This complication occurs readily in the presence of or shortly after a respiratory tract infection.

Malignant hyperthermia. Volatile agents, succinylcholine or amide-type local anaesthetic agents may trigger this syndrome in susceptible individuals (see Ch 43).

Raised intracranial pressure (ICP). All volatile agents may produce an increase in ICP and this is accentuated by retention of CO_2 which accompanies the use of volatile agents in the spontaneously breathing patient. A spontaneous ventilation technique is therefore contraindicated in patients with an intracranial space-occupying lesion or cerebral oedema.

Atmospheric pollution. The use of the appropriate scavenging apparatus helps to reduce levels of theatre pollution by volatile and gaseous agents (see Ch 20).

Delivery of Inhalational Agents – Airway Maintenance

Maintenance of the airway is one of the most important of the anaesthetist's tasks. Inhalational agents may be delivered via a face mask, a laryngeal mask airway (LMA) or another supraglottic airway device (SAD), or a tracheal tube.

Use of the Face Mask. Inhalational anaesthesia usually involves the use of a face mask. The face mask has many variants of type and size, and selection of the correct fit is important to provide a gas-tight seal.

For children, a mask with excessive dead space should be avoided. The patient's head position during mask anaesthesia is important; the mandible is held 'into' the mask by the anaesthetist using a bony contact point rather than pressing into the soft tissues, which may result in airway obstruction (especially in children). The mandible is held forward, helping to prevent posterior movement of the tongue and obstruction of the airway.

The importance of observation of the airway during mask anaesthesia cannot be overemphasized. Soft tissue indrawing in the suprasternal and supraclavicular areas is evidence of upper airway obstruction. Noisy ventilation or inspiratory stridor provides further evidence that airway obstruction is present and requires rapid correction. Maintenance of the airway may be assisted further by the use of an oropharyngeal (Guedel) airway. An appropriate stage of anaesthesia must be reached before insertion of the airway as stimulation of the pharynx at stage 2 or at light stage 3 produces coughing, laryngospasm or breath-holding. The use of local anaesthetic spray or jelly to coat the airway may permit its insertion at an earlier stage. A nasopharyngeal airway may be better tolerated.

The face mask is used in current practice only before tracheal intubation or insertion of the laryngeal mask or during short non-invasive procedures, e.g. dental anaesthesia and orthopaedic manipulations. To ensure patency of the airway, other airway adjuncts such as an oropharyngeal or a nasopharyngeal airway may be used.

Use of the Laryngeal Mask Airway and Other Supraglottic Airway Devices

INDICATIONS

- To provide a clear airway without the need for the anaesthetist's hands to support a face mask.
- To avoid the use of tracheal intubation during spontaneous ventilation.
- In a case of difficult intubation, to facilitate subsequent insertion of a tracheal tube via the intubating LMA.

CONTRAINDICATIONS

- A patient with a 'full stomach' or with any condition leading to delayed gastric emptying.
- A patient in whom the risk of regurgitation of gastric contents into the oesophagus is increased (e.g. hiatus hernia).
- Where surgical access (e.g. to the pharynx) is impeded by the cuff of the LMA.

Conduct of LMA insertion. An appropriate depth of anaesthesia is required for successful insertion of the LMA. Fewer difficulties are encountered after i.v. induction of anaesthesia with propofol than with thiopental because of the greater tendency of the former to suppress pharyngeal reflexes. The appropriate size of LMA is chosen according to the weight of the patient (Table 21.4). In general, the largest size possible is used to create a seal with a cuff inflation less than

TABLE 21.4		
Laryngeal Mask Airway Sizes		
Mask Size	*Patient Weight (kg)*	*Cuff Volume (mL)*
1	<5	2–5
1.5	5–10	5–7
2	10–20	7–10
2.5	20–30	12–14
3	>30	15–20
4	n/a	25–30
5	n/a	35–40

After Brimacombe et al. 1996

the maximum. In adults, the larger sizes are used according to inspection. The patient's head is extended, the mouth is opened and, if necessary, the mandible can be held down by an assistant. The LMA cuff is evacuated and the LMA is inserted into the pharynx in a direction along the axis of the hard palate so that the cuff encounters the posterior pharyngeal wall and is swept distally into the laryngopharynx. This may be assisted by use of the gloved fingers in the 'classic' technique. The cuff then lies posterior to the larynx. Air is injected into the cuff and the breathing system is attached via a catheter mount to the 22-mm proximal connector. The LMA is secured in place with tape or a bandage after confirmation of correct placement by observation of movement of the reservoir bag, or of the chest after a gentle manual inflation of the lungs. The reinforced LMA may be useful when the standard LMA may hinder surgical access or be prone to kinking.

Alternative SADs comprise the Igel, Pro-seal LMA, supreme LMA (SLMA), and the intubating LMA (ILMA) which may be used to facilitate tracheal intubation. These are described in Chapter 15. The anaesthetist should gain clinical experience with these types in order to appreciate the differences in insertion technique from that of the classic LMA.

Tracheal Intubation

Indications

- Provision of a clear airway, e.g. anticipated difficulty in using mask anaesthesia in the edentulous patient.
- An 'unusual' and prolonged position, e.g. prone or sitting. A reinforced non-kinking tube may be necessary.
- Operations on the head and neck, e.g. ENT, dental. A nasotracheal tube may be required.
- Protection of the respiratory tract, e.g. from blood during upper respiratory tract or oral surgery and from inhalation of gastric contents in emergency surgery or patients with oesophageal obstruction. The use of a cuffed tube for adults is mandatory in these circumstances.
- During anaesthesia using IPPV and muscle relaxants.
- To facilitate suction of the respiratory tract.
- During thoracic operations.

Contraindications. There are few contraindications. In emergency situations, hypoxaemia must be relieved if at all possible before insertion of a tracheal tube.

Preparation

Before starting, the anaesthetist must check the availability and function of the necessary equipment. He or she should have a 'dedicated', trained, experienced assistant. Laryngoscopes of the correct size are chosen and the function of bulb and batteries checked, the patency of the tracheal tube is checked and the integrity of the cuff ensured. Various aids to intubation must also be present (see Table 21.1).

Choice of Equipment

Laryngoscopes. Laryngoscopes are manufactured in many shapes and sizes. There are two basic types of blade – straight or curved. Straight-blade laryngoscopes (e.g. Magill) are favoured for children, in whom the epiglottis is floppy, and are designed to pass posterior to the epiglottis and to lift it anteriorly, exposing the larynx. The curved blade (e.g. Macintosh) is designed so that the tip lies anterior to the epiglottis in the vallecula, pressing on the hyoepiglottic ligament and moving it anteriorly to expose the larynx and vocal cords (Fig. 21.3). The McCoy blade incorporates a movable distal tip to facilitate a view of the glottis in appropriate patients.

Tracheal Tubes. Modern tracheal tubes are disposable and made from PVC which is 'implant tested' for its inert effect upon the tissues. In some circumstances, e.g. head and neck or throat surgery, the tracheal tube may be subject to direct or indirect pressure and standard tubes may kink or become compressed. It may be appropriate to use a tube which is reinforced with a nylon or steel spiral in such cases. Tracheal tubes are introduced usually through the mouth, although it may be preferable to pass the tube through the nose, particularly for oral surgery. The supplied length of disposable tubes exceeds that required normally for oral intubation and the tube should be cut to the appropriate length before use. During thoracic surgery, it may be necessary to ventilate the lungs independently and a bronchial tube, bronchial blocker or double-lumen tube is required (see Ch 33).

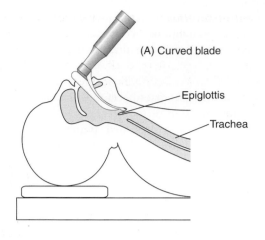

(A) Curved blade

Epiglottis

Trachea

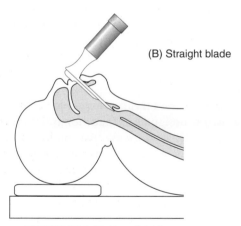

(B) Straight blade

FIGURE 21.3 ■ Use of the laryngoscope.

In order to seal the airway, most tracheal tubes are manufactured with an inflatable cuff at the distal end. The cuff may be of low or high volume; low-volume cuffs produce a seal over a smaller area of tracheal mucosa and tend to exert a high pressure on the mucosal cells, reducing the capillary blood supply and rendering the cells potentially ischaemic. High-volume cuffs cover a wide area of mucosa; the pressure exerted varies during the respiratory cycle, but on average is lower than that produced by a low-volume cuff. A medium-volume, low-profile cuffed tube represents a compromise and has some practical advantages.

Tracheal tubes of different sizes are required. The size quoted is the internal diameter (ID). Adult males normally require a tube of 9–9.5 mm ID and females

8–8.5 mm ID. For oral intubation, the tube should normally be 20–23 cm in length. The appropriate internal diameter of tube for paediatric use may be calculated from the following formula: (age/4)+4 mm. This is an approximation and a tube 0.5 mm smaller and 0.5 mm larger should also be prepared. The length of tube required for oral intubation in children is approximately equal to (age/2)+12 cm. A tube of slightly smaller ID may be required for nasal intubation and its length may be calculated from the formula (age/2)+15 cm.

An appropriate connector is required between the tracheal tube and the anaesthetic breathing system, e.g. curved connector for nasal tube, lightweight plastic with low dead space for children or a connector with a suction port for thoracic surgery. It is important before use to ensure the patency of breathing system connectors and the absence of foreign material occluding the lumen; vulnerable components of the breathing system should remain wrapped until just before their use.

Anaesthesia for Tracheal Intubation

Tracheal intubation may be performed under local anaesthesia (using topical spray, transtracheal spray and superior laryngeal nerve block) or under general anaesthesia (either i.v. or inhalation, with or without the use of muscle relaxation). The usual approach is to provide general anaesthesia and muscle relaxation, to perform laryngoscopy and direct vision intubation and then to maintain anaesthesia via the tracheal tube with spontaneous or controlled ventilation.

Inhalational Technique for Intubation. Adequate depth of anaesthesia is necessary to depress the laryngeal reflexes and provide a degree of relaxation of the laryngeal and pharyngeal muscles. Sevoflurane 8% provides rapid attainment of the necessary depth, which can be judged from the pattern of respiration with predominance of diaphragmatic breathing (a useful sign in children is the 'dissociation' of the thoracic and abdominal excursion). The mask is removed and laryngoscopy and intubation performed. The anaesthetic circuit is then connected to the tracheal tube and anaesthesia maintained at a depth appropriate for surgery.

Relaxant Anaesthesia for Intubation. After i.v. or inhalational induction of anaesthesia, the short-acting depolarizing muscle relaxant succinylcholine may be used to provide relaxation for tracheal intubation. After loss of consciousness, the patient breathes 100% oxygen or 50% nitrous oxide in oxygen and succinylcholine is administered in a dose of $1–1.5\,mg\,kg^{-1}$. Assisted ventilation is maintained via the face mask until muscle relaxation occurs (except in emergency patients and those likely to regurgitate) and laryngoscopy and intubation are performed. Inhalational anaesthesia may be continued with manual ventilation until the effects of the relaxant have ceased, whereupon spontaneous ventilation is resumed. Alternatively, non-depolarizing neuromuscular blockade is produced and ventilation controlled.

Conduct of Laryngoscopy

The position of the patient's head and neck is important. The neck should be flexed and the head extended with the support of a pillow; thus, the oral, pharyngeal and tracheal axes are brought into alignment (Fig. 21.4). The laryngoscope is designed for left-hand use and is introduced into the right side of the mouth while the right hand opens the mouth, parting the lips to avoid interposing them between laryngoscope and teeth. The teeth may be protected from blade trauma with the fingers or the use of a plastic 'guard'. The laryngoscope blade deflects the tongue to the left and the length of the blade is passed over the contour of the tongue. The laryngoscope is lifted upwards and forwards, avoiding a levering movement which can damage the upper anterior teeth. Using a straight blade, the tip is passed posterior to the epiglottis, which is lifted anteriorly, and the vocal cords are seen. With a curved blade, the tip is inserted into the vallecula and

pressure on the hyoepiglottic ligament moves the epiglottis to expose the vocal cords. External pressure on the thyroid cartilage by an assistant may aid laryngeal vision at this stage. Alternatively, using the McCoy adaptation of the Macintosh blade, the distal lever may be used to elevate the epiglottis to assist in viewing the larynx.

Conduct of Intubation

After laryngeal visualization, the supraglottic area and cords may be sprayed, if required, with local anaesthetic solution (lidocaine 4%). The tracheal tube is passed from the right side of the mouth (which may be held open by the assistant's finger if necessary, permitting a clear view of the midline) and between the vocal cords into the trachea until the cuff is below the vocal cords. A semirigid stilette may be used during intubation to provide the correct degree of curvature of the tracheal tube to facilitate intubation. This is useful particularly with reinforced tubes.

The tube cuff is inflated sufficiently to abolish audible gas leaks on inflation of the lungs. The correct position of the tube must now be confirmed. If the tube has been seen clearly at laryngoscopy to pass through the vocal cords into the trachea, then equal movement of both sides of the chest during ventilation should be confirmed and auscultation in each axilla for breath sounds should be performed to ensure that the tip of the tracheal tube has not passed too far distally to enter, or occlude, one of the main bronchi (see Ch 43); if there is unilateral air entry, the tube should be withdrawn slowly and carefully until air entry is equal in both lungs. If the tube has not been seen clearly to enter the trachea, or if there is any reason to suspect that its distal end is not in the trachea, then the steps outlined in Chapter 43 must be undertaken immediately to identify possible oesophageal intubation.

After its correct position has been determined, the tube is secured with cotton tape, bandage or sticking plaster strips. Correct fixation of the tube is important, particularly if the head is inaccessible during surgery, e.g. when the patient is in the prone position. On such occasions, extra security is gained using broad 'elastoplast' strapping over the primary fixing tape on the patient's face.

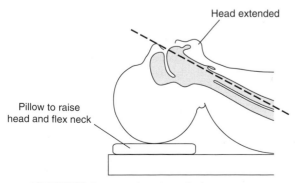

Head extended

Pillow to raise head and flex neck

FIGURE 21.4 ■ Head position for laryngoscopy.

Nasal Intubation

Nasal intubation may be used for dental operations, ENT operations, etc., and may be preferred for long-term intubation because it provides easier tube fixation, easier oral toilet and greater patient comfort.

A slightly smaller tube is used and is introduced preferentially into the right nostril, as the left-facing bevel of the tube favours this approach. The tube is passed along the floor of the nose and advanced *gently* into the pharynx, avoiding excessive force. Laryngoscopy takes place and the tube is advanced into the trachea by manipulation of the proximal end or by grasping the distal tip with Magill's intubating forceps to pass it between the cords.

Packing of the throat may be used after intubation, especially for oropharyngeal operations. The moist gauze pack is introduced using the laryngoscope and Magill forceps. The pharynx should be packed on each side of the tracheal tube. The pack should be applied gently to avoid abrasion of the mucosa. A 'tail' of the pack is left protruding from the mouth and the anaesthetist must accept responsibility for removal of the pack before extubation. A latex 'foam' pack may be used as an alternative to cotton gauze.

Difficult Intubation

The incidence of difficult intubation is reported as being one in 65 patients. In practice, most cases represent difficulty with laryngoscopy. Poor management of difficult intubation is a significant cause of anaesthetic morbidity and mortality. Sequelae include dental and airway trauma, pulmonary aspiration and hypoxaemia.

Aetiology. Table 21.5 shows the common causes of difficult intubation. The single most important cause is an inexperienced or inadequately prepared anaesthetist, often complicated by equipment malfunction. There are numerous causes of difficult laryngoscopy related to patient factors. The anatomical features associated with difficult laryngoscopy are listed in Table 21.6. Of these, the atlanto-occipital distance is the best predictor of difficulty but requires an X-ray examination. Many of these factors are normal anatomical variations; they may also be congenital or acquired.

Congenital. Many syndromes are associated with multiple anatomical abnormalities such as a small mouth, large tongue and cleft palate. Patients with encephalocele, cystic hygroma and hydrocephalus may have restricted head or jaw movement. Morquio and Down syndromes are associated with cervical spine instability.

Acquired. Acquired factors may affect jaw opening, neck movement or the airway itself. Reduced jaw movement is a common cause of difficult laryngoscopy. Trauma and infection may cause reflex spasm of the masseter and medial pterygoid muscles (trismus). This occurs typically with dental abscess or mandibular fractures and is usually relaxed by anaesthetic agents. In contrast, the reduced jaw movement associated with temporomandibular joint fibrosis is usually fixed. This may complicate chronic infection, rheumatoid arthritis, ankylosing spondylitis and radiotherapy. Any local soft tissue swelling or mass may also reduce jaw movement.

Reduced head and neck movement is an important cause of difficult laryngoscopy. Optimal positioning for laryngoscopy requires extension of the head at the atlanto-occipital joint; this joint may be damaged in patients with rheumatoid arthritis, osteoarthritis and ankylosing spondylitis. Cervical spine movement may be reduced by surgical fusion, fibrosis and soft tissue swellings of the head and neck. Cervical spine instability (e.g. fractures, tumours, rheumatoid arthritis) makes neck movement undesirable.

Disorders of the airway itself may pose a serious threat to ventilation in addition to preventing normal laryngoscopy. Soft tissue oedema of the face/upper airway from dental abscess, other infections, drug hypersensitivity, burns and trauma may cause considerable anatomical distortion with life-threatening airway obstruction. Foreign bodies, tumours and scarring after infection, burns and radiotherapy may also cause difficult laryngoscopy. Vocal cord apposition from recurrent laryngeal nerve palsy can hinder passage of the tracheal tube through the larynx. Positioning of the tracheal tube in the trachea may be difficult if there is compression or deviation caused by thyroid tumours, haematoma (traumatic, surgical) and thymic or lymph node tumours. Other rare disorders include vascular rings and laryngotracheomalacia. In clinical practice, the cause of difficult laryngoscopy is often multifactorial, for example in patients with morbid obesity, pregnancy and rheumatoid arthritis.

TABLE 21.5
Common Causes of Difficult Intubation

Anaesthetist
Inadequate preoperative assessment
Inadequate equipment preparation
Inexperience
Poor technique

Equipment
Malfunction
Unavailability
No trained assistant

Patient

Congenital	Syndromes (Down, Pierre Robin, Treacher Collins, Marfan's) Achondroplasia Cystic hygroma Encephalocele	
Acquired	Reduced jaw movement	Trismus (abscess/infection, fracture, tetanus) Fibrosis (postinfection/radiotherapy/ trauma) Rheumatoid arthritis, ankylosing spondylitis Tumours Jaw wiring
	Reduced neck movement	Rheumatoid/osteoarthritis Ankylosing spondylitis Cervical fracture/instability/fusion
	Airway	Oedema (abscess/infection, trauma, angio-oedema, burns) Compression (goitre, surgical haemorrhage) Scarring (radiotherapy, infection, burns) Tumours/polyps Foreign body Nerve palsy
	Others	Morbid obesity Pregnancy Acromegaly

Management. *Preoperative assessment.* Preoperative examination of the airway (Table 21.7) is essential. Identifying patients with a potentially difficult airway (see Tables 21.5 and 21.6) allows time for planning an appropriate anaesthetic technique. Previous anaesthetic records should always be consulted. However, a past record of normal tracheal intubation is no guarantee for future anaesthesia as airway anatomy may be altered. Pregnancy is a common example. The presence of stridor or a hoarse voice is a warning sign

for the anaesthetist. As it is impossible to identify all patients with a difficult airway during preoperative assessment, the anaesthetist must be prepared to manage the unexpected difficult laryngoscopy.

Many additional clinical tests to predict difficult laryngoscopy have been described. None of these tests is totally reliable, but their use may complement routine examination of the airway. The 'Mallampati' test is a widely used and simple classification of the pharyngeal view obtained during maximal mouth opening and

TABLE 21.6
Anatomical Factors Associated with Difficult Laryngoscopy

Short, muscular neck

Protruding incisors (buck teeth)

Long, high arched palate

Receding lower jaw

Poor mobility of mandible

Increased anterior depth of mandible

Increased posterior depth of mandible (reduces jaw opening, requires X-ray)

Decreased atlanto-occipital distance (reduces neck extension, requires X-ray)

TABLE 21.7
Preoperative Assessment of the Airway

General appearance of neck, face, maxilla and mandible

Jaw movement

Head extension and neck movement

Teeth and oropharynx

Soft tissue of neck

Recent chest and cervical spine X-rays

Previous anaesthetic records

tongue protrusion (Fig. 21.5). In practice, this test suggests a higher incidence of difficult laryngoscopy if the posterior pharyngeal wall is not seen. The predictive value of this test may be strengthened if the thyromental distance (thyroid cartilage prominence to the bony point of the chin during full head extension) is less than 6.5 cm. The Mallampati classification correlates with the view obtained at laryngoscopy (Fig. 21.6). The difficulty associated with a 'grade 3' laryngoscopy may usually be overcome by posterior laryngeal displacement and/or the use of a suitable bougie. A patient whose epiglottis is not visible at laryngoscopy ('grade 4') usually has obvious preoperative anatomical abnormalities. Management of these patients requires the use of special techniques such as fibreoptic laryngoscopy (see Ch 15).

Preoperative preparation. Premedication with an antisialagogue reduces airway secretions. This is advantageous before inhalational induction and essential for awake fibreoptic laryngoscopy to maximize the effectiveness of topical local anaesthesia. An anxiolytic may also be given but is contraindicated in patients with airway obstruction. The presence of a trained assistant is essential and the availability of an experienced anaesthetist and a special 'difficult intubation' trolley with a range of equipment such as bougies, laryngoscopes and tracheal tubes is desirable.

Regional anaesthesia. This should be used wherever possible in patients with a difficult airway although the patient, anaesthetist and equipment must be prepared for general anaesthesia should a complication arise.

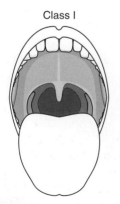
Class I

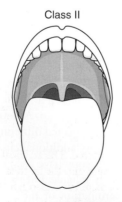
Class II

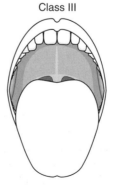
Class III

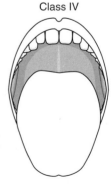
Class IV

FIGURE 21.5 ■ Classification of the pharyngeal view when performing the Mallampati test. The patient must fully extend the tongue during maximal mouth opening. Class I: pharyngeal pillars, soft palate, uvula visible. Class II: only soft palate, uvula visible. Class III: only soft palate visible. Class IV: soft palate not visible.

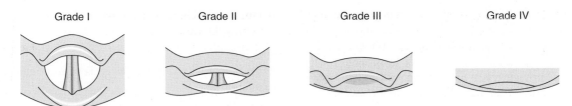

FIGURE 21.6 ■ Grading of the laryngoscopic view. Grade I: vocal cords visible. Grade II: arytenoid cartilages and posterior part of vocal cords visible. Grade III: epiglottis visible. Grade IV: epiglottis not visible. Note: the pharyngeal view (Fig. 21.5) is a clinical guide to the likely laryngoscopic view.

General anaesthesia. Unless tracheal intubation is essential for airway protection or to facilitate muscle relaxation and ventilation, the use of an artificial airway such as the laryngeal mask with spontaneous ventilation is a safe technique. If intubation is essential, the appropriate anaesthetic technique depends on the anticipated degree of difficulty, the presence of airway obstruction and the risk of regurgitation and aspiration. There is no place for the use of a long-acting neuromuscular blocker to facilitate intubation where difficulty is anticipated. Correct positioning of the head and neck is essential and the lungs should be preoxygenated after cannulation of a vein and appropriate monitoring. The safest anaesthetic technique may usually be chosen from the following clinical examples:

1. *Patients with an increased risk of regurgitation and aspiration (e.g. full stomach, intra-abdominal pathology, pregnancy).* An inhalational induction is inappropriate in these patients. Regional anaesthesia is preferable in the parturient (see Ch 35). Preoxygenation and a rapid sequence induction with succinylcholine can be used if there is little anticipated difficulty. If intubation is unsuccessful, no further doses of neuromuscular blocking drug should be used, the patient allowed to wake and further assistance sought. If there is a high degree of anticipated difficulty, an awake technique is recommended (see below).

2. *Patients with little anticipated difficulty and no airway obstruction (e.g. mild reduction of jaw or neck movement).* After a sleep dose of intravenous induction agent and confirmation of the ability to ventilate the lungs manually by mask, succinylcholine may be given to provide the best conditions for tracheal intubation. If difficulty is encountered, the patient is allowed to wake up and the procedure replanned. Where appropriate, anaesthesia is deepened by spontaneous ventilation using a volatile agent and alternative techniques to facilitate tracheal intubation used (see below).

3. *Patients with severe anticipated difficulty and no airway obstruction (e.g. severe reduction of jaw or neck movement).* Appropriate techniques include inhalational induction with sevoflurane or the use of fibreoptic laryngoscopy either in the awake patient or after inhalational induction. Neuromuscular blocking drugs must not be used until the ability to ventilate the lungs manually and view the vocal cords is confirmed.

4. *Patients with airway obstruction (e.g. burns, infection, trauma).* An inhalational induction may be used; otherwise an awake technique should be considered. Neuromuscular blocking drugs should not be used until tracheal intubation is confirmed.

5. *Extreme clinical situations.* Tracheostomy performed under local anaesthesia may be the safest technique.

Inhalational Induction. Premedication with an antisialagogue is desirable. Depth of anaesthesia is increased carefully by spontaneous ventilation of increasing concentrations of a volatile agent in 100% oxygen until laryngoscopy may be performed safely. Halothane may still be the agent of choice for this purpose. If the larynx is viewed easily intubation may be performed with or without succinylcholine. If the view is limited, the use of a suitable bougie assists passage of the tracheal tube through the larynx. This is confirmed by detecting tracheal rings or resistance when the smaller bronchi are encountered. The tracheal tube is then 'railroaded' over the bougie into the trachea, often made easier by rotating the tracheal tube through 90° in an anticlockwise direction to align the bevel as it passes through the larynx. If this is unsuccessful, anaesthesia may be maintained and the use of fibre-optic laryngoscopy can be considered.

Awake Intubation. Fibreoptic laryngoscopy and intubation require special equipment, skill and time. The procedure may be performed by the nasal or oral route after topical anaesthesia is achieved by spraying the nasal and oropharyngeal mucosa and/or gargling viscous preparations. The injection of 3–5 mL of lidocaine 2% through the cricothyroid membrane induces coughing and anaesthetizes the tracheal and laryngeal mucosa. Conventional laryngoscopy may also be performed in awake patients. After cricothyroid injection of lidocaine, laryngoscopy is performed in stages. The oropharynx is anaesthetized progressively with lidocaine spray until the patient tolerates deep insertion of the laryngoscope, enabling the larynx to be viewed.

Complications of Tracheal Intubation

Complications may be mechanical, respiratory or cardiovascular and may occur early or late.

Early Complications. Trauma may occur to lips and teeth or dental crowns. Jaw dislocation and dislocation of arytenoids may be produced. Trauma during intubation may result in damage to larynx and vocal cords. Nasal intubation may produce epistaxis, trauma to the pharyngeal wall or dislodgement of adenoid tissue. Obstruction or kinking of the tube may occur and carinal stimulation or bronchial intubation may take place if the tube is too long. Laryngeal trauma may produce postoperative croup, bronchospasm or laryngospasm, especially in children. Mechanical complications may be avoided with a careful technique. Broken teeth must be retrieved and the event documented. Immediate postoperative respiratory complications may be minimized by humidification of inspired gases. Cardiovascular complications of intubation include arrhythmias and hypertension, especially in untreated hypertensive patients.

Late Complications. These are more common after long-term intubation. Tracheal stenosis is rare, but damage to tracheal mucosa from a cuffed tube may be related to its design; high-volume, low-pressure cuffs may be preferred for long-term intubation. Trauma to vocal cords may result in ulceration or granulomata which may require surgical removal. Cord trauma may be more common in the presence of an upper respiratory tract infection.

Anaesthesia Using Neuromuscular Blocking Drugs

Indications

As an alternative to deep anaesthesia with spontaneous ventilation and volatile agents leading to multisystem depression, the triad of sleep, suppression of reflexes and muscle relaxation may be provided separately with specific agents. The use of a neuromuscular blocking agent provides muscle relaxation, permitting lighter anaesthesia with less risk of cardiovascular depression. Thus, the technique is appropriate for major abdominal, intraperitoneal, thoracic or intracranial operations, prolonged operations in which spontaneous ventilation would lead to respiratory depression, and operations in a position in which ventilation is impaired mechanically.

Conduct of Relaxant Anaesthesia

After induction of anaesthesia, neuromuscular blockade is produced by using either (a) a depolarizing neuromuscular blocker (NMB) (succinylcholine) followed, after its action has subsided, by a non-depolarizing NMB, or (b) in the case of an elective fasting patient with normal gastric emptying and no history of hiatus hernia or regurgitation, an intubating dose of a non-depolarizing NMB (see Ch 6). The choice of agent depends upon operative indications or the patient's condition (e.g. vecuronium and rocuronium produce little cardiovascular depression). The airway is then secured with a tracheal tube.

Controlled ventilation is commenced, first manually by compression of the reservoir bag and then by a mechanical ventilator delivering the appropriate tidal and minute volumes (see Appendix C). Anaesthesia and analgesia are provided by nitrous oxide/oxygen or air/oxygen, together with a volatile agent and i.v. analgesic. The inspired and end-expired concentrations of volatile agents should be monitored. Analgesia may also be supplemented by opioid pre-medication or by use of regional or local anaesthetic techniques.

Assessment of Relaxant Anaesthesia. Light anaesthesia with preservation of reflexes permits the use of physical signs for the continued assessment of the adequacy of anaesthesia.

Adequacy of anaesthesia. Autonomic reflex activity with lacrimation, sweating, tachycardia, hypertension or reflex movement in response to surgery indicate 'light' anaesthesia and response to surgical stimulation, and warn that the depth of anaesthesia should be increased or further increments of i.v. analgesic given.

Awareness during anaesthesia. The possibility of conscious or unconscious awareness exists in a patient who is under the influence of an NMB if nitrous oxide/oxygen anaesthesia is unsupplemented or is supplemented by an opioid with little or no volatile agent. The anaesthetist should ensure that this possibility is avoided by constant observation of the patient for clinical signs of light anaesthesia and by use of small concentrations of a volatile agent. Up to 1% of patients may recall intraoperative events spontaneously if a mixture of nitrous oxide 67% in oxygen is administered, even with an i.v. opioid, and a proportion of these patients experience pain. Awareness during anaesthesia is now a common source of litigation. An appropriate concentration of volatile anaesthetic agent should be used routinely during elective surgery. The use of the BIS monitor may decrease the incidence of awareness.

Adequacy of muscle relaxation. Clinical signs of return of muscle tone include retraction of the wound edges during abdominal operations and abdominal muscle, diaphragmatic or facial movement. An increase in airway pressure (with a time- or volume-cycled ventilator) may indicate a return of muscle tone. Quantitative estimation of neuromuscular status may be obtained with a peripheral nerve stimulator (see Ch 6). Small increments (e.g. 25–35% of the original dose) of NMB may be given to maintain relaxation; alternatively, an i.v. infusion may be a more convenient method of administration, but the use of a peripheral nerve stimulator is mandatory with this technique.

Adequacy of ventilation. Clinical signs of inadequate ventilation and an increase in $PaCO_2$ include venous dilatation, wound oozing, tachycardia, hypertension and attempts at spontaneous ventilation by the patient.

Measurement of airway pressure and end-expired PCO_2 with a capnograph are mandatory during anaesthesia. Monitoring expired gas volume provides useful information to adjust the degree of mechanical ventilation, and occasionally arterial PCO_2 measurement may be used.

Reversal of Relaxation

At the end of surgery, residual neuromuscular blockade is antagonized and spontaneous ventilation should begin before the tracheal tube is removed and the patient awakened. Residual neuromuscular blockade is antagonized with neostigmine 2.5–5 mg (0.05–0.08 mg kg^{-1} in children). Atropine 1.2 mg or glycopyrronium 0.5 mg (in adults) counteracts the muscarinic side-effects of the anticholinesterase and may be given before, or with, neostigmine. Care should be exercised in the use of an anticholinergic agent in the presence of existing tachycardia, pyrexia, carbon dioxide retention or ischaemic heart disease.

Resumption of spontaneous ventilation should occur if normocapnic ventilation has been used and assured by monitoring the end-expired PCO_2. Tracheobronchial suction (see below) has the beneficial side-effect of stimulating respiration if used at this stage.

OTHER TECHNIQUES

Total Intravenous Anaesthesia

Total intravenous anaesthesia (TIVA) techniques for induction and maintenance of anaesthesia are widely used. The pharmacokinetic and pharmacodynamic profile of agents such as propofol, alfentanil and remifentanil permit rapid titration of drug dose to the required effect in individual patients. Most general anaesthesia is still maintained using inhalational techniques, partly for historical reasons, but mainly because the non-invasive measurement of end-expired partial pressure of the agent gives a useful estimate of the partial pressure of the agent at the effector site in the central nervous system. However, drug delivery systems have been developed which give improved control of intravenous anaesthesia.

Target controlled infusion (TCI) devices (e.g. Diprifusor) enable the theoretical drug concentration in the plasma of propofol to be controlled continuously and administered without the need for complex calculation by the anaesthetist. The pharmacokinetic data for propofol have been obtained from measurements in patient populations of different age, sex and weight, to create a pharmacokinetic model; different models have been produced. The computer program in the TCI device continuously calculates the distribution and elimination of propofol and automatically adjusts the infusion rate to maintain a predicted (not measured) plasma drug concentration.

Advantages of TIVA include the avoidance of some of the complications of inhalational anaesthesia such as distension of gas-filled spaces, diffusion hypoxia and production of fluoride ions. It may be used safely in patients susceptible to malignant hyperthermia. There is also a reduced incidence of postoperative nausea and vomiting. The main disadvantages are that the plasma concentrations are predicted not measured, the actual plasma concentrations of the intravenous agent are subject to biological variability, and variations in the patient's physiological state reduce the model's predictive value. Therefore, the predicted plasma concentration must be adjusted to control the depth of anaesthesia assessed clinically, in the same way as the end-expired partial pressure would be adjusted when using an inhalational technique.

Opioid Infusions

Remifentanil, an ultra-short acting opioid may be used as an adjunct to inhalational anaesthesia or in total intravenous anaesthesia, as part of a balanced technique, therefore reducing the amount of anaesthetic agent required and/or avoiding the need for nitrous oxide. Remifentanil is an ester and undergoes rapid hydrolysis by esterases in the plasma. Its short duration of action is a useful property in specialities such as neurosurgery where analgesic requirements are high intraoperatively but where rapid recovery is needed postoperatively. Recommended infusion rates for remifentanil are published as part of its data sheet. Remifentanil is given by intravenous infusion titrated to patient response. Sometimes a slow bolus of 0.25–0.5 mcg kg^{-1} is given initially, though this can cause bradycardia and hypotension especially in frail or elderly patients. Where postoperative pain is likely to be significant, another type of analgesia *must* be given before discontinuation of remifentanil as its offset of action is rapid.

CONDUCT OF EXTUBATION

This may take place with the patient supine if the anaesthetist is satisfied that airway patency can be maintained by the patient in this position and there is no

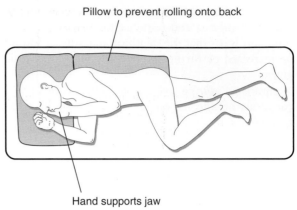

Pillow to prevent rolling onto back

Hand supports jaw

FIGURE 21.7 ■ Recovery position.

risk of regurgitation. In patients at risk of regurgitation and potential aspiration, the lateral position is preferred. However, it is safer to use the lateral recovery position after extubation (Fig. 21.7). Return of respiratory reflexes is signified by coughing and resistance to the presence of the tracheal tube.

Tracheobronchial suction via the tracheal tube is carried out using a soft sterile suction catheter with an external diameter less than half the internal diameter of the tube. Preoxygenation precedes suctioning, as the oxygen stores may be depleted by tracheal suction. The catheter is occluded during insertion and suction applied during withdrawal.

Pharyngeal suction is performed best under direct vision, avoiding trauma to the pharyngeal mucosa, uvula or epiglottis. This should take place before antagonism of residual neuromuscular blockade.

Oxygen 100% replaces the anaesthetic gas mixture before extubation to avoid the potential effects of diffusion hypoxia and to provide a pulmonary reservoir of oxygen in case breath-holding or coughing occurs.

Tracheal extubation is performed preferably during inspiration when the larynx dilates; the cuff is deflated and the tube is withdrawn along its curved axis, as careless withdrawal in a straight line may damage laryngeal structures. Some anaesthetists generate a positive pressure in the trachea during this manoeuvre by 'squeezing the bag' in order to propel secretions into the pharynx.

After extubation, the patient's ability to maintain the airway is ensured, the ability to cough and clear secretions is assessed and an oropharyngeal airway is inserted if required. Administration of oxygen is continued by face mask. Preparations are made for recovery.

Complications of Tracheal Extubation

Laryngeal Spasm

This may follow stimulation during extubation. Extubation during deep anaesthesia and subsequent maintenance with a mask may be used. Local anaesthetic spray to the larynx may block the reflex, and pharyngeal suction before extubation removes secretions which may cause stimulation.

Regurgitation/Inhalation

Aspiration via the nasogastric tube (if present) should be performed before tracheal extubation to remove gastric liquid. In emergency patients, extubation should be performed with the patient awake so that airway control is continuous. Partial incompetence of laryngeal reflexes may occur in the immediate post-extubation period, especially if local anaesthetic spray has been used. In this event, recovery should take place with the patient in the lateral head-down position, with facilities at hand for suction, oxygenation and reintubation.

Current practice is usually to extubate the trachea as the patient regains response to command as this minimizes the risks of both laryngospasm and inhalation of gastric material.

EMERGENCE AND RECOVERY

After completion of surgery, anaesthetic agents are withdrawn and oxygen 100% is delivered. Following removal of the tracheal tube or LMA, the patient's airway is supported until respiratory reflexes are intact. The patient's muscle power and coordination are assessed by testing hand grip, tongue protrusion or a sustained head lift from the pillow in response to command. Adequacy of neuromuscular transmission may also be assessed before the patient is conscious (see Ch 6). Return of adequate muscle power must be ensured before the patient leaves theatre. Full monitoring of the patient should not be discontinued before recovery of consciousness.

The patient is then ready for transfer from the operating table to a bed or trolley. Oxygen is delivered by face mask during transport, and further recovery takes place in a recovery area of theatre or in the recovery ward (see Ch 40).

The lateral recovery position (see Fig. 21.7) is adopted unless the anaesthetist is satisfied that this is unnecessary. The patient is turned on one side, upper leg flexed and lower extended; the head is on one side and the tongue falls forward under gravity, thus avoiding airway obstruction.

REFERENCES AND FURTHER READING

AAGBI (Association of Anaesthetists of Great Britain and Ireland), 2003. Suspected anaphylactic reactions associated with anaesthesia. AAGBI, London.

AAGBI (Association of Anaesthetists of Great Britain and Ireland), 2004. Checking anaesthetic equipment. AAGBI, London.

AAGBI (Association of Anaesthetists of Great Britain and Ireland), 2008. Infection control in Anaesthesia 2. AAGBI, London.

Ahmed, I., Russell, W., 2010. Jaw thrust: are we applying it correctly? Pediatr. Anesth. 20, 107–108.

Brimacombe, J.R., Brain, A.I.J., Berry, A.M., 1996. The laryngeal mask airway instruction manual, third ed. Intavent, Pangbourne.

Department of Health, 2004. Protecting the breathing circuit in anaesthesia – Report of an expert group on blocked anaesthetic tubing. http://webarchive.nationalarchives.gov.uk/20130107105354/http://www.dh.gov.uk/en/Publicationsandstatistics/Publications/PublicationsPolicyAndGuidance/DH_4081825.

Henderson, J.J., Popat, M.T., Latto, I.P., Pearce, A.C., 2004. Difficult Airway Society guidelines for management of the unanticipated difficult intubation. Anaesthesia 59, 675–694.

Latto, I.P., Vaughan, S., 1997. Difficulties in tracheal intubation, second ed. WB Saunders, London.

Martin, J.T., Warner, M.A., 1997. Positioning in anesthesia and surgery, third ed. WB Saunders, Philadelphia.

WHO Surgical Safety Checklist. http://www.nrls.npsa.nhs.uk/resources/clinical-specialty/surgery/?entryid45=59860.

22 MANAGEMENT OF THE DIFFICULT AIRWAY

This important topic can be divided into anticipated and unanticipated difficult airway management. Although both situations may require similar techniques, the approach, urgency and risk of adverse outcomes differ considerably between the two settings.

Difficulties arise most commonly at the start or end of anaesthesia, with the former the more common. Difficulty at the end of anaesthesia involves either airway obstruction or aspiration; when the problem is airway obstruction, difficulty may be categorized in the same manner as difficulty after induction. Difficult airway management may involve any of the four main categories of airway management:

- face-mask ventilation
- supraglottic airway device (SAD) placement and ventilation
- tracheal intubation
- emergency surgical airway (including cannula cricothyroidotomy and surgical techniques).

Airway management is usually routine and straightforward, but each of the above techniques may fail. Anaesthetists are used to high levels of success at what they do and routine airway management does not usually fail. The frequency of failure of routine airway management is as follows:

- face-mask ventilation   <1 in 700
- laryngeal mask ventilation   <1 in 100
- tracheal intubation   <1 in 1500
- tracheal intubation and
  mask ventilation (CICV)   ~1 in 5000.

CICV is an abbreviation for 'Can't intubate, can't ventilate'.

Failure rates probably vary depending on definitions used, operator experience and the group of patients examined. Novices may have failure rates more than 10-fold higher. Difficulty may arise at least 10 times more often than failure. For example, difficult laryngoscopy (and hence difficult intubation) occurs in about 6% of intubations in unselected patients but in selected groups, e.g. those presenting for cervical spine surgery, this may be as high as 20%. The urgency of a procedure also contributes to ease and success. During emergency intubation (with rapid sequence induction), intubation fails approximately eight times as often as during elective intubation.

About a quarter of major airway emergencies occur in the Intensive Care Unit (ICU) or the emergency department and it is necessary to ensure that the same response to airway difficulty can be provided in these locations as in the operating theatre. In the emergency department, tracheal intubation may be difficult in 1 in 12, fail as often as 1 in 50, and an emergency surgical airway has been reported to be needed as often as 1 in 200 intubation attempts.

Although it is important not to dismiss complications arising during uncomplicated airway management, the vast majority of complications occur during 'difficult airway management', however defined.

Airway management difficulties contribute to a large proportion of anaesthesia-related deaths and CICV accounts for over 25% of all anaesthesia-related deaths.

BEFORE MANAGING THE DIFFICULT AIRWAY

Preparedness

The key to safe management of the difficult airway is *preparedness*.

Organizational Preparedness

Guidelines. Organizational preparedness requires that those events which might reasonably be anticipated to occur can be managed appropriately in the organization. This in turn requires guidelines (or policies) and equipment. As a minimum, the guidelines should cover the following:

- management of unanticipated difficult tracheal intubation
- management of unanticipated CICV
- triggers and mechanisms for getting assistance when airway difficulty is anticipated or unexpectedly encountered
- information to provide to a patient after a difficult airway event.

Guidelines will also ideally include unexpected failed mask ventilation and unexpected failed insertion of a SAD. Guidelines might also address the indications for fibreoptic intubation and management of extubation of the difficult airway. These guidelines need not be created by every institution and there is much to be said for nationally accepted or published guidelines being adopted as local policy (e.g. the Difficult Airway Society [DAS] guidelines in the UK). There are several advantages to widespread adoption of this approach; for example, practice becomes based on available evidence and employees who move between hospitals will be immediately familiar with emergency protocols.

Equipment. Logic dictates that the equipment needed to satisfy institutional preparedness is that which is needed for all the guidelines to be carried out in their entirety. This equipment should be procured, stored, maintained and checked appropriately to ensure that it is readily available whenever and wherever it is required. Difficult airway equipment (perhaps better described as advanced airway equipment) is usually maintained in an airway trolley (Fig. 22.1). It is advisable for all

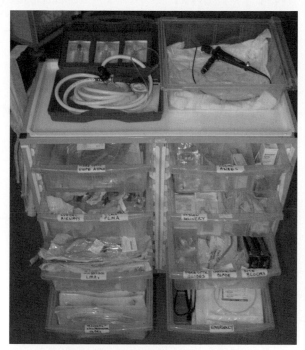

FIGURE 22.1 ■ A difficult airway trolley.

airway trolleys in an organization to have the same content and layout; this includes areas such as ICU and the emergency department. Organizing the airway trolley so that the layout of the equipment matches the flow of the airway guideline may improve compliance with the guideline and patient care; an example based on the DAS guideline is shown in Figure 22.2.

Communication and Training. The final aspect of institutional preparedness is communication and training. Guidelines are of limited value if they are not understood, accepted and practised by the relevant staff. Many hospitals have access to training in advanced airway management. Guidelines should be distributed widely. Training should involve the use of local guidelines and locally available equipment to ensure relevance. Where possible, those individuals who work together in teams should be trained together so that the chances of the team working well in an emergency are enhanced. The 'team' need not be limited to the anaesthetist and anaesthetic assistant, and some training (rather like a trauma team) allocates specific roles to surgeons, scrub nurses and other anaesthetists who attend to help in a crisis.

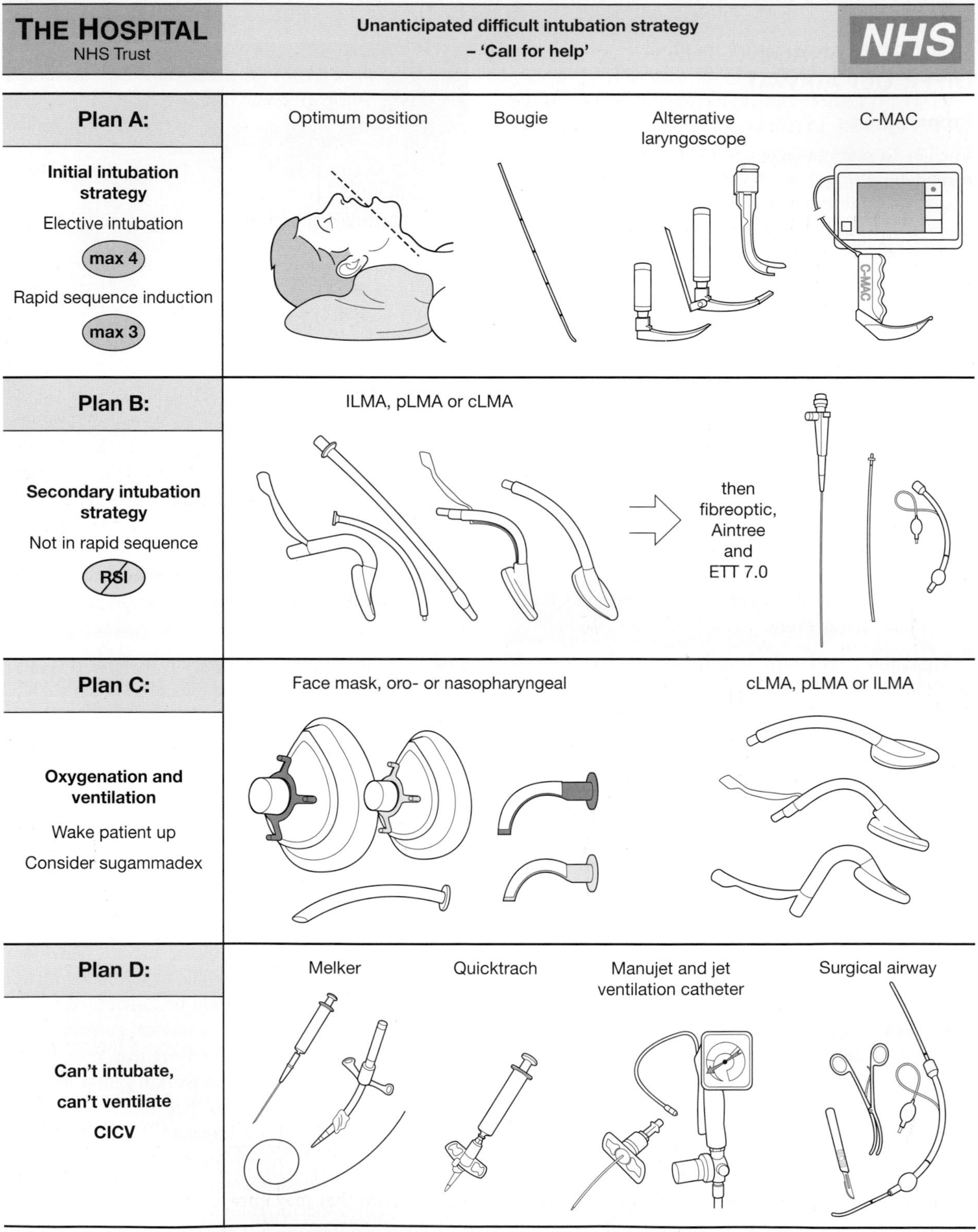

| THE HOSPITAL
NHS Trust | Unanticipated difficult intubation strategy
– 'Call for help' | NHS |

Plan A:

Initial intubation strategy

Elective intubation

(max 4)

Rapid sequence induction

(max 3)

Optimum position   Bougie   Alternative laryngoscope   C-MAC

Plan B:

Secondary intubation strategy

Not in rapid sequence

(RSI)

ILMA, pLMA or cLMA

then fibreoptic, Aintree and ETT 7.0

Plan C:

Oxygenation and ventilation

Wake patient up

Consider sugammadex

Face mask, oro- or nasopharyngeal   cLMA, pLMA or ILMA

Plan D:

Can't intubate,

can't ventilate

CICV

Melker   Quicktrach   Manujet and jet ventilation catheter   Surgical airway

FIGURE 22.2 ■ An example of a local protocol for management of unanticipated difficulty in securing the airway. (*Adapted from a figure provided by kind permission of Dr C Thompson.*)

While there is no evidence that such an approach improves outcome in real airway emergencies, it probably enables an organized, systematic approach and has the value of enabling a 'team leader' to oversee the management of the crisis, perhaps avoiding 'task fixation' and promoting 'situation awareness'.

Institutional preparedness is a process whereby the organization facilitates good difficult airway management by individuals. Such preparation usually requires that the organization has a nominated airway lead for this role, usually a consultant anaesthetist.

Personal Preparedness

Individual anaesthetists have a clear responsibility to be prepared to manage the difficult airway. At different stages of training and expertise the responsibilities will differ. The elements of individual preparedness are:

- education
- training
- patient assessment and planning.

Through appropriate education, individual anaesthetists should ensure that they have the appropriate knowledge and skills to deal with anticipated and unanticipated airway difficulties and emergencies which they may reasonably expect to encounter. It is also important that the less experienced know the limitations of their expertise and therefore when to call for assistance.

Individual training requires that each anaesthetist is familiar with local guidelines and is trained to find and use the locally available equipment according to local guidelines. Training should also include an understanding of how the less experienced anaesthetist seeks senior assistance. To the trained anaesthetist, management of the difficult airway should become a part of routine practice.

Appropriate individualized assessment and planning is a vital part of personal preparedness and is discussed below.

Assessment and Planning a Strategy.
While it is accepted that not all cases of airway difficulty can be anticipated (perhaps 50% are unanticipated), many can be. Airway assessment is discussed in detail in Chapter 21. Only principles are discussed here.

Airway assessment involves using patient history, previous notes and any other available documentation (e.g. alert bracelets) to identify:

- any previous airway problems
- any clinical symptoms or signs that predict difficulty
- any clinical symptoms or signs that predict ease.

Assessment should include an assessment of the likely ease or difficulty of performing the planned primary airway technique and potential rescue techniques. Assessment should also specifically assess the risk of aspiration. When difficulty with one technique is identified, particular attention is required in assessment of other techniques, first because that rescue technique is more likely to be required and second because in patients in whom one technique fails there is an increased likelihood that other techniques will also fail. Multiple airway problems tend to co-exist in the same patient.

While there are many features that may predict difficult airway management the following should raise particular concerns:

- obesity (BMI $>30\,kg\,m^{-2}$) and morbid obesity (BMI $>40\,kg\,m^{-2}$).
- obstructive sleep apnoea
- previous radiotherapy to the neck/floor of mouth
- mouth opening $<2.5\,cm$
- fixed flexed neck
- high risk of aspiration (this will severely restrict many options).

The importance of assessment and planning is underlined by the fact that several large studies examining major airway complications have identified failure to assess, failure to alter technique in the light of findings, and failure to have back-up plans as causes of poor outcomes.

A strategy is a logical sequential series of plans which aim to achieve oxygenation, ventilation and avoidance of aspiration and which are appropriate to the patient's specific features and condition. Airway management should not rely on the success of plan A and should be based on a clear strategy that is communicated to all. An aphorism that may encapsulate this is 'in order to succeed, it is necessary to plan for failure'. Guidelines are, in essence, a strategy for unexpected difficulty. The strategy should usefully identify a 'place of safety'; this is a pre-planned rescue plan when problems arise; for instance, if insertion of a laryngeal mask is known to be successful this may be the place of safety, but alternatively the safest option may be to allow the patient to wake.

Assessment is a pointless ritual unless the chosen technique is adjusted as necessary according to the findings. The strategy should be consistent with the findings at assessment.

MANAGEMENT OF THE DIFFICULT AIRWAY

Training, Teamwork and Human Factors

Many 'airway disasters' are associated with poor planning, use of techniques that are unfamiliar to the user (sometimes used incorrectly or sub-optimally), poor team-work and poor communication. Human factors associated with airway management complications include:

- misuse of equipment through lack of knowledge or training
- task fixation
- poor situation awareness
- communication problems
- lack of leadership
- poor team-working
- failure to follow guidelines.

Task fixation is the tendency, having started a task (e.g. tracheal intubation), to persevere with attempts to complete that task, even when it is not in the patient's interest (e.g. repeated attempts risking airway trauma and progression to CICV). Situation awareness should enable the anaesthetist (or someone else in the team) to realise that the task is failing and that another technique or approach is necessary, or perhaps that priorities have changed (e.g. from intubation to oxygenation and waking the patient). When a team works well together and hierarchical boundaries are broken down, communication within the team is enhanced. A level hierarchy should not be confused with lack of leadership; the ability of one person to step aside and observe the team behaviour may have value. Conversely, multiple individuals all pursing their own approach to managing the crisis is unlikely to be constructive or successful.

Good team-work and avoiding the pitfalls of human factors does not happen by accident and requires that a team works together and is trained in human factors and teamwork together.

Before Approaching the Difficult Airway

Several questions can usefully be considered before approaching any anticipated difficult airway. These questions are based on the preamble to the American Society of Anesthesiologists' (ASA) Difficult Airway algorithm.

- Will delivery of oxygen be difficult?
- Will face-mask ventilation be difficult?
- Will SAD placement be difficult?
- Will tracheal intubation be difficult?
- Will direct access to the trachea be difficult?
- Will there be problems with patient consent or co-operation?

Consider the relative merits of:

- securing the airway with the patient awake or anaesthetized
- making the initial approach to tracheal intubation direct or indirect
- maintaining spontaneous ventilation or ablating it during airway management.

The ASA also makes the recommendation to 'actively pursue opportunities to deliver supplemental oxygen throughout the process of difficult airway management'.

Securing the Airway Awake

When airway difficulty is anticipated, the point at which the anaesthetist risks loss of control and 'burning bridges' is likely when general anaesthesia is induced. At this point, respiratory drive is diminished or obliterated, airway reflexes are largely ablated and the loss of muscle tone of the airway means that the risk of airway obstruction increases dramatically. If general anaesthesia is induced, the time from cessation of administration to patient waking is often up to 10 min, which is more than sufficient to cause profound hypoxaemia, hypoxic tissue injury or even death.

Securing the airway awake should be considered actively whenever significant difficulty in intubation is predicted. The argument for this increases when mask ventilation is predicted to be difficult, when rescue techniques such as direct tracheal access are predicted to be difficult and when there is a high risk of aspiration.

Although awake fibreoptic intubation (AFOI) is generally considered the standard mode of awake intubation, there are several methods of awake intubation reported. These include:

- awake fibreoptic intubation via oral or nasal routes
- topical anaesthesia of the oral route followed by:
  - awake direct laryngoscopy (standard laryngoscope)
  - awake indirect laryngoscopy (rigid fibreoptic laryngoscope/videolaryngoscope)
  - awake intubation via an intubating LMA
  - awake intubation via another SAD
- awake tracheostomy or surgical cricothyroidotomy.

While not all anaesthetists currently have the skills and experience to perform AFOI, such skills must be available in every anaesthetic department at all times and should be deployed whenever indicated.

Administration of Muscle Relaxants in the Patient with a Difficult Airway

When general anaesthesia is administered, neuromuscular blocking drugs can be friend or foe during difficult airway management. It is notable that neuromuscular blockade is not usually necessary for mask ventilation or SAD insertion, but does facilitate tracheal intubation and probably insertion of an emergency surgical airway.

When mask ventilation is problematic, administration of a neuromuscular blocking agent usually makes ventilation easier. This has led some to promote the use of neuromuscular blockade when mask ventilation is difficult in patients with a difficult airway. However, it is important to note that the evidence of easier ventilation is derived from patients who are not particularly difficult in the first place. In contrast, there is no robust evidence that neuromuscular blockade makes ventilation *reliably* easy when dealing with patients with abnormal anatomy or an anticipated difficult airway. There is also no robust evidence that neuromuscular blockade reliably converts CICV to a situation in which ventilation is possible. The

disadvantage of inducing neuromuscular blockade in this situation is that it commits the anaesthetist to securing the airway promptly and eliminates the option of waking the patient. Patients who are difficult or impossible to ventilate using a face mask are also at increased risk of failed intubation. Thus administration of a neuromuscular blocker may be reasonable when difficult mask ventilation occurs and waking the patient is not desirable but the anaesthetist must be prepared to manage a critical airway if it does not improve the situation.

In contrast, when both mask ventilation and intubation have failed, if waking the patient is not possible, there is little to be lost and much to be gained by administering a neuromuscular blocker. If successful, it will avoid an unnecessary emergency surgical airway and may save the patient's life.

The subject remains controversial but can be summarized as follows:

- neuromuscular blockade often makes difficult mask ventilation easier
- this is not universal and is uncertain in anatomically abnormal patients
- administration of a neuromuscular blocker removes the possibility of waking the patient
- if neuromuscular blockade is used to manage difficult mask ventilation, the anaesthetist must be adequately prepared to secure the airway, including managing a CICV situation
- even if it was not part of the initial airway management strategy, if CICV occurs and waking the patient is not an option, a muscle relaxant should be given before determining the need to proceed to a surgical airway.

Selecting an Appropriate Size of Tracheal Tube

A couple of decades ago, the use of tracheal tubes as large as 10 mm internal diameter was routine. While smaller tracheal tubes are used by most anaesthetists, some persist in using tracheal tubes as large as 9 mm internal diameter. In the circumstance of difficult airway management, there is a strong argument for using small tracheal tubes. A smaller tracheal tube:

- passes though some narrow lumens which a larger tracheal tube will not pass

- passes through a narrow lumen with greater ease and with less risk of trauma to the airway
- is easier to 'railroad' over a bougie or exchange catheter with less risk of 'hold-up' during insertion.

Spontaneous ventilation is rarely required for prolonged periods after tracheal intubation and all but the most impaired patient can breathe with ease through a tracheal tube of 6 mm internal diameter. Selection of a tracheal tube of 6.0–6.5 mm internal diameter may make airway management easier and use of tubes larger than 7.0 mm is rarely indicated.

DIFFICULT AIRWAYS AND THEIR MANAGEMENT

The ASA and DAS Guidelines

Because problems relating to the management of a difficult airway are the leading cause of death related to anaesthesia, the need for guidelines to formalize and help in the management of the difficult airway has been recognized in many countries. Major complications arising from difficult airway management are relatively rare but they are frequent enough that almost all anaesthetists will encounter them in their careers.

The first guidelines were published in 1993 by the ASA. The introduction of guidelines in the USA has been demonstrated to have led to a reduction in death and brain damage claims (and therefore probably critical incidents) related to airway management, most notably at the time of induction of anaesthesia. Many European countries developed their own guidelines in subsequent years. While all these claim to be evidence-based, the paucity of robust evidence means that most guidelines differ significantly from each other, often reflecting local preferences. The UK guidelines were published by the Difficult Airway Society in 2004. The major differences between the guidelines published by the ASA and DAS are summarized in Table 22.1. Both emphasize the most important principles in airway management:

- to have devised a plan for airway management in the eventuality of it proving difficult, and a backup plan(s) which has been prepared for and practised

- priority must be given to ensuring oxygenation and preventing iatrogenic trauma to the airway at all times.

The ASA guidelines cover airway assessment and a number of different difficult airway situations. They offer the user a wide choice of options at each point of airway difficulty. They recommend multiple different techniques and it is likely that not all will be within the competence of all anaesthetists. They offer 'choices'. In contrast, the DAS guidelines are didactic and present a single recommended pathway arranged in plans A to D and differentiating between the patient undergoing routine intubation or rapid sequence induction. They do not prescribe any advanced techniques but recommend simple procedures using equipment that should be familiar to all anaesthetists in training. They also strongly emphasize the need for regular practice of the recommended techniques using simulators and manikins where appropriate. The DAS guidelines are shown in Figures 22.3–22.5.

Difficult Mask Ventilation

The first problem encountered in any difficult airway situation is often difficulty with face-mask ventilation. This is a vital step because it represents the basic and least invasive way of ensuring oxygenation of the patient. For mask ventilation to occur, a clear, sealed and patent airway from face mask to the lower airway is required. Difficulty can be diagnosed when there is inadequate chest movement despite high airway pressures (in the case of obstruction) or very low airway pressures (due to a leak during inspiration). Capnography and spirometry, both of which are available on most modern anaesthetic machines, can also identify poor ventilation before hypoxaemia occurs (Fig. 22.6).

Difficulties with Mask Ventilation can be due to:

- failure to maintain a patent upper airway (by far the most common problem)
- laryngeal obstruction (either spasm or pathology)
- obstruction below the larynx, in the trachea, bronchi or in patients with reduced pulmonary compliance.

TABLE 22.1

Comparison between the American Society of Anesthesiologists' and Difficult Airway Society's Guidelines Dealing with Management of the Difficult Airway

	ASA Guidelines 2012	DAS Guidelines 2004
Breadth of 'difficult airway' management covered	A clinical situation in which a conventionally trained anesthesiologist experiences difficulty with face mask ventilation of the upper airway, difficulty with tracheal intubation or both	A Cormack and Lehane grade 3 or 4 view despite optimal direct laryngoscopy, using an alternative laryngoscope and external laryngeal manipulation
Evaluation of the airway	11 non-reassuring findings	Not covered
Number of attempts at laryngoscopy allowed before moving to a different technique	>3, multiple attempts	Up to 4 during routine intubation and 3 during RSI. A further single attempt if a more experienced anaesthetist arrives.
Techniques recommended for difficult intubation	Multiple including AFOI, blind, retrograde, LMA used as conduit and invasive airway access	Optimal laryngoscopy with gum elastic bougie (Plan A), then LMA/ILMA as conduit using fibreoptic control (Plan B)* then invasive airway access (Plan D)
Order of techniques	None given	Clear flow chart
Recommendations for extubation	Yes	Published separately (2012)
Recommendations on training	None given	Should form part of all anaesthetist training

*Plan B is omitted during RSI.
RSI, rapid sequence induction; AFOI, awake fibreoptic intubation; LMA, laryngeal mask airway; ILMA, intubating laryngeal mask airway.

Face-mask ventilation requires the combination of: establishing a seal between the mask and the face; maintaining a clear upper airway; and ventilation of the lungs. Flexion of the lower cervical spine, extension of the upper cervical spine and mandibular protrusion are required, ideally with good quality facial soft tissues to enable an adequate seal with the mask. Using a 'C-grip', the thumb and first finger are used to hold the mask pushing downwards while the remaining three fingers pull the chin, jaw and soft tissues into the mask while also maintaining head and neck positions (Fig 22.7). Manual ventilation is performed with the anaesthetist's other hand. Problems with the upper airway can often be predicted by prior airway assessment. Patients for whom obtaining an adequate mask seal is often problematic include the edentulous elderly, bearded patients and those who require high ventilation pressures, such as the morbidly obese.

If there are problems with maintaining patency of the airway, the following simple measures should be employed:

- jaw thrust
- chin lift
- insertion of an appropriately sized oropharyngeal airway
- consideration of a nasopharyngeal airway
- a two-person technique (Fig. 22.8)
- a three-person technique (Fig 22.9).

In a two-person (four-handed) technique, the senior anaesthetist holds the mask with two hands, one on either side of the mask, maintaining the airway seal and head and neck position, while a second person performs manual ventilation. In the three-person (six-handed) technique, the third person acts solely to improve airway positioning and seal with jaw thrust. In an alternative technique, one or two people maintain the airway and the reservoir bag is squeezed by a foot, or mechanical ventilation is employed. If ventilation is still not possible and the depth of anaesthesia is adequate an appropriate SAD should be inserted. Ensure adequate depth of anaesthesia and muscle relaxation where appropriate.

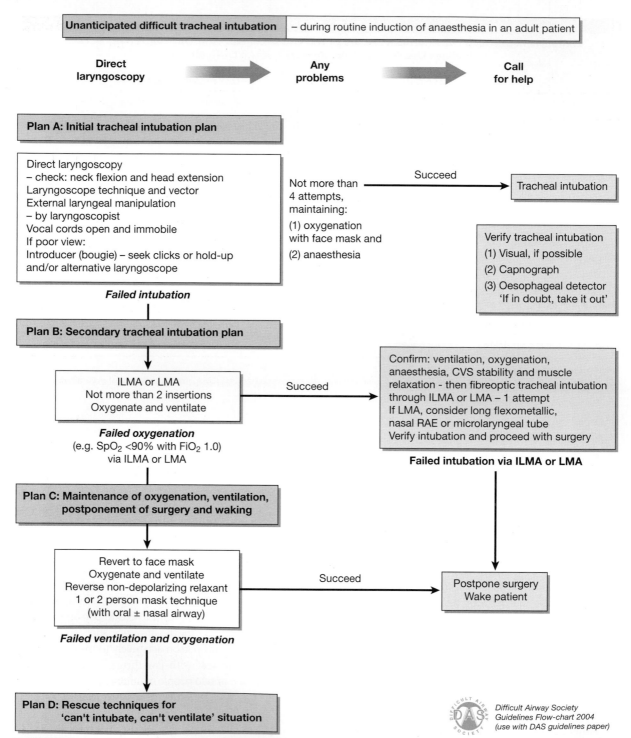

FIGURE 22.3 ■ Difficult Airway Society guideline for unanticipated difficult tracheal intubation during routine induction of anaesthesia in an adult patient. *(Adapted from Henderson JJ, Popat MT, Latto IP, Pearce AC. Difficult Airway Society guidelines for management of the unanticipated difficult intubation. Anaesthesia 2004; 59:675–964, with permission from Blackwell Publishing Ltd. LMA, laryngeal mask airway; ILMA, intubating laryngeal mask airway.)*

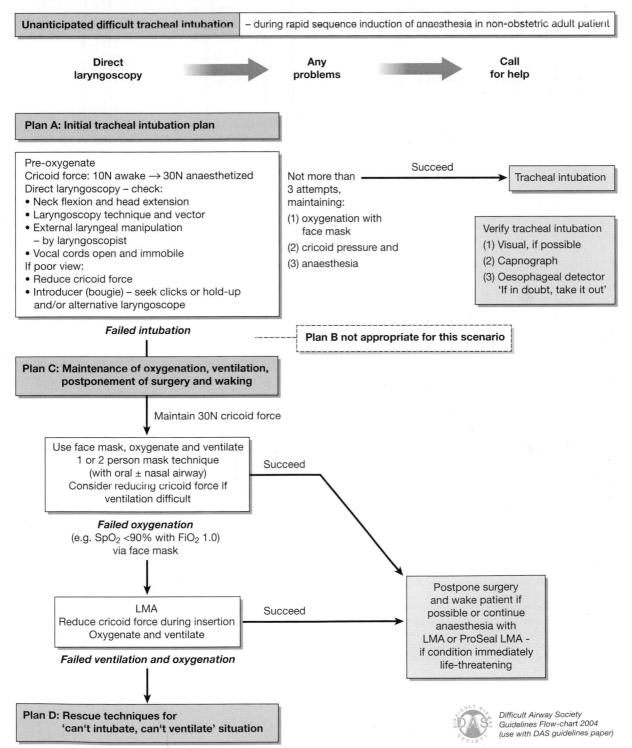

Unanticipated difficult tracheal intubation – during rapid sequence induction of anaesthesia in non-obstetric adult patient

Direct laryngoscopy → **Any problems** → **Call for help**

Plan A: Initial tracheal intubation plan

Pre-oxygenate
Cricoid force: 10N awake → 30N anaesthetized
Direct laryngoscopy – check:
• Neck flexion and head extension
• Laryngoscopy technique and vector
• External laryngeal manipulation
  – by laryngoscopist
• Vocal cords open and immobile
If poor view:
• Reduce cricoid force
• Introducer (bougie) – seek clicks or hold-up
  and/or alternative laryngoscope

Not more than 3 attempts, maintaining:
(1) oxygenation with face mask
(2) cricoid pressure and
(3) anaesthesia

Succeed → **Tracheal intubation**

Verify tracheal intubation
(1) Visual, if possible
(2) Capnograph
(3) Oesophageal detector
'If in doubt, take it out'

Failed intubation ------- Plan B not appropriate for this scenario

Plan C: Maintenance of oxygenation, ventilation, postponement of surgery and waking

Maintain 30N cricoid force

Use face mask, oxygenate and ventilate
1 or 2 person mask technique
(with oral ± nasal airway)
Consider reducing cricoid force if
ventilation difficult

Succeed →

Failed oxygenation
(e.g. SpO₂ <90% with FiO₂ 1.0)
via face mask

LMA
Reduce cricoid force during insertion
Oxygenate and ventilate

Succeed →

Postpone surgery and wake patient if possible or continue anaesthesia with LMA or ProSeal LMA - if condition immediately life-threatening

Failed ventilation and oxygenation

Plan D: Rescue techniques for 'can't intubate, can't ventilate' situation

Difficult Airway Society
Guidelines Flow-chart 2004
(use with DAS guidelines paper)

FIGURE 22.4 ■ Difficult Airway Society guideline for unanticipated difficult tracheal intubation during rapid sequence induction of anaesthesia in a non-obstetric adult patient. *(Adapted from Henderson JJ, Popat MT, Latto IP, Pearce AC. Difficult Airway Society guidelines for management of the unanticipated difficult intubation. Anaesthesia 2004; 59:675–694, with permission from Blackwell Publishing Ltd.)*

Failed intubation, increasing hypoxaemia and difficult ventilation in the paralyzed anaesthetized patient:

Rescue techniques for the 'can't intubate, can't ventilate' situation

**Failed intubation
and difficult ventilation**
(other than laryngospasm)

→

Face mask
Oxygenate and ventilate patient
Maximum head extension
Maximum jaw thrust
Assistance with mask seal
Oral± 6mm nasal airway
Reduce cricoid force – if necessary

Failed oxygenation
(e.g. SpO_2 <90% with FiO_2 1.0)
via face mask

call for help

↓

LMA Oxygenate and ventilate patient
Maximum 2 attempts at insertion
Reduce any cricoid force during insertion

→ Succeed →

Oxygenation
satisfactory
and stable:
Maintain
oxygenation
and wake
patient

**'can't intubate, can't ventilate'
situation with increasing hypoxaemia**

**Plan D: Rescue techniques for
'can't intubate, can't ventilate' situation**

or

Cannula cricothyroidotomy
Equipment:
• Kink-resistant cannula, e.g. Patil (Cook) or Ravussin (VBM)
• High-pressure ventilation system, e.g. Manujet III (VBM)

Technique:
1. Insert cannula through cricothyroid membrane
2. Maintain position of cannula - assistant's hand
3. Confirm tracheal position by air aspiration – 20mL syringe
4. Attach ventilation system to cannula
5. Commence cautious ventilation
6. Confirm ventilation of lungs, and exhalation through upper airway
7. If ventilation fails, or surgical emphysema or any other complication develops – convert immediately to surgical cricothyroidotomy

→ Fail →

Surgical cricothyroidotomy
Equipment:
• Scalpel – short and rounded (no. 20 or Minitrach scalpel)
• Small (e.g. 6 or 7 mm) cuffed tracheal or tracheostomy tube

4-step technique:
1. Identify cricothyroid membrane
2. Stab incision through skin and membrane
Enlarge incision with blunt dissection (e.g. scalpel handle, forceps or dilator)
3. Caudal traction on cricoid cartilage with tracheal hook
4. Insert tube and inflate cuff

Ventilate with low-pressure source

Verify tube position and pulmonary ventilation

Notes: 1. These techniques can have serious complications – use only in life-threatening situations
2. Convert to definitive airway as soon as possible
3. Postoperative management – see other difficult airway guidelines and flow-charts
4. 4mm cannula with low-pressure ventilation may be successful in patient breathing spontaneously

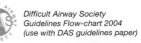

*Difficult Airway Society
Guidelines Flow-chart 2004
(use with DAS guidelines paper)*

FIGURE 22.5 ■ Difficult Airway Society guideline for management of failed intubation, increasing hypoxaemia and difficult ventilation in the paralysed, anaesthetized patient, with rescue techniques for the 'can't intubate, can't ventilate' situation. *(Adapted from Henderson JJ, Popat MT, Latto IP, Pearce AC. Difficult Airway Society guidelines for management of the unanticipated difficult intubation. Anaesthesia 2004; 59:675–694, with permission from Blackwell Publishing Ltd.)*

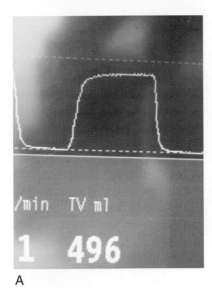 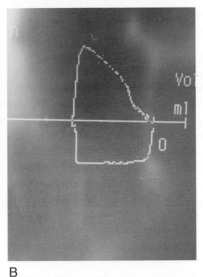

FIGURE 22.6 ■ (**A**) A normal capnograph trace. (**B**) A flow-volume loop from a patient with an unobstructed airway.

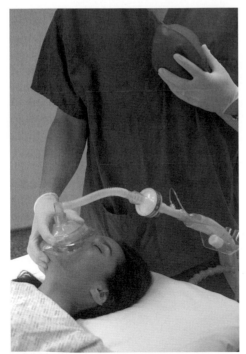

FIGURE 22.7 ■ Mask ventilation with one person. Note the C-grip of the fingers over the mask and the three fingers supporting the airway.

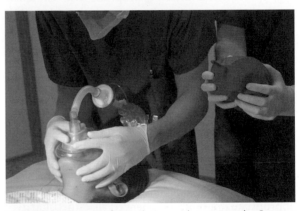

FIGURE 22.8 ■ Mask ventilation with two people. See text for details.

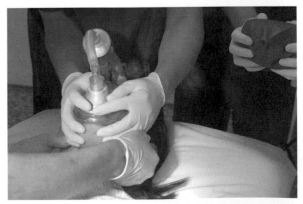

FIGURE 22.9 ■ Mask ventilation with three people. See text for details.

MANAGEMENT OF UNPREDICTED DIFFICULT INTUBATION

Every anaesthetist should have a strategy prepared for dealing with problems with intubation, including plans for the more serious situation of CICV. The DAS algorithm is a suitable approach and is shown in Figures 22.3–22.5. This, or another equally valid strategy, should be familiar to all anaesthetists who are practising without direct supervision.

Management is in four parts which should be approached in sequence in the event of deteriorating oxygenation and increasing difficulty with ventilation.

Plan A: Primary Intubation Attempt

This involves the first and best attempts at intubation. It requires good pre-oxygenation, optimal positioning, optimal anaesthesia, appropriate neuromuscular blockade and an appropriate laryngoscope blade. Use of external laryngeal manipulation and a (high quality) bougie are appropriate. If there is difficulty, the anaesthetist should call for help, but not send away their primary assistant. Attempts at intubation must be limited to no more than four (preferably fewer) as multiple attempts at laryngoscopy are associated with increased risk of airway trauma, failed rescue techniques, CICV, morbidity and mortality. The major concern is of converting a patient who cannot be intubated but can be ventilated into one who cannot be intubated or ventilated. A final attempt is deemed appropriate if a more experienced anaesthetist arrives and adequate face mask ventilation can be maintained.

There is no necessity to use the same laryngoscope blade for all attempts at intubation. Alternative blades include a long (size 4) Macintosh blade, the McCoy (levering laryngoscope) blade and a number of straight-bladed laryngoscopes (e.g. Miller, Henderson). Arguably, at least one attempt should be with a McCoy blade (Fig. 22.10) because it is recognized to move the fulcrum of the force applied to the airway distally and to improve the view when laryngoscopy is awkward. Use of a straight blade may offer the benefit of using an alternative approach to the laryngoscopy, such as a retromolar approach (Fig. 22.11), and this may be helpful, particularly if there is a small mandibular space.

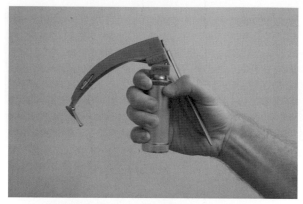

FIGURE 22.10 ■ The McCoy laryngoscope.

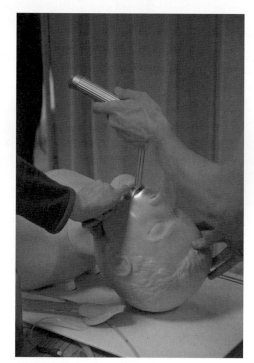

FIGURE 22.11 ■ A retromolar approach using a straight laryngoscope blade.

Rigid videolaryngoscopy is appropriate at this point for those with the appropriate skills and training. This is discussed below.

Plan B: Secondary Intubation Attempt

This is appropriate if adequate ventilation is possible and anaesthesia can be maintained. A classic (cLMA) or intubating (ILMA) laryngeal mask airway is inserted to enable ventilation and is then used as a conduit for intubation. Fibreoptic guidance of intubation is recommended.

Intubation Via a SAD. The cLMA is recommended because it is a device with which all anaesthetists are familiar. The cLMA does have several important limitations for such a use.

- The tube lumen is relatively narrow. To intubate through a size 3 cLMA requires a tracheal tube of maximum internal diameter of 6 mm (size 4, 6.5 mm; size 5, 7.0 mm).
- The LMA aperture bars can obstruct the passage of the tube.
- The length of the cLMA tube requires a long tracheal tube to ensure that the trachea is entered.
- Removal of the LMA may be awkward once the tracheal tube has been successfully inserted and may risk displacing the tracheal tube.

In view of these limitations, a microlaryngeal or long flexometallic tube is recommended.

Several of these issues may be overcome by the use of an alternative SAD as a conduit. The ProSeal LMA and i-gel have no aperture bars and may be better rescue devices. Current evidence, published since the publication of the DAS guidelines, supports use of the ProSeal and i-gel for fibreoptic guided intubation. Blind intubation via any standard SAD is extremely unlikely to be successful and cannot be recommended. The use of fibrescope through a SAD has a high success rate, is a relatively low-skill procedure and may be practised both in manikins and in patients in a non-emergency setting, with appropriate consent.

An important modification of this technique, which is not included in the DAS guidelines, is to use an Aintree Intubation Catheter (AIC). The AIC (internal diameter 4.6 mm) is slid over the fibrescope and fibreoptic intubation is then performed via the SAD (Fig. 22.12). The AIC is left in the trachea (close to the carina) while first the fibrescope and then the SAD are removed. If oxygenation is required, a connector is available to enable ventilation via a standard anaesthetic breathing system. A lubricated tracheal tube is then railroaded over the AIC into the trachea and the AIC removed. The AIC has an external diameter of approximately 7.0 mm, requiring a standard tracheal tube

of at least this size internal diameter to be inserted, although a 6.5 mm internal diameter ILMA tracheal tube is also accommodated. These techniques require practice and it is strongly recommended that, if such techniques are part of departmental guidance, then an appropriate regular training programme should be in place.

Intubation Via an ILMA. The ILMA is also an option for management of plan B. Unlike the other SADs, it is specifically designed for facilitating tracheal intubation. The ILMA has a mask end which is similar to a cLMA but the grille is replaced by an 'epiglottic elevating bar' which is a firm piece of silicone anchored at one end only. The stem of the ILMA is both shorter and wider than other LMAs and is rigid, with a handle attached on the concave side (Fig. 22.13); the stem passes through an angle of approximately 110°. The ILMA is supplied with a specifically designed ILMA tracheal tube (ILMA TT) which is straight, reinforced and has a soft bullet-shaped tip. The ILMA is supplied in three sizes (3–5, for patients of 30–100 kg) and each accommodates all sizes of ILMA TT from 6.0–8.0 mm internal diameter (Fig. 22.13).

The ILMA is inserted with the head in the neutral position by holding the handle, placing the bowl on to the hard palate and then advancing with a rotating movement until the ILMA is fully inserted into the airway.

The position of the ILMA over the airway must then be optimized using several steps.

- The anaesthetic circuit is attached and the patient's lungs are ventilated manually.
- The ILMA is advanced or withdrawn partially or lifted anteriorly until the optimal ventilation position is found.
- If ventilation is poor, the ILMA can be removed 6 cm and re-inserted to resolve epiglottic down-folding.

Once the optimal position is established it is maintained, the circuit is disconnected and a lubricated ILMA TT is inserted with the longitudinal line facing either backwards or forwards (as this places the bevelled tip in the optimal position).

If a blind technique is in use, the ILMA TT is advanced until the horizontal black line on the ILMA TT disappears into the ILMA stem indicating that the tip of the tube is about to exit the ILMA, and push

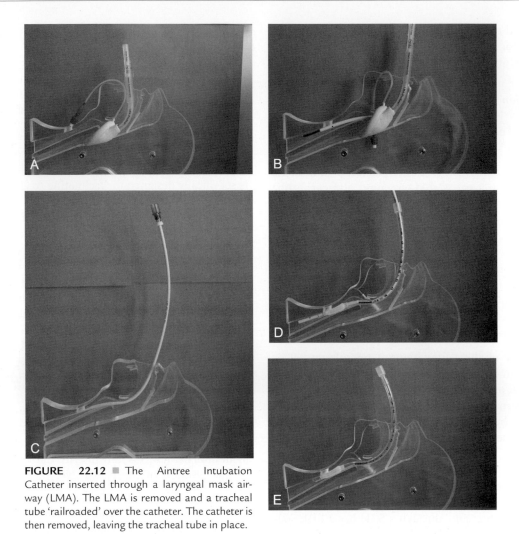

FIGURE 22.12 ■ The Aintree Intubation Catheter inserted through a laryngeal mask airway (LMA). The LMA is removed and a tracheal tube 'railroaded' over the catheter. The catheter is then removed, leaving the tracheal tube in place.

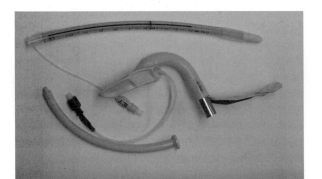

FIGURE 22.13 ■ The intubating laryngeal mask airway (ILMA) kit. See text for details.

the epiglottic elevating bar anteriorly to displace the epiglottis.

The ILMA TT can then be advanced into the trachea (Fig. 22.14). It should enter the trachea in no more than a further 6–8 cm.

The ILMA TT cuff is inflated and correct position confirmed with capnography and other routine tests.

The success rate of the blind technique is approximately 75% (compared to 10–15% when intubating blindly through other SADs). The success rate can be increased to close to 100% by use of a fibrescope within the ILMA TT to guide its direction; this is the technique advocated in the DAS guidelines. When this technique is used, the ILMA TT may be advanced ahead of the fibrescope so that the epiglottic elevator is moved out of the way ('tube first technique') or the scope may be negotiated around the elevator and the larynx intubated before the ILMA TT is advanced ('scope first technique').

Although all ILMAs accept an ILMA TT of up to 8.0 mm internal diameter, there is little to be gained by the use of the larger sizes and the use of a size 6.0 mm or 6.5 mm tube is probably easier and is certainly large enough. The re-usable (pink) ILMA TT has a high-volume high-pressure cuff; it is a common mistake to inflate the cuff to standard pressures and for a leak to persist (especially if a small tube is used). The solution is simply to inflate further until the airway is sealed. However, because, even if a fibrescope is used, the TT is not seen entering the trachea, it is important to ensure that the cuff is not placed at the level of the vocal cords; this is easily avoided by fibreoscopy through the tube and positioning the tip in the mid-trachea. The single-use ILMA TT (white-tipped) has a medium-volume medium-pressure cuff.

It is recommended that the ILMA TT is inserted whenever the ILMA is used because it maximizes success rates. A sharp-bevelled rigid PVC tracheal tube risks intubation difficulty, laryngeal trauma and, if intubation fails, oesophageal trauma.

When the trachea has been intubated, the ILMA should usually be removed. If left in place, it may cause minor morbidity because it exerts a moderate pressure against the pharyngeal wall. A 'tube stabilizer' is provided to facilitate this. The 15-mm connector of the ILMA TT is removed (ideally having been loosened before intubation) and the stabilizing rod is placed into the proximal end of the tube. The ILMA TT cuff is confirmed as inflated and the ILMA cuff is deflated (Fig. 22.14). The stabilizing rod is then used to maintain the ILMA TT position while the ILMA is withdrawn; at the point at which the ILMA is almost out of the mouth, the stabilizing rod is removed and the anaesthetist's gloved hand is inserted into the mouth to hold the tube in position. There are two important points: first, the stabilizing rod is not a 'pusher' and the ILMA TT should not be advanced during this procedure; second, if the stabilizing rod is not removed before the ILMA is withdrawn

completely, the pilot cuff of the ILMA TT is avulsed and the cuff deflates (this is problematic, but can be rescued by inserting an i.v. cannula into the cut end of the pilot tube to enable re-inflation, followed by clamping) (Fig. 22.14).

Most evidence on the efficacy of the ILMA is based on a re-usable device, although a single-use PVC device has recently been developed. Other SADs specifically designed for intubation are the intubating laryngeal airway and the Ambu Aura-i.

Plan C: Failed Intubation, Oxygenation and Waking

If intubation cannot be achieved using the above techniques then ventilation should be maintained using face-mask ventilation. The patient should be woken up. Surgery should then be postponed or the airway established using an awake technique. If neuromuscular blockade has been established, this must be allowed to wear off or be reversed; sugammadex may have an important role if rocuronium (or vecuronium) has been used to induce neuromuscular blockade but will not reverse CICV which has an anatomical or mechanical cause.

Management of Unanticipated Difficult Intubation During RSI. The principal differences in the guidelines for unanticipated difficult intubation during RSI are as follows:

- The patient is always fully pre-oxygenated, which creates more time before oxygen desaturation in the event of difficulties with intubation.
- Cricoid pressure is used to prevent pulmonary aspiration of any regurgitated gastric contents.
- Cricoid pressure should be reduced or briefly removed if it is impeding laryngoscopy. This should be done with 'sucker in hand' so that regurgitated material can be removed promptly.
- There is no plan B for secondary attempts at tracheal intubation because the patient is at risk of aspiration, and succinylcholine has a relatively short duration of action. Consequently, in all but life-threatening situations, the safest course of action is to postpone the surgery and allow the patient to wake. If rocuronium is used as part of a modified RSI technique, sugammadex

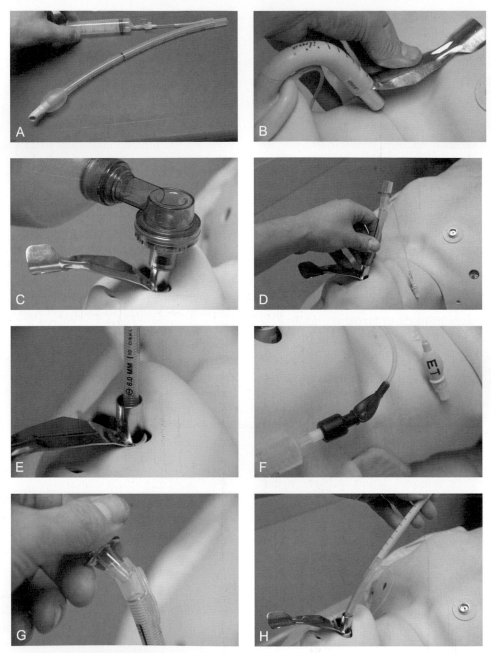

FIGURE 22.14 ■ The use of the intubating laryngeal mask airway (ILMA). (**A**) ILMA TT is checked; (**B**) ILMA is inserted; (**C**) ventilation is optimized; (**D**) ILMA TT is passed through ILMA; (**E**) ILMA TT inside ILMA and position confirmed; (**F**) cuff of ILMA is deflated while TT remains inflated; (**G**) TT connector is removed: (**H**) tube stabilizing rod inserted in end of TT; (**I**) position of stabilizing rod maintained in same position as ILMA withdrawn over TT and stabilizer; (**J**) TT stabilized in mouth before ILMA removed completely; (**K**) stabilizing rod removed to prevent cuff trapping of TT cuff between rod and ILMA and cuff avulsion; (**L**) ILMA removed completely.

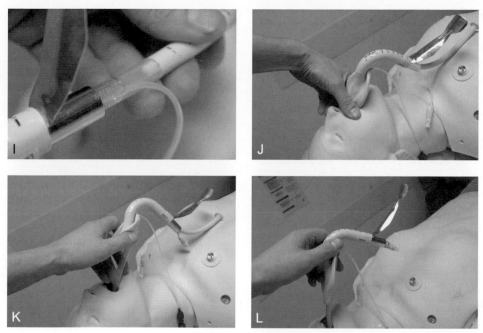

FIGURE 22.14 ■ Cont'd.

may be used to reverse it, although this can only be achieved in a timely fashion if the drug is immediately available *before* induction commences.

■ If (as is often the case) active airway management is required to maintain oxygenation while the patient wakes, the ProSeal LMA is also advocated as a rescue device.

In either situation, if, despite maximal efforts, adequate ventilation cannot be achieved with bag-mask ventilation or via a SAD and there is worsening oxygenation, plan D should be activated. This is the final common pathway of the DAS guidelines and describes a plan for managing the CICV situation.

Plan D: Management of the CICV Situation

As part of plan D, a laryngeal mask airway (or other SAD) should be re-inserted. This may rescue the airway and if it does not, it still maintains a patent upper airway which is important after narrow-bore cricothyroidotomy to provide a route of egress for gases during high pressure source ventilation (see below).

CICV can arise unexpectedly during routine anaesthesia but is probably more frequent when multiple attempts at laryngoscopy/intubation have changed a 'can't intubate, can ventilate' situation into CICV. Risk factors for difficult mask ventilation overlap with risk factors for difficult laryngoscopy (e.g. Mallampati classes 3–4) and patients who are difficult/impossible to ventilate by mask are more likely than others to be difficult or impossible to intubate.

Obesity is also an important factor when considering CICV. Obesity is certainly a risk factor for impossible mask ventilation but the evidence is less clear-cut as to whether it is a risk factor for failed intubation. The importance lies in the fact that, when airway problems occur in obese patients, the time available to secure the airway before profound hypoxaemia occurs is dramatically reduced and may be as little as 30–60 s, even after full preoxygenation. The presence of obstructive sleep apnoea in addition to obesity increases the risk of airway obstruction and rapid hypoxaemia after induction of anaesthesia.

All organizations should have a guideline (and individuals a plan) for the management of CICV. The DAS guideline is one option (Figs 22.3–22.5).

The principles behind management of CICV are:

1. Give 100% oxygen and call for help
2. Perform optimal face-mask ventilation

3. Insert an appropriate SAD
4. Wake the patient if this is feasible
5. If waking is not feasible and CICV persists, administer a neuromuscular blocking drug if not already administered
6. If the situation is not resolved, secure the airway with direct tracheal access.

Give 100% Oxygen and Call for Help. CICV is a life-threatening emergency. Oxygen should be delivered at high flow, maximum concentration. Even experienced anaesthetists require assistance in these circumstances. Call for the emergency airway trolley. However the main assistant should not be sent away – rather call on others to help and ensure all around understand clearly that the situation is a critical emergency.

Perform Optimal Face Mask Ventilation. This involves a tight-fitting appropriately sized mask. Continuous positive airways pressure (CPAP) and an anti-Trendelenburg position may be helpful. An oropharyngeal (and perhaps nasopharyngeal) airway should be inserted. Two-handed (one person) mask ventilation should be changed to four- or six-handed ventilation (Figs 22.8–22.9).

Insert an Appropriate SAD. The ideal SAD for rescuing the airway during CICV has several properties:

- reliable first-time insertion
- reliable ventilation of the lungs after insertion
- protection against aspiration of regurgitated material.

Based on risk factors and epidemiology, CICV might typically occur in an obese, paralysed patient at risk of aspiration and undergoing emergency surgery. The evidence base supports the use of a second generation SAD with a high seal pressure. The ProSeal LMA, inserted over a gum-elastic bougie placed in the oesophagus, is logically the best choice as this combines high first-time success with the best airway seal of all SADs and increased protection against aspiration (Fig. 22.15). Alternatives include the i-gel, LMA Supreme or laryngeal tube suction II.

Prospective studies suggest that the cLMA will rescue many cases of CICV (>90%), while studies of poor

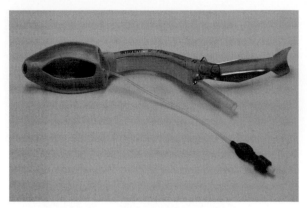

FIGURE 22.15 ■ The Pro-Seal laryngeal mask airway. See text for details.

outcomes from airway complications suggest that failure to rescue the airway with a SAD increases the risk of a poor outcome. Multiple attempts at laryngoscopy will probably lead to laryngeal trauma and reduce the success rate of airway rescue with a SAD. Obesity may also be a risk factor.

CICV should not be allowed to progress to a stage where the patient's life is at risk without attempted rescue with an appropriate SAD.

Wake the Patient if this is Feasible. If the airway cannot be rescued, the default option should be to seek a 'place of safety' which in most cases involves waking the patient up. As a rule of thumb, this should be considered actively in all cases of airway difficulty and, if it is feasible, it is the safest option. In cases where difficulty may be anticipated it is particularly useful to adopt a 'wake up trigger' as part of the airway strategy and communicate it to all around before commencing anaesthesia. The airway can subsequently be secured awake. This option is equally valid when the airway has been secured with a SAD.

However, waking the patient up is not practical in many emergencies, most commonly because either the patient has received a neuromuscular blocking drug or because of profound progressive hypoxaemia. Less commonly, the urgency of the surgery demands that it must proceed and the airway must be secured 'come what may'.

If Waking is not Feasible and CICV Persists, Administer a Neuromuscular Blocking Drug if not Already Administered. This may be considered by some to be controversial but we believe it is not; rather, it is entirely logical. It is well recognized that neuromuscular blockade may assist ventilation. The only strong argument for not administering a neuromuscular blocker when ventilation is difficult is the concern about how to manage the airway if ventilation is not improved. In the circumstance of CICV, where waking is not feasible, it is not possible for the situation to get worse and the realistic possibility that neuromuscular blockade may improve the airway means that it is entirely logical because it may prevent the need to provide an emergency surgical airway. Even if it does not enable ventilation, it is likely that performance of an emergency surgical airway will be easier after neuromuscular blockade.

If the Situation is not Resolved, Secure the Airway with Direct Tracheal Access. When CICV is not resolved by optimal face-mask ventilation, attempted SAD insertion and neuromuscular blockade, profound hypoxia and cardiac arrest occur rapidly (usually within 3–5 min) unless an airway is established and the blood is re-oxygenated. There are three options:

- narrow-bore cannula with high pressure source ventilation
- wide-bore cannula
- surgical technique.

Decision making in CICV. As, or arguably more important than, choosing the correct device to rescue the airway is making the decision that a rescue procedure is needed. There have been numerous studies which illustrate that many emergency surgical airways are performed too late to prevent hypoxic brain injury or death.

When CICV is unresolved and hypoxia is progressing, the decision should be made and communicated to those around, and prompt actions should be taken. Even in ideal circumstances, it is unlikely the airway will be secured after this decision is made in less than 3 min. An appropriate early decision may save a life.

EMERGENCY SURGICAL AIRWAY TECHNIQUES

Devices

Narrow-Bore Cannula with High Pressure Source Ventilation. A narrow-bore cannula (most are approximately 2 mm internal diameter) is usually inserted as a cannula-over-needle technique through the cricothyroid membrane. Once inserted, ventilation is based on two important principles: first, a high driving pressure is required to inflate the lungs due to the enormous resistance to flow through the cannula; second, expiration must take place though the patient's upper airway. It is appropriate to use specifically designed devices (e.g. Ravussin cannula; Fig. 22.16A) which sit against the neck correctly (Fig. 22.16B) and are less likely to kink. Similarly, a specifically designed ventilating device (e.g. Manujet injector; Fig. 22.17) is strongly recommended. Use of intravenous cannulae (which cannot be fixed securely and tend to kink) and 'Heath-Robinson' assemblies for ventilation are difficult to justify in settings such as operating theatres where it can be predicted that such a technique will be required from time to time: avoiding the need for such *ad hoc* devices is part of institutional and personal preparedness.

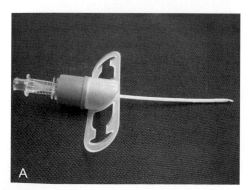 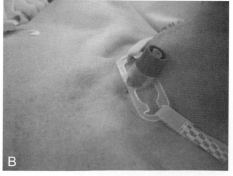

FIGURE 22.16 ■ **(A)** The Ravussin cricothyroid cannula. **(B)** The Ravussin cannula fixed to the skin after insertion.

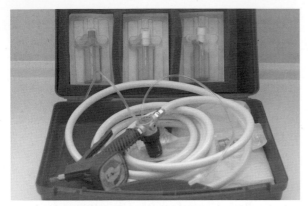

FIGURE 22.17 ■ The Manujet injector kit.

Wide-Bore Cannula (≥4 mm). Wide-bore cannulae may be cannula-over-needle devices (e.g. QuickTrach) or those requiring a Seldinger insertion technique (e.g. Melker cricothyroidotomy devices; Fig. 22.18).

Cannula-over-needle devices require a large sharp needle which risks significant tissue trauma if misplaced and such devices may be too short to reach the trachea in patients with an obese neck. Seldinger-type devices take somewhat longer to insert but the technique is familiar (and generally favoured) by anaesthetists.

The Melker 5.0 mm internal diameter cuffed cricothyroidotomy device is a Seldinger-type device which is generally inserted with ease, using a technique similar to a percutaneous tracheostomy. One option for rescuing the airway is to insert a Ravussin cannula and to ventilate the lungs with a Manujet to re-oxygenate, and then change this to a large bore cannula inserting the Seldinger wire from the Melker kit through the Ravussin cannula as the first step.

Surgical Airway. A surgical airway technique comprises four steps.

1. The cricothyroid membrane is identified.

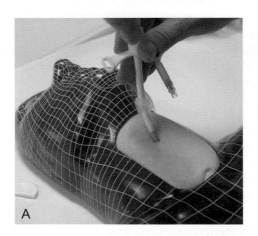
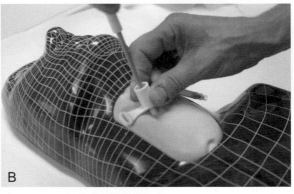
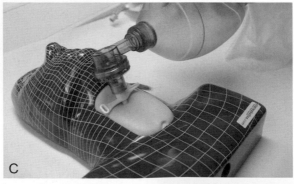

FIGURE 22.18 ■ The Melker cricothyroidotomy device. (**A**) The introducer and cannula are advanced over a Seldinger wire placed in the trachea (not shown). (**B**) The cannula is advanced over the introducer. (**C**) The introducer is withdrawn and ventilation is started after inflating the cuff.

2. An incision is made in the neck over the crico-thyroid membrane (a round-ended No. 20 blade is recommended) extending deep into the membrane and the scalpel is kept in place.

3. A 'cricoid hook' is inserted and the cricoid cartilage pulled forward.

4. A 6.0 mm internal diameter tracheal tube (or tracheostomy tube) is inserted.

Numerous variations are described and include the use of tracheostomy dilators instead of the cricoid hook or insertion of a bougie into the trachea instead of a tube. The important feature is to ensure that, once the trachea has been entered, something stays in it, keeping the tracheostomy tract open at all times.

Various simulation studies suggest that a surgical technique can be performed as rapidly as a Seldinger cannula technique, although these are typically performed in bloodless fields. However, studies from America, where the technique is probably used most commonly, suggest that the likelihood of saving a life with a surgical airway is considerably higher than mortality from the bleeding complications of an attempt.

In a recent study of major complications of airway management, more than 60% of cannula cricothyroidotomies inserted by anaesthetists to rescue the airway in an emergency failed. The causes were numerous and included use of inappropriate equipment, misuse of appropriate devices, device failure, poor technique and inappropriate ventilation via a correctly placed narrow-bore device. The chances of success are increased greatly if the correct equipment is used skilfully and correctly. This requires training. Training in such techniques fades after approximately three months and requires regular updating. Training should include both cannula and surgical techniques.

Ventilation and Expiration Via Cricothyroidotomy Devices

Narrow-Bore Cannula. When ventilating through a narrow-bore cannula, a high pressure source is needed to overcome the resistance of the cannula. However, the pressure changes in the trachea during this type of ventilation are similar to those during conventional ventilation. The technique should not be confused with 'jet ventilation' or 'oscillation'; what is achieved is 'high pressure source conventional ventilation'. Appropriate sources of the high pressure for such ventilation are either wall oxygen or an oxygen cylinder, both approximately 400 kPa (4 bar, 4000 cmH$_2$O, 58 psi). If wall oxygen is used, the flow rate should be set at greater than 15 L min^{-1}. When using an anaesthetic machine, pressure regulators and 'blow-off' valves reduce the pressure available; an attached anaesthetic breathing system with a conventional anaesthetic reservoir bag limits pressure to 6 kPa (60 cmH$_2$O), which is totally inadequate for ventilating through a narrow cannula. If the anaesthetic flush is deployed continuously, a pressure of 30–60 kPa (300–600 cmH$_2$O) can be achieved and this may be just sufficient to ventilate the lungs. Maximum flow rates from an anaesthetic machine are 15 L min^{-1} via a flowmeter and 30–60 L min^{-1} when the oxygen flush button is depressed. An anaesthetic machine cannot provide a reliably high pressure source unless a connection is made to a high pressure source outlet at the back of the machine, usually a 'mini-Schrader' connector which can then be used to drive an injector or similar device (Fig. 22.19). An oxygen 'injector' such as a Sanders or Manujet injector can deliver a high pressure source ranging from 0.5–4 bar (500–4000 kPa) at a flow rate of up to 1000 mL s^{-1}. Wall oxygen or the use of an injector may inflate the chest by 500 mL within 0.5 s. Using a Manujet, a driving pressure of 1 bar may be adequate to ventilate most slim patients, and reduces the risk of barotrauma. Neuromuscular blockade, and inserting a SAD to maximize the expiratory route, also increase the success of the technique.

However, when ventilating the lungs using a cricothyroid cannula in the presence of complete upper

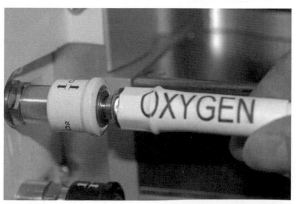

FIGURE 22.19 ■ A mini-Schrader oxygen connector on the back of an anaesthetic machine.

airway obstruction, the critical aspect is not lung inflation (inspiration) but lung deflation (exhalation). This is critical both to generating adequate minute ventilation and preventing complications. Exhalation of 500 mL via a 14-gauge cannula takes at least 30 s and therefore is of no practical use. There is a myth that a second cannula should be inserted into the airway to enable exhalation; to enable exhalation in 4 s would require 32–64 cannulae! Delivering further breaths through a misplaced cannula or without allowing full expiration leads inevitably to barotrauma, which can rapidly be life-threatening. However, even in CICV, exhalation through the upper airway is usually effective. During ventilation via the patient's normal airway, the upper airway is drawn inwards in inspiration and tends to collapse. In expiration, positive intraluminal pressure tends to expand and open the upper airway. As a result, inspiratory airway obstruction is more common than expiratory. Even in CICV situations, the airway is sufficiently patent during expiration to allow exhalation in up to 90% of patients. As a 'rule of thumb' during high pressure source ventilation via a small cannula, the operator should ensure that the chest falls completely before the next inspiration. A hand placed on the chest during ventilation can confirm that the chest is rising and falling, and detect early surgical emphysema if it develops. If exhalation is slow because of upper airway obstruction, the frequency of ventilation must be decreased appropriately. Ventilation can continue safely, albeit at a slower rate and with a reduced minute volume. Manually compressing the chest during expiration to augment exhalation may be of benefit. If expiration cannot be achieved, the gas flow should be reduced to basal flow (0.25–0.5 L min^{-1}) in an attempt to provide apnoeic oxygenation, without ventilation.

A device (Ventrain) has recently been developed which uses a driving gas that bypasses a cricothyroid/tracheal cannula during the expiratory phase and entrains gas from the cannula to achieve 'assisted exhalation' using the Venturi effect. It is not yet in widespread use but may solve some of the problems and confusion surrounding this mode of ventilation.

Wide-Bore Cannula and Surgical Techniques. Wide-bore cannulae are defined as those with an internal diameter of at least 4 mm because this is the minimum

calibre through which an adult can exhale with adequate speed to maintain a normal minute volume. This applies whether inspiration is mechanical or spontaneous, because expiration is a passive process.

After the device has been inserted, ventilation can be achieved with a low pressure gas source (e.g. a standard anaesthetic machine). In contrast to narrow bore cannulae, large bore cannulae require that the upper airway is obstructed during inspiration to avoid the ventilating gas being vented via the upper airway. This may be achieved by actively obstructing the upper airway (e.g. a SAD is inserted and the proximal end obstructed) or, preferably, by the use of a cuffed cannula. Spontaneous ventilation via a wide bore cannula is also possible.

To summarize, this is a complex and often confused topic. There are three methods of achieving oxygenation and ventilation via a cricothyroidotomy.

- ■ Small cannula (approx. 2 mm) techniques (usually inserted as cannula over needle) require a high pressure gas source to overcome device resistance and rely on a patent upper airway for exhalation. Entrainment may augment inspiratory flow.
- ■ Large cannula (≥ 4 mm) techniques enable ventilation with lower pressures but require either a tracheal cuff, or the upper airway to be obstructed, to prevent loss of driving gas through the upper airway. Entrainment is minimal or non-existent.
- ■ Surgical airway techniques allow insertion of a large tube into the trachea and conventional (low pressure) ventilation, as for large cannulae.

MANAGEMENT OF THE PREDICTED DIFFICULT AIRWAY

The main difference between management of the unanticipated and the predicted difficult airway is that the latter enables the anaesthetic team to plan and prepare more thoroughly and to fit a strategy to the specific needs of the patient rather than following a guideline designed to 'fit all situations'. Due to the limitations of airway assessment, many patients with a 'predicted difficult airway' will not prove to be difficult, but this is not a reason to ignore preoperative findings or history of difficulty. Many airway disasters are preceded by anaesthetists ignoring the history or signs of difficulty and then getting into avoidable trouble.

When airway management is predicted to be difficult, the strategy can be based around achieving:

- the right place
- the right time
- the right plan (strategy)
- the right person.

Ensuring the right place may require that the patient is transferred to a location where appropriate monitoring, equipment and skills are available to manage the airway safely. However, transfer of a patient with a critical airway is fraught with danger and an assessment of specific risks should be made, including a plan for management of deterioration during transfer. In the operating theatre setting, patients in whom airway difficulty is anticipated should usually be managed in the operating theatre rather than the anaesthetic room for reasons of space, visibility, monitoring, communication and teamwork.

The right time implies patients with anticipated difficulty should be managed at the time that is safest for the patient. Urgent and emergency patients must be managed with appropriate promptness but elective procedures should be managed with enough time for assessment, collecting all necessary information (e.g. retrieving notes and scans as necessary) and gathering the equipment and personnel needed for optimal management.

The right plan has been discussed earlier in the chapter in the section describing strategy. In patients with a predicted difficult airway, careful assessment is vital to determine which specific routes of access and techniques are likely to be problematic or successful, so that a logical individualized strategy can be constructed.

The right person may not be the anaesthetist to whom the patient presents. The right person may also not be one individual but a number of individuals with the skills to carry out specialized parts of the airway strategy. If possible, the right personnel should be present from the start of airway management. Most airway difficulties provide ample opportunity for teaching and these opportunities should be seized.

Although the detail may differ, the principles of managing the patient with predicted airway difficulty are no different to managing unanticipated problems (e.g. strategy, oxygenation, rescue techniques, good teamwork).

MANAGEMENT OF THE OBSTRUCTED AIRWAY

The management of the obstructed airway represents a very dangerous, although rare, situation. Obstruction may occur from the pharynx to any point distally and may be due to many causes including infection or trauma, but the most common cause is malignancy. The patient may present late or occasionally be referred incorrectly to the ICU team with a diagnosis of worsening asthma/COPD, having failed to respond to treatment and perhaps *in extremis*. To manage these patients safely and achieve a successful outcome requires careful preparation, planning and good communication between anaesthetists, ENT specialists, the operating theatre team and, in some situations, cardiothoracic surgeons.

Optimal management of the obstructed airway is controversial but it is generally the case that airway obstruction becomes worse during anaesthesia because of supine positioning and loss of airway tone and reflexes. All approaches may lead to life-threatening complications (e.g. complete obstruction after induction of anaesthesia, haemorrhage or swelling in the airway). Involvement of anaesthetists and surgeons with appropriate experience is essential and back-up plans should be established and communicated to all.

Precise management depends on the level and cause of the obstruction, the urgency for intervention and several other factors. Assessment should determine the following factors.

- What is the level of the obstruction?
- What is the degree of obstruction?
- Is it fixed or variable?
- What is its cause (e.g. tumour, haematoma, infection)?
- Is it friable or likely to bleed?
- Has there been previous airway or neck surgery, or radiotherapy? All place the patient in a higher risk category.
- Can the patient's airway be improved? If time allows, nebulized adrenaline (epinephrine) or steroids may improve the airway for short periods

of time. Heliox (a mixture of helium and oxygen) may be beneficial before anaesthesia in critical cases. Radiotherapy may improve the airway, although often this is impractical.

- Is there any important co-morbidity?
- What is the surgical plan and preferred route for anaesthetic access? These patients illustrate the complexity of a 'shared airway' and there is no point in planning an anaesthetic approach which is not compatible with an agreed surgical plan.
- What is the urgency of the intervention? It is important to differentiate patients in whom anaesthesia is planned to achieve surgery to improve the airway from those in whom anaesthesia is necessary to secure the airway in order to preserve life.

Important features of the history and clinical examination are noisy breathing and waking up in the middle of the night fighting for breath (having a panic attack), or having to sleep in an upright position. These features enable the anaesthetist to determine the patient's 'best breathing position' to be used during induction of anaesthesia. If a patient cannot tolerate lying flat when awake, that position is likely to be dangerous after induction of anaesthesia. Stridor (inspiratory noise) is a concerning sign as it represents significant upper airway narrowing; however, it is not always present and patients with chronic obstruction may can present with a very narrow airway and no stridor. Expiratory noise (wheeze) may indicate a lower level of obstruction.

Other than in the most urgent cases or if the patient's condition makes it impossible, full investigation is warranted. This usually involves CT or MRI, nasendoscopy and lung function tests. Imaging is vital to planning both the surgical and anaesthetic approaches and should be viewed together. Imaging is performed supine and is a static image; it does not necessarily reflect the airway in the sitting position or the dynamic nature of the obstruction. It is also important to note the date of any imaging; lesions may progress rapidly.

Nasendoscopy is underused by anaesthetists and, although discussion of the surgical findings may be useful, it is often sensible for the anaesthetist to perform awake nasendoscopy, even when a fibreoptic approach is not planned. Lung function tests including flow volume loops may help in assessing the extent of physiological compromise and the level of the obstruction. If these tests are not possible, a 'walk test' may be of value because it enables the accompanying anaesthetist to assess exercise tolerance and respiratory pattern, and may elicit signs such as noisy breathing which add information not acquired at the bedside.

Patients with an obstructed airway can be considered according to the level of obstruction.

Upper Airway Obstruction

In patients with upper airway obstruction, the cause is usually malignancy, trauma or infection affecting the larynx and other supraglottic structures such as the tonsils and tongue. Many approaches to the airway are possible. The management depends on whether or not it is judged that intubation from above the vocal cords is going to be possible. Usually an informed decision can be made after nasendoscopy and imaging.

If it is clear before surgery that intubation will not be possible due to excessive tumour reducing the laryngeal opening, no recognizable structures visible at nasendoscopy or any other reason that might make direct laryngoscopy difficult, the safest approach is to perform a tracheostomy under local anaesthesia. Lesions of the base of the tongue and floor of the mouth often interfere with laryngoscopy, particularly if there has been previous surgery or radiotherapy. Where there is doubt, awake fibreoptic intubation is a safe method for trying to secure the airway. Laryngeal lesions may interfere with all forms of tracheal intubation. Awake fibreoptic intubation may be an option but surgical technique may require unrestricted access to the larynx. Supraglottic (from above), transglottic (via a narrow 2–3 mm catheter placed through the cords) or transtracheal (via a catheter placed in the trachea) ventilation may all be options or necessities and each requires attention and good communication between the anaesthetist and surgeon.

Inevitably, some patients require general anaesthesia for airway management. The choices between intravenous and inhalational induction, and between spontaneous and controlled ventilation, are controversial. Whichever method is chosen, a clear plan for airway management and back-up is needed, with all relevant equipment and personnel present. Airway interventions should not be performed before the patient is adequately anaesthetized. A senior ENT surgeon should be in the operating theatre and prepared to carry out immediate surgical cricothyroidotomy or tracheostomy if the airway is lost. If intubation proves impossible but the airway is patent and the patient is stable, the patient may be woken or a tracheostomy undertaken, depending on the patient's needs.

Mid-Tracheal Obstruction

This presents an entirely different problem and is often caused by a retrosternal thyroid mass, although malignancies and infections may be the cause (Fig. 22.20). In the presence of a thyroid mass, the onset of airway compromise is usually slow and further radiological assessment is possible. A CT scan is vital to show the level and extent of the obstruction. Lesions below the larynx do not interfere with laryngoscopy (although the larynx and trachea may be displaced; Fig. 22.21) or the ability to use a face mask or SAD but they may interfere with ventilation after induction of anaesthesia and the ability to insert a tracheal tube.

There are several key issues which must be clarified before anaesthesia.

- How wide is the tracheal lumen and what size of tracheal tube may be used?
- Is there space below the obstruction and above the carina to accommodate the end of the tracheal tube and the cuff?

- Is the tracheal wall itself invaded? If so, there is a risk of collapse after any external mass has been removed.
- Would an emergency tracheostomy be possible and would a standard tracheostomy tube be long enough to bypass the obstruction?

If laryngoscopy is predicted to be straightforward, if there is no tracheal invasion and if there is a clear distance below the obstruction and above the carina, a standard anaesthetic induction technique followed by administration of a muscle relaxant can be considered. Otherwise, the safest way of securing the airway is likely to be awake fibreoptic intubation, although the problem of obstructing the airway while the obstruction is passed ('cork in a bottle') remains and may be distressing to the patient. Airway stimulation and coughing may lead to complete obstruction; an experienced operator is essential. Plan B in the situation in which a rapid tracheostomy would not be possible is the use of a rigid bronchoscope by a skilled operator.

Lower Tracheal or Bronchial Obstruction

This is a very difficult clinical problem and life-threatening complications may occur. The cause is usually a malignant mediastinal mass and obstruction of the superior vena cava often co-exists. Sudden

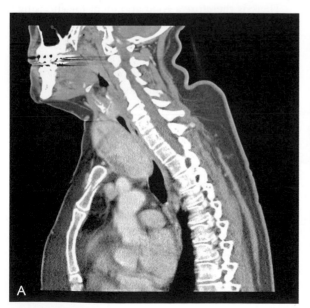
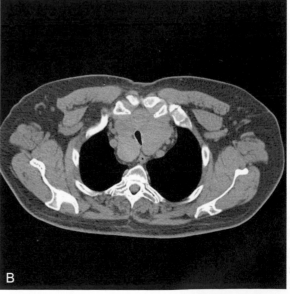

FIGURE 22.20 ■ Sagittal (**A**) and axial (**B**) images of a thyroid mass partly obstructing the mid-trachea.

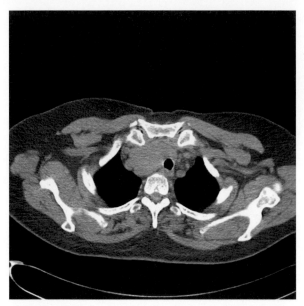

FIGURE 22.21 ■ Axial image of a large thyroid mass which has displaced but not compressed the trachea.

and total obstruction to ventilation can occur at any time, particularly if the patient becomes apnoeic or a muscle relaxant is used. Subatmospheric intrapleural pressure during inspiration may contribute to holding the airways open; if lost, the pressure from any mass external to the airway can cause airway collapse and complete obstruction. A tissue diagnosis should be obtained under local anaesthesia if possible and an emergency course of chemo/radiotherapy should be considered; stenting or laser resection may be surgical options. Management is complex and, if possible, the patient should be transferred to a cardiothoracic centre where rapid induction of anaesthesia and skilled rigid bronchoscopy may be the technique of choice. Extracorporeal oxygenation may be required.

SPECIFIC TECHNIQUES

Supraglottic Airway Devices for Airway Rescue

SADs are an important group of devices for airway rescue, in particular for failed mask ventilation or for CICV. Neuromuscular blockade is not required for insertion (unlike tracheal intubation) and success rates are high. Success rates for airway rescue are reported to be as high as 95% for the classic laryngeal mask airway. Whether rates are as high for PVC and other single-use laryngeal masks is not known.

Despite this high rate of success, there is a strong argument for selecting an alternative SAD as first choice. Patients who require airway rescue are often obese, male, scheduled to undergo emergency surgery and likely to have received a neuromuscular blocker either before or during the airway emergency. Many are at a significantly increased risk of regurgitation and aspiration of gastric fluid because of obesity, urgency of surgery and possible gastric inflation during attempts to ventilate by face mask. These are not the type of patients whom most anaesthetists would choose to manage with a standard laryngeal mask. In this circumstance, the requirements for a SAD to rescue the airway are:

- speedy and reliable insertion
- reliable ventilation (even if lung compliance is low)
- early detection of regurgitation and increased protection against aspiration
- ability to empty the stomach
- suitable as a conduit for subsequent fibreoptic guided tracheal intubation.

There is therefore a good argument for choosing a second generation SAD for airway rescue. Suitable devices include the ProSeal LMA (probably inserted over a bougie to increase success), i-gel. The Supreme LMA and Laryngeal Tube Suction II enable airway rescue but are less suited as conduits to intubation.

SADs as Conduits for Intubation

This has been discussed above.

'Videolaryngoscopes', Rigid Indirect Laryngoscopes, Optical Stilettes and Advanced Intubation Aids: (see also Chapter 15)

Numerous devices aimed at improving management of difficult direct laryngoscopy have been developed and marketed in the last decade. The main principle behind these devices is an intent to convert intubation that would previously have been blind (e.g. blind nasal, bougie-guided, light-wand guided) into a visualized technique. The devices can be described as videolaryngoscopes, rigid fibrescopes or indirect laryngoscopes, although none of these descriptions includes all devices. They can be divided into three major groups:

- bladed indirect laryngoscopes
- conduited intubation guides
- optical stilettes.

Bladed indirect laryngoscopes form the largest group. Older versions include the Bullard and Upsherscope and newer devices include the Glidescope, McGrath 5 and C-MAC. These devices move the viewing point beyond the curve of the laryngoscope blade, making it possible, effectively, to 'see round corners'. A much wider angle of view is achieved because the viewing point is distal.

Conduited intubation guides include several rigid fibreoptic laryngoscopes (Pentax AWscope, AP Advance laryngoscope) and the Airtraq (Fig. 22.22), which uses optical prisms rather than fibreoptics to illuminate the object and transmit an image.

Optical stilettes are metal rods with an internal fibreoptic or video system which enables the user to view the image from the distal end directly from the viewing port or on a remote screen. Most stilettes are rigid with a fixed angle (e.g. Bonfils, Levitan). The Shikani stilette (Fig. 22.23) is semi-malleable and the Sensascope has a flexible fibreoptic tip which allows some manipulation. Optical stilettes are placed within the lumen of the tracheal tube and then directed into the larynx before the tracheal tube is advanced into the airway. The main advantage of the stilettes is that they require minimal mouth opening (as little as 1 cm)

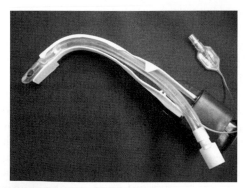

FIGURE 22.22 ■ An Airtraq conduited rigid fibreoptic laryngoscope with a tracheal tube mounted in the conduit.

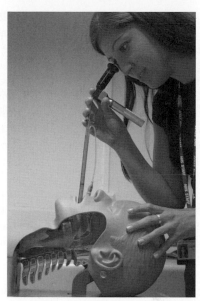

FIGURE 22.23 ■ A Shikani stilette inside an ILMA tracheal tube in use on a manikin.

and can be advanced with negligible tissue disruption. Their main disadvantage is the inability to manipulate and displace airway structures in the manner that a bladed instrument can.

The potential advantages of these devices include:

- ability to 'see round corners'
- reduced head and neck movement to achieve a view of the larynx
- reduced tissue distortion and haemodynamic responses to laryngoscopy
- ability to display the image on a remote screen, which permits:
  - improved supervision by trainers of intubation performed by trainees
  - an assistant to observe what the intubator sees (e.g. guiding cricoid pressure)
- recording for medical notes and medicolegal reasons
- recording of an objective image or video for presentation, teaching or research purposes.

Despite their obvious appeal, the benefits of these devices are less well proven than might be expected. Most research undertaken has been on patients with a normal airway and some is of poor quality. As a result, their efficacy in patients with a difficult airway is uncertain. The ability to move the viewing point distally in the airway is an obvious advantage but the fact the tracheal tube is not introduced under direct vision means that its insertion may be more difficult. The devices may improve the view of the larynx without making intubation easier and in easy intubations, these devices often prolong the time to intubation. To overcome this problem, many manufacturers advise the use of a rigid or semi-rigid stilette to pre-form the shape of the tracheal tube before insertion. There is a risk of damage to other tissues in the airway as the tracheal tube/stilette assembly is introduced (blindly). Conduited devices and stilettes have a potential advantage over bladed indirect laryngoscopes because the device guides the tracheal tube directly to the area being viewed through the device and there is no need for blind introduction of a tracheal tube/stilette assembly. There is no consensus on which device or group of devices performs best.

There is increasing evidence, for some of these devices, that videolaryngoscopy does offer a useful alternative to direct laryngoscopy in patients known, or found unexpectedly, to be difficult to intubate. In addition, they can be used awake after topical administration of local anaesthetic to the airway because less tissue distortion is needed in comparison to a conventional laryngoscope. It is likely that their use will become much more prevalent. All the devices are expensive and have a learning curve. If such a device is to be used, it is logical to acquire skills in the use of one device; if skills in the use of more than one device are needed, it is logical to select one device from each of the three groups.

EXTUBATION AND RECOVERY

Airway problems at extubation and in the recovery room account for approximately one-third of major airway complications of anaesthesia. Most involve airway obstruction, some with secondary aspiration of fluid into the lungs. At the time of extubation, there is a change from a controlled situation, with airway protection, suppressed airway reflexes and the ability to deliver 100% oxygen, to one of absent airway protection, partial recovery of airway reflexes and an ability to reliably deliver only much lower oxygen concentrations. In this respect, it contrasts markedly

with intubation. Airway obstruction which occurs during emergence and recovery needs to be rapidly recognized and resolved to prevent hypoxaemia and post-obstructive pulmonary oedema (POPO), which considerably worsen the situation.

Factors which increase the risk of problems at the time of extubation/emergence and recovery include:

- patients who had problems at intubation or induction
- blood in the airway from surgical or anaesthetic causes
- patients who may have airway oedema from anaesthetic or surgical interventions
- obese patients, particularly those with obstructive sleep apnoea
- intraoral or airway surgery (risks both oedema and aspiration of blood).

Management of at-risk extubation requires recognition of the potential problem, planning, preparation, preoxygenation and, sometimes, special procedures. Communication with the operating theatre team is important because there is a natural tendency for the surgical and nursing team members to relax and attend to other tasks at the end of surgery.

Planning involves creating a strategy for extubation (plan A and back-up plans), communicating this to assistants and colleagues and ensuring that the right equipment is immediately available and that personnel with the necessary skills are present. This may require the difficult airway trolley, summoning senior anaesthetic assistance or requiring the surgeon to remain in the event that an emergency surgical airway is required. Planning also includes making a clear decision as to whether the airway will be removed with the patient 'deep' or awake.

Pre-oxygenation is part of preparation but is separated for emphasis: it is the single most important preparatory step before extubation.

Preparation involves optimizing the patient for extubation. This includes (but is not limited to) ensuring full reversal of neuromuscular blockade, adequate offset of anaesthetic and opioid medication (choice of appropriate drugs at an early stage in the anaesthetic makes this easier), pharyngeal and bronchial suction as necessary and emptying the stomach if there is a risk of aspiration. Dexamethasone may be administered to minimize airway swelling although its effect is delayed and its administration does not influence the immediate consequences of extubation. Direct inspection of the airway may be necessary to assess oedema and is specifically indicated when there has been blood in the airway to ensure that there is no risk of aspiration of blood after extubation. A leak-test may be performed, in which the tracheal tube cuff is deflated and positive pressure applied while listening for an audible leak around the trachea. The test assesses only laryngeal swelling and is very dependent on the size of tracheal tube used and the pressure applied, so its efficacy in predicting safe extubation is limited.

Special procedures are non-routine actions at extubation performed to improve the safety of extubation and to facilitate re-intubation if that is necessary. Examples include insertion of a cricothyroid needle or airway exchange catheter (AEC) prior to extubation, exchange of the tracheal tube for a SAD immediately before or after extubation, or extubation followed immediately by CPAP. If an AEC is left in place it should be placed in strict accordance with manufacturer's instructions and the tip should not lie beyond the mid-trachea (i.e. no more than 26 cm from the lips in adults). Administration of oxygen through the AEC risks significant barotrauma if the catheter migrates distally and is unnecessary other than in exceptional circumstances. If it is considered that there is very high risk at extubation, an elective tracheostomy may be appropriate. Alternatively, extubation may be delayed and the patient transferred to ICU. In these circumstances, extubation on ICU will probably need the same processes of planning through to special procedures and it may be appropriate to return to the operating theatre specifically for safe extubation.

Problems occurring in the recovery room are particularly dangerous because the care of the patient's airway is delegated to a nurse and there may be limited access to equipment, personnel with advanced airway skills and capnography. The anaesthetist usually returns to the operating theatre and is involved in anaesthetizing the next patient within a few minutes. If the airway is at risk after surgery, the anaesthetist must either recover the patient in the operating theatre or remain with the patient until the airway is safe. A diagnosis of hypoventilation and airway obstruction in recovery may be masked by administration of oxygen because oxygen desaturation may not occur until the situation is advanced. Recovery staff should be skilled in the recognition of signs of airway obstruction and its early management. Capnography should be available and can be used with a SAD or face mask in place: its use is increasingly recommended during recovery. Where it is used the recovery room staff need to be trained in its interpretation.

Aspiration of blood and blood clots is a specific risk after intraoral surgery (e.g. maxillofacial, tonsillectomy, adenoidectomy). Good surgical technique and good surgical and anaesthetic communication are important in preventing problems. At the end of surgery, the surgeon and the anaesthetist together must ensure there is no blood, blood clots (including in the post nasal space) or bleeding before airway removal. If a throat pack has been used, recommended methods of communicating its presence and ensuring its removal are important. Positioning for extubation and transfer are important; extubation and transfer with the patient in the lateral position is recommended until consciousness and airway reflexes have returned. Aspiration of blood or blood clot can cause laryngospasm or tracheal obstruction. If tracheal obstruction occurs, the diagnosis may be missed unless it is actively considered; the clinical picture of hypoxaemia, inability to ventilate and high airway pressures may be mistaken for asthma, anaphylaxis or even oesophageal intubation. A flat capnograph trace in an intubated patient (even during CPR) indicates absence of ventilation; the tracheal tube or trachea may be obstructed or the tube is not in the trachea. Management may require bronchial suction, reintubation or rigid bronchoscopy.

Deaths still occur from aspiration of blood in the recovery period and all anaesthetists must be aware of the clinical signs and management.

Guidelines on Management of Extubation

There has been a steady increase in interest in the topic of extubation. In 2012, DAS published the first national guidance on extubation of adult patients (Fig. 22.24). This guidance divides extubation into four phases: plan, prepare, perform and post-extubation care. It recommends that an early assessment is made to determine whether extubation is low (fasted, uncomplicated airway, no other risk factors) or high risk (others). After taking the precautions described above, low risk extubation can

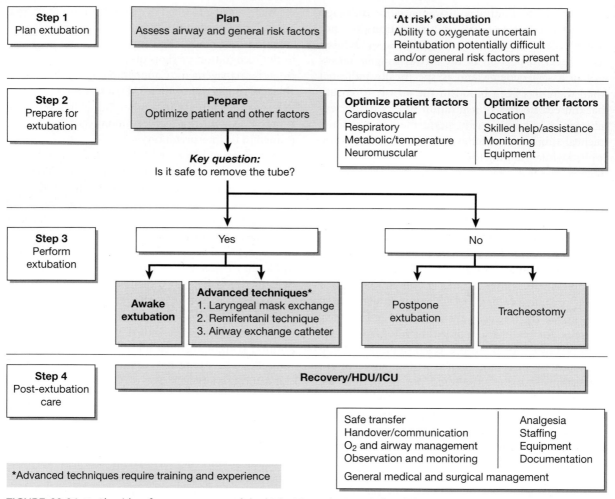

FIGURE 22.24 ■ Algorithm for management of the high risk extubation. *(Adapted from Popat M, Mitchell V, Dravid R, Patel A, Swampillai C, Higgs A. Difficult Airway Society Guidelines for the management of tracheal extubation. Anaesthesia 2012; 67:318–340, with permission from the Association of Anaesthetists of Great Britain & Ireland/Blackwell Publishing Ltd.)*

usually be managed awake or 'deep' according to the anaesthetist's preference and judgement, though making clear that the default method is awake. For patients requiring high risk extubation a number of options are offered: awake extubation, advanced techniques, delayed extubation and tracheostomy. Advanced techniques are conversion to a laryngeal mask with the tracheal tube *in situ* before extubation, a 'remifentanil extubation' or use of an AEC. Deep extubation in the high risk setting is not advocated. All the advanced techniques are described in detail but require expertise and practice before use in an acute situation.

THE DIFFICULT AIRWAY IN OTHER LOCATIONS

A difficult airway is encountered most commonly in the operating theatre suite around the time of surgery, but most deaths from airway management difficulty occur elsewhere. At least a quarter of major airway events occur outside theatres, with ICU and the emergency department being particularly important areas. When such events occur in these sites, the risk of injury is increased compared to the risk in the operating theatre environment.

The reasons for this are complicated. Patients on ICU are critically ill, with markedly reduced physiological reserve. Approximately 8% have a difficult airway. Most have pre-existing respiratory compromise and increased intrapulmonary shunt and therefore tolerate airway obstruction or apnoea very poorly. Initial tracheal intubation is often performed as an extreme emergency and allowing the patient to wake if difficulty occurs is often not an option. While intubation in the ICU is accepted to be very high risk, a large proportion of critical airway events in this setting occur at a time well after intubation. Dislodgement of tracheal tubes and particularly tracheostomies, followed by airway difficulty, especially in the obese, is a notable cause of morbidity and mortality. The airway is often oedematous for a considerable period after prolonged intubation and re-intubation may be more difficult.

In the emergency department, patients often have reduced physiological reserves as a result of the pathophysiological problem that led to admission. Trauma is a specific condition in the emergency department which often increases the difficulty of airway management. The combination of an at-risk cervical spine requiring immobilization of the neck, blood in the airway and multiple trauma with pulmonary injury and hypovolaemia is a major challenge.

There are also extrinsic factors which may lead to an increased likelihood of difficulty and to poor management of the difficult airway outside the operating theatre suite.

- Hazardous environment: an environment not designed for airway management and where this is sometimes not considered a main priority.
- Failure to recognize and plan for patients with a known or predictably difficult airway.
- A more limited range of equipment for management of the difficult airway than in theatres.
- Less skilled intubators if not from an anaesthetic background.
- Lack of experienced and skilled assistance.
- Absence of guidelines for management of routine airway problems (tracheostomy or tracheal tube displacement or failed RSI).
- Lack of routine use of capnography.

While some of these factors are unavoidable many are not. All staff who manage the airway in ICU, the emergency department and in remote hospital locations should recognize that both patient factors and extrinsic factors interact to increase the likelihood of difficult airway management. Preparation for such difficulty is vital.

MANAGEMENT OF THE DIFFICULT AIRWAY IN CHILDREN

The unexpected difficult airway in paediatric practice is rare in comparison with the adult population. Many difficulties are relatively easy to predict prior to induction and are associated classically with craniofacial problems such as those which occur in Pierre Robin, Treacher Collins and Goldenhar syndromes. Other types of craniofacial abnormality may also lead to difficult airway management. Congenital subglottic stenosis or tracheal abnormalities such as webs or haemangiomas are encountered occasionally. In most of these children, the small calibre of the airway and limited oxygen reserves mean that most airway difficulty occurs while the child is an infant. In contrast, the airway of a child with mucopolysaccharide storage diseases (Hunter and Hurler syndromes) becomes increasingly difficult to manage as the child grows and the soft tissues become infiltrated, leading to a risk of airway obstruction and difficulty in manipulation of the tissues. Other airway challenges in children may arise in the acute situations encountered with trauma, infections (e.g. epiglottitis, croup) or burns involving the airway. However, unexpected difficulties can also occur during routine surgery.

These were published in 2013 and are available on http://www.das.uk.com/content/paediatric-difficult-airway-guidelines and http://www.apagbi.org.uk/publications/apa-guidelines. The basic principles of difficult airway management described above apply equally in children but the airway management options are more limited.

- Awake techniques are generally impractical because of issues of co-operation.
- Anatomical differences mean that some techniques (e.g. cricothyroidotomy) are less suitable in children and infants.
- Newly developed equipment is often available only in adult sizes in the first instance. It can be many years before paediatric versions become available (e.g. videolaryngoscopes, second generation SADs) and some are not available at all (e.g. ILMA tracheal tubes, Aintree Intubation Catheter, several videolaryngoscopes).

Recent developments have increased the options for difficult airway management in children. These include second generation SADs, videolaryngoscopes and cuffed tracheal tubes that are appropriate for children. The focus of care for children and infants with airway difficulty is, as in adults, to take all steps to ensure adequate oxygenation (rather than becoming fixated on tracheal intubation) and all anaesthetists involved in the care of children must have a strategy which includes a plan and back-up plans. They should be familiar with the equipment which may be required and have practised using it. If a difficult airway is predicted, it is good practice to have a minimum of two experienced anaesthetists with appropriate paediatric experience present in the operating theatre.

The techniques used in adults are entirely appropriate for the older child (above 30 kg), using smaller equipment. The intubating LMA has a size 3 version and a number of SADs are available in small sizes; classic LMA, ProSeal LMA, Supreme LMA and i-gel now all have size ranges that include size 1.5 (suitable for infants 5–10 kg) and some even size 1 (for <5 kg). These devices have been shown to be effective in elective paediatric patients but are unproven for difficult airway management and are generally less easy to use and perhaps less reliable in comparison to those used in adult practice.

Inhalational induction is used widely in paediatric practice and is particularly favoured for management of the difficult airway. Gastric distension is a special problem in children and infants and is more likely if there has been respiratory distress before anaesthesia and if positive pressure is applied to the airway. It is sensible to decompress the stomach when an adequate depth of anaesthesia has been achieved. Anaesthesia can be maintained using a tracheal tube inserted partially into the nasopharynx but SADs are increasingly used to maintain the airway and provide a conduit for fibreoptic techniques (even in small babies). The ProSeal LMA and i-gel probably have the best features for this role. Specialized paediatric bronchoscopes are available with an external diameter as small as 2.2 mm (accommodating a 2.5 mm tracheal tube) but they are very fragile, have no facility for suction, can be harder to use than larger fibrescopes and are not available in most institutions. The absence of a suction channel is important because it prevents both clearance of the

airway and delivery of local anaesthesia to suppress airway reflexes. Larger adult bronchoscopes with an external diameter of 3.5–4 mm can still be used in children. For larger children, the fibrescope can be used in the standard manner to insert an appropriately sized tracheal tube. However, it may be difficult to remove the SAD safely because the tracheal tube is shorter than the length of the SAD; this is overcome by mounting two tracheal tubes (joined together) onto the fibrescope and removing the SAD over these before detaching the proximal tracheal tube. In smaller children, the fibrescope may be inserted into the trachea and a wire passed into the trachea via the working channel of the fibrescope. If the fibrescope is too large even to enter the trachea, it can be positioned above the larynx and a wire deployed under direct vision. The wire can then be 'stiffened' using an airway exchange catheter (or stiff fine-bore nasogastric tube) and then, when tracheal intubation has been confirmed using capnography, an appropriate tracheal tube can be railroaded into place.

Alternative devices available to facilitate intubation in children include:

- bladed videolaryngoscopes (Glidescope)
- conduited videolaryngoscopes (Airtraq)
- optical stilettes (several adult versions may be used for children)
- light-wand.

Management of the Child with an Inhaled Foreign Body

Although this is not necessarily a difficult airway problem, the need to maintain an airway compromised by an inhaled foreign body while sharing it with the surgeon makes it a considerable challenge. The procedure may be semi-elective or occasionally a critical emergency with the child *in extremis* from airway obstruction. Heliox may be beneficial before anaesthesia in critical situations.

Discussion of surgical plans is always necessary. Traditional anaesthetic priorities are to establish a deep plane of anaesthesia while maintaining spontaneous ventilation and avoiding complications that may require positive pressure ventilation. A calm inhalational induction is the usual technique and may be followed by surgical instrumentation of the pharynx and larynx (high foreign bodies) or use of a rigid bronchoscope (lower airway foreign bodies). Topical anaesthesia to the airway (under deep anaesthesia) may be beneficial. Because the procedure may be prolonged, it is important to use a rigid bronchoscope which enables continuous delivery of oxygen and anaesthetic gases. More recently the necessity of absolute avoidance of controlled ventilation has been questioned.

AIRWAY ALERT

HOSPITAL NAME AND ADDRESS
Tel
Fax

Name	
Date of birth Hospital number	
Home address Telephone	
GP address Tel	

To the patient:
Please keep this letter safe and show it to your doctor if you are admitted to hospital.
Please show this letter to the anaesthetic doctor if you need an operation.
This letter explains the difficulties that were found during your recent anaesthetic and the information may be useful to doctors treating you in the future.

To the GP:
Please copy this letter with any future referral.
READ CODE SP2y3

Summary of Airway Management
Date of operation:
Type of operation:

		Reasons/comments
Difficult mask ventilation?	**YES/NO**	
Difficult SAD insertion?	**YES/NO**	
Difficult direct laryngoscopy?	**YES/NO**	
Difficult videolaryngoscopy?	**YES/NO**	
Difficult tracheal intubation?	**YES/NO**	
Laryngoscopy grade	1 / 2a / 2b / 3a / 3b / 4	
Extubation		.
Further investigation		.

Equipment used:

Other information:

Is awake intubation necessary in the future?

Follow-up care (tick when completed)

Copies of letter
YES/NO One copy to patient
YES/NO One copy to GP
YES/NO One copy in case notes
YES/NO One copy in anaesthetic department

YES/NO Spoken to patient
YES/NO Anaesthetic chart complete
YES/NO Information on front of case notes
YES/NO Medic Alert or Difficult Airway
Society referral (Specify)

Name of anaesthetist:
Grade: Consultant   Date:

If you require further information please contact the Anaesthetic Department.

FIGURE 22.25 ■ An example of an airway alert form *(derived from one published by Dr D Ball for DAS).*

Airway swelling may occur after removal of the foreign body and infection may be present distally. Careful postoperative monitoring, dexamethasone, nebulized adrenaline and supplemental oxygen may all be needed.

AFTER DIFFICULT AIRWAY MANAGEMENT

Although there is often considerable focus on securing a safe airway in patients with a predicted or known difficult airway, it is equally important to establish a strategy for immediate management at the end of the procedure, and in the longer term if there is a need for further anaesthesia.

Immediate Management

The management of extubation is discussed above.

Long-Term Management

When the patient has recovered fully and before discharge from hospital, the senior anaesthetist involved should inform the patient of the relevant facts and the ways in which the difficulties experienced may affect airway management in future anaesthetics. It is probably appropriate that any patient whose airway is *likely to prove difficult to manage during RSI by a junior anaesthetist* is given written information to that effect. The anaesthetic record should contain a clear record of the problem, what was done, what did and did not work, and a judgement as to the likely problems and solutions in the future. This information should be given to the patient, sent to the patient's general practitioner and filed in the hospital records. An example of a proforma is shown in Figure 22.25. The general practitioner should be asked to include the information in any future referrals. The Read code for difficult intubation can usefully be included in such letters and is SP2y3. It may be appropriate for the patient to wear a medical alert bracelet.

FURTHER READING

Cook, T.M., Nolan, J.P., Cranshaw, J., Magee, P., 2007. Needle cricothyroidotomy. Anaesthesia 62, 289–290.

Cook, T.M., Woodall, N., Frerk, C., 2011. Major complications of airway management in the UK: results of the Fourth National Audit Project of the Royal College of Anaesthetists and the Difficult Airway Society. Part 1 Anaesthesia. Br. J. Anaesth. 106, 617–631.

Cook, T.M., Woodall, N., Harper, J., Benger, J., 2011. Major complications of airway management in the UK: results of the Fourth National Audit Project of the Royal College of Anaesthetists and the Difficult Airway Society. Part 2 Intensive Care and Emergency Department. Br. J. Anaesth. 106, 632–642.

Cook, T.M., McDougall-Davis, S.R., 2012. Complications and failure of airway management. Br. J. Anaesth. 109 (Suppl 1), i68–i85.

Harmer, M. 2005. Independent Review on the care given to Mrs Elaine Bromiley on 29 March 2005. Clinical Human Factors Group http://www.chfg.org/resources/07_qrt04/Anonymous_Report_Verdict_and_Corrected_Timeline_Oct_07.pdf.

Hawthorne, L., Wilson, R., Lyons, G., Dresner, M., 1996. Failed intubation revisited: 17-yr experience in a teaching maternity unit. Br. J. Anaesth. 76, 680–684.

Mihai, R., Blair, E., Kay, H., Cook, T.M., 2008. A quantitative review and meta-analysis of performance of non standard laryngoscopes and rigid fibreoptic intubation aids. Anaesthesia 63, 745–760.

Peterson, G.N., Domino, K.B., Caplan, R.A., et al., 2005. Management of the difficult airway: a closed claims analysis. Anesthesiology 103, 33–39.

Rose, D.K., Cohen, M.M., 1996. The incidence of airway problems depends on the definition used. Can. J. Anaesth. 43, 30–34.

Samsoon, G.L.T., Young, J.R.B., 1987. Difficult tracheal intubation: a retrospective study. Anaesthesia 42, 487–490.

Sheriffdom of Glasgow and Strathkelvin, 2010. Determination of sheriff Linda Margaret Ruxton in fatal accident inquiry into the death of Gordon Ewing. http://www.scotcourts.gov.uk/opinions/2010FAI15.html.

23 MANAGEMENT OF THE HIGH-RISK SURGICAL PATIENT

■ ■ ■ ■ ■ ■ ■ ■ ■ ■ ■ ■ ■

A high-risk surgical procedure can be considered as one in which there is an accepted postoperative mortality rate of more than 1%. This includes cardiothoracic surgery, vascular surgery and major intra-abdominal cancer surgery, either as elective or emergency procedures. There are a number of factors that can put a patient at risk from such procedures. These can be divided into two broad categories: first, the technical hazards of the surgical procedure itself, e.g. the construction of a gastrointestinal tract anastomosis and the potential for it to break down; and second, the presence of significant co-morbidities in the patient before surgery, usually of a cardiorespiratory nature, which are severe enough to cause impaired preoperative functional status. In most patients, poor outcome from major surgery arises from a combination of these factors, in which the patient with impaired physiological reserve is unable to cope with the physiological demands of the surgery, leading to multi-organ dysfunction syndrome (MODS), multi-organ failure (MOF), and death in the worst cases.

Cardiothoracic anaesthesia and emergency anaesthesia are considered elsewhere (Chs 33, 34 and 37), and this chapter will concentrate on the patient undergoing scheduled major non-cardiac surgery. However, the principles of treatment, particularly fluid management, generally apply also to the patient undergoing an emergency procedure.

WHAT MAKES AN OPERATION HIGH-RISK?

Major surgery generates a systemic inflammatory response which is driven by the release of pro-inflammatory cytokines such as tumour necrosis factor (TNF) and interleukin-6 (IL-6). The magnitude of the inflammatory response, as judged by the levels of pro-inflammatory cytokines in the circulation, is associated directly with postoperative outcome, with higher concentrations of circulating IL-6 associated with an increased incidence of postoperative complications.

Pro-inflammatory responses are particularly marked in surgery involving the gastrointestinal tract, major vascular surgery and cardiac surgery. Other factors which increase the inflammatory response include the need for major blood transfusion, emergency surgery and the presence of decreased tissue perfusion, particularly in the gastrointestinal tract.

The effect of the inflammatory responses is a postoperative increase in oxygen requirements of up to 50% above basal levels. This substantial increase in oxygen demand is met normally by increases in cardiac output and tissue oxygen extraction. Most patients can meet the increased oxygen demand by increasing cardiac output and usually recover well after surgery. However, there is a group who may not have the physiological reserve to increase cardiac output to the required level and these patients are at higher risk of complications after surgery.

In addition to the systemic inflammatory response, major surgery generates a neuroendocrine stress response. Although this stress response may be attenuated to a degree, it is difficult to modify an established systemic inflammatory response and treatment strategies for the high-risk patient have relied on identifying patients early and optimizing various aspects of patient care in order to reduce risk and improve outcome.

497

IDENTIFYING THE HIGH-RISK SURGICAL PATIENT

Large-scale audits of surgical deaths in the UK have found that patients at risk are usually elderly, and 60–70% have established cardiorespiratory disease. When cardiac output monitoring is used in patients undergoing major surgery, it has been found that patients are more likely to die if they are unable to increase their cardiac output spontaneously in response to the physiological demands of the procedure. Poor outcome after major surgery is also associated with other related physiological factors which are all markers of impaired tissue perfusion, either globally or more specifically.

- Pre-operative factors
  - Decreased exercise tolerance
  - Onset of myocardial wall abnormalities during stress echocardiography
- Intra-operative and postoperative factors
  - Inability to increase oxygen delivery after surgery
  - Reduced central or mixed venous oxygen saturation
  - Development of a base deficit during surgery
  - Reduced gastric mucosal pH indicating impaired gut microcirculation.

Because these abnormalities may manifest themselves only during surgery or in the postoperative period, the challenge for the anaesthetist is to identify high-risk patients before surgery, wherever possible.

RISK PREDICTION SCORING SYSTEMS

ASA Score

The American Society of Anesthesiologists' scoring system (ASA score) was developed as a guide to patient risk, and depends on a subjective assessment by an anaesthetist of the impact of co-morbidities on an individual patient's risk. The system has only 5 categories, and the subjective nature of the assessment means that there is a large degree of variability between anaesthetists when classifying patients. In practice, it has some limited use as a rough guide, but does not have specific risk-prediction value for individual patients.

Shoemaker's Criteria

In the 1980s, Shoemaker noted that a decreased oxygen delivery (DO_2) was associated with poor outcome, and described a list of clinical risk factors associated with decreased survival, known as the Shoemaker criteria.

- Previous severe cardiorespiratory illness (acute MI, COPD, stroke)
- Extensive ablative surgery planned for carcinoma
- Severe multiple trauma (more than three organs or two body cavities involved)
- Massive acute blood loss (more than 8 units)
- Age over 70 years with limited physiological reserve
- Shock (mean arterial pressure less than 60 mmHg)
- Septicaemia
- Respiratory failure
- Acute abdominal catastrophe with haemodynamic instability (pancreatitis, bowel infarction, perforated viscus, GI bleeding)
- Acute renal failure
- Vascular disease involving aorta.

These criteria have been used to select patients for therapeutic trials, and are a useful guide to highlight at-risk patients, but do not provide an individual-specific risk assessment.

POSSUM Score

The _P_hysiological and _O_perative _S_everity _S_core for the en_U_meration of _M_ortality and Morbidity (POSSUM score) was developed specifically to provide predicted risk scores for complications and death after surgery.

The score requires physiological data from the patient's condition prior to surgery, and intraoperative data from the surgical procedure itself.

POSSUM score physiological variables:

- age
- Glasgow coma score
- haemoglobin concentration
- white cell count
- serum sodium concentration
- serum potassium concentration
- serum urea concentration
- heart rate

- systolic blood pressure
- respiratory co-morbidity
- cardiac co-morbidity
- ECG abnormality.

POSSUM score surgical variables:

- operative severity
- degree of cancer spread
- peritoneal soiling
- number of procedures required
- blood loss
- urgency of surgery.

The POSSUM system assigns different scores to degrees of abnormalities demonstrated by the variables. The total scores for the physiological and operative components are entered into an equation which gives predicted percentage values for the risks of mortality and morbidity (a specified range of complications). The original POSSUM system was devised 20 years ago in a general surgical population and the values of predicted mortality and morbidity reflect the current standards of care at that time. Subsequent research has produced more procedure-specific and location-specific versions of the POSSUM score but the overall structure of the system remains unchanged. The requirement for intraoperative data severely limits the real-time use of POSSUM as a tool for predicting the risk of an individual patient prior to surgery, but it has been shown to be a useful tool for retrospective assessment of the risk of comparative patient groups for audit and research purposes.

Revised Cardiac Risk Index

The Revised Cardiac Risk Index (RCRI) is a more system-specific score, designed to predict the risk of a patient developing a cardiac-related complication following non-cardiac surgery. Six variables are identified as independent predictors.

- Ischaemic heart disease
- Congestive cardiac failure
- Cerebrovascular disease
- Requirement for insulin therapy
- Renal insufficiency (creatinine $>170\,\mu mol\,L^{-1}$)
- Requirement for major surgery.

The risk of cardiac events ranges from 0.4% without any factors to 11% if three or more factors are present. Although simple to use, the RCRI predicts only specific cardiac morbidity. In addition, the score was derived during the 1990s, and subsequent developments in treatment for secondary prevention of ischaemic heart disease are likely to have led to a reduction in the incidence of postoperative events, and to an over-prediction of risk.

POSTOPERATIVE PULMONARY COMPLICATION RISK PREDICTORS

Seven independent risk predictors for postoperative pulmonary complications (PPC) have been identified.

- Increasing age
- Low preoperative oxygen saturation
- Respiratory infection within last month
- Preoperative anaemia
- Type of surgical incision
- Duration of surgery
- Emergency procedure.

Weightings are given to different categories of the independent variables, and an overall score is calculated leading to a classification of low, intermediate or high risk for PPC.

LABORATORY INVESTIGATIONS FOR RISK ASSESSMENT

Routine Investigations

In patients presenting for elective surgery, investigations such as full blood count, or serum urea and electrolyte concentrations, will not, in general, be of any significant value in predicting risk, although they may be useful as components of more comprehensive scoring systems such as POSSUM (see above), and they may highlight specific abnormalities, such as severe anaemia, which should be corrected before surgery.

Plasma Biomarkers

Biomarkers are biochemical substances that can be assayed from plasma samples and abnormal levels of biomarkers may be associated with certain disease states. B-type natriuretic peptide (BNP) is a hormone secreted by cardiac cells in response to stretching of the myocardium. BNP results in increased sodium excretion and decreased systemic vascular resistance, with the net result of decreasing blood volume. BNP levels are raised in patients with heart failure and correlate with the degree of severity of the disease. In the patient undergoing major surgery, the presence of a raised concentration of BNP is associated with higher risks of adverse cardiac events and mortality after surgery, and normal levels are powerful negative predictors of complications.

Resting Echocardiography

Resting echocardiography in the elderly patient is useful in diagnosing and categorizing aortic stenosis, which has been highlighted as a significant problem in these patients. Normal left ventricular function in terms of ejection fraction or resting echocardiogram does not necessarily mean that the patient's risk of developing postoperative cardiac complications is low, as a significant proportion of patients with heart failure have a preserved ejection fraction. These patients may have diastolic dysfunction or heart failure and will also have an increased risk of adverse cardiac events after surgery.

Stress Echocardiography

If the demand on the myocardium is increased by an infusion of a positive inotropic agent such as dobutamine, the onset of wall-motion abnormalities indicates that a patient is at increased risk of postoperative cardiac-related complications. Conversely, a normal stress response is highly predictive of a very low risk of cardiac complications. However, dobutamine stress echocardiography is not readily available, interpretation is very user-dependent, and it is useful only in predicting specific cardiac risk.

Assessment of Functional Capacity

The physiological response to major surgery is a dynamic situation and assessment of the patient's preoperative functional capacity has been recognized as a useful test with some predictive value. A patient who has limitation of cardiorespiratory reserve on exercise may be less able to elevate cardiac output in response to postoperative demands, and therefore may be considered at greater risk of complications.

Traditionally it has been taught that patients are at higher risk of complications after surgery if they are unable to perform exercise to a level that equates to 4 metabolic equivalents (METs), where MET is the energy expenditure at rest of a 40-year-old, 70 kg male. The degree of exercise equating to 4 METs would be climbing two flights of stairs. Questionnaires have been devised which allow practitioners to estimate a patient's level of fitness, but these inevitably rely on the patient giving an accurate and honest appraisal of their levels of activity, and are therefore subject to bias.

Simple Exercise Testing

Objective testing of exercise capacity can provide a reasonable estimate of risk. This can vary from simple stair-climbing to more formal tests such as the shuttle walk test, in which the subject walks between two cones placed 10 m apart until unable to keep pace with a timed beep. The results of the test are expressed in metres walked, and the further the subject walks, the better the outcome after surgery is likely to be.

Although simple walking or climbing tests are useful in giving an overall impression of a patient's reserve, they have significant limitations; for example, some elderly patients have significant mobility problems of the lower limb due to osteoarthritis and may find walking difficult. The main value of these simple tests lies in their negative predictive value, which means that fit patients can be identified who are very unlikely to have complications after surgery. However, these tests give little useful information about the underlying causes of impairment of functional capacity in patients who do not perform well in the test. This is an important limitation, because some patients perform poorly due to an underlying disease state, most commonly cardiac impairment, whilst others perform poorly simply through being out of condition due to lack of physical activity. Recognition of the cause of decreased functional capacity may allow effective preoperative interventions to improve the patient's performance and reduce the risk of surgery. To evaluate patients in this way, more sophisticated testing is required.

Cardiopulmonary Exercise Testing (CPET)

During CPET, a patient undergoes exercise of increasing intensity which requires an increase in metabolic activity in the exercising muscles, which in turn demands increases in ventilation and cardiac output.

Limitations in either respiratory or cardiac function (or both) result in decreased oxygen uptake by the exercising muscles.

CPET is performed with the patient pedalling on a static bicycle with a flywheel to which increasing resistance is applied. During the test, oxygen uptake and carbon dioxide production are measured using a metabolic monitoring cart. A 12-lead ECG is recorded simultaneously. Cardiorespiratory performance during exercise is usually defined by the measurement of oxygen uptake by the tissues (oxygen consumption, VO_2), either as the maximum oxygen uptake measurable (VO_{2max}), or as the oxygen uptake at the onset of lactate production, commonly known as the anaerobic threshold (AT). Other useful parameters obtained include measures of ventilatory efficiency and the ability to diagnose myocardial dysfunction from heart failure or ischaemic heart disease.

Anaerobic Threshold

AT occurs usually at 50–60% of VO_{2max}, and is independent of patient motivation. If the AT is the prime objective of the CPET, the test can be stopped after it has been reached, and this may be advantageous in the frail or elderly surgical patient. This variant of CPET is known as a *submaximal* test, as the intention is not to test the patient to the maximum effort.

AT is identified as the point at which there is onset of lactate production through the activation of anaerobic pathways. The lactate produced is buffered by bicarbonate to produce water and carbon dioxide. The net effect is an increase in the slope of the graph of carbon dioxide production relative to oxygen uptake (Fig. 23.1)

Patients whose AT occurs at oxygen uptake values less than $11\,mL\,kg^{-1}\,min^{-1}$ are at 6–7 times increased risk of mortality after surgery compared with those who have a higher oxygen uptake at AT.

Ventilatory Efficiency

This is estimated from the ventilatory equivalent of carbon dioxide, which is the ratio of minute ventilation to carbon dioxide production, V_E/V_{CO_2}. A normal value is around 25–30, and increases in the ratio reflect impairment of V/Q mismatch, either from respiratory causes or from impaired cardiac function. In patients with heart failure, a value for V_E/V_{CO_2} greater than 34 is associated with a poor prognosis, particularly when combined with an AT less than $11\,mL\,kg^{-1}\,min^{-1}$. The same holds true for surgical patients, because the

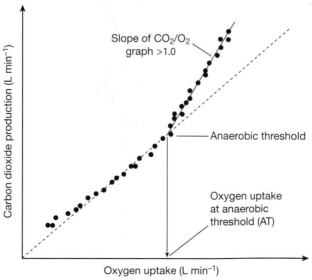

FIGURE 23.1 ■ V-slope method for estimating Anaerobic Threshold. Oxygen uptake increases as exercise intensity increases. During the initial aerobic phase the slope of the graph of CO_2 production vs. O_2 uptake is less than 1. After the onset of lactate production from anaerobic pathways (the Anaerobic Threshold), extra CO_2 is generated by the buffering of lactate with bicarbonate, and the slope of the CO_2/O_2 graph is greater than 1.

implication is that this combination reflects a patient with more severe underlying cardiac dysfunction. These patients are often asymptomatic at rest, but the mortality rate after surgery in this group of patients is elevated, reflecting abnormal cardiac function in response to the stress of surgery.

In a typical UK population of elderly surgical patients, approximately 30% have reduced AT combined with reduced ventilatory efficiency, and are therefore in a high-risk group for surgical intervention. This group of patients should be optimized medically before surgery if possible, and managed on high dependency care after surgery.

Identification of Myocardial Dysfunction

Two parameters derived from gas exchange data can be used to identify patients with underlying myocardial dysfunction.

- Oxygen uptake per heart beat (Vo_2/HR, also known as the 'oxygen pulse'). This should increase steadily during exercise as a reflection of increases in underlying stroke volume initially, followed by increases in oxygen extraction. Flattening of the slope of the graph during exercise may reflect underlying myocardial wall motion abnormalities.

- Oxygen uptake to work rate relationship (Vo_2/WR) (Fig. 23.2). For each 1 W increase in work rate, oxygen uptake should increase by $10 \, mL \, min^{-1}$.

A value of Vo_2/WR significantly less than $10 \, mL \, min^{-1} \, W^{-1}$ may indicate underlying heart failure. A sudden change of the Vo_2/WR relationship during exercise may indicate the onset of myocardial ischaemia with consequent myocardial wall motion abnormalities.

Changes in either oxygen pulse or the Vo_2/WR relationship occur usually 2–3 min before changes in the ST segment of the exercise ECG are observed. A patient who develops these abnormalities may benefit from referral for cardiological assessment if symptomatic and if other variables such as AT are significantly impaired, or from cardiac protection from cardioselective β-blockade if asymptomatic (see below).

REDUCING RISK BEFORE SURGERY

Information from preoperative assessment and investigations, particularly cardiopulmonary exercise testing, can help the clinician answer three important questions in an effort to reduce risk for an individual patient.

- Is the patient fit enough for the proposed surgery, or would a less invasive procedure, or even postponement of surgery, be more suitable?

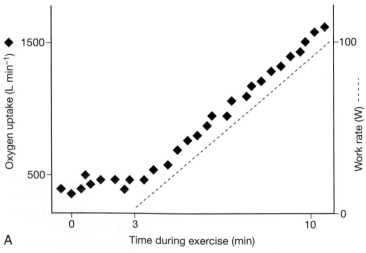

FIGURE 23.2 ■ Relationship between oxygen uptake and work rate (VO_2/WR). **(A)** Normal: for each 1 W increase in work rate intensity, oxygen uptake increases by $10 \, mL \, min^{-1}$. In this example, O_2 uptake is $500 \, mL \, min^{-1}$ at the onset of loaded cycling, and $1500 \, mL \, min^{-1}$ after 100 W, an increase of $10 \, mL \, min^{-1} \, W^{-1}$.

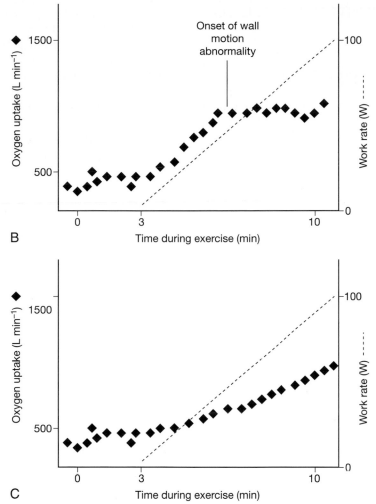

FIGURE 23.2 ■ Cont'd **(B)** Ischaemic heart disease: The VO_2/WR relationship starts normally, but O_2 uptake abruptly stops increasing at the critical ischaemic point as wall motion abnormalities develop. **(C)** Chronic heart failure: VO_2/WR is significantly decreased, as the myocardial pump does not respond normally to increasing exercise intensity.

- Can the patient's medical condition be improved before surgery, with consequent risk reduction?
- Does the patient need to go to a high dependency care or intensive care unit after surgery, or is postoperative care in a general ward appropriate?

ALTERNATIVES TO MAJOR SURGERY

The availability of different treatment options is influenced by the surgical condition. For instance, an abdominal aortic aneurysm can be treated by open repair or endovascular repair, or can even be left *in situ* in a particularly high-risk patient. For colorectal disease, the alternatives to curative-intent surgery are limited, but surgical risk can still be modified, for instance by choosing to perform a Hartmann's procedure in a very high-risk patient with a rectal tumour rather than risking an anastomotic leak in a patient with limited reserve. Such decisions need to be taken on a case-by-case basis, with all other factors taken into account.

PREOPERATIVE INTERVENTIONS TO REDUCE RISK

β-Blockade

The purpose of cardioselective β-blockade is to reduce the risk of myocardial ischaemia after surgery through the prevention of tachycardia and the consequent decrease in myocardial oxygen demand and improvement in myocardial perfusion time. β-Blockers are now also used widely in the treatment of heart failure as well as the prevention of ischaemic events, but in heart failure, it is necessary to establish β-blockade over a period of time for full effect, starting with a low dose.

In practice, the introduction of β-blockers has not always shown clinical benefit. The use of bisoprolol (a cardioselective β-blocker) in patients with demonstrable wall motion defects on stress echocardiography significantly reduces the risks of death and myocardial infarction after surgery. However, it may be necessary to start treatment with bisoprolol several weeks before surgery. Metoprolol started immediately before surgery results in a small but significant reduction in cardiac events, but at the expense of increased hypotension, an increase in cerebrovascular events and an increase in overall mortality.

Retrospective studies have shown that the protective effect of β-blockade is greater in patients who have an increased number of RCRI cardiac risk factors, and there is even a suggestion that β-blockade in patients with no cardiac risk factors may be harmful.

Many patients are already established on long-term β-blockade, and it is important that β-blockade is continued around the time of surgery, as sudden cessation is definitely associated with a worse outcome. Parenteral preparations of atenolol and metoprolol are available for the patient who is 'nil by mouth' and there is some suggestion that the longer-acting atenolol may be more beneficial.

Statin Therapy

Many surgical patients are already established on long-term statin therapy as part of secondary prevention of cardiovascular disease. If so, it is important that this treatment is continued around the time of surgery, as withdrawal can cause a rebound effect.

Long-term statin use has been shown to reduce the risk of mortality after surgery in patients undergoing aortic surgery. Although more evidence is required, introducing statins before surgery may have some beneficial effect, possibly through their anti-inflammatory actions, and is unlikely to cause harm because side-effects are rare. There is no parenteral preparation of statins, but it may be useful to use a longer-acting preparation such as fluvastatin, taken on the morning of surgery.

Coronary Revascularization

A cardiological evaluation is required for patients with unstable angina, or severe exercise limitation accompanied by ischaemia. These patients are at risk of adverse cardiac events irrespective of their surgical disease, but in practice constitute a small proportion of surgical patients.

There is a much larger group of patients who are asymptomatic, but have cardiac risk factors, and in whom coronary lesions can be identified on angiography. Prophylactic revascularization of such lesions before non-cardiac surgery has not been shown to have any overall benefit when the morbidity of the revascularization is taken into account.

Surgery may be further complicated in patients who have undergone percutaneous coronary intervention (PCI) with stenting because they need to take dual anti-platelet therapy for a minimum of 6 weeks in the case of bare metal stents, and 12 months for drug-eluting stents. In patients who are known to require surgery after their PCI, a bare metal stent should be used to minimize the time on dual anti-platelet therapy.

Smoking Cessation

A benefit in terms of reduced pulmonary complications occurs only after 2–3 months of smoking cessation. However, there may be some immediate gains in the patient at high risk of cardiovascular complications because smoking causes a hypercoagulable state which increases myocardial work, decreased oxygen delivery through increased occupancy of haemoglobin by carbon monoxide, vasoconstriction and catecholamine release.

Chest Physiotherapy

Preoperative chest physiotherapy may be beneficial in reducing atelectasis after surgery in patients at risk of developing pulmonary complications (see above).

Correction of Anaemia

Most healthy patients tolerate a haemoglobin concentration of $8\,g\,dL^{-1}$, but the high-risk patient is more likely to be elderly and to have ischaemic heart disease, and may therefore require a higher haemoglobin concentration.

The patient may already be anaemic due to the nature of the surgical disease, particularly tumours of the right colon, stomach and urogenital tract, and anaemia is an independent risk factor for the development of complications after colonic surgery.

In patients with limited reserve, the anaemia should be reversed, if not completely corrected, in the first instance with either oral or parenteral iron administration. In more severe cases, the clinician needs to decide whether a preoperative transfusion is justified, although with improving parenteral iron therapy, the need for transfusion should be reduced.

IDENTIFYING PATIENTS IN NEED OF POSTOPERATIVE CRITICAL CARE

High-dependency care unit (HDU) and intensive care unit (ICU) beds are expensive resources in all hospitals, and demand usually outstrips supply. Some patients are admitted automatically to an HDU bed after major surgery such as open aortic aneurysm repair or upper gastrointestinal cancer surgery. However, after other more common surgical procedures, such as colorectal cancer surgery, weight reduction surgery or complex orthopaedic surgery, it is often unclear which patients are more likely to benefit from the extra monitoring and additional supportive measures which the HDU can provide.

A reduced value of anaerobic threshold (AT), measured from cardiopulmonary exercise testing (CPET), has been used to define groups at higher risk of complications after surgery. A protocol for triage of patients to ICU, HDU or to ward care after surgery based on CPET results was described by Older in 1999. Mortality rates were very low among patients who were allocated to ward care on the basis of good AT values, indicating that CPET was accurate in identifying patients who did not need HDU care, irrespective of clinical history or age. This model of care is now becoming established in hospitals with access to preoperative CPET. A typical protocol is shown in Figure 23.3.

The usefulness of this approach is emphasized by the results from a recent large audit of surgical outcomes in a UK tertiary centre, which showed that clinical judgement alone does not identify high- or low- risk surgical patients with the same degree of accuracy.

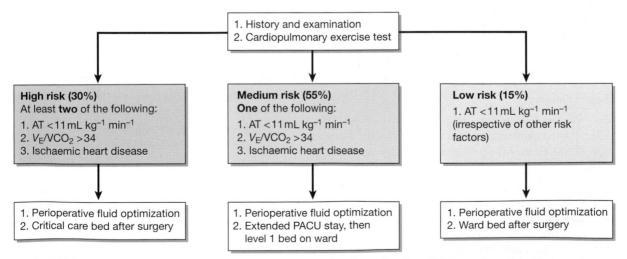

FIGURE 23.3 ■ Triage flowchart for perioperative care. An example of how data from CPET as well as clinical information can lead to a rational approach to allocation of postoperative critical care.

PERIOPERATIVE MANAGEMENT OF THE HIGH-RISK PATIENT

Ideally, the high-risk patient presents for surgery having been identified as being at increased risk, and having had medical co-morbidities optimized as much as possible at the preoperative assessment clinic stage.

This section concentrates on the anaesthetic management of the patient, with emphasis on haemodynamic monitoring and optimization of the circulation.

Choice of Anaesthetic Technique

General anaesthesia is usually necessary for patients who undergo major body cavity surgery, whereas a regional anaesthetic technique may be considered advantageous for peripheral surgery in a high-risk patient, although there is little evidence that the risk of developing complications is significantly reduced by use of regional anaesthesia.

In many patients who undergo body cavity surgery, general anaesthesia is supplemented by a neuraxial block technique, usually using a thoracic epidural catheter inserted before induction. The main purpose is to provide a high quality of pain relief after surgery, but a carefully managed epidural also reduces the need for systemic opioid analgesia during surgery. However, an epidural block is likely to produce a sympathetic block which causes peripheral vasodilatation and hypotension, and this can lead to decreased tissue perfusion, which may be significant in the compromised patient.

Haemodynamic Monitoring, Fluid Therapy, and Optimization of Oxygen Delivery

Oxygen Delivery

Many studies have shown that patients are more likely to develop complications after surgery if they show signs of impaired tissue perfusion and oxygen delivery during the perioperative period.

Oxygen delivery (DO_2) is dependent upon cardiac output and the oxygen content of arterial blood.

- DO_2 = cardiac output × O_2 content (haemoglobin × O_2 saturation × 1.34)

Additionally, there is a small but clinically insignificant amount of dissolved oxygen.

Assuming that the haemoglobin concentration is satisfactory ($>8\,g\,dL^{-1}$), the variable most likely to alter during anaesthesia is the cardiac output.

Cardiac output (CO) depends on the stroke volume (SV, volume of blood ejected during systole) and the heart rate (HR).

- $CO = SV \times HR$

Cardiac output is usually expressed as an indexed value, where the absolute value of cardiac output ($L\,min^{-1}$) is divided by the body surface area, which allows closer comparison between individuals of different sizes.

Oxygen Consumption

Oxygen consumption can be estimated by measuring the difference in oxygen contents of arterial blood (before oxygen is delivered to the tissues) and mixed venous blood (blood returning to the lungs from the tissues), and multiplying by cardiac output:

- $VO_2 = CO \times (SaO_2 - S_{cv}O_2) \times 1.34 \times Hb$

Stroke Volume

Stroke volume is dependent on cardiac preload, afterload and cardiac contractility, factors which can all change during anaesthesia and surgery.

- Preload decreases if the patient becomes hypovolaemic, either through blood loss, insensible losses or relative hypovolaemia through excessive vasodilatation and capacitance increase of the circulation.
- Afterload is dependent on systemic vascular resistance (SVR), which can decrease through the vasodilator effects of anaesthetic agents on the peripheral circulation, or epidural-induced sympathetic blockade. SVR can increase if sympathetic tone is increased, for example by circulating catecholamine increases in response to surgical stimulation.
- Contractility can decrease through direct action of anaesthetic agents or circulating inflammatory cytokines, or increase if sympathetic activity increases.

In clinical practice, the most important of these variables is the volume of preload, and its effect on stroke volume. The Frank–Starling law states that increasing venous return to the left ventricle increases left ventricular end-diastolic pressure and volume, resulting in an increase in stroke volume. Increasing the preload increases the active tension developed by the muscle fibre and increases the velocity of fibre shortening, assuming that afterload and inotropic states remain constant (if the afterload is changed or inotropic activity changes, the shape of the Frank–Starling curve alters).

Figure 23.4 shows the effect of boluses of fluid on stroke volume at different points on the Frank–Starling curve. On the lower portion of the curve, when preload is low, a fluid bolus is likely to produce an increase in stroke volume of greater than 10%. As preload increases, the increases in stroke volume reduce, until a rise of less than 10% is obtained, indicating that the plateau of the Frank–Starling curve has been reached, and that further fluid boluses are not required.

The high-risk surgical patient benefits from measures which aim to optimize oxygen delivery through the careful administration of fluid, guided by careful monitoring of circulatory flow and preload.

The techniques used to measure stroke volume or preload, and the protocols used for fluid therapy, vary, but essentially fall into one of three categories:

- preoperative optimization of oxygen delivery
- intraoperative stroke volume optimization
- preload responsiveness optimization.

All of these approaches have been shown to improve outcome through reductions in mortality and complication rates.

Preoperative Optimization of Oxygen Delivery

Early studies of outcome after high-risk surgery used the observation from Shoemaker in the 1980s that survival after surgery was associated with a DO_2 index of greater than $600\,mL^{-1}\,min^{-1}\,m^{-2}$. Patients were admitted to critical care beds before surgery and a pulmonary artery catheter was inserted to measure cardiac index. A DO_2 of $600\,mL^{-1}\,min^{-1}\,m^{-2}$ was targeted using fluid boluses initially, and an infusion of an inotropic drug was started if the target oxygen delivery was not achieved with fluid alone.

In trials in which the patients were at very high risk, as shown by mortality in the control group, this approach produced significant reductions in mortality. However, further studies of patients who were at lower risk failed to show benefit. In addition, the use of the pulmonary artery catheter to measure cardiac output has largely fallen out of favour due to its invasive nature and the need for expert interpretation. New techniques for measurement of cardiac output

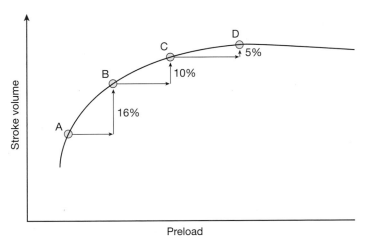

FIGURE 23.4 ■ Optimizing stroke volume with fluid: the Frank–Starling curve. At point A on the curve, the patient is significantly hypovolaemic and responds to a fluid bolus with a 16% increase in stroke volume at point B. The second bolus (B to C) produces a smaller but still significant increase, but the third bolus (C to D) produces only a small (<10%) increase in SV, signifying that the plateau portion of the Frank–Starling curve has been reached and that further fluid boluses will not lead to an increase in stroke volume.

have now been developed which are less invasive than the pulmonary artery catheter, and easier to use in the general surgical patient.

Intraoperative Stroke Volume Optimization

The development of the oesophageal Doppler device has allowed direct measurement of the stroke volume. Placed in the oesophagus after induction of anaesthesia, the Doppler probe is focused on the optimal waveform in the descending portion of the thoracic aorta.

The measured parameters of the Doppler waveform (Fig. 23.5) include:

- corrected flow time (FTc, ms)
- peak velocity (PV), considered a surrogate marker of contractility
- stroke distance, the distance which a column of blood moves in the aorta during systole, from which stroke volume is calculated using a nomogram based on the patient's height, weight and age.

A value for corrected flow time of less than 330 ms indicates hypovolaemia, and stroke volume usually increases if a bolus of fluid is given. Flow time increases if systemic vascular resistance decreases, which is usually the case in the anaesthetized patient; administration of vasoconstrictors increases systemic vascular resistance and decreases flow time. Because of these confounding influences on flow time, most practitioners use the derived estimate of stroke volume to guide fluid therapy.

Figure 23.6 shows a typical protocol for Doppler-guided fluid administration in which boluses of fluid are given until no further increases in stroke volume occur.

Doppler-guided fluid strategies have been shown to reduce complication rates and hospital length of stay in cardiac, general and orthopaedic surgery. Doppler-guided stroke volume optimization is associated with

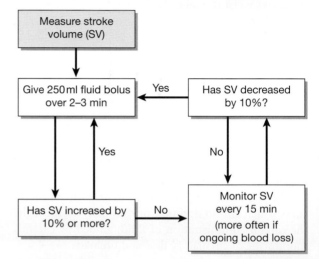

FIGURE 23.6 ■ Protocol for administering fluid guided by oesophageal Doppler. In the anaesthetized patient, stroke volume is the optimal parameter to guide fluid therapy when using the oesophageal Doppler. The approach followed in this example aims to optimize the patient's Frank–Starling curve (see Fig. 23.4) by sequential boluses of fluid until no further increases in stroke volume are observed.

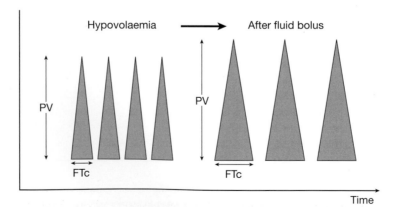

FIGURE 23.5 ■ Oesophageal Doppler trace with response to fluid. The height of the trace represents the peak velocity (PV), a marker of contractility. The corrected Flow Time (FTc) is the systolic ejection time in milliseconds; a value less than 330 ms indicates hypovolaemia. The hypovolaemic patient responds to a fluid bolus by increasing both flow time and peak velocity.

improved perfusion of the gut mucosa, and with reduced interleukin-6 concentrations after surgery. These studies suggest that correcting occult hypovolaemia at an early stage during surgery has an important beneficial role through improvement of gut perfusion with consequent reduction in the magnitude of the inflammatory response.

The oesophageal Doppler has some limitations. For consistent measurements, the patient needs to be either anaesthetized or deeply sedated. The technique is contraindicated in patients with oesophageal pathology, and the values are inaccurate during clamping of the aorta.

Preload Responsiveness to Guide Fluid Therapy

Stroke volume can be measured through analysis of the arterial pulse waveform (pulse contour analysis). This requires insertion of an arterial line, but this should be considered routine monitoring in the high-risk patient. A patient who has a sustained increase in stroke volume after a fluid challenge can be described as being preload responsive. As an alternative to direct observation of stroke volume responses to a fluid challenge, preload responsiveness can be estimated by assessing changes in the arterial pressure or plethysmographic waveform during mechanical ventilation. To date, several preload responsiveness variables have been described:

- systolic pressure variation (SPV)
- pulse pressure variation (PPV)
- stroke volume variation (SVV)
- plethysmogram variability index (PVI).

SPV, PPV and SVV all require insertion of an arterial line, whereas PVI is derived from analysis of the pulse oximeter waveform and is therefore non-invasive.

The ability of these variables to determine preload responsiveness is based on observation of the cyclical changes which occur in stroke volume in response to mechanical ventilation (Fig. 23.7).

- Right ventricular stroke volume decreases due to a decrease in preload as raised intrathoracic pressure causes decreased flow in the inferior vena cava and increased afterload.
- Left ventricular stroke volume increases initially as increased alveolar pressure causes an increase in flow of blood already in the low-pressure pulmonary capillary system returning to the left atrium.
- Left ventricular stroke volume subsequently decreases as the decrease in right ventricular stroke volume causes a decrease in left ventricular preload.

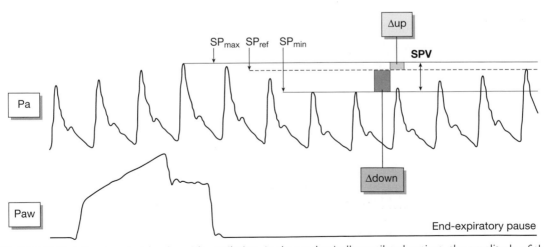

FIGURE 23.7 ■ Variation in arterial pulse with ventilation. In the mechanically ventilated patient, the amplitude of the arterial pulse varies during the ventilatory cycle. Variations in the systolic pulse (SPV) greater than 12–14% indicate that a patient is hypovolaemic and likely to respond to fluid by increasing stroke volume. *(Adapted from: Michard F. Changes in arterial pressure during mechanical ventilation. Anesthesiology 2005; 103:419–428.)*

Respiratory variations in stroke volume are the main determinant of the respiratory change in pulse pressure, as long as arterial compliance remains the same. In hypovolaemia, SVV and PPV are increased as the under-filled right atrium and vena cavae are more compliant, and hence collapsible during inspiration, and the heart is generally more sensitive to changes in preload because of the position on the steeper portion of the Frank–Starling curve. Consequently, variations in stroke volume, pulse pressure and, to a lesser extent, systolic pressure increase in hypovolaemic conditions. A pulse pressure or stroke volume variation greater than 12–13% is highly sensitive and specific for hypovolaemia, and a patient with this degree of variability normally responds to a fluid challenge with an increase in stroke volume.

Most studies of preload responsiveness have been conducted in patients undergoing cardiac surgery or in the ICU. Some surgical outcome studies have been undertaken and show that a fluid administration protocol based on stroke volume or pulse pressure variation can lead to a reduction in postoperative complications, although the evidence base is smaller compared with that for stroke volume optimization guided by Doppler, which has been available for longer.

PVI is obtained using recent technology in which the variation of the amplitude of the plethysmogram waveform during the respiratory cycle is analysed. It has been shown that values of PVI in excess of 14% are associated with hypovolaemia in stable cardiac surgical patients.

Preload responsiveness monitoring variables share the same significant limitations in that they require a stable heart rhythm, and are only validated in patients whose lungs are ventilated mechanically. It is unlikely that one technique is superior to the other, as long as the principles of measuring the response to a fluid challenge are adhered to, with the aim of ensuring that the patient has an optimal preload, and is on the plateau portion of the Frank–Starling curve.

Choice of Fluid

Both colloid and crystalloid solutions are used regularly for fluid therapy in the high-risk surgical patient. Although some anaesthetists express strong views in favour or against one or other of these types of fluid, it is likely that a combination of both fluids, used for different purposes, is the optimal solution.

Crystalloids should be used for provision of maintenance fluid until the patient is able to tolerate oral fluid. This should be given at a rate of at least $1.5\,mL\,kg^{-1}\,h^{-1}$, although larger doses are often used. Crystalloids are also the vehicle for electrolyte replacement therapy. Surgical patients need $1–2\,mmol\,kg^{-1}$ of sodium daily and $1\,mmol\,kg^{-1}$ of potassium. Solutions which contain dextrose only, or a mixture of dextrose and hypotonic saline (0.18%), lead to hyponatraemia and hypokalaemia, and should be avoided.

Colloid solutions should be reserved for correction of hypovolaemia and optimization of tissue perfusion, given as fluid challenges guided by flow-based measurements such as stroke volume or the preload responsiveness variables described above. Two types of colloid have been used in anaesthetic practice, the gelatins and starches. Gelatins are generally cheaper and provide a plasma volume expansion effect for 2–3 h. Starch-based colloids have now been withdrawn in the UK following after results from large randomised clinical trials and a meta-analysis reported an increased risk of renal dysfunction and mortality in critically ill or septic patients who received hydroxyethyl starch compared with crystalloids.

Infusion of large volumes of 0.9% sodium chloride ('normal saline') has been associated with the development of a hyperchloraemic metabolic acidosis. This acidosis is usually mild, and the clinical consequences are unclear. The most significant problem is probably the potential for erroneous interpretation of metabolic acidosis, and administration of unnecessary treatment in an otherwise normal patient. There may even be some benefit to a mild acidosis as it induces a leftward shift in the oxygen dissociation curve leading to increased oxygen delivery to the tissues.

It remains clinically unproven whether physiologically balanced crystalloids, such as Ringer's lactate, or colloids suspended in physiologically balanced solutions, have a clear clinical advantage over those containing saline.

Fluid Restriction Regimens

There is some evidence that giving patients unrestricted amounts of crystalloid solutions around the time of surgery can lead to increased complications.

Although crystalloid fluids have some immediate volume expansion effects when given as a fast bolus, these effects are short-lasting because crystalloid solutions (Ringer's lactate or 0.9% saline) are largely dispersed throughout the extracellular fluid compartment, which is 14 L in the average adult. Of 1 L of crystalloid solution administered, approximately only 25–30% remains within the circulation, with the remainder adding to the interstitial fluid volume.

The net effect is to increase the likelihood of tissue oedema, which, in the lungs, can cause impairment of gas exchange and, in the gut, can lead to ileus and increased gut permeability, with a delay in return of normal gut function.

Some studies of regimens in which crystalloid use has been restricted have shown improved outcome, but the wide range of regimens used, the lack of the use of goal-directed fluid therapy and the results of other studies showing no benefit, has led to uncertainty over the benefits of true 'restrictive' fluid regimens.

In summary, the important factor is how carefully intravenous fluids are administered. Crystalloids should not be given in large volumes, but used for maintenance support, and the use of colloid should be restricted to optimization of circulating volume and replacement of circulatory losses until the point at which blood component therapy is required, which is usually when the haemoglobin concentration decreases to below $8\,g\,dL^{-1}$.

POSTOPERATIVE MANAGEMENT

Successful management strategies for the high-risk surgical patient are based on preventing complications where possible through appropriate cardiovascular support as described above, and early recognition and treatment of situations in which surgical complications or unforeseen medical problems cause deteriorating organ function.

The level of monitoring required depends on the risk status of the patient, hopefully identified prior to surgery, so that the appropriate arrangements can be made in advance. Major elective surgery in a high-risk patient should proceed only if it has been confirmed that the appropriate level of postoperative care is available.

A patient previously identified as high-risk should be managed in a critical care bed after surgery, usually a High Dependency Unit (HDU, level 2 care) bed, unless mechanical ventilation or renal support is necessary, in which case an Intensive Care Unit (ICU, level 3 care) bed is required.

It may be possible to manage patients who undergo major surgery but who are not considered as being at high risk in the Post-Anaesthesia Care Unit (PACU) for a few hours after surgery before returning to the surgical ward. Some surgical wards have an 'enhanced care' area (level 1 care), in which patients can have an additional level of continuous monitoring, usually ECG, pulse oximetry and non-invasive blood pressure, as well as additional nursing support to assist mobilization and physiotherapy.

Monitoring on the General Ward

General ward monitoring is normally restricted to standard clinical observations, although some wards may be able to monitor central venous pressure (CVP) as well. The same principles of monitoring apply to both general ward patients and critical care patients in that the clinician is using the monitoring to detect organ dysfunction and decreased tissue perfusion at the earliest possible stage. The variables shown in Table 23.1 should be monitored routinely. These variables are usually combined into a scoring system known as a 'patient at risk' (PAR) score, or 'early warning system' (EWS) score. A particular PAR or EWS score value, or change in value, is pre-defined as a trigger point for nursing staff to summon medical assistance so that a potentially deteriorating patient can be identified early and appropriate treatment can be given, including transfer to critical care if indicated.

Monitoring in the Critical Care Unit

Critical care provides an environment in which the invasive monitoring used in the operating room can continue to be used safely after surgery. This applies particularly to the use of arterial cannulae, which should never be used on the general ward because an unobserved disconnection can lead to profound blood loss. Information gained from invasive monitoring in the postoperative critical care unit can be used to detect organ dysfunction at an early stage.

Central Venous Catheter

- *Central venous pressure (CVP)*. This can be used to assess circulating volume status *if* the response to a carefully administered fluid challenge is observed.

TABLE 23.1

Routine Observations for the High-Risk Surgical Patient

	POTENTIAL CAUSES OF ABNORMALITY	
	Elevated	*Depressed*
Level of consciousness	Agitation can be due to poor pain relief or hypoxaemia.	Hypotension and poor cerebral perfusion Over-sedation from opiate analgesia (systemic or epidural) Cerebrovascular accident
Heart rate	Hypotension Arrhythmia Inadequate pain relief	Heart block Drug effect – sedation, β-antagonist, ACEI
Blood pressure	Inadequate pain relief Omission of anti hypertensive medication	Bleeding (until proven otherwise) Hypovolaemia (untreated) Sepsis Sympathetic blockade from epidural or spinal
Respiratory rate	Metabolic acidosis from poor tissue perfusion from bleeding, hypovolaemia or sepsis Hypoxia from primary pulmonary complication, e.g. infection, atelectasis	Opiate overdose
Urine output	-	Less than $0.5\,mL\,kg^{-1}\,h^{-1}$ of *ideal* body weight suggestive of hypovolaemia

- *Central venous oxygen saturation* $(S_{CV}O_2)$. Oxygen saturation of blood returning to the heart of less than 70% has been associated with an increased risk of complications. Decreased $S_{CV}O_2$ reflects decreased oxygen delivery and a consequent increase in oxygen extraction.

Arterial Cannula

- Adequacy of oxygenation and ventilatory function through measurement of PaO_2 and $PaCO_2$.
- Assessment of pH and identification of causes of abnormalities, e.g. whether an acidosis is metabolic, respiratory or hyperchloraemic in origin.
- Assessment of tissue perfusion using lactate and bicarbonate, with an elevated lactate, decreased bicarbonate ('base deficit') and decreased pH indicating that tissue perfusion is inadequate, and that treatment with fluids and possibly inotropic drugs may be required.
- Cardiac output monitoring using a pulse contour analysis device. Using this technology, stroke volume and cardiac output can be estimated in the awake patient without the need for pulmonary artery catheterization. Fluid challenges can be given to increase stroke volume, and subsequent improvements in tissue perfusion can be assessed using base deficit, lactate or central venous oxygen saturation as described above.

INOTROPIC SUPPORT FOR THE HIGH-RISK SURGICAL PATIENT

Protocols which target an oxygen delivery value have usually incorporated the use of an inotropic agent to increase cardiac contractility if the oxygen delivery target has not been achieved with fluid loading alone. Adrenaline (α_1-, β_1- and β_2-agonist), dobutamine (β_1-agonist) and dopexamine (β_2-, DA_1- agonist) have all been used in this context.

There has been particular interest in the use of dopexamine in this group of patients, as it has splanchnic vasodilator and anti-inflammatory properties in addition to a mild inotropic activity. Early work suggested that dopexamine was associated with a reduction in complications after surgery, but more recent studies have shown that when fluid is given in a goal-directed manner, targeting either stroke volume or stroke volume variation, the routine use of dopexamine does not confer an additional significant clinical advantage.

Some patients may require inotropic or vasoconstrictor support if, despite adequate fluid loading, they still have signs of inadequate tissue perfusion (large base deficit, increased lactate concentration, decreased central venous oxygen saturation, etc.). In these situations, cardiac output monitoring should ideally be used to help guide treatment.

FURTHER READING

Canet, J., Galart, L., Gomar, C., et al., 2010. Prediction of postoperative pulmonary complications in a population-based surgical cohort. Anesthesiology 113, 1338–1350.

Copeland, G.P., Jones, M.W., 1991. POSSUM: a scoring system for surgical audit. Br. J. Surg. 78, 355–360.

Davies, S.J., Wilson, R.J.T., 2004. Preoperative optimisation of the high-risk surgical patient. Br. J. Anaesth. 93, 121–128.

Davies, S.J., Wilson, R.J.T., 2009. Rationalising the use of surgical critical care: the role of cardiopulmonary exercise testing. In: Vincent, J.L. (Ed.), Yearbook of Intensive Care and Emergency Medicine. Springer-Verlag, Berlin.

Grocott, M.P.W., Mythen, M.G., Gan, T.J., 2005. Perioperative fluid management and clinical outcomes in adults. Anesth. Analg. 100, 1093–1106.

Lee, T.H., Marcantonio, E.R., Mangione, C.M., et al., 1999. Derivation and validation of a simple index for prediction of cardiac risk of major noncardiac surgery. Circulation 100, 1043–1049.

Loftus, I. (Ed.), 2010. Care of the critically ill surgical patient, third ed. Hodder Arnold, London.

McConachie, I. (Ed.), 2009. Anaesthesia for the high-risk patient, second ed. Cambridge University Press, Cambridge.

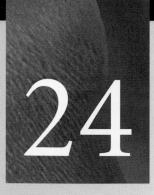

24   LOCAL ANAESTHETIC TECHNIQUES

L ocal anaesthetic techniques are used for both operative anaesthesia and for postoperative analgesia. They are becoming more popular as a result of advances in drugs, equipment and improved techniques of anatomical localization, including nerve stimulation and ultrasonic location. In addition, there is a greater appreciation of the need to improve postoperative pain control using techniques that not only reduce pain but have the ability to abolish it and potentially improve outcome. This chapter outlines the basic principles of patient management and the methods used in the performance of a variety of blocks which are commonly undertaken by the trainee anaesthetist. Regional techniques for obstetrics and dental surgery are described in other chapters.

FEATURES OF LOCAL ANAESTHESIA

Regional anaesthetic techniques may be used alone or in combination with sedation or general anaesthesia, depending on individual circumstances. Advantages of regional techniques include:

- *Avoidance of the adverse effects of general anaesthesia.* These may range from relatively minor postoperative nausea and vomiting, sore throat or myalgia to major issues such as respiratory impairment, awareness, airway complications or aspiration pneumonitis. In addition, the management of many patients with significant medical co-morbidity such as diabetes, obesity, or chronic pulmonary disease, can be improved or simplified. In elderly patients, acute perioperative cognitive impairment may be limited by

reducing or avoiding psychoactive drugs and maintaining contact with their surroundings.

- *Postoperative analgesia.* Local anaesthetic techniques can be used to provide effective prolonged postoperative analgesia whilst avoiding the systemic effects of other analgesic drugs, especially opioids. This can be provided using long-acting agents or by utilizing continuous catheter techniques, either neuraxial or peripheral. Some patients may be distressed by the accompanying numbness and motor block, but adequate preoperative explanation should minimize this concern. In addition, it is important that both nursing staff and patient are aware of the risk of tissue damage to any blocked area whether from direct trauma or indirect pressure from poor positioning or prolonged immobility. Simple techniques such as supporting the arm in a sling after brachial plexus block may help prevent injury and encourage earlier mobilization.

- *Preservation of consciousness during surgery.* The ability to assess neurological status continuously may be an advantage in patients with a head injury, diabetes or those undergoing carotid endarterectomy. Patient positioning may be safer, more comfortable and damage to pressure areas or joints avoided if the patient is awake. Airway and neck manipulation can be avoided; this may be especially important in a patient with severe rheumatoid arthritis or an unstable cervical spine. The awake patient undergoing caesarean section under regional anaesthesia is able to protect her own airway and experience the birth of the child.

- Sympathetic blockade and attenuation of the stress response to surgery.
- Improved gastrointestinal motility and reduced nausea and vomiting. This can allow earlier feeding and more rapid mobilization and discharge.
- Simplicity of administration.

There are now several studies suggesting that the net effect of these features may lead to a reduction in the incidence of major postoperative respiratory complications, though claims of other pathophysiological benefits remain unproven.

However, some patients may be unhappy at the prospect of being awake during surgery. In this situation the combination of a regional block with target-controlled intravenous sedation or general anaesthesia may be valuable. Similarly, this combination works well for prolonged surgery, where patient positioning may be compromised by generalized discomfort or where operation at several sites is necessary.

COMPLICATIONS OF LOCAL ANAESTHESIA

The incidence of complications may be minimized by ensuring adequate supervision and training in local anaesthetic techniques and by exercising care in the performance of each block. Many anaesthetists recommend performing all blocks in the awake (or lightly sedated) patient. The advantages of this are:

- It encourages careful, meticulous practice
- It provides the anaesthetist with valuable information on block onset and efficacy
- It alerts the anaesthetist to early complications such as inadvertent intravenous injection or intraneural injection.

Sufficient expertise and equipment must always be available to deal with potential complications. Complications common to many techniques are discussed in this section; more specific problems are considered later.

Local Anaesthetic Toxicity

LA toxicity usually results from accidental intravascular injection, an excessive dose of local anaesthetic or faulty technique, particularly during performance of Bier's block.

Clinical Features and Treatment

The clinical features and treatment of LA toxicity are described in Chapter 4.

Prevention

The following precautions are useful to minimize the risk of LA toxicity:

- slow injection of drug
- meticulous and correct technique
- careful, repeated aspiration using fractionated injections
- the use of a test dose.

Of these, the main safety measure is slow injection. This prevents rapid production of very high plasma concentrations even if the injection is intravascular. By this means, toxicity may be diagnosed early, the injection discontinued and a major reaction avoided. Rapid injection of local anaesthetic is not necessary for the performance of any block. The use of ultrasound-guidance to visualize local anaesthetic spread may be a useful addition to reduce intravascular injection with peripheral nerve block techniques.

Test Dose

This may be used before administration of the main dose of local anaesthetic drug. It is indicated particularly for epidural block, where it should be capable of demonstrating inadvertent intravenous (i.v.) or subarachnoid injection. A test dose of 4 mL plain lidocaine 2% is sufficient to cause mild symptoms in most patients after accidental i.v. injection, and any features of local anaesthetic blockade 2 min after injection are good evidence of accidental subarachnoid block. No test dose is infallible; the most important factor in avoiding local anaesthetic toxicity is slow administration of the main dose.

Hypotension

There are several possible mechanisms by which a local anaesthetic technique may cause hypotension. The anaesthetist must always remember that surgical factors may be responsible.

Sympathetic Blockade

A limited sympathetic block may be produced by peripheral nerve anaesthesia, but only central blocks are likely to produce hypotension by this mechanism.

Total Spinal Blockade

This occurs occasionally during subarachnoid block if excessive spread of local anaesthetic solution occurs, and is a recognized complication of epidural block if the dura has been penetrated (see below). Apnoea may occur if local anaesthetic solution reaches the cerebrospinal fluid (CSF) from perforation of a dural cuff during interscalene brachial plexus block, or the ventricular system during retrobulbar nerve block.

Vasovagal Attack

This is more likely to occur in an anxious patient with a rapidly ascending spinal block. Symptoms are pallor, nausea, and bradycardia associated with hypotension. It can occur with the patient in the supine position and usually resolves rapidy if i.v. atropine 0.3–0.6 mg or ephedrine 5–6 mg is administered. Cautious i.v. sedation (e.g. midazolam 1–2 mg) may be helpful.

Anaphylactoid Reaction

This is very rare with amide local anaesthetics.

Local Anaesthetic Toxicity

This is considered above and in Chapter 4.

Motor Blockade

To avoid unnecessary distress, patients must be warned of the possibility of limb weakness or paralysis which may persist for some time after operation.

Pneumothorax

This is a potential hazard of supraclavicular brachial plexus, intercostal and paravertebral blocks. Hence these techniques should not be performed as bilateral blocks or in outpatients.

Urinary Retention

This may follow the use of central neuraxial blocks. It is important to avoid overhydration, as bladder distension may require catheterization. The use of large volumes of crystalloid in the treatment of hypotension often has a very transient effect and predisposes patients to urinary retention, or worse, pulmonary oedema, when the block regresses.

Neurological Complications

Carefully performed blocks rarely result in neurological complications. Risk factors include obesity, diabetes and the perioperative use of potent anticoagulants. The incidence of neurological complications resulting from central neuraxial blocks is likely to be less than 4 per 10 000 or 0.04%.

Neuritis with persisting sensory changes and/or weakness may result from trauma to the nerve, intraneural injection or bacterial, chemical or particulate contamination of the injected solution. Injection of the incorrect solution has caused some of the most severe neurological complications. To avoid this, all drugs must be checked personally and labelled by the anaesthetist immediately before injection.

Anterior spinal artery syndrome may follow an episode of prolonged, severe hypotension and results in painless permanent paraplegia. *Adhesive arachnoiditis* has been described after subarachnoid and epidural blockade and may lead to permanent pain, weakness and bladder or bowel dysfunction. It is suspected that this complication results from injection of the incorrect solution. *Haematoma* or *abscess* formation in the spinal canal after subarachnoid or epidural anaesthesia results in weakness and sensory loss below the level of spinal cord compression. It is associated with intense back pain and is a neurosurgical emergency which demands immediate decompression to avoid permanent disability.

Equipment Problems

Needles are most likely to break at the junction with the hub and therefore should never be inserted fully. Catheters may also break, but exploratory surgery to find small pieces of catheter is inappropriate, as complications are very unlikely.

GENERAL MANAGEMENT

Patient Assessment and Selection

Careful preoperative evaluation is as important before a local anaesthetic technique as it is before general anaesthesia, and the same principles of preoperative management apply. Therapy to improve the patient's condition before surgery should be commenced if appropriate. It is inappropriate to proceed with surgery under local anaesthesia for the sake of convenience in the poorly prepared patient. A decision should be made on the need for immediate surgical intervention before the anaesthetic technique is chosen.

The preoperative visit should be used to establish rapport with the patient. A clear description of the proposed anaesthetic technique should be given in simple terms, but there is rarely a need for excessive detail. Patients require an explanation of the reasons for selecting a regional technique along with its advantages and potential disadvantages, but there should be no attempt at coercion to accept a particular technique.

Potential problems related to the intended block should be anticipated and sought. Anatomical deformities or pain affecting patient positioning may render some blocks impractical. A history of allergy to amide local anaesthetics is rare, but is an absolute contraindication, as is infection at the site of needle insertion. For most blocks, recent anticoagulant therapy and bleeding diatheses are also absolute contraindications, and the use of major blocks in patients with distant infection or receiving low molecular weight heparin, rivaroxaban or potent anti-platelet drugs such as clopidogrel, requires careful consideration. The use of non-steroidal anti-inflammatory drugs is not generally considered to be a contraindication to neuraxial block unless combined with other anticoagulant agents. The decision to perform spinal or epidural anaesthesia and the timing of catheter removal in a patient receiving antithrombotic therapy should be made on an individual basis, weighing the small, but definite risk of spinal haematoma against the benefits of regional anesthesia for a specific patient. The patient's coagulation status should be optimized at the time of spinal or epidural needle/catheter placement and indwelling catheters should not be removed in the presence of therapeutic anticoagulation because this seems to significantly increase the risk of spinal haematoma. Close monitoring is vital to allow early evaluation of neurological dysfunction and allow prompt intervention where necessary.

Sympathetic blockade with consequent vasodilatation may lead to profound hypotension in patients with significant aortic or mitral stenosis because of the relatively fixed cardiac output. Hypovolaemia must be corrected before contemplating subarachnoid or epidural anaesthesia.

There is no evidence that neuromuscular disorders or multiple sclerosis are adversely affected by local anaesthetic techniques, but most anaesthetists use regional anaesthesia in such patients only if there are obvious benefits to be gained; any perioperative deterioration in the neurological condition may be associated by the patient with the local anaesthetic procedure. Raised intracranial pressure is a contraindication to central neuraxial blockade but peripheral techniques may be considered.

Selection of Technique

Local anaesthetic drugs may be administered by:

- single dose
- intermittent bolus:
    - repeated injections
    - indwelling catheter for repeat administration
- continuous infusion (with optional bolus doses) via a catheter.

If regional anaesthesia has been selected primarily to provide analgesia during and after surgery under general anaesthesia, a more peripheral technique may be more appropriate to provide a more selective motor and sensory blockade with less functional impairment.

Because a local anaesthetic technique renders only part of the body insensible, it is essential that the method employed is tailored to, and sufficient for, the planned surgery. Account must be taken of the duration of surgery, its site (which may be multiple, e.g. the need to obtain bone grafting material from the iliac crest) and the likelihood of a change of procedure in mid-operation. The problem of multiple sites of surgery may be met by one block which covers both sites, or by more than one regional anaesthetic procedure where indicated. The duration of anaesthesia may be tailored to the anticipated duration of surgery by selection of an appropriate local anaesthetic agent, or may require the use of a technique which allows further administration of drug.

Premedication

Manipulation of fractures and other short emergency procedures are often carried out using a local anaesthetic technique in the unpremedicated patient, as rapid recovery is desirable. However, premedication is helpful before inpatient elective or emergency surgery.

An oral benzodiazepine allays anxiety, but an opioid (e.g. morphine) alleviates the discomfort of prolonged immobility which may be required during a long procedure. Preoperative analgesia may be required before definitive surgical fixation. A nerve block may be useful in these circumstances, e.g. a femoral block may be performed in the Emergency Department to alleviate the pain from a fractured femoral shaft. Patients should be fasted for all but the most minor peripheral nerve blocks.

Timing

It is essential that sufficient time is allowed to perform the block without undue haste on the part of the anaesthetist. This is largely a matter of organization and the experienced practitioner seldom causes delay to an operating list. Any preoperative delay is compensated for by the ability to return the patient to bed immediately after completion of surgery.

Resuscitation Equipment

A full range of resuscitation equipment must be immediately available and in working order whenever a local anaesthetic technique is used. This includes:

- an anaesthetic breathing system through which oxygen may be administered under pressure via a face mask or tracheal tube
- a laryngoscope with two sizes of blade, a range of tracheal tubes and an introducer
- a table which may be rapidly tilted head-down

- suction apparatus
- intravenous cannulae and fluids
- thiopental or propofol to control convulsions
- drugs to treat bradycardia or hypotension, especially atropine, ephedrine and metaraminol or phenylephrine
- lipid emulsion 20% for treating serious systemic toxicity (see Ch 4).

An intravenous cannula must be sited before any local anaesthetic block is performed, in case emergency therapy is required.

Regional Block Equipment

Regional anaesthesia may be used with basic equipment, but some special items increase the success rate and reduce the risk of complications.

Needles

The use of very fine spinal needles (26G) has significantly reduced the incidence of post-spinal headache as has the use of pencil-point 25G Whitacre and 24G Sprotte needles (Fig. 24.1A). The 27G Whitacre needles appear to be associated with the lowest incidence of post-spinal headache but confident and successful use of these needles requires greater expertise than is needed for the use of larger needles. For peripheral blocks, short-bevelled needles allow greater tactile appreciation of fascial planes and appear to reduce the likelihood of nerve damage. A variety of insulated needles are available for plexus and peripheral

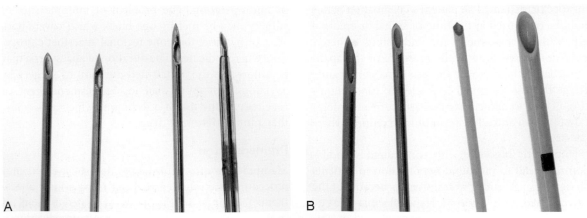

FIGURE 24.1 ■ **(A)** Left to right: Quincke, Whitacre, Sprotte and Spinocath needles. **(B)** Left to right: standard-bevelled, short-bevelled, insulated short-bevelled and insulated Tuohy needles.

nerve blockade using a nerve stimulator (Fig. 24.1B). Ultrasound needle visibility may be improved by using echogenic needles which have 'corner stone' reflectors positioned at the distal end of the cannula shaft (Fig. 24.11C).

A recent patient safety initiative aimed at reducing drug administration errors, has recommended the development and evaluation of spinal needles and catheter infusion systems with non-Luer connectors that cannot therefore attach to intravenous equipment or standard syringes. This should help prevent wrong route intrathecal injection and stop the accidental intravenous administration of drugs intended for epidural or regional block.

Immobile Needle Technique

For plexus and major nerve blocks, local anaesthetic drug is drawn into labelled syringes and connected to the block needle by a short length of tubing (Fig. 24.2). This allows the anaesthetist to hold the needle steady while aspiration tests are performed and syringes changed. The system must be primed to prevent air embolism and also to avoid image artefact when using ultrasound-guidance.

Catheters

Continuous administration of local anaesthetic drugs has been made possible by the development of high-quality catheters, which are introduced through a needle (or occasionally over a needle; Fig 24.1A) and

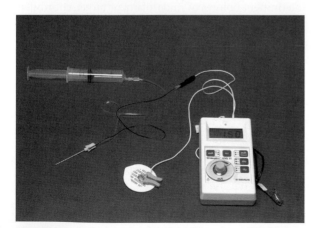

FIGURE 24.2 ■ Nerve stimulator and insulated stimulating needle attached to syringe.

may be left in position for hours or even days. Careful fixation is essential to maintain the position of the catheter in the postoperative period. Catheters, in particular spinal (subarachnoid) catheters, should be labelled clearly to prevent accidental overdosage.

Nerve Stimulators

Few anaesthetists now aim to deliberately elicit paraesthesiae when performing a major nerve block; many still use the nerve stimulator (Fig. 24.2) but an increasing number now use ultrasound-guidance. It is important to explain to the patient the sensation elicited by nerve stimulation. It causes little discomfort unless the contracting muscle crosses a fracture site, when duration of stimulation should be kept to the absolute minimum necessary to confirm needle position. The incidence of paraesthesia with short-bevelled insulated needles is very low because of their ability to stimulate without direct neural contact. They are also more likely to displace nerves rather than penetrate them.

Stimulators that deliver a constant current and give a digital display of the current used are readily available. One lead is attached to an electrocardiogram (ECG) electrode on the patient's skin, and the other to the needle. After skin puncture, the stimulator is set to a frequency of 1 Hz and an initial current of 1–2 mA. Most stimulators have a visual display to confirm a complete circuit when needle touches patient. If this fails, connections should be checked or the ECG electrode replaced. Failure to confirm a complete circuit could result in unwanted paraesthesiae or potential nerve injury from repeated needling.

As the nerve is approached, motor fibre stimulation causes muscle contraction in the appropriate distribution. The current is reduced until maximal contraction is still present at a current of, optimally, around 0.5 mA. At this point, a gentle aspiration test is performed and 2 mL of local anaesthetic solution slowly injected. Muscle contraction should cease immediately due to nerve displacement. If it does not, and an insulated needle is being used, the tip may have moved, be beyond the nerve or placed intravascularly; gentle aspiration should be repeated, the needle withdrawn slightly and the procedure repeated. Severe pain on injection suggests intraneural injection, in which case the needle should be repositioned. When the correct position has been found, the remainder of the anaesthetic solution should be injected slowly with repeated aspiration tests. Performance of the block in the awake patient allows better assessment of early intravascular toxicity and intraneural injection in addition to encouraging gentle and careful technique.

Ultrasound

The most significant recent change in the practice of regional anaesthesia has been the introduction of ultrasound guidance. A variety of high quality scanners and probes are now available and vast improvements in image quality have contributed greatly to advances with these techniques. The ultrasound transducer functions as both a transmitter and receiver with the beam reflected, refracted and scattered after it encounters structures of different acoustic impedance, returning to the transducer to produce the target image. Production of a clear target image as well as location and safe needle guidance in real time, requires sound cross-sectional anatomical knowledge along with excellent technical skills, which develop only following adequate training and repetitive hands-on practice. Transducers can be either linear or curved array, with higher frequency probes (8–12 MHz) generally used to produce superficial images of high resolution, such as would be required for interscalene or axillary block. Lower frequency probes (4–7 MHz) provide improved penetration to visualize deeper structures but with reduced resolution. Using the curved array probe for deeper blocks will provide a broader field of view for appreciation of surrounding anatomical structures and landmarks, for example during performance of a subgluteal sciatic block or an infraclavicular brachial plexus block. Most nerves exhibit a distinctive 'honeycomb' appearance on scanning, a combination of nerve fascicles and connective tissue, which varies in appearance depending on the individual nerve, its location and the angle of incidence of the probe. More proximal nerve roots, such as with interscalene imaging, tend to appear hypoechoic or dark, due to reduced amounts of connective tissue compared with the axilla and peripherally. As well as visualizing the target nerve structures, ultrasound guidance is useful to identify other important structures such as blood vessels and pleura in order to avoid complications and also allows visualization of local anaesthetic spread. Needle advancement can be tracked in real time, allowing subtle adjustment of needle position to ensure optimal local anaesthetic distribution.

Asepsis

A 'no-touch' technique is essential. Drapes should be used for all major blocks and gloves and gown should be worn by the novice. Gown, gloves, hat and mask are recommended for all central blocks even with a 'no-touch' technique, especially when a catheter is inserted either centrally or peripherally. Taking precautions seriously fosters good practice. For all ultrasound-guided blocks a sterile field should always be prepared using antiseptic solution and the probe covered with a sterile sheath or adhesive dressing before commencing the block. It is vitally important to cover the skin with sterile conductivity gel to remove the air-skin interfaces and allow good ultrasound wave penetration.

Monitoring

It is essential that the anaesthetist remains with the patient throughout the operative procedure. Monitoring equipment should be appropriate to the anaesthetic technique and surgical procedure, with a minimum of ECG, non-invasive blood pressure and pulse oximetry.

Supplementary Techniques

A local anaesthetic may be the only drug administered to the patient, or it may form part of a balanced anaesthetic technique. During surgery, patients may be awake, or sedated by i.v. or inhalational means. Intermittent boluses of midazolam, or target-controlled infusion of propofol are commonly used. General anaesthesia may be used as a planned part of the procedure. A combination of regional and general anaesthesia may be useful to obtain advantages from both, particularly for prolonged procedures or where positioning is difficult because of additional trauma or significant arthritis.

When a surgical tourniquet is used, the chosen block must extend to the tourniquet site unless the procedure is brief. Discomfort from prolonged immobility on a hard table is relieved by the administration of an opioid either as a premedicant or i.v. during surgery. This type of discomfort is not relieved by sedative drugs, which often result in the patient becoming agitated, confused and uncooperative. An i.v. infusion of remifentanil is being used increasingly for this purpose although this technique is not for the beginner and requires careful respiratory monitoring, preferably by continuous nasal capnography in addition to pulse oximetry.

After-Care

Clear instructions should be given to the nurses caring for the patient.

After day-case surgery, the patient must be in a safe condition at the time of discharge. Plexus blockade with a long-acting agent is inappropriate because of the risk of the patient injuring the anaesthetized limb, but is suitable for postoperative pain relief in supervised inpatients following major surgery, particularly when the limb is immobilized or conversely when continuous passive mobilization is required. Patients who have received central nerve blockade should have routine nursing observations at least until the block has worn off.

Continuous infusion techniques are suitable for use only by experienced anaesthetists. When used correctly, administration by infusion is safer than repeated bolus injection of drug, but regular observations are essential and the nursing staff must have an adequate level of knowledge to appreciate possible complications. An anaesthetist must be available within the hospital at all times.

INTRAVENOUS REGIONAL ANAESTHESIA

Ideally, intravenous regional anaesthesia (IVRA) (Bier's block) should be the first local anaesthetic technique learnt by a trainee, because its technical simplicity allows the trainee to concentrate on acquiring the skills of patient management. In practice, however, this technique is being used increasingly by Emergency Department staff and less frequently by anaesthetists, who often prefer to block the brachial plexus. Bier's block is simple, safe and effective when performed correctly using an appropriate drug in correct dosage. Deaths from IVRA have resulted from incorrect selection of drug and dosage, incorrect technique and the performance of the block by personnel unable to treat toxic reactions. The drug involved in these deaths, bupivacaine, was not the most suitable agent and is now contraindicated. The lessons to be learned from these deaths are applicable to all local anaesthetic techniques, and emphasize that expert guidance is essential even when learning the most basic blocks.

Indications

Intravenous regional anaesthesia is suitable for short procedures when postoperative pain is not marked, e.g. manipulation of Colles' fracture or carpal tunnel decompression. Recovery is rapid, and the technique is appropriate for outpatient surgery. Premedication may delay patient discharge and a reassuring visit preoperatively from the anaesthetist is usually sufficient in these circumstances.

Method

Intravenous regional anaesthesia involves isolating an exsanguinated limb from the general circulation by means of an arterial tourniquet and then injecting local anaesthetic solution intravenously. Analgesia and weakness occur rapidly and result predominantly from local anaesthetic action on peripheral nerve endings.

An orthopaedic tourniquet of the correct size is applied over padding on the upper arm. All connections must lock, and the pressure gauge should be calibrated regularly. An intravenous cannula is sited in the contralateral arm in case administration of emergency drugs is required. An indwelling cannula is inserted into a vein of the limb to be anaesthetized. A vein on the dorsum of the hand is preferred; injection into proximal veins reduces the quality of the block and increases the risk of toxicity. Exsanguination by means of an Esmarch bandage improves the quality of the block and increases the safety of the technique by reducing the venous pressure developed during injection. In patients with a painful lesion (e.g. Colles' fracture), elevation combined with brachial artery compression is adequate. The tourniquet should be inflated to a pressure 100 mmHg above systolic arterial pressure.

In an adult, 40 mL prilocaine 0.5% is injected over 2 min with careful observation that the tourniquet remains inflated. Analgesia is complete within 10 min, but it is important to inform the patient that the feeling of touch is often retained at this time. The anaesthetist must be ready to deal with toxicity or tourniquet pain throughout the surgical procedure. The tourniquet should not be released until at least

20 min after injection, even if surgery is completed. This delay allows for diffusion of drug into the tissues so that plasma concentrations do not reach toxic levels after release of the tourniquet. The technique of repeated reinflation and deflation of the cuff during release has little effect on plasma concentrations and is not necessary.

Tourniquet Pain

This may be troublesome if the cuff remains inflated for longer than 30–40 min. It is sometimes alleviated by inflating a separate tourniquet below the first on an area already rendered analgesic by the block; the first cuff is then deflated. Failing this, general anaesthesia is preferable to administration of large and often ineffective doses of opioids and sedatives.

Choice of Drug

The agent of choice for this procedure is prilocaine 0.5% plain. It has an impressive safety record with no major reactions reported after its use, although minor side-effects such as transient light-headedness after release of the tourniquet are not uncommon. Prilocaine has distinct pharmacokinetic advantages for IVRA and does not cause methaemoglobinaemia in the doses used for IVRA.

Lower Limb

Intravenous regional anaesthesia of the foot may be produced using the same dose of prilocaine and a calf tourniquet positioned carefully at least 10 cm below the tibial tuberosity to avoid compression of the common peroneal nerve on the fibular neck.

CENTRAL NERVE BLOCKS

Spinal anaesthesia is a term that may be used to denote all forms of central nerve blockade, although it usually refers to intrathecal administration of LA. The term subarachnoid block (SAB) avoids ambiguity. The technique of SAB is basically that of lumbar puncture, but knowledge of factors which affect the extent and duration of anaesthesia, and experience in patient management are essential. Epidural nerve block may be performed in the sacral (caudal block), lumbar, thoracic or cervical regions, although lumbar block is used most commonly. Local anaesthetic solution is injected through a needle after the tip has been introduced into the epidural space, or may be injected through a catheter placed in the space.

Physiological Effects of Subarachnoid Block

Differential Nerve Blockade

Local anaesthetic solution injected into the CSF spreads away from the site of injection and the concentration of the solution decreases as mixing occurs. A differential blockade of fibres occurs because small fibres are blocked by weaker concentrations of local anaesthetic solution. Sympathetic B fibres are blocked to a level approximately two segments higher than the upper segmental level of sensory blockade. Motor blockade may be several segments caudal to the upper level of sensory block. A sensory level to T3 with SAB may be associated with total blockade of the T1–L2 sympathetic outflow.

Respiratory System

Low SAB has no effect on the respiratory system and the technique is an important part of the anaesthetist's armamentarium for patients with severe respiratory disease. However, motor blockade extending to the roots of the phrenic nerves (C3–5) causes apnoea and blocks which reach the thoracic level cause loss of intercostal muscle activity. This has little effect on tidal volume (because of diaphragmatic compensation), but there is a marked decrease in vital capacity resulting from a significant decrease in expiratory reserve volume. The patient may experience dyspnoea, and difficulty in taking a maximal inspiration or in coughing effectively. A thoracic block may lead to a reduction in cardiac output and increased ventilation/perfusion imbalance, resulting in a decrease in arterial oxygen tension (PaO_2). Awake patients with a high spinal block should always be given oxygen-enriched air to breathe.

Cardiovascular System

The cardiovascular effects are proportional to the height of the block and result from denervation of the sympathetic outflow tracts (T1–L2). This produces dilatation of resistance and capacitance vessels and results in hypotension. In awake patients, vasoconstriction above the height of the block may compensate almost completely for these changes, thereby maintaining arterial pressure, but general anaesthetic agents may reduce this compensatory response, with consequent profound hypotension. Hypotension is exacerbated by:

- the use of head-up posture
- any degree of hypovolaemia – pre-existing or induced by surgery
- administration of sedatives, opioids or especially induction agents which should be given in greatly reduced dosage
- positive pressure ventilation.

Prevention of Hypotension

Both the incidence and the degree of hypotension are reduced by limiting the height of the block and, in particular, by keeping it below the sympathetic supply to the heart (T1–4).

It is common practice to attempt to minimize hypotension during SAB or epidural anaesthesia by preloading the patient with 500–1000 mL of crystalloid solution i.v. before or during the performance of the block. These volumes are usually ineffective even in the short term, may risk causing pulmonary oedema in susceptible individuals either during the procedure or when the block wears off, and may lead to postoperative urinary retention. Appropriate fluid should be given to replace blood and fluid losses and prevent dehydration.

Bradycardia may occur because of:

- neurogenic factors, particularly in awake patients, i.e. vasovagal syndrome
- paradoxical Bezold-Jarisch reflex; decreased venous return and heightened sympathetic tone leads to forceful contraction of a near empty left ventricle, with consequent parasympathetically mediated arterial vasodilatation and bradycardia
- block of the cardiac sympathetic fibres (T1–4).

Careful patient positioning, maintenance of a normal circulating volume and the use of pharmacological agents (see later), if required, should minimize the incidence of hypotension.

SAB has no direct effect on the liver or kidneys, but reductions in hepatic and renal blood flow occur in the presence of hypotension and reduced cardiac output associated with high spinal blocks.

Gastrointestinal System

The vagus nerve supplies parasympathetic fibres to the whole of the gut as far as the transverse colon. Spinal blockade causes sympathetic denervation (proportional to height of block), and unopposed parasympathetic action leads to a constricted gut with increased peristaltic activity. This is regarded by some as advantageous for surgery.

Nausea, retching or vomiting may occur in the awake patient and are often the first symptoms of impending or established hypotension. If nausea or retching occurs, the anaesthetist must assess arterial pressure and heart rate immediately and take appropriate measures.

Physiological Effects of Epidural Block

The physiological effects of epidural blockade are similar to those following SAB, but may develop more slowly. Additional effects may occur from the much larger volumes of anaesthetic solutions used, as there may be appreciable systemic absorption of local anaesthetic and adrenaline if an adrenaline-containing solution is used.

Indications for Subarachnoid Block

Blockade is produced more consistently and with a lower dose of drug by the subarachnoid route than by epidural injection. Duration of analgesia is usually limited to 2–4 h depending on surgical site and may be prolonged by catheter techniques. Catheter techniques may also be used to establish block height more carefully in more compromised patients. SAB is most suited to surgery below the umbilicus and in this situation the patient may remain awake. Surgery above the umbilicus using SAB is less appropriate and would necessitate addition of a general anaesthetic, in order to abolish the unpleasant sensations from visceral manipulation resulting from afferent impulses transmitted by the vagus nerves.

Types of Surgery

Urology. Subarachnoid block is commonly employed for urological procedures such as transurethral prostatectomy, but it should be remembered that a block to T10 is required for surgery involving bladder distension. Perineal and penile operations may also be carried out using a low 'saddle block', peripheral blockade or caudal anaesthesia.

Gynaecology. Minor procedures such as dilatation and curettage may be performed reliably with a block to T10. Pelvic floor surgery and vaginal hysterectomy may also be carried out readily with an SAB extending to T6, but for procedures requiring laparoscopic assistance, general anaesthesia is usually necessary.

Obstetrics. The widespread introduction of the pencil-point spinal needle with a reduction in the incidence of post-lumbar-puncture headache has led to the common use of SAB in obstetric practice to the extent that this is considered the technique of choice for the majority of elective caesarean sections and a large proportion of emergency ones. SAB may also be used for evacuation of retained products of conception, avoiding the risks of general anaesthesia. Further details of obstetric practice are discussed in Chapter 35.

Any Surgical Procedure on the Lower Limbs or Perineum.

For patients with the following medical problems, low SAB may be the anaesthetic technique of choice:

Metabolic disease. Diabetes mellitus.

Respiratory disease. Low SAB has no effect on ventilation and obviates the requirement for anaesthetic drugs with depressant properties and instrumentation of the airway. There is some evidence that SAB may reduce the incidence of chest infection and atelectasis as well as improving postoperative oxygenation.

Cardiovascular disease. Low SAB may be valuable in patients with ischaemic heart disease or congestive cardiac failure, in whom a small reduction in preload and afterload may be beneficial. SAB is effective in preventing cardiovascular responses to surgery (e.g. hypertension, tachycardia) which are undesirable, particularly in patients with ischaemic heart disease.

Pain management. SAB allows the simultaneous administration of intrathecal opioids. Preservative-free morphine 0.1 mg provides optimal postoperative analgesia of long duration for total hip arthroplasty. There is minimal risk of serious side effects such as respiratory depression but nausea and urinary retention are not uncommon. These patients should be adequately monitored in the postoperative period.

Indications for Epidural Blockade

The indications for epidural anaesthesia are widespread, because it is an extremely versatile technique which may be tailored to suit a variety of situations. The duration of analgesia may be prolonged as necessary by means of an indwelling catheter and the use of intermittent top-ups or a continuous infusion. Bupivacaine, levobupivacaine or ropivacaine are the drugs of choice when one of these continuous techniques is used. Their pharmacokinetic properties are such that, with the doses necessary to maintain adequate blockade, systemic accumulation of drug is slow and the risk of systemic toxicity is low. Ropivacaine and levobupivacaine are considered to be safer alternatives to racemic bupivacaine, particularly with regard to cardiotoxicity after inadvertent intravenous administration. Either local anaesthetic drugs or opioids, or frequently a combination of both, may be used for epidural analgesia. Opioids are most suited for postoperative analgesia and are inadequate alone for surgery in most circumstances. Almost all opioids have been tried by the epidural route with success but diamorphine or fentanyl are the most common additives in the UK. Clonidine combined with local anaesthetic has also been used successfully.

Contraindications to Subarachnoid Block and Epidural Anaesthesia

Most contraindications are relative, but the following are best regarded by the trainee as absolute:

- bleeding diathesis
- hypovolaemia
- sepsis – local or systemic
- severe stenotic valvular heart disease and in particular aortic stenosis – the patient may be unable to compensate for vasodilatation because of a fixed cardiac output
- pre-eclamptic toxaemia – epidural block is used with great benefit in this condition but a platelet count $<100 \times 10^9 \, L^{-1}$ usually precludes epidural or subarachnoid anaesthesia
- acute neurological diseases/raised intracranial pressure
- lack of patient consent.

Performance of Subarachnoid Block

Intravenous Access

Intravenous access must be secured before lumbar puncture is performed.

Positioning the Patient

Lumbar puncture for SAB may be performed with the patient sitting or in the lateral decubitus position (Table 24.1, Fig. 24.3). If it is anticipated that lumbar puncture may be difficult, the midline is usually more discernible with the patient in the sitting position, but the risk of hypotension in the sedated patient or following development of the block is increased. The technique of lumbar puncture for the patient in the lateral position is described in the next section.

Technique of Lumbar Puncture

For the right-handed anaesthetist, the patient is positioned on the operating table in the left lateral position. The patient's back should lie along the edge of the table and must be vertical. A curled position opens the spaces between the lumbar spinous processes. An assistant stands in front of the patient to assist with positioning and to reassure the patient. The anaesthetist must inform the patient before performing each part of the procedure.

A line between the iliac crests lies on the fourth lumbar spinous process; lumbar puncture should be performed at the L3/4 or L4/5 space. A full sterile technique (with gown, gloves and surgical drapes) is adopted. All drugs should be drawn into syringes directly from sterile ampoules using a filter needle to prevent the injection of glass particles into the subarachnoid space. A selection of spinal needles (22–27 gauge) should be available.

The skin and subcutaneous tissues are infiltrated with local anaesthetic using a small needle. The spinal needle is inserted in the midline, midway between two spinous processes. In the well-positioned patient, the needle is directed at right angles to the skin. Passage through the interspinous ligament and ligamentum flavum into the spinal canal is appreciated easily with a 22-gauge needle (Fig. 24.4A), but these needles are now rarely used because of the high incidence of postdural puncture headache. With some practice, these structures are usually discernible with a 25G or 27G pencil-point needle, which all anaesthetists should aspire to use. The use of an introducer (19-gauge needle) is advisable to brace the smaller needles, which are very flexible. When the needle tip has entered the spinal canal, the stilette is withdrawn from the needle and the hub is observed for flow of CSF; a needle with a transparent hub makes this easier. A gentle aspiration test should be performed if a free flow of CSF is not observed, or the needle carefully rotated through 90°.

The three most common reasons for difficulty are poor patient positioning, failure to insert the needle in the midline and directing the needle laterally (Fig. 24.4B). This last fault is seen most easily from one side and is usually apparent to onlookers, but not to the anaesthetist, who looks only along the line of the needle.

	TABLE 24.1		
	Techniques of Subarachnoid Block		
Type of Block	*Upper Level of Analgesia*	*Position During Lumbar Puncture*	*Volume of Solution*
Saddle block	S1	Sitting 5 min	1 mL hyperbaric solution
Low thoracic	T10–12	Sitting/lateral decubitus	3–4 mL isobaric solution*
Mid thoracic	T4–6	Lateral decubitus/sitting (immediately supine)	2–3 mL hyperbaric solution

Unilateral: A unilateral block, or at least a differential block between limbs, may be achieved by the slow injection of small volumes (1–1.5 mL) of hyperbaric solution in the lateral position. This position then has to be maintained for at least 15 min to minimize spread. On return to the supine position there may still be some contralateral spread and the necessity for smaller volumes and dosage may increase block failure rate.

*Plain bupivacaine is slightly hypobaric at body temperature and although it usually results in a low thoracic block, it may occasionally be unpredictable.

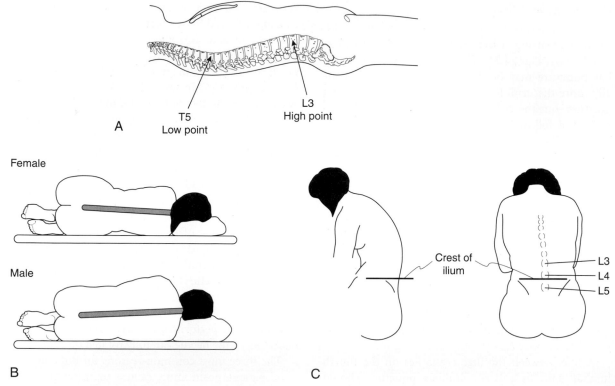

FIGURE 24.3 ■ Spinal curvature. **(A)** Supine position. **(B)** Lateral position. **(C)** Sitting position.

When CSF is obtained, the syringe containing the local anaesthetic solution should be carefully attached firmly to the needle, taking care not to displace the needle. Gentle aspiration confirms the needle position and the solution is injected at a rate of 1 mL every 5–10 s. Aspiration after injection confirms that the needle tip has remained in the correct place. Needle and introducer are withdrawn together and the patient placed supine.

Factors Affecting Spread

The most important factor which affects the height of block in SAB (Table 24.2) is the baricity of the solution, which may be made hyperbaric (i.e. denser than CSF) by the addition of glucose. The specific gravity (SG) of CSF is 1.004. The addition of glucose 5% or 6% to a local anaesthetic produces a solution with SG of 1.024 or greater. A patient who assumes the sitting position for 5 min after injection of 1 mL of hyperbaric solution develops a saddle block which affects the perineum only. Conversely, a patient placed supine immediately after injection of 2–3 mL develops a block to the mid-thoracic region. Slightly larger volumes are advisable to ensure spread above the lumbar curvature (see Fig. 24.3).

Within the range normally used for SAB (2–4 mL), the volume of solution has only a minor effect on spread. Obesity, pregnancy and a high site of injection are minor factors which increase the height of the block; lower volumes may be desirable in these situations. Barbotage and rapid injection may produce high blocks, but increase the unpredictability of spread.

Factors Affecting Duration

The duration of anaesthesia depends on the drug used and the dose of drug injected. Vasoconstrictors added to the local anaesthetic solution significantly increase the duration of action of tetracaine, which is widely used in the USA, but this is not so for other agents.

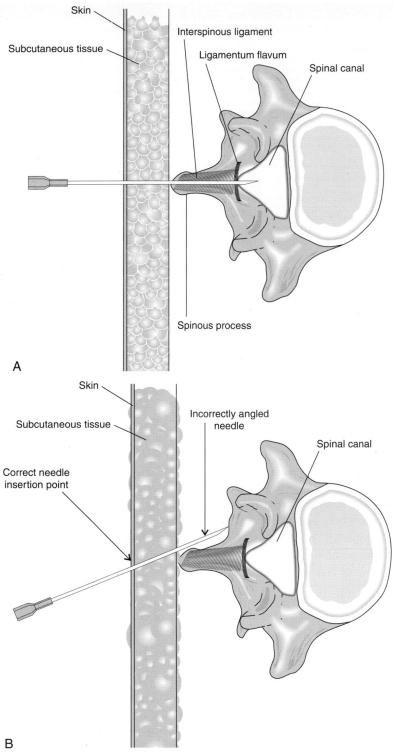

FIGURE 24.4 ■ Midline approach for subarachnoid block. **(A)** Correctly angled. **(B)** Incorrectly angled.

TABLE 24.2

Factors Influencing Spread of Hyperbaric Spinal Solutions

Factor	Effect
Position of patient	Sitting position produces perineal block only, provided that small volumes are used
Spinal curvature	With standard volumes (2–3 mL) the block often spreads to T4. With small volumes (1 mL) the block may affect only the perineum even when the patient is placed supine immediately
Dose of drug	Within the range of volumes usually employed (2–4 mL), increasing the dose of drug increases the duration of anaesthesia rather than the height of the block
Interspace	Minor factor affecting height of block
Obesity	Minor factor affecting height of block. Obese patients tend to develop higher blocks
Speed of injection	Rapid injection makes the height of block more variable
Barbotage	No longer used. Makes the height of block more variable

Agents

Four agents are currently available for SAB in the UK: plain bupivacaine, heavy bupivacaine, plain levobupivacaine and the recently introduced formulation of hyperbaric prilocaine. Ropivacaine is currently undergoing evaluation and seems to have a shorter duration of action compared with both racemic bupivacaine and levobupivacaine. Plain bupivacaine 0.5% is slightly hypobaric at body temperature and spread tends to be more unpredictable, although it does tend to produce a lower maximal block height when used in the lateral position, making it a popular choice for lower limb orthopaedic and vascular surgery. It is used in volumes of 3–4 mL and lasts 2–3 h. Hyperbaric bupivacaine 0.5% is more predictable for abdominal procedures and consistently produces a block to the umbilicus (and usually to T5) in supine patients. As with all hyperbaric solutions, hypotension is encountered more frequently because of higher levels of sympathetic blockade. Volumes of 2–3 mL are used and a duration of 2–3 h is usually assured. Hyperbaric prilocaine 2% has a duration of action of 100–130 minutes and is now available for use in ambulatory surgery. A volume of 2–3 mL can be used for surgical procedures anticipated to last up to 1 hour, allowing mobilization at around 4 hours after injection.

Complications

Acute. *Hypotension.* Significant hypotension is common with SAB and should be anticipated. Changes in position, e.g. turning the patient from the supine to the prone position, may result in a sudden increase in

TABLE 24.3

Management of Hypotension

5° head-down tilt	
Maintain blood volume	
Heart rate:	
<60 beats min^{-1}	Atropine 0.3 mg
60–80 beats min^{-1}	Ephedrine 3 mg
>80 beats min^{-1}	Metaraminol 0.5 mg

the height of block, with consequent extension of sympathetic blockade. This may occur even after 15–20 min. Treatment (Table 24.3) may not be necessary; moderate hypotension may help to reduce operative blood loss and is tolerated well by most patients. Severe or unwanted hypotension may be treated by i.v. fluids or drugs. The use of large volumes of crystalloid or colloid in this situation is not recommended, as urinary retention may occur postoperatively or circulatory overload may result when the block wears off. However, it is essential that operative blood losses are replaced promptly, and when blood losses are expected (e.g. caesarean section) it is wise to administer fluid in advance of the loss. Hypotension is associated commonly with bradycardia, and ephedrine 5–6 mg i.v. is the most appropriate treatment. Atropine may be useful, but sympathomimetic drugs are usually more effective than vagolytics.

Oversedation. This may occur when sedative drugs have been administered before performance of SAB. When the block is established, the previously satisfactory level of sedation may become excessive, with the attendant risks of respiratory obstruction or aspiration. Some reports of cardiac arrest associated with SAB may be related to hypoxaemia produced in this manner.

Postoperative. Headache. This is more common in young adults and particularly in obstetric patients. It may present up to 2–7 days after lumbar puncture, and may persist for up to 6 weeks. Characteristically it is worse on sitting, occipital in distribution and very disabling. The incidence is reduced by using small-gauge or pencil-point needles and may be reduced by aligning the bevel of the needle to penetrate the dura in a sagittal plane. Simple analgesics may be the only treatment required, but occasionally an epidural blood patch is necessary. The incidence of post-spinal headache is not reduced by keeping the patient supine for 24 h; the patient should remain supine only until the anaesthetic has worn off and the risk of postural hypotension is minimal. If headache is severe and persistent, an epidural blood patch may be performed by removing 20 mL of the patient's own blood under aseptic conditions and injecting it epidurally at the same interspace as SAB was performed. Injection should be stopped if discomfort is experienced. This is 70–80% effective for lumbar puncture headache and appears to be remarkably free from adverse effects.

Other complications. These include:
- Urinary retention – this may be associated with the surgical procedure. Large volumes of i.v. fluids may increase the frequency of this complication.
- Labyrinthine disturbances.
- Cranial nerve palsy – sixth nerve palsy may occur and is usually temporary. This complication is more common with larger needles.
- Meningitis and meningism.
- Spinal cord trauma caused by inserting the needle at too high an interspace – fortunately these conditions, giving rise to permanent neurological damage or paraplegia, are rare.

Continuous Spinal Anaesthesia

Subarachnoid blockade can be produced incrementally or the duration prolonged by using an indwelling spinal catheter. It may be performed using either a small catheter passed through a 19-gauge Tuohy needle or using a purpose-made catheter-over-wire kit such as the Spinocath (see Fig 24.1A). With the latter, the epidural space is located using a loss of resistance technique with a Crawford-type epidural needle and the 22-gauge Spinocath with guide wire, inserted through it to puncture the dura. The guide wire is then withdrawn, leaving the catheter in the subarachnoid space. Therefore there is minimal CSF leak around the catheter, reducing the risk of post-dural-puncture headache.

Spinal catheter techniques fell out of favour in the early 1990s following reports of cauda equina syndrome occurring in association with the use of 28-gauge and 32-gauge microcatheters and large doses of hyperbaric lidocaine 5%. It is postulated that the problem arose through pooling of high concentrations of lidocaine around the sacral nerve roots because of a slow injection rate, leading to permanent neurological damage. Hyperbaric lidocaine 5% and catheters finer than 24-gauge should be avoided and, because of the additional technical difficulty and potential for infection, the technique should be limited to more experienced practitioners in specific circumstances.

Performance of Epidural Block

By virtue of its great versatility, epidural analgesia is probably the most widely used regional technique in the UK. It may be used for procedures from the neck downwards and the duration of analgesia can be tailored to meet the needs of surgery and postoperative pain relief by using a catheter system.

The major differences between SAB and epidural block are summarized in Table 24.4. Further expansion of the technique has taken place with the advent of epidural administration of opioids and other agents such as clonidine or ketamine may have a place in providing postoperative epidural analgesia.

Equipment

Epidural anaesthesia is usually performed using a Tuohy needle (Fig. 24.5). The needle is marked at 1 cm intervals and has a Huber point which allows a catheter to be directed along the long axis of the epidural space. Disposable catheters are available with a single end-hole or with a sealed tip and three side-holes distally.

TABLE 24.4
Differences between Subarachnoid and Epidural Block

	Subarachnoid	*Epidural*
Dose of drug used	Small: minimal risk of systemic toxicity	Large: possibility of systemic toxicity after intravascular injection or total spinal blockade after subarachnoid injection
Rate of onset	Fast: 2–5 min for initial effect, 20 min for maximum effect	Slow: 5–15 min for initial effect, 30–45 min for maximum effect
Intensity of block	Usually complete anaesthesia	Often not complete anaesthesia for all segments
Pattern of block	May be dermatomal for first few minutes, but rapidly develops appearance of cord transection	Dermatomal
Addition of vasoconstrictor	Reliably prolongs block with tetracaine, but not with other drugs	Reliably prolongs block with lidocaine. May prolong block with bupivacaine, but not in all patients

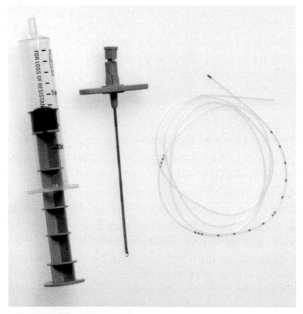

FIGURE 24.5 ■ 16-Gauge Tuohy extradural needle with loss of resistance syringe and catheter.

Technique

Epidural block may be performed at any level of the vertebral column to provide segmental analgesia over an area that can be predetermined with reasonable success. Initial experience should be gained in the lumbar region before progressing to sites above the termination of the spinal cord.

The pressure in the epidural space was originally considered to be subatmospheric, particularly in the thoracic region. In fact, it is slightly positive, but negative pressures are induced by tenting of the epidural space from the Tuohy needle and account for the rapid inward entry of saline using the hanging-drop method. Some older methods of identifying the epidural space (e.g. Odom's indicator, Macintosh's balloon) relied on detection of this *subatmospheric* pressure in the epidural space. However, methods which depend on loss of resistance to injection of air or saline as the tip of the needle penetrates the ligamentum flavum and enters the epidural space have become more popular. A midline lumbar approach is described here, using loss of resistance to saline to detect the epidural space.

The patient is positioned as for SAB and the vertebral level is identified from the iliac crests. The skin and subcutaneous tissues of the third lumbar interspace are infiltrated with local anaesthetic solution in the midline. A sharp needle is used to puncture the skin and the round-ended epidural Tuohy needle is introduced through the skin puncture, subcutaneous tissue and supraspinous ligament. The common reasons for difficulty are the same as those for SAB. When inserted into the interspinous ligament, the unsupported needle remains steady. The stilette is withdrawn and a 10 mL plastic syringe filled with saline is attached and advanced using firm but gentle pressure on the plunger. The needle must be gripped tightly at all times (Fig. 24.6) to prevent sudden forward movement.

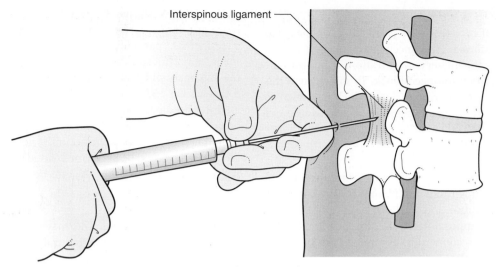

Interspinous ligament

FIGURE 24.6 ■ Loss of resistance technique to identify the epidural space. See text for details.

When the needle penetrates the ligamentum flavum, there is a sudden loss of resistance to pressure on the plunger, but the needle must not be allowed to advance further. The needle must not be rotated after its tip has entered the epidural space, as this increases the risk of penetration of the dura.

Single-Dose Technique

The syringe containing local anaesthetic is connected to the epidural needle, and after aspiration a test dose is administered to detect intravascular or subarachnoid placement. After an appropriate pause, the remainder of the solution is injected at a rate not exceeding 10 mL min^{-1} while verbal contact is maintained with the patient.

Catheter Insertion

An epidural catheter should pass freely through the needle into the epidural space. If the catheter does not thread easily, the needle should be repositioned, as forcing the catheter into the epidural space makes intravascular placement more likely. When a sufficient length of catheter (3–5 cm) is in the space, the needle is carefully withdrawn over the catheter. After ensuring that there is no flow of blood or CSF down the catheter, the hub is attached and an aspiration test performed; if blood or CSF is obtained, the catheter should be reinserted in an adjacent space.

A filter is connected and a test dose given. If this is satisfactory, the catheter is fixed to the patient's back with adhesive strapping and the main dose is administered.

Factors Affecting Spread

Epidural spread varies widely among individuals and the initial injection site will govern the pattern of distribution relative to this injection site. The most important determinant of spread appears to be the total mass of drug injected with the same mass of drug given in different concentrations and volumes producing similar spread of sensory blockade. Higher concentrations of drug will tend to increase the intensity of block including motor block. Posture has a minimal effect on spread; in the lateral position the dependent side will have block levels approximately 0–3 segments higher, whereas a supine Trendelenburg position of 15° will result in higher sensory block levels in pregnant women. Patients who are pregnant, obese or aged over 60 years may have an increased likelihood of a high block with a given dose of LA.

Factors Affecting Onset

Onset time may be reduced by increasing the concentration of the LA and by the addition of adrenaline 1:200 000.

Factors Affecting Duration

The choice of LA agent has a major effect on the duration of anaesthesia. The concentration of the drug also has an effect; the higher concentrations of bupivacaine produce a more prolonged block. To some extent this is a reflection of increased dose, which is known to increase the duration of anaesthesia. The addition of adrenaline 1:200 000 to lidocaine increases duration.

Agents

Lidocaine. Lidocaine is used in concentrations of 1.5–2% with or without adrenaline 1:200 000. Without adrenaline, the duration of action is approximately 1 h; a duration of approximately 1–2.5 h may be expected when solutions containing adrenaline are used, depending on surgical site.

Bupivacaine. Bupivacaine is available in concentrations of 0.25% and 0.5%. Increasing the concentration to 0.75% results in a faster onset, a denser block, more profound motor block (and therefore muscle relaxation) and increased duration of anaesthesia, but this concentration is not now freely available for use in the UK.

Levobupivacaine. Levobupivacaine is the pure S-isomer of bupivacaine and is less cardiotoxic than the racemic mixture, but otherwise appears equipotent in terms of sensory and motor blockade. Levobupivacaine is available as a 0.25%, 0.5% and 0.75% solution. The advantages of a 0.75% solution as described above may be broadly applicable to the use of levobupivacaine although clinical and research experience is more limited. A block lasting more than 4 h may be achieved with a 0.75% solution.

Ropivacaine. Ropivacaine is a long-acting agent that is less cardiotoxic than bupivacaine and may produce less motor block for a similar degree of sensory blockade. It is usually regarded as being less potent than bupivacaine and slightly higher concentrations/doses are usually employed.

Complications

Intraoperative. *Dural tap.* The incidence should be less than 0.5% in experienced hands. It usually occurs with the needle rather than the catheter and is immediately obvious because of the free flow of CSF. If this occurs, epidural block should be instituted at an adjacent space and managed cautiously, although experienced anaesthetists, particularly in the obstetric environment, may choose to pass the 'epidural' catheter into the subarachnoid space and manage as a continuous SAB (see Ch 35). Puncture of the dura with a large epidural needle leads to a high incidence of headache, of up to 70%. Simple analgesics and adequate hydration may suffice if headache occurs; if not, an epidural blood patch should be performed. Accidental total spinal anaesthesia (see below) is rare because the dural tap is usually obvious.

Total Spinal Anaesthesia. This may occur if the large volume of solution used for epidural anaesthesia is injected into the subarachnoid space. The consequences may be:

- profound hypotension
- apnoea, unconsciousness and dilated pupils secondary to local anaesthetic action on the brainstem.

Paralysis of the legs should alert the physician to the possibility of subarachnoid injection. When using a test dose, motor function should be tested by asking the patient to raise the whole leg and not merely to wiggle the toes; movement of the toes may not be abolished for 20 min after SAB, if at all. It should be noted that relatively large volumes of local anaesthetic solution, e.g. 10 mL of bupivacaine 0.25%, may be injected into the subarachnoid space without total spinal anaesthesia occurring.

Provided that skilled resuscitation is undertaken rapidly, a total spinal should be followed by complete recovery. Appropriate personnel and equipment should be present before epidural analgesia is undertaken and whenever top-up injections are administered.

Massive Epidural Block and Subdural Block. A very high block may occur in the absence of subarachnoid injection. This may be associated with Horner's syndrome.

Other complications. These include:

- intravenous toxicity (see Ch 4)
- hypotension
- urinary retention
- shivering

- nausea/vomiting – this may result from hypotension or visceral manipulation in the awake patient.

Postoperative

- *Headache* following dural tap.
- *Epidural haematoma.* The spinal canal acts as a rigid box, and an expanding haematoma within the canal compresses the spinal cord, resulting in loss of neurological function unless the compression is relieved surgically at a very early stage. Decompression within 6 h is completely effective in virtually all patients, but after 12 h it is almost totally ineffective.
- *Epidural abscess.*
- *Other neurological complications,* e.g. damage to a single nerve root or paraplegia following accidental administration of potassium chloride.

Anticoagulants and Subarachnoid Block or Epidural Anaesthesia

Oral Anticoagulants

Anticoagulation should be stopped at an appropriate time before surgery if SAB or epidural anaesthesia is planned. The degree of anticoagulation most appropriate for the patient depends on a balance between the risk of withholding anticoagulation and the nature of the surgery, in particular the associated risk of bleeding.

Platelets

The platelet count should ideally be $>150 \times 10^9 \, L^{-1}$.

Antiplatelet Agents

Concern has been expressed about the antiplatelet effect of aspirin, NSAIDs and dipyridamole with respect to increased risk of vertebral canal haematoma. There is little evidence to support this concern but clopidogrel should be stopped at least 7 days before surgery unless there are overwhelming clinical circumstances, as reports of both serious surgical bleeding and vertebral canal haematoma have been associated with its use.

Heparin

The half-life of heparin given i.v. is 50–160 min, depending on dose. When given s.c., blood concentrations vary widely; in some patients plasma concentrations are in the anticoagulant range. At present, it is regarded as imprudent to use SAB or epidural analgesia when subcutaneous heparin has already been given, especially the low-molecular-weight variety. Removal of an epidural catheter should be timed to precede, rather than follow, administration of a further dose of subcutaneous heparin.

Guidelines for the use of low-molecular-weight heparin and epidural anaesthesia are given in Table 24.5.

TABLE 24.5
Guidelines for the Insertion and Removal of Epidural Catheters in Association with Low-Molecular-Weight Heparins (LMWH)

1	Patients who need DVT prophylaxis before theatre should receive LMWH the day before at approximately 18.00 h.
2	LMWH should not be given on the day of surgery – this allows 12 h before catheter placement; although the LMWH is providing DVT prophylaxis at this time, plasma concentrations are below peak activity and therefore less likely to create a problem.
3	LMWH may be given 2 h after placement of an epidural catheter.
4	The epidural catheter should be removed 12 h after the last dose of LMWH and the next dose should not be given until 2 h have elapsed.
5	Antiplatelet drugs and anticoagulant drugs should not be used concurrently with LMWH.
6	The smallest effective dose of LMWH should be used.
7	Patients should have regular (every 4 h) neurological examination after removal of the epidural catheter. This should include sensation, power and reflexes.
8	In cases of traumatic or repeated epidural puncture, administration of LMWH should be delayed for more than 24 h; an alternative method of DVT prophylaxis should be used.
9	Epidural mixtures should contain a low concentration of local anaesthetic so that motor function may be assessed.
10	If the patient develops a neurological abnormality either during epidural infusion or within 48 h of epidural catheter removal, an urgent MRI scan is required and a neurosurgical opinion should be obtained.

Intraoperative Heparinization

Epidural analgesia and SAB offer advantages for major vascular surgery, but the routine use of heparin introduces the theoretical risk of haemorrhage if an epidural catheter is in place. The precise risk is unknown, as prospective trials would require in excess of 10 000 cases. Some large series (3000 patients) have been conducted under epidural analgesia without haematoma formation.

Caudal Anaesthesia

Caudal block involves injection of local anaesthetic into the epidural space through the sacral hiatus to obtain anaesthesia of sacral and coccygeal nerve roots. Injection of very large volumes to obtain anaesthesia of lumbar and thoracic roots, although described, is seldom practised because of a high incidence of side-effects and failure to achieve a sufficiently high block. With appropriate volumes, caudal blockade affects the lower limbs infrequently, does not cause sympathetic blockade and has a low risk of dural puncture. The anatomy is variable and difficulty is experienced in approximately 5% of subjects.

Indications

Caudal anaesthesia is suitable for perineal operations, e.g. haemorrhoidectomy, although in practice a subarachnoid saddle block is usually preferred. It is frequently used in paediatric practice for postoperative analgesia following circumcision, orchidopexy and inguinal hernia and hypospadias repairs.

Method

Caudal blockade may be performed with the patient in the prone position, but the left lateral position is usually more acceptable to the patient and easier in the anaesthetized paediatric patient. Palpation down the sacral spine leads to the depression of the sacral hiatus at S5, flanked by the sacral cornua, through which the needle is inserted. A 21-gauge hypodermic needle or 22-gauge cannula is introduced through skin and sacrococcygeal ligament in a cephalad direction at 45° to the skin (Fig. 24.7). When the membrane is penetrated, injection may be performed or the needle hub may be depressed toward the natal cleft, and inserted a further

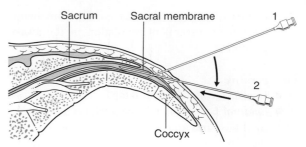

FIGURE 24.7 ■ Needle position for caudal anaesthesia.

2–3 mm along the sacral canal; it must be remembered that the dura may extend to S3. Lidocaine 2%, with or without adrenaline, and bupivacaine 0.5% are suitable agents. In an adult, 10 mL of solution blocks anal sensation consistently.

In conjunction with general anaesthesia, caudal anaesthesia provides smooth operating conditions and good postoperative analgesia. With this combined technique, the advantages of performing caudal block before induction of general anaesthesia are as follows:

- The patient does not need to be repositioned while anaesthetized.
- Subperiosteal injection is reported by the patient.
- Accidental i.v. injection may be detected before the full dose is given.

For patients undergoing haemorrhoidectomy, many surgeons rely on the tone in the anal sphincter to identify it accurately and avoid damage. In these patients, general anaesthesia may be supplemented by a short-acting opioid such as alfentanil for the intraoperative period, and caudal anaesthesia given following the procedure. Extremely effective postoperative analgesia lasting several hours is provided.

Complications

Misplaced needle. Injection into subcutaneous tissue causes a swelling with fluid, or surgical emphysema with 2–3 mL of air. Intraosseous or subperiosteal injection results in marked resistance to injection. Penetration of rectum and fetal head (in obstetric practice) have been reported but should not occur if the technique is performed carefully.

Dural tap. This is rare, but the procedure should be abandoned if CSF is aspirated.

PERIPHERAL BLOCKS

Head and Neck Blocks

Superficial cervical plexus block is now commonly used for carrying out awake carotid endarterectomy but other specialized blocks are mostly used in ophthalmic and plastic surgery. Only the technique of local anaesthesia for awake intubation is described here. Blocks used in ophthalmic surgery are discussed in Chapter 30.

Awake Intubation

This may be the safest option in a patient with known or anticipated difficulty with intubation from a variety of causes, anatomical or otherwise. Pretreatment with an antisialagogue such as glycopyrrolate 0.2 mg may be useful to decrease secretions and improve anaesthesia obtained with topical application. Sedation with midazolam or a combination with fentanyl or a target-controlled remifentanil infusion is desirable, if this is not likely to exacerbate airway obstruction. A blind, fibreoptic or retrograde technique may be used, and experience and training in these techniques are now more widespread.

The nose is prepared with topical lidocaine 2% with or without a vasoconstrictor such as phenylephrine. The patient may then either suck a benzocaine lozenge, or the posterior tongue and pharynx are sprayed with lidocaine 4%. For laryngeal analgesia, either a 'spray as you go' technique through the scope under direct vision is used, or a cricothyroid injection is performed through either a 23-gauge needle or 22-gauge cannula inserted through the cricothyroid membrane (Fig. 24.8A, B) with air aspirated to confirm the position. Two millilitres of lidocaine 4% are injected and the needle is withdrawn immediately. A vigorous cough results and spreads the solution. Although absorption of lidocaine from mucous membranes is rapid, in practice, significant amounts tend to be lost or swallowed and rarely cause systemic toxicity.

Upper Limb Blocks

The upper limb is well suited to local anaesthetic techniques and these remain among the most useful and commonly practised peripheral regional techniques. The pattern of blockade is partly determined by the approach used and because each technique has its own limitations in regard to the extent of block and the risk of side-effects, it is important to relate the surgical requirements to the benefits and risks of the intended block for each individual patient. Interscalene block is the most useful approach for shoulder surgery as it successfully blocks the cervical plexus as well as the proximal brachial

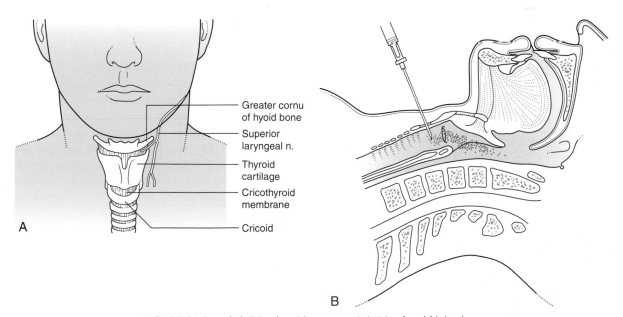

FIGURE 24.8 ■ **(A)** Cricothyroid anatomy. **(B)** Cricothyroid injection.

plexus, whilst axillary, supraclavicular and infraclavicular blocks can all be used for elbow, forearm and hand surgery. These techniques are commonly used as the sole technique for surgery and the recent introduction of ultrasound-guidance has led to an upsurge of interest in this area with many potential benefits.

The aim with all of these techniques, whether using peripheral nerve stimulation or ultrasound, is to achieve rapid and complete blockade with the lowest possible failure rate and with minimal complications. With appropriate training, these techniques may now be expected to provide successful surgical anaesthesia in more than 90% of patients using a variety of anatomical approaches. The majority of the remainder can be managed with additional local infiltration or the addition of a peripheral 'rescue' block before resorting to general anaesthesia.

Anatomy of the Brachial Plexus

A sound anatomical knowledge is essential to the practice of peripheral regional anaesthesia. The nerve supply of the upper limb is derived mainly from the brachial plexus, which is formed from the anterior primary rami of the fifth to eighth cervical and first thoracic nerve roots. The roots of the plexus divide repeatedly and recombine to form trunks, divisions, cords and terminal nerves (Fig. 24.9). The roots emerge from the intervertebral foramina and combine into three trunks above the first rib. Each trunk separates above the clavicle into anterior and posterior divisions; anterior divisions supply the flexor structures of the arm and posterior divisions the extensor structures. The divisions recombine into three cords, which surround the second part of the axillary artery behind pectoralis minor and then form the terminal nerves.

The roots lie between the anterior and middle scalene muscles and are invested in a sheath, derived from the prevertebral fascia, which splits to enclose the scalene muscles. The cutaneous and deep nerve supplies of the upper limb are depicted in Figure 24.10.

Part of the cutaneous nerve supply of the upper limb is not derived from the brachial plexus; the upper medial part of the arm is supplied by the intercostobrachial nerve (T2) whilst the skin over the shoulder tip is supplied by the supraclavicular nerves of the cervical plexus. The reader is referred to standard texts for a more detailed anatomical description.

Ultrasound-Guidance

Ultrasound-guidance has been greatly increasing in popularity over the last 10 years, particularly for the performance of peripheral upper and lower limb blocks. For the first time, the anaesthetist has been able to visualize anatomical structures and variants, allowing accurate needle placement and importantly, visualization of local anaesthetic spread around these target structures. Potential advantages of these techniques remain a source of debate (Table 24.6). Although definitive outcome studies comparing ultrasound-guidance with nerve stimulation are not available, there is increasing evidence that ultrasound offers a number of advantages including greater block success, faster onset time, reduced procedure-related pain, reduced local anaesthetic dosage and reduced adverse effects such as inadvertent intravascular injection and phrenic nerve paresis with interscalene block.

Axillary Block

This technique represents perhaps the safest approach to the brachial plexus for the trainee to learn whether using peripheral nerve stimulation or ultrasound-guidance. It is useful for elbow, forearm and hand surgery and safe for out-patients, but traditional single-injection approaches are limited by high failure rates of both musculocutaneous and radial nerves. This is due to the anatomical positions of the nerves and the presence, in some individuals, of fibrous septae within the brachial plexus sheath which prevent circumferential spread of local anaesthetic. The most common orientation of nerves around the axillary artery is shown in Figure 24.11A, as are the needle positions necessary for successful complete blockade using nerve stimulation. Ultrasound visualization allows both the detection of anatomical variation and the optimization of local anaesthetic spread around these structures. Dense, complete blockade can often be achieved within 10–15 min using multiple injection techniques.

Positioning. The patient lies supine with the arm to be blocked abducted to no more than 90° and the elbow bent to 90° (see Fig. 24.11B). Further abduction with the hand placed behind the head is convenient, but the axillary vessels become stretched and distorted, and performance of the block is more difficult.

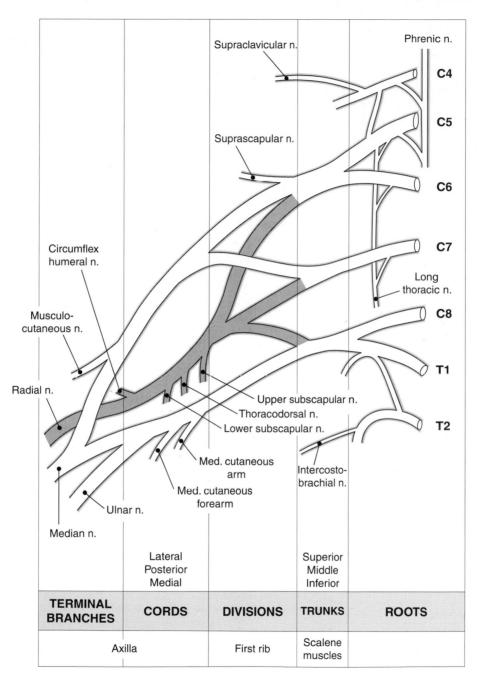

FIGURE 24.9 ■ Formation of the brachial plexus.

Inside figure labels:

Supraclavicular n.

Phrenic n.

C4

C5

Suprascapular n.

C6

Circumflex humeral n.

C7

Long thoracic n.

Musculo-cutaneous n.

C8

Radial n.

T1

Upper subscapular n.

Thoracodorsal n.

Lower subscapular n.

T2

Med. cutaneous arm

Intercosto-brachial n.

Med. cutaneous forearm

Ulnar n.

Median n.

TERMINAL BRANCHES	CORDS	DIVISIONS	TRUNKS	ROOTS
	Lateral Posterior Medial		Superior Middle Inferior	
Axilla		First rib	Scalene muscles	

Method. The axillary artery is palpated and traced to a point 1–2 cm distal to the lateral border of pectoralis major. A 2 mL subcutaneous wheal of local anaesthetic is raised superficial and inferior to the artery at this point, which also blocks the intercostobrachial nerve. A 22-gauge insulated short-bevelled needle is introduced through this wheal after puncturing the skin with a standard needle. The nerve stimulator is set

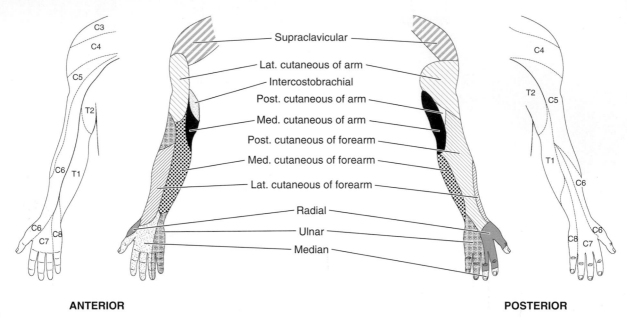

ANTERIOR   POSTERIOR

FIGURE 24.10 ■ Innervation of the upper limb: outer, dermatomal innervation of the skin; inner, cutaneous nerve supply to the upper limb.

TABLE 24.6
Potential Advantages of Ultrasound-Guided Nerve Blockade

Visualization of target structure

Visualization of surrounding anatomical structures

Accuracy of needle placement

Visualization of local anaesthetic spread in real time

Compensation for anatomical variation

Avoidance of intraneural or intravascular injection

Variety of approaches (not landmark dependent)

Rapid block onset

Reduced local anaesthetic dosage

Reduced procedure-related pain

Reduced complications

to deliver a current of 2 mA and the needle directed immediately above the artery (almost parallel to the floor). Stimulation of the musculocutaneous nerve causes biceps contraction and flexion of the elbow. The current should then be reduced until optimal contraction is obtained at a current of around 0.5 mA; 5 mL of the LA is injected following gentle aspiration. The needle is then withdrawn and redirected through the same puncture, in a more inferior direction with the current again set to deliver 2 mA. Flexion of wrist and fingers occurs following a distinct fascial click as the needle enters the sheath and stimulates the median nerve. Current is again reduced to optimize muscle contraction at 0.5 mA and 15 mL of LA solution injected in 5 mL increments, each preceded by careful aspiration. Finally, the needle is withdrawn and redirected below the artery until extension of the fingers is obtained and again current reduced from 2 mA to 0.5 mA. Ten mL of LA is then injected in two 5 mL increments. A total of 30 mL of local anaesthetic solution is therefore used. For most routine upper limb surgery, lidocaine 1.5% with adrenaline 1:200 000 is used, but for major painful procedures, ropivacaine or levobupivacaine 0.5% may be substituted. After completion of injection, the arm should be returned to the patient's side.

Ultrasound-guidance: The plexus of most individuals can be visualized using a linear 10 MHz probe set to a depth of 3 cm. An anatomical survey is carried out to demonstrate the positions of the nerves (Fig 24.11C). The musculocutaneous nerve is generally

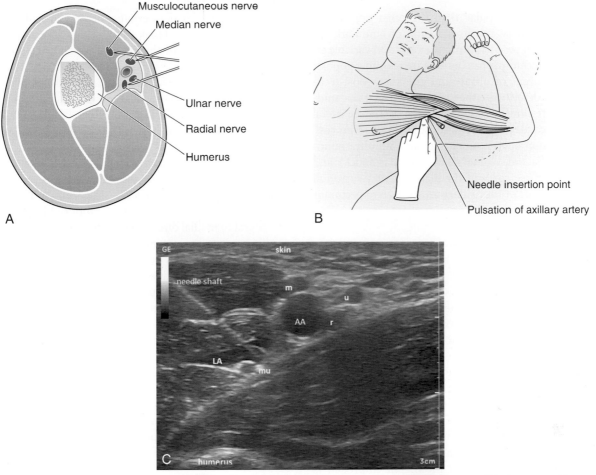

FIGURE 24.11 ■ **(A)** Cross-sectional relationship of the brachial plexus nerves to the axillary artery. **(B)** Correct position and approach for axillary block. **(C)** Ultrasound image of distal axilla showing echogenic needle targeting the musculocutaneous nerve (mu). AA, axillary artery; m, median nerve; u, ulnar nerve; r, radial nerve; LA, local anaesthetic.

seen lying between biceps and coracobrachialis muscles lateral to the artery, the median nerve is usually located adjacent to the artery in the '9–12 o'clock' position with the ulnar nerve often seen in the corresponding '12–2 o'clock' position, a discrete distance from the artery and often just below the axillary vein. The radial nerve is the most difficult to visualize and tends to lie beneath the ulnar nerve in the '5 o'clock' position. The block needle is introduced either in-plane or out of plane, following local anaesthetic infiltration. Local anaesthetic is then distributed around the individual nerves as described above and additionally around the ulnar nerve.

Disadvantages. Access is occasionally problematic if arm abduction and external rotation are limited by either additional shoulder trauma or severe arthritis. This approach rarely blocks the axillary nerve unless large volumes of solution are used. If blockade of this nerve is required, a more proximal approach to the plexus should be considered. Puncture of the axillary artery is rarely a problem, but may lead to haematoma formation or inadvertent intravascular injection. Nerve damage occurs rarely and is more likely to result from malposition of the anaesthetized limb or failure to recognize a compartment syndrome postoperatively.

Infraclavicular Block

Historically less popular than the other approaches due to the variety and imprecision of landmark approaches, high vascular puncture rates and variable efficacy, this technique has become increasingly popular since the advent of ultrasound-guidance. Most techniques are described either below the clavicular midpoint (vertical infraclavicular block) or a more lateral approach caudal and medial to the coracoid process. The latter approach is more popular with ultrasound-guidance (lateral sagittal infraclavicular block) and blocks the three cords of the plexus as they surround the second part of the axillary artery deep to pectoralis minor muscle.

Advantages. The block can be performed with the arm at the side and may therefore be useful when access for axillary block is prevented by limitation of shoulder abduction. Using ultrasonic location and ensuring local anaesthetic spread posterior and medial to the axillary artery, excellent efficacy and complete block within 10–15 min can be achieved from a single injection site. For best images and ease of needle placement in the limited space below the clavicle, a small curved array probe is used. This probe not only shows the important vascular structures with which the nerves are intimately related, but with experience also demonstrates the three neural cords and the local anaesthetic spread around them. The approach is useful for elbow, forearm and hand surgery and is particularly useful if a catheter is sited for postoperative use, because of greater ease of secure fixation below the clavicle. Blockade of the phrenic nerve is unlikely with the lateral approach.

Disadvantages. Pneumothorax has been reported although the risk appears to be low. Vascular puncture is fairly common using nerve stimulator techniques because of the close proximity of nerves to both axillary artery and vein in this location. Ultrasonic location reduces this to a minimum. Success rates decrease with inadequate spread, but administering 35–40 mL rather than 30 mL of LA solution may improve medial spread with a single-injection approach, providing this remains within the safe recommended dosage of the local anaesthetic agent.

Supraclavicular Block

This approach provides perhaps the best overall efficacy of complete arm block from a single injection as the trunks/divisions of the brachial plexus are closely related at this point.

The key to successful and safe nerve stimulation approaches is accurate palpation of the interscalene groove (see Fig. 24.12) above the clavicle, which helps delineate the position of the first rib and lateral border of pleura as well as locating the plexus. Popularity has been increasing since the introduction of ultrasound-guidance as plexus, subclavian artery, pleura and first rib are all usually straightforward to visualize (Fig 24.13). The needle is introduced in-plane, in a lateral to medial direction and should be visualized continuously to prevent inadvertent pleural puncture.

Advantages. The arm does not require to be abducted for access and complete upper limb local anaesthesia, including axillary nerve block, is possible from a single injection. Onset time may be as short as 10–15 min and 30 mL of solution is sufficient to produce a dense block in most adults. It is suitable for proximal humeral surgery as well as more distal upper limb surgery.

Disadvantages. The risk of pneumothorax is always present, but is very small (<0.5%) in experienced hands even when using peripheral nerve stimulation.

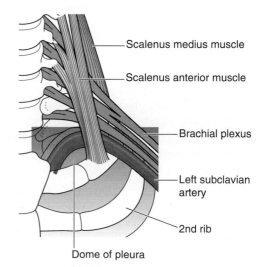

Scalenus medius muscle

Scalenus anterior muscle

Brachial plexus

Left subclavian artery

2nd rib

Dome of pleura

FIGURE 24.12 ■ Relationships of the brachial plexus in the neck.

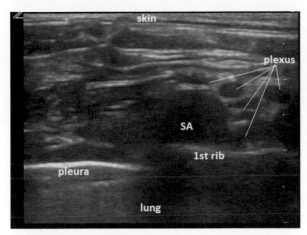

FIGURE 24.13 ■ Ultrasound image of supraclavicular brachial plexus. SA, subclavian artery.

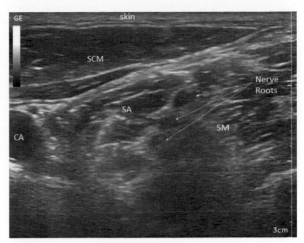

FIGURE 24.14 ■ Ultrasound image of C5 & C6 nerve roots for interscalene block. CA, carotid artery; SCM, sternocleidomastoid muscle; SA, scalenus anterior; SM, scalenus medius.

The safety and success depend on the accurate localization of the interscalene groove which may not always be straightforward, particularly in the obese. Pleural puncture should be preventable using ultrasound-guidance but has been reported. Phrenic nerve paralysis may occur in around one-third of patients, but is usually asymptomatic. Axillary block is the method of choice if there is diminished respiratory reserve. Sympathetic block is relatively common and results in Horner's syndrome. The technique is still not recommended routinely for out-patients.

Interscalene Block

Advantages. This is the most proximal approach to the brachial plexus and the only approach which reliably blocks the plexus above C5. With adequate volume (25–30 mL) interscalene injection usually extends to block the cervical plexus roots C3 and C4 and is therefore most suitable for shoulder and upper arm surgery.

Disadvantages. Block of the C8 and T1 roots may prove difficult and make the technique rather less suitable for hand surgery. Complications are similar to those for supraclavicular block but phrenic nerve block occurs almost universally with the volumes of local anaesthetic described. Ultrasound guidance, targeting the C5 and C6 nerve roots (Fig 24.14) allows much smaller volumes of LA (as little as 5–10 mL) to be used for postoperative analgesia, reducing the incidence of phrenic paresis to around 50%. Pneumothorax, vertebral artery puncture,

total spinal and direct intraspinal injection are also possibilities. Seizures may occur from direct vertebral artery injection with as little as 1–2 mL of LA solution.

Agents

Lidocaine 1.5%, with adrenaline 1:200 000, bupivacaine, ropivacaine or levobupivacaine 0.2–0.5% are all suitable agents. The more dilute solutions are necessary when larger volumes or additional nerve blocks are required, or may be used when the block is combined with general anaesthesia, particularly if a postoperative local anaesthetic infusion is planned.

Blocks in the Trunk

Intercostal and paravertebral blocks are useful in providing analgesia following abdominal, breast and thoracic surgery and also provide good analgesia for rib fractures. The analgesic area may be extended using multiple injections or by spread of a larger single bolus, usually via an indwelling catheter, which may then be employed for repeat administrations. There is a significant risk of pneumothorax when these blocks are performed by unskilled personnel. Paravertebral block can be a relatively straightforward procedure particularly with ultrasound-guidance, but is only suitable for the more experienced anaesthetist. It is gaining popularity for analgesia following breast and inguinal hernia surgery, but is not considered further here.

Intercostal Nerve Block

Anatomy. Intercostal nerves are formed from the ventral rami of segmental thoracic nerves after communicating with the associated sympathetic ganglia through white and grey rami communicantes (Fig. 24.15). An intercostal nerve has three main branches: the lateral cutaneous branch divides into anterior and posterior branches; the anterior terminal branch supplies the anterior thorax, rectus muscle and overlying skin; and a collateral branch arises from most nerves in the posterior intercostal space. This may rejoin the main nerve or form a separate anterior cutaneous nerve. Fibres from T1 join the brachial plexus, T2 and T3 supply fibres to form the intercostobrachial nerve, and T12, together with L1, contribute to the iliohypogastric, ilioinguinal and genitofemoral nerves.

Method. The optimal place to block the intercostal nerve is proximal to the formation of the lateral cutaneous branch, posterior to the mid-axillary line. With the patient in the lateral position, nerve blocks may be conveniently performed immediately following surgery for unilateral procedures such as open biliary and gallbladder surgery. In awake patients, for example

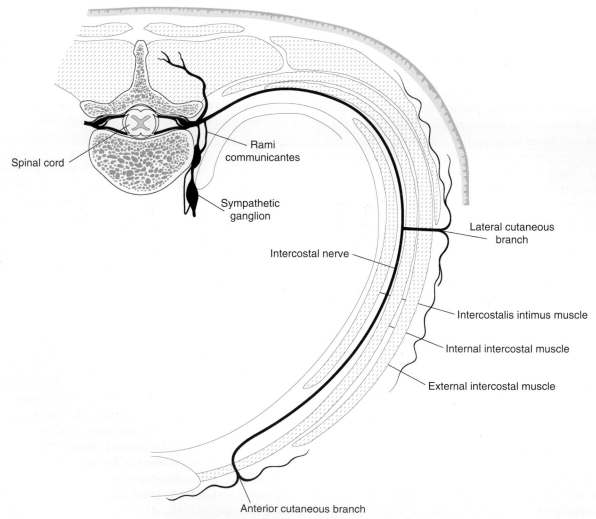

Spinal cord

Rami communicantes

Sympathetic ganglion

Intercostal nerve

Lateral cutaneous branch

Intercostalis intimus muscle

Internal intercostal muscle

External intercostal muscle

Anterior cutaneous branch

FIGURE 24.15 ▪ Anatomy of the intercostal nerve.

following unilateral rib fractures, a sitting position with the patient leaning forward to abduct the scapulae is often convenient. A 23-gauge needle is inserted perpendicular to the skin to make contact with an appropriate rib. The needle is then 'walked' caudally until it can be inserted under the lower border of the rib, through the external intercostal muscle (a depth of 2–3 mm). Following a negative aspiration test, 3–5 mL of local anaesthetic solution is then injected. Rapid absorption of LA solution may produce high systemic concentrations after multiple intercostal nerve blocks and the dose and concentration of drug need to be chosen carefully; 0.25–0.5% levobupivacaine or ropivacaine 0.2–0.5% is recommended, depending on the number of intercostal nerves being blocked. A single injection of 20 mL using a catheter technique may block up to five adjacent segments (approximately two above and three below). Pneumothorax and haemorrhage are the most likely complications after intercostal nerve block.

Ilioinguinal and Iliohypogastric Blocks

The main nerves which supply the groin are the subcostal (T12), iliohypogastric (L1) and ilioinguinal (L1). Ilioinguinal and iliohypogastric blocks are used for postoperative analgesia after inguinal hernia surgery, hydrocoele repair and orchidopexy, but can also be used to reduce opioid requirements after gynaecological and obstetric surgery. They are frequently used in paediatric practice and can provide analgesia comparable with caudal analgesia for paediatric day case surgery. Block efficacy can be improved and dosage reduced by using ultrasound-guidance. Local anaesthesia is used routinely as the sole anaesthetic for adult inguinal hernia surgery in some centres and may be the method of choice in the unfit patient or in the day-case unit, but only when surgeons are experienced with this technique. When used as the sole anaesthetic technique for adult inguinal hernia repair, supplementary infiltration along the line of skin incision and around the internal ring and hernial sac, is usually necessary to provide complete analgesia.

The traditional 'blind' approach requires a short-bevelled needle to be inserted 1.5 cm medial and inferior to the anterior superior iliac spine. The fascial click on penetrating external oblique aponeurosis is readily appreciated as the needle is advanced. A total volume of fifteen to twenty millilitres of local anaesthetic are injected under the aponeurosis to block the iliohypogastric nerve followed by a deeper injection within the internal oblique muscle, to ensure blockade of the ilioinguinal nerve as it penetrates this muscle. Another 5 mL of solution can be deposited superficial to the external oblique aponeurosis medially from this point to obtain blockade of cutaneous T12 fibres. A more proximal injection point, cranial and posterior to the anterior superior iliac spine has been recommended with ultrasound-guidance, as the nerves are easier to visualize and they each tend to lie in the same plane between transversus abdominis and internal oblique at this point. Levobupivacaine or ropivacaine 0.2–0.5% are suitable agents for postoperative analgesia.

Transversus Abdominus Plane (TAP) Block

This block provides analgesia of the anterior and lateral abdominal wall by blocking the T6–L1 afferent fibres as they lie within the neurofascial plane between the transversus abdominis and internal oblique muscles. Injection is made in the mid-axillary line above the iliac crest and can be performed blindly or ideally with ultrasound-guidance. It is suitable as part of a postoperative analgesic strategy following unilateral lower abdominal surgery such as hernia repair and appendicectomy or performed bilaterally for procedures such as retropubic prostatectomy or total abdominal hysterectomy. Local anaesthetic volumes of at least $0.3 \, mL.kg^{-1}$ are required to ensure adequate spread and dilute solutions will therefore be required if blocks are performed bilaterally, to ensure that dosage is kept within recommended safe limits.

Penile Block

The dorsal nerves to the penis are derived from the pudendal nerves and are blocked with 5–10 mL of LA solution injected inferior to the symphysis pubis in the midline at a depth of 3–4 cm. Care must be taken to avoid intravascular injection in this area and vasoconstrictors *must not* be used. Plain bupivacaine or levobupivacaine 0.5% are suitable agents. The base of the penis is innervated by the genital branch of the genitofemoral nerve, which may be blocked if necessary by s.c. infiltration around the penis.

Penile block is quick and simple, produces a limited effect and is the block of choice for circumcision or other minor penile surgery such as meatotomy. It is commonly used in combination with light general anaesthesia and provides good postoperative pain relief. However, a simpler technique is to smear lidocaine jelly over the wound on a regular 4 to 6-hourly basis in the postoperative period.

Lower Limb Blocks

Lower limb blocks are practised less frequently than upper limb blocks for three reasons:

- It is not possible to block the whole of the lower limb with one injection.
- Subarachnoid or epidural anaesthesia may prove simpler.
- There is an impression among some anaesthetists that lower limb blocks are difficult and unreliable.

However, new approaches to the peripheral nerves of the lower limb and the use of ultrasound-guidance have simplified the subject and the blocks considered below are appropriate for the trainee anaesthetist.

Sciatic Nerve Block

Anatomy. The sciatic nerve (L4, L5, S1–3) arises from the sacral plexus, passes through the great sciatic foramen and descends in the posterior thigh to the popliteal fossa, where it divides into the tibial and common peroneal nerves. In the thigh, it supplies muscles and the hip joint. The posterior cutaneous nerve of the thigh (S1–3) may run with the sciatic nerve or separate from it proximally; this nerve supplies the skin of the posterior thigh and upper calf. The tibial and common peroneal nerves, together with the saphenous nerve, supply all structures below the knee.

Method. There are several approaches to the sciatic nerve; with ultrasound-guidance the nerve is best visualized where it is most superficial either subgluteal or in the popliteal fossa (Fig. 24.16) With nerve stimulation, the posterior approach described by Labat is the most straightforward but requires the patient to be turned to a lateral semi-prone position; the limb to be blocked is uppermost and flexed at the knee. A line is drawn from the posterior superior iliac spine to the tip of the greater trochanter of femur. At the midpoint, a second perpendicular line is drawn caudally for 4–5 cm to mark the point of needle insertion

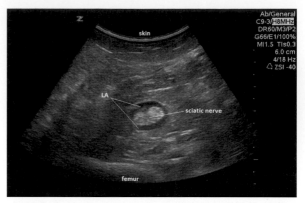

FIGURE 24.16 ■ Ultrasound image of sciatic nerve surrounded by local anaesthetic (LA), in the popliteal fossa.

(Fig. 24.17). Following aseptic preparation, the skin is infiltrated with 2 mL of local anaesthetic and a 100 mm, 21G insulated block needle inserted perpendicular to skin with the stimulator set to deliver 2 mA. After some initial twitches in the gluteal area, further advancement usually results in hamstring contraction. The current is then best reduced to 0.5–1 mA before further subtle advancement produces either dorsiflexion or, ideally, plantar flexion of the foot at a current of 0.5 mA. Fifteen to 20 mL of local anaesthetic is then injected in 5 mL aliquots after negative aspiration.

This block has a high success rate with few complications, although intravascular placement may be difficult to detect because of the length of the needle. The posterior cutaneous nerve of thigh is usually blocked with this approach. Sciatic block may often be used alone for several procedures in the foot, e.g. hallux valgus operations, using a below-knee tourniquet. This must be positioned at least 10 cm below the tibial tuberosity to avoid compression of the common peroneal nerve as it courses around the fibular neck. The block is particularly useful for the medically compromised, arteriopathic patient requiring peripheral or forefoot amputation. This may require additional saphenous block at the ankle to complete cutaneous analgesia on the medial aspect of the foot. Sciatic block may also be combined with either lumbar plexus or femoral block to allow use of a thigh tourniquet or to complete analgesia of the lower limb.

Lidocaine 1.5–2% with adrenaline 1:200 000, or ropivacaine, levobupivacaine or bupivacaine 0.375–0.5% are suitable agents. Fifteen to 20 mL of solution

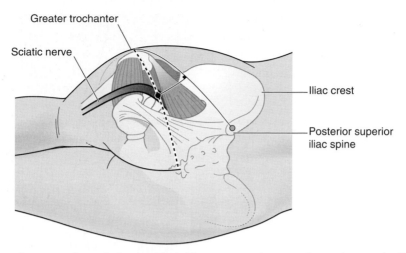

FIGURE 24.17 ■ Posterior approach to sciatic nerve block. The greater trochanter and posterior superior iliac spine are marked.

is necessary. The more dilute solutions are required when other blocks are performed concurrently.

Femoral Nerve Block

Anatomy. The femoral nerve (L2–4) arises from the lumbar plexus and runs between psoas and iliacus to enter the thigh beneath the inguinal ligament, 1–2 cm lateral to the femoral artery and at a slightly greater depth. Branches of the anterior division include the intermediate and medial cutaneous nerves of the thigh and the supply to the sartorius. The posterior division supplies the quadriceps and the hip and knee joints and terminates as the saphenous nerve, which supplies the skin of the medial side of the calf as far as the medial malleolus and sometimes the medial side of the dorsum of the foot.

Method. The patient lies supine and the inguinal ligament and femoral artery are identified. The skin is anaesthetized lateral to the femoral artery, 1 cm below the inguinal ligament. A 22-gauge, short-bevelled insulated needle is inserted parallel to the artery in a cephalad direction of approximately 45° with respect to skin (Fig. 24.18). With the nerve stimulator set to deliver 2 mA, two distinct fascial pops are generally appreciated before muscle contractions occur. Patellar ascension or 'tapping' is observed when the femoral nerve is accurately located with the current reduced to around 0.5 mA. Observation of this patellar movement should prevent confusion with the contractions obtained by direct stimulation of the sartorius muscle. Fifteen to 20 mL of solution is required for satisfactory blockade. Ultrasound-guidance, either in-plane or out of plane, can be used to locate the nerve and confirm spread of local anaesthetic around it and below the fascia iliaca.

Femoral nerve block is usually combined with sciatic block for operative procedures. Analgesia following femoral fracture or knee surgery may be satisfactory with femoral nerve block alone, although complete analgesia following knee replacement is best achieved initially with additional sciatic block.

The inguinal perivascular technique of lumbar plexus anaesthesia (the so-called '3-in-1 block') was reported to provide anaesthesia in the distribution of the femoral, lateral cutaneous and obturator nerves from the single injection of 20–30 mL of solution with distal digital pressure. In practice, however, careful assessment has shown that the obturator nerve is not blocked routinely by this approach.

Suitable LA agents for femoral or '3-in-1' block are the same as for sciatic nerve block.

Lumbar Plexus Block

A paravertebral approach to the lumbar plexus provides, in many ways, a more logical approach to blockade of the three main terminal branches: femoral, obturator and lateral cutaneous nerve of thigh, than

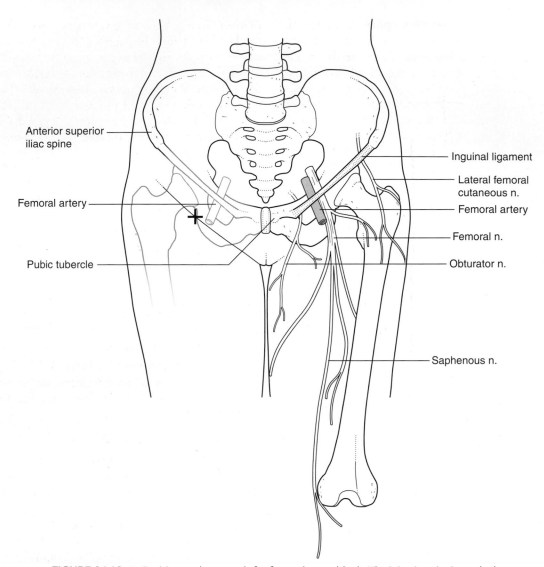

FIGURE 24.18 ■ Position and approach for femoral nerve block. The injection site is marked.

the inguinal 3-in-1 approach mentioned above. It may be used in combination with sciatic block to complete analgesia of the lower limb and has been used as the sole technique for femoral neck surgery in addition to providing postoperative analgesia after major hip or revision surgery carried out under general anaesthesia or central neuronal blockade.

Anatomy. The lumbar plexus is formed from the ventral rami of the first three and large part of the fourth lumbar nerves. The nerves run from the vertebral column in an inferolateral direction within the posterior part of the psoas muscle. The femoral and lateral cutaneous nerves then emerge from the lateral aspect and the obturator from the medial aspect of this muscle and all three nerves may be blocked with LA within the psoas muscle at the L3/4 level or L4/5 level.

Method. The patient is positioned either sitting or more commonly in the lateral decubitus position with operative side uppermost. The spine of the fourth lumbar vertebra is identified by palpating the iliac crests. A 21-gauge,100-mm insulated needle is inserted at the junction of the lateral third and medial two thirds of a line drawn between the spinous process of L4 (approximately 1 cm cephalad to the upper edge of the iliac crests) and a perpendicular line, parallel to the spinal column passing through the posterior superior iliac spine. After contact with the lumbar transverse process is made, the needle is withdrawn and redirected in a cephalad direction (or occasionally in a caudad direction) until the needle glides over the transverse process. The depth from skin is variable but contact with the plexus, resulting in quadriceps contraction, is usually found at a depth of 1.5–2 cm from the transverse process. Following careful aspiration, 15–20 mL of local anaesthetic, usually levobupivacaine 0.375–0.5% or ropivacaine 0.4–0.5%, is injected in 5 mL increments.

Complications. Care must be taken in selecting an appropriate concentration of LA, particularly when combined with sciatic block, to ensure maximum dosage is not exceeded, resulting in systemic toxicity. Epidural spread, usually unilateral, has been reported particularly in paediatric practice. Penetration of the retroperitoneum leading to haematoma formation, kidney or bowel puncture is possible. Central nervous system toxicity, epidural and intrathecal spread leading to respiratory failure and cardiac arrest have all been reported.

Ankle Block

Anatomy. Five nerves supply the forefoot. The medial and lateral plantar nerves are the terminal branches of the posterior tibial nerve, which enters the foot posterior to the medial malleolus; they supply deep structures within the foot and all of the sole. The common peroneal nerve divides into deep and superficial branches; the deep peroneal nerve supplies the web space between first and second toes and the superficial branch supplies the dorsum of the foot. The saphenous nerve may supply a variable area of skin on the medial side of the dorsum of the foot. The sural nerve is a branch of the tibial nerve; it runs posterior to the lateral malleolus and supplies skin over the lateral side of the foot and 5th toe.

Method. To block the posterior tibial nerve, the posterior tibial artery is palpated behind the medial malleolus as far distally as possible. Injection of 3 mL of LA to each side of it, below deep fascia, blocks medial and lateral plantar nerves. Alternatively, the posterior tibial nerve may be blocked with 5 mL of local anaesthetic injected at a point distal and posterior to the sustentaculum tali, particularly when there is no vascular landmark. Injection of 2 mL of LA to each side of the dorsalis pedis artery, below deep fascia, blocks the deep peroneal nerve. The saphenous and superficial peroneal nerves are blocked by s.c. infiltration at the level of the ankle joint in a line extending from a point anterior to the medial malleolus to the lateral malleolus. The sural nerve is blocked with a subcutaneous infiltration behind the lateral malleolus. A complete block of the foot requires 15 mL of solution; ropivacaine, levobupivacaine or racemic bupivacaine are most suitable for postoperative analgesia. It is probably advisable to avoid all five nerve blocks when the circulation to the foot is impaired although selective blockade is useful for vascular amputations. A single injection sciatic block is often therefore more appropriate as the sole technique for significant foot surgery.

Continuous Peripheral Nerve Block

These techniques are growing in popularity for both upper and lower limb blocks, as a method of prolonging postoperative analgesia and facilitating rehabilitation without the side-effects associated with opioids and with fewer unwanted cardiorespiratory complications and the urinary difficulties associated with epidural analgesia. Postoperative care is simplified and may usually be carried out in a general ward environment. The anaesthetist should be proficient in single-shot peripheral blocks – brachial plexus, femoral, lumbar plexus and sciatic – before advancing to catheter techniques. Some of the most popular techniques would include continuous femoral infusion following total knee replacement, sciatic infusion following below knee amputation, interscalene infusion following major shoulder surgery and infraclavicular infusions for elbow replacement or arthrolysis. Equipment has improved greatly in recent years and insulated Tuohy needles (see Fig. 24.1) and facet-tipped needles are available to assist catheter placement. Local

anaesthetic agents, usually levobupivacaine or ropivacaine, because of their reduced systemic toxicity,
are most commonly used in concentrations of 0.1–
0.25% although much lower concentrations of levobupivacaine have been used by infusion for femoral
nerve blockade following total knee arthroplasty in
an attempt to minimize motor blockade and promote
earlier and safer ambulation. Alternatively, local anaesthetic top-ups can be administered by intermittent
bolus either by appropriately trained staff, or as part
of a patient-controlled system with or without a background infusion.

Intra-Articular Techniques

Intra-articular and wound infiltration techniques, particularly following knee replacement surgery, are becoming increasingly popular as part of a multimodal
analgesic strategy aimed at minimizing side effects of
parenteral opioids, improving analgesia and promoting early ambulation by avoiding significant motor
block. Although at an early stage of development, it
appears to be cheap, simple and safe and has recently
been suggested to improve early outcomes and reduce
hospital stay. The technique for knee replacement surgery involves infiltrating the entire surgical site with
100–120 mL of dilute LA solution such as ropivacaine
0.1% and then leaving an intra-articular catheter for
subsequent top-ups.

SPECIAL SITUATIONS

Paediatric Techniques

Most nerve blocks used in adult practice are suitable for use in children, but because of the nature
of most paediatric surgery and the understandable
difficulties that may be experienced with patient co-
operation, only a limited, but increasing, number of
techniques are commonly used. Many of these are
used for postoperative analgesia and are performed
after induction of general anaesthesia; they should
only be performed by experienced anaesthetists.
Ultrasound-guidance may be useful for peripheral
blockade due to the variation in depth and position
of nerves and to avoid intraneural injection in the
anaesthetized child. The accurate placement of LA
can also significantly reduce the dosage required for
many blocks.

The disposition of local anaesthetic agents in children differs from that in adults. In children of less
than 1 year of age, and particularly in the neonate,
very high plasma concentrations of LA may ensue
after standard doses based on weight. In children
exceeding 1 year of age, plasma concentrations are
consistently lower than would be expected from
adult data.

Agents and doses for paediatric blocks are shown
in Table 24.7. Caudal block for subumbilical surgery
may be prolonged usefully in the postoperative period
by the addition of preservative-free S (+)-ketamine
0.5 mg kg^{-1}.

Topical Anaesthesia

This may be achieved with either EMLA (eutectic
mixture of local anaesthetics) or Ametop (tetracaine)
cream, held in place with an occlusive dressing. Both
provide anaesthesia of intact skin which is particularly
useful before venepuncture in children. EMLA cream

TABLE 24.7
Agents and Doses of Local Anaesthetics used in Paediatric Practice

Caudal Anaesthesia

0.25% bupivacaine	
0.5 mL kg^{-1}	Sacral block
1.0 mL kg^{-1}	Low thoracic block

0.19% bupivacaine (three parts bupivacaine 0.25%:one part saline)	
1.25 mL kg^{-1}	Mid-thoracic block

Penile Block

0.5% bupivacaine *plain*	
Body weight	*Dose*
2.5 kg	0.5 mL
10 kg	1.0 mL
20 kg	2.0 mL
40 kg	4.0 mL

Axillary Block

0.25% bupivacaine	
Body weight	*Dose*
10 kg	6 mL
20 kg	12 mL
30 kg	18 mL
40 kg	24 mL

must remain in contact with the skin for at least 1 h to be effective and may be left in place for up to 5h. Ametop is generally effective within 30–45 min, after which time the cream and occlusive dressing should be removed and the site marked.

FURTHER READING

Brull, R., McCartney, C.J.L., Chan, V.W.S., El-Beheiry, H., 2007. Neurological complications after regional anesthesia: contemporary estimates of risk. Anesth. Analg. 104, 965–974.

Chelly, J.E., Casati, A., Fanelli, G., 2001. Continuous peripheral nerve block techniques; an illustrated guide. Mosby, London.

Cook, T.M., Counsell, D., Wildsmith, J.A., 2009. Royal College of Anaesthetists Third National Audit Project 2009. Major complications of central neuraxial block: report on the Third National Audit Project of the Royal College of Anaesthetists. Br. J. Anaesth. 102, 179–190.

Ellis, H., Feldman, S., Harrop Griffiths, W., 2004. Anatomy for anaesthetists, eighth ed. Blackwell Publishing, Oxford.

Horlocker, T.T., Wedel, D.J., Rowlingson, J.C., et al., 2010. Regional anesthesia in the patient receiving antithrombotic or thrombolytic therapy: American Society of Regional Anesthesia and Pain Medicine Evidence-Based Guidelines (3rd edn). Reg. Anesth. Pain Med. 35, 64–101.

Marhofer, P., 2008. Ultrasound guidance for nerve blocks: principles and practical implementation. Oxford University Press, Oxford.

Neal, J.M., Gerancher, J.C., Hebl, J.R., et al., 2009. Upper extremity regional anesthesia: essentials of our current understanding 2008. Reg. Anesth. Pain Med. 34, 134–170.

Rigg, J.R.A., Jamrozik, K., Myles, P.S., et al., MASTER Anaesthesia Trial Study Group, 2002. Epidural anaesthesia and analgesia and outcome of major surgery: a randomised trial. Lancet 359, 1276–1282.

Wildsmith, J.A.W., Armitage, E.N., McClure, J.H., 2003. Principles and practice of regional anaesthesia, third ed. Churchill Livingstone, Edinburgh.

25

ANAESTHESIA FOR THE BARIATRIC PATIENT

INTRODUCTION

An estimated 63% of British adults are above normal weight; 26% of these are obese and around 2.5% are morbidly obese or higher. These figures are projected to rise, with nearly 50% of adults in the obese category by 2030. Britain's obesity rates are not as high as in some other developed and developing countries. The scale of the demographic changes and the associated multisystem comorbidity mean that the obese patient is likely to present across the spectrum of healthcare and not simply to the specialist in the bariatric field.

MEASURING OBESITY

A patient's mass varies with size and shape. Absolute mass can be important when considering factors such as equipment safety limits. However, it is more important to reference a person's expected mass to height. The most widely used technique is calculation of Body Mass Index (BMI).

$$BMI = \{mass(kg) / height^2(m^2)\}$$

BMI has limitations and may not be representative in certain ethnic groups, or in those of athletic build. It cannot describe the distribution of weight, nor discriminate the nature of the excess tissue. However, calculation of BMI, from two ubiquitous measurements, requires the minimum equipment and expertise. Hence, it is likely to remain the measure of choice as a shorthand to express obesity (Table 25.1, Fig. 25.1).

The limitations of BMI may account for some of the variability in obesity research. Other difficult

measures such as hip to abdominal girth ratio and skin fold thickness may be better at describing more dangerous patterns of fat distribution. Central obesity ('apple-shaped', predominantly male) carries more associated risks than peripheral obesity (gluteofemoral or 'pear-shaped') often seen in females.

OBESITY PATHOPHYSIOLOGY, COMORBIDITY AND THE METABOLIC SYNDROME

Obesity is a multi-system disorder. The aetiology is complex and has long been oversimplified. The network of contributing factors includes socio-economic, ethnic, societal, social and psychological. The underlying and acquired pathophysiology cross the traditional boundaries of medicine to include endocrine, cardiovascular, respiratory, GI tract, locomotor and psychiatric disorders.

TABLE 25.1	
WHO Obesity Classes by BMI (Other Nomenclatures Included)	
Category	*BMI (kg m⁻²)*
Underweight	<18.5
Normal	18.5–24.9
Overweight (pre-obese)	25–29.9
Obese Class I	30–34.9
Obese Class II (severe to morbid)	35–39.9
Obese Class III (morbid to super)	40+
(Super obesity)	45–50+

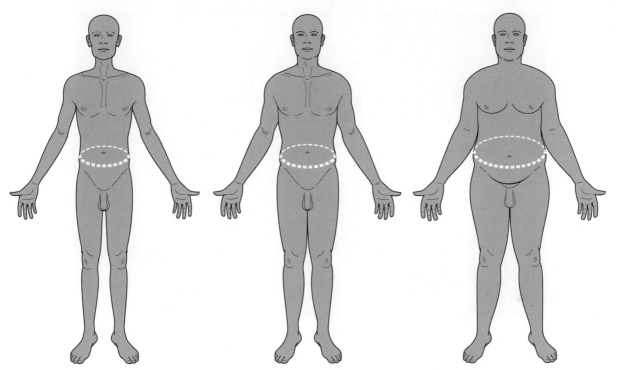

FIGURE 25.1 ■ Body habitus and silhouettes by category. Left to right – normal, overweight and obese.

The Adipose Organ

The traditional view of fat tissue has been as a metabolically inert triglyceride energy store, with insulation from physical and temperature stress as a useful secondary effect. However, fat tissue actually exists as a continuum. In particular, hepatic and intra-abdominal visceral fat tissue is much more active than previously thought. It is known to excrete over 20 mediators. The observed effects are pro-inflammatory (cytokines, adipsin), pro-coagulant (plasminogen activator inhibitor 1) and endocrine (leptin, resistin, adiponectin).

The underlying biochemical state is probably responsible for the common patterns of accelerated comorbidity observed in morbid obesity. The 'metabolic syndrome' is the name applied to the pattern of central obesity associated with at least two of the following:

- Hypertension
- Hyperglycaemia/insulin resistance
- Dyslipidaemia and atherogenesis
- Non-alcoholic fatty liver disease
- Pro-thrombotic and inflammatory state

COMORBIDITY AND ANAESTHETIC MANAGEMENT

Airway

The airway of the obese patient should be regarded with caution. Traditional teaching and audits of national practice predict that the management of the obese patient's airway is likely to be difficult. However, a number of studies have demonstrated that, in experienced hands, certain aspects of airway management, in particular tracheal intubation, may be no more difficult than normal.

Anatomy. In the obese patient, the airway undergoes progressive adipose infiltration. This occurs at all levels from the oropharynx through to the glottis and vocal cords. Adipose infiltration causes progressive narrowing and reduction in airway diameter, which may reduce by 50% or more from the physiological male normal of about 20 mm in the hypopharynx.

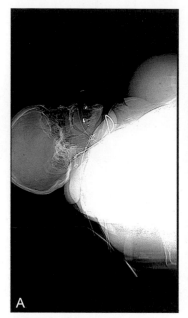
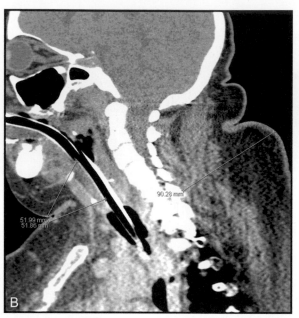

FIGURE 25.2 ■ **(A)** Lateral CT Scout (supine, female, BMI 59 kg m⁻²). Note neck position, 'free-floating' head and the potential for neck, chest and breast adipose tissue to hinder airway management. **(B)** Sagittal cross-section (BMI 55 kg m⁻²). Note depth of both anterior and posterior airway structures and the extent of airway soft tissue around the 7.5 tracheal tube.

The effect of adipose deposition on airway anatomy is not simply internal. External factors also need to be considered. The presence of a thoracic 'hump' can significantly affect supine posture, resulting in extension of the neck and flexion at the atlanto-occipital (AO) joint. Moreover, posterior adipose deposition between the occiput running inferior to the spine of T1, can hinder atlanto-occipital extension. Hence, in an unsupported supine position, the airway of the obese patient can easily become the opposite of ideal; neck extension and fixed AO flexion.

Careful positioning is key to successful management of the bariatric airway. This can be achieved either using specifically designed equipment, or special modifications to normal equipment. In urgent situations a number of aids to achieving the position have been suggested including multiple towels, fluid bags or inflatables. The key is to ensure true neck flexion and AO extension. This is best achieved by ensuring that the patient posture, in particular neck/head position is viewed from the side (Fig. 25.2A and B).

Airway Adjuncts. A range of products to assist in the management of difficult airways exists. Simple adjuncts such as oral and nasopharyngeal airways, and the use of CPAP can help to splint the airway open. Laryngeal mask airway products retain their role in airway salvage. Their routine use in the morbidly obese patient remains controversial, focusing on concerns around pulmonary aspiration and optimization of pulmonary function.

Standard laryngoscopes and blades remain the default equipment for tracheal intubation, particularly when combined with careful positioning. Video devices may help if additional risk factors exist. Many are designed with short-handled bodies, useful if a large chest and fixed neck posture limit space.

Respiratory Pathophysiology

Anatomy

Lung size is predicted by height or ideal body mass, rather than gross weight. The lung fields of obese patients often look small when assessed by chest radiography (Fig. 25.3). This is an artefact of accommodating the patient on the chest X-ray. Total lung capacity is usually nearly normal and it is functional spirometry which reveals the associated pathology (Fig. 25.4).

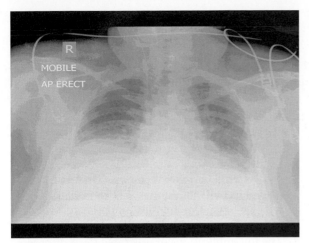

FIGURE 25.3 ■ Anteroposterior chest X-ray of a morbidly obese patient.

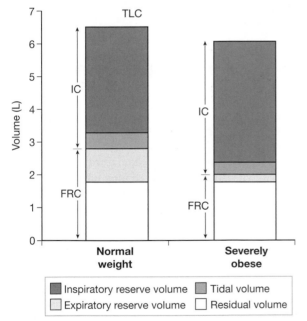

FIGURE 25.4 ■ Spirometric changes with obesity. Note the significant reduction in FRC. TLC, total lung capacity; IC, inspiratory capacity; FRC, functional residual capacity.

In obesity, there is heavy adipose infiltration of the chest wall and breast tissue, which leads to decreased chest wall compliance and damping of natural recoil expansion of the chest wall. This is further exacerbated by abdominal wall infiltration and a raised intra-abdominal pressure. Additionally, there is peribronchial

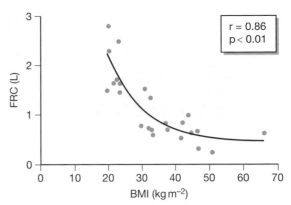

FIGURE 25.5 ■ Changes in functional residual capacity (FRC) with increasing body mass index (BMI). *(Adapted from Pelosi et al (1998).)*

parenchymal fat infiltration. Respiratory muscles demonstrate fat infiltration and the effect of inflammatory mediators. Diminished muscle power and respiratory endurance result.

Pathophysiology

Total lung capacity and vital capacity reduce in a gentle, linear manner with rising weight. The spirometric observations reflect the change in the balance between chest wall and parenchymal forces with rising obesity.

- Functional residual capacity decreases (Fig. 25.5) and closing volume increases. Resulting atelectatic shunt reduces PaO_2. At higher levels of morbid obesity, tidal ventilation may impinge on closing volume even in the standing position.
- FEV_1 decreases, although the FEV_1/FVC ratio is often preserved, particularly with central obesity patterns.
- Work of breathing increases by 70% from low levels of obesity to an energy cost 300% higher in complicated, high BMI states. The energy cost of maintaining adequate minute ventilation is mitigated by a reduction in tidal volume, resulting in rapid, shallow breathing at rest.

The elastic load increases (reduced static compliance; Fig. 25.6). This is a reflection of both the reduced elastance of chest wall and parenchymal tissue and tidal ventilation occurring at lower lung volumes. Dynamic compliance (i.e. resistance to gas movement)

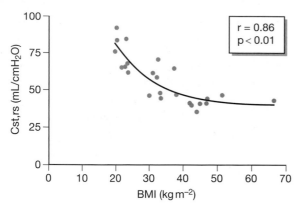

FIGURE 25.6 ▪ Changes in static respiratory system compliance (Cst,rs) with increasing body mass index (BMI). *(Adapted from Pelosi et al (1998).)*

also falls. In the lower airway, there is narrowing of the small conducting airways. This may be due to multiple factors:

- External compression from parenchymal fat deposition
- A reduction in the part of the lung volume at which tidal breathing occurs.
- Chronic inflammatory changes and increased smooth muscle reactivity/bronchospasm.

CLINICAL RESPIRATORY COMORBIDITY

Asthma

About 5% of the general population are diagnosed as asthmatic. Asthmatic symptoms such as wheezing, dyspnoea and reduced exercise capacity are reported by around 25% of the obese population; however, bronchodilator reversibility may not be found. Contradictions in the epidemiological data linking obesity and asthma may relate to exacerbating comorbidities in obesity such as gastro-oesophageal reflux or the interplay of the proinflammatory and endocrine mediators previously described.

Sleep-Disordered Breathing

Sleep-disordered breathing describes the spectrum of obstructive sleep apnoea, central sleep apnoea, obesity hypoventilation syndrome and pathological patterns of nocturnal ventilation.

Obstructive sleep apnoea can be diagnosed in 4% of the general population. However, 60% of these are in patients with a BMI $>30 \, kg \, m^{-2}$. Weight loss of a magnitude such as achieved with weight loss surgery is associated with symptomatic reduction or resolution in approximately 75% of patients. Clinical screening tools such as the self-assessed Epworth (sleepiness) score and the STOP–BANG criteria are helpful to target more specific investigations such as sleeping oximetry or full flow and effort-sensitive sleep studies.

Sleep-disordered breathing is associated with a number of comorbid conditions and their sequelae. These include systemic hypertension, pulmonary hypertension and the cardiovascular consequences of each.

The full implications of untreated sleep-disordered breathing on the perioperative patient are unresolved. Presentation as patients who display significant sensitivity to ventilatory depressants is well recognized. Prolonged apnoea/hypoventilation and narcolepsy can be found after relatively small doses of opioid.

ANAESTHETIC MANAGEMENT POINTS

All respiratory and sleep-related comorbidities should be identified, investigated and treated. At induction of anaesthesia, the use of the reverse Trendelenburg (head-up) or tipped beach chair positions maximize spontaneous and anaesthetized lung function. FRC on induction of anaesthesia can reduce by up to 50%.

Ventilation volumes should be calculated from ideal body weight. Recruitment manoeuvres and PEEP of 10 cmH$_2$O maximize lung function and minimize shunt. Pneumoperitoneum diminishes the benefit of postural changes.

Postoperatively, balanced analgesia, rapid mobilization, incentive spirometry and physiotherapy may help to avoid respiratory morbidity.

CARDIOVASCULAR PATHOPHYSIOLOGY

In common with other organs, cardiovascular changes in obesity are part of a continuum. The nature and extent of the pathophysiology relate to the extent and duration of being overweight and also the sequential effects of associated comorbid processes in other organs.

Oxygen Demand and Delivery

Oxygen demand increases in proportion to the increase in fat-free mass (FFM) rather than in relation to the patient's BMI. FFM increases with total body weight (TBW), but with a decreasing curve gradient, to a ceiling of approximately 1 kg per centimetre of height.

Blood volume describes an inverse hyperbolic relationship with increasing BMI. The blood volume:TBW ratio decreases from around $70\,mL\,kg^{-1}$ to $40\,ml\,kg^{-1}$ at a BMI of $70\,kg\,m^{-2}$.

Cardiac output increases with BMI in proportion to the square root of the ratio between actual BMI and ideal BMI. The increase is linear in relation to body surface area and fat-free mass gain. Indexed to adipose tissue mass, fat perfusion decreases as BMI increases. This decrease highlights the relatively poor vascular supply to peripheral adipose tissue ($<150\,mL\,kg^{-1}\,min^{-1}$). Early stage increases in cardiac output appear to be achieved by blood volume-related preload increases in stroke volume, mediated by β-natriuretic peptide inhibition and aldosterone. The contribution of increased heart rate remains relatively minor.

Cardiac Pathophysiology

The heart of the obese patient may exhibit a number of pathological changes (Fig. 25.7). These may be related to either the primary obesity or associated comorbidity, e.g. hypertension, diabetes, hyperlipidaemia or sleep apnoea.

Echocardiographic evidence suggests that three pathological patterns predominate in obesity. Concentric remodelling (LV wall thickening short of hypertrophy), concentric hypertrophy (hypertrophy with increased relative wall thickness) and eccentric dilated hypertrophy (thickened hypertrophic LV wall, but reduced wall:cavity ratio secondary to dilatation) occur. The practical application of these states is the recognition of the early existence of reduced ventricular wall compliance and ventricular diastolic dysfunction. As compensatory cardiac dilatation occurs, there is a progressive reduction in systolic contractility. The observed paradox of these states is discussed below.

Electrophysiology

A number of ECG changes may be recorded in obese patients. These may be related to habitus or pathology.

- Atrial fibrillation is the commonest arrhythmia associated with obesity and the prevalence increases exponentially with BMI.
- Voltage magnitudes vary and QRS complex size is not reliable for diagnosis.
- Conduction axis is frequently left-shifted, but this may be caused by physical displacement of the heart from the normal position and rotation.

Conduction anomalies are relatively common and may relate either to fatty infiltration and fibrosis of the conduction system or underlying coronary artery disease. PR and QRS prolongation, through fascicle block to bundle branch block, are seen and may be benign. QTc prolongation appears to have a negative prognostic value.

Right Ventricular Pathophysiology

Right ventricular dysfunction is associated in particular with sleep-disordered breathing. The combined effects of chronic pulmonary hypertension (nocturnal hypoxaemia), with the effects of chronic volume overload (obesity) and progressive left ventricular changes lead to right-sided dilatation, systolic and diastolic dysfunction and failure.

VASCULAR DISEASE

Arterial disease is associated with both primary obesity and its comorbid diseases (hyperlipidaemia, diabetes mellitus, etc.). Some trials have suggested that there may be an absolute risk increase in coronary arterial disease of 50% between normal and overweight individuals, rising to a hazard ratio of >2.5 in the severely morbidly obese. However, confusingly, lower cardiac mortality rates are reported in the mildly obese. The contradiction may lie partly in the limitations of BMI as a measure of the dangerous central obesity pattern. For example, controlled for comorbid conditions, peripheral vascular disease shows no correlation with BMI. However, obesity expressed as waist circumference, waist:hip ratio or waist:thigh ratio has a raised vascular risk profile. This unresolved effect is known as the obesity paradox. This is the term given to the lower mortality observed in obese patients in a number of conditions. These include critical illness, congestive cardiac failure and eccentric compared to concentric cardiac hypertrophy.

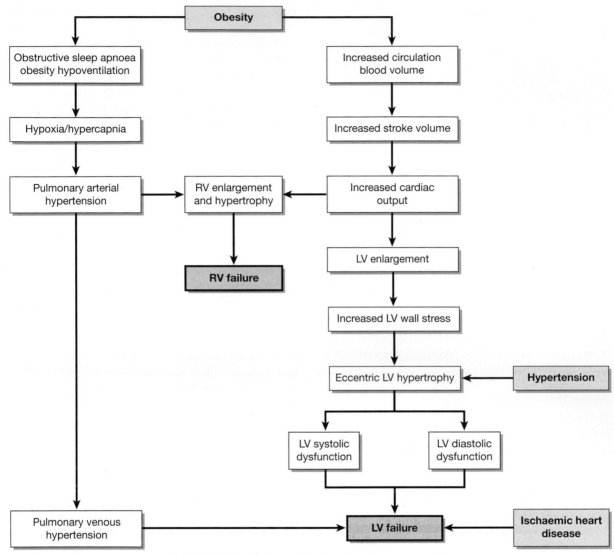

FIGURE 25.7 ■ Effects of obesity-related cardiomyopathy.

LIVER

Adipose tissue in the liver is highly metabolic endocrine and paracrine tissue. There is a close relationship between liver fat content and insulin resistance. In early obesity, insulin sensitivity returns with weight loss. Weight loss of 8% reduces liver fat content by 80%. Non-alcoholic steatohepatitis (NASH) or higher grades of non-alcoholic fatty liver disease (NAFLD) appear to uniformly precede the development of type 2 diabetes. Insulin resistance contributes to

dyslipidaemia, hyperglycaemia and eventual pancreatic islet cell burn-out. The available data suggests that 20% of patients with NASH will progress to cirrhotic liver disease.

NAFLD alone, or as part of the metabolic syndrome (see above) is associated with accelerated atherogenesis, ischaemic heart disease and raised cardiovascular mortality.

Intra-abdominal pressure is raised in obesity and increases with BMI. Resting pressure is usually around twice normal, at 10 mmHg (Fig. 25.8). During

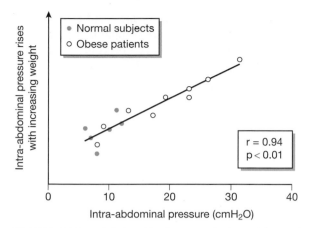

FIGURE 25.8 ■ Relationship between body weight and intra-abdominal pressure. *(Adapted from Pelosi et al (1999).)*

TABLE 25.2	
Factors Which Affect the Pharmacokinetic and Pharmacodynamic Properties of Drugs in Obesity	
Kinetic Property	*Effect of Increasing Obesity*
Blood volume and cardiac output	Increase
Adipose and lean body mass	Increase
Hepatic blood flow and glucuronidation rate	Increase
GFR and renal excretion	Increase
Cytochrome P450 isoenzymes	Variable
Renal tubular reabsorption	Decrease

laparoscopic procedures, the pneumoperitoneal pressure may need to be high to allow adequate vision. Care should be taken because pressures of 15 mmHg or higher have been shown to significantly reduce femoral vein, gut, visceral and portal blood flows. Measures such as positioning and adequate relaxation should be addressed first.

Gastro-Oesophageal Reflux

Meta-analysis supports the traditional view that increasingly obese patients are at higher risk of gastro-oesophageal reflux. The direct causal nature of the relationship is ill-defined. However, reported symptoms are present 2–3 times more frequently in the obese compared to the general population. Detrimental factors such as higher gradient pressures, residual volumes and dysmotility may outweigh factors such as enhanced gastric emptying.

PHARMACOLOGY

Patients who are obese may display altered pharmacokinetics and pharmacodynamics (Table 25.2). These factors have clinical relevance. The application of basic concepts such as drug solubility, compartment volumes, transportation and metabolism may be helpful. However, the interactions are complex and reference to published data should be made. For these reasons, controversy remains and particular care should be taken with the use of target controlled infusion algorithms developed for patients of normal weight.

Intravenous Induction Agents

Blood volume, cardiac output and vessel-rich tissue (approximates to fat-free mass/lean body mass) are enlarged in the obese. A bolus of intravenous induction agent based on ideal body weight is therefore likely to exhibit lower peak plasma concentration and a faster redistributive decay, i.e. less likely to reach effective anaesthetic brain tissue concentrations and have effect for a shorter duration. For this reason, in general, the dose of an intravenous induction agent in the obese should be calculated allowing for the increases in cardiac output and lean body mass.

Inhalational Agents

There are a number of theoretical concerns regarding the use of inhalational agents. Decreased FRC, increased cardiac output, lipid solubility and adipose mass might be predicted to affect both wash-in and wash-out curves. However, these do not appear to translate into clinical problems. A majority of bariatric practitioners have a preference for lower lipid solubility agents such as desflurane and sevoflurane. However, the 63% alveolus:fat equilibrium times are 22 h for desflurane and 35 h for isoflurane. This would suggest that, in routine use, the build-up of an adipose store has little clinical relevance.

Muscle Relaxants

Suxamethonium. Suxamethonium has traditionally been the drug of choice for facilitating tracheal intubation in the obese. This has largely been driven by concerns about the need for rapid sequence induction, the potential for difficult intubation and the difficulty of managing the airway with a face mask and airway adjuncts. Morbidly obese patients have been shown to have increased pseudocholinesterase activity and a larger immediate distribution volume. Dosing based on $1\,mg\,kg^{-1}$ total body weight has been demonstrated to give better intubating conditions than dosing by ideal body weight or lean body weight, but at the expense of approximately 90 additional seconds before return of spontaneous breathing.

Non-Depolarizing Agents. The quaternary ammonium group makes non-depolarizing relaxants highly ionized and generally poorly lipophilic. This limits their distribution to extracellular fluid. Dosing based on total body weight uniformly leads to a prolonged duration of action. Consensus suggests that dosing on the basis of ideal body weight is predictable and acceptable, although some authorities suggest that correction for body surface area may be more precise.

Reversal Agents. Limited data exists for the most appropriate dose of neostigmine in the morbidly obese. Dosing studies suggest that if a suboptimal ceiling effect is observed with neostigmine, full twitch height recovery from this point in the morbidly obese patient is prolonged.

Sugammadex. The cyclodextrin sugammadex rapidly and selectively binds rocuronium (and vecuronium to a lesser extent) to form inactive complexes. Consequently, there is an agent-specific alternative to neostigmine and, because of the speed of the reversal, the possibility for a two-agent alternative to suxamethonium for rapid sequence induction. Dosing of sugammadex by total body weight is currently advised in all patients. However, some emerging data suggests that a dose based on a modification of lean body mass may be effective.

BARIATRIC OPERATIONS

Control of weight, appetite and calorific balance is complex, multisystem and multifactorial. Dietary measures alone are often an ineffective longer term solution and lead to weight oscillation. Weight-loss surgery encompasses a number of techniques. Some simply restrict the passage of food and create a feeling of gastric fullness; more complicated procedures have dramatic hormonal effects on comorbidity such as diabetes. These latter procedures may be referred to as metabolic surgery.

Gastric Banding

Gastric banding is a restrictive technique. The band restricts the passage of food moving from the oesophagogastric junction. This causes early dilation and stretch of the junction. Usually, this occurs only when the stomach is absolutely full. The stretching of this area sends inhibitory signals to the thalamic satiety centre, inhibiting appetite.

A tract is formed by blunt dissection around the back of the top of the stomach and an inflatable silicone strip is inserted, and fixed to form a ring around the fundus. A port site is inserted underneath the skin and attached to the band by tube. By adjusting the degree of inflation of the band with saline, delivered transcutaneously to the port site, the degree of restriction of eating and the speed of weight loss can be controlled effectively. The ability to adjust the band means that the technique is more effective than, and has therefore replaced, techniques such as vertically banded gastroplasty.

Sleeve Gastrectomy

Sleeve gastrectomy achieves approximately 50% excess weight loss. The operation involves surgical removal of the greater curve of the stomach, including the fundus. The effect on appetite of stretch of the oesophagogastric junction at low volumes is similar to that of banding. However, there is a further hormonal effect. The removal of the fundus causes a reduction in the level of ghrelin production. Ghrelin is a positive orexigenic hormone which ultimately acts via YR_1 receptors on the arcuate nucleus. The lack of ghrelin shifts the arcuate signal balance towards anorexia and increased metabolism.

Malabsorbtive Procedures

Many procedure variations exist, having been refined over time. In this type of surgery, a restrictive pouch is formed from the stomach (approx. 4 or 5 mouthfuls of food) and food is diverted away from the pancreas, biliary tree and duodenum, mixing with the digestive juices only at a distal small bowel anastomosis forming a short (approx. 100 cm) common limb before the colon. The commonest of these procedures is now probably the roux-en-Y gastric bypass.

Improvement and resolution of comorbid conditions such as type II diabetes and hypertension occur much faster and more frequently than would simply occur with the expected 70% excess weight loss.

POSTOPERATIVE CARE OF THE OBESITY SURGERY PATIENT

It has proved difficult to establish exactly how many bariatric weight loss operations are carried out each year in the UK. It is likely that this figure is around 6000 per year. Consequently, it is increasingly likely that anaesthetic practice will encompass those who have had previous surgery.

Presentations associated with the surgical procedure include the following.

- Band slippage, band erosion, band infection
- Perforation (early and late)
- Fistula formation
- Obstruction herniation (bypass)

Weight Loss and Malnutrition

Patients who undergo weight-loss surgery submit to undergo life-long follow-up. They will receive continuing dietetic advice and dietary supplementation, as required. Patients who are outside follow-up programmes are at higher risk of failed weight loss, and dietary difficulty and complications.

To achieve sustainable weight loss after bariatric surgery, it should be achieved gradually, over a period of six months to around two years. Rates of weight loss in excess of this may give a higher risk of failure.

When dealing with a patient who has undergone bariatric surgery, the following points should be considered.

- A careful history should be taken, including obtaining information about the operating centre, follow-up arrangements and weight history.
- It is prudent to consult an expert centre for advice. Consider band deflation and be aware of post-surgery anatomical alterations.
- Care should be taken in the use of modified-release medications. Mechanisms differ and may be severely affected in patients who have undergone bariatric surgery.

FURTHER READING

Alvarez, A., Brodsky, J.B., Lemmens, H.J.M., Morton, J.M. (Eds.), 2010. Morbid obesity. Cambridge University Press, Cambridge.

Ortiz, V.E., Wiener-Kronish, J. (Eds.), 2010. Perioperative anaesthetic care of the obese patient. Informa Healthcare.

Pelosi, P., Croci, M., Ravagnan, I., et al., 1998. The effects of body mass on lung volumes, respiratory mechanics, and gas exchange during general anesthesia. Anesth. Analg. 87, 654–660.

26

DAY-CASE ANAESTHESIA

■ ■ ■ ■ ■ ■ ■ ■ ■ ■ ■ ■ ■

A day-case patient is one who is admitted for investigation or operation on a planned non-resident basis. Patients are usually discharged from the hospital or unit later on the day of the procedure. The procedure may require general, regional or local anaesthesia, sedative techniques or a combination of these.

The NHS plan predicts that 75% of all elective operations will be carried out as day cases. According to the British Association of Day Surgery (BADS), patients support day surgery because it provides timely treatment, less risk of cancellation, a lower incidence of hospital-acquired infection and an earlier return to normal activities. Procedures commonly selected for day-case care are those which take <60 min to complete and which do not cause severe haemorrhage or produce excessive amounts of postoperative pain (Table 26.1). Increasingly complex cases are now performed as day-case procedures, including laparoscopic cholecystectomy and tonsillectomy. By extending day surgery opening hours and using staggered admission times, patients who would normally require hospital admission may be treated as day cases. The British Association of Day Surgery (BADS) publishes guidelines and protocols for the management of specific issues: for example, day surgery for patients with diabetes. BADS has also published a list of 25 procedures which should normally be undertaken as day cases. The NHS Modernisation Agency audited current day surgery rates for these procedures and set target rates for individual hospitals.

Achievement of a pain-free ambulant patient requires skilful patient selection and experienced anaesthetists and surgeons working within a day surgery unit. Large-scale reports have indicated that day surgery represents a safe, cost-effective and efficient practice. Advantages include decreased risks of nosocomial infection and deep venous thrombosis, less social disruption to patients and their families and minimal need for inpatient hospital resources. Therefore we now face the challenge of providing faster recovery, more rapid discharge and better pain relief for these patients.

PATIENT SELECTION

The selection of patients for day-case surgery is of vital importance if maximum use is to be made of the resources in the day-case unit and also to facilitate smooth running of the unit. The selection of patients must take into account two separate aspects: firstly, the patient's state of health, and secondly, his or her social circumstances. Patients should normally be ASA I or II, or medically stable ASA III. Recent reviews have shown that patients with a body mass index of >35 kg m^{-2} do not have an increase in unplanned admission rates or postoperative complications. The Association of Anaesthetists of Great Britain and Ireland has recommended that obese patients should not be excluded from day surgery based on their BMI measurement alone. There is no evidence of significant morbidity in the immediate postoperative period when treating morbidly obese patients as day-cases. Although an increased risk of adverse events occurring intraoperatively and in the immediate recovery period in obese patients has been reported, these have not been shown to increase the incidence of unplanned admission significantly.

TABLE 26.1
A Selection of Surgical Procedures Commonly Undertaken as Day Cases

Gynaecology

Dilatation & curettage, laparoscopy, vaginal termination of pregnancy, colposcopy, hysteroscopy

Plastic Surgery

Dupuytren's contracture release, removal of small skin lesions, nerve decompression

Ophthalmology

Strabismus correction, cataract surgery, lacrimal duct probing, examination under anaesthesia

ENT

Adenoidectomy, tonsillectomy, myringotomy, insertion of grommets, removal of foreign body, polyp removal, submucous resection

Urology

Cystoscopy, circumcision, vasectomy, transurethral bladder resection

Orthopaedics

Arthroscopies, carpal tunnel release, ganglion removal, bunion operation, removal of metalwork

General Surgery

Breast lumps, herniae, varicose veins, endoscopy, laparoscopic cholecystectomy, haemorrhoidectomy, anal fissure dilatation

Paediatrics

Circumcision, orchidopexy, squint, dental extractions

TABLE 26.2
Guidelines for Patient Selection for Day-Case Surgery Under General Anaesthesia

ASA 1 or 2 and medically stable ASA 3
Age: >52 weeks post-conceptual age
Weight: body mass index=weight/height^2 (kg m^{-2})
　≤35: acceptable
　>35: discuss with anaesthetic department
Generally healthy, i.e. can climb two flights of stairs

Exclusions

Cardiovascular
　MI/TIA/CVA within 6 months
　Hypertension: persistent diastolic pressure >110 mmHg
　Unstable angina
　Arrhythmias
　Heart failure
　Poor exercise tolerance
　Symptomatic valve disease
Respiratory
　Acute respiratory tract infection
　Asthma requiring regular β_2-agonists or steroids
Metabolic
　Alcoholism /narcotic addiction
　Insulin-dependent diabetes
　Renal failure
　Liver disease
Neurological/musculoskeletal
　Severe arthritis of jaw or neck
　Cervical spondylosis/ankylosing spondylitis
　Myopathies/muscular dystrophies/ myasthenia gravis
　Advanced multiple sclerosis
　Epilepsy >3 fits per year
Drugs
　Steroids
　Monoamine oxidase inhibitors
　Anticoagulants
　Antiarrhythmics
　Insulin

Evidence has shown that many elderly patients cope better at home. Careful preoperative assessment should highlight patients who will require an extended time in hospital. Elderly patients are more likely to have comorbidities and these patients should be assessed according to their physiological rather than their chronological age. Careful medical and social preoperative assessment is required to help elderly patients to benefit from shorter hospital stays with less risk of postoperative confusion. The patient should stay a minimum of a 1-h drive from the hospital on the night following surgery and they should have an adult escort available for the first 24 h. An example of guidelines used for patient selection for day-case anaesthesia is shown in Table 26.2.

The selection of patients for day-case surgery is made at the time of outpatient consultation and routine measurement of pulse rate and blood pressure, urine analysis and other relevant investigations (e.g. ECG, full blood count and sickle cell testing) are performed; performance of these routine tests minimizes the number of problems when patients are admitted on the day of surgery. A standardized patient health/anaesthesia questionnaire and preliminary nurse assessment with appropriate referral for anaesthetic consultation minimize difficulties encountered on the day of surgery. Pre-assessment clinics provide an opportunity to educate patients and have been shown to reduce both cancellations by patients and unnecessary preoperative investigations. Children should be treated as day cases if possible and children scheduled for day-case procedures should be healthy and usually ASA I or II. Premature babies who have not reached 52 weeks post-conceptual age should not be considered for day-case surgery because of the risk of postoperative apnoea, and special consideration should be given to babies who have been receiving ventilatory support. The parent must be able to cope with the pre-procedure instructions and with the care of the child following treatment. The parent must agree to day treatment and be available to stay throughout the day although there may be exceptions for older children who attend regularly. Home facilities and travelling conditions should be taken into account. Following a general anaesthetic, the use of public transport is inappropriate.

Following selection of a patient for day-case surgery, the nature of the operation and the routine of management are explained fully to the patient and the consent form may be signed. Many units issue the patient with explanatory leaflets, CDs/DVDs or even podcasts explaining the procedure. A date for surgery can then be arranged and registration completed, as for an in-patient admission. It is wise to book any pathological or radiological investigations which are required well in advance of the day of admission.

The patient should be given written instructions detailing the date and time of attendance at the day unit, with written instructions relating to preoperative starvation and the patient's regular medication, e.g. antihypertensives, should be taken as usual but oral hypoglycaemics must be omitted on the morning of surgery. These instructions should be written clearly in plain English (or another appropriate language). The patient is usually advised not to eat anything from midnight for a morning operating list.

Recent clinical studies suggest that overnight fasting may not be required in adults or children. Pulmonary aspiration occurs usually in emergency abdominal and obstetric procedures where there may be complicating factors such as recent food and fluid intake, trauma or administration of opioid analgesics. These factors do not normally apply to healthy elective day-case patients. The universal order of nil by mouth from midnight should apply only to solids. Clear fluids should be allowed until 3 h before the scheduled time of surgery. The effect of giving patients 150 mL of clear fluid 2 h before general anaesthesia for termination of pregnancy has been studied; the results showed that clear fluids do not increase the incidence of regurgitation or vomiting during anaesthesia and the postoperative period and that preoperative thirst was decreased in the clear fluid group. It is advisable to ask patients who smoke to refrain from smoking for 4–6 weeks before the operation. Patients should be asked to bring with them all tablets and medicines which they take regularly.

ORGANIZATION OF THE DAY-CASE UNIT

Types Of Unit

In order to help improve the number of day-case operations, BADS has produced a directory of 160 procedures. Attached to each of these procedures are four possible management options.

- Procedure room; an operation which can be performed in a suitable clean environment outside the operating theatre.
- Day surgery; traditional day surgery.
- 23-h stay; patient admitted and discharged within 24 h.
- Under 72-h stay; patient admitted and discharged within 72 h.

There are three common types of day-case unit.

- A unit within a hospital complex, but with separate staff, wards and operating theatre; this is functionally the most flexible type as it may be adapted to the varying requirements of day-case patients.
- A unit with a separate ward, but using the hospital's main operating theatre complex.
- Outside the UK, it is common for a separate centre to have its own operating theatres and wards remote from a conventional hospital. This type of unit has now been introduced into the UK.

Ideally, day surgical units should not be freestanding but situated on in-patient hospital sites. The ward area should be close to the operating theatre to reduce portering time, particularly when short operations are performed. This arrangement also enables parents to accompany their children to the anaesthetic room if this is desirable.

Preferably, the unit should be near a car park and well signposted to facilitate the prompt arrival of patients and to avoid unnecessary delays.

Facilities Available

The accommodation should ideally include the following.

- *An admission area,* which includes reception, treatment and examination rooms, a nurses' station, lavatories, a playroom and a discharge area.
- *An anaesthetic room,* fully equipped and large enough to allow free access around the patient's trolley to permit the use of local or general anaesthesia. There should be good lighting, scavenging, piped gases and suction equipment, anaesthetic machine and monitoring equipment. The hazards and risks of general anaesthesia for day surgery are no less than those associated with elective in-patient surgery; indeed, in some respects they may be greater and the facilities provided must be at least comparable.
- *An operating theatre,* which should be of the same specification as the in-patient equivalent. A good operating light, air conditioning and piped services are required, in addition to the usual scrub-up and autoclave facilities. There is always the possibility of a minor operation developing unexpectedly into a major operation and this demands that the theatre is equipped to deal with that eventuality.
- *A fully equipped recovery room,* which must always be equipped and staffed for the safe recovery of patients following general anaesthesia. Piped gas supplies and resuscitation equipment are mandatory and the full range of monitoring and ventilation equipment must be readily available.

Other facilities which should be available include office space, an equipment store, staff changing and locker rooms, a staff room, a pantry to make drinks and lavatories for patients, parents and staff.

Admission

Patients should be admitted to the day ward in adequate time for history-taking and examination. The results of any investigation requested as an outpatient should be available and noted. Patients should receive an identity bracelet and their name should be entered into the nursing record. The surgeon should ensure that the indication for surgery is still present, e.g. presence or absence of lumps to be removed, because it may be several weeks since the clinic appointment. The consent form should be signed if not already done during the outpatient appointment, and the operation site clearly marked.

Venous thromboembolism prophylaxis should be provided according to local hospital policy based on the risk factors which are present. It is also important that careful attention is paid to WHO checklists and procedures, to maximize patient safety in the day-case environment.

A pregnancy test in women of fertile age may need to be performed if there is any risk of pregnancy. Staggering patient admissions decreases waiting times and improves the efficiency of the unit. Using dedicated paediatric day-case lists ensures an appropriate staffing mix for these patients. The use of separate operating lists for local anaesthesia and general anaesthesia may improve throughput, as does the introduction of day-surgery operating trolleys.

ANAESTHESIA

Premedication

Most anaesthetists do not routinely prescribe premedication for day-case surgery because it is usually unnecessary and for fear of delaying recovery and discharge. Premedicant drugs that may be used if required include the following.

Benzodiazepines

It is thought that sedative premedication may prolong the recovery time and delay the patient's discharge from hospital. However, a double-blind study of temazepam premedication for day surgery found effective anxiolysis in the patients who received temazepam 10 or 20 mg; there was no delay in recovery times as measured by memory test cards and all patients were discharged from the day unit within 3 h after administration of general anaesthesia. Oral midazolam has been used as a premedicant in day surgery, but it was found that it produced a delay in immediate and late recovery compared with temazepam.

Antiemetics

If patients are at high risk of postoperative nausea and vomiting (PONV), antiemetics may be administered orally before operation, or via the intravenous or rectal routes perioperatively. Apfel et al (2002) developed a simplified PONV risk score and suggested the use of prophylactic antiemetics for any patient with two or more of the following: female gender; past history of motion sickness or PONV; non-smoker; and use of postoperative opioids. However, risk scores such as this have no more than a 70% chance of predicting PONV.

Antacids

If there is a risk of acid reflux, H_2-antagonists are commonly prescribed as a premedication in day surgery.

Analgesics

Oral non-steroidal anti-inflammatory drugs (NSAIDs) and paracetamol may be given preoperatively. Some day-case units administer paracetamol routinely to all patients unless there are specific contraindications. Oral COX II inhibitors have better gastrointestinal side-effect profiles than NSAIDs and less antiplatelet effects. Dermal application of tetracaine (amethocaine) over a vein has a useful role preoperatively for children and nervous adults or those with a needle phobia because it acts within 20 min and does not cause local vasoconstriction.

General and Regional Anaesthesia

General, local or regional anaesthesia may be administered safely to day-case patients. The choice of technique should be determined by surgical requirements, anaesthetic considerations and the patient's physical status and preference.

General Anaesthesia

The choice of induction and maintenance agent depends upon the requirements of the patient and the preferences of the anaesthetist. The anaesthetic induction agent used in day-case anaesthesia should ensure a smooth induction and good immediate recovery with minimal postoperative sequelae and a rapid return to street fitness.

Propofol is the induction agent used routinely in day-case anaesthesia. One of its main advantages is the ease and rapidity with which patients recover. Patients are clear-headed and have a low incidence of PONV. The inhalational agent sevoflurane may be used for induction of anaesthesia. It is non-irritant to the airways and has the advantages of rapid induction in both children and adults, minimal cardiovascular side-effects and a rapid recovery profile. However, sevoflurane causes more PONV than propofol.

Both sevoflurane and desflurane have been marketed as ideal agents for maintenance of anaesthesia for day-case surgery, with favourable recovery profiles and more rapid awakening than those associated with isoflurane. However, both sevoflurane and desflurane have been associated with emergence delirium because of rapid awakening, especially in children. In addition, desflurane is less suitable for spontaneously breathing subjects because it is more irritant to the airways than either sevoflurane or isoflurane. The use of nitrous oxide for maintenance of anaesthesia has been shown to increase the risk of PONV; however, its use does reduce the requirements for volatile agents and may reduce the risk of intraoperative awareness. Target-controlled infusion (TCI) of propofol with or without an infusion of the ultra-rapid-acting opioid remifentanil minimizes the risk of PONV and results in short recovery times; however, the analgesic effect of remifentanil is very short and other analgesic drugs must be administered to deal with analgesia for anticipated postoperative pain.

A clear airway is a fundamental requirement of safe anaesthesia. The laryngeal mask airway (LMA) is used widely, avoids the need for tracheal intubation and extubation, and thus improves turnaround time between cases. Many anaesthetists use the LMA for procedures which were thought formerly to need tracheal intubation, such as tonsillectomy or laparoscopy. The ProSeal LMA provides a higher pressure seal than a conventional LMA and has an internal lumen which aids the escape of gastric contents if necessary. There is now a wide choice of alternative supraglottic airway devices available. However, a rapid-sequence induction technique with tracheal intubation is still required for patients identified as being at risk of regurgitation and aspiration of gastric fluid; this is not a contraindication to day surgery.

The choice of muscle relaxant depends on the anticipated duration of surgery. Succinylcholine is associated with muscle pains, especially in ambulant patients, and for all but the shortest procedures is not ideal in the day-case setting (except when rapid-sequence induction is required). Of the non-depolarizing muscle relaxants (NDMRs) currently available, atracurium and vecuronium have relatively short durations of action when used in appropriate doses and are readily antagonized after 15–30 min. Mivacurium has an even shorter duration of action because it undergoes rapid hydrolysis by plasma cholinesterase, but a small number of patients may suffer prolonged muscle paralysis following the use of mivacurium because of a plasma cholinesterase deficiency. Rocuronium may have a role to play because it has a more rapid onset of action than any of the other NDMRs, providing good intubating conditions within 60–90 s following a dose of 0.6 mg kg^{-1} and a duration of action of 30–45 min. Cisatracurium, the stereoisomer of atracurium, has a slightly longer duration of action compared with that of atracurium but without the side-effect of histamine release.

The relatively new reversal agent sugammadex is now available for the reversal of the effects of rocuronium and vecuronium. Sugammadex is able to reverse profound rocuronium-induced muscle relaxation. This has advantages over the more conventional reversal agent neostigmine if reversal is required soon after the administration of vecuronium. There may be specific advantages associated with the use of this agent in obese patients, or those with a difficult airway, in whom rapid return of neuromuscular function is desirable.

Regional Anaesthesia

Spinal anaesthesia has been used for day-case anaesthesia, but the side-effects of post-dural puncture headache (PDPH) and motor weakness may delay discharge. Smaller-gauge pencil-point spinal needles have reduced the incidence of PDPH to <1% in patients aged >40 years. Shorter-acting local anaesthetics may increase the use of day-case spinals in the future; however, intrathecal lidocaine has been associated with transient neurological symptoms and is not licensed

for intrathecal use in the UK. Prilocaine, mepivacaine and pethidine have also been used for outpatient spinals in other countries, including the United States, and hyperbaric prilocaine is now available in the UK. The new preservative-free preparation of 2-chloroprocaine may provide acceptable anaesthesia and discharge times with low potential for transient neurological symptoms, but more clinical trials are needed. Low-dose bupivacaine (3 mL of 0.17%) has been used successfully for knee arthroscopy with times to discharge of 190 min. The addition of fentanyl 10 μg increases the duration of sensory blockade without affecting discharge times.

Local anaesthetic blocks are an excellent choice for day-case patients because of the low incidence of PONV and the provision of good postoperative analgesia. Many anaesthetists now use ultrasound-guided nerve blockade routinely to improve success rates, reduce the volume of local anaesthetic required and hopefully reduce the incidence of complications. Inguinal hernia repair is performed commonly under an ilioinguinal nerve block and local infiltration. For operations on the hand or arm, axillary or mid-humeral approach to brachial plexus block is preferable to the supraclavicular approach to minimize the risk of producing a pneumothorax, which may become apparent only after discharge. Intravenous regional anaesthesia (Bier's block) is another alternative for hand operations provided that effective exsanguination of the arm is achieved before performing the block.

Caudal block is used to reduce pain in paediatric patients after circumcision, herniorrhaphy, hypospadias or orchidopexy, using 0.25% plain bupivacaine; this provides excellent postoperative analgesia. Whenever a caudal block is administered for analgesia, care must be taken to ensure that motor strength is not compromised. There does not appear to be any advantage in using more concentrated solutions than 0.25% bupivacaine. Penile block and the application of local anaesthetic cream are also effective for circumcision.

Intra-articular local anaesthetics are useful following arthroscopy of the knee or shoulder. Femoral nerve block has been found to give superior analgesia to patients going home after anterior cruciate ligament repair and, combined with sciatic nerve block, reduces admission rates for complex knee surgery. Regional catheter techniques such as continuous interscalene brachial plexus block using a portable infusion pump allow a local anaesthetic infusion to continue at home. Analgesia is improved and side-effects from opioids are minimized. Guidance from community outreach teams improves efficacy and patient satisfaction. New elastomeric pumps which slowly infuse local anaesthetic solution at a fixed rate and which incorporate an air filter have been used safely on an outpatient basis. These pumps do not need a power source and deliver local anaesthetic directly to the surgical site.

POSTOPERATIVE CARE

Recovery from anaesthesia is an important aspect of day-case anaesthesia. The recovery area should be provided with the same range of monitoring equipment and resuscitation facilities as available in an in-patient facility. Many day surgery units in the UK now have three separate recovery areas: the first stage is for the immediate postoperative period, when patients require one-to-one nurse-to-patient care and monitoring; the second involves lower nursing dependency care where the patient is not attached to monitoring, but is mobilizing and usually given food and drink; and the third stage is the discharge area. The overall responsibility for assessing when patients are ready to go home is that of the clinicians involved. Often, experienced nursing staff who work regularly in the day unit become very good at detecting potential problems with day-case patients.

Postoperative pain control should be started pre- or intraoperatively by supplementing intravenous or inhalational anaesthesia with a combination of a non-steroidal anti-inflammatory drug (NSAID), paracetamol (especially in children), a short-acting opioid analgesic and local/regional block intraoperatively. Awakening is smoother and discharge home is quicker. The most frequently used drugs to provide intraoperative analgesia are fentanyl and alfentanil; the relatively short duration of action of these drugs makes them suitable for use in day-case anaesthesia. The provision of good postoperative analgesia is primarily the responsibility of the anaesthetist. Anaesthetists may do little to limit the number of patients requiring admission for surgical complications, but do play a major role in reducing admissions caused by pain or vomiting. NSAIDs, e.g. diclofenac, are useful for provision of postoperative

analgesia in day-case patients. COX II inhibitors are available as intravenous or oral preparations and have better gastrointestinal side-effect profiles than NSAIDs and fewer antiplatelet effects. An intravenous preparation of paracetamol is available and provides good analgesia without side-effects. Multimodal analgesia reduces the requirement for postoperative opioids.

Factors contributing to postoperative nausea and vomiting include a previous history of PONV, gender (females are more susceptible), the use of longer-acting opioid analgesic drugs such as morphine, the choice of anaesthetic technique or agents, operative procedure, pain, sudden movement or position change, history of motion sickness, hypotension, obesity, day of menstrual cycle and high oestrogen levels. A relationship between pain and the frequency of nausea and vomiting in the postoperative period has been established. There is controversy regarding the use of opioid analgesics in the day-case patient because they may increase PONV. Several studies have shown that, if an opioid-nitrous oxide anaesthetic is given, the occurrence of PONV is greater compared with an inhalational anaesthetic. In contrast, there are studies that have demonstrated that an opioid-supplemented anaesthetic technique results in earlier ambulation and discharge. PONV may be treated with intravenous 5-HT$_3$ antagonists, dexamethasone or cyclizine, and intramuscular prochlorperazine. Adequate hydration and analgesia are also of paramount importance.

In general, discharge of the patient should not take place until the patient is able to sit unaided, walk in a straight line and stand still without swaying. Usually, patients have been able to drink and eat (this also demonstrates the absence of nausea). A responsible person should be present to escort the patient home and both the responsible person and the patient should be given verbal and written discharge instructions and an adequate supply of oral analgesic drugs for at least 3 days. The patient should be advised to refrain from activities such as driving a car, operating machinery and drinking alcohol for 24 h. Communication with the patient's general practitioner is very important to ensure awareness of the operation performed and the requirements for postoperative follow-up. A follow-up telephone call to the patient after discharge should highlight any specific problems. Table 26.3 displays typical discharge criteria for day-case patients.

TABLE 26.3
Discharge Criteria for Day-Case Patients

Stable vital signs for at least 1 h

Orientated in time, place and person

Adequate pain control

Minimal nausea, vomiting or dizziness

Adequate oral hydration

Minimal bleeding or wound drainage

Able to pass urine

Responsible escort

Discharge authorized by appropriate staff member

Written and verbal instructions given to patient

Suitable analgesia provided

Patient hotels are a relatively new concept. The patient spends the first postoperative night in a hotel near to the day surgery unit where there is a resident nurse. These have been used so far for patients who have had, for example, a tonsillectomy. Patient hotels are cheaper than an in-patient overnight stay and are useful for patients who live too far from the day unit to be considered under normal circumstances for day surgery.

Each day-care unit should have an established system for audit of outcomes related to anaesthesia and include these outcomes in quality assurance and peer review processes. Reasons for non-attendance, cancellation and unplanned overnight admission should be assessed.

REFERENCE
Apfel, C.C., Kranke, P., Eberhart, L.H.J., 2002. Comparison of predictive models for PONV. Br. J. Anaesth. 88, 234–240.

FURTHER READING
British Association of Day Surgery, www.bads.co.uk.

Chung, F., Mezei, G., Tong, D., 1999. Pre-existing medical conditions as predictors of adverse events in day-case surgery. Br. J. Anaesth. 83, 262–270.

Davies, K.E., Houghton, K., Montgomery, J.E., 2001. Obesity and day case surgery. Anaesthesia 56, 1090–1115.

Duncan, P.G., Cohen, M.M., Tweed, W.A., et al., 1992. The Canadian four centre study of anaesthetic outcomes: III Are anaesthetic complications predictable in day surgical practice? Can. J. Anaesth. 39, 440–448.

Ilfeld, B.M., Morey, T.E., Wright, T.W., 2003. Continuous interscalene brachial plexus block for postoperative pain control at home: a randomized, double-blinded, placebo controlled study. Anesth. Analg. 96, 1089–1095.

Millar, J.M., Rudkin, G.E., Hitchcock, M., 1997. Practical anaesthesia and analgesia for day surgery. BIOS Scientific Publishers, Oxford.

Modernisation Agency Day Surgery Programme, www.wise.nhs.uk.

The Association of Anaesthetists of Great Britain & Ireland, 2007. Perioperative management of the morbidly obese patient. http://www.aagbi.org/sites/default/files/Obesity07.pdf.

Urmey, W.F., 2003. Spinal anaesthesia for outpatient surgery. Best Pract. Res. Clin. Anesthesiol. 17, 335–346.

White, P.F., Issioui, T., Skrivanek, G.D., 2003. The use of continuous popliteal sciatic nerve block after surgery involving the foot and ankle: does it improve the quality of recovery? Anesth. Analg. 97, 1303–1309.

Williams, B.A., Kentor, M.L., Vogt, M.T., 2003. Femoral-sciatic nerve blocks for complex outpatient knee surgery are associated with less postoperative pain before same day discharge: a review of 1200 consecutive cases from the period 1996–1999. Anesthesiology 98, 1206–1213.

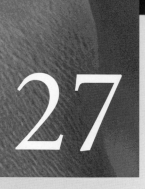

27 ANAESTHESIA FOR GYNAECOLOGICAL AND GENITOURINARY SURGERY

T here are many techniques and considerations which are common to both urological and gynaecological anaesthetic practice. As in other areas of surgery, increasing numbers of older, and often more frail, patients require surgery. In both specialities, the need for pelvic or perineal surgical access requires positioning of the patient which is associated with specific complications. In both specialities, there is widespread adoption of endoscopic surgical techniques and there is increased emphasis on the need for anaesthetic techniques which allow for day-case surgery, or surgery involving fast-track recovery programmes.

GENERAL CONSIDERATIONS

Positioning

Perineal, per urethra and per vaginal surgery mostly require the patient to be supine with the hips flexed and abducted and the knees bent. Lloyd Davies and lithotomy are the two common positions in which this is achieved. The main difference between them is the greater degree of flexion of the hips and knees in the lithotomy position. Because of the risk of nerve damage as a result of either direct compression or excessive stretching, care should be taken to avoid extreme hip flexion (femoral nerve compression, sciatic or obturator nerve stretching) and to avoid any prolonged pressure against the femoral and tibial condyles (common peroneal or saphenous nerve compression). When the patient is first put into either position, care should also be taken to avoid trapping the hands in the operating table mechanism. Calf compression leading to compartment syndrome has been associated with both

positions and if the position needs to be adopted for many hours it is advisable to lower the legs intermittently to allow reperfusion to occur.

Hypotension from blood loss or regional anaesthesia may be masked by the legs being raised and may become apparent only after they are lowered at the end of surgery.

The Trendelenburg (head-down) position is often required during pelvic surgery and is associated with decreased functional residual capacity (FRC), increased risk of passive regurgitation and raised intracranial and intraocular pressures. Transperitoneal laparoscopic surgery (for example, laparoscopic prostate surgery or hysterectomy) may require steep Trendelenburg positioning (30–45°) for prolonged periods of time and careful attention to preoperative conditions such as glaucoma is necessary. There have been concerns that prolonged steep Trendelenburg position combined with the hypercapnia which often occurs during laparoscopy might cause a raised intracranial pressure (as much as a 150% rise in animal models) and anecdotal evidence suggests that patients are at risk of developing acute confusional states on emergence from anaesthesia. In order to reduce this risk, some anaesthetists have advocated the routine use of parenteral dexamethasone or mannitol intraoperatively. Studies measuring the degree of intraoperative cerebral oxygenation in urological patients positioned in this way suggest that it is well preserved.

Tracheal intubation is required in most patients who require prolonged head-down positioning in order to maintain adequate ventilation, and in patients who are at high risk of passive regurgitation it should be considered even for short procedures. If passive regurgitation occurs in the head-down position, gastric acid can pool around the eyes leading to corneal burns unless it is washed out rapidly, and the patient should be positioned such that the anaesthetist is able to see the face in case this occurs.

Renal surgery most often requires the patient to be in a lateral position with the table 'broken' in the middle in order to extend the flank. Cardiorespiratory stability is maintained in most patients despite one lung being dependent, although temporary hypotension sometimes occurs as a result of decreased venous return. Padding of the legs and arms is required to avoid peroneal, saphenous and ulnar nerve damage and care should be taken to avoid lateral neck flexion which may result in brachial plexus injuries. Corneal abrasions are surprisingly common in the lateral position, mostly as a result of inadvertent contact with apparatus near the head (for example HME filters).

Prone positioning is required only for percutaneous nephrolithotomy. For this procedure, patients require general anaesthesia with tracheal intubation and mechanical ventilation. In this position, it is essential that the tracheal tube is well secured. Careful attention should be paid to the position of the head, eye-padding, avoidance of abdominal compression and pressure-point protection (nose, chin, genitals, knees).

Laparoscopic Procedures

As in other areas of surgery, there has been an increase in the number of urological and gynaecological procedures which are performed laparoscopically, including surgery for hysterectomy, oophorectomy, cystectomy, nephrectomy and prostatectomy. Laparoscopic surgery is associated with lower intraoperative blood loss, lower postoperative analgesia requirements and faster postoperative recovery times. There is also less potential for heat loss than during open surgery.

Most laparoscopic surgery involves a transperitoneal approach and requires a pneumoperitoneum. The exceptions to this include renal surgery, in which a retroperitoneal approach is also possible, and radical prostate surgery, in which anteroperitoneal gas insufflation may be used. It has been suggested that anteroperitoneal and retroperitoneal approaches allow for faster postoperative recovery.

The pneumoperitoneum required for laparoscopic surgery is accomplished by the insufflation of carbon dioxide to a pressure of 10–15 mmHg. This can be performed after the insertion of a laparoscopic port or a Veress insufflation needle. In both cases, there is the potential for inadvertent damage to major blood vessels, or for subcutaneous insufflation resulting in surgical emphysema. Very rarely, venous gas embolism occurs as a result of insufflation directly into a blood vessel.

The cardiovascular effects of peritoneal insufflation include increases in venous return and cardiac output, accompanied by an increase in systemic vascular resistance. If higher pressures are required, compression of the vena cava may occur, resulting in a decrease in venous filling. Occasionally, the peritoneal stimulation which occurs during gas insufflation can cause a vagal bradycardic response requiring rapid deflation and the administration of an anticholinergic.

Pneumoperitoneum also results in decreased functional residual capacity, and when combined with the Trendelenburg position, there is an increased risk of atelectasis and V/Q mismatch. Tracheal intubation and mechanical ventilation can help to minimize the effects, particularly if positive end-expiratory pressure is applied, but in patients with marked respiratory disease, a prolonged pneumoperitoneum may not be tolerated well. On rare occasions, a congenital diaphragmatic fistula or a surgical breach of the diaphragm may result in a pneumothorax or pneumomediastinum which can interfere with ventilation.

Carbon dioxide is absorbed through the peritoneum during laparoscopic surgery, resulting in a raised $PaCO_2$, tachycardia and increased myocardial contractility. Retroperitoneal insufflation often results in a greater degree of gas absorption which may persist after surgery. Anteroperitoneal radical prostate surgery is worth a special mention because it can result in severe surgical emphysema in the scrotal area and/ or chest and face. The surgical emphysema is caused by carbon dioxide spreading throughout the subcutaneous tissues where it is readily absorbed, resulting sometimes in severe hypercapnia. Methods to decrease the degree of surgical emphysema and hypercapnia include ensuring adequate muscle relaxation (for example by using an infusion of muscle relaxant) and by increasing the minute volume achieved by mechanical ventilation both intraoperatively and sometimes for a short period after surgery has ended. The use of nitrous oxide is not recommended during anteroperitoneal surgery because it exacerbates the degree of surgical emphysema.

The frequency with which laparoscopic procedures are converted to open operation depends on the operation and the experience of the operator. It may be appropriate to ask the surgeon beforehand whether conversion to an open procedure is likely.

Other Endoscopic Surgery

Urethral or transcervical endoscopic approaches can be used to perform bladder, prostate, ureteric and intra-uterine surgery. Flexible endoscopes may be used for some procedures, such as surveillance cystoscopy, in which case topical anaesthesia may be sufficient. If surgical resection is necessary, it is probable that a rigid endoscope will be required, facilitated by general or spinal anaesthesia. The rigid endoscope allows the use of rigid instruments, such as a resection diathermy loop, and fluid irrigation which allows visualization of the surgical field and washes away blood and resected tissue.

The choice of irrigation fluid is determined by the surgical technique. If monopolar diathermy equipment is used, a relatively non-conducting irrigating fluid is required so that current is not dissipated away from the point at which the diathermy equipment comes into contact with the body. In contrast, bipolar equipment works better with an irrigating fluid which conducts charge from the active part of the instrument to the nearby return electrode. Until recently, most diathermy equipment used by urologists was monopolar and the irrigation fluid of choice was glycine, which combined good optical properties with poor electrical conduction. Saline irrigation is used with the more recently developed bipolar resectoscopes.

Endoscopic resection with continuous irrigation requires the fluid to be under pressure, achieved usually by hanging the fluid reservoir from a drip-stand. Fluid can be forced under pressure into tissue planes as well as veins or sinuses opened by the diathermy process. In this manner, a large amount of fluid can be absorbed, which can result in fluid overload in susceptible patients. If the irrigating fluid is glycine, TUR (transurethral resection) syndrome may also develop (see below).

Lasers can also be used for transurethral resection and are used commonly for prostatic resection. There are various techniques available using different lasers, including holmium and Greenlight lasers. Smaller instrumentation of the urethra may be possible, including the use of flexible endoscopes, and there is minimal blood loss with faster postoperative recovery times.

TRANSURETHRAL RESECTION (TUR) SYNDROME

Despite the name, TUR syndrome is not exclusive to transurethral surgery. It is sometimes known as TURP (trans-urethral resection of the prostate) syndrome, and, as the name implies, it is most commonly associated with endoscopic prostatic surgery in which prostatic sinuses and veins are cut during resection, allowing irrigating fluid to be absorbed. Less commonly, TUR syndrome has been reported after other procedures, including bladder tumour resection, cystoscopy, various forms of lithotripsy and transcervical endometrial resection.

TUR syndrome occurs if a large volume of hypotonic irrigating solution is absorbed rapidly, resulting in rapid changes in serum osmolality and electrolyte concentrations. Glycine solution is the most commonly used hypotonic irrigating fluid in the UK, and commercial solutions have an osmolality of approximately $200\,mosmol\,L^{-1}$. In high concentrations, glycine can exhibit toxic effects on the cardiovascular and central nervous systems (including retinal neurotransmission) in addition to the effects of altered blood chemistry. The clinical findings associated with TUR syndrome are shown in Table 27.1.

TUR syndrome usually occurs only after more than 2 L of irrigating fluid have been absorbed into the circulation, but because this may occur as a result of fluid redistribution from perivesicular tissue planes into the vasculature, the onset of TUR syndrome may be delayed until some hours after surgery. In addition to the potential effects of fluid overload, the clinical features of TUR syndrome are those of decreased or altered consciousness and cardiovascular compromise. The most obvious biochemical abnormality is acute hyponatraemia. Acute haemolysis has also been associated with TUR syndrome, but is unlikely to occur with modern glycine solutions.

TABLE 27.1
Clinical Features of TUR Syndrome

Symptoms in the Awake Patient	Clinical Signs and Investigation Results
Vertigo	Confusion or agitation
Nausea and/or vomiting	Decreased consciousness
Abdominal pain	Seizures
Visual disturbance/blurred vision	Pupillary dilatation
	Papilloedema
Dyspnoea	Bradypnoea/hypopnoea
Chest tightness	Pulmonary oedema
	Cyanosis
	Oliguria
	Hypotension (although there may be initial hypertension)
	Bradycardia or other dysrhythmias
	Widened QRS and/or ST changes on ECG
	Cardiac arrest
	Hyponatraemia
	Decreased serum osmolality
	Hyperammonaemia

TUR syndrome is more likely to occur when higher irrigation pressures are used or if surgical resection is prolonged or extensive (e.g. if the prostate is very large or if perforation of the prostatic capsule occurs during surgery). Various attempts have been made to monitor the degree of fluid absorption, including adding ethanol to the irrigation fluid (in order to monitor exhaled ethanol concentrations), strict fluid input/output measurement, and semi-continuous weighing of the patient. None of these techniques has gained widespread acceptance because of the inherent difficulties associated with their use.

The risk of TUR syndrome can be minimized by limiting the duration of surgery, decreasing the irrigation pressure (by limiting the height of the reservoir above the patient to 60–80 cm above the operating field), ensuring that glycine irrigation is converted to saline as soon as surgery is complete and the judicious use of diuretics if surgery is prolonged. The use of bipolar resection with saline irrigation exposes the patient to the risk of fluid overload alone, rather than to the biochemical derangement of TUR syndrome.

The use of spinal anaesthesia is thought to make earlier identification of TUR syndrome possible because the initial signs are most commonly agitation and restlessness.

If TUR syndrome is suspected, the operation should be concluded as rapidly as possible. The treatment of TUR syndrome consists of supportive measures combined with diuretics such as furosemide or mannitol. Hypertonic saline (i.e. 3% solution) may be required in patients who develop extreme neurological or myocardial dysfunction. Sodium replacement must be performed in a controlled manner in order to avoid pontine demyelination; an increase in serum sodium concentration of $1–2\,mmol\,L^{-1}\,h^{-1}$ is widely accepted to be within safe limits (to a maximum of $12\,mmol\,L^{-1}$ within a 24-h period). Fortunately, the sodium changes which occur in TUR syndrome are so acute that this complication of treatment is unlikely to occur. A commonly quoted formula to guide sodium replacement is [body weight $\times 1.2$] $mL\,h^{-1}$ of 3% saline, which increases the serum sodium concentration by about $1\,mmol\,L^{-1}\,h^{-1}$. High-dependency monitoring is required.

REGIONAL ANAESTHESIA

Regional anaesthesia, either alone or in combination with general anaesthesia, is often the preferred technique for many gynaecological and genitourinary procedures. It provides excellent intraoperative and postoperative analgesia and is perceived as being associated with decreased risks of respiratory and airway dysfunction in patients with significant comorbidities. Epidural anaesthesia is often combined with general anaesthesia in procedures in which there is likely to be prolonged abdominal pain postoperatively, or if it is anticipated that there may be significant disturbance to bowel or other intraperitoneal organs; examples include open surgery for cystectomy, Wertheim's hysterectomy or nephrectomy. Spinal anaesthesia may be combined with general anaesthesia for procedures in which postoperative pain is likely to be severe, but not as prolonged, e.g. operations involving Pfannenstiel or lower midline abdominal incisions, such as hysterectomy or open prostate surgery. The addition of an intrathecal opioid to spinal anaesthesia can extend the duration of spinal analgesia further into the postoperative period, but careful monitoring is required to avoid complications as there is an increased risk of delayed respiratory depression (particularly if a parenteral opioid is also prescribed) and increased incidences of nausea, vomiting and pruritus. If spinal anaesthesia is used in combination, it should be performed before induction of general anaesthesia in order to minimize the risk of inadvertent nerve or spinal cord damage. Sympathetic nerve blockade occurs in association with spinal or epidural anaesthesia, and profound hypotension can result when this is combined with the cardiovascular effects of general anaesthetic agents. This is particularly true of 'one-shot' techniques such as spinal anaesthesia performed immediately before induction of general anaesthesia.

Spinal anaesthesia without general anaesthesia is often the preferred anaesthetic technique for TURP and cystoscopic procedures. Not only is it perceived as being safer in patients with significant respiratory or airway comorbidities but it also offers the potential for early identification of TUR syndrome when monopolar resection techniques are used. For procedures which require bladder irrigation, anaesthesia with a sensory block of up to up to at least the T10–12 dermatomes is needed to prevent discomfort caused by distension of the bladder. Occasionally, spinal anaesthesia results in penile tumescence, which makes penile surgery and instrumentation of the urethra difficult. Intravenous ketamine has been used to treat this complication but its efficacy is probably limited and side-effects may occur. Intracorporeal administration of a low-dose α-adrenergic agonist (e.g. phenylephrine 100–200 μg) is likely to be more effective, with little risk of systemic side-effects.

More localized regional or infiltrative techniques may provide adjunctive analgesia for other gynaecological or genitourinary procedures. Local anaesthetic infiltration is often used during perineal surgery, and the addition of a vasoconstrictor may reduce local bleeding. Anaesthetists should be aware that a vasoconstrictor used by the surgeon has the potential to cause systemic effects as it is absorbed.

Other techniques include the use of caudal block to provide saddle analgesia, and transversus abdominis plane (TAP) blocks to provide analgesia of the abdominal wall. A penile ring block provides excellent analgesia for penile operations such as circumcision, but must be performed using a plain local anaesthetic solution to avoid vasoconstriction.

PERIOPERATIVE INFECTIONS

There is a high incidence of occult urinary tract infections in patients with urinary tract stones or an indwelling catheter. Antimicrobial prophylaxis can be used to help to prevent bacteraemia, particularly during surgery in which the urinary tract mucosa is likely to be breached (e.g. stone extraction, bladder tumour or prostate resection). Antimicrobial prophylaxis may also be required in surgery in which there is a risk of bowel perforation, e.g. cystectomy or radical prostate surgery.

OTHER CONSIDERATIONS

Postoperative nausea and vomiting occur more commonly after gynaecological surgery and the preemptive use of antiemetics is often advisable in these patients.

Venous thromboembolic events are strongly associated with pelvic and renal cancers and surgery. Appropriate prophylaxis should always be considered, but special attention should be paid to the possibility that venous thrombosis may already be present before surgery, necessitating preoperative anticoagulation and possibly the insertion of a filter in the inferior vena cava (IVC).

Blood conservation strategies should be considered before operations associated with major blood loss. This may include the routine use of anti-fibrinolytic medications such as tranexamic acid. Cell salvage technology may also be of benefit, but its use may be limited in cancer surgery because of the theoretical risk of haematogenous metastasis. Currently, many centres infuse cell-salvaged blood through white cell filters for cystectomy and radical prostate operations, but not for gynaecological malignancies. Cell salvage should be stopped immediately before planned bowel incision, for example at the time of ileal conduit formation.

A urinary catheter is often required in the postoperative period, particularly if ongoing bladder irrigation is required. Care should be taken when moving the patient to avoid undue tension and accidental displacement, particularly after a urethral anastomosis has been created. Bladder spasm is a common problem in the postoperative period, often occurring in previously catheter-naïve patients who may benefit from the addition of a muscarinic receptor antagonist such as hyoscine butylbromide.

Active warming measures are necessary during many gynaecological and urological surgical procedures, particularly during open procedures or those which require continuous fluid irrigation.

ANAESTHETIC IMPLICATIONS OF SPECIFIC SURGICAL TECHNIQUES

Pelvic Surgery

Surgery for cystectomy, hysterectomy and oophorectomy is performed with the patient head-down and either supine or in the lithotomy/Lloyd Davies position. For open abdominal and laparoscopic approaches, tracheal intubation and mechanical ventilation are required. For open approaches, combined general and regional anaesthesia provide good intraoperative and postoperative analgesia. The choice of technique depends on the incision used, with Pfannenstiel incisions being more amenable to spinal anaesthesia. Alternatively, postoperative patient-controlled analgesia (PCA) regimens can be used, and there is increasing use of postoperative local anaesthetic wound infusion catheters. Laparoscopic approaches are likely to require less analgesia postoperatively, but this depends on any final incision required to remove the resected viscera.

Cystectomy and large gynaecological resections are often prolonged surgical procedures with the potential for marked physiological derangements to occur intraoperatively which are likely to necessitate the use of invasive arterial and/or central venous monitoring. Surgery for gynaecological pelvic cancers can sometimes be very extensive, requiring the excision of multiple structures at once, e.g. pelvic exenteration surgery. There is the potential for very large blood loss. In such cases, high-dependency monitoring is likely to be needed in the postoperative period.

Chronic blood loss relating to the disease process requiring cystectomy or hysterectomy may mean that the patient is anaemic before surgery. Other preoperative considerations include the potential for large pelvic cancers to affect renal function as a result of either chemotherapy or ureteric obstruction/compression. Preoperative chemotherapy, especially for ovarian cancer, can also result in systemic complications such as cardiac impairment. The physical effects of large pelvic tumours can include abdominal mass effects such as abdominal compartment syndrome, obstruction of the IVC and diaphragmatic splinting. The extent of any preoperative nerve compression should be documented before regional anaesthesia is performed.

Cystectomy requires the formation of an ileal conduit into which the ureters are diverted. Generally, this does not impact on renal function, and potentially nephrotoxic drugs such as NSAIDs can be used once there is minimal risk of postoperative hypotension. One of the commonest complications of ileal conduit formation is postoperative ileus, which can present many days after surgery. Epidural analgesia has been suggested as a means of promoting earlier recovery of gut function (probably by reducing postoperative use of opioids), as has the avoidance of insertion of a nasogastric tube during surgery.

Vaginal hysterectomy causes less surgical trauma than open abdominal surgery and is less painful postoperatively. Depending upon the patient, a general anaesthetic with a laryngeal mask airway, or spinal anaesthesia alone, may be sufficient. There is the potential for perioperative occult bleeding to occur because of the impaired surgical view.

Laparoscopic sterilization requires general anaesthesia but is normally relatively short and can often be performed using a laryngeal mask airway. The degree of postoperative pain as a result of placing clips around the fallopian tubes is often hard to predict, although most patients require only oral analgesics.

Emergency surgery for ectopic pregnancy may be either semi-urgent surgery as a result of early detection, or, if rupture and haemorrhage have occurred, a true emergency requiring immediate resuscitation and surgery. Patients are usually young and fit and the signs of haemorrhage are often masked, but if bleeding is suspected there should be minimal delays in proceeding to open surgery; if possible, two large-bore venous cannulae should be inserted and intravenous fluid resuscitation started as soon as possible. A rapid-sequence induction (RSI) technique should be employed because of the risk of a full stomach. If the patient is grossly hypovolaemic, hypotension may occur on induction and this may require fluids and/or vasopressors. Blood should be cross-matched and transfused as required, and any coagulopathy corrected aggressively.

If there is no evidence of haemorrhage, a laparoscopic technique may be used; tracheal intubation and artificial ventilation are required and RSI may be indicated. Both procedures are likely to be painful post-operatively requiring both simple analgesics and opiates, such as a patient-controlled opiate analgesia infusion.

Nephrectomy and Renal Surgery

The indications for nephrectomy include the presence of a renal tumour, intractable infection, trauma, calculous disease, renovascular hypertension or as a living donor. Renal tumours are associated with a high incidence of preoperative renal tract blood loss and the patient may be anaemic before surgery. Paraneoplastic syndromes are also common in patients with a renal tumour and may cause hypercalcaemia, hypertension, polyneuropathy and fever. As in other surgery for malignant disease, anaesthetic assessment should take into account the possibility of metastatic spread, particularly to the lungs. The extent of local spread is also important because tumours which impinge on the inferior vena cava may require it to be clamped during surgery.

If a tumour is very large or vascular, endovascular embolization under radiological guidance may be performed a day or so before surgery. Preoperative analgesia is required, and an epidural block is often inserted before the embolization.

The removal of a kidney does not necessarily impact on postoperative renal function, particularly if the kidney was functioning poorly beforehand, but indices of renal function should be reviewed by the anaesthetist. Potentially nephrotoxic drugs such as NSAIDs and aminoglycosides can often be used provided that renal function is adequate and perioperative hypotension avoided.

Clearly, in patients whose final functioning kidney is being removed, dialysis will be required postoperatively and care should be taken to avoid large doses of drugs which are likely to accumulate, such as morphine. Care should also be taken if possible to avoid placing venous cannulae in areas such as the forearm because these are likely to be needed for future fistula formation. A partial nephrectomy may be considered as a means of preserving some renal function, but these have a lower rate of tumour clearance and a higher incidence of intraoperative or postoperative haemorrhage.

The anaesthetic requirements for pyeloplasty are very similar to those for nephrectomy except that the patient may be positioned in the lithotomy position first, whilst a ureteric stent is inserted.

Renal surgery may be performed using open or laparoscopic surgery and the choice of surgical technique is often dependent on the size of the tumour or the complexity of the resection. In both eventualities, tracheal intubation and artificial ventilation are necessary to allow surgical access and to minimize complications. If open surgery is performed, epidural analgesia usually provides good postoperative pain relief, although patient-controlled analgesia regimens with morphine are also appropriate. Intercostal or intrapleural nerve blocks can be used but are relatively short-acting and risk the development of a pneumothorax. After laparoscopic procedures, a parenteral opioid should generally be sufficient to provide analgesia.

Occasionally, a pneumothorax develops if the pleura is breached during renal surgery. Pneumothoraces are generally self-limiting and resolve after laparoscopic insufflation is discontinued, or are maintained at a small size by the use of positive pressure ventilation during open surgery. It is rare to need to insert an intrapleural drain.

In patients whose cardiovascular system is unstable, or if major blood loss is expected, invasive arterial and/or central venous monitoring should be employed.

Prostate Surgery

Prostatic surgery may be required either for cancer or for benign prostatic hypertrophy. In both cases, the incidence of disease increases with age and patients may be frail or affected by comorbidities. In addition, many patients with benign prostatic hypertrophy present after an episode of acute urinary retention which has been triggered by another medical insult such as recent major surgery. The most prevalent group for acute urinary retention is men aged 75–84 years, in whom the one-year mortality after presentation is approximately 13% if the retention occurred spontaneously and 18% if the episode of retention was precipitated by an acute event. These figures are more than doubled if comorbidities are also present.

Preoperative assessment should aim to identify significant comorbidities, especially those affecting the cardiovascular or respiratory systems. In addition to the risks inherent in anaesthetizing patients with cardiovascular disease, the significant fluid shifts involved in transurethral resection of the prostate (TURP) may result in fluid overload in susceptible individuals. Any pre-existing metabolic derangement, such as hyponatraemia resulting from diuretic use or other causes, is likely to be exacerbated. Prostatic disease may also affect renal function and this should be assessed preoperatively.

Complications associated with TURP include blood loss, which can often be difficult to quantify because of the use of irrigation fluid. Other complications include hypothermia, sepsis and TUR syndrome. Although general anaesthesia using a laryngeal mask airway can be used, spinal anaesthesia is often the preferred anaesthetic technique for TURP because of the decreased risks of respiratory and airway dysfunction. Spinal anaesthesia may also provide the potential for early identification of TUR syndrome when monopolar techniques are used because confusion and agitation are amongst the earliest clinical signs (see Table 27.1).

If the prostate is very large, a retropubic prostatectomy (Millen's procedure) may be required. This approach uses a Pfannenstiel-type incision, and because of the size of the prostate is an increased risk of major blood loss during the procedure.

Curative prostatic cancer surgery (radical prostatectomy) requires transperitoneal or anteroperitoneal resection which can be performed using open or laparoscopic techniques. Both require general anaesthesia and tracheal intubation, with or without spinal or epidural analgesia. During laparoscopic radical prostatectomy, the urethra is resected at the base of the bladder during the procedure and it must be borne in mind that a large diuresis during this time may obscure the surgical field. There is the potential for major haemorrhage using either approach.

Newer transrectal ultrasound treatments (high-intensity focussed ultrasound, HIFU) have been developed and are used in some centres. These procedures cause minimal physiological disturbance with much less postoperative pain. Anaesthesia for these simply requires the patient to lie still in the lateral position for 1–2 h.

Intrauterine and Transurethral Bladder Surgery

Suction termination of pregnancy (STOP) requires dilatation of the cervix and instrumentation of the uterus under general anaesthesia. A volatile anaesthetic agent can be used to maintain anaesthesia but may result in uterine relaxation and is therefore avoided by many anaesthetists. The procedure is often very short and intermittent propofol can be used, accompanied by a short-acting opioid analgesic. Deep anaesthesia is necessary at the time of cervical dilatation because this can be very stimulating and may result in a profound vagal response or laryngospasm.

Evacuation of retained products of conception (ERPC) has similar anaesthetic requirements and both procedures are associated with the risk of haemorrhage and uterine perforation requiring further surgery.

Oxytocin is often administered at the end of these procedures to promote uterine contraction and decrease postoperative bleeding. The administration of oxytocin may result in transient hypotension and tachycardia. Simple oral analgesics are usually sufficient to control postoperative pain.

Donor egg retrieval (as part of fertility treatment) is performed using transvaginal aspiration under ultrasound guidance. It can be performed under sedation or using a general anaesthetic with a laryngeal mask airway. Complications during egg retrieval (e.g. haemorrhage or damage to intervening structures) are rare.

Cervical and transcervical surgery includes resection of tumours, endometrial ablation for menorrhagia (performed using thermal or electrocautery), hysteroscopy and cervical dilatation and uterine curettage. General and regional anaesthetic techniques are both suitable.

Brachytherapy may be used to insert radioactive sources directly into cancerous areas such as the prostate, uterus or cervix. Anaesthesia is usually required for gynaecological brachytherapy. Prolonged postoperative analgesia may be needed, for example if a vaginal pack is inserted, and spinal, epidural or caudal techniques can be used. Institutions undertaking brachytherapy have specific protocols designed to protect staff from ionizing radiation.

Patients with a bladder tumour are often elderly and may have a history of cigarette smoking (the same is also true for cervical and vulval cancer); cardiorespiratory comorbidities should be identified preoperatively.

Bladder tumours often require many years of regular surveillance and intermittent resection. Anaesthesia for cystoscopy has to facilitate bladder irrigation but not always bladder tumour resection; it is often difficult to predict the extent of surgery preoperatively. General anaesthesia with a laryngeal mask airway is generally sufficient as these procedures are often short.

Spinal anaesthesia is a good alternative for higher risk patients, although patients with respiratory disease may be more prone to coughing when lying supine with legs raised in the lithotomy position, and coughing can make surgery difficult and potentially hazardous. Resection of tumours from the lateral bladder wall may result in obturator nerve stimulation, which can also be hazardous as a result of sudden leg movements. In some patients, there may be a surgical request for administration of a neuromuscular blocking drug in order to avoid this complication.

Complications of transurethral resection of bladder tumours (TURBT) include TUR syndrome, haemorrhage and bladder perforation. Bladder perforation may not be immediately obvious in the postoperative period, especially while the continuing effects of spinal anaesthesia mask pain. Blood clots may cause postoperative obstruction of the bladder catheter and urinary retention, even if an irrigating catheter is used.

Postoperative pain associated with TURBT and transcervical surgery is often relatively easy to control with simple analgesics, accompanied by intermittent administration of an opioid if required.

Perineal, Penile and Testicular Surgery

Testicular surgery, e.g. repair of hydrocoele or investigation of a suspected testicular torsion, involves a scrotal incision, and general or spinal anaesthesia can be used. Supplemental infiltration of local anaesthetic may provide additional analgesia. Orchidectomy is often performed using an inguinal incision, and local infiltration or an ilioinguinal nerve block may be of benefit. If orchidectomy is performed for testicular cancer, the possibility of distant metastases should be considered. Para-aortic node dissection may also be required, which carries with it all the implications of major abdominal surgery.

General and spinal anaesthesia are both appropriate for most penile or perineal procedures. An additional penile ring block can provide good analgesia, and may be used as the sole anaesthetic for circumcision. Vulval operations may benefit from local anaesthetic infiltration. Antibiotic prophylaxis is not routinely required, but is indicated if a penile implant is inserted or for repair of penile fracture. Radical vulvectomy and penile amputation are both used for the resection of cancers and are likely to include lymph node dissection. Both have the potential for more severe blood loss.

Fournier's gangrene (fasciitis of the perineum) requires extensive debridement of the scrotum and perineum. Postoperative pain may be quite severe and significant blood loss may occur. Patients with this condition are septic and postoperative HDU care is recommended. Broad-spectrum antimicrobial treatment should be started before surgery.

Continence Surgery

Various procedures can be performed to promote continence. Pelvic floor repair and transvaginal tape (TVT, in which a tape is inserted transvaginally around the bladder neck with both ends coming out on to the abdominal skin) can both be performed under general or spinal anaesthesia, and supplemental local anaesthetic infiltration may be used. Postoperative analgesia requirements are generally low.

Abdominal procedures such as colposuspension can be performed using open or laparoscopic approaches and are associated with slightly more postoperative pain. Although spinal anaesthesia can be sufficient for open procedures using a Pfannenstiel incision, it is more usual to use general anaesthesia with tracheal intubation and mechanical ventilation. If surgery involves the insertion of a bladder-neck prosthesis, prophylactic antibiotics are required.

Surgical techniques to increase the bladder capacity include Helmstein's procedure and Clam cystoplasty. Helmstein's procedure is performed rarely and consists of forced bladder distension using fluid which can then be kept in place using a clamped catheter for 4–6 h. This results in prolonged discomfort and epidural anaesthesia is usually employed until the catheter is released. Clam cystoplasty requires the bladder to be incised and a 'patch' of small bowel to be sutured to the edges of the incision in order to increase bladder volume. The anaesthetic requirements are very similar to those for cystectomy.

Surgery for Renal Tract Stones

Stones within the bladder or ureter can often be removed using cystoscopy with or without ureteroscopy. Mechanical or laser instruments may be used for removal of the stones; if a laser is used during surgery, the general precautions for their use should be followed. Ureteric stents (JJ stents) may be inserted around the time of surgery, and on-table X-ray imaging is often needed. General or regional anaesthesia may be used; although urethral stimulation during the procedure occasionally necessitates supplemental analgesia if spinal anaesthesia is employed.

Occasionally, bladder stones are too large for this approach and a mini-Pfannenstiel incision is required. This has similar anaesthetic requirements to a retropubic prostatectomy.

Percutaneous nephrolithotomy/lithotripsy (PCNL) is performed when extracorporeal shockwave lithotripsy has failed. The procedure is performed in two stages, the first stage being cystoscopy and insertion of a ureteric balloon. During the second stage, the patient is placed in the prone position, a percutaneous tract is formed down to the renal pelvis under X-ray guidance and a nephroscope is inserted. Ultrasonic fragmentation or nephroscopic forceps are used to break up the stone. Irrigation with saline is used to flush out fragments of stone. Fluid can be forced into the retroperitoneal or peritoneal spaces, and this can occasionally be very severe, resulting in a 'tense abdomen' with diaphragmatic splinting. Haemorrhage from the kidney or nearby organs is also possible, and it is sometimes difficult to differentiate between irrigation fluid effects and retroperitoneal haematoma or haemoperitoneum. Pneumothoraces can also occur.

All surgery for renal tract stone removal carries the risk of postoperative bacteraemia and sepsis, and, as with other procedures which require irrigation, there is the potential for significant cooling to occur.

Tracheal intubation and mechanical ventilation are necessary for PCNL surgery because of the need for prone positioning.

FURTHER READING

Armitage, J.N., Sibanda, N., Cathcart, P.J., et al., 2007. Mortality in men admitted to hospital with acute urinary retention: database analysis. Br. Med. J. 335, 1199–1202.

Conacher, I.D., Soomro, N.A., Rix, D., 2004. Anaesthesia for laparoscopic urological surgery. Br. J. Anaesth. 93, 859–864.

Cousins, J., Howard, J., Borra, P., 2005. Principles of anaesthesia in urological surgery. Br. J. Urol. 96, 223–229.

Knight, D.J.W., Mahajan, R.P., 2004. Patient positioning in anaesthesia. Continuing Education in Anaesthesia, Critical Care and Pain 4, 160–163.

Midgley, S., Tolley, D.A., 2006. Anaesthesia for laparoscopic surgery in urology. European Association of Urology Update Series 4, 241–245.

Moore, J., McLeod, A., 2009. Anaesthesia for gynaecological oncology surgery. Current Anaesthesia & Critical Care 20, 8–12.

O'Donnell, A.M., Foo, I.T.H., 2009. Anaesthesia for transurethral resection of the prostate. Continuing Education in Anaesthesia, Critical Care and Pain 9, 92–96.

Park, E.Y., Koo, B.N., Min, K.T., Nam, S.H., 2009. The effect of pneumoperitoneum in the steep Trendelenburg position on cerebral oxygenation. Acta Anaesthesiol. Scand. 53, 895–899.

Vijayan, S., 2011. TURP syndrome. Trends in Anaesthesia and Critical Care 1, 46–50.

28 ANAESTHESIA FOR ORTHOPAEDIC SURGERY

■ ■ ■ ■ ■ ■ ■ ■ ■ ■ ■ ■

O ne in five operations in the United Kingdom is for orthopaedic, spinal or trauma surgery. Anaesthesia for trauma surgery is discussed in Chapter 37. This chapter provides a framework for the conduct of anaesthesia for orthopaedic surgery.

THE PATIENT POPULATION

A large proportion of patients presenting for orthopaedic surgery are young and healthy. Sporting injuries and disease processes without systemic impact are common and these patients are at low risk of complications relating to anaesthesia or surgery. However, several disease processes are more common in patients presenting for orthopaedic surgery than in the general surgical population, and these are discussed below.

Comorbidities

Rheumatoid Arthritis

Rheumatoid arthritis is a chronic inflammatory disease of unknown aetiology, affecting women more often than men. Rheumatoid factor is found in 90% of affected patients and there exists a genetic predisposition with associated human leucocyte antigen HLA-DR4. It is a multisystem disease which may present the anaesthetist with problems of a difficult airway, cervical spine instability (and cervical cord vulnerability) and widespread vasculitis-induced organ dysfunction. Additionally, drug therapy for rheumatoid disease frequently produces severe and widespread side-effects. These are detailed below. The airway of the rheumatoid patient may present

problems because of stiffness of the temporomandibular joint, stiffness or instability of the neck and cricoarytenoid arthritis. Radiological examination shows involvement of the cervical spine in 80% of patients, and 30% have neurological symptoms suggesting instability of the neck. Atlantoaxial subluxation, subaxial subluxation and cervical spine ankylosis are common, and should be investigated through history-taking, clinical examination and cervical X-ray. Flexion-extension views may be necessary to observe instability. Magnetic resonance imaging provides good assessment of the rheumatoid neck. Systemic disease is very common, and includes pericardial effusion, constrictive pericarditis, heart block, aortic and mitral valve disease, pleural effusion, interstitial fibrosis, anaemia, thrombocytopaenia and renal and hepatic dysfunction.

A thorough history and examination are important for patients with rheumatoid disease. Careful assessment of the airway and cervical spine should be performed. The range of neck movement should be assessed, and any associated neurological symptoms should be noted. A full blood count and serum urea and electrolyte concentrations should be measured, and an ECG and chest X-ray should be considered. Additionally, a lateral cervical X-ray, preferably with flexion-extension views, should be considered, particularly if tracheal intubation is planned. Systemic disease may indicate the need for arterial blood gas analysis, lung function tests, echocardiogram or liver function tests to be undertaken. Suspicion of cricoarytenoid involvement should prompt preoperative indirect laryngoscopic examination.

Regional anaesthesia should be used if possible. It has the advantage of avoiding airway and neck manipulation, and may be safer than general anaesthesia in patients with severe systemic disease. However, epidural and spinal anaesthesia may be very difficult because of spinal ankylosis and osteophyte formation. If general anaesthesia is used, patients with an unstable neck should be managed by an experienced anaesthetist, especially if tracheal intubation is planned. Tracheal intubation is made more difficult if movement of the temporomandibular joint is restricted. The need for tracheal intubation should be considered carefully in patients with severe disease because of the associated risks and difficulty. For many procedures, the use of a laryngeal mask airway is a suitable and a potentially less traumatic alternative. If tracheal intubation is required, intubation aids such as the intubating laryngeal mask airway or fibreoptic-guided intubation may be safer alternatives to tracheal intubation using direct laryngoscopy.

Osteoarthritis

A reduced range of joint movement may present problems in positioning, airway management, regional blockade and vascular access. Concurrent analgesic therapy may cause increased bleeding and renal dysfunction (non-steroidal anti-inflammatory drugs; NSAIDs) or tolerance to opioid analgesia (opioids).

Ankylosing Spondylitis

Ankylosing spondylitis causes rigidity of the entire spinal column, and may present problems with tracheal intubation. Unlike rheumatoid arthritis, cervical spine instability does not occur, but the fixed flexion deformity may render direct laryngoscopy utterly impossible. The use of a laryngeal mask airway is a suitable option for many procedures, and fibreoptic laryngoscopy is usually fairly straightforward unless the disease process is advanced. The normal routes of escape of local anaesthetic solution from the epidural space may be obstructed in patients with ankylosing spondylitis, and spinal cord ischaemia with permanent nerve damage has been reported after rapid injection of local anaesthetic into the epidural space in patients suffering from this condition.

Concurrent Drug Therapy

Many young healthy patients presenting for orthopaedic surgery do not take concurrent medication. However, use of analgesics is very common in the orthopaedic population because of the painful nature of their disease process. Concurrent therapy with antihypertensive, antianginal, antidepressant or cholesterol-lowering medication is common in older patients presenting for orthopaedic surgery. These patients often present for arthroplasty and this major procedure may place significant demands upon their physiological reserves. Preparation of the patient taking these drugs is discussed in detail in Chapter 18. Patients may also be using orthopaedic disease-modifying drugs such as methotrexate, steroids and gold.

Non-Steroidal Anti-Inflammatory Drugs

Thromboxane A_2 and prostaglandin endoperoxide, which are needed for the haemostatic function of platelets, are synthesized from arachidonic acid by the cyclo-oxygenase (COX) enzyme system. Non-steroidal anti-inflammatory drugs (NSAIDs) inhibit this enzyme system, impairing the formation of clots and, consequently, haemostasis. There are two COX isoforms: COX-1 synthesizes prostaglandins, which protect the gastric mucosa; COX-2 is involved with inflammatory responses. Inhibition of these systems ceases rapidly when administration of NSAIDs is stopped. However, the effects of aspirin persist for up to 10 days after treatment because of its covalent bonding with cyclo-oxygenase. Although NSAIDs taken up to the time of surgery may increase surgical blood loss, this does not imply that preoperative administration should be avoided. NSAIDs are valuable in providing analgesia pre- and postoperatively, and increased surgical blood loss is usually modest. Of more concern is gastroduodenal ulceration, of which the first symptom may be life-threatening upper gastrointestinal haemorrhage. The risk of ulceration is dose-related, commoner as age advances and even commoner if corticosteroids are also used to control inflammation. This complication stimulated the production of specific COX-2 inhibitors, but their use has been curtailed following reports of increased cardiovascular and cerebrovascular complications. NSAIDs should be avoided in patients who have a history suggestive of gastrointestinal ulceration or bleeding.

Opioid Analgesics

Chronic opioid use results in tolerance to the analgesic effects of the drugs and to their undesirable side-effects. When patients have used opioids for more than a few days before surgery, postoperative administration of an opioid becomes less effective than normal, and a larger dose is required than would be expected in the opioid-naïve patient. A useful guide is to provide the regular intake of opioid *in addition* to that prescribed for acute, postoperative pain relief. It is mandatory that frequent observations are made of these patients, and the involvement of an acute pain team is advisable.

Corticosteroids

Regular medication with glucocorticoid drugs (e.g. prednisolone, hydrocortisone, dexamethasone) produces suppression of endogenous glucocorticoid production. There is an increase in glucocorticoid concentration as part of the stress response after surgery, and these patients are at risk of an Addisonian crisis, including a precipitous fall in blood pressure because they may not be able to synthesize sufficient endogenous glucocorticoid. Patients who have taken doses of steroids greater than the equivalent of prednisolone 10 mg daily during the past 3 months require replacement corticosteroid therapy. Corticosteroid therapy may cause poor wound healing and gastrointestinal ulceration; consequently, low-dose replacement therapy is currently favoured. For patients undergoing minor surgery under general anaesthesia, the usual oral dose of corticosteroid should be given on the morning of surgery or a single dose of hydrocortisone 25–50 mg intravenously at induction. For patients undergoing moderate or major surgery, the usual morning dose of corticosteroid should be given and 25–50 mg of intravenous hydrocortisone at induction followed by further doses of 25–50 mg intravenously three times daily for 24 h after moderate surgery or for 48–72 h after major surgery. The patient's usual corticosteroid regimen is then re-established.

Immunosuppressant Drugs

Drugs such as methotrexate inhibit the immune system, damping the inflammatory response that causes distressing symptoms from some joint diseases. The induced immunosuppression may also render the patient at increased risk of hospital-acquired infection, and strict aseptic techniques should be used during any invasive procedures.

Other Drugs

A large variety of potentially toxic drugs is used to reduce the symptoms and retard the disease process in rheumatoid arthritis. Antimalarials, such as chloroquine, may cause retinopathy and cardiomyopathy. Gold and penicillamine cause undesirable side-effects in up to 40% of patients; these include nephrotic syndrome, thrombocytopaenia, agranulocytosis, marrow aplasia, hepatitis and pneumonitis. Sulfasalazine may cause haematological toxicity and fibrosing alveolitis. Administration of azathioprine may result in gastrointestinal side-effects, cholestatic hepatitis, leucopaenia, thrombocytopaenia and anaemia.

It should be apparent that the provision of anaesthesia for any patient with rheumatoid arthritis must be associated with a thorough search for the potentially dangerous side-effects of concurrent drug therapy.

TECHNIQUES OF ANAESTHESIA

General Anaesthesia

This is appropriate for all types of orthopaedic surgery, but regional anaesthesia may be the preferred technique for many procedures, for reasons discussed below. Patients undergoing procedures of long duration (e.g. hip revision) often require general anaesthesia because of the discomfort incurred by remaining in the same position for a prolonged period of time. In many countries, including the United Kingdom, patients often expect to receive general anaesthesia, and may not have been aware in advance of their surgery that regional anaesthesia represents a viable option. Thus, the use of general anaesthesia offers the benefit to patients of familiarity. General anaesthesia causes the greatest loss of control for the patient and many patients are pleasantly surprised to find that regional anaesthesia is an option for their operation.

Regional Anaesthesia

Central neuraxial block (spinal or epidural anaesthesia) reduces the stress response to surgery and has been shown to reduce some serious complications following many types of surgery. Benefits may include a reduction in the incidences of deep vein thrombosis, blood loss, myocardial infarction, respiratory and renal complications, and possibly pulmonary embolism. There is a high incidence of thromboembolic events in patients undergoing major lower limb arthroplasty, which makes this type of anaesthesia an attractive option.

Lower limb arthroplasty and minor lower limb procedures are frequently carried out using central neuraxial block. For longer procedures, such as hip

TABLE 28.1	
Peripheral Regional Anaesthesia and Analgesia	
Site of Surgery	*Block*
Shoulder	Interscalene brachial plexus
Upper arm	Interscalene and medial cutaneous nerve of the arm or supraclavicular brachial plexus. Plus intercostobrachial after either of these
Forearm and hand	Infraclavicular or axillary brachial plexus, IVRA, elbow or wrist
Fingers	Metacarpal or digital nerve
Hip	Posterior lumbar plexus (psoas compartment), 3-in-1 femoral sheath, proximal sciatic nerve
Knee	Femoral and sciatic nerve (popliteal fossa or above)
Ankle	Sciatic (popliteal fossa) ± saphenous nerve or IVRA
Foot	Sciatic (popliteal fossa) ± saphenous nerve or ankle or IVRA
Toes	Ankle, metatarsal or digital nerve

IVRA, intravenous regional anaesthesia.

arthroplasty, sedation or light general anaesthesia may be added. The combination of general anaesthesia with a central neuraxial block has not been shown to reduce the benefits attributable to this form of regional anaesthesia.

Following central neuraxial block, the patient is usually pain-free in the immediate postoperative period. Careful thought should be given to administration of analgesia after the nerve block has worn off (see below). There is a higher incidence of urinary retention in patients who have undergone joint arthroplasty under central neuraxial block and this leads to an increased risk of urinary tract infection. Patients may be managed by prophylactic urethral catheterization or monitoring of bladder volume postoperatively using ultrasound.

Peripheral nerve block is commonly used as a sole technique for many procedures, with the advantages of excellent pain relief, reduction of surgical stress, avoidance of complications of general anaesthesia and earlier discharge in the day-case setting. Peripheral surgery in 'high-risk' patients may also be carried out under peripheral nerve block to avoid the potential complications of general anaesthesia or central neuraxial block. Patients report a high degree of satisfaction following surgery carried out using this form of anaesthesia. Table 28.1 shows the sites at which surgery may be performed in association with specific nerve blocks. This form of anaesthesia requires a high level of expertise and an understanding of the issues of managing a conscious patient during surgery.

Intravenous regional anaesthesia (IVRA) is suitable for manipulation of fractures and brief operations (less than 30 min) on the forearm and lower leg. It is technically easy to perform but fatalities have occurred as a result of a large dose of local anaesthetic reaching the systemic circulation. Before performing IVRA, it is essential to understand how the risk of complications may be minimized and how they may be treated if they occur. Details of the technique and safety precautions are described in Chapter 24.

POSTOPERATIVE ANALGESIA

Oral and Intravenous Agents

Many patients are already taking regular analgesics for pre-existing bone and joint pain. Paracetamol is very useful in reducing the dose requirements of other analgesics, and may occasionally be sufficient analgesia alone. It is virtually free from side-effects in standard doses, and is contraindicated only in patients with liver dysfunction. If gastric motility is impaired, it may be administered rectally. The addition of NSAIDs, in the absence of contraindications, is usually useful and reduces the requirement for opioid analgesia.

NSAIDs inhibit the formation of prostaglandins and are widely used as analgesics in the treatment of acute bone-related pain. The newer COX-2 inhibitors potentially widened the number of patients who could benefit from these agents by reducing the potential for gastroduodenal ulceration, although as mentioned above, their use has been curtailed due to reports of increased incidences of myocardial infarction and stroke in patients taking long-term COX-2 inhibitors, leading to the withdrawal of rofecoxib in September 2004.

Prostaglandins are known to have an important role in bone repair and homeostasis. Animal studies have demonstrated that both non-specific and specific inhibitors of COX impair fracture healing. Some studies have suggested that this impairment results from

COX-2 inhibition. This has raised concerns regarding the use of NSAIDs as anti-inflammatory or analgesic drugs in patients undergoing orthopaedic procedures; however, the clinical implications of this are probably minimal and NSAIDs remain extremely important analgesic agents for orthopaedic patients.

NSAIDs also affect platelet function and would therefore be expected to increase perioperative blood loss. The clinical evidence for increased blood loss in major arthroplasty surgery patients receiving NSAIDs is minimal.

Intravenous opioids are frequently used following major joint arthroplasty. Patient-controlled analgesia systems are the most commonly used delivery systems. The doses of opioid required are much reduced by the other analgesic agents prescribed, thus minimizing the risk of side-effects.

Central Neuraxial Drugs

Single-dose spinal or epidural anaesthesia using local anaesthetic alone usually provides analgesia for only a relatively short period of time after operation. An adjuvant administered into the intrathecal or epidural space with the local anaesthetic improves the quality of the block and extends the duration of analgesia. Table 28.2 describes some of the more commonly administered drugs.

An epidural (or, rarely, intrathecal) infusion of local anaesthetics may be combined with an opioid to produce excellent analgesia. The combination of local anaesthetic and opioid is synergistic, reducing the side-effects of both and minimizing motor block. However, relatively high incidences of itching, nausea and urinary retention are encountered. It is routine practice in most hospitals to insert a urethral catheter in the anaesthetic room to avoid urinary retention in the postoperative period.

Epidural infusions are commonly used for up to 5 days following major orthopaedic surgery. Careful observation for signs of inadequate analgesia (often a result of catheter migration) and infection is required. The involvement of an acute pain team is very useful in this regard. Many units manage these patients in an extended recovery or high-dependency setting to increase the level of nursing care and to facilitate early detection and prompt management of complications.

Peripheral Nerve Blocks

Peripheral nerve block, with or without a central neuraxial block or general anaesthesia, often provides excellent pain relief for a number of hours postoperatively, allowing transition to oral or intravenous analgesia when required. The use of continuous 3-in-1 (femoral sheath) nerve block after knee replacement surgery results in better pain relief, faster postoperative rehabilitation and earlier discharge from hospital than opioid analgesia alone. Posterior lumbar plexus block (psoas compartment) or 3-in-1 femoral sheath block combined with proximal sciatic nerve block (e.g. Labat's approach or a parasacral approach) can be used for hip surgery, although it is difficult to obtain analgesia of the entire surgical area with peripheral blocks

TABLE 28.2			
Central Neuraxial Block Adjuvants			
Drug	*Action*	*Duration*	*Side-Effects*
Morphine	Opioid receptor agonist	Long	Itching, nausea, urinary retention, respiratory depression
Diamorphine	Opioid receptor agonist	Medium	Itching, nausea, urinary retention, respiratory depression
Fentanyl	Opioid receptor agonist	Short	Itching, nausea, urinary retention, respiratory depression
Clonidine	α_2-adrenoceptor agonist	Extends block duration	Sedation, hypotension, respiratory depression
Ketamine	N-methyl D-aspartate receptor antagonist	Long	Dysphoria, sedation, possible intrathecal toxicity
Adrenaline	Adrenoceptor agonist	Extends block duration	Systemic sympathetic activation (tachycardia, hypertension), myocardial ischaemia

alone. More recently, the introduction of enhanced recovery programmes, involving extensive local anaesthetic infiltration around the joint capsule and early mobilization following surgery, has reduced the use of formal peripheral nerve blockade following lower limb arthroplasty.

Single-dose peripheral nerve blocks using a long-acting local anaesthetic such as levobupivacaine may last for over 16h. Additives such as clonidine may be used to prolong the duration of single-dose blocks, although few additives have been shown clearly to be effective in this regard. Alternatively, a catheter may be inserted, allowing an infusion of a low concentration of a local anaesthetic drug (e.g. 0.2% ropivacaine) to allow selective return of motor power.

Nerve injury due to peripheral nerve block is rare (see Ch 43); it occurs in 1:5000 to 1:10 000 blocks performed, and patients with concurrent comorbidity, such as diabetes or vascular disease, may have an increased risk. However, the incidence of nerve injury secondary to orthopaedic surgery (direct trauma, tourniquet or positioning) is more frequent and often occurs in the sensory distribution of the nerve block. This reduces the popularity of peripheral nerve blocks in some institutions lest the block is blamed for nerve damage.

SURGICAL CONSIDERATIONS

Positioning

Patients with arthritis frequently have restricted mobility of joints. Positioning at the extremes of the range of movement of diseased joints may cause severe postoperative pain in addition to the pain resulting from the operation. Consequently, a patient's ability to assume the position required for operation must be assessed carefully; it is often useful to ask the patient to adopt that position before induction of anaesthesia if there is concern that mobility of joints may be an issue. Orthopaedic surgery often requires the use of unusual positions, some of which carry risks of nerve damage, soft tissue ischaemia, electrical and thermal injury, and joint pain. Care must be taken in protecting areas at risk of injury. These include bony promontories, sites of poor tissue viability and locations where nerves run close to the skin or close to the surface of a bone.

Forceful movement of the patient by the surgeon is often inevitable during orthopaedic surgery. When such movement occurs, it is advisable to re-check the patient's position, ensuring that soft tissues, nerves, eyes and venous access sites are protected. Although some procedures may be performed under regional anaesthesia alone, long operations may result in discomfort related to posture, and when the block wears off there may be significant discomfort if positioning has been poor during the procedure.

Some positions adopted during orthopaedic surgery are associated with venous air embolism. These postures include the lateral position for hip surgery, the sitting position for shoulder surgery and the prone position for spinal surgery. Monitoring for, and treatment of, air embolism are discussed in detail in Chapter 43.

Prophylaxis Against Infection

Prophylactic intravenous antibiotics are often used during orthopaedic surgery. Infection of bone is particularly threatening to the patient and is very difficult to eradicate; consequently, prevention is a high priority. Allergic reactions to antibiotics may occur and facilities must be available to treat such a reaction when intravenous antibiotics are used.

Laminar flow is used commonly in orthopaedic theatres to provide a constant flow of microscopically filtered air over the surgical field, and to minimize the risk of wound infection by environmental pathogens. This high flow of air over the patient's body surface greatly speeds convective heat loss, and precautions should be taken to avoid hypothermia.

Various in-theatre rituals exist for the prevention of cross-infection. These include the wearing of face masks and hats; however, the evidence supporting their use is scant.

Prophylaxis Against Hypothermia

Following induction of general or regional anaesthesia, heat is redistributed from the core to the peripheries. Following induction of general anaesthesia, there is typically a reduction in core temperature of 1°C in the first 30 min of anaesthesia. Core temperature reduces more slowly after this initial redistribution phase, typically by approximately 0.5°C per hour, although the rate of fall is heavily dependent upon ambient temperature, exposure and insulation, and the use of warming devices (see Ch 11).

Hypothermia is known to be associated with increased blood loss because of the narrow temperature range in which enzyme-dependent systems work, and perhaps because of platelet sequestration in the spleen. Hypothermia is also associated with poor postoperative wound healing and postoperative hypoxaemia.

The most effective method of reducing heat loss is forced air warming. However, warmed intravenous and surgical irrigation fluids and impermeable surgical drapes to reduce heat loss by evaporation are also useful.

Prophylaxis Against Thromboembolism

Deep venous thrombosis (DVT) may complicate any surgery, but is associated particularly with surgery involving the pelvis, hip and knee. Pulmonary embolism (PE) may be fatal and accounts for 50% of all deaths after surgery for hip replacement. Although an infusion of dextran has been shown to reduce the incidence of PE after surgery, there is a relatively high risk of anaphylaxis associated with its administration, and low-dose heparin regimens have become the norm. There is evidence that heparin reduces the incidence of fatal PE in high-risk groups, including patients who undergo surgery on the pelvis, hip or knee. Compared with unfractionated heparins (UFH), low molecular weight heparins (LMWH) inhibit the coagulation enzyme Xa and bind antithrombin-3 to a similar extent, but bind less to thrombin. The use of LMWH might be expected to result in less surgical bleeding than when UFH is used. LMWH probably protects better against DVT after hip replacement but the evidence for better prophylaxis against PE is less firm. The simplicity of once-daily administration of LMWH is an added advantage compared with UFH. Newer oral agents have the potential to provide patients with an even simpler postoperative prophylaxis treatment. This topic is discussed in detail in Chapter 13.

Dehydration and immobility increase the risk of the development of postoperative DVT. Consequently, adequate hydration and encouragement of early postoperative mobilization are advisable. Good analgesia improves mobilization and regional anaesthesia may be particularly helpful in this regard.

Epidural anaesthesia reduces fibrinolysis and activation of clotting factors, reduces the risk of DVT and may reduce the risk of PE. These advantages, and the very small risk of epidural haematoma in patients who have received heparin, must be considered in an overall risk–benefit assessment of the use of epidural anaesthesia or analgesia during and after surgery. Current practice is to wait at least 12 h after the administration of LMWH before insertion of an epidural catheter. A similar interval should be used between administration of LMWH and removal of the epidural catheter.

Correctly applied graduated stockings and intermittent calf compression devices reduce the incidence of DVT, but there may be no extra benefit for patients who receive heparin.

Arterial Tourniquets

Effective exsanguination of a limb and application of an arterial tourniquet greatly improve the visibility of the surgical field, as well as minimizing surgical blood loss. Exsanguination may be performed by elevation of the limb or by wrapping it in a rubber bandage. The tourniquet cuff should be 20% wider than the diameter of the limb; this correlates to approximately one-third of the circumference of the limb. To avoid damage by shearing and compression of skin, nerves and other tissues, the tourniquet should be lined with padding and applied over muscle bulk. To avoid injury from chemical burns, entry of spirit-based cleansing lotions under the cuff must be prevented. This is achieved usually by wrapping adhesive tape round the distal edge of the tourniquet and the adjacent skin.

The pressure in the arterial tourniquet should, in all cases, exceed arterial pressure, but, for reasons explained below, pressures are required that significantly exceed arterial pressure if arterial ooze is to be prevented. For the lower limb, this pressure is typically 300 mmHg (or 150 mmHg above systolic arterial pressure) and for the upper limb, 250 mmHg (or 100 mmHg above systolic arterial pressure). These rather wide margins are used for two reasons. First, the pressure on the measuring gauge is not the same as the effective tourniquet pressure; the narrower the cuff, the greater is the difference. Second, blood pressure commonly increases about 30 min after the tourniquet is inflated. This is not caused by the autotransfusion during exsanguination or by the increased systemic vascular resistance caused by tourniquet inflation, but results probably from activation of C-fibres by ischaemia (mediating 'slow' pain). This pain may be difficult to relieve, and patients whose operation is conducted under regional anaesthesia may find the pain intolerable, and may therefore require general anaesthesia. Some temporary tolerance may be achieved by administration of a short-acting opioid (e.g. alfentanil 250 µg), inhaled nitrous oxide or intravenous ketamine (e.g. 0.2 mg kg^{-1}). Dense regional anaesthesia, whether spinal, epidural or nerve block, may prevent tourniquet pain. However, despite an apparently adequate block, occasions may arise in which the patient becomes intolerant of the tourniquet after some time. The noxious stimulation of tourniquet pain is also apparent during general anaesthesia, when the arterial pressure often increases progressively until the tourniquet is deflated.

Electromyographic and histological changes which follow prolonged application of a tourniquet reverse after deflation. The maximum period of safe ischaemia is unknown. Lasting damage is unlikely if a tourniquet time of 90–120 min is not exceeded. Current practice is that 2 h represents the absolute upper limit of tourniquet inflation time. Brief deflation followed by re-inflation of a tourniquet that has been in place for 2 h is not adequate 'rest' for the limb; several hours are required for restoration of metabolic normality within the limb.

When the tourniquet is deflated, the products of anaerobic metabolism in the limb are released. A bolus of cold, acidic, hypercapnic and hypoxic blood is returned to the circulation. The systemic vascular resistance suddenly decreases, and venous volume increases. This may result in transient cardiovascular changes, including cardiac arrhythmias, myocardial ischaemia and changes in arterial pressure. There may also be an increase in intracranial pressure (which is of importance in patients with reduced intracranial compliance, e.g. as a result of recent head injury). Bleeding may also occur at the operative site. Tourniquets on more than one limb should never be deflated (or inflated) simultaneously.

Tourniquets may cause damage to peripheral tissues, to the tissue underlying the cuff and to the patient as a whole due to the release of altered blood once the tourniquet is deflated. They are contraindicated to differing degrees in patients with poor peripheral circulation, crush injuries, infection and sickle cell disease or trait. The use of a tourniquet in a patient with sickle cell disease may result in within-limb sickling and subsequent ischaemia or thrombosis.

Blood Conservation

An arterial tourniquet is used during a large proportion of orthopaedic operations. Consequently, intraoperative blood loss is often slight. However, tourniquets cannot be used for some procedures, such as hip arthroplasty and shoulder surgery, which may result in significant blood loss. Spinal surgery, in particular, is frequently associated with very extensive blood loss; bleeding from epidural veins is often responsible, and the techniques of blood conservation described below have made possible several spinal surgical procedures which were previously too dangerous to contemplate. Transfusion of donated blood carries significant risks, including cross-infection, hypothermia, clotting dysfunction, electrolyte disturbances, mismatched transfusion and allergic reactions. Donor blood is also a very expensive and rapidly dwindling resource. For these reasons, it is considered appropriate to avoid blood transfusion where possible. Various techniques are in popular use.

Avoidance of Red Cell Loss

The use of a tourniquet significantly reduces blood loss associated with limb surgery (see above). Isovolaemic and hypervolaemic haemodilution have been proposed as methods of reducing the requirement for donor blood, but the evidence for these practices is tenuous. Careful positioning may reduce venous bleeding through the assurance of adequate venous drainage at the surgical site. The maintenance of normothermia avoids hypothermia-induced clotting dysfunction. Epidural and spinal anaesthesia are associated with reduced intraoperative blood loss; this association is probably related to reductions in both arterial and venous pressures.

Cell Salvage

The collection and retransfusion of blood lost during surgery has become popular in recent years. Few contraindications exist, although some of these are relevant in patients presenting for orthopaedic surgery.

- Salvage and retransfusion of blood from a wound containing malignant cells is contraindicated because of the risk of dissemination of tumour cells. Malignant cells are incompletely removed by washing and filtration.

■ Contamination with bowel contents or infection at the site of blood retrieval is a contraindication to salvage and retransfusion. Washing with antibiotic solutions has been shown to be ineffective in neutralizing all bacteria.

■ Salvaged blood which contains topical haemostatic agents such as collagen, cellulose, gelatin and thrombin should not be retransfused as it may result in intravascular coagulation.

■ Salvaged blood which contains surgical irrigants, liquid methylmethacrylate or antibiotics not licensed for parenteral use (e.g. neomycin) should not be retransfused.

Modified Transfusion Triggers

Most modern clinical practice guidelines recommend restrictive red blood cell transfusion practices with the goal of minimizing transmission of blood-borne pathogens. The haemoglobin concentration used as a trigger for transfusion has reduced progressively in recent years as awareness has increased that patients are relatively tolerant of anaemia if they do not have any organs with perfusion or oxygenation problems, and if an adequate cardiac output (and therefore an adequate circulating intravascular volume) is present. The context of the patient's anaemia is also of importance; if the patient is still losing blood, a haemoglobin concentration of $8\,g\,dL^{-1}$ is less tolerable than if bleeding has ceased. Independent of the patient's coexisting pathology, anaemia is less acceptable half-way through a hip arthroplasty than it would be at the end of a knee arthroscopy. Thus, the patient's haemoglobin concentration is relevant, but must be considered together with coexisting organ function and oxygenation (e.g. angina, renal dysfunction, transient ischaemic attacks), the nature of the operation and the timing of the measurement in relation to the progress of the procedure.

Healthy patients tolerate a haemoglobin concentration of $7\,g\,dL^{-1}$ well if they have no additional requirements for physiological reserve. It may be safer to use a higher trigger than this for patients with known organ malperfusion. The adoption of lower transfusion triggers for patients undergoing surgery mandates that intravascular volume is maintained meticulously, because anaemia is tolerated poorly in the presence of a reduced cardiac output. It is also necessary to check the patient's haemoglobin concentration frequently during the operation and in the early postoperative period; this is performed easily using a HemoCue® haemoglobinometer.

Hypotensive Anaesthesia

Intentional reduction of the systemic arterial pressure is rarely indicated in orthopaedic surgery. The risk of poor perfusion of vital organs makes this a potentially dangerous technique, and other options exist to avoid donor blood transfusion and to maintain a clear surgical field.

SPECIFIC SURGICAL PROCEDURES

Primary Hip Arthroplasty

The operation is performed in either a supine or a modified lateral position. The femoral head is removed, and the new cup and femoral components are fixed to prepared bone with polymethylmethacrylate cement. Application and hardening of the cement, particularly after its insertion into the femoral shaft, are sometimes accompanied by sudden reductions in end-tidal CO_2 concentration and arterial pressure. Although attributable in part to toxic monomers released as the cement polymerizes, the high incidences of these changes reported when the technique was relatively new were probably related to a high frequency of air embolism; air was forced into the circulation as the prosthesis was pushed into the femoral shaft. Techniques such as filling the shaft with cement from the bottom upwards, or venting the shaft with a cannula, have dramatically reduced the incidence of adverse events. However, insertion of cement may still cause embolism of marrow, fat or blood clots. Embolization of air is also possible if the intramedullary pressure increases above venous pressure. Intramedullary pressure reaches its highest values when intact bone is first opened and reamed.

Regional anaesthesia is regarded by many anaesthetists as the preferred technique for hip replacement (see above) and immediate postoperative pain may be controlled by the addition of a spinal opioid to the local anaesthetic used. Blood loss is rarely large during primary replacement but vigilance is required, as assessment is made difficult by the large volumes of irrigation fluid used during the operation. Temperature homeostasis should be maintained by the use of active warming devices such as a warm air blanket.

To reduce the risk of dislocation of the new joint, the patient is placed supine in an abduction splint at the end of the procedure. This device makes it difficult to move the patient, and extra assistance is needed if the patient needs to be turned during the immediate recovery phase. After the first few postoperative hours, analgesic requirements are usually fairly low, irrespective of the anaesthetic technique employed. Newer enhanced recovery strategies involve extensive infiltration of the whole joint capsule with a large volume of dilute local anaesthetic (plus a variety of adjuvant agents), to allow early mobilization and encourage rapid recovery following surgery.

Hip Resurfacing Arthroplasty

This is a more recently developed surgical technique for primary hip arthroplasty with the advantage that only the joint surfaces are removed during surgery. Most of the normal bone is preserved, including the femoral head and neck. The medullary canal is not opened and no femoral stem prosthesis is necessary. It is an operation designed to postpone definitive joint replacement in younger patients with progressive disease. The operation is intended to interfere minimally with the normal mechanics of the joint and it is also anticipated that the longevity of the prosthesis should be greater than when a rigid stem prosthesis is placed in elastic bone. The anaesthetic management for this procedure is essentially the same as for traditional primary hip arthroplasty. The risk of embolic events is low because of the reduced bone destruction and lack of exposure of the femoral medullary canal.

Revision of Hip Replacement

Hip prostheses have a finite life, and increasing numbers of patients present for removal of the original prosthesis and insertion of a new one. This procedure is of longer duration and usually involves greater blood loss than primary hip replacement. General anaesthesia, often combined with a regional block, is used commonly. In addition to the precautions for primary hip replacement, central venous and invasive arterial pressure monitoring may be considered. A bladder catheter should be inserted to monitor urine output. Greater heat loss is experienced because of the increased length of the procedure and particular attention needs to be paid to maintenance

of core temperature to reduce intraoperative coagulation abnormalities and postoperative complications. The use of blood conservation techniques such as intraoperative cell salvage should be considered. Replacement clotting factors may be required to correct abnormalities of coagulation if major blood loss occurs. Patients who have undergone revision of a hip replacement may require a period of high-dependency care postoperatively.

Dislocation of a Prosthetic Hip

This needs manipulation and reduction to relieve pain and is more urgent if posterior dislocation threatens the sciatic nerve; this is more likely after trauma. Usually, a brief general anaesthetic without neuromuscular blockade suffices; if reduction is difficult, muscle relaxation may be required. It is often unrealistic to move the patient from the bed before inducing anaesthesia, but precautions against regurgitation and aspiration of gastric fluid, including antacids and rapid sequence induction, may be indicated if urgent reduction is required or if the patient has been receiving systemic opioid analgesics (which delay gastric emptying). Usually, the patient wakes up with less pain than before manipulation.

Knee Replacement

Spinal or general anaesthesia are appropriate techniques for this operation. Knee replacement is performed with the patient in the supine position. Pain after knee replacement is more severe than after most other major joint replacements. Administration of a spinal opioid or performance of sciatic and 3-in-1 (femoral sheath) blocks results in prolonged analgesia. Paracetamol and NSAIDs should be prescribed on a regular basis (if there are no contraindications), together with an opioid. Again, newer enhanced recovery strategies involve extensive infiltration of the whole joint capsule with a large volume of dilute local anaesthetic (plus a variety of adjuvant agents) to allow early mobilization and encourage rapid recovery following surgery.

There is less risk of thromboembolism after knee replacement than after other major joint replacements. Close observation for evidence of hypotension and cardiac arrhythmias, particularly in frail patients, is required following deflation of the tourniquet as the products of cellular metabolism are washed out of the tissues into the circulation. Significant blood loss may occur when the tourniquet is deflated and it may be necessary to reassess fluid and blood transfusion needs in the early recovery period. Specialized drains, which collect postoperative blood loss and allow immediate retransfusion, are often inserted by the surgeon.

Manipulation under anaesthesia is sometimes needed in the postoperative period. Muscle relaxants are not required. Depending on the extent of manipulation, intravenous opioid analgesia may be required to control pain, especially in the first hour after the procedure. Nerve blocks may be given to aid passive mobilization of the joint following the procedure.

Shoulder Replacement

Patients undergoing shoulder replacement are often younger than those requiring hip or knee arthroplasty. They usually mobilize more rapidly in the postoperative period and rarely require a prolonged infusion of intravenous fluids or blood transfusion.

During surgery, the patient is placed in a lateral or 'deckchair' position. The patient's head is relatively inaccessible during the procedure; tracheal intubation with a reinforced tube provides a secure airway. Surgery often involves vigorous manipulation of the arm, so the head needs to be fixed firmly to the operating table. To avoid sudden hypotension, elevation to the deckchair position should be undertaken with a freely running intravenous infusion, with vasopressors available. Because the shoulder is above the heart during surgery, there is a risk of air embolism. Interscalene brachial plexus block with insertion of a catheter provides effective analgesia after surgery; indeed, it is possible to carry out the whole procedure under this block in combination with judicious sedation. Transient neuropraxia may be attributed to these blocks but, as with lower limb surgery, this is more likely to be caused by the surgical procedure. After other operations on the shoulder, when no prosthesis is inserted and the infection risk is lower, intermittent injections of local anaesthetic through a subacromial catheter may be used for pain management. More peripheral blockade of the nerve supply to the shoulder (suprascapular and axillary) may also be carried out to provide postoperative analgesia.

Spinal Surgery

Spinal surgery is a major orthopaedic subspecialty. It provides several challenges for the anaesthetist; these include massive blood loss, difficult airway management, single-lung ventilation and consideration of a variety of pathologies seldom seen outside this surgical population. Spinal surgical procedures include trauma surgery, vertebral fusion, laminectomy and correction of scoliosis. The very young and the very old may present for spinal surgery.

Active warming is required during most procedures to prevent hypothermia caused by extensive surgical exposure through a long wound, blood transfusion and laminar airflow systems.

Airway management may be difficult in patients with cervical spine instability; these patients may have external spinal fixation. Patients with a cervical spinal cord injury may develop autonomic hyperreflexia and cardiovascular instability. Succinylcholine may produce a dangerous increase in serum potassium concentration in patients who have a denervating spinal cord injury which is more than 24 h old. This is caused by a proliferation of nicotinic cholinergic receptors at the neuromuscular junction. Difficult airway management skills are often needed to achieve tracheal intubation in patients with an anatomical abnormality of the spine, e.g. ankylosing spondylitis or scoliosis.

Scoliosis is associated with neuromuscular diseases in many patients. There is some evidence that such diseases (e.g. muscular dystrophies) may be associated with an increased risk of malignant hyperthermia or a malignant hyperthermia-like syndrome of abnormal metabolism in muscles, with a rapid and progressive increase in core temperature. There may also be increased difficulty with spontaneous ventilation in the postoperative period because of muscle weakness.

Patients with scoliosis may have severely limited respiratory function (e.g. a restrictive defect due to scoliosis) and may be at risk of increased intraoperative bleeding. Single-lung ventilation is often required to achieve adequate surgical access during the correction of thoracic scoliosis.

Spinal cord function may be compromised during correction of scoliosis because of ischaemia caused by excessive straightening of the spine. Spinal cord integrity may be tested using an intraoperative wake-up test. This requires preoperative psychological preparation of the patient and a suitable anaesthetic technique. However, the wake-up test has been superseded almost entirely by advances in spinal cord monitoring techniques including somatosensory and motor evoked potential recording, which give an early warning of compromised spinal cord blood supply during surgery to correct scoliosis.

Peripheral Surgery

Most peripheral orthopaedic surgery may be carried out in the day-case setting. If general anaesthesia is required, a simple inhalational technique usually suffices. Regional techniques provide excellent analgesia postoperatively and reduce the degree of disability which the patient suffers. Regional techniques may obviate the need for general anaesthesia and may lead to earlier discharge and a high level of patient satisfaction. There is increasing interest in the use of regional techniques for both intraoperative and postoperative management; one or more catheters are inserted at the time of operation, and used to infuse a local anaesthetic. It is easy to underestimate the degree of pain and disability that the patient may experience following peripheral orthopaedic operations. Analgesia should be prescribed on a regular basis postoperatively and additional 'as required' analgesia should be made available. Regular paracetamol, NSAIDs and opioids, if required and not contraindicated, should be prescribed. At the end of many procedures, a plaster cast is applied. If anaesthesia ends before the plaster hardens, the patient may move, break the cast and need to be reanaesthetized.

FURTHER READING

Auroy, Y., Narchi, P., Messiah, A., et al., 1997. Serious complications related to regional anesthesia: results of a prospective survey in France. Anesthesiology 87, 479–486.

British Medical Association and Royal Pharmaceutical Society. Cautions and contra-indications of corticosteroids. In: British National Formulary, June 2013. http://www.medicinescomplete.com/mc/

Singelyn, F.J., Deyaert, M., Joris, D., et al., 1998. Effects of intravenous patient-controlled analgesia with morphine, continuous epidural analgesia, and continuous three-in-one block on postoperative pain and knee rehabilitation after unilateral total knee arthroplasty. Anesth. Analg. 87, 88–92.

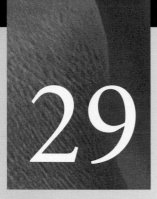

29

ANAESTHESIA FOR ENT, MAXILLOFACIAL AND DENTAL SURGERY

■ ■ ■ ■ ■ ■ ■ ■ ■ ■

E ar, nose and throat (ENT), maxillofacial and dental surgical procedures account for a significant proportion of work in most anaesthetic departments. Recent cost-benefit and evidence-based analyses have reduced the number of common procedures performed such as tonsillectomy, insertion of grommets and removal of impacted wisdom teeth. Bodies such as the National Institute for Health and Clinical Excellence (NICE) have reviewed the evidence relating to many procedures and developed rigorous guidelines for referral and intervention.

Other trends in surgical practice have offset this reduction, e.g. the prevalence of alcohol-related facial trauma and the increasing use of surgery in the treatment and palliation of cancer of the head and neck. The incidence of these cancers, particularly of the oral cavity, presents a significant and increasing global burden of disease.

The development of anaesthetic practice in these areas has therefore been concentrated on increasing the use of day-case surgery for more minor procedures and facilitating long and technically challenging operations to remove tumours and reconstruct defects. The effect of surgical pathology on the upper airway continues to require meticulous attention to airway management and has led to the proliferation of new devices and techniques to overcome difficult intubation.

ENT SURGERY

The Shared Airway

Special problems are caused when the airway is shared by both anaesthetist and surgeon (Table 29.1). If bleeding is anticipated, the airway *must* be protected and the oropharynx may be packed to avoid contamination of the larynx with blood, pus and other debris. If a pack is

TABLE 29.1
Potential Problems Associated with the Shared Airway
Disconnection of tracheal tube
Dislodgement of tracheal tube
Access for surgeon or anaesthetist
Airway soiling
Tube damage, e.g. laser
Lack of visual confirmation of ventilation
Eye care

used, it should either be labelled or the tail left obviously emerging from the mouth as a reminder that it must be removed at the end of the operation. The anaesthetic circuit connections are usually hidden under the drapes and may well be 'knocked' by the surgeon during the procedure. Anaesthetic disconnections are, therefore, a constant threat. It is important to realize that disconnections on the machine side of the capnograph sampling tube, in a patient who is breathing spontaneously, does not lead to a loss of the capnograph trace and so careful observation of the reservoir bag is mandatory.

At the end of the procedure, the pack, if present, must be removed and the pharynx cleared of blood and debris before the trachea is extubated with the patient in a head-down lateral position. The fact that a pack was used and has been removed should be recorded.

Tonsillectomy

The number of tonsillectomy operations has decreased by about a third since 1996, but there are still approximately 50 000 procedures performed annually

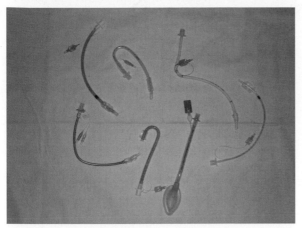

FIGURE 29.1 ■ Various tubes used in ENT and oromaxillofacial surgery. Clockwise from top left: armoured tracheal tube, south-facing moulded tracheal tube, north-facing moulded tracheal tube, microlaryngoscopy tube, armoured LMA, laryngectomy tube, laser tube.

in England, just under half of which are in children. Almost all are performed under general anaesthesia, with 34% undertaken as day-case surgery.

Premedication is frequently impractical with modern admission practices but robust preoperative assessment is mandatory, in particular to obtain any history of obstructive sleep apnoea or other airway problems. Often, the patient is young and otherwise fit, and routine investigations are unnecessary.

Surgical access to the pharynx requires the insertion of a Boyle Davis gag. To facilitate this, a secure airway is usually maintained with a 'south-facing' moulded tracheal tube (Fig. 29.1). Alternatively, a reinforced laryngeal mask airway (LMA) can be used successfully provided that the surgeon carefully avoids displacement of the LMA during the insertion and removal of the gag.

Spontaneous ventilation following the use of a short-acting muscle relaxant can be used to facilitate deep extubation in the lateral head-down position to protect the airway from soiling during emergence. Alternatively, positive pressure ventilation can be maintained throughout the procedure, with extubation fully awake in the sitting position. Various surgical techniques can be employed including cold steel dissection, electrodiathermy, laser and coblation. Blood loss can be significant and vigilance must be

maintained regarding fluid replacement; however, blood transfusion is rarely necessary.

Tonsillectomy is painful and requires adequate postoperative analgesia. This frequently involves a multimodal approach with an initial dose of intravenous morphine together with paracetamol and a non-steroidal anti-inflammatory drug (NSAID). The latter can be given orally before surgery or parenterally during the procedure. Some evidence may point towards an increased risk of bleeding associated with the use of NSAIDs, but this is not clear-cut and most centres use this combination of drugs to facilitate early discharge. Multimodal antiemetic therapy should also be used because postoperative nausea and vomiting is a frequent cause of delay in discharge. There is also evidence to support the use of steroids for control of emesis and pain, usually as a single dose of dexamethasone. Some evidence supports the use of topical or locally infiltrated local anaesthetic. The early establishment of oral intake of food, fluids and analgesia encourages early discharge and should enable most operations to be performed as a day-case.

Adenoidectomy

This is a commonly performed operation in children to improve the symptoms of otitis media with effusion, and chronic rhinosinusitis. It is often combined with tonsillectomy and insertion of grommets. Recent systematic reviews have questioned the evidence of efficacy of adenoid surgery and therefore the frequency is decreasing. Adenoidectomy is also performed occasionally in adults for glue ear.

As in tonsillectomy, good access to the pharynx is required, usually with a Boyle Davis gag, and therefore airway control with a 'south-facing' tracheal tube or reinforced LMA is employed. Adenoidectomy as a sole procedure is usually rather quicker and less painful than tonsillectomy and may not require long-acting opioid pain control.

Rigid Endoscopy and Microlaryngoscopy

Rigid endoscopy is performed commonly in ENT to facilitate examination, biopsy and treatment of abnormalities of the upper aerodigestive tract.

General anaesthesia is required, usually with tracheal intubation to provide a safe airway during surgery. Provided that no difficulty with intubation is

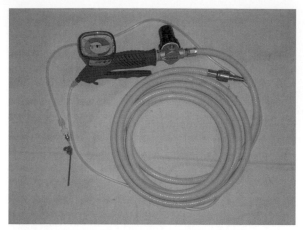

FIGURE 29.2 ■ Jet insufflator (note connection to attach to rigid endoscope).

predicted, intravenous or gaseous induction is followed by the administration of a muscle relaxant dependent on the anticipated duration of the procedure. In general, a small cuffed (microlaryngoscopy) tube with internal diameter 4–6 mm is inserted into the trachea to allow the surgeon greater access to the pharynx. This should be placed in the left side of the mouth to allow passage of the rigid endoscope down the right.

Examination, with or without biopsy, is usually of a short duration and mivacurium or suxamethonium is often used. Increasingly however, the operating microscope is used to resect neoplasms of the upper airway, especially laryngeal carcinoma, allowing less invasive damage to voice function. These operations may be prolonged, requiring attention to normothermia and fluid balance. Microlaryngeal tumour resection is often carried out using a precision laser cutting tool which requires either a tube specifically designed to tolerate lasers or extreme care on the part of the surgeon to avoid the risk of damage to the tube and potential airway fire. Short-acting opioids provide balanced anaesthesia but morphine may be required for longer operations. Blood loss is not usually significant and is often controlled by the topical application of adrenaline with or without local anaesthetic. Safe extubation is normally achieved with full emergence and recovery of airway reflexes, and careful pharyngeal suction prior to the removal of the tube.

Occasionally, the surgeon requires access to the larynx without the presence of a tracheal tube. In this situation, oxygenation can be provided by jet insufflation of the lungs via a subglottic catheter or an attachment to the endoscope (Fig. 29.2). The catheter can be inserted into the trachea either down the endoscope or through the cricothyroid membrane. Anaesthesia is maintained using an intravenous agent, usually propofol.

Thyroid Surgery

Thyroid surgery is increasingly performed by specialist ENT surgeons although some general surgeons still undertake the operation.

Preoperative assessment of the anatomy of any goitre, usually by computed tomography, is vital to predict any impact on the ease of intubation of the trachea or ventilation of the lungs. Preoperative assessment also allows the surgical access route to be planned; this is usually via the neck, but may require intrathoracic access such as a sternal split if significant retrosternal extension of the tumour exists. Medical management of thyroid disease must be optimized preoperatively because abnormalities such as a thyroid storm can cause gross physiological problems intraoperatively.

For routine thyroid surgery via the neck, it is sufficient to provide balanced general anaesthesia usually, using a reinforced tracheal tube to allow the operative area to be draped safely without risking occlusion of the tube. If the goitre is causing significant subglottic stenosis without stridor, a small tube must be available which will pass easily through the stenosed area. If the stenosis extends into the chest towards and beyond the carina, specialized thoracic techniques such as bronchial intubation may be required. If any difficulty is anticipated in securing ventilation or if stridor exists, intravenous hypnotics and muscle relaxants are contraindicated until a definitive airway has been established.

Tracheostomy

Surgical tracheostomy is usually performed in a sedated or anaesthetized intubated patient. Occasionally, emergency tracheostomy is required in the unintubated patient, for example in stridor, and may even take place under local anaesthetic if general anaesthesia with a secure airway cannot be performed (see ENT emergencies below). Many procedures now take place percutaneously on the intensive care unit. If surgical tracheostomy is required, the patient is stabilized and the lungs ventilated in thc operating theatre with the head and neck extended to allow access. When the surgeon has dissected down to the trachea, the lungs are ventilated with 100% oxygen and the tracheal tube is withdrawn carefully into the proximal trachea to allow the tracheal window to be excised without perforating the cuff. At this point, positive pressure ventilation of the lungs becomes impossible but in the event of surgical failure to insert the tracheostomy tube, the anaesthetic tracheal tube can be advanced back down the trachea past the defect to allow ventilation to be reinstituted. After the tracheostomy tube has been inserted, the breathing system is connected to it and ventilation confirmed with visualization, auscultation and capnography. The anaesthetic tube may be removed and discarded after the tracheostomy tube has been secured.

Nasal and Sinus Surgery

Various operations are performed on the nose and sinuses to treat and prevent epistaxis, to improve the nasal airway, to reduce the symptoms of chronic rhinosinusitis or to improve the external appearance of the nose. Nearly all can be performed as day-case procedures. Major invasive access to the nasal sinuses such as the Caldwell Luc procedure have largely been replaced by the use of endoscopic sinus surgery which is more cost-effective in terms of symptom relief.

Most nasal procedures in the UK are performed under general anaesthesia and range from simple diathermy of the inferior turbinates to prolonged cosmetic external rhinoplasty. The application of a mixture of topical local anaesthetic agents and other adjuncts (e.g. Moffat's solution, which is a mixture of cocaine, adrenaline and bicarbonate) provides vasoconstriction before surgery. The airway must be secured to allow the delivery of oxygen and a volatile anaesthetic agent and also to protect the trachea from soiling by blood from the operative site. This can be achieved satisfactorily by the use of a reinforced LMA if there are no specific indications for tracheal intubation such as obesity or the expectation of a prolonged operation. Special attention must be paid to avoid disconnection or occlusion of the breathing system by the surgeon, or soiling of the trachea. Balanced anaesthesia is achieved using increments of a short-acting

opioid or a longer-acting drug for prolonged or painful procedures. Careful pharyngeal suction is performed at the end of surgery to ensure the removal of blood and other debris which may have accumulated. The use of a pharyngeal pack is generally unnecessary but, if used, it is vital to ensure that it has been removed before emergence. Serious complications, including death, have been reported after failure to remove a throat pack. The usual principles applying to day-case anaesthesia are adhered to including preoperative assessment and postoperative care (see Ch 26).

Ear Surgery

Examination under anaesthetic, suction clearance and myringotomy with insertion of grommets are extremely common operations, particularly in children, and are performed to relieve the symptoms of chronic otitis media with effusion and to improve hearing. They may be combined with adenoidectomy and tonsillectomy for recurrent tonsillitis or chronic rhinosinusitis. Recent guidance published by NICE may reduce the prevalence of surgical management of these conditions. In general, these are quick operations requiring attention to the principles of paediatric day-case anaesthesia. Postoperative pain is usually managed with a combination of paracetamol and an NSAID to allow early discharge.

More complex procedures are performed on the structures of the ear using a microscope (Fig. 29.3), such as tympanoplasty to repair defects in the tympanic membrane, mastoidectomy to reduce the risk of abscess and infection in the mastoid air cells and stapedectomy to improve hearing in otosclerosis. These are performed under general anaesthesia, increasingly as day-case procedures. Moderate hypotension has been employed to minimize bleeding in the operative field but hypotensive agents such as β-blockers and vasodilators have largely been superseded by the use of short-acting narcotic agents given by intermittent bolus or infusion. These provide smooth anaesthesia without variations in blood pressure associated with surgical bleeding, which can obscure the surgeon's view through the microscope. If hypotensive anaesthesia is to be employed, care should be taken to maintain vital organ perfusion and keep the mean arterial pressure above the lower limit of autoregulation of about 55 mmHg. In general, these techniques

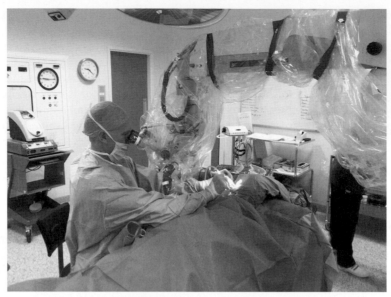

FIGURE 29.3 ■ Ear surgery.

require positive pressure ventilation with an element of muscle relaxation. A 'south-facing' moulded tracheal tube or reinforced LMA can be used. Nitrous oxide is avoided in the gas mixture because it can increase the pressure in the middle ear, thereby increasing the risk of graft failure. Postoperative pain is not usually severe and can usually be managed using oral analgesia, often allowing same-day discharge.

ENT Emergencies

Bleeding Tonsil

Primary haemorrhage occurs in the immediate postoperative period, usually in the recovery room, whereas secondary haemorrhage occurs at home some days later and may present via the Emergency Department. Blood loss may be profound and, occasionally, death still occurs as a result of post-tonsillectomy haemorrhage. Initial treatment involves attention to the primary goals of life support with the establishment of good intravenous access and volume resuscitation as well as the administration of oxygen. A blood sample must be sent for urgent cross-match. Emphasis has been placed on restoration of blood volume and pressure before induction of anaesthesia but in the face of profuse active bleeding, urgent surgical haemostasis is of paramount importance. Most experienced practitioners advocate a rapid sequence induction of

anaesthesia with cricoid pressure because the stomach may be full of blood. Preoxygenation is often difficult with the patient sitting up regularly spitting out blood, but it is vital. As soon as loss of consciousness has been achieved, the patient is placed in the supine position and the trachea is intubated as quickly as possible, with suction readily available. Alternatively, gaseous induction can take place in the left lateral head-down position and the trachea intubated under deep inhalational anaesthesia. When haemostasis has been achieved, full resuscitation takes place. Restoration of normal blood pressure must be ensured to reveal all potential bleeding points. Consideration can then be given to postoperative management, which will depend on the condition of the patient.

Epistaxis

Common causes of epistaxis include surgery, trauma and spontaneous epistaxis, the last particularly in elderly hypertensive patients. Blood loss can be profound and resuscitative measures may be necessary. General anaesthesia may be required to facilitate anterior or posterior packing of the nose, ligation of the sphenopalatine or anterior ethmoid arteries (often done endoscopically) and occasionally exploration of the neck to tie off the external carotid artery. Elderly patients are often on long-term anticoagulant therapy which may require urgent reversal using vitamin K and/or plasma derivatives, and blood samples must be sent for cross-matching. The patient has usually ingested significant amounts of blood and rapid sequence induction with tracheal intubation is mandatory. If haemorrhage is swift and ongoing, preoxygenation may take place in the sitting position with immediate transition to the supine position with the application of cricoid pressure as soon as consciousness is lost. When surgical control has been achieved, normal blood pressure must be restored to reveal any further bleeding points prior to emergence and extubation fully awake. Occasionally, if surgical control is incomplete or tenuous, it may be prudent to keep the patient sedated with the trachea intubated to allow for full correction of clotting abnormalities and for clots to form and organize before extubation.

Epiglottitis and Stridor

Epiglottitis is an acute life-threatening illness characterized by inflammation of the epiglottis and surrounding structures which can progress rapidly to complete airway obstruction. Previously, it was considered to be primarily a disease of childhood but since the introduction of routine *H influenzae* type B vaccination, it is now seen less frequently in children and is more common in adults. Presentation commonly involves a combination of one or more of drooling, dysphagia and distress, often with other signs of systemic illness such as fever. The onset of respiratory symptoms such as breathlessness or stridor indicates an extreme emergency and action should be taken to secure the airway. The cause is usually *H influenzae* type B bacterial infection (even in previously immunized individuals) and treatment involves airway support and intravenous antibiotics. If progression of airway compromise is anticipated, intubation of the trachea is indicated. Airway management may be very difficult and senior anaesthetic and ENT support must be summoned urgently. Tracheal intubation should take place if possible in an operating theatre environment with ENT surgical support and equipment immediately available, including facilities for rigid bronchoscopy and emergency tracheostomy. Fear and stimulation are known to worsen the airway compromise, and it is recommended that attempted venous access should not be undertaken in a child before induction of anaesthesia.

Intubation may be difficult because of distortion of the laryngeal anatomy and most experts advocate inhalational induction with laryngoscopy under a deep plane of anaesthesia, with equipment for difficult intubation readily to hand. In the adult, fibreoptic-assisted intubation has been recommended. The trachea must remain intubated on an intensive care unit until it is confirmed that the swelling has largely subsided, usually by fibreoptic nasendoscopy. If ventilation becomes compromised before intubation, creation of an emergency surgical airway may be necessary.

Stridor, defined as a harsh high-pitched noise of breathing usually on inspiration, may also be due to other pathologies. Treatment is aimed at resolving the cause but in the face of worsening respiratory distress, emergency intubation of the trachea may be required. The anaesthetic management principles are as above; senior anaesthetic and ENT personnel must be available and intubation should take place in an operating theatre environment. In general, supraglottic stridor caused by neoplasm or abscess may cause extreme difficulty in rigid laryngoscopy and specialized methods must be available such as flexible fibreoptic endoscopy or retrograde intubation. In the event of failure, rapid surgical access to the airway may be necessary. In the presence of periglottic stridor, e.g. caused by laryngeal neoplasia, or subglottic stridor, e.g. due to thyroid disease, tracheal intubation can usually be achieved using a rigid laryngoscope under deep inhalational anaesthesia. Intravenous hypnotics or muscle relaxants must *never* be administered to a stridulous patient before securing the airway.

ORAL AND MAXILLOFACIAL SURGERY

Oral Surgery

The scope of modern oral surgical practice under anaesthesia continues to encompass primarily the removal of impacted teeth and treatment of associated dental pathology which cannot be dealt with under local anaesthesia by either the dentist or the oral surgeon due to the severity of the disease or the inability of the patient to tolerate dental procedures. Referral guidelines now restrict the removal of impacted third molar teeth only to patients who are symptomatic, which has reduced the incidence of those operations.

Consideration must be given to the principles of management of the shared airway and often nasotracheal intubation is required to allow a safe airway with good surgical access to the mouth. Careful attention is paid to the correct length of tube, and visualization of the reservoir bag and capnography. The muscle relaxant used is determined by the anticipated length of the procedure and whether the anaesthetist prefers to use a spontaneous breathing technique or positive pressure ventilation. In simple surgery, the anaesthetist and surgeon may elect to work around a laryngeal mask airway but vigilance is required to avoid displacement or disconnection, leading to ventilation problems. The use of a throat pack is largely historical because the surgeon should pay close attention to pharyngeal toilet at all times and the airway used should protect the trachea from soiling. Extubation may occur either under deep anaesthesia in the lateral head-down position, or fully awake. Most procedures are undertaken as day-cases and the principles of pain control involve a multimodal combination of local anaesthetic infiltrated by the surgeon, simple analgesics, and NSAIDs. Strong opioids are rarely required.

Orthognathic Surgery

Patients with severe facial architecture abnormalities or bite asymmetry problems may present for treatment requiring mandibular or maxillary osteotomy and advancement procedures. This occurs generally at a young age with minimal comorbidities but requires a general anaesthetic, usually lasting for several hours. Difficult laryngoscopy may be anticipated in patients with a severely retrognathic mandible and can require flexible fibreoptic intubation. Nasotracheal intubation is necessary and attention must be paid to fluid balance and intraoperative temperature control. Prophylactic intravenous antibiotics are given because microplates and screws are inserted to fix the skeleton into the new position. Postoperative pain and swelling can be severe and patients are often monitored on a high dependency unit and given ice packs and morphine if required. Postoperative jaw wiring is rarely indicated but multimodal antiemetic therapy is still important, including dexamethasone, which may reduce swelling as well as emesis. Paediatric orthognathic surgery, e.g. for cleft lip or palate repair, may also be performed by oromaxillofacial surgeons.

Facial Trauma and Fractures

In the field of maxillofacial trauma, the anaesthetist may be called upon to provide help in the treatment of the acutely injured patient in the Emergency Department or, more commonly, in the operating theatre for scheduled repair of facial fractures sustained previously.

Facial trauma due to road traffic accidents became less common after the implementation of legislation relating to seat belts and driving while intoxicated, but this has been more than offset in the UK by the increase in alcohol-related violent injury. The management of trauma follows the principles of resuscitation of airway, breathing and circulation and this is the primary goal particularly in victims of polytrauma. In facial trauma, airway difficulties may result from obstruction, disruption of normal anatomy, intoxication and cervical spine immobilization. Emergency tracheal intubation may be required if the clinical features of respiratory obstruction, hypoxaemia or coma are progressing and also if the anticipated course of events is likely to lead to airway compromise, e.g. facial burns. In these circumstances, rapid sequence induction of anaesthesia with rigorous preoxygenation and cricoid pressure is the technique of choice if extreme difficulty in intubation is not anticipated. Equipment must be available for difficult laryngoscopy such as the gum elastic bougie and McCoy laryngoscope, and senior anaesthetic personnel familiar with these techniques must be present. In the event of failure to intubate the trachea, a plan must be in place to maintain oxygenation if bag-mask ventilation is difficult. This may involve the laryngeal mask airway followed by cricothyroid airway access if that fails. If intubation using direct laryngoscopy is predicted to be extremely difficult or impossible, awake intubation may be necessary, or tracheostomy can be performed under local anaesthesia. Either technique can be challenging in the intoxicated and combative individual. Some advocate the 'awake look' which involves gentle insertion of the laryngoscope before anaesthesia to ascertain whether a good view of the posterior pharyngeal structures can be obtained. If this is satisfactory, intravenous induction of anaesthesia may be attempted safely.

Patients with facial fractures usually present for reduction and fixation 24–48 h after injury, when swelling has subsided, intoxication is no longer present and the presence of a significant head injury has been excluded. Depending on the mechanism of injury, the fracture may be mandibular, mid-face or isolated fractures of the zygoma or orbit. General anaesthesia is required and tracheal intubation is necessary in all but the simplest zygomatic elevation in a starved patient. Attention must be paid to the principles of the shared airway and consideration given to the optimal route of access to allow surgical intervention to proceed. Rarely, difficult intubation may be encountered because of anatomical disruption or residual swelling. Reduced mouth opening is usually caused by pain and stiffness. Most repairs of the mandible or mid-face involve intraoperative intermaxillary fixation to optimize postoperative function and nasotracheal intubation is required. Isolated orbital or zygomatic repairs can be managed with a 'south-facing' oral tube. Occasionally, nasotracheal intubation is not possible if complex repairs involving the naso-ethmoidal bony skeleton are also to be undertaken, or if a fracture of the base of the skull is suspected (which may occur in Le Fort III fractures of the mid-face). In these circumstances, tracheostomy may be required or, alternatively, submental intubation in which the tube is passed via an incision in the floor of the mouth through the oral cavity and into the trachea.

When the operation has been completed, the tracheal tube can be removed safely and the patient should be nursed in an environment in which postoperative pain and swelling can be monitored and treated.

ANAESTHESIA FOR HEAD & NECK CANCER SURGERY

Tumours of the head and neck can arise from the lips, oral cavity, salivary glands, nose or nasal sinuses, oropharynx, hypopharynx or larynx. Worldwide, cancer of the mouth and oropharynx is the tenth most commonly occurring form of cancer. The tumours are most commonly squamous cell carcinomas which metastasize to lymph nodes in the neck. Neck disease may present with an unknown primary which can often be identified by examination or radiological scanning. Squamous cell carcinomas are known to be associated with alcohol and tobacco use, and increase in incidence with age. However in the UK and other developed countries, for reasons which are unclear, there has been

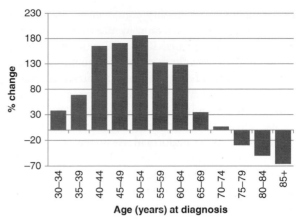

FIGURE 29.4 ■ Percentage changes in incidence of oral cancer in different age groups in the UK 1975–2007. *Prepared by Cancer Research UK. Original data sources:*
1. *Office for National Statistics. Cancer Statistics: Registrations Series MB1. http://www.statistics.gov.uk/statbase/Product.asp?vlnk=8843.*
2. *Welsh Cancer Intelligence and Surveillance Unit. http://www.wcisu. wales.nhs.uk.*
3. *Information Services Division Scotland. Cancer Information Programme. www.isdscotland.org/cancer.*
4. *N. Ireland Cancer Registry. www.qub.ac.uk/nicr.*

a recent increase in the incidence of oral cancer in the age group 40 to 65 years, particularly in men (Fig. 29.4). Surgery, radiotherapy or chemotherapy may be the primary treatment modality depending on patient factors and the staging of the disease. Combinations are often used. Surgical resection may be performed by ENT surgeons or maxillofacial surgeons depending on the site of the tumour, and the expertise of plastic surgeons may be used for the reconstruction of defects. Anaesthesia must create conditions which allow surgery to take place safely, ensuring physiological support of all systems, lack of awareness, pain control and excellent surgical access.

Laryngectomy

Small superficial tumours of the larynx are treated surgically by laser microlaryngoscopy (see above) or by partial or hemilaryngectomy. Total laryngectomy is performed for more advanced disease, usually without neck dissection because tumours of the glottis rarely metastasize to the neck. Preoperative assessment of patients for laryngectomy must establish whether there is any evidence of respiratory compromise, which may be due to airway obstruction by the tumour or concurrent smoking-related illness. Flexible endoscopic examination of the glottis and CT staging of the neck can be used to predict difficulty in direct laryngoscopy. Tumours at the glottic level rarely present difficulty in intubation and, if no respiratory obstruction exists, intravenous induction followed by tracheal intubation can be performed. A smaller non-cuffed tube may be required if there is significant glottic or subglottic stenosis. If respiratory obstruction with stridor is present, inhalational induction and laryngoscopy under deep inhalational anaesthesia should be performed. Fibreoptic intubation may be necessary if difficult laryngoscopy is encountered or predicted, e.g. because of radiation-induced scarring of the floor of the mouth. During surgery, an end-tracheostomy is fashioned and a tracheostomy tube is inserted after the trachea has been divided below the larynx. To facilitate the division, the oral tracheal tube must first be withdrawn proximally and the lungs ventilated with 100% oxygen. The operation usually lasts for several hours and attention must be paid to intraoperative warming, monitoring and fluid balance.

Excision of Salivary Glands

Access may be intra- or extra-oral; in the former, nasotracheal intubation may be required. Otherwise, standard general anaesthesia using an orotracheal tube is appropriate. Operations on the parotid gland may be prolonged and it may be necessary to reverse neuromuscular blockade during surgery so that the surgeon can use a peripheral nerve stimulator to identify branches of the facial nerve. An infusions of a potent short-acting narcotic analgesic such as remifentanil can facilitate this.

Neck Dissection

This may be performed as a curative procedure or for local control of disease. It is usually combined with excision of the primary lesion, which may be oropharyngeal or nasal, but it is performed occasionally as a sole procedure if the primary is unknown or has been treated using another modality such as radiation. Cervical lymph tissue is dissected out, preserving blood vessels and nerves if possible. The tissue can then be examined microscopically to stage the disease

and guide further treatment and prognosis. The neck dissection is often followed by creation of a free tissue graft pedicle with anastomoses to the blood vessels in the neck. General anaesthesia with tracheal intubation is required, using a reinforced tube facing away from the neck to allow access. A long procedure should be anticipated. In radical neck dissection, the internal jugular vein may be ligated; if this is performed bilaterally, severe oedema of the face and neck may develop and tracheostomy may be necessary to protect the airway.

Surgery for Oral, Nasal and Oropharyngeal Cancer

If surgery is used, it generally consists of wide excision of the primary tumour, dissection of the cervical lymph nodes (depending on the staging of the disease) and reconstruction of the resulting defect. Procedures include glossectomy, pharyngectomy, maxillectomy and mandibular resection. Operations can be extremely prolonged (up to 15 h), particularly if microvascular tissue transfer is performed.

Preoperative assessment may reveal significant comorbidities, particularly in the elderly, and these may influence the anaesthetic technique and postoperative care. Supraglottic tumours can cause difficult intubation and this should be anticipated by careful examination of the patient and radiological investigations. Techniques such as awake fibreoptic intubation or the use of other difficult airway devices may be required.

The functions of airway control and ingestion are usually secured by insertion of a tracheostomy and gastrostomy feeding tube which can be removed after bleeding and swelling have resolved and healing has produced a stable and secure tract. Prolonged operations require careful attention to fluid balance and warming, and blood loss may be significant.

Reconstruction of defects is an important element of surgery. This commonly involves the insertion of a tissue graft into the defect. The graft may be swung on a vascular pedicle (e.g. pectoralis major flap) or a free tissue graft may be anastomosed with the blood vessels of the neck. A free flap tends to give a more favourable cosmetic and functional result but is extremely time-consuming. Grafts may be soft tissue only (e.g. radial forearm skin) or composite for bony defects (e.g. fibula). A free jejunal graft or a pull-up of the stomach from the abdomen may be required to restore integrity of the gastrointestinal tract if total pharyngectomy has been performed. Both will require laparotomy. Consideration should be given to allowing adequate rest breaks for the entire theatre team, including the anaesthetist. Postoperatively, the patient should be nursed on a high dependency unit where monitoring can continue and pain can be controlled effectively.

DENTAL ANAESTHESIA

Anaesthesia and dentistry have a strong historical association. The development of both disciplines and the increasing awareness of the benefits of dental care and oral hygiene resulted in the uncontrolled proliferation of the use of anaesthesia in dental practice, often by dentists themselves, who had had minimal training in anaesthesia, sedation and resuscitation. At its peak in the 1950s, over 2 million outpatient dental anaesthetics were given annually in the UK. Disquiet relating to the possible risks of death associated with the use of anaesthesia in dentistry resulted in the Department of Health commissioning a report in 1990 which recommended that general anaesthesia should be avoided if possible and that pain and anxiety associated with dental procedures should be ameliorated by local anaesthesia and conscious sedation. Further reports and guidelines since then have reinforced this viewpoint and general anaesthesia is now reserved almost exclusively for small children, and adults with learning difficulties. General anaesthesia for dental procedures must be administered in a hospital setting with full theatre resources and anaesthetic support. Conscious sedation can be used in the dental surgery if anxiolysis is required. This is administered by an anaesthetist or trained sedationist. The traditional dental chair anaesthetic has ceased to exist.

General Anaesthesia

In paediatric practice, the vast majority of procedures are for the extraction of carious teeth. There is a low incidence of systemic disease but upper respiratory tract infections are common. Premedication may consist of topical local anaesthetic cream together with an oral analgesic and, if necessary, a sedative such as oral midazolam. Psychological preparation is an important element and is best carried out in a specialized paediatric environment. The majority of procedures are extremely short. Induction may be intravenous or inhalational, and airway support is commonly provided using a face mask, nasal mask or laryngeal mask airway delivering a combination of oxygen, nitrous oxide and a volatile anaesthetic agent. The principles of care of the shared airway must be observed and good communication between the anaesthetist and dentist is essential. Full anaesthetic monitoring is required, although it may be necessary to wait until after induction of anaesthesia in unco-operative patients. A combination of simple analgesics and NSAIDs is generally used for pain control and allows early discharge.

In the adult, general anaesthesia for simple dentistry is indicated only for patients who are unable to tolerate local anaesthesia with sedation for psychological reasons or those unable to co-operate, e.g. because of severe learning difficulties. The vast majority of dental procedures under general anaesthesia in adults are performed when it is technically difficult to achieve the result without general anaesthesia, e.g. severely impacted third molar teeth or roots, or if poorly controlled carious disease has resulted in significant infection or anatomical derangement. These operations take place on oral surgery lists, commonly as day-case procedures. Nasotracheal intubation may be required for more difficult operations (see above). Patients are generally young and fit but concurrent disease may be present in patients undergoing a total dental clearance before treatment for head and neck cancer or cardiac valve surgery.

Sedation

The greatly reduced use of general anaesthesia in dental surgery has resulted in an increase in the use of sedative techniques to allow surgery to take place comfortably in anxious patients or when complex dental work is undertaken. Sedation is defined as the use of a drug or drugs to render a state of reduced consciousness to allow treatment to be carried out but in which verbal contact is maintained with the patient throughout the period of sedation. The drugs and techniques used should carry a margin of safety large enough to make loss of consciousness unlikely. In the UK, intercollegiate working parties from dentistry and anaesthesia have developed guidance relating to the safe conduct of sedation in dental surgery, stressing the need for adequate equipment, training, and documentation. It is recognized that potentially life-threatening complications may occur rarely.

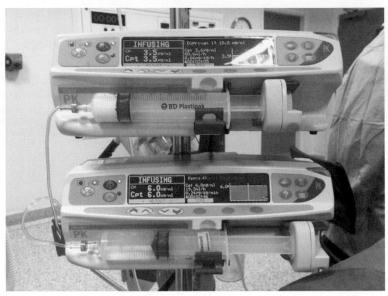

FIGURE 29.5 ■ Target-controlled infusion devices may be used for sedation and total intravenous anaesthesia in ENT and dental practice.

Common techniques involve the administration of an intravenous benzodiazepine or the use of nitrous oxide. Sedation may be administered by the operator before surgery or there may be a dedicated sedationist. Anaesthetists are often asked to take on this role and may use more complex techniques such as a continuous infusion of propofol using a target-controlled infusion device (Fig. 29.5).

FURTHER READING

Chesshire, N.J., Knight, D.J.W., 2001. The anaesthetic management of facial trauma and fractures. BJA CEPD Reviews 1, 108–112.

Chester, A.C., Antisdel, J.L., Sindwani, R., 2009. Symptom-specific outcomes of endoscopic sinus surgery: a systematic review. Otolaryngol. Head Neck Surg. 140, 633–639.

Goldman, A.C., Govindaraj, S., Rosenfeld, R.M., 2000. A meta-analysis of dexamethasone use with tonsillectomy. Otolaryngol. Head Neck Surg. 123, 682–686.

Grainger, J., Saravanappa, N., 2008. Local anaesthetic for post tonsillectomy pain: a systematic review and meta-analysis. Clin. Otolaryngol. 33, 411–419.

http://eng.mapofmedicine/evidence/map/epiglottitis_adult_2.html.

http://guidance.nice.org.uk/CG60.

http://guidance.nice.org.uk/TA1.

http://rcoa.ac.uk/docs/SCSDAT.pdf.

http://www.hesonline.nhs.uk.

http://www.rcoa.ac.uk/docs/GPAS-headneck.pdf.

Marret, E., Flahault, A., Samama, C.M., et al., 2003. Effects of postoperative, nonsteroidal, anti-inflammatory drugs on bleeding risk after tonsillectomy: meta-analysis of randomized, controlled trials. Anesthesiology 98, 1497–1502.

Mehanna, H., Paleri, V., West, C.M., Nutting, C., 2010. Head and neck cancer – Part 1: epidemiology, presentation, and prevention. Br. Med. J. 341, 663–666.

Murphy, M.F., Walls, R.M., 2004. Identification of the difficult and failed airway. In: Walls, R.M. (Ed.), Emergency airway management, second ed. Lippincott Williams & Wilkins, USA, pp. 70–82.

Ravi, R., Howell, T., 2007. Anaesthesia for paediatric ear, nose, and throat surgery. Continuing Education in Anaesthesia Critical Care and Pain 7, 33–37.

Somerville, N., Fenlon, S., 2005. Anaesthesia for cleft lip and palate surgery. Continuing Education in Anaesthesia Critical Care and Pain 5, 76–79.

Van den Aardweg, M.T., Schilder, A.G., Herkert, E., Boonacker, C.W., Rovers, M.M., 2010. Adenoidectomy for otitis media in children. Cochrane Database Syst. Rev. Jan 20 (1):CD008282.

30

OPHTHALMIC ANAESTHESIA

■ ■ ■ ■ ■ ■ ■ ■ ■ ■ ■ ■ ■ ■ ■ ■

P atients who present for eye surgery are frequently at the extremes of age. Neonatal and geriatric anaesthesia both present special problems. Some eye surgery may last many hours and repeated anaesthetics at short intervals are often necessary. The anaesthetic technique may influence intraocular pressure (IOP), and skilled administration of either local or general anaesthesia contributes directly to the successful outcome of the surgery. Close co-operation and clear understanding between surgeon and anaesthetist are essential. Risks and benefits must be assessed carefully and the anaesthetic technique selected accordingly.

Ophthalmic surgery can be classified into subspecialties and intraocular or extraocular procedures may be performed (Table 30.1); each has different anaesthetic requirements.

PHYSIOLOGY OF THE EYE

The perception of light requires function of both the eye and its central nervous system connections. The protective homeostatic mechanisms of the eye are interfered with by anaesthesia in a similar way to the effects of anaesthesia on the central nervous system. The sclera and its contents are analogous to the skull and its contents. There is a similar elastance curve, but for slightly different reasons. This is due to the sclera being an elastic but completely full container unlike the rigid, but slightly empty, cranium which has some room for expansion of its contents.

TABLE 30.1
Categorization of Ophthalmic Surgery

Ophthalmology Subspecialities
Paediatric
Oculoplastic
Vitreoretinal
Anterior segment
Glaucoma
Neuro-ophthalmology

Extraocular Operations
Globe and orbit
Eyebrow and eyelid
Lacrimal system
Muscles
Conjunctiva
Cornea, surface

Intraocular Operations
Iris and anterior chamber
Lens and cataract
Vitreous
Retina
Cornea, full thickness

Control of Intraocular Pressure

The factors controlling IOP are very complex and include external pressure, volume of the arterial and venous vasculature (choroidal volume) and the volumes of the aqueous and vitreous humour.

Intraocular pressure depends on the rigidity of the sclera as well as any external pressure. Functionally, it is a balance between the production and removal of aqueous humour (approximately $2.5\,\mu L\,min^{-1}$). Factors which affect IOP are shown in Table 30.2. Chronic changes in IOP (normally 10–25 mmHg (mean 15)), either upwards or downwards cause structural effects and loss of function. There is a relationship between increasing axial length and increasing IOP. Low pressure results in blood–aqueous barrier breakdown, cataract, macular oedema and papilloedema. High pressure causes iris sphincter paralysis, iris atrophy, lens opacities and optic nerve atrophy.

Pressure is distributed evenly throughout the eye and the pressure is generally the same in the posterior vitreous body as it is in the aqueous humour, despite the fact that the pressure is generated in the anterior segment. Each eye may have a different pressure. The aqueous is produced by an active secretory process in the non-pigmented epithelium of the ciliary body. Large molecules are excluded by the so-called blood–aqueous barrier between the epithelium and iris capillaries. The Na^+/K^+ ATPase pump is involved in the active transport of sodium into the aqueous. Carbonic anhydrase catalyses the conversion of water and carbon dioxide to carbonic acid, which passes passively into the aqueous. Acetazolamide, an inhibitor of carbonic anhydrase used in the treatment of raised IOP, reduces bicarbonate and sodium transport into the aqueous to produce its therapeutic effect.

In addition to this active secretory production, there is a less important hydrostatic element dependent on ocular perfusion pressure. The ciliary body is highly vascular and supplied directly by the ciliary arteries. Aqueous production is related linearly to blood flow. Flow and vascular pressure are controlled by the autonomic nervous system and autoregulation exists, similar to cerebral blood flow. Aqueous removal is inhibited by pressure within the pars plana, and episcleral venules restrict the vascular outflow, as does the IOP.

The aqueous flows from the ciliary body through the trabecular meshwork into the anterior chamber before exiting through the angle of Schlemm (Fig. 30.1). The sum of the hydrostatic inflow and the active aqueous production minus the active resorption and passive filtration must equal zero to achieve balance. Alteration of any individual feature can lead to changes in IOP.

TABLE 30.2
Factors Which Affect Intraocular Pressure (IOP)

IOP	Increase IOP	Decrease IOP
Systemic	Age	Exercise
	Large increase in blood pressure	Large decrease in blood pressure
	Increased carotid blood flow	Decreased carotid blood flow
	Increased central venous pressure	Decreased central venous pressure
	Valsalva manoeuvre	Parasympathetic stimulation
	Carotid-cavernous fistula	Pregnancy
	Plasma hypo-osmolality	Hypothermia
	Hypercapnia	Acidosis
	Sympathetic stimulation	Plasma hyperosmolality
		Adrenalectomy
		General anaesthesia
Local	Increased episcleral venous pressure	Decreased episcleral venous pressure
	Blockage of ophthalmic vein	Decreased ophthalmic artery blood flow
	Blockage of trabecular meshwork	Prolonged external pressure
	Contraction of extraocular muscles	Retrobulbar anaesthesia
	Restricted extraocular muscle	Ocular trauma
	Acute external pressure	Intraocular surgery
	Forced blinking	Retinal detachment
	Relaxation of accommodation	Choroidal detachment
	Prostaglandin release (biphasic)	Inflammation
	Hypersecretion of aqueous	Prostaglandins (biphasic)
		Accommodation
		Increased aqueous outflow

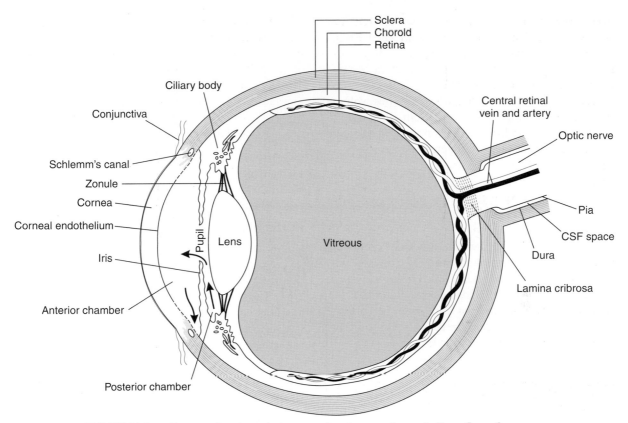

FIGURE 30.1 ■ Cross-section through the eye and optic nerve. Arrows indicate flow of aqueous.

External Pressure

Pressure from squeezing the eyes closed or the injection of a volume of local anaesthetic into the orbit is transmitted to the eyeball and increases the IOP.

Venous Pressure

Venous congestion increases vascular volume within the eye and reduces aqueous drainage through the canal of Schlemm, causing an increase in IOP. During anaesthesia, venous pressure is influenced mainly by posture and transmitted intrathoracic pressure. A 15° head-up tilt causes a significant decrease in IOP.

Raised arterial pressure, anxiety, restlessness, full bladder, coughing, retching and airway obstruction cause an increase in venous pressure which is reflected immediately in the IOP. Intermittent positive-pressure ventilation (IPPV) produces a small increase in venous pressure secondary to the increase in mean intrathoracic pressure, but is compensated for by control of arterial PCO_2.

Arterial Blood Gas Tensions

Arterial PCO_2 is an important determinant of choroidal vascular volume and IOP. A reduction in $PaCO_2$ constricts the choroidal vessels and reduces IOP. Elevation of $PaCO_2$ results in a proportional and linear increase in IOP. Increases in $PaCO_2$ may also increase central venous pressure. Hypoxaemia produces intraocular vasodilatation and an increase in IOP.

Arterial Pressure

Stable values of arterial pressure within the physiological range maintain normal IOP. Sudden increases in systolic arterial pressure above the normal autoregulatory range increase choroidal blood volume and consequently IOP. Reduction in arterial pressure below normal physiological levels reduces IOP, but the response is unpredictable in old age when arterial capacitance is reduced.

Aqueous and Vitreous Volumes

A decrease in either aqueous or vitreous volume reduces IOP. Osmotic diuretics are sometimes used to reduce aqueous and vitreous volume. Acetazolamide reduces the production of aqueous.

Sodium Hyaluronate

Sodium hyaluronate is used as a soft viscous retractor during surgery. Sodium hyaluronate is a large-molecular-weight, clear viscoelastic polysaccharide. It augments the effect of general anaesthesia by controlling vitreous bulge and compensates for small changes in IOP. The manufactured product is injected by the surgeon at the time of incision and helps to maintain the shape of the anterior chamber and the work space. Hyaluronate with lidocaine admixture may be used when cataract surgery is conducted under topical anaesthesia.

OCULAR BLOOD FLOW

Ocular blood flow and IOP are intrinsically linked, as are cerebral blood flow and intracranial pressure. The control mechanisms are similar, although there are differences in the anatomy. Ocular perfusion pressure (OPP) equals the mean arterial pressure (MAP) minus the intraocular pressure:

$$OPP = MAP - IOP$$

This is subject to autoregulation within the range 60 to 150 mmHg (Fig. 30.2).

OCULOCARDIAC REFLEX

The oculocardiac reflex is a triad of bradycardia, nausea and syncope. Classically precipitated by muscle traction, it may also occur in association with stimulation of the eyelids or the orbital floor, and pressure on the eye itself. Apnoea may also occur. The ophthalmic division of the trigeminal nerve is the afferent limb, passing through the reticular formation to the visceral motor nuclei of the vagus nerve.

The risk of development of the oculocardiac reflex is highest in children undergoing squint surgery and patients receiving explant surgery for retinal

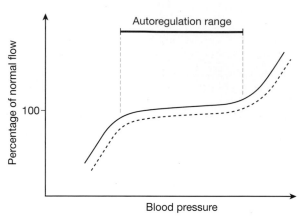

FIGURE 30.2 ■ Auto-regulation of intraocular pressure (IOP).

detachment. Treatment requires either a cessation of the stimulus or an appropriate dose of an anticholinergic drug such as atropine or glycopyrrolate. Some anaesthetists consider it mandatory to use prophylaxis against this reflex in susceptible patients, using the same agents.

CONDITIONS FOR INTRAOCULAR SURGERY

For most intraocular operations, the eye must be pain-free and preferably immobile. Except for glaucoma surgery, the pupil should be dilated and intraocular pressure reduced.

Expulsive Haemorrhage

In the presence of markedly raised IOP, sudden reduction in pressure on incision of the globe may lead to the expression of the contents. The balance between venous and intraocular pressure is crucial. An increase in venous pressure causes fluid to pool in the choroid and may progress to cause rupture of the ciliary artery with prolapse of the iris. On rare occasions, disastrous expulsive haemorrhage may result in the loss of the entire contents of the eyeball.

Effect of Anaesthetic Drugs on Intraocular Pressure

Premedication

Drugs used for premedication have little effect on intraocular pressure, and the commonly used anxiolytic and antiemetic drugs may be used as preferred.

Induction Agents

Most of the intravenous induction agents, with the exception of ketamine, reduce intraocular pressure and may be used as indicated clinically. Ketamine should be avoided if intraocular surgery is planned.

Muscle Relaxants

Succinylcholine increases intraocular pressure, with a maximal effect 2 min after i.v. administration, but the pressure returns to baseline values after 5 min. This effect is thought to be caused by the increase in tone of the extraocular muscles and intraocular vasodilatation. Pretreatment with a small dose of a non-depolarizing muscle relaxant does not obtund this response reliably. The problems involved with the use of succinylcholine in the patient with penetrating eye injury are discussed on page 616.

Non-depolarizing muscle relaxants have no significant direct effects on IOP.

Volatile Anaesthetic Agents

All the volatile anaesthetic agents in use today decrease intraocular pressure. Nitrous oxide has no effect on IOP in the absence of air or a therapeutic inert gas bubble in the globe (see below).

Opioids

Opioids cause a moderate reduction in IOP in the absence of significant ventilatory depression. They contribute to postoperative nausea and vomiting and are not often required for postoperative analgesia following eye surgery.

CHOICE OF ANAESTHESIA

Ophthalmic surgery can be carried out under either local or general anaesthesia provided that there is both consent and compliance. The type of surgery, its urgency and the age and fitness of the patient influence the choice (Table 30.3). Local anaesthesia is preferred for older and sicker patients, because the stress response to surgery is diminished and complications such as postoperative confusion, nausea, vomiting and urinary retention are mostly eliminated. Younger patients may sometimes be too anxious for local anaesthesia and are usually managed with general anaesthesia.

TABLE 30.3
Preferred Anaesthetic Technique for Common Surgical Procedures in Ophthalmology

Local Anaesthesia
Cataract
Glaucoma techniques
Minor extraocular plastic surgery
Laser dacrocystorhinostomy
Minor anterior segment procedures
Simple vitrectomies

General Anaesthesia
Paediatric surgery
Squint surgery
Major oculoplastic surgery
Dacrocystorhinostomy
Penetrating keratoplasty
Orbital trauma repair
Penetrating eye injuries
Complex vitreoretinal surgery

Risks and benefits of the available techniques must be assessed carefully and anaesthesia selected accordingly. There is a need to maintain homeostasis in the eye if intraocular surgery is planned. For the purposes of patient comfort, it may also be necessary to consider the duration of the procedure and the patient's ability to stay immobile for a period longer than a short cataract operation. However all types of ophthalmic surgery have been carried out with local anaesthesia in compliant patients, including repair of ocular trauma. As a general rule, patients who require general anaesthesia are usually children and special needs adults, or adults scheduled to undergo potentially complex ophthalmic surgery. It is important to understand the basic physiology and anatomy of the eye before embarking on anaesthesia, irrespective of whether general or local anaesthesia is chosen.

General Anaesthesia

Indications for General Anaesthesia

General anaesthesia is indicated when the patient is unwilling or unable to tolerate local anaesthesia. The length and complexity of the operation are important determinants. Surgical experience and the need for education and training of medical staff in a suitable environment are also relevant considerations.

Contraindications to General Anaesthesia

Contraindications to general anaesthesia are related to risk/benefit analysis. Cardiovascular, respiratory and neurological diseases increase in frequency with age. Adverse cardiac outcome, respiratory failure and postoperative cognitive dysfunction leading to admission to a Critical Care Unit can occur after either local or general anaesthesia. If a simple and safer anaesthetic solution exists and the opinion of the anaesthetist is that there is a significant risk of death or serious neurological morbidity from general anaesthesia, the balance may shift towards local anaesthesia or cancelling surgery. There are no absolute contraindications and it is not uncommon for patients with serious comorbidities which cannot be improved preoperatively to say that the risk of death associated with proceeding with surgery and general anaesthesia is worth it when the desired outcome is maintenance or improvement of vision.

Assessment and Preparation

Standard preoperative assessment should be carried out for all patients irrespective of the chosen anaesthetic technique. Multiprofessional teamwork is the norm and the Joint Royal Colleges' guidelines offer appropriate advice. Appropriately trained nursing staff undertake pre-assessment and preoperative preparation of most patients, under the guidance of a lead ophthalmic anaesthetist. A thorough history is required and, with input from the surgeon, a decision can be made about the most appropriate choice of anaesthetic to be offered to the patient. Investigations should be based on the examination findings and NICE guidance. Increasing age, comorbidity (such as cardiorespiratory disease) and chronic drug treatments make routine investigations such as ECG, full blood count and measurement of serum urea and electrolyte concentrations potentially useful tests. However, if local anaesthesia is planned, investigations are usually reserved for very specific indications. Particular thought needs to be given to management of patients with hypertension, ischaemic heart disease, diabetes mellitus or chronic obstructive pulmonary disease. It is important that the preoperative preparation includes consideration of whether the patient will be able to lie flat for up to an hour without becoming uncomfortable, claustrophobic, hypoxaemic or suffering ischaemic cardiac problems, or coughing.

Chronic anticoagulation presents potential complications which are more relevant to the surgeon or those practising local anaesthesia (see below).

It is imperative to make sure that the patient understands and consents to the choice of anaesthetic by taking part in an informed discussion. Patients (and surgeons) often request anaesthetic choices which appear contrary to the anaesthetic risk/benefit assessment.

Induction of Anaesthesia

A smooth induction is the goal of all anaesthetists and is particularly important in the ophthalmic setting. Avoidance of coughing, straining and accidental increases in intrathoracic pressure which cause venous congestion are important so that optimal eye conditions are maintained. The choice of induction drug is of much less importance than how it is used. However, propofol has a number of ideal qualities in this setting, especially related to the ease of insertion of the laryngeal mask airway. In equipotent doses, propofol has a greater depressant effect on IOP than thiopental, but also causes more hypotension. Succinylcholine, in isolation, causes an increase in IOP due to muscular contractions and intraocular vasodilatation but this effect is more than balanced out by the effect of the induction agent.

Short-acting opioids such as fentanyl act synergistically with the induction agent and obtund cardiovascular responses to airway manipulation.

Airway Management

Management of the airway is particularly important in head and neck surgery. The airway may remain inaccessible throughout surgery and any need to adjust or reposition an airway device during surgery could cause disruption to surgery, with potentially sight-threatening consequences in ophthalmic surgery. Thus, the safest option was traditionally felt to be to intubate the trachea and maintain ventilation and neuromuscular blockade throughout the operation. Topical and intravenous lidocaine during laryngoscopy (and during emergence) can help to reduce stimulation of the trachea and larynx. A south-facing RAE tracheal tube which is well stabilized with hypo-allergenic tape (avoiding ties) is the best choice and, along with mechanical ventilation, provides ideal conditions for nearly all types of ophthalmic surgery. Guaranteed paralysis with the use of neuromuscular monitoring avoids the risks of movement during surgery. However, tracheal intubation can be associated with a risk of increasing IOP as a result of coughing and bucking during laryngoscopy, the pressor response to laryngoscopy and intubation, laryngospasm or coughing after extubation, and postoperative nausea and vomiting related to the use of neostigmine. All of these complications assume much greater importance in open eye surgery.

The use of propofol followed by insertion of a laryngeal mask airway (LMA) has therefore become popular, particularly for short ophthalmic procedures, reducing many of the risks associated with tracheal intubation but carrying an additional risk that maintenance of the airway is less certain if the LMA is poorly positioned or inadequately secured. The use of neuromuscular blockade with the LMA may aid mechanical ventilation and tighter control of ocular physiology but is considered by some anaesthetists as carrying a significantly increased risk of aspiration.

Therefore a risk/benefit assessment should be made by the anaesthetist, taking into account the relative importance of the following factors: body mass index, history of gastro-oesophageal reflux, hiatus hernia, predicted ease of insertion of tube or LMA, length of operation, open eye operation and fasting time.

Maintenance of Anaesthesia

The choice of technique for maintenance of anaesthesia is influenced by personal preference and the method of airway management. The use of a volatile anaesthetic agent is commonest because of familiarity, controllability and cost. Inhalational anaesthesia causes a dose-dependent reduction in IOP. However, virtually all sedative and hypnotic drugs reduce IOP. There are, in practice, few clinical differences between the effects of different volatile anaesthetic agents, or between inhalational and intravenous anaesthesia.

The use of nitrous oxide depends on local availability of medical air and personal preference. The benefits of nitrous oxide are well known but two particular risks must be considered in relation to ophthalmic anaesthesia: the increased risk of postoperative retching and vomiting, and the effect on IOP when intraocular gas mixtures are used for vitrectomy (see below).

Relative hypotension during anaesthesia combined with normoxia and normocapnia provide a soft, well-perfused eye. A 15° head-up tilt may improve conditions. However, excessive hypotension may prompt questions from the ophthalmologist because of absence of flow in the retinal arteries during some ocular procedures. Maintenance of an adequate blood pressure is a greater challenge in elderly patients in the absence of significant surgical stimulation. Avoidance of an increased IOP is necessary to avoid loss of ocular contents during open surgery.

The systemic physiological disturbance associated with most eye surgery is low. There is little, if any, alteration in body fluid status and care should be taken not to be too liberal with intravenous fluids to avoid overloading the myocardium or inducing urinary retention in the elderly. The elderly are also more susceptible to the adverse effects of hypothermia and attention should be given to maintaining body temperature during all but very short procedures. Appropriate measures should be taken to minimize the risk of venous thromboembolism. Ophthalmic surgery is performed commonly on patients with diabetes due to complications of the disease. If general anaesthesia is required, local euglycaemia protocols must be followed. Analgesia requirements are based on the intraoperative use of a short-acting opioid and paracetamol. Non-steroidal anti-inflammatory drugs (NSAIDs) may be useful if there are no contraindications. Local anaesthesia with a longer-duration local anaesthetic drug is particularly useful provided that eye protection is maintained for the duration of action. It is unusual to require potent long-acting opioids and a cause for severe postoperative pain should be sought because this can be a sign of ophthalmic complications. Ophthalmic patients are particularly prone to suffer from nausea and vomiting despite the absence of long-acting opioids. Dexamethasone and ondansetron are useful as prophylaxis.

Local Anaesthesia for Eye Surgery

An experienced ophthalmic surgery team can achieve a safe and efficient service with prompt patient turnaround and excellent operating conditions based on the use of local anaesthesia. However, serious complications of ophthalmic local anaesthesia can and do occur. A detailed knowledge of the anatomy of the eye and the relevant pharmacology is of paramount importance.

NOMENCLATURE OF BLOCKS

The terminology used for ophthalmic block varies but the widely accepted nomenclature is based on the anatomical location of the needle tip. The injection of local anaesthetic agent into the muscle cone behind the globe formed by the four rectus muscles and the superior and inferior oblique muscles is known as intraconal (retrobulbar) block whereas in the extraconal (peribulbar) block, the needle tip remains outside the muscle cone. Multiple communications exist between the two compartments and it is difficult to differentiate whether the needle is intraconal or extraconal after insertion. Injected local anaesthetic agent diffuses easily across compartments and, depending on its spread, anaesthesia and akinesia may occur. A faster onset of akinesia suggests that the block is intraconal. A combination of intraconal and extraconal block is described as a combined retro–peribulbar block. In sub-Tenon's block, local anaesthetic agent is injected under the Tenon's capsule and this block is also known as parabulbar block, pinpoint anaesthesia or medial episcleral block.

Relevant Anatomy

The orbit is a four-sided irregular pyramid with its apex pointing posteromedially and its base anteriorly. The annulus of Zinn is a fibrous ring which arises from the superior orbital fissure. Eye movements are controlled by four rectus muscles (inferior, lateral, medial and superior), and the superior oblique and inferior oblique muscles (Fig. 30.3). These muscles arise from the annulus of Zinn and insert on the globe anterior to the equator to form an incomplete cone. The distance from annulus to inferior temporal orbital rim ranges from 42 to 54 mm. It is very important that the needle should not be inserted too far, close to the annulus, where the vital nerves and vessels are tightly packed.

The optic nerve (II), oculomotor nerve (III, containing superior and inferior branches), abducent nerve (VI), nasociliary nerve (a branch of nerve V), ciliary ganglion and vessels lie in the cone (Fig. 30.4). The ophthalmic division of the oculomotor nerve divides into superior and inferior branches before emerging from the superior orbital fissure. The superior branch supplies superior rectus and levator palpebrae superioris muscles. The inferior branch divides into three to supply the medial rectus, the inferior rectus and the

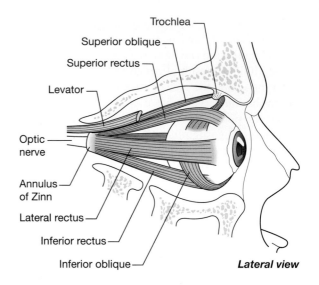

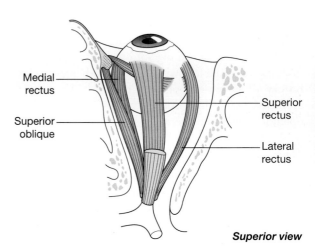

FIGURE 30.3 ■ Extraocular muscles of the eye. See text for details. *(Adapted from Gray, Henry. Anatomy of the human body. Lea & Febiger, Philadelphia 1918; Bartleby.com, 2000.)*

inferior oblique muscles. The abducent nerve emerges from the superior orbital fissure beneath the inferior branch of the oculomotor nerve to supply the lateral rectus muscle. The trochlear nerve (IV) courses outside the cone but then branches and enters the cone to supply the superior oblique muscle. An incomplete block of this nerve leads to retained activity of the superior oblique muscle and this occurs frequently. Squeezing and closing of the eyelids are controlled by the zygomatic branch of the facial nerve (VII), which supplies

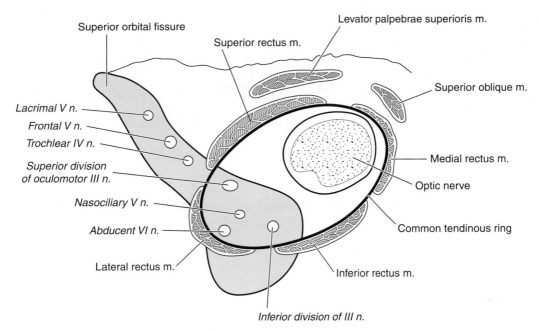

FIGURE 30.4 ■ Anatomy of the right orbit: relationship of the four rectus muscles and the apex of the cone to the orbital nerve supply.

the motor innervation to the orbicularis oculi muscle. This nerve emerges from the foramen spinosum at the base of the skull, anterior to the mastoid and behind the earlobe. It passes through the parotid gland before crossing the condyle of the mandible, and then passes superficial to the zygoma and malar bone before its terminal fibres ramify to supply the deep surface of the orbicularis oculi. The facial nerve also supplies secretomotor parasympathetic fibres to the lacrimal glands, and glands of the nasal and palatine mucosa.

Tenon's capsule or bulbar fascia is a membrane which envelops the eyeball from the optic nerve to the sclerocorneal junction, separating it from the orbital fat and forming a socket in which it moves (Fig. 30.5). The capsule originates at the limbus and extends posteriorly to the optic nerve and as sleeves along the extraocular muscles. Tenon's capsule is divided arbitrarily by the equator of the globe into anterior and posterior portions. Anterior Tenon's capsule is adherent to episcleral tissue from the limbus posteriorly for about 5–10 mm and is fused with the intermuscular septum of the extraocular muscles and overlying bulbar conjunctiva. The conjunctiva fuses with Tenon's capsule in this area and the sub-Tenon space can be accessed easily through an incision 5–10 mm behind the limbus. The posterior sub-Tenon's capsule is thinner

and passes round to the optic nerve, separating the globe from the contents of the retrobulbar space. Posteriorly, the sheath fuses with the openings around the optic nerve.

Sensation to the eyeball is supplied through the ophthalmic division of the trigeminal nerve (V). Just before entering the orbit, it divides into three branches: lacrimal, frontal and nasociliary. The nasociliary nerve is sensory to the entire eyeball. It emerges through the superior orbital fissure between the superior and inferior branches of the oculomotor nerve and passes through the common tendinous ring. Two long ciliary nerves give branches to the ciliary ganglion and, with the short ciliary nerves, transmit sensation from the cornea, iris and ciliary muscle. Some sensation from the lateral conjunctiva is transmitted through the lacrimal nerve and from the upper palpebral conjunctiva via the frontal nerve. Both nerves are outside the cone. Intraoperative pain may be experienced if these nerves are inadequately blocked.

The superomedial and superotemporal quadrants have abundant blood vessels but the inferotemporal and medial quadrants are relatively avascular and are safer places to insert a needle or cannula.

To achieve adequate anaesthesia and akinesia, the cranial and sensory nerves described above must be

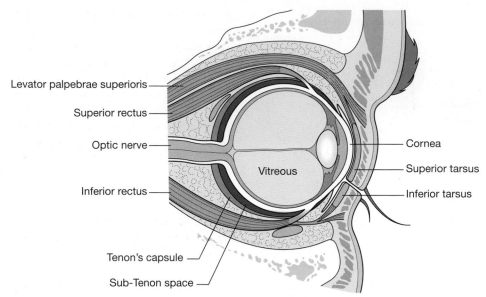

Levator palpebrae superioris

Superior rectus

Optic nerve

Vitreous

Inferior rectus

Cornea

Superior tarsus

Inferior tarsus

Tenon's capsule

Sub-Tenon space

FIGURE 30.5 ■ A sagittal section through the right orbital cavity, showing Tenon's capsule and the sub-Tenon space. *(Adapted from Gray, Henry. Anatomy of the human body. Lea & Febiger, Philadelphia 1918; Bartleby.com, 2000.)*

blocked. However, it is very difficult to target these nerves individually and an adequate volume of local anaesthetic should be injected safely either into the retrobulbar or peribulbar space; subsequent diffusion will ultimately block the relevant nerves.

Selection of Patients and Blocks

Numerous published studies confirm the preference of ophthalmologists, anaesthetists and patients for local anaesthetic techniques. However, the preferred technique varies from topical anaesthesia, through cannula-based block to needle-based blocks. There is conflicting evidence about whether there are real differences in effectiveness of blocks, suggesting that peribulbar and retrobulbar anaesthesia produce equally good akinesia and equivalent pain control. There is insufficient evidence in the literature to make a definitive statement concerning the relative effectiveness of sub-Tenon's block in producing akinesia when compared with peribulbar or retrobulbar block. The technique chosen depends on a balance between the patient's wishes, the operative needs of the surgeon, the skills of the anaesthetist and the type of surgery.

Preoperative assessment is generally limited to medical history, drug history and physical examination. According to the UK Joint Colleges Guidelines 2012, routine investigations are unnecessary if local anaesthesia is to be employed and these are performed only if it is thought that the results may lead to improved general health of the patient. Patients are not fasted and this is particularly helpful in managing patients with diabetes mellitus who can receive all their normal medications and achieve better glycaemic control in the perioperative period. The blood sugar concentration should still be checked. Patients receiving anticoagulants and antiplatelet agents are advised to continue their usual medications unless told otherwise. Warfarin therapy is not considered an absolute contraindication to local anaesthesia provided that the preoperative INR value is in the therapeutic target range; a sub-Tenon's block or topical anaesthesia is preferred. The axial length of the eye is usually measured before cataract surgery and serious caution in the use of needle blocks is required if the axial length exceeds 26 mm (Fig. 30.6) or if the axial length is unknown, e.g. in surgery for glaucoma. Antibiotics are not necessary in patients with valvular heart disease. Premedication is not usually necessary but, if needed, may be given intravenously just before the local anaesthetic block is inserted.

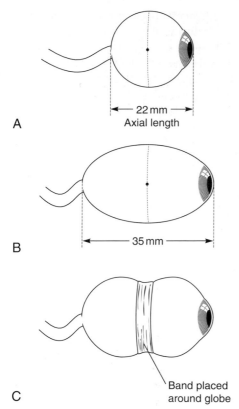

A

←— 22 mm —→
Axial length

B

←————— 35 mm —————→

C

Band placed
around globe

FIGURE 30.6 ■ Eyeballs of various shapes. **(A)** Normal eyeball. **(B)** High myope. **(C)** Scleral buckle applied after surgery for retinal detachment.

OPHTHALMIC REGIONAL BLOCKS

Insertion of an intravenous cannula is good practice and must be established if a sharp-needle technique is planned. Full cardiopulmonary resuscitation equipment and trained staff should be immediately available. Appropriate cardiorespiratory monitoring should be used. Ophthalmic regional anaesthesia should provide conditions appropriate for the surgeon's needs and planned surgery.

Needle-Based Blocks

Atkinson described the classical retrobulbar block in 1936. In this technique, the patient is asked to look upward and inward. A needle 38 mm in length is inserted at the junction of the medial ⅔ and lateral ⅓ of the inferior orbital margin after raising a wheal of skin with local anaesthetic. The needle is directed towards the apex and 2–3 mL of local anaesthetic is injected

close to the optic nerve. Akinesia and analgesia result quickly but a facial nerve block is essential to block the orbicularis oculi muscle. Both classical retrobulbar and facial nerve blocks are associated with significant sight- and life-threatening complications and these techniques have been replaced by the modern retrobulbar block.

Modern Retrobulbar Block. Surface anaesthesia is obtained with local anaesthetic drops (oxybuprocaine 0.4% or similar). The conjunctiva is cleaned with aqueous 5% povidone iodine. Evidence-based literature suggests that the eye should be kept in the neutral (primary) gaze position at all times and a needle length shorter than 31 mm is inserted through the skin or conjunctiva in the inferotemporal quadrant as far lateral as possible below the lateral rectus. The needle is directed upwards and inwards, with the needle always tangential to the globe. A volume of 4–5 mL of local anaesthetic agent of choice such as 2% lidocaine is injected. A separate facial nerve block is not required.

Inferotemporal Peribulbar Block. Surface anaesthesia and asepsis are obtained as above. The globe is kept in a neutral gaze position and a needle of less than 31 mm in length is inserted as far as possible in the extreme inferonasal quadrant through the conjunctiva or lower lid. A peribulbar block is essentially similar to a modern retrobulbar block but the needle is not directed upwards and inwards and the needle always remains tangential to the globe along the inferior orbital floor (Fig. 30.7). A volume of 5–6 mL of local anaesthetic agent is injected. However, more than 60% of patients require a supplementary injection in the form of a medial peribulbar block.

Medial Peribulbar Block. A supplementary injection is often required either in the same quadrant or through an injection in the medial compartment and is called a medial peribulbar block. A needle is inserted between the caruncle and the medial canthus to a depth of 1–1.5 cm and 3–5 mL of local anaesthetic is injected. A single medial peribulbar block with 6–8 mL of local anaesthetic has been advocated if akinesia is essential in patients with myopic eyes.

In practice, the differentiation between retrobulbar and peribulbar block is more semantic than actual. If

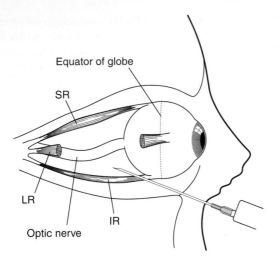

Equator of globe

SR

LR

IR

Optic nerve

FIGURE 30.7 ■ Intraconal injection is placed between the inferior border of the lateral rectus and the inferior rectus. SR, superior rectus; LR, lateral rectus; IR, inferior rectus.

the onset of anaesthesia is rapid with a peribulbar anaesthetic, then the chances are that it has found a direct pathway or been injected directly into the cone.

The gauge of needle should be the finest that can be used comfortably but this is usually limited to a 25- or 27-gauge needle. Finer needles are difficult to manipulate but larger needles may cause more pain and damage. Sharp needles are used because blunt needles are painful to insert and cause vasovagal syncope. The operator should consistently use the same volume syringe with the same gauge needle, because it is then easier to feel and judge the resistance to injection. A correctly placed injection has minimal resistance.

Gentle digital pressure and massage around the globe help to disperse the anaesthetic and reduce IOP. Alternatively, a pressure-reducing device such as Honan's balloon can be used. The maximum pressure should be limited to 25 mmHg in order to avoid compromise to the globe's blood supply.

Sub-Tenon's Block. Sub-Tenon's block involves a minor surgical procedure, and although it avoids some of the complications of the other two techniques, its use is associated with some specific problems.

Surface anaesthesia and asepsis are obtained as above. The lower eyelid is retracted or a speculum used. The patient is asked to look upwards and outwards. The conjunctiva and Tenon's capsule are

gripped together with a non-toothed forceps 5–10 mm from the limbus in the inferonasal quadrant. A small incision is made through these layers with Westcott scissors until the white sclera is seen. A sub-Tenon cannula (19-gauge, curved, 2.54-cm long, metal, opening at the end) is inserted gently along the curvature of the globe and should pass easily without resistance. In the posterior capsule, 3–5 mL of local anaesthetic of choice is injected slowly. The injected local anaesthetic agent diffuses around and into the intraconal space leading to anaesthesia and akinesia. Inferotemporal, superotemporal and medial quadrants may also be used to access the sub-Tenon's space. A variety of cannulae, both flexible and shorter lengths, are available. This method reduces the risk of CNS spread, optic nerve damage and global puncture but may be more likely to cause superficial haemorrhage. Akinesia may take longer to achieve.

Local Anaesthetic Agents and Adjuncts

The ideal local anaesthetic agent should be safe and painless to inject. It should block motor and sensory nerves quickly. The duration of action should be long enough to perform the operation but not so long as to cause persistent postoperative diplopia.

Lidocaine 2% remains the gold standard. It is safe and produces effective motor and sensory blocks. Bupivacaine has largely been superseded by its isomer levobupivacaine, which has less propensity to cause cardiovascular side-effects. It may be used in concentrations of 0.5% or 0.75%. Its onset of action is slower than that of lidocaine but it has a longer duration of action. The more concentrated solution may cause prolonged diplopia or myopathy if accidentally injected directly into one of the extraocular muscles. Prilocaine 2–4% has a rapid onset of action, few side-effects and a duration of action comparable with that of bupivacaine. Ropivacaine 1% has also been shown to be effective.

Hyaluronidase is an enzyme which reversibly liquefies the interstitial barrier between cells by depolymerization of hyaluronic acid to a tetrasaccharide, thus enhancing diffusion of molecules through tissue planes. The amount of hyaluronidase powder mixed with the local anaesthetic varies from 5 to 150 IU mL^{-1}. The use of hyaluronidase for ophthalmic blocks is controversial and its use for sub-Tenon's block is questioned for a short operation such as cataract surgery. Side-effects are rare but include allergic reactions, orbital cellulitis and formation of pseudotumours.

A vasoconstrictor such as adrenaline is commonly added to local anaesthetic solutions to increase the intensity and duration of block and minimize bleeding from small vessels. Absorption of local anaesthetic is reduced, which avoids any surge in plasma concentrations. Adrenaline may cause vasoconstriction of the ophthalmic artery, compromising the retinal circulation, and has also been implicated in complications in the elderly with cardiovascular and cerebrovascular comorbidities.

Commercial preparations of lidocaine and bupivacaine are acidic in solution and the basic local anaesthetic exists predominantly in the charged ionic form. The non-ionized form of the local anaesthetic agent which traverses the lipid membrane of the nerve produces the conduction block. At higher pH values, a greater proportion of local anaesthetic molecules exist in the non-ionized form and this allows more rapid influx into the neuronal cells. Adjustment of the pH of levobupivacaine and lidocaine by the addition of sodium bicarbonate allows more of the local anaesthetic solution to exist in the uncharged form. Alkalinization has been shown to decrease the onset time and prolong the duration of action after needle blocks but its use in clinical practice is probably unwarranted.

Complications of Ophthalmic Regional Blocks

Reported complications of needle blocks abound. They range from mild to serious, and may affect the eye or be systemic. Orbital complications include failure of the block, corneal abrasion, chemosis, subconjunctival haemorrhage, orbital haemorrhage, globe damage, optic nerve damage and extraocular muscle malfunction. Systemic complications such as local anaesthetic agent toxicity, brainstem anaesthesia and cardiorespiratory arrest may occur as a result of intravenous injection or spread or misplacement of drug in the orbit during or immediately after injection.

Sub-Tenon's block is considered a safe alternative to needle block but a number of minor and major complications have been reported. Minor and frequent complications such as pain during injection, reflux of local anaesthetic, chemosis and subconjunctival haemorrhage occur with varying incidences. Visual analogue pain scores are typically low but even minor discomfort in the orbit may be interpreted as severe and unpleasant pain. Smaller cannulae may afford a marginal benefit. Anterograde reflux and loss of local anaesthetic on injection occurs if the dissection is oversized relative to the gauge of the cannula. Inadequate access into the sub-Tenon's space can also promote chemosis. The incidence of chemosis varies with the volume of local anaesthetic, dissection technique and choice of cannula. Shorter cannulae are associated with an increased likelihood of conjunctival chemosis. Conjunctival haemorrhage is common. In one study of patients taking drugs with the potential to impair coagulation, conjunctival haemorrhage occurred in 19% of the control group, 40% of patients taking clopidogrel, 35% of those taking warfarin and 21% of patients taking aspirin. The incidence can be reduced with careful dissection, application of topical adrenaline or, controversially, the use of handheld cautery.

Orbital Haemorrhage

Orbital haemorrhage is a sight-threatening complication of intraconal and extraconal anaesthesia as well as, rarely, sub-Tenon's block (Fig. 30.8). It occurs with a frequency of between 0.1 and 3% following needle-based blocks. The haemorrhage may be venous or arterial in origin and may be concealed or revealed. Venous bleeding is slow and usually stops. Venous haemorrhage usually presents as markedly bloodstained chemosis and raised IOP. It may be possible to reduce the IOP by digital massage and cautious application of an IOP-reducing device to such an extent that surgery can proceed safely. Before the decision is made to proceed with surgery or postpone it for a few days, it is advisable to measure and record IOP. Arterial bleeding is rapid, with blood filling the periorbital tissues, increasing tissue volume and pressure. This is transmitted to the globe, raising the IOP. Urgent measures must be taken to stop the haemorrhage and reduce IOP. Firm digital pressure usually stops the bleeding and, when it has been arrested, consideration must be given to reducing the IOP so that the blood supply to the retina is not compromised. Lateral canthotomy, acetazolamide or mannitol, or even paracentesis, may need to be considered in consultation with the ophthalmologist.

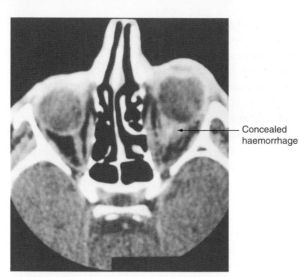

FIGURE 30.8 ■ CT scan taken in coronal section of a patient following an intraconal haemorrhage. Note the marked proptosis of the right eye and the confined space occupied by the haemorrhage. This was a concealed haemorrhage because, despite elevated intraocular pressure and proptosis, no signs of bleeding or bruising were evident until the next day.

Prevention of Haemorrhage. Straining due to anxiety during the block leads to engorgement and potential puncture of vessels around the eye. Sedation may help and the patient should be encouraged to breathe quietly through an open mouth and so prevent a Valsalva manoeuvre. The fewer injections that are made into the orbit, the less are the chances of damaging a blood vessel. Cutting and slicing movements at the needle tip should be avoided. Fine needles are less traumatic than thicker ones. Deep intraorbital injections must be avoided. The inferotemporal quadrant has fewer blood vessels and is less hazardous. It is advisable to apply firm digital pressure to the orbit as soon as the needle is withdrawn after any intraorbital injection, as this reduces any tendency to ooze.

Central Spread of Local Anaesthetic Agent

Mechanism. The cerebral dura mater provides a tubular sheath for the optic nerve as it passes through the optic foramen. This sheath fuses to the epineurium of the optic nerve, providing a potential conduit for local anaesthetic to pass subdurally to the brain. Central spread can occur on injection if the needle tip has entered the optic nerve sheath. Central spread following sub-Tenon's block has also been reported. Even

an injection of a small volume of local anaesthetic may enter the central nervous system and/or cross the optic chiasma to the opposite eye and may cause life-threatening sequelae, e.g. catastrophic cardiorespiratory collapse. The time of onset of symptoms is variable but usually appears in the first 15 min after injection. Central spread may occur on rare occasions if an orbital artery is cannulated by the needle tip, resulting in retrograde spread up the artery until it meets a branch, where it can then flow in a cephalad direction; in addition to orbital haemorrhage, systemic collapse is almost instantaneous.

Signs and Symptoms of Central Spread. The symptomatology of central spread is varied and depends upon which part of the central nervous system is affected by the local anaesthetic. Because of the anatomical proximity of the optic nerve to the midbrain, it is usual for this area to be involved. Signs and symptoms involving the cardiovascular and respiratory systems, temperature regulation, vomiting, temporary hemiplegia, aphasia and generalized convulsions have been described. Palsy of the contralateral oculomotor and trochlear nerves with amaurosis (loss of vision) is pathognomonic of central nervous system spread and should be sought in any patient whose response to questions following block are not as crisp as they were beforehand.

Treatment of Central Spread. Cardiorespiratory arrest may occur and should be treated as at any other arrest. Bradycardia requires treatment with an anticholinergic drug. Asystole has been reported rarely, but if it occurs, intravenous vasoactive drugs are required. Respiratory depression or apnoea necessitates ventilatory support, intravenous fluid therapy and administration of supplemental oxygen. Convulsions are treated with an intravenous induction agent such as propofol, or a benzodiazepine.

Prevention of Central Spread. Intraconal or extraconal injections should always be undertaken with the patient looking in the neutral or the primary gaze position. The optic nerve is a C-shaped structure and there is slackness in the primary gaze position so that it lies out of the way of the advancing needle (Fig. 30.9). If the needle encounters the optic nerve in this position,

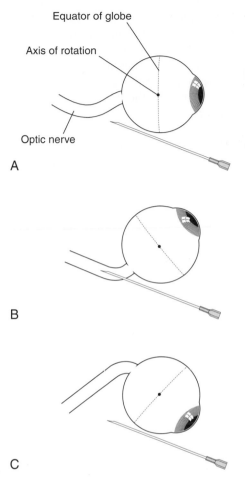

A

B

C

FIGURE 30.9 ■ Movements of the optic nerve in relation to eyeball movement when the needle is introduced into the cone from the inferotemporal quadrant. **(A)** Primary gaze. **(B)** Upwards and inwards. **(C)** Downwards and outwards.

it is unlikely to damage or perforate its sheath because slackness in the structure allows the nerve to be pushed aside. The most dangerous position is when the patient looks upwards and inwards, as this presents the stretched nerve to a needle directed from the inferotemporal quadrant. The injection should not be made deep into the orbit, where the optic nerve is likely to be tethered.

Damage to the Globe

Global puncture is a serious complication of ophthalmic blocks. It has been reported following both intraconal and extraconal blocks and even following sub-Tenon's and subconjunctival injection.

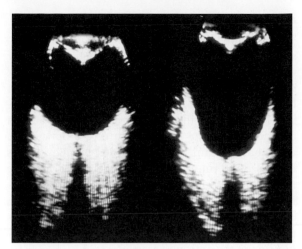

FIGURE 30.10 ■ Ultrasound scan of a normal eyeball (left) and a high myope.

Perforation of the globe has entry and exit wounds whereas penetration of the globe has only the wound of entry. With appropriate care, it should be a very rare complication because the sclera is a tough structure and, in most patients, is not perforated easily. Puncture of the eyeball is most likely to occur in patients with high myopia, previous retinal banding, posterior staphyloma or a deeply sunken eye in a narrow orbit. Not all globes are the same length and not all orbits are the same shape. In most patients who present for cataract surgery, axial length of the eyeball is measured with ultrasound (Fig. 30.10) to calculate the power of the intraocular lens. Normal globes have an axial length of 20–24 mm. Patients with high myopia have much longer axial lengths and extreme caution with needle blocks should be exercised in these patients.

Puncture of the globe is usually recognized at the time of surgery and presents as an exceptionally soft eye with a loss of red reflex. In cataract surgery, if the block is good, the surgeon should be encouraged to proceed with the lensectomy but to stitch up the eye with twice as many sutures as normal. Without lensectomy, it may not be possible to observe the damage to the posterior segment of the eye. It can be expected that the needle track through the vitreous will form a band of scar tissue. If this is not excised, it contracts and detaches the retina, sometimes causing sudden total blindness in the affected eye.

Optic Nerve Damage

This is a rare but late complication which usually results from obstruction of the central retinal artery or direct trauma following classical retrobulbar block with a long needle. This artery is the first and smallest branch of the ophthalmic artery arising from that vessel as it lies below the optic nerve. It runs for a short distance within the dural sheath of the optic nerve and, about 35 mm from the orbital margin, pierces the nerve and runs forward in the centre of the nerve to the retina. Damage to the artery may cause bleeding into the confined space of the optic nerve sheath, compressing and obstructing blood flow. If the complication is recognized soon enough, surgical decompression of the optic nerve is performed.

Extraocular Muscle Malfunction

The inadvertent injection of a long-acting local anaesthetic into any extraocular muscle mass may result in muscle damage manifesting as prolonged weakness, fibrosis or even necrosis of the muscle. The old-fashioned classical retrobulbar technique in which the needle was inserted between the lateral ⅓ and medial ⅔ junction of the inferior orbital rim predisposed to this complication. The safest site for inferotemporal injection is the extreme temporal area just below the lateral rectus. Recent evidence suggests that the addition of hyaluronidase to the local anaesthetic agent helps to disperse the agent before lasting damage can be done. Persistent diplopia following local anaesthesia should be investigated with a suitable scan because urgent surgical intervention to the affected muscle may be required.

OPHTHALMIC DRUGS RELEVANT TO THE ANAESTHETIST

β-Adrenergic blockade (e.g. timolol) decreases IOP by reduction of production of aqueous humour. Topical administration of drugs can cause clinically significant concentrations in the plasma via nasal drainage and the systemic side-effects of timolol including hypotension, bradycardia and bronchospasm are well reported. Phenylephrine applied to the eye intraoperatively to dilate the pupil can cause myocardial ischaemia and hypertension. Prostaglandin analogues (e.g. latanoprost) increase the uveoscleral outflow of aqueous,

reducing intraocular pressure. α-Adrenergic drugs (e.g. clonidine) have the same effect.

Carbonic anhydrase inhibitors (e.g. acetazolamide) reduce aqueous formation and are used orally or intravenously to treat or prevent increases in IOP. These are sulphonamides without bacteriostatic actions and should not be used in patients with a relevant allergy. They can cause an acidosis (renal loss of bicarbonate) and a diuresis as a result of their effects on the renal tubules. The acidosis can be made worse in the perioperative period if the effect of opioids and anaesthesia reduce respiratory compensation.

Hypertonic mannitol increases aqueous outflow. Initial increases in blood pressure and systemic blood volume are followed by a diuresis. The use of intraoperative diuretics necessitates the use of urinary catheterization. Ecothiopate is of historical interest as a treatment for intraocular hypertension because it irreversibly bound to cholinesterase and could last for a week; the duration of action of succinylcholine was therefore prolonged significantly.

ANAESTHESIA FOR SPECIFIC OPHTHALMIC PROCEDURES REQUIRING GENERAL ANAESTHESIA

Penetrating Eye Injury

The penetrating open eye injury attracts first place in the list, if only because of its perceived importance in examinations undertaken by trainee anaesthetists. Eye injuries may be difficult to inspect in detail because of swelling and pain and exploration under general anaesthesia may be required at the earliest opportunity. The potential for loss of intraocular contents exists even if penetration is not obviously present preoperatively. Eye injury may also coexist with other major head injuries or polytrauma. The incidence of penetrating eye injury is highest in young adult males although the introduction of seatbelt legislation brought about a significant reduction. As with any trauma, there may be a short fasting time before the injury and subsequent delay in gastric emptying, especially if alcohol was consumed before the injury or if an opioid was administered in the Emergency Department. The situation may therefore exist of anaesthesia for a patient with a potentially full stomach.

In patients with penetrating eye injury alone or associated with other trauma, general anaesthesia is routine. Orbital regional anaesthesia has been used successfully in some centres. The classical dilemma of rapid tracheal intubation to prevent aspiration using succinylcholine and the subsequent risk of increased IOP causing loss of eye contents is a balance of anaesthesia risk versus surgical risk. The overwhelming importance is to choose the anaesthetic technique which minimizes the risk of pulmonary aspiration of gastric contents most effectively throughout the perioperative period, but consideration should be given to reducing the IOP until the eye is made safe. In principle, therefore, the use of succinylcholine as the muscle relaxant with the fastest onset of good or excellent intubating conditions, in association with cricoid pressure, is first choice. However, large retrospective studies of penetrating eye injury have not shown vitreous loss to be clinically significant.

The urgency of surgery has the greatest influence on the anaesthesia decision-making process. Ophthalmologists are currently more likely to choose to wait for 6 h after the last meal or often, due to the time of day, wait until morning before exploring the eye. This is dependent on the severity of the injury as well as the potential to produce a good ocular outcome. There is little incentive to risk aspiration and death if there is little likelihood of preserving vision as the benefit. If appropriate fasting delays have been followed, the anaesthetist is in a position to make whatever anaesthetic choice is suitable for any other intraocular surgery with similar airway risk factors.

Surgery may be bilateral and lengthy and subsequent return to theatre for repeated procedures is also common. Loss of vision in one or both eyes following accidental injury in the young population understandably heightens preoperative anxiety.

Cataract Surgery

Cataract surgery has been revolutionized in recent decades and the need for complex anaesthesia has diminished. Phacoemulsification surgery is increasingly performed with smaller gauge probes and the procedure can be performed under topical anaesthesia, although many ophthalmologists prefer a block technique. The use of sub-Tenon's block is common and needle-based block is avoided in many countries. General anaesthesia is almost a rarity.

Vitreoretinal (VR) Surgery

VR surgery covers a range of intra- and extraocular procedures which may involve lengthy periods of time in the dark. Anaesthetic considerations relating to length of procedure and individual choices of technique and airway are described above. The use of a local block is common, with both needle- and cannula-based blocks in use. General anaesthesia is used in younger patients or if surgery is expected to exceed the patient's ability to remain comfortable. Of particular interest is the relevance of the use of nitrous oxide in general anaesthesia. Vitrectomy removes all the vitreous from the eye with the purpose of clearing cloudy or bloody vitreous, as well as performing intraocular procedures on the retina. The integrity and pressure of the vitreal cavity is determined by the surgeon throughout the procedure whilst the structured jelly-like apparatus is removed. The cavity may then be filled with an air/gas mixture (commonly perfluoropropane or sulphur hexafluoride) or silicone. The surgeon may make a decision on which of these to use towards the end of surgery and therefore it is sensible to avoid the use of nitrous oxide for vitrectomy surgery because, if an air/gas mixture is used by the surgeon, nitrous oxide in equilibrium in the eye cavity may diffuse out quickly at the end of the procedure, leaving a lower pressure in the eye than surgically intended. This can cause detachment or re-detachment of the retina. If nitrous oxide has been used, it should be switched off well before the insertion of surgical gas into the vitreal cavity. Gases may persist in the eye for up to three months postoperatively and the non-ophthalmic anaesthetist needs to be aware of the relevance of ophthalmic gases. A wrist band is placed on the patient after surgery to alert any subsequent anaesthetist to avoid nitrous oxide; nitrous oxide would diffuse into the cavity faster than nitrogen would diffuse out and the IOP could increase, with serious consequences. Likewise, flying can cause the bubble to expand. The gas diffuses out of the eye slowly over time. Silicone oil used for the same purpose needs to be removed surgically at a later stage. Nitrous oxide use is of no relevance if silicone oil has been used.

Retinal surgery can also be performed from outside the sclera. Buckling, bands, cryotherapy and laser therapies are used to repair breaks. The eye requires a lot of surgical manipulation during these procedures and the oculocardiac reflex can be profound and recurrent. Anticholinergic prophylaxis may be helpful. The VR anaesthetist may find that the operating list is very flexible because some detachments (e.g. macular detachment) require urgent surgery and are therefore common additions to the list at the end of the day.

Subsequent repeated operations are very common. General anaesthetic considerations remain the same; however, local anaesthesia may become complicated by adhesions related to the original surgery.

Strabismus Surgery

This is the most commonly performed paediatric ophthalmic procedure and is usually undertaken as a day-case. Airway considerations of head and neck procedures apply but a laryngeal mask airway is the most commonly selected technique, particularly in older children. Long-acting opioids are not required and are likely to increase an already high risk of postoperative nausea and vomiting. Surgery itself requires tension to be applied to the extraocular muscles. Steady deep anaesthesia with or without muscle relaxation (to guarantee immobility) allows the surgeon to gauge how much muscle repositioning is required. However, it is the tension applied by the surgeon to the muscle which can cause severe bradycardia, especially in the vagally responsive child. Prophylaxis with glycopyrronium is recommended. Strabismus surgery in children has been linked to a first presentation of malignant hyperthermia and temperature measurement is mandatory. Standard measures to control postoperative pain and reduction of nausea and vomiting should be considered.

Glaucoma Surgery

If general anaesthesia is required, most of the considerations are the same as for cataract surgery. However, unlike most ocular surgery, intraoperative miosis is required although this is not a contraindication to the use of intravenous atropine. A still, soft eye makes the surgical procedure easier to perform. Neuromuscular blockade and good anaesthetic control over IOP variables produce ideal conditions.

Dacrocystorhinostomy

Dacrocystorhinostomy (DCR) is a procedure performed for watery eyes. There is surgical exposure of the tear duct and a new opening is created into the nasal cavity. This is a relatively stimulating procedure. General anaesthesia is suitable although local anaesthesia (with or without sedation) has gained popularity. The operation may be performed with an open technique or through a nasal endoscope although, in relation to anaesthesia, the considerations are similar. All normal ophthalmic anaesthetic considerations apply. However, there is the additional risk of blood in the airway during and immediately after the procedure. Tracheal intubation and the safe use of a throat pack offer airway protection. Measures to prevent blood ooze at the site of surgery can aid the surgeon and these include hypotension, head-up position and the use of vasoconstriction in the surgical field. Xylometazoline or cocaine provides vasoconstriction in the nose. Endoscopic laser DCR is another surgical operation and the anaesthetist should have additional training in the practicalities of laser airway surgery. The laser safety officer will provide the correct eye protection for the anaesthetist.

Other Oculoplastic Procedures

The range of surgery for this subspecialty relates to the lid, socket or adnexae. Many procedures are short and lid surgery is generally performed under local anaesthesia. Longer procedures such as enucleation and tumour surgery are generally performed under general anaesthesia and appropriate measures are taken to provide postoperative pain relief. Bilateral blepharoplasties for cosmetic reasons are increasingly frequent and, in common with all oculoplastic surgery, the requirements for a bloodless field are best met with controlled relative hypotension and surgical site vasoconstriction.

Paediatric Procedures

In addition to strabismus surgery, children, including infants and neonates, may require other ophthalmic procedures. Although the majority of children are ASA I or II and may be managed as day cases, there are a number of patients with associated comorbidities who require detailed examinations or ocular surgery. Congenital cataracts, glaucoma, vascular and lens disorders can occur in diseases such as Down's, mucopolysaccharidoses, craniofacial and connective tissue disorders. Retinopathy of prematurity may require treatment in sick neonatal patients outside the theatre suite. Anaesthetic considerations relevant to the condition balanced with the surgical requirements guide anaesthesia choices. An infant with airway anomalies may require a complex anaesthetic skill-set simply to undergo ophthalmoscopy.

Sedation and Ophthalmic Blocks

Sedation is used commonly in conjunction with topical anaesthesia. Selected patients in whom explanation and reassurance have proved inadequate may benefit from sedation. Short-acting benzodiazepines, opioids and small doses of intravenous anaesthetic induction agents are favoured but the dosage must be minimal. The routine use of sedation is discouraged because of an increased incidence of adverse intraoperative events. It is essential that, when sedation is administered, a means of providing supplementary oxygen is available. Equipment and skills to manage any life-threatening events must be immediately accessible.

CONCLUSION

The practice of anaesthesia has seen preferences for local or general anaesthesia for ophthalmology repeatedly swing in both directions since Koller introduced a choice, using cocaine almost 130 years ago. Currently, the preference is firmly in favour of local anaesthesia and a practising ophthalmic anaesthetist should possess skills in a range of different techniques to deal with the needs of different operations, operators and, most importantly, patients. There is no place for *ad hoc* attendance in the eye unit or occasional practice.

FURTHER READING

Kumar, C.M., Dodds, C., 2006. Sub-Tenon's anesthesia. Ophthalmol. Clin. North Am. 19, 209–219.

Kumar, C.M., Dowd, T.C., 2006. Complications of ophthalmic regional blocks: their treatment and prevention. Ophthalmologica 220, 73–82.

Kumar, C.M., Dodds, C., Fanning, G.L. (Eds.), 2002. Ophthalmic anaesthesia. Swets and Zeitlinger, Netherlands.

Joint guidelines from the the Royal College of Anaesthetists and the Royal College of Ophthalmologists: 2012. http://www.rcoa.ac.uk/system/files/LA-Ophthalmic-surgery-2012.pdf. Accessed 24.06.13.

31

ANAESTHESIA FOR VASCULAR, ENDOCRINE AND PLASTIC SURGERY

MAJOR VASCULAR SURGERY

Many aspects of vascular surgery have changed during the last two decades, largely as a result of advances in radiological practice and cardiology. Examples include improvements in the treatment of myocardial infarction, the development of endovascular aortic surgery and lower limb angioplasty; such progress is likely to continue. However, anaesthesia for major vascular surgery remains a challenging area of practice. In addition to general considerations, the specific features of the commoner vascular procedures are described in this chapter: elective and emergency repair of abdominal aortic aneurysm (AAA), endovascular AAA repair, lower limb revascularization and carotid endarterectomy.

General Considerations

Peripheral vascular disease is a manifestation of generalized cardiovascular disease, and therefore coronary artery disease is present to some degree in almost all patients presenting for major vascular surgery. Most patients are elderly and have a high incidence of other coexisting medical disease, in particular:

- ischaemic heart disease
- hypertension
- congestive cardiac failure
- chronic obstructive pulmonary disease
- renal disease
- diabetes mellitus.

Most of these are considered independent risk factors for perioperative cardiac complications after major surgery (see Ch 18).

The broad aims of preoperative evaluation before vascular surgery are to:

- assist risk assessment, permit further investigation if appropriate and allow optimization of co-existing medical conditions
- evaluate and discuss the risks with the patient and surgical team
- establish the best surgical options (e.g. non-invasive or endovascular surgery) for an individual
- plan the anaesthetic technique, perioperative monitoring and postoperative care, and allow required facilities (e.g. ICU) to be organized.

Vascular surgery is associated with a high morbidity and mortality, resulting mostly from cardiac complications (myocardial infarction, arrhythmias and cardiac failure) (see Chs 18 and 43). It is therefore vital that cardiac function is assessed preoperatively and that the risks of surgery are evaluated and discussed with the patient. Although the outcome of subsequent vascular surgery is improved in those who have previously undergone coronary revascularization by coronary artery bypass grafting (CABG), this is associated with additional risks. Percutaneous coronary interventions (insertion of bare metal or drug-eluting intracoronary stents (ICS)) are being used increasingly as an alternative to CABG in suitable patients. There is a risk of stent thrombosis after ICS so patients receive dual antiplatelet therapy (aspirin and clopidogrel) for 6 weeks after bare metal and 1 year after drug-eluting stent insertion. The risks of perioperative cardiac events or stent thrombosis are very high if surgery is performed during the period when dual antiplatelet drugs are needed because of increased haemorrhage if antiplatelet therapy is continued, or acute thrombotic events if it is interrupted. The most recent guidelines suggest that elective surgery should be postponed for at least 4–6 weeks after bare metal stent insertion (and ideally delayed for 3 months) and for 1 year after drug-eluting stent insertion, unless surgery is more urgent. It should be remembered that coronary revascularization should be performed only if indicated because of the severity of coronary disease and is not justified simply to improve outcome from subsequent vascular surgery.

Preoperative Medical Therapy in Vascular Surgical Patients

The preoperative assessment clinic is an ideal opportunity to assess concurrent medication. Drugs particularly relevant to the patient with vascular disease are β-blockers, antiplatelet drugs and statins.

β-Blockers are used extensively in patients with angina, and improve the long-term survival after myocardial infarction and in patients with heart failure. Some studies have shown beneficial effects of perioperative β-blockade in high-risk patients undergoing major vascular surgery although the benefits in lower risk patients are less clear. Current guidelines suggest that β-blockers may be commenced in patients with inducible ischaemia (documented on preoperative stress testing), or proven coronary artery disease, who are undergoing major vascular surgery. The optimum duration, dose and role of individual regimens for β-blockade are not established, but if they are used, bisoprolol 2.5–10 mg or atenolol 25–100 mg daily should be started 1–2 weeks preoperatively, titrated towards a heart rate of 60–70 beats min^{-1}. Conversely, the perioperative discontinuation of β-blockers may be harmful, and they should be continued when already being used to control angina, arrhythmias or hypertension.

Current UK recommendations are that all patients undergoing major vascular surgery should be receiving antiplatelet therapy with aspirin unless there is a contraindication. Clopidogrel or dipyridamole are alternatives. Some clinicians consider that clopidogrel should be stopped 5 days before aortic surgery, but this should be discussed with the surgeon and prescribing physician. Aspirin should be continued throughout the perioperative period. Statin therapy should also be considered in all vascular surgical patients, and if

prescribed it should be continued throughout the perioperative period.

Minimum investigations before major vascular surgery should include ECG, chest X-ray, full blood count and serum urea and electrolyte concentrations, but more invasive or specialized tests may be required (see Ch 18), including cardiopulmonary exercise testing where available. Some assessment of exercise tolerance should be made in all patients because it is a useful indicator of functional cardiac status, although many vascular patients are limited by intermittent claudication or old age and may have a sedentary lifestyle. In this case, a patient with severe coronary artery disease may have no symptoms of angina and a normal resting ECG. In some patients (e.g. those with limited functional capacity or life expectancy because of severe intractable coexistent medical conditions), the risks of elective vascular surgery may outweigh the overall potential benefits and invasive surgery may not be appropriate.

Abdominal Aortic Aneurysm

Abdominal aortic aneurysms (AAAs) occur in 2–4% of the population over the age of 65 years, predominantly in males. Approximately 90% of AAAs arise below the origin of the renal arteries and they tend to expand over time. The risk of rupture increases exponentially when the aneurysm exceeds 5.5 cm in diameter and elective surgery is then indicated. The mortality from elective AAA repair is decreasing and is now 5–8%, but overall mortality from a ruptured AAA is up to 90%, and is 50% in those who survive until emergency surgery can be performed. Consequently, screening programmes are in place to identify patients with a small asymptomatic aneurysm and to offer intervention when the aneurysm reaches a diameter of 5.5 cm. Open surgery involves replacing the aneurysmal segment with a tube or bifurcated prosthetic graft, depending on the extent of iliac artery involvement. In all cases, the aorta must be cross-clamped (see below) and a large abdominal incision is required. Surgery is prolonged and blood loss may be substantial. Patients are usually elderly, with a high incidence of coexisting disease. These factors contribute to the high morbidity and mortality of this procedure. Endovascular aortic aneurysm surgery avoids some of these problems (see below).

Elective Open AAA Repair

Preoperative evaluation and risk assessment are paramount. All vasoactive medication (except perhaps ACE inhibitors and angiotensin-II receptor blockers) must be continued up to the time of surgery and an anxiolytic premedication may be advantageous. The patient may have recently undergone arteriography and the injection of large volumes of radiopaque dye may cause renal dysfunction. Maintenance of hydration with intravenous crystalloids is advisable the night before surgery. Some patients with severe chronic obstructive pulmonary disease may benefit from regular nebulizers and chest physiotherapy before surgery to decrease the incidence of respiratory complications.

An intra-arterial and two large intravenous cannulae should be inserted before induction of anaesthesia, with monitoring of ECG and pulse oximetry. Cardiovascular changes at induction may be diminished by preoperative hydration and careful titration of the intravenous induction agent. After neuromuscular blockade, the trachea is intubated (see below) and anaesthesia continued using a balanced volatile/opioid technique. Perioperative epidural analgesia is useful and may be undertaken before or after induction of anaesthesia.

Several important considerations apply to patients undergoing aortic surgery (Table 31.1). The following are required:

- two large (14-gauge) cannulae for infusion of warmed fluids
- arterial catheter for intra-arterial pressure monitoring and blood sampling for acid-base and blood gas analysis

TABLE 31.1
Major Anaesthetic Considerations for Patients Undergoing Aortic Surgery
High incidence of coexisting cardiovascular and respiratory disease
Cardiovascular instability during induction of anaesthesia, aortic cross-clamping and declamping
Large blood loss and fluid shifts during and after surgery
Prolonged major surgery in high-risk patients
Marked heat and evaporative fluid losses from exposed bowel
Potential postoperative impairment of respiratory, cardiac, renal and gastrointestinal function

- multilumen central venous catheter for drug administration and determination of right atrial pressure
- continuous ECG monitoring for ischaemia (CM_5 position) preferably with ST-segment analysis
- oesophageal or nasopharyngeal temperature probe
- urinary catheter
- nasogastric tube.

In the more compromised patient, e.g. with ischaemic heart disease and poor left ventricular function, an additional cardiac output monitor (e.g. trans-oesophageal echocardiography or other non-invasive device) should be used to monitor cardiac index and guide fluid management. A pulmonary artery catheter may be indicated in some patients. All possible measures should be undertaken to maintain body temperature, including heated mattress and overblanket, warmed intravenous fluids, and warmed and humidified inspired gases. The ambient temperature should be warm and the bowel may be wrapped in clear plastic to minimize evaporative losses.

Three specific stimuli may give rise to cardiovascular instability during surgery:

- *Tracheal intubation.* Laryngoscopy and tracheal intubation may be accompanied by marked increases in arterial pressure and heart rate which may precipitate myocardial ischaemia in susceptible individuals. This response may be attenuated by the i.v. administration of a β-blocker (e.g. esmolol $1.5\,mg\,kg^{-1}$) or a rapidly-acting opioid (e.g. alfentanil $10\,\mu g\,kg^{-1}$) before intubation.
- *Cross-clamping of the aorta.* Clamping of the aorta causes a sudden increase in aortic impedance to forward flow and hence left ventricular afterload. This increases cardiac work and may result in myocardial ischaemia, arrhythmias and left ventricular failure. Arterial pressure proximal to the clamp increases acutely even though left ventricular ejection fraction and cardiac output are reduced. The effects on preload are variable. The degree of cardiovascular disturbance is greater when the clamp is applied more proximally (greater at the supracoeliac>suprarenal>infrarenal levels). A vasodilator, e.g. glyceryl trinitrate (GTN), is often infused just before

clamping (and continued up to clamp release) to obviate these problems. Deepening of volatile anaesthesia or an additional dose of an opioid may also be used at aortic clamping. While the aorta is clamped, blood flow distal to the clamp decreases, and distal organ perfusion is largely dependent on the collateral circulation. The lower limbs, pelvic and abdominal viscera suffer variable degrees of ischaemia during which inflammatory mediators are released from white blood cells, platelets and capillary endothelium. These mediators include oxygen free radicals, neutrophil proteases, platelet activating factor, cyclo-oxygenase products and cytokines.

- *Aortic declamping.* Declamping of the aorta causes sudden decreases in aortic impedance, systemic vascular resistance and venous return with reperfusion of the bowel, pelvis and lower limbs and redistribution of blood. Inflammatory mediators are swept into the systemic circulation causing vasodilatation, metabolic acidosis, increased capillary permeability and sequestration of blood cells in the lungs. This is a critical period of anaesthesia and surgery because hypotension after aortic declamping may be severe and refractory unless circulating volume has been well maintained. If relative hypervolaemia is produced during the period of clamping by infusion of fluids to produce a CVP of greater than 12–14 mmHg (and perhaps administration of GTN until shortly before clamp release), declamping hypotension is less of a problem and metabolic acidosis may be diminished. Declamping hypotension usually resolves within a few minutes but vasopressors or positive inotropes are often required; these can be given before clamp release in anticipation. Good communication with the surgeon and slow or sequential clamp release helps the anaesthetist to manage aortic declamping. Renal blood flow decreases even when an infrarenal cross-clamp is used, and steps to maintain renal function are often required. The single most important measure is the maintenance of extracellular fluid volume (i.e. CVP >12–14 mmHg). Prophylactic mannitol 0.5–1.0 g kg^{-1} i.v. or furosemide may also be administered, although the evidence for their efficacy is conflicting.

Bleeding is a problem throughout the operation, often after aortic clamping when back bleeding from lumbar vessels occurs, but may be particularly severe at aortic declamping as the adequacy of vascular anastomoses is tested. A red cell salvage device should be used routinely in aortic surgery when it is available, but other modes of autologous blood transfusion (predonation, normovolaemic haemodilution) may be valuable. In addition to red cells, specific clotting factors are often required. It is often preferable to reserve the use of clotting factors until the anastomoses are complete and most of the anticipated blood loss has occurred. Many surgeons request the administration of heparin (usually 5000 units i.v.) before insertion of the graft and occasionally it may be appropriate to reverse its effects with protamine (0.5 mg per 100 units of heparin). Point-of-care haemostatic testing (thromboelastography or thromboelastometry) are very useful to diagnose coagulopathy and guide the use of clotting products.

Epidural analgesia is usually provided through a catheter placed at the mid-thoracic level, unless there is a contraindication. There is some debate as to whether epidural local anaesthetics are best administered during surgery (to attenuate cardiovascular and stress responses) or at the end of surgery (because sympathetic blockade may cause hypotension and make cardiovascular management more difficult during the procedure). A popular technique is to use combined volatile general anaesthesia with boluses of fentanyl or an infusion of remifentanil for intraoperative analgesia; epidural analgesia is then established after aortic declamping and once cardiovascular stability is ensured, using a combination of local anaesthetic and fentanyl.

Most patients are elderly and are unable to tolerate the large heat loss occurring through the extensive surgical exposure, which necessitates displacement of the bowel outside the abdominal cavity. Hypothermia causes vasoconstriction, which may cause myocardial ischaemia, delayed recovery and difficulties with fluid management during rewarming, because large volumes of intravenous fluid may be required. Therefore, all measures should be taken to prevent hypothermia.

The Postoperative Period. Postoperatively, the patient should be transferred to a high-dependency or intensive care unit. The decision to continue artificial ventilation or to extubate the trachea after surgery depends on the patient's previous medical condition and physiological stability during and at the end of surgery. Artificial ventilation should be continued until body temperature and acid-base status are normalized, cardiovascular stability restored and effective analgesia provided. Patients have a high incidence of postoperative cardiovascular and respiratory complications; renal dysfunction and ileus are also common. Close monitoring is required for several days.

Emergency Open Repair

The principles of management are similar to those discussed above. However, the patient may be grossly hypovolaemic and arterial pressure is often maintained only by marked systemic vasoconstriction and the action of abdominal muscle tone acting on intra-abdominal capacitance vessels. Resuscitation with intravenous fluids before the patient reaches the operating theatre should be judicious; permissive hypotension (maintaining systolic pressure at 80–100 mmHg) limits the extent of haemorrhage and improves outcome. The patient is prepared and anaesthesia induced on the operating table. While 100% oxygen is administered by mask, an arterial and two large-gauge i.v. cannulae are inserted under local anaesthesia. The surgeon then prepares and towels the patient ready for surgery and it is only at this point that anaesthesia is induced using a rapid-sequence technique. When muscle relaxation occurs, systemic arterial pressure may decrease precipitously and immediate laparotomy and aortic clamping may be required. Thereafter, the procedure is similar to that for elective repair.

The prognosis is poor for several reasons. There has been no preoperative preparation and most patients have concurrent disease. There may have been a period of severe hypotension, resulting in impairment of renal, cerebral or myocardial function. Blood loss is often substantial and massive transfusion of red cells and clotting factors is usually required. Postoperative jaundice is common because of haemolysis of damaged red cells in the circulation and in the large retroperitoneal haematoma which usually develops after aortic rupture. In addition, postoperative renal impairment and prolonged ileus often occur. Artificial ventilation and organ support are required for several days and the cause of death is usually multiorgan failure.

Endovascular Aortic Aneurysm Repair

Endovascular aortic aneurysm repair (EVAR) is now an established alternative to open surgery. A balloon-expandable stent-graft is inserted under radiological guidance via the femoral or iliac arteries into the aneurysm to exclude it from the circulation. It is performed via groin incisions and the aortic lumen is temporarily occluded from within, rather than being cross-clamped. The cardiovascular, metabolic and respiratory consequences are reduced in comparison with conventional open surgery. Perioperative blood loss, transfusion requirements, postoperative pain, hospital stay and morbidity are lower compared with open surgery. Perioperative morbidity is 1–2% although long-term (>8 years) survival after EVAR is similar to that after open surgery because of deaths from cardiovascular and respiratory diseases. Despite advances in stent-graft technology, the morphology of the aneurysm in some patients renders it unsuitable for EVAR (based on the site, shape, degree of angulation and the size of iliac arteries). Repeated radiological procedures (e.g. angioplasty) are required in up to 20% of patients. The procedure usually takes 1–2 h and may be performed by radiologists and/or surgeons but the patients have the same coexisting diseases and some of the anaesthetic considerations are similar. In some cases, EVAR may be preferred as a less invasive technique in patients judged unfit for open surgery. Access to the iliac vessels is often possible using infra-inguinal incisions in the groin and postoperative pain is therefore minimal compared to open surgery. In many centres, EVAR is performed in the radiology suite, in which case the anaesthetist must ensure that anaesthetic facilities for high-risk patients are adequate.

EVAR may be performed under general, regional or local anaesthesia with or without sedative adjuncts. In all cases, direct arterial pressure monitoring is mandatory because rapid fluctuations in arterial pressure may occur during stent-graft deployment. In awake patients, hyoscine 20 mg i.v. may be useful to decrease bowel motility during stent-graft placement. CVP monitoring is not usually necessary unless dictated by the patient's medical condition (e.g. moderate/severe cardiac disease). Short periods of apnoea are needed during insertion of the device; this is easy when ventilation is controlled but requires the patient's co-operation if a regional or local anaesthetic technique is used. The devices are positioned under angiographic control and large volumes of radiocontrast may be used, predisposing to contrast-induced nephropathy (CIN). It is important to avoid hypotension and hypovolaemia, both of which can contribute to CIN; sodium bicarbonate, N-acetylcysteine or mannitol may be administered, although the evidence of their benefit is limited. Brisk haemorrhage is unusual during EVAR and, although bleeding may be significant, it is usually insidious. However, large-diameter cannulae should be inserted and vasoactive drugs readily available because if endovascular repair is not technically feasible, conversion to open surgery may be required. EVAR may also be used to repair contained ruptured or leaking AAAs, and has an increasing role in the management of thoracic aortic aneurysms.

Surgery for Occlusive Peripheral Vascular Disease

Peripheral reconstructive surgery is performed in patients with severe atherosclerotic arterial disease causing ischaemic rest pain, tissue loss (ulceration or gangrene), severe claudication with disease at specific anatomical sites (aorto-iliac, femoropopliteal, popliteal or distal) or failure of nonsurgical procedures. Most patients are heavy smokers, suffer from chronic pulmonary disease and have widespread arterial disease. Most patients present with intermittent claudication. Consequently, exercise tolerance is limited and severe coronary artery disease may be present despite few symptoms. Surgical revascularization is performed to salvage the ischaemic limb, but arterial angioplasty is a less invasive alternative and is increasingly performed as a first-line procedure in suitable patients. Patients presenting for surgical reconstruction are often those in whom angioplasties have failed and who may have more severe vascular disease. Short-term mortality after lower limb revascularization is comparable to that following AAA repair and long-term outcome is worse as a consequence of associated cardiovascular disease. Acute limb ischaemia which threatens limb viability requires rapid intervention comprising full anticoagulation, intrathrombus thrombolysis after arteriography, analgesia and revascularization via embolectomy, angioplasty or bypass surgery as indicated. The clinical findings of sensory loss and muscle weakness necessitate intervention within 6 h and therefore preoperative evaluation and correction of risk factors may be limited.

Bypass of Aorto-Iliac Occlusion

Aortic bifurcation grafting is performed to overcome occlusion in the aorta and iliac arteries and to restore flow to the lower limbs. Because the disease evolves gradually, a considerable collateral circulation usually develops. Normal surgical practice is to side-clamp the aorta, maintaining some peripheral flow, and to declamp the arteries supplying the legs in sequence. Thus, the cardiovascular and metabolic changes are less severe than those seen during open AAA surgery, but the anaesthetic considerations and management are similar.

Peripheral Arterial Reconstruction

The commonest procedures involve the insertion of an autologous vein or synthetic vascular graft between axillary and femoral, or femoral and popliteal, arteries. Axillofemoral bypass surgery is performed in those not considered fit for open aortic surgery, and these patients are often particularly frail. All these operations are prolonged and an IPPV/relaxant balanced anaesthetic technique is suitable. A meticulous anaesthetic technique is paramount, with particular attention to the maintenance of normothermia and administration of i.v. fluids. Hypothermia or hypovolaemia may cause peripheral vasoconstriction, compromising distal perfusion and postoperative graft function. Blood loss through the walls of open-weave grafts may continue for several hours after surgery and cardiovascular status should be monitored closely during this time. Epidural analgesia may be used alone or as an adjunct to general anaesthesia for lower limb procedures. Despite theoretical advantages, epidural anaesthesia has no effect on graft function *per se* but it does provide effective postoperative analgesia. However, i.v. heparin is usually administered during and after surgery (see below) and the risks of epidural haematoma should be considered. Oxygen therapy should be continued for at least 24 h after surgery, and monitoring in a high-dependency unit is often required.

Carotid Artery Surgery

Despite advances in the medical treatment of patients with stroke, it remains a significant cause of death and disability. Carotid endarterectomy is performed to prevent disabling embolic stroke in patients with atheromatous plaques in the common carotid bifurcation, or internal or external carotid arteries. Most patients are elderly, with generalized vascular disease. Cerebral autoregulation may be impaired and cerebral blood flow is therefore much more dependent upon systemic arterial pressure. The main risk of surgery is the production of a new neurological deficit (which may be fatal or cause permanent disability), although cardiovascular complications account for 50% of the overall morbidity and mortality.

Carotid endarterectomy is unusual in that it is a preventative operation with well-defined indications based on the results of large-scale, randomized studies performed in Europe and the USA. In patients with a previous stroke and a carotid stenosis >70%, the benefits of surgery outweigh the risks, whereas in those with mild stenosis (<30%), the risks outweigh the benefits and medical treatment with antiplatelet drugs is preferred. Therefore, the patients presenting for surgery are those with the most severe disease, and the potential benefits are only realized if the overall perioperative mortality and morbidity are low (<5%). Specific perioperative risk factors are age >75 years, female sex, systolic hypertension, peripheral vascular disease (probably as a marker for coronary artery disease), experience of the surgeon and ipsilateral cerebral symptoms. Longer-term outcome is also worse in smokers and those with diabetes or hyperlipidaemia. Carotid artery angioplasty is a less invasive alternative to surgical endarterectomy, although its place is yet to be established. It is now clear that the risks of major stroke are highest within the first few days after a transient ischaemic attack (TIA) or minor stroke. Consequently, carotid endarterectomy should be performed as soon as is feasible (within 1 week and ideally within 48 h) after a minor stroke or TIA when indicated (embolic stroke, significant carotid stenosis). This limits the time available for preoperative preparation, investigation and risk reduction.

During surgery, the internal, external and common carotid arteries are clamped and the atheromatous plaque removed. During application of the clamps, cerebral perfusion is dependent on collateral circulation via the circle of Willis. Many surgeons insert a temporary shunt to bypass the site of obstruction, minimizing the period of potential cerebral ischaemia. Several methods are available to assess cerebral blood flow during clamping, before proceeding with the endarterectomy; if flow is adequate, some surgeons prefer not to use a temporary shunt. Monitoring of neurological status in an awake patient is considered by many to be the 'gold standard', but other methods used in practice include:

- transcranial Doppler ultrasonography of the middle cerebral artery flow velocity
- measurement of arterial pressure in the occluded distal carotid segment (the 'stump' pressure)
- EEG monitoring.

Although most strokes related to surgery are associated with thromboembolism rather than hypo- or hypertension, and the majority of these are caused by inadvertent technical surgical error, the anaesthetist has a crucial role in the maintenance of cardiovascular stability before, during and after surgery. Rapid swings in arterial pressure are common because of the direct effects of surgical manipulation, plaque removal and carotid cross clamping in patients with impaired baroreceptor function due to carotid atheroma and cardiovascular disease.

The main aims of anaesthesia for carotid endarterectomy are maintenance of oxygen delivery to the brain, cardiovascular stability, airway protection, provision of neurological protection and rapid recovery. Most intraoperative strokes are apparent on recovery from anaesthesia and early postoperative neurological assessment is important. Any residual postoperative effects of anaesthesia may confuse the diagnosis of intraoperative embolism or ischaemic change, so a technique that permits rapid return of function is required. These aims may be achieved using general, local or regional anaesthetic techniques, with or without sedative or analgesic adjuncts. In all cases, an intra-arterial cannula is mandatory for monitoring of arterial pressure, which should be maintained particularly during carotid clamping, and attention paid to maintain normothermia.

Local infiltration of the surgical field may be used alone or in combination with superficial and intermediate or deep cervical plexus blockade. Superficial cervical plexus block is performed by infiltration of local anaesthetic along the entire length of the posterior border of the sternomastoid muscle, using 10–15 mL local anaesthetic (e.g. levobupivacaine 0.25%). The intermediate block involves injection of 5 mL of local anaesthetic 1–2 cm deep to the midpoint of the sternomastoid. Advantages of locoregional techniques include definitive neurological monitoring (therefore allowing selective use of shunts), preservation of cerebral and coronary autoregulation, and the maintenance of higher cerebral perfusion pressures during the procedure (Table 31.2). These techniques rely on good cooperation between the patient, the surgeon and the anaesthetist. Many patients find it difficult to lie still and supine for the duration of the procedure, particularly those with heart failure or respiratory disease; this may be compounded by diaphragmatic compromise because phrenic nerve paralysis may accompany deep cervical plexus blockade. Sudden loss of consciousness or seizures may occur if cerebral perfusion is inadequate after clamping, and subsequent airway control may be very difficult because access is limited.

Performing surgery under general anaesthesia avoids these problems. Both propofol and volatile agents (at low doses) preserve cerebral and coronary autoregulation, reduce cerebral oxygen requirements and, in theory, may provide some degree of neuroprotection. General anaesthesia with artificial ventilation allows $PaCO_2$ to be manipulated but hypotension may be more common compared with regional anaesthesia. The airway is not accessible during surgery and tracheal intubation with a well-secured reinforced tracheal tube is advisable. Anaesthesia should be induced cautiously using an i.v. agent and maintained with a balanced technique using an inspired oxygen concentration of 50% in air or nitrous oxide (100% inspired oxygen produces cerebral vasoconstriction) with isoflurane, sevoflurane or desflurane. All anaesthetic agents should be short-acting, and remifentanil, alfentanil or low-dose fentanyl (100–200 µg) are useful adjuncts. Hypotension may potentially occur after induction and during the placement of cerebral monitoring, but it should be treated promptly. Vasopressors (e.g. ephedrine 3–6 mg or phenylephrine 25–50 µg increments) are frequently required and should be

---

TABLE 31.2
Suggested Advantages and Disadvantages of Local or General Anaesthesia for Carotid Surgery

Advantages	Disadvantages
Local Anaesthesia	
Definitive CNS monitoring	Technical difficulties
Maintenance of higher cerebral perfusion pressure	Patient discomfort lying supine during prolonged procedure
Maintenance of cerebral autoregulation	Sedative or analgesic supplementation usually required
Allows selective shunting	Lack of airway protection
Arterial pressure usually higher so less vasopressors required compared with GA	Difficult access to patient if intraoperative neurological or cardiac complications occur
Avoids 'minor' complications of general anaesthesia	
General Anaesthesia	
Patient comfort	Some method of monitoring of cerebral blood flow required
Airway protection	'Minor' complications of general anaesthesia (e.g. sore throat, sedation, nausea, vomiting)
Reduced $CMRO_2$ and theoretical cerebral protection	
Cerebral autoregulation maintained using low doses of volatile agents	Tendency towards intraoperative hypotension; requiring treatment with vasopressors
Therapeutic manipulation of arterial CO_2 possible	

drawn up before induction of anaesthesia. A high PaO_2, normocapnia and normothermia should be maintained. Blood loss and fluid requirements are usually modest. Postoperatively, significant pain is unusual and the combination of wound infiltration with local anaesthetic with a nonsteroidal anti-inflammatory analgesic during surgery is effective.

Data from the GALA trial (general anaesthesia vs. local anaesthesia) and systematic reviews have shown no difference in overall outcome with any specific anaesthetic technique.

Patients should be monitored in a high-dependency environment for several hours postoperatively. Hypertension is common in the early postoperative period because of impaired circulatory reflexes; pain from the wound or from bladder distension may also contribute. Hypertension is associated with adverse neurological outcomes because it may compromise the graft or cause intracranial haemorrhage. Arterial pressure should be controlled to achieve systolic pressures <165 mmHg and diastolic pressures <95 mmHg, accounting for the range of individual preoperative values. Intravenous α- or β-blockers or an infusion of a vasodilator (e.g. GTN or hydralazine) may be required as prophylaxis or treatment.

The other main postoperative complication is the development of a haematoma. Initial treatment involves local pressure and reversal of heparin with protamine. However, local oedema and the presence of a large haematoma may cause airway compromise and hypoxaemia requiring urgent surgical exploration. Induction of general anaesthesia in these circumstances is particularly hazardous and evacuation of the haematoma under local infiltration is usually preferable. Recurrent laryngeal nerve damage is a recognized complication of carotid endarterectomy. In most cases, this simply causes a hoarse voice but in patients who have had a previous contralateral carotid endarterectomy, specific preoperative evaluation of vocal cord function should be performed before surgery.

Cardioversion

Direct current (DC) cardioversion is an effective treatment for some re-entrant tachyarrhythmias, which may produce haemodynamic instability and myocardial ischaemia and which do not respond to other measures. Atrial fibrillation of less than 6 months'

duration, atrial flutter, supraventricular tachycardia and ventricular tachycardia may be converted to sinus rhythm, although maintenance of sinus rhythm depends usually on subsequent antiarrhythmic drugs. Cardioversion has little effect on contractility, conductivity or excitability of the myocardium, and has a low incidence of side-effects or complications.

Pre-Anaesthetic Assessment

Patients may present with a chronic arrhythmia for elective cardioversion or as an emergency *in extremis* with a life-threatening arrhythmia. They may have other serious cardiovascular pathology such as rheumatic disease, ischaemic heart disease, recent myocardial infarction or cardiac failure. Digoxin therapy predisposes to postcardioversion arrhythmias; it is often withheld for 48 h before cardioversion. If DC cardioversion is required in a patient receiving digoxin, the initial DC dose should be low (e.g. 10–25 J) and increased if necessary. In some patients there is a significant risk of embolic phenomena, e.g. those with:

- mitral stenosis and atrial fibrillation of recent onset
- atrial fibrillation and a dilated cardiomyopathy
- a prosthetic mitral valve
- a history of embolic phenomena.

These patients should receive prophylactic anticoagulants for 2–3 weeks before cardioversion, and anticoagulation should be continued afterwards. Accurate knowledge of the medical and drug history and thorough clinical examination are essential before anaesthesia.

Cardioversion

Direct current (DC) electrical discharge passed through the heart depolarizes all excitable myocardial cells and interrupts abnormal pathways and foci. The electrodes are usually positioned on the anterolateral chest with the patient supine, but the anteroposterior arrangement, with the patient in the lateral position, is sometimes used. The paddles should not be sited over the scapula, sternum or vertebrae and the skin must be protected with electrolyte jelly, saline-soaked gauze or any type of conducting pad.

The ECG monitoring lead chosen should demonstrate a clear R wave in order to synchronize the discharge away from the T wave and thus reduce the risk of development of ventricular fibrillation. If the arrhythmia does not convert after the first 50 J discharge, further shocks are given, using an increased energy discharge of up to 200 J.

Despite the use of synchronized discharge, ventricular fibrillation may be produced in the presence of hypokalaemia, ischaemia, digoxin toxicity and QT prolongation (e.g. caused by quinidine or tricyclic antidepressants).

Anaesthesia

Treatment should be carried out only in areas specifically designed for the purpose and with a full range of drugs, resuscitation and monitoring equipment available. These must be checked by the anaesthetist, and patients prepared as for a surgical procedure.

ECG monitoring, pulse oximetry and measurement of arterial pressure are instituted. A vein is cannulated and the patient's lungs are preoxygenated before i.v. induction of anaesthesia. The choice of drug is determined by the cardiovascular stability and recovery period required. If the patient is clinically shocked, precautions to prevent aspiration of gastric contents should be taken and a rapid-sequence induction with cricoid pressure and tracheal intubation should be used. However, many patients are admitted for elective cardioversion on a day-case basis, and a technique using i.v. propofol and spontaneous ventilation is suitable.

As soon as the patient is unconscious, the airway is secured and oxygenation maintained with a suitable breathing system. Before activation of the defibrillator, it is important to check that the patient is not in contact with any person or metal object. If repeated shocks are required, incremental doses of the anaesthetic may be given. The patient should be monitored carefully both during anaesthesia and after recovery of consciousness, in particular for evidence of recurrent arrhythmia, hypotension, pulmonary oedema, or systemic or pulmonary embolism.

SURGERY FOR TUMOURS OF THE ENDOCRINE SYSTEM

Amine precursor uptake and decarboxylation (APUD) cells originate from neuroectoderm and are distributed widely throughout the body. They synthesize and store neurotransmitter substances, including serotonin, ACTH, calcitonin, melanocyte-stimulating hormone (MSH), glucagon, gastrin and vasoactive intestinal polypeptide (VIP). Neoplastic change within these cells produces the group of tumours termed apudomas, e.g. carcinoid, pancreatic islet cell tumour, pituitary and thyroid adenoma, medullary carcinoma of thyroid and small cell carcinoma of the lung. These may be orthoendocrine or paraendocrine – the former produce amines and polypeptides associated normally with the constituent cells, while the latter secrete substances produced usually by other organs. Two orthoendocrine apudomas in particular may produce significant problems for the anaesthetist.

Carcinoid Tumour

Carcinoid tumours are rare tumours derived from enterochromaffin cells of the intestinal tract, most commonly the small bowel or appendix. However, they may arise at any site in the gut and rarely in the gallbladder, pancreas or bronchus. They are usually benign. Malignant change occurs in 4% and may produce hepatic metastases. Carcinoid tumours may secrete a number of vasoactive peptides and amines (e.g. serotonin, histamine, kinins and prostaglandins) which have a variety of effects on vascular, bronchial and gastrointestinal smooth muscle activity. These compounds are normally metabolized in the liver and carcinoid tumours are usually asymptomatic unless the mediators reach the systemic circulation from hepatic metastases, an extra-abdominal primary (e.g. bronchus), or if the tumour is large and hepatic metabolism is exceeded. In these cases, the clinical symptoms of carcinoid syndrome occur. These are variable but include flushing, increased intestinal motility, abdominal pain, bronchospasm and dyspnoea. Flushing, bronchospasm, increased intestinal motility, hypotension and oedema are related to the production of kallikrein, which is metabolized to bradykinin, a potent vasodilator. Adrenergic stimulation and alcohol ingestion increase the production of bradykinin. Serotonin (5-hydroxytryptamine, 5-HT) causes abnormal gut motility, diarrhoea and bronchospasm. It has positive inotropic and chronotropic effects and produces vasoconstriction. It may cause endocardial fibrosis, leading to pulmonary and tricuspid stenosis or regurgitation (although bronchial carcinoid tumours may lead to left-sided cardiac valvular lesions). Histamine secretion may cause bronchoconstriction and flushing. Acute attacks of carcinoid syndrome may also be precipitated by fear or hypotension.

Diagnosis is confirmed by high urinary excretion of 5-hydroxyindoleacetic acid (5-HIAA), a metabolite of 5-HT. Urinary 5-HIAA concentrations correlate with tumour activity and perioperative complications.

Primary and secondary tumours are localized by CT, MRI, ultrasound, combined PET/CT scans or radionuclide scans. Although medication may alleviate some symptoms, the definitive treatment of carcinoid tumours is surgery, including excision of the primary tumour and resection or radiofrequency ablation of hepatic metastases. The main anaesthetic considerations are perioperative prevention of mediator release and preparation for control of carcinoid crises. Systemic release of carcinoid mediators can be exacerbated or precipitated by anxiety, tracheal intubation, inadequate analgesia, tumour manipulation or the administration of catecholamines or drugs which cause histamine release. In severe cases, acute intraoperative cardiovascular instability (arrhythmias and extreme fluctuations in arterial pressure) and resistant bronchospasm may occur.

Management

Patients may be taking drugs to diminish symptoms of diarrhoea, flushing and bronchospasm, but specific agents are used to inhibit synthesis, prevent release or block the actions of the mediators released by the tumour. The most important drug is the somatostatin analogue octreotide, which improves both symptoms and biochemical indices, and which is useful in the prevention and management of perioperative hypotension and carcinoid crisis. Somatostatin (half-life 1–3 min) is secreted naturally by the pancreas and regulates gastrointestinal peptide production by inhibiting the secretion of growth hormone, thyroid-stimulating hormone (TSH), prolactin and other exocrine and endocrine hormones. Octreotide, the octapeptide analogue of somatostatin, has a longer half-life, high potency and low clearance, and may be given i.v. or s.c. The usual s.c. dose is 50–200 μg every 8–12 h. It is useful for symptom relief in other conditions, notably acromegaly, VIPoma and glucagonoma. It may cause gastrointestinal side-effects, gallstones and impaired glucose tolerance.

5-HT antagonists (ketanserin, methysergide) and antihistamines, e.g. ranitidine, chlorphenamine (chlorpheniramine), are also used. Cyproheptadine has both antihistamine and anti 5-HT actions.

Conduct of Anaesthesia

Perioperative management should be in close cooperation with both physician and surgeon, and the patient's regular medication should be continued up to the time of surgery. The possibility of cardiac valvular lesions should be considered. Hypovolaemia and electrolyte disturbance should be corrected before operation. Anxiolytic premedication with minimal cardiovascular disturbance is desirable; an oral benzodiazepine is often used alone or together with an antihistamine, although oversedation should be avoided. Octreotide must be continued as premedication 50–100 μg s.c. 1 h preoperatively. It may also be administered during surgery as an i.v. infusion at 50–100 μg h^{-1}. A smooth anaesthetic technique is essential, and techniques which may cause hypotension, including epidural and subarachnoid block, should be used with extreme caution. Drugs which release histamine (e.g. thiopental, morphine, pethidine, atracurium, mivacurium) should be avoided.

Continuous monitoring of ECG and direct arterial pressure should be started before careful induction of anaesthesia with etomidate or propofol, accompanied by measures to obtund the potentially exaggerated pressor response to tracheal intubation. Succinylcholine is best avoided because it may cause peptide release and nondepolarizing muscle relaxants with minimal histamine release (e.g. rocuronium or vecuronium) are preferable. Anaesthesia should be maintained with opioids (e.g. fentanyl or remifentanil), inhaled nitrous oxide and a volatile agent. Total intravenous anaesthesia with propofol has also been used. Bronchospasm may be severe and should be treated with octreotide or aminophylline rather than adrenaline, and a flow-generator type of ventilator capable of delivering the inspired gases at high pressure should be used. Major fluid shifts may occur during surgery and the effects of circulating peptides may distort the physiological response to hypovolaemia. Central venous pressure measurement is advisable when large blood loss is likely and pulmonary artery catheterization may be required in patients with cardiac complications. Intraoperative hypotension may be severe and should be treated with intravenous fluids and octreotide 100 µg i.v. Sympathomimetic drugs may cause α-mediated peptide release and are not recommended for the treatment of bronchospasm or hypotension. Hypertension is usually less severe and usually responds to increased depth of anaesthesia, β-blockade or ketanserin.

Close cardiovascular monitoring and good analgesia are required postoperatively and the patient should be observed in a high-dependency or intensive therapy unit. The use of epidural analgesia is controversial, but an epidural infusion of fentanyl alone or with bupivacaine 0.1% has been used successfully.

Phaeochromocytoma

Phaeochromocytomas are derived from chromaffin cells which secrete catecholamines (predominantly noradrenaline, but also adrenaline and occasionally dopamine) and occur in less than 0.1% of hypertensive patients. The majority present in middle-aged adults but they may be found in childhood. Most are found as a single benign tumour of the adrenal medulla, but 10% occur in ectopic sites, e.g. paravertebral sympathetic ganglia. Approximately 10% of phaeochromocytomas are malignant, and 10% are bilateral. Genetic factors are frequently involved and they may be associated with multiple endocrine neoplasia (MEN) and other syndromes (Table 31.3).

The clinical features depend on the quantity of hormones secreted and on which is predominant, although episodes may be paroxysmal and clinical findings may be normal between attacks. Noradrenaline-secreting tumours tend to cause severe refractory hypertension, headaches and glucose intolerance; circulating blood volume is reduced and vasoconstriction occurs. Adrenaline-secreting tumours trigger palpitations, anxiety and panic attacks, sweating, hypoglycaemia, tachycardia, tachyarrhythmias and occasionally high-output cardiac failure. Malaise, weight loss, pallor and psychological disturbances may occur, and end-organ damage (e.g. retinopathy, nephropathy, dilated cardiomyopathy) may arise as a consequence of hypertension. They present several problems to the anaesthetist (Table 31.4).

TABLE 31.3
Associations of Phaeochromocytoma with Other Syndromes

Von Hippel-Lindau disease (retinocerebral haemangioblastoma)

MEN IIa (Sipple's syndrome)
    Phaeochromocytoma
    Medullary cell thyroid carcinoma
    Hyperparathyroidism

MEN IIb (mucosal neuroma syndrome)
    Phaeochromocytoma
    Medullary cell thyroid carcinoma
    Mucosal neuromata
    Marfanoid habitus

Phaeochromocytoma-paraganglionoma syndrome

Von Recklinghausen's disease (multiple neurofibromatosis)

TABLE 31.4
Anaesthetic Considerations in Patients with Phaeochromocytoma

Preoperative

Hypertension

Hypovolaemia (vasoconstriction with reduced circulating volume)

Pharmacological stabilization
    α-blockade
    β-blockade
    Control of catecholamine synthesis

End-organ damage

Anxiolytic/sedative premedication

Intraoperative

Severe cardiovascular instability, particularly:
    at induction of anaesthesia and tracheal intubation
    during pneumoperitoneum (laparascopic procedures)
    during tumour handling
    following ligation of venous drainage

Hypoglycaemia after tumour removal

Postoperative

Hypotension

Hypoglycaemia

Somnolence, opioid sensitivity

Hypoadrenalism

LV dysfunction

Diagnosis

Diagnosis is important because the mortality of patients undergoing unrelated surgery with an unsuspected phaeochromocytoma is up to 50%. Diagnosis is confirmed by measurement of high plasma and urine concentrations of free catecholamines. Random 1-h or 24-h urinary excretion of catecholamine metabolites (metanephrines and 3-methoxy-4-hydroxymandelic acid (HMMA; also known as vanillylmandelic acid [VMA])), are an alternative. In some cases a clonidine suppression test may be required to distinguish between hypertensive patients and those with phaeochromocytoma. MRI of the abdomen is probably the investigation of choice to localize tumours greater than 1 cm in diameter. Computed tomography (performed without intravenous contrast media, which may precipitate release of hormone) is an alternative. Confirmation of the identity and position of an adrenal mass is by uptake of [^{131}I] m-iodobenzylguanidine (MIBG) monitored by gamma camera. MIBG scanning or 18 F-fluorodopamine positron emission tomography may be useful for the localization of small or extra-adrenal tumours not detected by other means.

Preoperative Preparation

Medical treatment of the effects of the tumour must be achieved before surgery. α-Adrenergic antagonists counteract the increased peripheral vascular resistance and reduced circulating volume, and phenoxybenzamine (noncompetitive, nonselective antagonist), prazosin and doxazosin ($α_1$-selective, competitive antagonists) have been used successfully. Noncompetitive α-antagonists are preferable because surges of catecholamine concentrations, occurring particularly during tumour handling, do not overwhelm the effects of a noncompetitive drug. Phenoxybenzamine is given in increasing titrated doses over 2–3 weeks before surgery, starting from 10 mg b.d. up to a usual dose of 40–50 mg b.d. In this way, the circulating volume expands gradually with normal oral intake of fluid. Adverse effects include initial postural hypotension, tachycardia, blurred vision and nasal congestion. A β-adrenergic antagonist may be required later to control tachycardia, but acute hypertension, cardiac failure and acute pulmonary oedema may occur if β-blockade is introduced first because of unopposed α-mediated vasoconstriction. Propranolol, metoprolol and atenolol

are useful agents if β-blockade is required. Labetalol is favoured by some physicians, but its β-effect predominates and α-antagonists should be administered first. Occasionally, phenoxybenzamine or phentolamine may be given by i.v. infusion (e.g. for 48–72 h preceding surgery). In this event, intravascular volume must be monitored by measurement of CVP and i.v. colloids are often required to maintain a normal circulating volume. Alternatively, catecholamine synthesis may be suppressed actively by administration of alpha-methyl-p-tyrosine, a tyrosine hydroxylase inhibitor. This drug may be very successful in controlling catecholamine effects but may cause severe side-effects, including diarrhoea, fatigue and depression and is usually reserved for long-term medical treatment in patients considered unsuitable for surgery.

Preoperative investigations depend on the patient's physical condition; the presence of end-organ damage should be determined. Nephrectomy may be required to remove the tumour completely and renal function should be assessed preoperatively. Echocardiography may also be useful.

Conduct of Anaesthesia

Sudden, severe hypertension (due to systemic release of catecholamines) may occur during tumour mobilization and handling, particularly if preoperative preparation has been inadequate. Severe hypotension may occur after ligation of the venous drainage of the tumour (when catecholamine concentrations decrease acutely). Marked fluctuations in arterial pressure may also occur during induction of anaesthesia and tracheal intubation.

Sedative and anxiolytic premedication is useful and both α- and β-adrenergic antagonists should be continued up to the day of surgery. Monitoring of ECG, CVP and direct arterial pressure must be started before induction of anaesthesia. Intraoperative monitoring should include temperature, blood gas tensions and glucose concentration; transoesophageal echocardiography or pulmonary artery catheterization may be required if significant cardiomyopathy is present. Anaesthetic drugs should be selected on the basis of cardiovascular stability and agents which have the ability to provoke histamine (and hence catecholamine) release are best avoided (Table 31.5). The exact choice of individual anaesthetic drugs is

TABLE 31.5
Drugs Which Should be Avoided in Patients with Phaeochromocytoma

Atropine

Succinylcholine

d-Tubocurarine

Atracurium

Pancuronium

Droperidol

Morphine

Halothane

less important than careful conduct of anaesthesia, which may be induced by slow administration of thiopental, etomidate or propofol and maintained with nitrous oxide in oxygen, supplemented by sevoflurane or isoflurane. Desflurane has the theoretical disadvantage of causing sympathetic stimulation if the inspired concentration is increased too rapidly. The use of moderate doses of an opioid (e.g. fentanyl $7–10 \mu g \, kg^{-1}$) may aid cardiovascular stability. Drugs should be immediately available to treat acute hypertension (e.g. SNP, phentolamine or nicardipine), tachycardia or arrhythmias (e.g. esmolol). Hypotension is treated with fluids initially but vasopressors (e.g. ephedrine, phenylephrine or noradrenaline) may be required. Intravenous magnesium sulphate may be useful: it suppresses catecholamine release from the tumour and adrenergic nerve endings, is a direct-acting vasodilator and has antiarrhythmic effects but has a narrow therapeutic window and plasma Mg^{2+} concentration should be monitored. Perioperative epidural analgesia may attenuate some of the cardiovascular responses, except during tumour handling, and is useful for postoperative analgesia. However, it should be used judiciously to avoid hypotension. Postoperative problems may include hypoglycaemia, somnolence, opioid sensitivity, hypotension and hypoadrenalism. Invasive monitoring should be continued for 12–24 h after surgery and the patient must be nursed in a high-dependency or intensive care unit.

Laparoscopic adrenalectomy is now the surgical treatment of choice for adrenal phaeochromocytoma.

It is performed via the transperitoneal or retroperitoneal routes. These laparascopic techniques are associated with less postoperative pain, and earlier mobilization and recovery, compared with open surgery. Overall, cardiovascular disturbance may be less, but the creation of a pneumoperitoneum during transperitoneal laparoscopy may cause large surges in catecholamine concentrations in addition to those occurring during tumour mobilization. Consequently, similar anaesthetic considerations apply as for open surgery.

PLASTIC SURGERY

Plastic surgery includes the reconstitution of damaged or deformed tissues (congenital abnormalities or resulting from trauma, burns or infection), removal of cutaneous tumours or cosmetic alteration of body features. Division or removal of the abnormality often necessitates skin grafting. Major plastic surgery includes the formation and repositioning of free and pedicle grafts and the movement of skin flaps.

General Considerations

Many of these procedures have important common features. Patients may be physically deformed and attention should be directed to their psychological state. This is influenced by long periods of confinement and rehabilitation, concern over disfigurement or loss of limb function, and occasionally chronic pain. The presence of local or generalized infection and the patient's state of nutrition are important factors in postoperative outcome and should be considered. Conversely, cosmetic surgery of the face, tattoo removal, breast augmentation and removal of unwanted adipose tissue are usually performed on healthy patients. Surgery is often prolonged, requiring special attention to blood and fluid replacement therapy, and maintenance of body temperature. Pain is usually peripheral in origin but may be severe, particularly from donor skin graft sites; local anaesthetic techniques (nerve or plexus blockade, or local infiltration) are very effective.

Anaesthesia for prolonged procedures should be administered using humidified gases in a warmed theatre environment, employing a technique which minimizes protracted recovery from anaesthesia. A remifentanil-based technique supplemented by a relatively insoluble volatile agent (e.g. isoflurane, desflurane or sevoflurane) is effective. Alternatively, a total intravenous technique may be employed, although the vasodilatation produced by volatile agents may be beneficial to surgical outcome. Nitrous oxide may produce bone marrow depression with exposure of more than 8 h duration and an oxygen/air mix should be substituted. Fluid balance should be maintained scrupulously. Significant haemorrhage is common during plastic surgery. Blood transfusion is frequently required, although microvascular flow is optimal with a haematocrit of approximately 0.3 and overtransfusion should be avoided. The outcome of microvascular surgery depends on adequate blood flow through a patent graft. Volatile anaesthetic agents and regional or sympathetic blockade cause vasodilatation, which may be helpful. However, graft blood flow may be impaired by hypotension, venous congestion or vasoconstriction caused by hypovolaemia, hypothermia, hypocapnia or pain. Therefore, maintenance of normal arterial pressure, circulating volume and cardiac output, normothermia, and provision of good analgesia are important to maximize peri- and postoperative perfusion of the surgical site. Vascular spasm may be diminished by the use of local vasodilators.

The patient must be positioned to avoid ligament strain, and lumbar support is useful during long procedures. Pressure areas should be protected with soft padding to prevent pressure injury, particularly over bony prominences, and a pressure-relieving mattress used. Measures should be taken to prevent DVT formation. When surgery has been completed, wound dressing and bandaging may be lengthy procedures. Bandages may be applied around the trunk and the patient must be lifted carefully to avoid injury.

Head and Neck

Tracheal intubation using a reinforced tube is recommended for surgery in this area. Tumours or scarring of the neck, deformity of facial bones and cleft palate can make tracheal intubation particularly difficult. The airway should be assessed carefully before anaesthesia, any difficulties anticipated and a complete range of equipment should be available. The administration of muscle relaxants in such patients may be unwise before the airway is secured by intubation; awake fibreoptic intubation under local anaesthesia or an inhalational technique should be considered. The method of maintenance is determined by the condition of the patient, the type and duration of surgery (frequently prolonged) and the experience and preference of the anaesthetist. Venous drainage is improved and bleeding reduced in head or neck surgery if the patient is positioned in a 10–15° head-up tilt. Hypotensive techniques may also be indicated, in which case an arterial cannula is advisable for measurement of arterial pressure. It is important to protect the eyes from pressure, the ears from blood and other fluids and the tracheal tube and anaesthetic tubing from dislodgement. It may be difficult to monitor chest movement, and access to the arms may be impossible. An i.v. infusion with extension tubing is essential; there should be access to a three-way tap for injection of drugs.

Trunk

Surgery performed on the trunk may be prolonged and require unusual patient positioning, e.g. hip flexion during and after abdominoplasty. Specific considerations include potential haemorrhage during breast reduction surgery, and the use of restrictive dressings applied after surgery.

Limbs

Local anaesthesia (e.g. by blockade of nerve plexuses in the neck, axilla or groin) may be an advantage in terms of analgesia and vasodilatation for surgery on upper or lower limbs. The duration of some plastic surgical operations and the use of a surgical tourniquet to provide a bloodless field may preclude some techniques, but prolonged neural blockade may be achieved using a catheter technique and by selection of an agent with a prolonged duration of action (e.g. bupivacaine or ropivacaine). Intravenous sedative drugs or light general anaesthesia are useful adjuncts to help the patient tolerate a prolonged procedure. Specific nerve blocks may be useful; for example, blockade of the femoral and lateral cutaneous nerve of the thigh provides good analgesia for skin graft donor sites during and after operation. Bier's block is of limited value because of tourniquet pain, and cuff deflation may be required by the surgeon to identify bleeding points.

Surgical techniques of reimplantation and microsurgical repair of the limbs are well established and make specific demands upon the anaesthetist. These include maintenance of general anaesthesia for up to 24 h, control of vascular spasm and provision of optimum conditions for postoperative recovery.

BURNS

Thermal burn injuries are common, and despite improvements in outcome over the last few decades, can still result in significant morbidity and mortality. Factors associated with death include increased age, the surface area and depth of the burn and the presence of inhalational injury. The anaesthetist may be involved with victims of thermal burns at an early stage during basic resuscitation and airway management, during transfer to, or management in, a critical care or specialized burns unit, or for the provision of general anaesthesia for:

- excision of damaged tissue and escharotomies
- excision of granulation tissue and subsequent grafting
- changes of dressing
- reparative plastic procedures to relieve contractures, permit limb function or correct deformities.

Surgeons now perform debridement of burns with escharotomies at an earlier stage because infection and sepsis are reduced, and cosmetic results are better.

Burns are classified according to the depth of burn and percentage of body surface area (BSA) involved. Partial-thickness burns may be confined to the epidermis (superficial epidermal or first-degree burns), or extend to the superficial or deeper layers of the dermis (superficial or deep dermal, second-degree burns). Typical features of first-degree burns include severe pain, lack of blistering and erythema which blanches on palpation. They heal spontaneously in a few days and should not be included in estimates of burn size. Superficial epidermal burns include blistering and also blanch, but usually heal naturally within 2 weeks. Deep dermal burns also cause blistering but do not blanch and are less painful than superficial burns. Full-thickness (third-degree) burns extend through the dermis into the subcutaneous tissues and appear white, red, brown or black, and do not blanch. They usually cause sensory loss because of superficial nerve injury. Both deep dermal and full-thickness burns require excision and grafting. The Wallace 'rule of nines' may be used to assess the area of burns in order to guide fluid management but is inaccurate in children. Lund and Browder charts are more accurate and are widely available. In clinical practice, the area of significant burn injury is often overestimated.

Pathophysiology

Early death in victims of fire is usually caused by hypoxaemia, resulting either from a reduction in inspired oxygen concentration in a smoke-filled atmosphere or from poisoning by products of combustion, e.g. carbon monoxide, hydrogen cyanide, hydrogen sulphide and ammonia. The affinity of carbon monoxide for haemoglobin is 200 times greater than that of oxygen, and in the presence of high carboxyhaemoglobin concentrations, arterial oxygen content is reduced. The oxygen dissociation curve is also distorted and shifted to the left, resulting in reduced oxygen delivery to the tissues. Inhalation of hot gases causes direct thermal upper airway burns with supraglottic oedema which may lead to airway obstruction within a few hours. Inhalation of smoke particles and toxic products of combustion can cause an inhalational injury comprising mucosal oedema, mucociliary damage, bronchospasm and loss of surfactant with the development of pneumonitis over the next 1–4 days. In addition to the local inflammatory response at the site of the burn, major burns also cause the widespread systemic release of cytokines, notably TNFα, interleukin-1 (IL-1) and IL-6, and reactive oxygen species. These may mediate the development of the systemic inflammatory response syndrome and contribute to the acute lung injury. Persistently high IL-6 concentrations are associated with a poor prognosis.

Cardiovascular changes after burn injuries include increased microvascular permeability with extravasation of plasma proteins, reduced plasma oncotic pressure and interstitial oedema. This is most marked at the site of the burn but also occurs throughout the vasculature, leading to marked hypovolaemia within hours. Myocardial contractility and cardiac output decrease independently of the reduction in circulating volume because of circulating depressant factors and diastolic dysfunction. Systemic vascular resistance is increased. If resuscitation is adequate, cardiac output may increase markedly after the first 24 h. Plasma potassium and urea concentrations increase initially because of cell tissue necrosis and haemolysis; muscle breakdown results in rhabdomyolysis. Renal failure may occur early after major burns primarily because of inadequate fluid resuscitation, but haemolysis or rhabdomyolysis may contribute.

The sympatho-adrenal response to burns includes enormous increases in plasma concentrations of catecholamines, aldosterone, ACTH and arginine vasopressin (AVP). These result in marked retention of sodium and water, with increased excretion of potassium, calcium and magnesium, so that hypokalaemia and anaemia are common after the first 48 h post-burn. There is also a hypercatabolic state with tachycardia, hyperpnoea and hyperpyrexia which may persist for several weeks or months. Muscle breakdown occurs in association with decreased protein synthesis, increased lipolysis and glycogenolysis so that nutritional and calorie requirements are increased markedly. Sepsis frequently develops following severe burns, often leading to widespread metabolic derangement, multiorgan failure and death. The outcome of sepsis in patients with burns is worse than in sepsis after trauma.

Recovery from burns trauma may be protracted. The anaesthetist must be aware of the probable requirement for multiple administrations of general anaesthesia, frequent use of opioid analgesics in the early stages and the importance of psychological support throughout the patient's stay in hospital.

Initial Management

The initial assessment and management of acute burn injuries are similar to those applied to other victims of trauma and are summarized in Table 31.6. The aim of immediate treatment is to secure the airway and administer high-flow humidified oxygen through a non-rebreathing system; tracheal intubation and IPPV with 100% oxygen may be required to maintain an adequate PaO_2. Fluid resuscitation should be started. Intravenous fluids guided by a formal protocol are required if the burn exceeds 10–15% of total BSA and central venous access is usually required with burns greater than 20% BSA. Early warning signs of upper airway burns include facial or intra-oral burns, singed facial or nasal hair, carbonaceous sputum, hypoxaemia, dyspnoea, cough or wheeze, although these are not universally present in the early stages and airway

TABLE 31.6
Initial Management of Patients with Severe Burns

1. History – time, extent and mechanism of burn, age and weight of patient, brief medical history
2. Airway assessment
3. Breathing – administer 100% humidified oxygen via a non-rebreathing mask
4. Circulation – establish two large-bore i.v. cannulae and commence fluid resuscitation
5. Assess neurological status
6. Exposure with environmental control
7. Analgesia – i.v. opioids
8. Formally assess burn area and re-evaluate fluid requirements
9. Monitoring – vital signs, urine output
10. Investigations – ABG, COHb, U&E, FBC, clotting screen, cross-match blood, ECG, CXR
11. Secondary survey to exclude other injuries
12. Burns dressings

ABG, blood gas analysis; COHb, carboxyhaemoglobin; U&E, urea and electrolyte concentrations; FBC, full blood count; CXR, chest X-ray.

obstruction may develop later. A history of burns in an enclosed space is highly suggestive. A high index of suspicion for airway burns should be maintained in all cases and prophylactic tracheal intubation is often justified, particularly in children or if interhospital transfer is required. However, the decision to secure the airway by tracheal intubation may be difficult and a senior anaesthetist should be involved. Hoarseness or stridor may indicate impending airway obstruction and tracheal intubation in these cases is mandatory. Pulse oximeters are unreliable in the presence of carboxyhaemoglobin because they cannot distinguish between oxyhaemoglobin and carboxyhaemoglobin and therefore overestimate true oxygen saturation; arterial blood gas analysis is required. Burns are extremely painful and carefully titrated intravenous opioids should be administered. Indications for ICU admission include potential airway problems, burns involving > 20% BSA and the presence of other injuries.

Tissue burns produce rapid fluid shifts and oedema formation, particularly during the first 36 h. The resulting depletion of intravascular volume is greatest in the first few hours and it is essential that a fluid replacement regimen is started as early as possible to avoid hypovolaemic shock and acute renal failure. Crystalloid-based regimens such as the Parkland formula are

TABLE 31.7
Fluid Regimens for Burned Patients

1. Estimate/measure weight

2. Estimate percentage area of burn using 'rule of nines' for adults and 'rule of tens' for children

3. Proceed with regimen if >15% burns in adults or >10% in children

4. Parkland formula:
   Requirements in first 24 h (mL) = body weight × % burn × 4
   Fluids given as Ringer's lactate alone, 50% within first 8 h,
   50% between 8 and 24 h
   Colloids administered only after first 24 h

5. Muir & Barclay formula:
   Requirements in each time period (mL) = body weight (kg) × % burns × 0.5
   Fluids (human albumin solution 4.5%) according to formula in *each* of the following periods:
   > 0–4 h
   > 4–8 h
   > 8–12 h
   > 12–18 h
   > 18–24 h
   > 24–36 h

In addition, water as 5% dextrose is required at $1-2\,mL\,kg^{-1}\,h^{-1}$.

N.B. These formulae should only be used as a guide to fluid requirements and individual prescriptions should be adjusted according to response.

used commonly (Table 31.7) although mixed colloid–crystalloid regimens based on that of Muir and Barclay are sometimes used. Many advocate administration of crystalloid solutions only in the first 24 h, with colloids added thereafter. However, the pathophysiology of fluid shifts is complex and these formulae should be used only as a guide to fluid therapy. Recent studies have shown that the type of resuscitation fluid used (crystalloid or colloid) does not affect mortality. Vital signs, urine output and body temperature should be observed closely, and volume replacement titrated to achieve a urine output of $0.5-1.0\,mL\,kg^{-1}\,h^{-1}$ ($1.0-1.5\,mL\,kg^{-1}\,h^{-1}$ in children). Non-invasive methods of cardiac output monitoring may also be used to guide fluid replacement and resuscitation. Haematocrit, base deficit and serum lactate, and urea and electrolyte concentrations should be monitored. It is important to be aware that excessive volumes of fluid for resuscitation can predispose to some complications including abdominal and extremity compartment syndromes. Bladder pressure monitoring (to detect intra-abdominal hypertension)

has been recommended for all patients with major burns of >30% BSA.

Anaesthetic Problems

Airway

It is vital to secure the airway in a patient with head and neck burns but this may be extremely challenging. In the initial stages, airway obstruction may occur, particularly in children where the airway is smaller. Many anaesthetists prefer to use an inhalational induction in the conscious patient, although raw, painful tissues may render proper application of a face mask difficult. Awake fibreoptic intubation may be preferable in adults. A rapid-sequence induction using succinylcholine may be inadvisable (see below). In all cases, facilities and expertise for emergency cricothyroidotomy or tracheostomy should be available, although elective tracheostomy is generally undesirable because of the risk of subsequent pulmonary sepsis and local infection in damaged skin. Later, as soft tissues fibrose and distort, the range of movement in the neck and temporomandibular joints may become grossly restricted and render laryngoscopic intubation impossible.

It may be difficult to secure the tracheal tube in patients with facial burns. Marked facial and neck swelling may occur which may result in dislodgement of tracheal tubes. Tubes should generally be left 'long'. Several ingenious methods have been devised, such as suspension of the anaesthetic breathing system from the ceiling, the use of umbilical tape to tie the tube in place and wiring the tube to the upper teeth. Tracheal intubation is often necessary for several days until airway oedema subsides. In this situation, or after prolonged surgery, the pharynx should be examined closely before tracheal extubation because laryngopharyngeal oedema may cause respiratory obstruction when the tracheal tube is removed.

Ventilation

Mechanical ventilation should be used in the severely burned patient and careful monitoring of ventilation is required. Humidification of inspired gas, physiotherapy and bronchial toilet are mandatory; bronchodilators and PEEP may be necessary. Acute lung injury developing over the first 4 days after burns causes alveolar oedema and hypoxaemia. This may be exacerbated by the administration of large volumes of fluid during resuscitation, but fluid restriction is associated with a worse outcome. Newer techniques include bronchial lavage, nebulized heparin, tissue plasminogen activator, acetyl cysteine and nitric oxide. The hypermetabolic state in large burns results in large increases in oxygen consumption and carbon dioxide production; i.v. nutrition increases the latter. The principles of artificial ventilation in burns patients are identical to those in acute lung injury from other causes: low tidal volume and minimal airway pressure (plateau pressure <35 cmH$_2$O, positive end-expiratory pressure titrated to maintain oxygenation) should be used and permissive hypercapnia tolerated if necessary; a sophisticated ventilator may be required for patients undergoing relatively simple surgical procedures. If significant inhalational injury has occurred, other ventilator modes such as airway pressure release ventilation or high frequency oscillation may be used.

Fluid Balance

Enteral feeding is established as soon as possible. The modern practice of early tissue excision is accompanied by extensive and rapid blood loss, and it is essential to establish adequate venous access with facilities for warming infused fluids; cross-matched blood must be available before surgery. Surgeons frequently use adrenaline during burn debridement to minimize blood loss and the anaesthetist should take measures to counteract any cardiovascular effects. Blood loss is particularly difficult to monitor during burns surgery, and should be measured as accurately as possible. Vascular access may be difficult and it is often necessary to utilize veins in less conventional sites which have escaped injury (e.g. axilla or scalp).

Monitoring

Cutaneous burns may make conventional monitoring (e.g. application of ECG electrodes or blood pressure cuff) difficult. Invasive arterial pressure monitoring is indicated during early-phase surgery where there is potential for rapid blood loss. Urine output and body temperature should be monitored. Central venous catheterization may be required in the presence of extensive burns, although catheter-related sepsis is a hazard. Non-invasive monitors of cardiac output may also be useful.

Patient Positioning

Burns surgery may require the patient to be positioned in unusual postures (e.g. prone or lateral), and the anaesthetist should be prepared because changes of position may be required during a procedure.

Temperature Loss

Heat loss is increased from a burned area by evaporation and inability of cutaneous vessels to constrict and prevent radiation. The anaesthetist should minimize heat loss during anaesthesia and surgery by use of a warming blanket, foil blanket, blood warmer, gas humidifier and an ambient theatre temperature and humidity of 27 °C and 50%, respectively.

Anaesthetic Drugs

Personal preference and the problems of repeated administration of anaesthesia govern the choice of anaesthetic agent. An inhaled nitrous oxide/oxygen mixture (Entonox) and i.v. ketamine are useful for analgesia during burns dressings. However, it is not safe to assume that the airway is preserved during ketamine anaesthesia and antisialagogue premedication is useful to diminish salivation. Diazepam may control the emergence hallucinations suffered by some patients who receive ketamine. Intravenous opioids (by infusion, boluses or patient-controlled analgesia) are effective alternatives. Supplementary analgesics are required in the short- and long-term, e.g. paracetamol, non-steroidal anti-inflammatory drugs. Adjunctive therapies include clonidine, tricyclic antidepressants, topical and systemic local anaesthetics or transcutaneous electrical nerve stimulation. For surgical procedures, a balanced technique using a volatile agent and opioid is indicated. The disposition and action of many drugs are affected following burns, e.g. there is marked resistance to the effects of nondepolarizing muscle relaxants from 1 week after major burns.

Succinylcholine should be not be administered from 24 to 48 h after the burn. In the presence of muscle damage, it may cause acute hyperkalaemia in concentrations sufficient to cause cardiac arrest. The mechanism involves upregulation of cholinergic receptors with the proliferation of immature receptor isoforms and extrajunctional receptors. The most dangerous period in this regard is probably between 4 days and 10 weeks after thermal injury.

FURTHER READING

Hines, R.L., Marschall, K.E., 2008. Stoelting's anesthesia and co-existing disease, fifth ed. Churchill Livingstone, Philadelphia.

Kaplan, J.A., Lake, C.L., Murray, M.J., 2004. Vascular anesthesia, second ed. Elsevier, New York.

Kasten, K.R., Makley, A.T., Kagan, R.J., 2011. Update on the critical care management of severe burns. J. Intensive Care Med. 26, 223–236.

MacLennan, A., Heimbach, D.M., Cullen, B.F., 1998. Anesthesia for major thermal injury. Anesthesiology 89, 749–770.

Mancuso, K., Kaye, A.D., Boudreaux, J.P., et al., 2011. Carcinoid and perioperative anesthetic considerations. J. Clin. Anesth. 23, 329–341.

Thompson, J.P., Telford, R.J., Howell, S.J., 2013. Oxford specialist handbook of vascular anaesthesia. OUP, Oxford.

Neurosurgical procedures include elective and emergency surgery of the central nervous system, its vasculature and the cerebrospinal fluid (CSF), together with the surrounding bony structures, the skull and spine. Almost all require general anaesthesia. In addition to a conventional anaesthetic technique which pays meticulous attention to detail, the essential factors are the maintenance of cerebral perfusion pressure and the facilitation of surgical access by minimizing blood loss and preventing increases in central nervous tissue volume and oedema.

APPLIED ANATOMY AND PHYSIOLOGY

Anatomy

Brain

The brain comprises the brainstem, the cerebellum, the midbrain and the paired cerebral hemispheres. The brainstem is formed from the medulla and the pons, with the medulla connected to the spinal cord below and to the cerebellum posteriorly. The medulla contains the ascending and descending nerve tracts, the lower cranial nerve nuclei and the respiratory and vasomotor (or 'vital') centres. Running through the brainstem is the reticular system which is associated with consciousness. A lesion or compression of the brainstem secondary to raised intracranial pressure produces abnormal function of the vital centres which is rapidly fatal ('coning'). The cerebellum coordinates balance, posture and muscular tone. The midbrain connects the brainstem and cerebellum to the hypothalamus,

the thalamus and the cerebral hemispheres. The cerebrum consists of the diencephalon containing the thalamus, hypothalamus and the two cerebral hemispheres. The thalamus contains the nuclei of the main sensory pathways. The hypothalamus coordinates the autonomic nervous system and the endocrine systems of the body. Below the hypothalamus is the pituitary gland. Pituitary tumours may produce the signs of a space-occupying lesion, restrict the visual fields by compressing the optic chiasma or give rise to an endocrine disturbance. The cerebral hemispheres comprise the cerebral cortex, the basal ganglia and the lateral ventricles. A central sulcus or cleft separates the main motor gyrus (or fold) anteriorly from the main sensory gyrus posteriorly. Each hemisphere is divided into four areas or lobes. The function of the different lobes is incompletely understood. However, the frontal lobe contains the motor cortex and areas concerned with intellect and behaviour. The parietal lobe contains the sensory cortex, the temporal lobe is concerned with auditory sensation and the integration of other stimuli, and the occipital lobe contains the visual cortex. Lesions of the cerebral hemispheres give rise to sensory and motor deficits on the opposite side of the body.

Spinal Cord

The spinal cord is approximately 45 cm long and passes from the foramen magnum, where it is continuous with the medulla, to a tapered end termed the conus medullaris at the level of the first or second lumbar vertebrae. At each spinal level, paired anterior (motor) and posterior (sensory) spinal roots emerge on each side of the cord. Each posterior root has a ganglion containing the cell bodies of the sensory nerves. The two roots join at each intervertebral foramen to form a mixed spinal nerve.

Cerebrospinal Fluid

Cerebrospinal fluid (CSF) fills the cerebral ventricles and the subarachnoid space around the brain and the spinal cord. The CSF acts as a buffer, separating the brain and spinal cord from the hard bony projections inside the skull and the vertebral canal. It is produced by the choroid plexus in the lateral, third and fourth ventricles by a combination of filtration and secretion (Fig. 32.1). The total volume of CSF is 150–200 mL. CSF passes back into the venous blood through arachnoid villi. Blockages which obstruct the normal flow of CSF through the ventricular system or prevent its reabsorption lead to a build-up in CSF pressure, dilation of the ventricles and hydrocephalus.

Meninges

Three meninges or membranes surround the brain and the spinal cord. These are the dura mater, the arachnoid mater and the pia mater. Around the brain, the dura mater is a thick, strong, double membrane which separates into its two layers in parts to form the cerebral venous sinuses. The outer or endosteal layer is adherent to the skull bones and is the equivalent of the periosteum. The inner layer is continuous with the dura which surrounds the spinal cord. The major artery supplying the dura mater in the head is the middle meningeal artery, which may be damaged in a head injury and skull fracture, leading to the formation of an extradural haematoma. The arachnoid mater is a thin membrane normally adjacent to the dura mater. Cortical veins from the surface of the brain pass through the arachnoid mater to reach dural venous sinuses and may be damaged by relatively minor trauma, leading to the formation of a subdural haematoma. The pia mater is a vascular membrane closely adherent to the surface of the brain and follows the contours of the gyri and sulci. The space between the pia and arachnoid maters is the subarachnoid space and contains CSF.

The dura mater forms a sac which ends below the cord, usually at the level of the second sacral segment. The dura extends for a short distance along each nerve

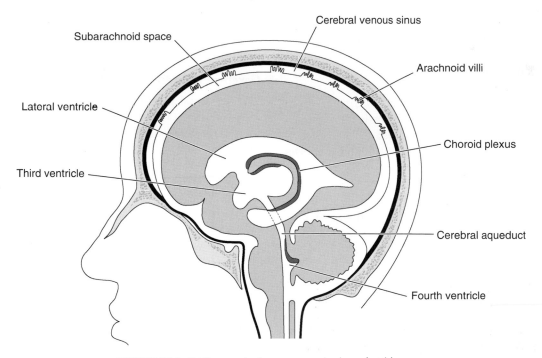

FIGURE 32.1 ■ The ventricular system and subarachnoid space.

root and is continuous with the epineurium of each spinal nerve. There is an extensive subarachnoid space between the arachnoid mater and the pia mater. The space between the dura and the bony part of the spinal canal (the extradural or epidural space) is filled with fat, lymphatics, arteries and an extensive venous plexus.

Vascular Supply

The arterial blood supply to the brain is derived from the two internal carotid arteries and the two vertebral arteries. The vertebral arteries are branches of the subclavian arteries and pass through foramina in the transverse processes of the upper six cervical vertebrae. They join together anterior to the brainstem to form the single basilar artery, which then divides again to form the two posterior cerebral arteries. These vessels and the two internal carotid arteries form an anastomotic system known as the circle of Willis at the base of the brain. The main arteries supplying the cerebral hemispheres are the anterior, middle and posterior cerebral artery for each hemisphere. The majority of cerebral aneurysms are of vessels that are part of, or very close to, the circle of Willis. Other important vessels supplying the brainstem and the cerebellum branch from the basilar artery. Venous blood drains into the cerebral venous sinuses, whose walls are formed from the dura mater. These sinuses join and empty into the internal jugular veins.

The blood supply to the spinal cord comes from the single anterior spinal artery formed at the foramen magnum from a branch from each of the vertebral arteries, and from the paired posterior spinal arteries derived from the posterior inferior cerebellar arteries. The anterior artery supplies the anterior two-thirds of the cord. There are additional supplies from segmental arteries and also a direct supply from the aorta, usually at the level of the eleventh thoracic intervertebral space. The blood supply to the spinal cord is fragile, and infarction of the cord may result from even minor disruption of the normal arterial supply.

Autonomic Nervous System

The autonomic nervous system is classified on anatomical and physiological grounds into the functionally opposing sympathetic and parasympathetic nervous systems. The central areas responsible for coordinating the autonomic nervous system are mostly in the hypothalamus and its surrounding structures, and in the frontal lobes. The sympathetic nervous system cells arise from the lateral horn of the thoracic and first two lumbar segments of the spinal cord. The neurones of the parasympathetic nervous system exit the central nervous system with the third, seventh, ninth and tenth cranial nerves and from the second to the fourth sacral segments of the spinal cord.

Intracranial Pressure

With normal cerebral compliance (the correct physiological parameter is elastance, which is the reciprocal of compliance), the intracranial pressure (ICP) is 7–15 cmH$_2$O (5–11 mmHg) in the horizontal position. When moving to the erect position, the ICP decreases initially, but then, because of a decrease in reabsorption of CSF, the pressure returns to normal. ICP is related directly to intrathoracic pressure and has a normal respiratory swing. It is increased by coughing, straining and positive end-expiratory pressure. In the presence of reduced cerebral compliance, small changes in cerebral volume produce large changes in ICP. Such critical changes may be induced by drugs used during anaesthesia (e.g. volatile anaesthetic agents and vasodilators), elevations in PaCO$_2$ and posture, as well as by surgery and trauma (Fig. 32.2).

Cerebral Blood Flow

Under normal conditions, the brain receives about 15% of the cardiac output, which corresponds to a cerebral blood flow (CBF) of approximately

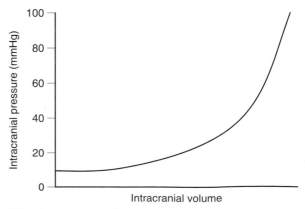

FIGURE 32.2 ■ The intracranial pressure/volume relationship.

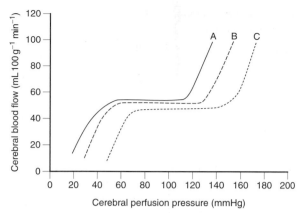

FIGURE 32.3 ■ Autoregulation of cerebral blood flow. **(A)** Drug-induced vasodilatation. **(B)** Normal. **(C)** Hypertension or haemorrhagic hypotension.

$50 \, \text{mL} \, 100 \, \text{g}^{-1}$ tissue min^{-1} or $600–700 \, \text{mL} \, \text{min}^{-1}$. The cerebral circulation is able to maintain an almost constant blood flow between a mean arterial pressure of 60 and 140 mmHg by the process of autoregulation. This is mediated by a primary myogenic response involving local alteration in the diameter of small arterioles in response to changes in transmural pressure. Above and below these limits, or in the traumatized brain, autoregulation is impaired or absent, so that cerebral blood flow is closely related to cerebral perfusion pressure (CPP) (Fig. 32.3). This effect is also seen in association with cerebral hypoxia and hypercapnia, in addition to acute intracranial disease and trauma. Cerebral perfusion pressure may be reduced as a result of systemic hypotension or an increase in ICP; CBF is maintained until the ICP exceeds 30–40 mmHg. The Cushing reflex increases CPP in response to an increase in ICP by producing, first, reflex systemic hypertension and tachycardia and then bradycardia, despite these compensatory mechanisms also contributing to an increase in ICP. In the treatment of closed head injuries, if both ICP and mean arterial pressure are being monitored, it is essential to maintain the resultant CPP with vasopressor therapy if cerebral perfusion is borderline because even transient absence of flow to the brain may produce focal or global ischaemia with infarction. Figure 32.3 also demonstrates that haemorrhagic hypotension associated with excess sympathetic nervous activity results in a loss of autoregulation at a higher CPP than normal, while the use of vasodilators to induce hypotension shifts the curve to the left, maintaining flow at lower levels of perfusion pressure. Vasodilators also differ in their effects; autoregulation is preserved at a lower CPP with sodium nitroprusside than with autonomic ganglionic blockade (however, vasodilators are rarely used during neuroanaesthesia). Cerebral blood flow is closely coupled to cerebral metabolic rate. Local increases in cerebral metabolic rate are associated with very prompt increases in CBF. The increased electrical activity associated with convulsions produces an increase in lactic acid and other vasodilator metabolites. This, together with an increase in CO_2 production, produces an increase in CBF. Conversely, cerebral metabolic depression, in association with either deliberate or accidental hypothermia or induced by drugs, reduces CBF.

Cerebral Metabolism

The energy consumption of the brain is relatively constant, whether during sleep or in the awake state, and represents approximately 20% of total oxygen consumption at rest, or $50 \, \text{mL} \, \text{min}^{-1}$. Anaesthesia results in a decrease in cerebral metabolic rate. Cerebral metabolism relies on glucose supplied by the cerebral circulation because there are no stores of metabolic substrate. Other substrates which the brain can use are ketone bodies, lactate, glycerol, fatty acids and some amino acids including glutamate, aspartate and γ-aminobutyric acid (GABA). The brain can tolerate only short periods of hypoperfusion or circulatory arrest before irreversible neuronal damage occurs. The brain also releases and subsequently inactivates neurotransmitters.

The energy production of the brain is related directly to its rate of oxygen consumption, and the cerebral metabolic rate for oxygen ($CMRO_2$) is often used to quantify cerebral activity. By the Fick principle, $CMRO_2$ is equal to the CBF multiplied by the arteriovenous oxygen content difference. Barbiturates have been used to reduce cerebral metabolic rate, and propofol and benzodiazepines have a similar, although less profound, effect. All are used in the sedation of patients with head injury, and the choice is related more to the anticipated duration of sedation than to differences in the effects of the drugs, with the exception of prolonged barbiturate coma induced by infusion of thiopental.

Hypothermia is associated with a reduction in cerebral metabolic rate, with a decrease of approximately 7% for every 1 °C decrease in temperature.

Effects of Oxygen and Carbon Dioxide on Cerebral Blood Flow

Physiologically, carbon dioxide is the most important cerebral vasodilator. Even small increases in $PaCO_2$ produce significant increases in CBF and, therefore, ICP. There is an almost linear relationship between $PaCO_2$ and CBF (Fig. 32.4). Over the normal range, an increase of $PaCO_2$ by 1 kPa increases CBF by 30%. Conversely, hyperventilation to produce a $PaCO_2$ of 4 kPa produces cerebral vasoconstriction and a decrease in ICP, although this is compensated for by an increase in CSF production over a more prolonged period of hyperventilation, such as that used in the treatment of head injuries. This is why there is no advantage in aggressive hyperventilation regimens in head injury management. Hypocapnia below a $PaCO_2$ of 4 kPa has little acute effect on ICP, and hyperventilation beyond this point to lower ICP should be avoided except as a last resort because the vasoconstriction induced may be associated with a reduction in jugular bulb oxygen saturation, suggesting hypoperfusion and ischaemia. At a $PaCO_2$ above 10 kPa, the vessels are maximally dilated and there is little, if any, further increase in CBF.

Reduction in blood oxygen content also leads to cerebral vasodilation such that cerebral oxygen delivery remains approximately constant. In the normal physiological range, alterations in PaO_2 have little effect on CBF over the normal range. It is only when PaO_2 decreases below about 7 kPa that cerebral vasodilatation occurs. Reduction in cerebral blood oxygen content due to anaemia has similar effects.

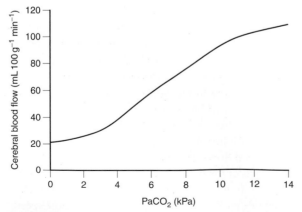

FIGURE 32.4 ■ The effect of increasing $PaCO_2$ on cerebral blood flow.

GENERAL PRINCIPLES OF NEUROSURGICAL ANAESTHESIA

Most intracranial operations involve a craniotomy, i.e. removal of a piece or flap of bone to gain access to the meninges and brain substance beneath. In many procedures, the size of the craniotomy can be 4–5 cm diameter or less (for example, for tumour biopsy, evacuation of a chronic subdural haematoma, insertion of an external ventricular drain or ventricular shunt catheter). Some procedures still require a large craniotomy (e.g. evacuation of acute subdural, extradural or intracerebral haematoma, meningioma resection, aneurysm surgery). A smooth anaesthetic technique is essential, avoiding increases in arterial and venous pressures and changes in carbon dioxide concentration while at the same time avoiding a decrease in cerebral oxygenation.

Most anaesthetists maintain hypnosis with either an inhalational anaesthetic agent, usually sevoflurane, or with a continuous infusion of propofol. Intraoperative analgesia is provided by a short-acting opioid such as remifentanil by infusion or intermittent doses of fentanyl (for short or minor procedures). Neuromuscular blockade and IPPV are usually employed. It is extremely important to ensure adequate fixation of the tracheal tube and intravascular cannulae and to protect the eyes, because access to the head and limbs is severely restricted during the operation. Continuous monitoring of the electrocardiograph and arterial pressure is essential; direct arterial pressure and temperature monitoring are normally used, together with continuous measurement of oxygen saturation, and end-tidal carbon dioxide and inspired anaesthetic agent concentrations. At the end of the procedure, the patient must be transferred to the recovery room with no residual neuromuscular blockade or opioid-induced respiratory depression because both may produce critical increases in ICP related to hypercapnia and hypoxaemia. Long-acting drugs with a marked sedative action are used with caution perioperatively so that a pathological failure of return to consciousness is not masked.

Induction of Anaesthesia

An intravenous infusion of an isotonic electrolyte solution should be started through a large-gauge intravenous cannula before induction. Intravenous induction should be used whenever possible. However, inhalational induction may be appropriate in children if the risk of a crying, distressed child is more likely to increase ICP than the vasodilator effects of a high inspired concentration of a volatile anaesthetic agent. Both thiopental and propofol reduce ICP and are suitable induction agents. The intravenous anaesthetic should be given with an appropriate dose of short-acting opioid and a neuromuscular blocking agent to facilitate a smooth induction and tracheal intubation, avoiding hypoxaemia and hypercapnia. A nerve stimulator should be used to ensure complete muscle paralysis before attempting direct laryngoscopy, to prevent any coughing or straining. It is important to remember that cerebral perfusion may be reduced when the ICP is raised, and an induction technique which produces significant hypotension may critically reduce cerebral perfusion in patients with a space-occupying lesion (SOL) or an intracranial or subarachnoid haemorrhage associated with vasospasm.

The most commonly used techniques to reduce the hypertensive response to laryngoscopy and tracheal intubation are supplementary short-acting opioids (fentanyl, alfentanil) or short-acting β-adrenoceptor blockade (e.g. esmolol). If remifentanil is used as a co-induction agent, an infusion is usually started immediately after the induction dose and acts to control the hypertensive response; alternatively, a target-controlled infusion (TCI) is used for both induction and maintenance during the intubation. A reinforced disposable tracheal tube is used. Careful positioning of the tube is vital because any intraoperative flexion of the neck may result in intubation of the right main bronchus if the tip of the tube is initially placed too close to the carina. After the tube has been secured, the neck should be flexed gently while listening for the presence of breath sounds in both axillae. The tube should be secured in place with several layers of sticky tape to prevent it peeling away after application of surgical 'prep' solution to the scalp. Cotton ties should not be used because they may compress the internal jugular veins, increasing venous pressure and leading to a reduction in cerebral perfusion pressure and increased intraoperative haemorrhage. Many anaesthetists routinely insert a pharyngeal throat pack to help to stabilize the tracheal tube in the mouth, but it is only essential if transnasal surgery (e.g. trans-sphenoidal hypophysectomy) is planned. A nasogastric tube is inserted in patients who are going to be prone for prolonged periods, or if surgery around the brainstem is planned (which might lead to a postoperative bulbar palsy).

The eyes are protected by applying paraffin gauze, padding with a folded swab and then covering with a waterproof tape. Skin cleaning ('prep') solutions must be prevented from entering the eyes. Low-molecular-weight heparin is not used preoperatively, but is started after surgery when the risk of perioperative haemorrhage has reduced. There is a significant risk of deep venous thrombosis (DVT) in this group of patients. Thromboembolism (TED) stockings are used pre- and postoperatively and intermittent pneumatic compression devices are used intra-operatively.

Positioning

Many neurosurgical operations are long and positioning of the patient to facilitate optimal access, while preventing hypothermia, pressure sores and peripheral nerve injury, is important. Supratentorial cranial surgery involving the frontal or frontotemporal areas is performed with the patient supine, while parietal and occipital craniotomies are carried out in the lateral or three-quarters prone ('park bench') position. In all cases, care must be taken to avoid neck positions such as marked rotation or flexion which might impede venous drainage. The fully prone position is used for surgery on the posterior fossa and around the foramen magnum, and the spine. The prone position is discussed in more detail in the section on spinal surgery (page 652). For some procedures, it is necessary to tilt or roll the table during the operation. The patient must be positioned securely with supports to prevent slipping if the table is moved. Some neurosurgical operations are prolonged and, whatever position is used, it is essential that all pressure points are protected adequately. During long operations, the pulse oximeter probe should be moved every 4 h, at least.

Heat Loss

Temperature should be maintained using a forced warm air blanket. It is important to prevent heat loss during prolonged surgery. Although there are theoretical benefits of allowing the body to cool intraoperatively (to around 35 °C) if cerebral ischaemia is likely or after head injury, well-controlled studies have failed to support such an approach. However, hyperthermia should be avoided.

Maintenance of Anaesthesia

The basis of anaesthesia for neurosurgery is ventilation of the lungs with air and oxygen to produce a $PaCO_2$ of around 4.5 kPa, using either a volatile anaesthetic agent or a propofol infusion supplemented by an opioid analgesic (remifentanil infusion or fentanyl boluses). Unless used carefully, remifentanil may produce hypotension, and when it is stopped, there may be rebound hypertension and the sudden onset of pain or agitation. Sevoflurane is the volatile agent of choice, given that its effects on the cerebral vasculature are much less than those of isoflurane. At clinical concentrations, sevoflurane has no effect on cerebral autoregulation and causes only a minimal increase in ICP. Alternatively, total intravenous anaesthesia with propofol TCI may be used. There is no evidence that one technique is associated with a better outcome compared with any other.

The choice of neuromuscular blocking agent depends usually on personal preference. In most cases, these drugs should be given by infusion. A peripheral nerve stimulator should be used and the infusion rate titrated to maintain an adequate degree of block (one twitch of the train-of-four stimulus pattern should be present), while preventing overdosage so that the block can be completely reversed shortly (10–15 min) after stopping the infusion and administering an anticholinesterase.

The initial part of a craniotomy is painful, but after the bone flap has been reflected and the dura incised, pain is not a significant feature again until closure of the wound. For this reason, supplementary intra-operative opioids in large doses are unnecessary. Use of opioids during maintenance does allow use of less hypnotic agent. Reflex vagal stimulation can occur, particularly following stimulation of the cranial nerve roots or during vascular surgery around the circle of Willis and the internal carotid artery. This may necessitate immediate administration of an anticholinergic agent to avoid severe bradycardia or even asystole.

Maintenance of normal arterial pressure is important in all patients, but may be a particular problem during induction in very sick or elderly patients. Hypotension, with the consequent reduction in cerebral perfusion, should be treated by infusion of a moderate volume of fluid, but it is advisable to administer a vasopressor such as ephedrine at an early stage.

Use of techniques permitting rapid recovery (for example sevoflurane, propofol, remifentanil) are particularly valuable in situations in which the patient is required to wake up and move to command intra-operatively, e.g. during spinal surgery or trigeminal nerve radiofrequency lesion generation.

Fluid Replacement Therapy

Most patients who present for elective intracranial operations are satisfactorily hydrated preoperatively. Patients with acute conditions such as trauma, those with a high ICP associated with nausea and vomiting and patients with general debility and cachexia may be dehydrated. The main intra-operative distinctions between patients are related to the underlying pathology. Cerebral tumours are associated with oedema and raised ICP, and therefore such patients may have been fluid-restricted preoperatively However, intra-operative hypotension must be avoided and careful perioperative fluid administration is essential. Cerebrovascular surgery is associated with vasospasm and maintaining an adequate cerebral blood flow is the prime prerequisite. A normal circulating blood volume is essential if the perfusion pressure is to be maintained, and although a slight reduction in haematocrit to about 0.30 is optimal for perfusion, adequate fluid replacement must be given.

All hypotonic fluids are avoided. Isotonic crystalloids are the standard maintenance fluids. There is no evidence for a specific role for colloid solutions, although blood is used if the haemoglobin falls below 8–9 g dL^{-1}. During significant haemorrhage or in patients with multiple injuries, careful attention to haemostasis is essential.

Supplementary Drug Therapy

Patients with a tumour or some other lesions may already be receiving an antiepileptic, and others may require intravenous phenytoin perioperatively, depending on the site of surgery. Patients receiving high-dose steroids need peri- and postoperative dexamethasone; the normal dose is 4 mg 6-hourly with 8–16 mg as an intra-operative bolus. Depending on local microbiological flora and surgeons' preferences, perioperative antibiotics are administered to many patients; a common choice is cefuroxime 1.5 g, which should be repeated 3-hourly during long operations.

Monitoring During Neurosurgical Anaesthesia

Standard monitoring should be started before induction. In patients in whom cardiovascular instability may be a problem, including the very elderly and frail or following subarachnoid haemorrhage, this should include direct arterial pressure monitoring started before induction. Arterial cannulation is now used routinely in all patients undergoing an intracranial operation, for surgery on the cervical spine, and in other situations in which rapid fluctuations in arterial pressure may occur. It also facilitates arterial sampling for blood gas analysis. Use of central venous pressure (CVP) catheters varies greatly among different practitioners and different neurosurgical units. They are used when major blood loss is expected, such as surgery for very vascular meningiomas, and for clipping of a cerebral aneurysm. They may be used in other operations in which there is a high risk of air embolism. A precordial or oesophageal stethoscope may be used to auscultate cardiac and respiratory sounds and also abnormal flow murmurs produced by air embolism. An oesophageal stethoscope is used more frequently in children.

Cerebral oximetry, transcranial Doppler, electroencephalography and evoked potentials are used in specific situations.

Mechanisms for Reducing Intracranial Pressure

The methods used commonly to reduce ICP (or to limit increases) are drugs, ventilation, posture and drainage. Adequate cerebral venous drainage must be assured by ensuring the neck veins are not compressed by ties, tapes or excessive neck rotation or flexion. Diuretics such as mannitol 10% or 20% ($0.5–1.0\,g\,kg^{-1}$) or furosemide (20–40 mg) deplete the intravascular fluid volume and subsequently reduce CSF production. A bolus of an intravenous anaesthetic agent such as propofol or thiopental may be used to reduce the cerebral metabolic rate, causing a reduction in cerebral blood flow and therefore decreases in cerebral blood volume and ICP. Direct

drainage of CSF may be accomplished either by lumbar puncture or by direct puncture of the cisterna magna or lateral ventricles. A move to an increased head-up position reduces venous congestion and ICP, but arterial hypotension must be avoided. Hypercapnia must be prevented by the use of IPPV, while short-term use of moderate hyperventilation produces cerebral vasoconstriction and a reduction in cerebral blood volume. If in doubt, an arterial blood gas analysis should be performed to verify adequate lung ventilation.

Elective Hypotension

Induced hypotension was formerly one of the mainstays of cerebrovascular surgery, but its use has diminished considerably in recent years because of the appreciation that cerebral perfusion is all-important. Most aneurysm surgery in now carried out at normotension; indeed, if the patient has an element of cerebral vasospasm, any reflex hypertension should be maintained. Hypotension is now a therapy of last resort if bleeding is torrential and it is otherwise impossible for the surgeon to regain control. If hypotension is required, the choice of technique is determined by the anticipated duration of induced hypotension. The alternatives are a short-acting β-adrenoceptor blocker such as esmolol, or increasing the depth of anaesthesia with a volatile agent. Direct vasodilators are rarely used because of the risk of 'steal' away from areas of poor perfusion, and the possibility of increasing cerebral blood volume and affecting the ICP. Hypotensive anaesthesia is used more frequently in spinal surgery, although the risks of inducing ischaemia in the cord substance are the same as in the brain. In this situation, evoked potentials may be used to assess spinal cord function during periods of hypotension.

Recovery from Anaesthesia

The majority of patients are allowed to wake up as usual at the end of operation, preferably in a dedicated neurosurgical recovery room. The Glasgow Coma Scale (Table 32.1) or an equivalent for children is recorded. Patients should return rapidly to at least their preoperative level of consciousness. A failure to achieve this, or a deterioration after an initial awakening, should alert carers to possible ischaemia or

TABLE 32.1
The Glasgow Coma Scale

Clinical Sign	Response	Score
Eyes open	Spontaneously	4
	To verbal command	3
	To pain	2
	No response	1
Best motor response to verbal command or to painful stimulus	Obeys	6
	Localizes pain	5
	Flexion withdrawal	4
	Abnormal flexion (decorticate rigidity)	3
	Extension (decerebrate rigidity)	2
	No response	1
Best verbal response	Orientated, converses	5
	Disorientated, converses	4
	Inappropriate words	3
	Incomprehensible sounds	2
	No response	1
	Total (minimum 3, maximum 15)	

raised ICP. Re-imaging or immediate wound exploration is then required. Seizures after elective intracranial neurosurgery are surprisingly rare and, if they occur, should be treated immediately and the cause identified.

Complete reversal of nondepolarizing neuromuscular blockade must be achieved and judicious use of intra-operative opioids should remove the need for administration of naloxone. Paracetamol is used, but non-steroidal anti-inflammatory drugs are avoided because of the risk of inhibiting platelet function and precipitating a postoperative intracranial bleed.

POSTOPERATIVE CARE

Although many patients who have undergone spinal or intracranial surgery are awake and conscious in the immediate postoperative period, some still require active, intensive treatment. This is important particularly in patients who have raised ICP (or when ICP is liable to rise) and in those who have undergone cerebral aneurysm surgery, when postoperative vasospasm may

be a problem. Ideally, all patients who have undergone intracranial surgery should be cared for in a high-dependency unit environment. Elective postoperative sedation and lung ventilation with continuous monitoring of both arterial and intracranial pressures is rarely necessary unless severe oedema is likely or when there is damage to critical structures such as the respiratory centre.

Fluid therapy is required to replace ongoing losses and while the patient is not drinking; only isotonic fluids should be used. Patient who have undergone craniotomy or major spinal surgery have a urinary catheter in place. Neurosurgical patients are at high risk of DVT and low molecular weight heparin should be started as soon as it is safe to do so (usually the day after surgery).

Historically, long-acting opioids were used very cautiously after craniotomy or upper cervical spine surgery. However, moderate to severe pain is common after craniotomy and most patients can be given an opioid intravenously or orally in addition to paracetamol. Surgery of the thoracic and lumbar spine is associated with significant postoperative pain and non-steroidal anti-inflammatory drugs and patient-controlled analgesia are used.

ANAESTHESIA FOR ELECTIVE INTRACRANIAL SURGERY

The preoperative condition of patients who present for craniotomy varies enormously. Some patients are confused, disorientated, euphoric or aggressive and in many cases the surgery is not truly elective.

Intracranial Tumours

Gliomas usually grow quickly and the history is often short (days or weeks); meningiomas are slow-growing and the history may be slow and insidious. Unlike gliomas, the volume effect of a meningioma is usually minimal because a reduction in the volume of the other intracranial contents compensates. However, the volume effects may eventually become apparent, especially if there is bleeding into the meningioma.

Patients with an intracranial tumour are usually taking steroids (normally dexamethasone 4 mg every 6 h), which may precipitate a latent diabetic state, requiring insulin during the acute episode. Most patients have some symptoms of raised ICP, such as headache, nausea, vomiting or visual disturbances. Anticonvulsant therapy may have been prescribed to patients who have presented with fitting or who are thought to be at risk. Some patients may be frankly dehydrated, and while it is important to avoid aggressive preoperative fluid therapy, hypovolaemia must be treated before induction of anaesthesia.

For slowly growing tumours such as meningiomas and less aggressive gliomas, as near total excision as possible is attempted. However, total excision of all the macroscopically identifiable glioma tissue is now considered futile for fast-growing lesions. Large portions of tumours are excised if pressure symptoms are the main presenting feature. For aggressive tumours, the greatest need is for a tissue diagnosis. If lesions are small, deep-seated or near critical areas (such as the motor strip or speech centre), a radiologically-guided biopsy or awake surgery (see section on functional surgery below) is appropriate. Stereotactic biopsy involves a CT scan with a rigid metal frame firmly attached to the skull. Trigonometry is then used to find co-ordinates, relative to the frame, which describe the exact site of the lesion (to within 1 mm). A biopsy needle is then passed through the brain to sample tissue from this site. The frame is applied after induction of anaesthesia and, because small changes in brain volume causes the lesion to move, the $PaCO_2$ should be maintained at a constant level for both the CT scan and the biopsy. Frameless image-guided surgery can be performed, in which a scan of the brain (and skull) is compared with topographical features of the head in theatre to guide a biopsy needle or small craniotomy biopsy and excision.

There is a small (~1%) risk of haemorrhage after a biopsy. Following surgery, patients should be assessed for neurological defects related to the excised tissue. There is a risk of postoperative haemorrhage after any craniotomy and a deterioration in conscious state should be investigated urgently. After retraction of normal brain tissue to access a tumour (e.g. retraction of the frontal lobes to excise an olfactory groove meningioma), reperfusion injury can lead to swelling and infarction during the first 24 h.

Cerebrovascular Lesions

Patients with a vascular lesion such as an intracranial aneurysm or arteriovenous malformation (AVM) may

TABLE 32.2		
World Federations of Neurosurgeons (WFNS) Grading of Subarachnoid Haemorrhage		
WFNS Grade	*GCS*	*Motor Deficit*
1	15	Absent
2	13–14	Absent
3	13–14	Present
4	7–12	Present or absent
5	3–6	Present or absent

GCS, Glasgow Coma Scale.

present acutely with a subarachnoid or intracerebral haemorrhage. Congenital lesions are seen frequently in young and previously healthy patients. Intracranial aneurysms occur in the older age group and may be associated with other, more widespread cardiovascular disease. Subarachnoid haemorrhage is now graded using the World Federation of Neurosurgeons' (WFNS) scale (Table 32.2). Although application of clips ('clipping') at craniotomy should prevent the risk of further bleeding, significant perioperative morbidity and mortality can result from vasospasm, which may occur pre- or postoperatively The current trend is to undertake emergency cerebral angiography and clipping of an aneurysm in good-grade patients, but to delay surgery in the poor-grade patients until their condition improves. The calcium channel blocker nimodipine is used to reduce or prevent vasospasm. By preference, it is given orally because the hypotensive effects are less.

An alternative method of treating intracranial aneurysms is by interventional neuroradiological 'coiling' (see below). This was used initially for inaccessible posterior circulation aneurysms but has now become the technique of choice for most aneurysms in many centres.

The conscious state in patients with intracerebral haemorrhage ranges from completely lucid to confused, and the preoperative assessment must take this into account. Those in the older age group may be receiving drugs with cardiovascular effects and are also frequently receiving aspirin or warfarin, which may be a contraindication to urgent craniotomy.

As flow is more pressure-dependent in areas with vasospasm, it is necessary to avoid both hypotension and hypertension. Similarly, hypocapnia should be avoided. A normal cerebral perfusion pressure should be maintained. Although fluid replacement therapy may be all that is required, the careful use of a vasopressor may be necessary in the interval between induction and incision. Nimodipine therapy interacts with inhalational anaesthetic agents to enhance their hypotensive effects. Postoperatively, nimodipine therapy is continued for several days until the risk of vasospasm has passed. Blood entering the CSF either as a result of the initial haemorrhage or during operation is an extreme irritant. Its presence may cause large increases in plasma catecholamine concentrations, with consequent hypertension and vasospasm. Blood which clots in the aqueduct of Sylvius causes obstruction to CSF flow and non-communicating hydrocephalus, necessitating temporary ventricular drainage or insertion of a ventriculo-peritoneal shunt.

Intra-operative temporary clipping of feeding vessels (or to prevent anastomotic backflow from tributaries) may be required to allow safe application of the permanent clip to the neck of the aneurysm. Temporary clips may also be required if the aneurysm bursts, to allow the surgeon to stop the haemorrhage. These clips cause temporary ischaemia in the territory supplied by that vessel. Attempts are usually made to reduce the risk of permanent ischaemic damage. Metabolic suppression with intravenous anaesthetic agents and mild hypothermia have been used. There is, however, no evidence that these techniques have any effect on outcome.

Anaesthesia for Interventional Neuroradiology

In addition to coiling of intracranial aneurysms, radiologists treat a variety of other lesions including AVMs, carotid-cavernous sinus fistulae and dural arteriovenous fistulae in the head or spine. These procedures use several techniques including detachable coils and glue placed within vessels to interrupt blood supply. The blood vessels supplying some tumours, e.g. meningiomas, may also be occluded before surgical excision. Most of these procedures are not painful, although headache may occur. However,

to allow precise localization of the lesion and accurate positioning of the intravascular catheters, the patient has to lie very still, sometimes for several hours, and general anaesthesia is commonly used. Many of the risks of open aneurysm surgery apply equally in this situation, and a full, conventional neurosurgical anaesthetic technique should be used, including direct arterial pressure monitoring both to monitor arterial pressure and to enable blood sampling for coagulation studies. Heparin is used during the procedure. If thrombus starts to form in the feeding vessels, antiplatelet treatment is started. Rupture of the aneurysm may require immediate craniotomy, clot evacuation and open clipping of the neck of the aneurysm. It is important not to underestimate the need for a full neuroanaesthetic technique, simply because a craniotomy is not being performed.

Pituitary Surgery (Hypophysectomy)

The pituitary fossa is sometimes approached through a frontotemporal craniotomy for large suprasellar tumours, or more usually through the nose (transsphenoidal). The majority of pituitary adenomas are non-functioning and cause pressure symptoms – usually on the optic chiasm. However, there may be preoperative endocrine abnormalities such as acromegaly or Cushings's disease. Acromegalic patients who present for pituitary surgery may pose considerable difficulties in tracheal intubation and are at risk of obstructive sleep apnoea. Glucocorticoid replacement is required in the immediate perioperative period; mineralocorticoid requirements increase only slowly over the subsequent days. Diabetes insipidus may present in the immediate postoperative period and requires stabilization with vasopressin until the degree of the imbalance is known. It usually resolves over the first few days. If the nasal approach is used, a pharyngeal pack must be inserted and the airway protected to prevent aspiration of blood and CSF.

CSF Shunt Insertion and Revision

The majority of patients who present for insertion or revision of a ventriculo-peritoneal shunt are children with congenital hydrocephalus, often resulting from spina bifida or from intraventricular haemorrhage after premature birth. Older patients may require a permanent shunt after intracranial haemorrhage or head injury or to treat normal pressure hydrocephalus. The major anaesthetic considerations lie in the presentation of a patient with severely raised ICP who may be drowsy, nauseated and vomiting, with resultant dehydration. Compensatory systemic hypertension to maintain cerebral perfusion may also be present. Rapid-sequence induction may be indicated to avoid aspiration; the increase in ICP caused by succinylcholine is of secondary importance. Artificial ventilation to control $PaCO_2$ is essential to prevent further increases in ICP, and a volatile anaesthetic agent should be used with care for the same reason. When the ventricle is first drained, a rapid decrease in CSF pressure may result in an equally rapid reduction in arterial pressure, which no longer needs to be elevated to maintain cerebral perfusion. Adequate venous access is important to allow rapid resuscitation in response to this severe but temporary hypotension. Shunt surgery may be painful, particularly at the site of insertion into the peritoneum or from the tunnelling of the catheter under the skin. Use of long-acting opioids has to be balanced against the need to have the patient achieve at least the preoperative level of consciousness.

An endoscopic technique may be used to create a new passage for the flow of CSF. The endoscope is passed through a small burr-hole into the lateral and then the third ventricles. The sudden changes in ICP from the use of irrigating fluid and the passage of the neuroendoscope near to vital structures may result in dramatic changes in heart rate and arterial pressure.

Functional Surgery

Surgery for Parkinson's disease and epilepsy is performed in an awake patient. The initial exposure may be made under general anaesthesia, but the mapping of the brain, and the surgery itself (e.g. inducing a lesion in the basal ganglia), are performed awake under local anaesthesia only. Surgery to remove slow-growing or benign tumours from the 'eloquent' or critical areas near the main motor and sensory gyri may also be performed in this way, to guide the surgeon and avoid damage to these areas. Careful assessment and selection of patients is essential to ensure that patient knows what to expect and can co-operate during long periods of awake surgery. Careful positioning (to avoid neck strain), urethral catheterization and temperature control are also required.

Treatment of Trigeminal Neuralgia

This extremely debilitating condition is usually treated pharmacologically with large doses of antiepileptic drugs. However, surgical lesions of the trigeminal ganglion are performed when the side-effects of medical treatment become unacceptable. A lesions of the ganglion is induced by radiofrequency ablation or injection of either phenol or alcohol. All these techniques are very painful and require general anaesthesia. The patient is anaesthetized while the ganglion is identified radiologically, awakened to allow identification of correct positioning of the needle, and then re-anaesthetized for generation of the lesion or neurolytic injection. If the CSF is encountered during localization of the ganglion, nausea frequently occurs and vomiting with the patient in the supine position should be anticipated. Some cases of trigeminal neuralgia are caused by an abnormal vascular loop compressing the trigeminal nerve in the posterior fossa. A small craniotomy and decompression of the nerve by placing a Teflon pad between the nerve and vessel is often successful in curing the symptoms; the problems of anaesthesia and surgery in this area are highlighted below.

Posterior Fossa Craniotomy

Surgery in the posterior cranial fossa involves lesions of the cerebellum and fourth ventricle. The lateral 'park bench' position may be used for some lesions such as vestibular schwannoma (acoustic neuroma). The prone position facilitates operations on the cerebellum, foramen magnum and upper cervical spine. Bone is usually removed as a craniectomy in the posterior fossa rather than by raising a bone flap.

In the past, some surgeons favoured the sitting position because this produced good venous drainage, relative hypotension and excellent operating conditions. The patients were frequently allowed to breathe a volatile anaesthetic agent (usually trichloroethylene) spontaneously so that changes in the respiratory pattern could be used to monitor the progress of fourth ventricular surgery in the region of the respiratory centre. This posed several major anaesthetic problems. Patients in the sitting position are prone to hypotension, which results inevitably in poor cerebral perfusion. Air embolism is also a severe potential problem because when the skull is opened many of the veins within the bone are held open and, if the venous pressure at this point is subatmospheric, air may enter the veins, leading to systemic air embolism. For these reasons, the sitting position is no longer used other than in exceptional circumstances. Although this change has diminished the risks of cerebral hypoperfusion and consequent hypoxia, air embolism is still a potential problem. The operative site, particularly with a moderate head-up tilt, is still above the level of the heart and the veins are held open by the surrounding structures.

Detection and Treatment of Air Embolism

The mainstay of detection is vigilance and a high index of suspicion. The main period of risk during surgery in the prone position is when the posterior cervical muscles are cut and the craniectomy is being performed. Air embolism may occur in the supine position because the patient is often placed slightly head-up to encourage venous drainage. Surgery near the dural venous sinuses may result in a sinus being opened. This may lead to torrential bleeding, but if the head is raised it may alternatively lead to air entrainment as the walls of the sinuses, formed by the dura, are held apart. The severity of the effects of air embolism depend upon the volume of air entrained and the time course of the accumulation of the air in the central circulation.

The main practical method of detection is by end-tidal carbon dioxide monitoring, because the 'airlock' produced in the pulmonary circulation results in a rapid reduction in CO_2 excretion (usually together with a reduction in oxygen saturation). Arterial pressure decreases and cardiac arrhythmias are frequently seen. The use of an oesophageal stethoscope permits auscultation of the classic 'mill wheel' murmur with large quantities of air, but requires continuous listening. Doppler ultrasonography is probably the most accurate method of early detection before the embolus leaves the heart, but frequently suffers from interference. Unfortunately, there are many false positives with more sensitive techniques such as Doppler ultrasonography. In practice, provided that the sitting position is not used, large air emboli are uncommon. Treatment consists of preventing further entry of air by telling the surgeon, who immediately floods the operative field with saline, lowering the level of the head and increasing the venous pressure by jugular compression. Ideally, the air should be trapped in the right atrium by placing the patient in the left lateral position; it is then occasionally possible to aspirate air through a central venous catheter. Vasopressors may be required until the circulation is restored; occasionally, full cardiopulmonary resuscitation is necessary.

ANAESTHESIA FOR SURGERY OF THE SPINE AND SPINAL CORD

Many neurosurgical procedures involve surgery around or on the spinal cord, usually either for decompression of nerves as a result of a prolapsed intervertebral disc or degenerative arthritis, or for decompression of the cord when the spinal canal is occupied by tumour. Some cervical spine surgery is performed supine (see below) but most spinal procedures require the patient to be positioned prone. The patient can be supported on a Montreal mattress, bolsters or blocks placed under the upper chest and iliac crests, or a purpose-built frame, all of which allow unimpeded respiratory movements and avoid abdominal compression. In the prone position, pressure areas may develop over the facial bones, particularly around the eyes; careful padding is vital. The neck should be kept in a neutral position, if possible, to avoid stretching the brachial plexus and if it is necessary to have the arms up above the head, they should not be abducted excessively nor should there be anything pressing into the axillae.

Anaesthesia for Cervical Spine Surgery

The cervical spine may be approached from either the anterior or the posterior route, depending largely upon the site of cord or root compression. Although the posterior approach is less likely to damage vital structures, the patient must lie prone, and hypotension, blood loss and access, particularly in a large individual, may cause problems.

In most patients, the neck is relatively stable. Bony degeneration from osteoarthritis can produce severe cord compression. However, rheumatoid arthritis can produce neck instability, particularly in flexion. It is essential to assess the range of neck movement in addition to the assessment of the ease of tracheal intubation. It is doubly unlucky to have a difficult intubation in a patient with an unstable neck! If problems are anticipated, the normal 'difficult intubation' drill should be followed, using the methods with which the anaesthetist is most familiar. Severe ankylosing spondylitis involving the neck probably presents the most awkward problem, caused by the rigid immobility of the cervical spine. Additional factors which apply particularly in rheumatoid patients include anaemia, steroid therapy, fragile skin, and renal and pulmonary problems.

Anterior Cervical Decompression

This technique involves exposing the anterior aspect of the cervical vertebral bodies and their interposing discs through a collar incision, removing the intervertebral disc and decompressing the cord while distracting the disc space mechanically. The vertebral bodies are then kept separated with a prosthetic spacer, artificial disc or sometimes a bone graft taken from the iliac crest. Single or multiple levels may be involved and the neck may be quite rigid for future intubation if several adjacent levels are decompressed.

Apart from the potential problems of tracheal intubation, anaesthesia is relatively straightforward, although pneumothorax is a potential problem with operations at the C7–T1 level. Retraction of the oesophagus and, more particularly, the carotid sheath and sinus, may produce severe temporary cardiovascular disturbance (usually sinus bradycardia). Postoperative haemorrhage may lead to acute airway obstruction.

Posterior Cervical Laminectomy

Patients are usually placed prone, with the neck flexed, and in a slightly head-up posture to reduce haemorrhage. Bleeding from the nuchal muscles is often a problem and air embolism remains a risk. The main difficulties, as in all spinal surgery in the prone position, arise from epidural venous bleeding, and the changes in intrathoracic pressure from IPPV can have a significant effect. In addition, prolonged cord compression can result in an autonomic neuropathy which may produce significant hypotension both at induction and when the patient is turned into the prone position. Cervical laminectomy may be accompanied by posterior fusion with either bone or metal, which results in immediate postoperative stability.

Anaesthesia for Thoracic and Lumbar Decompression

Lumbar microdiscectomy for sciatica and one-level laminectomy are usually quite minor procedures. Patients with severe sciatica may gain instant pain relief postoperatively. However, multiple-level laminectomies are more major operations and direct arterial blood pressure measurement may be required in elderly or debilitated patients. Thoracic discs and tumours such as neurofibromata are approached occasionally by the transthoracic route, involving thoracotomy and a combined approach with the patient in the lateral position. Bronchial intubation and one-lung anaesthesia may be needed to facilitate access in this situation.

Correction of spinal deformities such as scoliosis and surgery to stabilize vertebrae damaged by trauma or destroyed by metastatic tumour are often associated with significant bleeding and the need for massive blood transfusion. Hypotensive anaesthesia is used occasionally to decrease bleeding, and particularly the venous ooze in the operative field. Cell salvage reduces the need for blood transfusion, although its role in tumour surgery is unclear. Spinal cord monitoring using somatosensory- or motor-evoked potentials allows identification of spinal cord ischaemia during surgery. These potentials are affected by many anaesthetic agents, particularly the volatile anaesthetic agents, and a TIVA-based technique is preferred. Children with congenital scoliosis associated with other conditions (such as Duchenne muscular dystrophy) represent a significant anaesthetic challenge as a result of their co-morbidities, in particular their lung function, and the volume of blood loss.

ANAESTHESIA FOR EMERGENCY INTRACRANIAL SURGERY

The main indication for emergency intracranial surgery is bleeding as a result of trauma, which may be exacerbated in patients treated with anticoagulant drugs, including aspirin and clopidogrel. Intracranial haematomata may arise epidurally (extradurally), subdurally or intracerebrally and may accumulate either rapidly or slowly. Patients receiving warfarin may develop a subdural haematoma after a very minor head injury. Many patients who present for anaesthesia and surgery are unconscious or semiconscious and irritable as a result of raised ICP and cerebral compression. Virtually all patients with head injury have had an emergency CT scan as part of their initial management. Many have undergone tracheal intubation and ventilation of the lungs for this procedure and are subsequently kept anaesthetized and taken straight to the operating theatre for surgery to decompress the brain. It is important to remember that, with an expanding intracranial haematoma, speed is of the essence if cerebral damage is to be minimized or avoided. While adequate anaesthetic time must be taken to ensure safety, excessive delays may seriously affect the overall result of decompression and make the difference between a good and merely a moderate recovery.

The anaesthetic maintenance technique is similar to that used for elective intracranial surgery, consisting of careful use of a hypnotic, a short-acting intravenous opioid, neuromuscular blockade and IPPV to a $PaCO_2$ of 4.5 kPa. Tracheal intubation in patients at risk of regurgitation and aspiration of stomach contents should be facilitated with succinylcholine. If the patient is unconscious, the initial anaesthetic requirements may be small. Most acute haematomas are evacuated through a full craniotomy, because, if necessary, the bone flap may be left out or allowed to 'float' free, providing a method of decompression in the case of severe oedema.

Chronic subdural collections may be evacuated via burr holes. These are usually performed under general anaesthesia, but may be undertaken with local anaesthesia alone in frail, elderly patients. Many chronic subdural haematomas recur and underlying brain substance injury is common. As the patient's brain is decompressed, the level of consciousness may lighten considerably and it may be necessary to deepen anaesthesia to prevent the patient becoming aware. It is important to avoid long-acting opioid analgesics because these may mask the level of consciousness, which is used to follow the progress of cerebral trauma postoperatively.

MANAGEMENT OF THE HEAD-INJURED PATIENT

Head-injured patients, their subsequent treatment and rehabilitation represent a considerable proportion of neurosurgical practice. The immediate management requires meticulous attention to the prevention of secondary brain injury from ischaemia; little can be done about the primary insult to the brain or spinal cord. In recent years, the awareness of both the medical profession and the general public has had a profound effect on general resuscitation simply by improving airway management in the unconscious patient. The resuscitation and immediate care of all head-injured patients uses the same A-B-C principles taught on ATLS and ALS courses for care of all trauma victims and other seriously ill patients. Particular points to note for head injury care are as follows:

1. *Initial airway maintenance,* remembering that patients with craniofacial injuries often have associated damage to the cervical spine. Tracheal intubation is usually necessary, must be accomplished without excessive neck manipulation and should be performed by an experienced person. It is important to make intubation as atraumatic as possible; consequently, sedation and neuromuscular blockade should be used irrespective of the level of consciousness, except in the most severe situation. The benefits of succinylcholine usually outweigh the potential risks. Nasotracheal intubation is contraindicated because of the possibility of a basal skull fracture.

2. *Maintenance of adequate ventilation* with oxygen-enriched air. Avoidance of hypoxaemia and hypercapnia is essential.

3. *Maintenance of an adequate circulating volume and arterial pressure.* Hypotension after head injury greatly worsens outcome. Other injuries which may affect the circulatory state must be identified while resuscitation is being performed.

4. *Sedation and analgesia, and neuromuscular blockade,* are usually continued to allow management of other injuries, CT scanning and possible inter-hospital transfer.

5. *Detailed assessment of thoracic, abdominal and limb injuries* and appropriate therapy to stabilize the patient's cardiovascular and respiratory systems are required before transfer to the CT scanner and X-ray room. Other life-threatening injuries must be dealt with to prevent secondary brain injury caused by hypoxaemia or hypotension.

6. *Invasive arterial pressure monitoring,* together with ECG, capnography and pulse oximetry are all important in the early detection of deterioration in ICP, cardiovascular stability or

respiratory function. A contused, oedematous and non-compliant brain tolerates only minimal changes in oxygen supply or carbon dioxide tension before ICP increases still further.

7. *After the CT scan,* many patients are transferred directly to the neurosurgical operating theatre for evacuation of haematoma or insertion of an intraventricular catheter or pressure transducer. Patients who are scanned in peripheral hospitals have their scans relayed to the main neurosurgical centre. The patient is then transferred directly by ambulance to the neurosurgical operating theatre, but both cardiovascular and neurological stability must be achieved before the journey. Realistically, this involves the transfer of a sedated, intubated and ventilated patient, often pretreated with mannitol to minimize acute increases in ICP.

INTENSIVE CARE MANAGEMENT OF HEAD-INJURED PATIENTS

The main benefits of intensive care are in the provision of optimal conditions to allow recovery from the primary cerebral injury while minimizing any secondary damage.

Sedation

Sedation is usually achieved with an infusion of either propofol or midazolam together with an opioid (usually morphine or alfentanil). Thiopental may be beneficial in the presence of severely compromised cerebral blood flow and metabolism, or status epilepticus. Neuromuscular blockade is frequently used in addition to sedative drugs.

Ventilation

Mechanical lung ventilation is particularly important in patients suffering from multiple trauma, especially with the combination of head and chest injuries, to ensure optimal oxygenation in the face of pulmonary contusion. This is normally achieved by the use of IPPV and may involve the use of small amounts of positive end-expiratory pressure (PEEP). There is evidence to suggest that hyperventilation worsens outcome, and the main benefits of mechanical ventilation are the prevention of hypercapnia and the provision of adequate cerebral oxygenation.

Detailed Neurological Assessment

The Glasgow Coma Scale (Table 32.1), which is based upon eye opening, and verbal and motor responses, is used in non-sedated patients. Brain function may also be assessed by use of the electroencephalogram (or a processed EEG monitor such as the cerebral function analyzing monitor [CFAM]), transcranial Doppler and near-infrared spectroscopy.

ICP Monitoring

It is very helpful to be able to monitor the effectiveness of therapy used to manage intracranial hypertension, and in particular to achieve an effective cerebral perfusion pressure. The ICP is monitored using a transducer inserted either extradurally, subdurally or into the brain parenchyma. This may be undertaken in the ICU or in the operating theatre. ICP often increases in response to stimulation, physiotherapy, tracheal suction, etc., but should return to the pre-stimulation value within 5–10 min. Frequent and prolonged increases in ICP demonstrate a low cerebral compliance and the need for further sedation and ventilation. If weaning from mechanical ventilation is started and the ICP increases and remains elevated, the patient should be re-sedated and the lungs ventilated for a further 24-h period. It is beneficial to nurse head-injured patients in a 15° head-up tilt to assist in control of ICP, provided that coexisting conditions permit.

Adequate Fluid Therapy and Nutrition

Although otherwise healthy patients with an isolated head injury have very low metabolic requirements, many fail to absorb from the gastrointestinal tract because of the effects of sedative and opioid drugs or simply secondary to head trauma; associated hypoxaemia exacerbates the problem. It is sometimes necessary to introduce parenteral nutrition, particularly in patients who are catabolic from coexisting injuries. As in elective patients at risk from elevated ICP caused by cerebral oedema, head-injured patients are also at risk from excessive intravenous fluid therapy, particularly if hypotonic solutions are used. Fluid restriction may be appropriate, and if large amounts of fluid have been given during initial resuscitation, a gentle drug-induced diuresis with furosemide to create an overall negative fluid balance (or at least to prevent a positive balance) may be appropriate. Fluid overload also impairs oxygenation further in potentially hypoxaemic patients with combined head and chest injuries, or following aspiration at the time of head injury. The use of mannitol tends to be reserved for the emergency treatment of raised ICP rather than the treatment of simple fluid overload.

High-Dependency Nursing Care

Provision of appropriate care for the unconscious patient, even when breathing spontaneously, is difficult, and demands a high intensity of nursing care. Intensive or high-dependency care centralizes nursing, medical and monitoring resources to provide optimal care of the head-injured patient.

ANAESTHESIA FOR CT AND MRI SCANNING

This is discussed in Chapter 38.

FURTHER READING

Cold, G.E., Dahl, B.L. (Eds.), 2002. Topics in neuroanaesthesia and intensive care. Springer-Verlag, Berlin.

Matta, B.F., Menon, D.K., Smith, M. (Eds.), 2011. Core topics in neuroanaesthesia and neurointensive care. Cambridge University Press, Cambridge.

33 ANAESTHESIA FOR THORACIC SURGERY

■ ■ ■ ■ ■ ■ ■ ■ ■ ■ ■ ■

Thoracic anaesthesia offers a number of anaesthetic challenges:

- Control of the airway during bronchoscopy.
- Protection of the airway in patients with oesophageal disease, lung abscess, bronchopleural fistula or haemoptysis.
- Positioning a double-lumen tracheal tube to maintain safe anaesthesia in the lateral position with the chest opened and one lung collapsed.
- Postoperative care of a patient after lung tissue resection.

In common with major surgery at other sites, thoracic patients frequently:

- have parenchymal lung disease in addition to their presenting complaint
- experience severe pain after surgery
- are at risk of substantial haemorrhage
- need fluids intravenously after surgery.

Diagnosis, staging and resection of intrathoracic malignant disease occupy a large part of thoracic surgical practice. There is also a need for drainage and obliteration of an expanded pleural space to remove infection, or to prevent lung collapse and re-accumulation of air or liquid in the pleural space. Resection of bullous lung disease may improve the respiratory mechanics of the chest if there is parenchymal lung disease elsewhere.

PREOPERATIVE ASSESSMENT

History and Examination

Thoracic patients often exhibit respiratory symptoms of cough, sputum, haemoptysis, breathlessness, wheeze and chest pain, or oesophageal symptoms of dysphagia, pain and weight loss. Other common chest features include hoarseness, obstruction of the superior vena cava, pain in the chest wall or arm, Horner's syndrome, cyanosis and pleural effusion. Lung tumours may cause extrathoracic features by metastatic spread, principally to brain, bone, liver, adrenals and kidneys, or by endocrine effects such as finger clubbing, hypertrophic pulmonary osteoarthropathy, Cushing's syndrome, hypercalcaemia, myopathies (e.g. Eaton–Lambert syndrome), scleroderma, acanthosis and thrombophlebitis. Anaemia, cardiac disease and lung disease may cause breathlessness.

To distinguish between loss of lung tissue and reversible airways disease, the patient's own history of daily activity may reveal diurnal variation in breathlessness and associated symptoms of sputum, stridor and wheeze. Symptoms may conflict with the results of pulmonary function tests, which require voluntary effort, if the tests have been performed ineffectively. Wheeze during expiration and stridor during inspiration are likely to result from airway obstruction below and above the thoracic inlet, respectively.

Production of sputum is the most common stimulus to cough, which is therefore almost universal in cigarette smokers. A dry cough may result from tumour or external compression of the upper airways. Oesophageal tumours are associated with dysphagia. The restriction on ingestion of food exacerbates the cachexia of malignant disease. At induction of anaesthesia, patients are at risk of regurgitation of food and secretions from above the oesophageal obstruction.

Preoperative features of weight loss, protein-calorie malnutrition and hypoalbuminaemia make postoperative pulmonary infection, multi-organ failure and delayed wound healing more likely. Patients with pre-existing chronic lung disease are more likely to suffer postoperative pulmonary complications. Cyanosis may result centrally from intrapulmonary shunting caused directly by diseased tissue or because of lung collapse consequent to proximal airway obstruction. Peripheral cyanosis is possible in the face and arms if the superior vena cava becomes obstructed by mediastinal spread.

Many major thoracic surgical procedures are preceded by rigid bronchoscopy which requires clinical assessment of upper airway patency at the preoperative visit. Forced ventilatory effort by the patient may elicit stridor or wheeze, and palpation of the neck and inspection of the airway demonstrated on chest radiograph may reveal tracheal abnormality.

Differential Diagnosis

Preoperative investigations are required to confirm a diagnosis and stage the disease, in order to assess whether the disease is resectable. Tumours are staged by assessing the spread of the primary tumour, presence of local lymph node spread and distant metastases (TNM staging). Further tests to assess physiological reserve are required to determine if the patient is operable.

Investigations

A variety of preoperative investigations are performed to determine resectability. The chest radiograph may reveal changes months before symptoms are manifest. Of symptomatic patients, 98% have chest radiograph abnormalities. Lung tumours are central in 70% of patients and may show collapse or cavitation more peripherally in the lung. Tumours are commonly 3–4 cm in size by the time of presentation. Other features include tracheal deviation, obstruction of the superior vena cava, pleural effusions and air-filled cavities.

Tumour diagnosis and staging involve sputum cytology, bronchoscopy, needle biopsy, mediastinoscopy and mediastinotomy. Computed tomography (CT) and magnetic resonance imaging (MRI) of the chest may reveal the spread of disease. Biochemistry, bone scans and ultrasound scans of the abdomen may detect metastatic disease. Barium studies and oesophageal ultrasound are similarly able to diagnose and stage carcinoma of the oesophagus.

Investigations are used to quantify physiological reserve by measuring mechanical and parenchymal function, and cardiopulmonary interaction. Assessment should be on physiological reserve rather than chronological age. Rather than to deny surgery to patients, this is done to allocate resources to borderline patients to minimize their postoperative complications. Investigations to diagnose lung collapse, oedema, infection and bronchospasm allow patients to be presented in the best possible state on the day of surgery.

Whole-Lung Testing

Spirometry using voluntary effort, pulse oximetry and arterial blood gas tensions breathing air are influenced by the function of the whole lung.

Mechanical testing. Spirometry tests only the mechanical bellows function of the lung. Testing relies on voluntary effort and effective technique by the patient. From total lung capacity, the patient exhales to residual volume to measure the forced vital capacity (FVC). This is reduced in restrictive lung disease, such as cryptogenic alveolar fibrosis. The volume of gas exhaled forcibly in the first second gives the forced expiratory volume in 1 s (FEV_1). By definition, FEV_1 measures function when the lung is expanded well. In health, patients can exhale 70–80% of their vital capacity in 1 s, the FEV_1%. The remainder of the vital capacity may take another 2 s to exhale. With obstructive lung disease, the FEV_1% is reduced below 70% and the time taken to exhale the vital capacity is prolonged. The FEV_1% of patients with restrictive lung disease is preserved, although the absolute value of FVC, and therefore the volume exhaled in 1 s, is reduced. Values of 2 L for FVC and 1.5 L for FEV_1 offer a lower limit when screening for pneumonectomy. An FEV_1 of 1.0 L is cautionary for single lobectomy because a whole-lung FEV_1 >800 mL after surgery is required to avoid dependence on mechanical ventilation.

Predicted postoperative (PPO) lung function may be calculated using lung segments. From a total of 19 segments (three in the upper lobes, two in both the middle lobe and lingual and four in the left and five in the right lower lobes; Fig. 33.1), the fraction of lung remaining is multiplied by the preoperative spirometry measurement to give the predicted postoperative measurement of spirometry (PPO FEV_1 = preoperative $FEV_1 \times (1 - ($resected segments$/19)))$. Using whole-lung spirometry to predict postoperative lung function may be invalidated if the regional function of the lung is not known. For example, a patient with an FEV_1 of 1.5 L

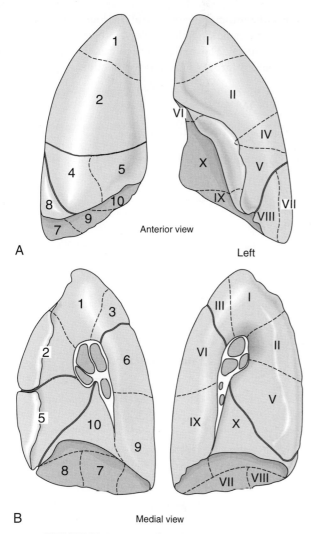

A   Anterior view   Left

B   Medial view

FIGURE 33.1 ■ Bronchopulmonary segments.

the same way as for mechanical function. PPO D_{LCO} values<40% of predicted in health – normal range 100–150 mL min⁻¹ mmHg⁻¹ – correlate with increased postoperative respiratory complications.

Cardiopulmonary interaction. Cardiopulmonary exercise testing requires a patient to be able to pedal a bicycle ergometer and breathe through a mouthpiece. Increasing exercise to a peak allows calculation of maximum oxygen uptake expressed in mL kg⁻¹ min⁻¹. Patients with VO_2max >10 mL kg⁻¹ min⁻¹ have been able to withstand lobectomy, whereas a PPO VO_2max >15 mL kg⁻¹ min⁻¹ is required to contemplate pneumonectomy.

Regional Lung Function

Ventilation/perfusion lung scans offer an indication of regional lung function. The relative contribution of the two separate lungs may be determined horizontally but regions are indicated as upper, middle and lower zones vertically within a lung rather than individual lobes or lung units.

Invasive Assessment

In patients with borderline lung function for whom surgical resection offers great prognostic advantage, the risks and discomfort of invasive assessment of regional lung function may be worth the information obtained about likely residual function after surgery. Balloon occlusion of a main pulmonary artery before surgery or clamping a pulmonary artery during surgery allows some assessment of pulmonary artery pressures and oxygenation after resection. Inadequate blood oxygenation, arterial carbon dioxide tension greater than 6.0 kPa and mean pulmonary artery pressure greater than 25 mmHg at rest, or greater than 35 mmHg with exercise, indicate inadequate function and increased operative risk.

Any intrathoracic operative procedure places an immediate burden on the right ventricle. Using echocardiography, magnetic resonance scanning or direct pressure measurement, diagnosis of a failing right ventricle or coexisting pulmonary artery hypertension may render a patient's chest pathology inoperable.

Treatment

Before surgery, patients should be motivated to stop smoking and lose excess weight. Reversible airway narrowing should be treated with bronchodilators such as salbutamol, terbutaline, theophylline, inhaled

may have the same or better FEV_1 after lobectomy if the main bronchus of the affected lobe was occluded completely at the time of testing before surgery. The oxygenation of blood of such a patient may be improved by the removal of a non-functioning lung or lobe through which considerable right-to-left shunt existed.

Parenchymal lung function. Arterial oxygen tension <8 kPa or carbon dioxide tension >6 kPa indicate increased risk for lung resection. The diffusing capacity of carbon monoxide (D_{LCO}) correlates with the total functioning area of the alveolar capillary membrane. Predictive postoperative values may be calculated in steroids or sodium cromoglycate. By giving antibiotics to treat chest infection, and loosening and removing bronchial secretions with inhaled nebulized water aerosols, chest physiotherapy and postural drainage, the incidence of pulmonary complications is reduced. Collapse in lung segments not intended for resection should be expanded, and pulmonary oedema treated by improving heart failure. Pulmonary hypertension should be treated where feasible. Overnight, stopping smoking improves bronchial reactivity and reduces carboxyhaemoglobin concentration. Eight weeks after cessation of smoking, the excessive production of mucus is reduced. This makes tracheobronchial clearance easier and improves small airway function.

ANATOMY

The bronchial tree and the views obtained when facing the patient are illustrated in Figure 33.2 and the bronchopulmonary segments are shown in Figure 33.1. The

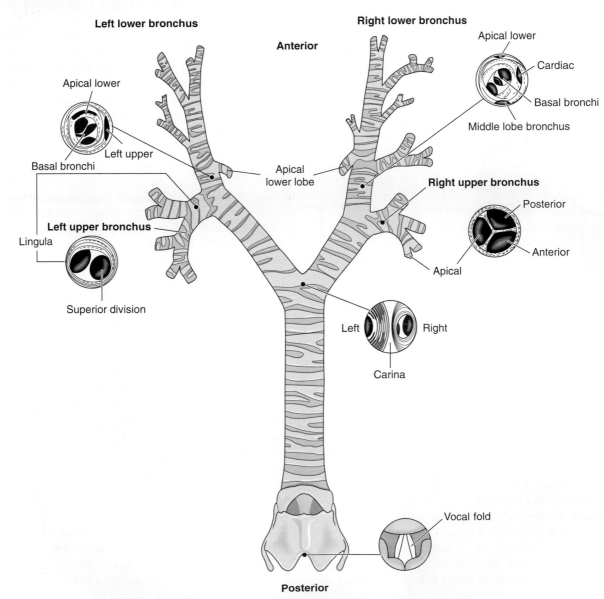

FIGURE 33.2 ■ Larynx, trachea, main and lobar bronchi.

trachea leads from the cricoid cartilage below the larynx at the level of the sixth cervical vertebra (C6) and passes 10–12 cm in the superior mediastinum to its bifurcation at the carina into left and right main bronchi at the sternal angle, T4/5. During inspiration, the lower border of the trachea moves inferiorly and anteriorly. The trachea lies principally in the midline, but is deviated to the right inferiorly by the arch of the aorta. The oesophagus is immediately posterior to the trachea and behind it is the vertebral column. The wall of the trachea is held patent by 15–20 cartilaginous rings deficient posteriorly where the trachealis membrane, a collection of fibroelastic fibres and smooth muscle, lies. It is wider in transverse diameter (20 mm) than anteroposteriorly (15 mm). The trachea passes from neck to thorax via the thoracic inlet at T2.

The right main bronchus is larger and less deviated from the midline than the left. The origin of the right upper lobe bronchus arises laterally 2.5 cm from the carina, whereas the origin of the left upper lobe arises laterally after 5 cm. These dimensions determine the relative ease of isolating and ventilating each lung independently using double-lumen bronchial tubes.

The oesophagus is a continuation of the pharynx at the level of the lower border of the cricoid cartilage (C6) 15 cm from the incisor teeth. It passes immediately anterior to the thoracic spine and aorta and descends through the oesophageal hiatus of the diaphragm at T10, to the left of the midline at the level of the seventh rib. There are four slight constrictions, at its origin, as it is crossed by the aorta and left main bronchus, and at the diaphragm, at 15, 25, 27 and 38 cm from the incisors.

Radiographic Surface Markings

The apices of the lungs extend 2.5 cm above the point at which the middle and inner thirds of the clavicle meet. Lung borders descend behind the medial end of the clavicle to the middle of the manubrium. The lung border is behind the body of the sternum and xiphisternum before sweeping inferiorly and laterally down to the level of the eleventh thoracic vertebra. On the left, at the level of the horizontal fissure at the fourth costal cartilage (T7), the medial border of the lung is displaced to the left of the sternal edge in the cardiac notch. The oblique fissure descends from 3 cm lateral to the midline at T4, inferiorly and anteriorly to the sixth costal cartilage 7 cm from the midline. The diaphragmatic reflection of the pleura extrudes below the lung to the lower border of T12.

INDUCTION AND MAINTENANCE OF ANAESTHESIA

All currently available anaesthetic agents have been used for thoracic surgery. They are used to maintain anaesthesia and haemodynamic stability during the procedure, while allowing the patient to breathe spontaneously in reasonable comfort immediately after surgery is complete. Large doses of i.v. opioid drugs are unlikely to achieve all these aims. Thoracic surgery patients may demonstrate sensitivity to drugs used in anaesthesia because of debility from the extent of their disease or from systemic effects, such as prolonged effects of neuromuscular blocking drugs in patients with Eaton–Lambert syndrome associated with carcinoma of the bronchus.

Lateral Thoracotomy

Many thoracic procedures are performed through a posterolateral thoracotomy incision between fifth and eighth ribs. Patients have to be positioned on their side with the neck flexed, dependent shoulder brought forward and the arm raised under the pillow to protect the shoulder and brachial plexus. The upper shoulder is flexed to 90° and the arm supported. Hips and knees are flexed together with a pillow between the legs. Padding, strapping, lower leg compression devices and diathermy pad complete the preparation for surgery (Fig. 33.3). Positioning with the chest flexed laterally

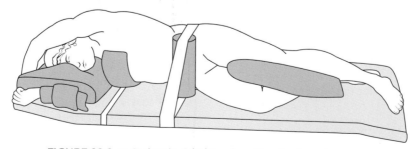

FIGURE 33.3 ■ Patient in right lateral position for thoracic surgery.

away from the operative side on a beanbag which is then aspirated of air, or breaking the operating table, may improve surgical access. The upper wrist has a tendency to flex, so radial artery cannulae cause less trouble when on the dependent side. Peripheral and jugular veins are more accessible on the operative side.

The Lateral Position

In health, with the chest erect, the right lung takes 55% of the pulmonary blood flow and the left lung 45%. In the right lateral position, the right lung takes 65% and the left lung 35% because of the influence of gravity. In the left lateral position, differences are reversed; the right lung takes 45% and left lung 55%. These changes persist under anaesthesia. However, anaesthesia does affect the changes to ventilation of the two lungs in the lateral position. Awake, there is more ventilation to the dependent lung; similarly, the bases receive proportionately more ventilation than the apices when the chest is erect. The dependent lung has a less negative intrapleural pressure than the upper lung and is on a more favourable part of the pressure–volume curve. A change in pressure produces a greater change in volume in the dependent lung than in the upper lung. Under anaesthesia, conditions for ventilation between the two lungs are reversed. Functional residual capacity is reduced. With paralysis of the diaphragm, the mechanical advantage of the greater curve of the lower diaphragm is lost and the lower lung is compressed by the mediastinum and abdominal contents. Awkward positioning on the operating table may further impede the lower lung. The lower lung is now in a less favourable position on the pressure–volume curve and any change in pressure produces greater change in the volume of the upper lung than the dependent lung. Anaesthesia therefore produces much worse ventilation/perfusion mismatch in the lateral position, with more blood going to the dependent lung and more ventilation going to the upper lung. Application of positive end-expiratory pressure up to 10 cmH$_2$O improves the changes in ventilation and tends to restore ventilation to the dependent lung.

One-Lung Anaesthesia

The principal indications for one-lung anaesthesia are:

- isolation of the lungs
- ventilation of one lung alone

- bronchopulmonary alveolar lavage
- collapse of one lung to allow surgical access to other structures.

Isolation of a diseased lung with sepsis or haemorrhage may be necessary to protect the healthy lung. When there is inadequate ventilation of both lungs because of a large bronchopleural or bronchocutaneous fistula, a large unilateral bulla or because the compliance of two lungs is so different that they require independent ventilation, satisfactory oxygenation may be obtained by ventilation of one lung alone. Pulmonary alveolar proteinosis may be treated by bronchoalveolar lavage. This requires that only one lung be lavaged with liquid at a time, whilst the other is protected. Video-assisted pulmonary and pleural surgery, and intrathoracic, non-pulmonary surgery such as oesophageal, aortic and spinal surgery, may require the lung to be collapsed to allow access to the operative structures.

Ventilation of one lung alone may require a double-lumen tracheal tube (Fig. 33.4), a bronchial blocker (Fig. 33.5) or a bronchial tube. The double-lumen tube has greatest flexibility to allow changes from ventilation of two lungs to one lung then back to two lungs during or at the end of surgery. It allows aspiration of the main bronchi independently, and insufflation of oxygen to the non-ventilated lung. It has a larger external diameter than the bronchial blocker or bronchial tube and may be difficult to position correctly if tracheal and bronchial anatomy is distorted. The two separate lumens are narrow and present a high resistance to spontaneous ventilation. This is overcome by positive pressure ventilation, but a single-lumen tube may have to be substituted at the end of surgery if resumption of spontaneous ventilation is not immediate.

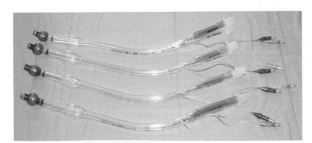

FIGURE 33.4 ■ Four left-sided Bronchocath double-lumen endobronchial tubes with balloons inflated, from 35 FG (uppermost) to 41 FG (lowest).

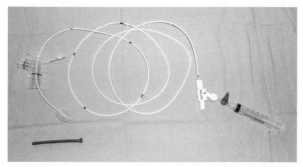

FIGURE 33.5 ■ A Rüsch 6 FG bronchial blocker (360601) – balloon is inflated with 5 mL air. The balloon guard is below the balloon and the stem passes through the 1.8 mm seal in the connector for the anaesthetic circuit. Luer-lock fittings (labelled 'balloon') to inflate the balloon and aspirate/inflate down the central lumen are on the right.

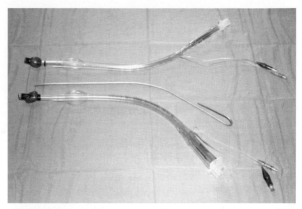

FIGURE 33.6 ■ Left (upper) and right (lower) 39 FG double-lumen bronchial tubes are shown with a flexible introducer, which may be used to shape the tube to facilitate insertion.

A bronchial blocker with a hollow lumen allows insufflation of oxygen, some suctioning and may be used with a jet ventilator, which overcomes some of the disadvantages of the technique. The Rüsch bronchial blocker illustrated in Figure 33.5 has a 170 cm long, 2 mm stem (outside diameter) with a central lumen to a 2.75 mm diameter balloon, which accepts 5 ml of air. It may be passed down a bronchoscope with a lumen greater than 2.8 mm diameter or through the 15 mm tapered connector with a 1.8 mm seal shown.

Positioning Double-Lumen Bronchial Tubes

Double-lumen bronchial tubes provide an effective means of isolating each lung to protect the other from blood and secretions. They allow ventilation of one lung only, or both lungs independently. Being longer and with lumens more narrow than single-lumen tracheal tubes, they have a greater resistance to air flow. They are therefore not usually suitable for spontaneous ventilation. Disposable polyvinyl chloride tubes (Fig. 33.6) have substantially replaced the re-usable red rubber Robertshaw double-lumen tubes. Sizes of tube in common use in adult practice range from 35 to 41 French gauge (FG). Sizes 37–39 are usually suitable for men and 37 for women, but sizes 41 and 35 are available for individuals at extremes of the range of adult build. Left- and right-sided versions of double-lumen bronchial tubes are necessary (Fig. 33.6) because the tracheal portions are curved antero-posteriorly, and the balloon of the right bronchial tube is fenestrated to

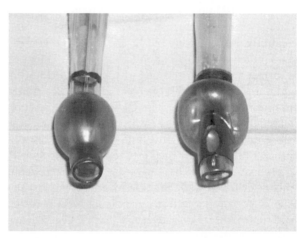

FIGURE 33.7 ■ Bronchial balloons inflated on left-sided (left) and right-sided (right) bronchial double-lumen tubes. The right tube is eccentric and shows the side lumen to allow inflation of the right upper lobe.

conduct gases to the right upper lobe bronchus, which would otherwise be occluded by the cuff of the tube (Fig. 33.7). The left upper lobe bronchus arises 2.5 cm further down the main bronchus than the right, so it is less likely to be occluded by the balloon of the bronchial tube.

Positioning a double-lumen bronchial tube correctly is a skill learned quickly with practice. The task is usually straightforward, but however experienced the anaesthetist, great difficulties may be encountered in some patients. An incorrectly positioned double-lumen bronchial tube may rapidly compromise the supply of oxygen to the lungs during thoracic surgery, with disastrous results. The correct position of double-lumen bronchial tubes may be assessed by clinical technique or confirmed using an intubating fibreoptic laryngoscope.

Clinical Assessment

The patient lies supine on a level operating table with the head supported on a single pillow pulled clear of the shoulders to flex the neck and extend the head. After induction of anaesthesia and muscle relaxation, the larynx is identified by laryngoscopy. The double-lumen bronchial tube is held at 90° to its eventual anatomical position on the non-operative side, to align the curve of the bronchial lumen anteroposteriorly. The bronchial lumen is passed between the cords until it rests within the trachea. The double-lumen bronchial tube is then rotated 90° back to point the bronchial lumen towards its intended bronchus. The head is turned away from the side of the bronchial lumen and the double-lumen bronchial tube advanced gently until resistance is encountered and the bronchial tube is thought to be in the correct position. The tracheal cuff is then inflated and the lungs ventilated manually through both lumens of the tube. Visible movement of both sides of the chest, detection of a recognizable trace of exhaled carbon dioxide, breath sounds auscultated in both axillae and an unchanging pulse oximeter reading reassure the anaesthetist that oxygen is being supplied to the lungs. Difficulties encountered whilst isolating individual lungs may be addressed after returning to this position of control.

The tracheal lumen of the breathing circuit is then clamped and the breathing system distal to the clamp opened to air. Breath sounds are confirmed on the bronchial side. Two or more millilitres of air are then injected into the bronchial cuff until the leak of air from the tracheal tube is no longer audible or palpable, and breath sounds auscultated over the side opposite to the bronchial lumen cease. The tracheal lumen is then closed, and the clamp is released and applied to the bronchial system; the circuit is opened and the procedure is repeated to confirm that chest movement and air entry occur to the tracheal side and not the bronchial side and that there are no air leaks from the anaesthetic system. The double-lumen bronchial

tube is then secured with a tracheostomy tape at the teeth by a clove hitch, and the tube tie is knotted round the neck by a bow to enable its release quickly when required.

During volume controlled ventilation, when each lumen of the double-lumen tube (DLT) is clamped, there should be a detectable increase in airway pressure during the breathing cycle when the tidal volume is directed down one lung. The peak airway pressure may then be controlled below 30 cmH_2O by reducing the tidal volume and increasing the ventilatory rate while maintaining the minute volume of ventilation. If there is no change on the ventilator or airway pressure gauges when one lumen of the tube is clamped, the bronchial lumen is likely to end in the trachea or else there is a substantial leak past the bronchial cuff. The position of the DLT should always be re-checked after the patient has been subjected to any changes in position, e.g. from supine to lateral.

Using the Fibreoptic Intubating Laryngoscope

Confirming the correct position of a double-lumen bronchial tube using a fibreoptic intubating laryngoscope should avoid problems encountered by malposition of the DLT. However, if parenchymal lung disease is so extensive that one lung is insufficient to keep tissues oxygenated, if pneumothorax develops on the side of the ventilated lung or if the double-lumen tube is subsequently dislodged, problems with ventilation and oxygenation may still be encountered.

Positioning the double-lumen tube often leaves the orifice of the right upper lobe bronchus covered by the tip of the bronchial tube (Fig. 33.8).

■ The tracheal cuff is then deflated, the laryngoscope is held fixed relative to the patient and the double-lumen tube advanced. The blue bronchial cuff then occludes sight of the orifice of the right upper lobe bronchus until the side hole in the bronchial cuff lies over it. Sight of bronchial rings of the right upper lobe bronchus confirms the correct position of the double-lumen bronchial tube (Fig. 33.9).

■ The double-lumen tube is then held firm and the bronchial cuff inflated with 2 mL of air. Uninterrupted sight of the right upper lobe bronchus confirms that this manoeuvre has not

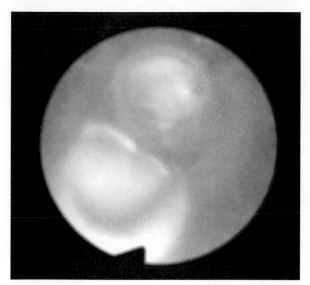

FIGURE 33.8 ■ Distal opening of bronchial lumen at 12 o'clock shows right middle and lower bronchi. The side opening of the bronchial lumen at 7 o'clock is against the wall of the right main bronchus and is not over the right upper lobe bronchus. The patient is lying on the right. Orientation: left, cephalad; upper, left; right, caudad; lower, right.

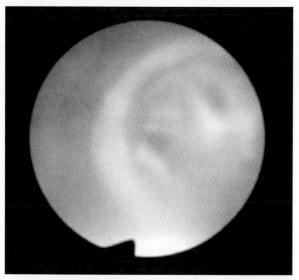

FIGURE 33.10 ■ Distal opening of bronchial lumen at 3 o'clock shows right lower and middle lobe bronchi. The dark colour at 9 o'clock is the bronchial lumen cuff. The patient is lying on the right. Orientation: left, cephalad; upper, left; right, caudad; lower, right.

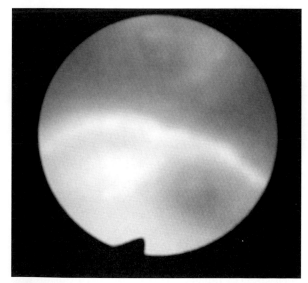

FIGURE 33.9 ■ The double-lumen tube has been repositioned so that the side opening of the bronchial lumen at 6 o'clock is now over the right upper lobe bronchus. The patient is lying on the right. Orientation: left, cephalad; upper, left; right, caudad; lower, right.

moved the side hole of the bronchial tube relative to the bronchus. The bronchi to the right middle and lower lobes may be seen through the distal lumen of the bronchial tube (Fig. 33.10). Withdrawing the intubating laryngoscope may give a view of the origins of all three lobar bronchi (Fig. 33.11).

■ The double-lumen tube is then held against the teeth or gums of the maxilla, the mark on the tube there is noted and the laryngoscope is removed from the bronchial lumen. Without moving it, the tube is tied with a clove hitch over this mark and the tube tie tied round the neck with a bow.

■ The tracheal cuff is then inflated with 5 mL of air and the fibreoptic laryngoscope is passed down the tracheal lumen until the carina is identified again. The bronchial lumen is seen to pass down the correct main bronchus and the bronchial cuff in its main bronchus is seen to be inflated, but not herniating to impinge over the lumen of the other main bronchus (Fig. 33.12).

■ The laryngoscope is removed from the tracheal lumen and both lungs are ventilated.

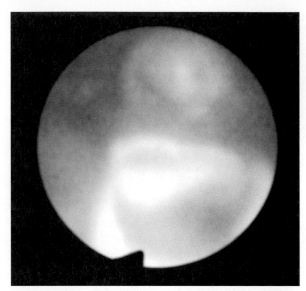

FIGURE 33.11 ■ The intubating laryngoscope is withdrawn to show the right middle and lower lobe bronchi through the distal opening at 12 o'clock and the right upper lobe bronchus through the side opening at 6 o'clock. The patient is lying on the right. Orientation: left, cephalad; upper, left; right, caudad; lower, right.

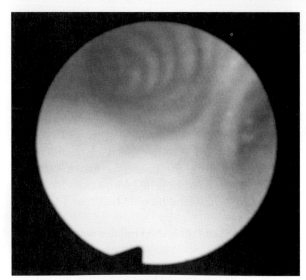

FIGURE 33.12 ■ The intubating laryngoscope has been passed down the tracheal lumen. The carina passes from 2 o'clock anteriorly to 6 o'clock posteriorly. The left main bronchus is to the left at 10–12 o'clock. On the other side of the carina, the dark crescent confirms that the inflated bronchial cuff is not herniating over the left main bronchus and the bronchial tube to the right of the cuff passes down the right main bronchus. The patient is lying on the right. Orientation: left, cephalad; upper, left; right, caudad; lower, right.

■ Bronchial and tracheal lumens are clamped in turn, observing airway pressures, leaks and the extent of ventilation of each lung.

The fibreoptic bronchoscope is necessary to position bronchial blockers through an endotracheal tube. Once inflated in position, gas can be aspirated through the central channel of the blocker to hasten collapse of the operative lung. When deflated, blockers have a propensity to move and may need to be rechecked using bronchoscopy when re-inflated. Blockers can achieve segmental collapse, leaving other parts of the lung still performing gas exchange.

Passing a suction catheter down the bronchial lumen before starting removes secretions faster than is possible through the suction port of the fibreoptic intubating laryngoscope. Lubrication of the laryngoscope with water-soluble jelly aids its passage down both lumens and prevents the tube being dislodged when the laryngoscope is withdrawn. A bottle of irrigation fluid aspirated through the suction port helps to prevent it being blocked by encrusted aspirate before there is an opportunity to clean the laryngoscope.

Clinical testing is specific – a problem detected with the position of the bronchial double-lumen tube is likely to predict a real problem if left uncorrected before surgery begins. However, it is not sensitive. Inadequate isolation of one lung and excessive airway pressures may be encountered after apparently successful positioning of the tube. Correct alignment of the fenestration in the bronchial cuff over the origin of the right upper lobe bronchus is particularly difficult to predict by clinical means alone, but demonstrable using fibreoptic bronchoscopy.

Mode of Ventilation

Breathing spontaneously through a surgical thoracotomy wound causes the same problem as trauma patients experience with a large open chest wound. The pleural space with the chest open is at atmospheric pressure. During inspiration, gas flows from trachea and lung in the open chest into the dependent lung. During expiration, the flow is reversed, causing the lung in the open chest to inflate. Gas is transferred from lung to lung during the paradoxical ventilation of the lung in the open chest, preventing excretion of carbon dioxide and rendering gas inspired into the dependent lung hypoxic. An occlusive dressing over the chest, or isolation of the lung in the open chest with a blocker or bronchial double-lumen tube, may stop paradoxical ventilation of the lungs. Both devices increase the resistance to gas flow to the dependent lung, and so mechanical one-lung ventilation is usual during thoracic surgery.

Physiological Changes

With one lung perfused but not ventilated, a substantial right-to-left shunt should produce significant hypoxaemia. Because of the greater solubility of carbon dioxide and its more linear dissociation curve, the gradient from arterial to alveolar partial pressure of carbon dioxide is smaller than that for oxygen. Increasing alveolar ventilation of the ventilated lung reduces arterial carbon dioxide tension without substantially increasing arterial oxygen tension. Because of the flat portion of the oxygen dissociation curve when haemoglobin is fully saturated, a further increase in alveolar oxygen tension results in only a small increase in oxygen content in solution, and has no effect on the oxygenation of the blood in the non-ventilated lung. Consequently, a high inspired oxygen fraction does not improve hypoxaemia caused by right-to-left shunt.

The severity of hypoxaemia observed is much less than that expected if regional perfusion remained unchanged. The lateral position directs more blood to the dependent lung due to gravity. In the non-ventilated lung, alveolar hypoxia results in increased vascular resistance, which directs more blood to the dependent ventilated lung, further reducing shunt and hypoxaemia – hypoxic pulmonary vasoconstriction (HPV). HPV is impaired by anaesthetic agents. However, in clinical practice, there are other compensatory mechanisms in the intact human lung to reduce shunt.

HPV has no effect if the alveolar oxygen tension is either 100% or 0%, or if the alveolar oxygen tension is the same throughout all lung units. It is more likely to have an effect with the 20–30% of cardiac output which shunts through the non-ventilated lung during one-lung anaesthesia. HPV effects are also maximal when pulmonary artery pressures and mixed venous oxygen saturation tensions are normal. The results of excessively high or low pulmonary artery pressures exceed the marginal changes in pulmonary artery pressures obtained by HPV. Similarly, an abnormally low mixed venous oxygen tension caused by low cardiac output or high oxygen consumption, for example by hyperthermia or shivering, has a greater influence than any changes

possible with HPV. High peak and end-expiratory ventilation pressures in the dependent lung increase its pulmonary vascular resistance and overcome any benefits of HPV in the non-ventilated lung. Excessive alveolar pressures may increase dead space by producing a region of lung which is ventilated but not perfused.

Volatile anaesthetic agents and pulmonary vasodilators such as glyceryl trinitrate, sodium nitroprusside, isoprenaline, dobutamine and nitric oxide have been shown to inhibit HPV. However, there are far more variables clinically than in the controlled conditions of the experimental laboratory bench. Poor positioning of the patient which compromises blood flow to the dependent lung, malposition of a double-lumen bronchial tube, low cardiac output caused by inadequate blood volume replacement or impediment to blood flow by surgical manipulation may have a greater influence on hypoxaemia than the effects of changes in HPV.

Hypoxaemia during one-lung anaesthesia may be minimized by:

- correct positioning of the bronchial tube
- increasing inspired oxygen concentration to 50%
- a tidal volume of 5–7 mL kg^{-1} or less to avoid increasing dead space
- positive end-expiratory pressure of no more than 5–10 cmH$_2$O to minimize dependent lung collapse without increasing vascular resistance
- maintaining cardiac output and pulmonary artery pressures near the normal range.

Insufflation of oxygen to the non-ventilated lung either at atmospheric pressure or with continuous positive alveolar pressure of 5 cmH$_2$O should avoid the need for pharmacological intervention such as inhaled nitric oxide to the ventilated lung. When the pulmonary artery is clamped during lung resection, the adequacy of gas exchange should be reassessed. The loss of shunt through diseased lung tissue may improve oxygenation and result in better function than expected after removal of lung tissue.

ANAESTHESIA FOR THORACIC SURGERY PROCEDURES

Rigid Bronchoscopy

Rigid bronchoscopy in thoracic surgery is performed most often to obtain tissue diagnosis and determine if a lesion may be resected. Other indications include removal of foreign bodies and secretions, and control of haemorrhage. Therapeutic procedures such as laser therapy, tracheal or bronchial stenting and alveolar lavage may be performed through a rigid bronchoscope.

Anaesthesia should permit the passage of a straight rigid bronchoscope of up to 9 mm external diameter, allow oxygenation and removal of carbon dioxide, avoid awareness, and control movement, coughing and reflex haemodynamic responses to mechanical stimulation of the tracheobronchial tree. This may be achieved by spontaneous ventilation, apnoeic oxygenation or, more usually, positive pressure jet ventilation. Spontaneous ventilation avoids inhaled foreign bodies being propelled more distally into the bronchial tree. However, it offers much less control than when neuromuscular blockade is used, and anaesthesia sufficient to cause respiratory depression is required to control reflex responses to bronchoscopy. Apnoeic oxygenation may be achieved by delivering oxygen into the conducting airways by a catheter and relying on diffusion down a concentration gradient from oxygenated airways to the alveoli, where oxygen is absorbed continuously. Although effective in maintaining oxygenation measured by pulse oximetry, arterial carbon dioxide tension increases by about 0.5 kPa min^{-1}. Using apnoeic oxygenation, enough time may be available to complete the surgical procedure, but eventually, assisted or spontaneous ventilation has to resume to ventilate the alveoli.

Positive pressure ventilation may be performed by intermittent occlusion of the bronchoscope or, more conveniently, by high-pressure jet ventilation using a Sanders Venturi technique. Oxygen at 400 kPa is released by a trigger held by the anaesthetist through a narrow orifice of 18–14 gauge. The gas is directed through the jet at the operator end of the bronchoscope towards the patient end. The high-pressure jet entrains atmospheric air and inflates the chest. Care must be taken to avoid pulmonary barotrauma by limiting delivery of oxygen under pressure to short intermittent bursts according to the chest movement observed and ensuring that there is a large unobstructed opening at the observer end of the bronchoscope to allow gas under pressure to escape from the conducting airways. Oxygenation may be monitored by pulse oximetry. Intermittent ventilation can usually be restricted to times when the operator is not looking down the bronchoscope.

With the patient supine, removal of the pillow or extension of the neck by lowering the head of the operating table may be necessary to allow the bronchoscope to pass down the trachea. Antisialagogue premedication dries oropharyngeal secretions and aids visibility. Induction of anaesthesia by inhalation of a volatile anaesthetic agent may be necessary occasionally to confirm that adequate ventilation can be achieved under anaesthesia where there is some obstruction to the upper airways. Depolarizing or competitive neuromuscular blocking agents may be used according to the needs of the patient or intended procedure. Topical local anaesthetic and a systemic opioid with a rapid onset of action help to obtund the haemodynamic response to bronchoscopy. Intermittent positive pressure ventilation with a Venturi device requires a total intravenous anaesthetic technique.

Local trauma and bleeding are the most common complications. Ventilation after bronchoscopy may be impaired by persisting effects of anaesthetic drugs, or compromise to the upper airway. A chest radiograph in the recovery room may provide early detection of pneumothorax or air in the mediastinum.

Rigid Oesophagoscopy

Fibreoptic oesophago-gastroduodenoscopy is performed usually as an outpatient procedure under sedation, without demands for anaesthetic assistance. Rigid oesophagoscopy under general anaesthesia presents the anaesthetist with patients who are at risk of aspirating gastric contents. Patients with achalasia may have a large volume of fetid fluid accumulated in their oesophagus. All oesophagoscopy patients should undergo rapid sequence induction with the suction catheter to hand and suction switched on. In patients with achalasia, there should be an attempt to drain the oesophagus before anaesthesia, which should be induced in a steep head-up tilt or in the left lateral position.

When anaesthesia has been induced and the cuff of the tracheal tube inflated to protect the airway, the tracheal tube should be passed to the left-hand side of the tongue to allow the oesophagoscope to be inserted behind where the tracheal tube usually lies. The tracheal tube is taped or tied securely, and then held at all times by the anaesthetist. This prevents the tracheal tube being dislodged by the operator on withdrawal of the oesophagoscope on most occasions, and makes the anaesthetist aware immediately of dislodgement of the tracheal tube, regurgitation of fluid into the oropharynx or requests for the tracheal cuff to be deflated as the oesophagoscope is passed through the cricopharyngeal sphincter.

Manipulations to the head or neck may be required to pass the oesophagoscope. Damage to the teeth or mucosal surfaces may occur. When the oesophagoscope has passed down the oesophagus, anaesthesia may be maintained with the patient breathing spontaneously. At the end of the procedure, patients should be awake and able to cough and protect the airway before tracheal extubation, which takes place with the patient lying on the left side with suction apparatus and trained assistance ready to hand as at induction of anaesthesia.

Perforation of the oesophagus is an unusual but serious complication. Patients should have been awake for 1 h after oesophagoscopy without complaint of chest discomfort and have an unchanged chest radiograph before ingestion of oral fluids resumes.

Cervical Mediastinoscopy and Anterior Mediastinotomy

Both procedures are used to stage the extent of spread of intrathoracic malignancy or obtain a tissue diagnosis. Ventilation of both lungs through a single-lumen tracheal tube is usually adequate and surgical access may be improved by resting the shoulders on a sandbag and the head on a head ring.

Analgesia after surgery may be helped by infiltration of the wound by local anaesthetic, or transverse superficial cervical plexus and intercostal nerve blocks. Although the procedures are usually straightforward, there is always the potential for significant haemorrhage, damage to surrounding structures and compromise to the airway from haematoma after surgery.

Video-Assisted Thoracoscopic Surgery

Improvements in imaging and thoracoscopic instruments have allowed more elaborate procedures than biopsy, such as lung resection, lung reduction surgery, pleurectomy and sympathectomy to be undertaken by video-assisted thoracoscopic surgery (VATS). The video image is magnified on monitors, but so too is movement and there is little space within the chest for instruments and camera lenses. A collapsed motionless lung may be essential, requiring one-lung anaesthesia.

As more extensive procedures are now performed using VATS, so some more minor VATS procedures are being performed by chest physicians using pleuroscopy under local analgesia.

Pain after VATS procedures is less intense and prolonged than after posterolateral thoracotomy. Patients are much more comfortable after the chest drain is removed than thoracotomy patients at the same stage after surgery. A single paravertebral block at the level of the chest drain and intercostal incisions with 20 mL of bupivacaine 0.5% followed by oral analgesia may be sufficient to allow patients to take deep breaths and cough after thoracoscopic surgery.

Pulmonary Lobectomy

One-lung anaesthesia allows dissection in a field disturbed only by the movement of the mediastinum. Inflation of the lung temporarily may help to identify the lung fissures. Passive insufflation of the collapsed lung either through a suction catheter or with $5\,cmH_2O$ continuous positive airways pressure may augment oxygenation achieved by one-lung anaesthesia. Surgical traction on mediastinal structures and disturbance to the mediastinum by surgeons' hands, instruments or retractors may cause bradycardia, interruption of the venous return to the heart or compression of the chambers of the heart.

When the bronchial stump is closed and haemostasis has been secured, the chest may be filled with warm saline and the airway pressure held at $40\,cmH_2O$ to test the integrity of the stump.

When chest drains are in position, re-inflation of the remaining lobe(s) is achieved by applying gentle positive pressure to the anaesthetic breathing system. Observing the pleural surface confirms if all superficial lung tissue is re-inflated. As the chest is closed, a subatmospheric pressure of 5 kPa is applied to the chest drains via an underwater seal. A significant air leak through damaged lung becomes apparent immediately if the ventilator reservoir collapses or if a reduction in the expired minute volume is detected by the ventilator alarm. The suction is then disconnected from the chest drains and reapplied when the patient resumes spontaneous breathing. Chest drains are then left without being clamped until the remaining lung has re-expanded fully, drainage has ceased and there is no air leak, when the chest drains are removed.

Pneumonectomy

The operative lung should be collapsed as soon as skin disinfection and draping begin. Problems with oxygenation may then be apparent early in the procedure. Borderline oxygenation may improve when the pulmonary artery is clamped and shunt through the lung to be resected is interrupted. Intrapericardial dissections for tumours that have extensive local spread pose a risk of sudden, substantial haemorrhage. After such dissection, cardiac herniation is a rare but serious cause of complications. The integrity of the stump of the main bronchus may be tested when the lung has been removed, as in lobectomy.

When the chest is closed at the end of surgery, the remaining lung is fully inflated and the chest drain to the pneumonectomy space is clamped. Clamps are released for 5 min every hour to ensure that no air, blood or excess fluid accumulates in the pneumonectomy space. Leaving the chest drains open continuously may lead to a reduction in the pneumonectomy space and the mediastinum being shifted to the operative side as the remaining lung becomes hyperinflated, with consequent respiratory embarrassment. The pleural space fills with serosanguinous fluid after pneumonectomy and fibroses subsequently, reducing the size of the space.

Pleurectomy and Pleurodesis

Recurrent pneumothorax or pneumothorax which fails to respond to conservative measures may require pleurectomy to re-expand the lung and prevent recurrence. Pleurectomy and talc pleurodesis are usually possible by thoracoscopy. Pain after pleurectomy is much greater than after diagnostic thoracoscopic procedures even with the same number of intercostal wounds. Patients may require the same analgesia as if the procedure had been performed via a thoracotomy wound.

Empyema

Patients may remain remarkably well despite a large collection of purulent material in the pleural space. Collections may arise after pulmonary infection, oesophageal rupture, or following thoracoscopy or thoracotomy. Chest drainage before surgery may reduce the volume of pleural fluid, but organized infection has to be removed by open surgery. There may be considerable blood loss during decortication of an empyema.

Lung Cysts and Bullae

Bullae are thin-walled, air-filled cavities within the lung which communicate slowly with the bronchial tree. In the presence of bullae, there is always the potential for tension pneumothorax under positive pressure ventilation, and the creation of a bronchopleuro-cutaneous fistula after insertion of a chest drain.

Similar changes in size may occur during anaesthesia with liquid-filled cysts. There is the added risk of soiling parenchymal lung tissue elsewhere with the liquid should the cyst rupture.

Bronchopleural Fistula

Although most common after lung resection surgery, bronchopleural fistulae may occur after acute respiratory distress syndrome (ARDS), or any intrathoracic sepsis. The chest should be drained before induction of anaesthesia to reduce the amount of purulent fluid in the chest cavity and avoid the prospect of tension pneumothorax. Anaesthesia should be induced with the affected side dependent, followed by prompt bronchial intubation of the main bronchus on the unaffected side, in order to isolate the healthy lung from contamination by purulent secretions from the affected side. After turning, one-lung ventilation allows surgery on the affected side. Should there still be lung tissue on the affected side, high-frequency jet ventilation can keep lung tissue inflated and ventilated in the presence of a large air leak, with mean intrathoracic pressures lower than with conventional intermittent positive pressure ventilation.

Tracheal Surgery

Unless cardiopulmonary bypass is used, there must be a changing sequence of means of ventilating the lungs during surgery, and measures to keep the neck flexed after surgery to avoid tension on the tracheal repair before it heals. Carinal surgery is one of the few remaining indications for a single lumen endobronchial tube.

Until the tracheal lesion is resected, airway obstruction must be overcome during the early stages of anaesthesia. Maintaining spontaneous ventilation initially allows assessment of the adequacy of assisted ventilation under anaesthesia. With the lesion exposed, ventilation of one or both lungs through an incision in the trachea distal to the lesion allows resection of the lesion and repair of the posterior wall of the trachea. A narrow tracheal or bronchial tube is passed through the larynx beyond the anastomotic site, and must allow space for repair of the anterior wall of the trachea. Suturing the chin to the skin over the sternum keeps the neck in flexion until the tracheal anastomosis heals.

Tracheostomy

The neck is extended by placing a sandbag under the shoulders and securing the head on a head ring. The pharynx should be aspirated when surgical dissection of the trachea is complete, because incision of the second and third tracheal rings frequently bursts the cuff on the tracheal tube. The tracheal tube is then withdrawn sufficiently far to allow insertion of the tracheostomy tube, but is not withdrawn from the trachea. This retains a means of ventilating the lung and a conduit into the trachea to replace the tracheal tube over a bougie if initial attempts to introduce the tracheostomy tube are unsuccessful. When the tracheostomy tube is positioned correctly, it is connected to a sterile catheter mount within the draped area and then to the anaesthetic breathing system. The sandbag is removed before the neck wound is sutured.

Pneumomediastinum and pneumothorax may occur intraoperatively because of damage to the posterior tracheal wall. Haemorrhage and damage to other structures may occur immediately, or later as a result of the effects of pressure from a malpositioned tracheostomy tube.

Oesophageal Surgery

Oesophagectomy is often preceded by oesophagoscopy with all the attendant risks of pulmonary aspiration. Thoracic approaches to the oesophagus may require one-lung ventilation to provide access for surgery. Oesophagectomy may take some hours and be associated with considerable fluid loss into the wound and surrounding tissues. After surgery, effective analgesia is necessary to enable the patient to expand the chest and cough effectively. Patients should be nursed sitting or supported on pillows to avoid regurgitation of gastrointestinal fluid and subsequent aspiration. Total parenteral nutrition is not required as a routine, but may be necessary in the presence of postoperative complications such as mediastinitis from an anastomotic leak. Judicious use of i.v. fluids after surgery is required.

POSTOPERATIVE CARE

Pulmonary function is impaired after thoracic surgery beyond any changes expected after lung resection. There is a 35% reduction in functional residual capacity after lung resection, which takes 6–8 weeks to recover to preoperative values. However, thoracic surgery patients should be able to breathe spontaneously immediately after anaesthesia and surgery. A need for mechanical ventilation after surgery is likely to result from problems in patient selection or during surgery and anaesthesia intraoperatively. A mini-tracheostomy tube may be inserted through the cricothyroid membrane at the end of surgery, with the trachea extubated and the lungs ventilated through a laryngeal mask, to help aspiration of the trachea of patients unable to cough effectively. Prolonged mechanical ventilation exposes thoracic patients to regional lung collapse and nosocomial pulmonary infection.

A high inspired oxygen concentration to overcome hypoxaemia is usually required for the first 24 h after surgery and during sleep at night until chest drains are removed. Patients breathing air with a $PaCO_2$ greater than 6.0 kPa before surgery are at increased risk of ventilatory failure after surgery and require oxygen therapy tailored to response. Most other patients benefit from oxygen 40–60% by plastic face mask or nasal prongs.

The posterolateral thoracotomy wound is exceedingly painful. Untreated, each breath provokes pain. To minimize pain, ventilation is rapid and shallow. Analgesia sufficient to permit deep inspiration and productive coughing without respiratory depression is necessary to restore adequate spontaneous ventilation after thoracic surgery. Continuous epidural analgesia or, if that is contraindicated, paravertebral nerve blockade is more likely to achieve these aims than systemic opioid analgesia. Epidural local anaesthetic or opioids, or mixtures of the two, may be infused through a catheter introduced between the fifth and eighth thoracic vertebrae, depending on the sites of wound and chest drains, and the size and alignment of the intervertebral spaces. Bupivacaine 0–15 mg h^{-1}, or fentanyl 0–50 μg h^{-1}, alone or in combination, may be given as continuous infusions or background infusions with additional patient-controlled demands. Paravertebral block delivering local anaesthetics through a catheter inserted at the end of surgery has been demonstrated to be at least as effective as epidural analgesia, with fewer side-effects such as hypotension, urinary retention, itch and respiratory depression.

After oesophageal surgery, oral fluids are withheld for some days while a nasogastric tube drains the stomach. After lung resection in the morning, patients may be able to manage some food in the evening. Intravenous fluids are required for the first 24 h, although less is given than after other forms of major surgery. Maintenance fluids are restricted to avoid pulmonary oedema in remaining lung tissue that has been handled or through which there is a relatively increased pulmonary artery flow after lung resection. Ringer lactate solution $10\,mL\,kg^{-1}\,h^{-1}$ in theatre and $1\,mL\,kg^{-1}\,h^{-1}$ thereafter provides maintenance fluids. Blood and colloid may be added to replace further losses and support the circulation.

Patients are likely to be cold after thoracic surgery as a result of lying in theatre covered only by sterile drapes and with the chest open during surgery. Simple means to conserve heat during surgery by warming i.v. fluids and humidification of inspired gases, followed by convective warming blankets in the recovery room, may restore body temperature to normal soon after surgery is finished.

Arrhythmias are common after thoracotomy, especially atrial tachyarrhythmias, which may affect 9–33% of patients over 60 years of age. They occur often 2–3 days after surgery and increase the risk of hypotension and stroke. Prophylaxis has proved ineffective and 85% resolve during hospital stay. Of the remainder, almost all resolve within 2 months.

OUTCOME

Despite best practice and standardized protocols, patients respond heterogeneously to thoracic surgery, in part due to genetic makeup. A better description of the influence of genomics may improve the explanation of risk to patients presenting for thoracic surgery.

FURTHER READING

Ambrosino, N., Gabbrielli, L., 2010. Physiotherapy in the perioperative period. Best Pract. Res. Clin. Anaesthesiol. 24, 283–289.

Banki, F., 2010. Pulmonary assessment for general thoracic surgery. Surg. Clin. North Am. 90, 969–984.

Bastin, R., Moraine, J.J., Bardocsky, G., et al., 1997. Incentive spirometry performance – a reliable indicator of pulmonary function in the early postoperative period after lobectomy? Chest 111, 559–563.

Bernstein, W.K., Deshpande, S., 2008. Preoperative evaluation for thoracic surgery. Sem. Cardiothorac. Vasc. Anesth. 12, 109–121.

Brister, N.W., Barnette, R.E., Kim, V., Keresztury, M., 2008. Anesthetic considerations in candidates for lung volume reduction surgery. Proc. Am. Thorac. Soc. 5, 432–437.

Brodsky, J.B., Lemmens, H.J.M., 2007. The history of anesthesia for thoracic surgery. Minerva Anestesiol. 73, 513–524.

Campos, J.H., 2009. Update on selective lobar blockade during pulmonary resections. Curr. Opin. Anaesthesiol. 22, 18–22.

Campos, J.H., 2009. Update on tracheobronchial anatomy and flexible fiberoptic bronchoscopy in thoracic anesthesia. Curr. Opin. Anaesthesiol. 22, 4–10.

Campos, J.H., 2010. An update on robotic thoracic surgery and anesthesia. Curr. Opin. Anaesthesiol. 23, 1–6.

Castillo, M.D., Heerdt, P.M., 2007. Pulmonary resection in the elderly. Curr. Opin. Anaesthesiol. 20, 4–9.

Daly, D.J., Myles, P.S., 2009. Update on the role of paravertebral blocks for thoracic surgery: are they worth it? Curr. Opin. Anaesthesiol. 22, 38–43.

Duggan, M., Kavanagh, B.P., 2010. Perioperative modifications of respiratory function. Best Pract. Res. Clin. Anaesthesiol. 24, 145–155.

Fischer, G.W., Cohen, E., 2010. An update on anesthesia for thoracoscopic surgery. Curr. Opin. Anaesthesiol. 23, 7–11.

Hernandez, G., Fernandez, R., Lopez-Reina, P., et al., 2010. Noninvasive ventilation reduces intubation in chest trauma-related hypoxemia: a randomized clinical trial. Chest 137, 74–80.

Jaklitsch, M., Billmeier, S., 2009. Preoperative evaluation and risk assessment for elderly thoracic surgery patients. Thorac. Surg. Clin. 19, 301–312.

McKevith, J.M., Pennefather, S.H., 2010. Respiratory complications after oesophageal surgery. Curr. Opin. Anaesthesiol. 23, 34–40.

Mineo, T.C., 2007. Epidural anesthesia in awake thoracic surgery. Eur. J. Cardio-Thorac. Surg. 32, 13–19.

Nagendran, J., Stewart, K., Hoskinson, M., Archer, S.L., 2006. An anesthesiologist's guide to hypoxic pulmonary vasoconstriction: implications for managing single-lung anesthesia and atelectasis. Curr. Opin. Anaesthesiol. 19, 34–43.

Ng, J.M., 2008. Perioperative anesthetic management for esophagectomy. Anesthesiol. Clin. 26, 293–304.

Pompeo, E., Tacconi, F., Mineo, T.C., 2010. Awake video-assisted thoracoscopic biopsy in complex anterior mediastinal masses. Thorac. Surg. Clin. 20, 225–233.

Rodrigo, J.L., Edguez-Panadero, F., 2008. Medical thoracoscopy. Respiration 76, 363–372.

Ross, A.F., Ueda, K., 2010. Pulmonary hypertension in thoracic surgical patients. Curr. Opin. Anaesthesiol. 23, 25–33.

Round, J.A., Mellor, A.J., 2010. Anaesthetic and critical care management of thoracic injuries. J. R. Army Med. Corps 156, 145–149.

Scarci, M., Joshi, A., Attia, R., 2010. In patients undergoing thoracic surgery is paravertebral block as effective as epidural analgesia for pain management? Interact. Cardiovasc. Thorac. Surg. 10, 92–96.

Schroeder, D., 1999. The preoperative period summary. Chest 115, 44S–46S.

Shaw, A., 2007. Exploring the perioptome: the role of genomics in thoracic surgery and anaesthesia. Curr. Opin. Anaesthesiol. 20, 32–36.

Sherry, K.M. (Ed.), 1996. Management of patients undergoing oesophagectomy. The report of the National Confidential Enquiry into Perioperative Deaths 1996/1997. Nuffield Provincial Hospitals Trust, London, pp. 57–61.

Shimizu, T., Abe, K., Kinouchi, K., Yoshiya, I., 1997. Arterial oxygenation during one lung ventilation. Can. J. Anaesth. 44, 1162–1166.

Slinger, P., 2009. Update on anesthetic management for pneumonectomy. Curr. Opin. Anaesthesiol. 22, 31–37.

Slinger, P.D., Johnston, M.R., 2001. Preoperative assessment for pulmonary resection. Anesthesiol. Clin. North America 19, 411–433.

Zibrak, J.D., 1990. Preoperative pulmonary-function testing. Ann. Intern. Med. 112, 763–771.

34 ANAESTHESIA FOR CARDIAC SURGERY

■ ■ ■ ■ ■ ■ ■ ■ ■ ■ ■

In the United Kingdom and much of the developed world, more than half of all cardiac surgical procedures are undertaken to revascularize ischaemic myocardium. Of the remainder, surgery for acquired valvular disease, congenital anomalies and disorders of the great vessels comprise the majority. Impaired ventricular function is not uncommon in this group of patients, the severity of which may greatly affect the conduct of anaesthesia and surgery as well as outcome. The combination of underlying cardiac pathology, comorbid conditions and concomitant medications – such as β-blockers and angiotensin converting enzyme (ACE) inhibitors – make many patients with cardiac disease susceptible to the adverse haemodynamic effects of anaesthetic agents, particularly peripheral vasodilatation. Regardless of the disease process or state, all efforts should be made to maintain haemodynamic stability and promote a positive myocardial oxygen balance during anaesthesia and throughout the postoperative period.

Undoubtedly, there is more equipment and technology on show in the cardiac surgical theatre than in other operating theatres, and the number of staff present is often large. This makes familiarity with equipment and multidisciplinary team working imperative, as well as a specialist knowledge of cardiovascular and respiratory physiology. The replacement of the functions of the heart and lungs by cardiopulmonary bypass (CPB) is often required, although some coronary surgery can be performed on the beating heart (off pump). Indeed, novel 'minimally invasive' methods may allow repair of various structures within the heart and even valve replacement or repair without CPB, and this is an exciting area of development.

TRENDS IN SURGICAL PRACTICE

The 6th National Adult Cardiac Surgical Database Report, published in 2009 by the Society for Cardiothoracic Surgery (SCTS) in Great Britain and Ireland, provides detailed information about trends in UK cardiac surgical practice. Although the total number of cardiac surgical procedures carried out in the UK in the period 2001–2008 increased year-on-year, coronary artery bypass graft (CABG) surgery plateaued at just under 23 000 operations per year, possibly due to advances in percutaneous intervention. Coincidentally, the number of elderly patients undergoing cardiac surgery of all types increased such that patients over the age of 75 years now make up more than 20% of the cardiac surgical population, and over 5% are over 80 years of age. Despite this, crude mortality rates decreased significantly between 2001 and 2008: 2.3% to 1.5% for isolated CABG; 5.2% to 3.5% for isolated valve surgery and 8.3% to 6.1% for combined procedures.

Ischaemic Heart Disease

The concept of aorto-coronary bypass grafting for the relief of coronary ischaemia was conceived and performed in animals in the early 1900s. It was not until the 1960s, following development of the heart-lung machine and the chance discovery of coronary angiography, that direct revascularization of the ischaemic myocardium using the autologous saphenous vein (Fig. 34.1) replaced indirect therapies such as sympathectomy, thyroidectomy and pericardial poudrage.

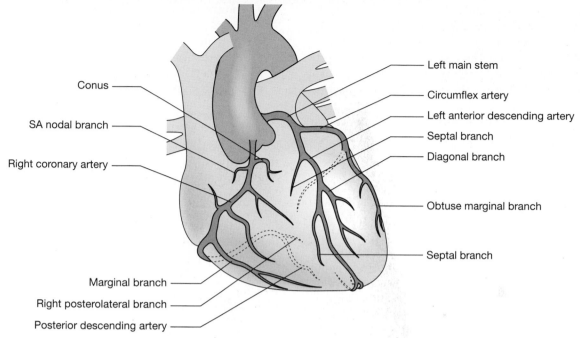

FIGURE 34.1 ■ Diagrammatic representation of coronary arteries. *(Adapted from JH Mackay and JE Arrowsmith (2012) Core topics in cardiac anesthesia. Cambridge University Press.)*

Since being popularized in the late 1960s, coronary artery bypass grafting (CABG) has become the most commonly performed cardiac operation. The internal mammary artery is used routinely as a graft conduit, and there is good evidence that this provides good survival benefit. Complete arterial revascularization is possible using arteries such as the radial and epigastric arteries. Improved surgical techniques have increased the popularity of off-pump coronary artery surgery but its precise role remains uncertain and any advantages over surgery using CPB have not yet been proven. Technological advances in coronary stent technology, especially coated (drug eluting) stents have led to a huge expansion in the use of percutaneous coronary intervention (PCI; angioplasty, atherectomy and stenting) in the cardiac catheter laboratory. These procedures are typically performed under sedation, and length of stay in hospital and return to normal activities is undoubtedly markedly improved. However, the long-term efficacy of stenting has recently been called into question, and traditional CABG, once thought to be in terminal decline, remains a popular procedure.

Valve Disease

Stenosis or incompetence (regurgitation or insufficiency) most commonly involves the mitral and aortic valves. The most common diseases are calcific degeneration (causing aortic stenosis, with or without regurgitation), chronic rheumatic disease (affecting mitral and aortic valves) and myxomatous disease (most often causing mitral regurgitation). It should be borne in mind that valve dysfunction may occur as the result of systemic disease (e.g. carcinoid syndrome, infective endocarditis) and disruption of nearby anatomical structures (e.g. aortic regurgitation in acute dissection of the ascending aorta and mitral regurgitation following papillary muscle rupture).

Surgery usually entails repair or prosthetic replacement, guided by intraoperative transoesophageal echocardiography (TOE). The use of bioprosthetic or 'tissue' (porcine, bovine, cadaveric homograft) valves obviates the necessity for, and risks associated with, life-long anticoagulation but exposes the patient to the prospect of reoperation within 15–20 years. In contrast, mechanical (tilting disc) valves tend to last longer than bioprostheses and are therefore better suited to younger patients and those already anticoagulated for other reasons (e.g. chronic atrial fibrillation). Improvements in technology have led to some prostheses lasting more than 20 years, especially in patients aged >70 years at the time of surgery. Minimally invasive transcatheter aortic valve replacement (TAVR) is now possible, making 'redo' sternotomy unnecessary in case of valve failure, by inserting a new tissue valve within the old prosthesis.

Congenital Heart Disease

Congenital heart disease has an incidence of 6–8 per 1000 live births. The majority of lesions requiring surgery are repaired during childhood in specialist paediatric cardiac surgical centres. Conditions such as a small atrial septal defect, partial anomalous pulmonary venous drainage or a bicuspid aortic valve may not present until adulthood. As a result of improvements in paediatric surgical and medical care, many patients now survive well into adulthood, and may require repeat surgery or other cardiac procedures. Specialist grown-up congenital heart (GUCH) disease centres have been created to cater for the often complex needs of this group of patients. A further description of these procedures is beyond the scope of this chapter.

Cardiopulmonary Bypass

The essential components of a cardiopulmonary bypass (CPB) circuit (Fig. 34.2) are:

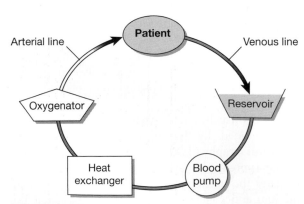

FIGURE 34.2 ■ Components of a cardiopulmonary bypass circuit. (*Adapted from JH Mackay and JE Arrowsmith (2012) Core Topics in Cardiac Anesthesia. Cambridge University Press.*)

- venous reservoir
- pump
- oxygenator
- heat exchange unit
- cardioplegia delivery system
- connecting tubes and filters.

Full anticoagulation of the patient, typically with unfractionated heparin, is required to prevent coagulation in the CPB circuit caused by contact between the blood and the plastic components, which would otherwise lead to potentially lethal CPB/oxygenator blockage and failure. Despite anticoagulation, blood/plastic contact leads to the release of a number of active substances which cause vasodilatation, consumption of clotting factors and fibrinolysis. These include cytokines, thromboxane A2 and leukotrienes, and they are responsible for the hypotension and increased bleeding associated with CPB.

Blood from the venous side of the circulation, the venae cavae or right atrium, is drained by gravity to a venous reservoir, from where it is pumped into a gas exchange unit (oxygenator) where oxygen is delivered to, and carbon dioxide removed from, the blood. The blood can also be cooled or warmed efficiently at this point, using water pumped through a countercurrent heat exchanger located within the oxygenator. Oxygenated or 'arterialized' blood is then delivered into the systemic circulation, usually via a cannula in the ascending aorta. The heart and lungs are thus 'bypassed' or isolated and their function maintained temporarily by mechanical equipment remote from the body. Any blood in or around the bypassed heart (whether spilt or drained) may be drained and returned to the venous (cardiotomy) reservoir for filtration, oxygenation and subsequent return to the circulation.

Venous Reservoir

A 500–2000 mL reserve of circulating volume permits the delivery of a constant system flow during times when venous drainage is inadvertently reduced or deliberately impeded. Clinical systems are described as being 'open' (blood in contact with air) or 'closed' (blood in a soft, flexible container not in contact with air). In order to prevent air entrainment, most systems incorporate a critical level alarm which automatically stops the CPB pump if the reservoir becomes empty.

Pumps

Roller pumps displace blood around the circuit by intermittent, semi-occlusive compression of the circuit tubing during each rotation. Intermittent acceleration of the roller head can be used to produce a 'pulsatile' pressure waveform although there is little evidence that a more physiological flow pattern improves outcome. Alternatively, a centrifugal pump may be used. Movement of a disc at very rapid speeds (>3000 revolutions per minute) leads to exertion of gravitational force on blood and results in propulsion at a flow which is dependent on the resistance (afterload) offered by the arterial tubing and the patient's systemic vascular resistance. There is some evidence that centrifugal pumps cause less blood component damage and activation, but this has not translated into improved outcome, and their use is usually confined to prolonged or complex surgery. Unlike roller pumps, which impede all flow when stopped, centrifugal pumps permit passive retrograde blood flow when switched off.

Oxygenator

Membrane oxygenators comprise a semi-permeable membrane which separates gas and blood phases and through which gas exchange occurs. Commercially available devices have an effective exchange area of around 7 m^2 – one tenth of the alveolar surface area of an adult.

Connecting Tubes, Filters, Manometer, Suction

These must be sterile and non-toxic and should damage blood as little as possible. A filter should also be incorporated in the arterial line to remove particulate and gaseous emboli which would otherwise pass directly to the aorta and cause blood vessel occlusion. Low-pressure suction pumps are supplied to vent blood collecting in the pulmonary circulation or left ventricle during bypass and also to remove shed blood from the surgical field. The blood is collected in the 'cardiotomy' reservoir, filtered and returned to the main circuit. Cardiotomy suction causes damage to blood components.

Fluid Prime

The CPB circuit must be primed with fluid (de-aired) prior to use. When CPB is commenced and the patient's blood is mixed with the clear fluids which prime the bypass circuit, the haematocrit decreases by approximately 20–25%. Although oxygen content is reduced, oxygen availability may be increased by improved organ blood flow resulting from reduced blood viscosity. In some patients (low body weight, children or preoperative anaemia, when dilution would reduce the haematocrit to below 20%), blood may be added to the prime. In the normal adult, 'clear' primes are used almost exclusively (usually a crystalloid/colloid mixture). Most units have individual recipes for addition to the prime (e.g. mannitol, sodium bicarbonate and potassium) to achieve an isosmolar solution at physiological pH.

PREOPERATIVE ASSESSMENT

In recent years, there has been a trend towards the assessment of elective patients in pre-admission clinics, typically one to two weeks before surgery. This allows routine paperwork, laboratory tests and radiological imaging to be completed before admission, which may not be until the day of surgery. Despite undergoing an extensive array of specialized investigations to diagnose and quantify cardiac disease, there is evidence that a significant number of cardiac surgical patients have additional and hitherto undocumented pathology. Thorough preoperative evaluation by the anaesthetist remains an essential component of perioperative care. This should, at the very least, include confirmation of the documented history and symptoms, documentation of current drug therapy, a review of the results of diagnostic investigations and a physical examination focused on the cardiovascular and respiratory systems.

Exercise Electrocardiography

Exercise (treadmill) testing is frequently used as a screening test before coronary angiography. Various stress protocols are used, in which a standard exercise test provokes ischaemic changes and symptoms. Changes in rhythm, rate, arterial pressure and conduction are recorded. Although it has relatively low sensitivity and specificity (60–70%) for coronary artery disease, it does provide some indication of effort tolerance.

Cardiac Catheterization

Left heart catheterization typically comprises coronary angiography, aortography, left ventriculography and manometry. This provides the following information (Table 34.1):

TABLE 34.1
Cardiac Catheterization

Technique	Procedure	Parameter
Manometry	Pressure measurement with catheter in aortic root and LV	Aortic valve gradient LV end-diastolic pressure
Angiography	Coronary arteries selectively cannulated, contrast injected	Coronary anatomy
Ventriculogram	Catheter in LV, contrast injected very rapidly	LV size and function Ejection fraction Severity of mitral regurgitation
Aortogram	Catheter in aortic root, contrast injected	Severity of aortic regurgitation

LV, left ventricle.

TABLE 34.2
Measurements Obtained During Cardiac Catheterization

	Parameter	Normal Values
Left heart	Systemic arterial/aortic pressure	<140/90 (mean 105) mmHg
	LV pressure	<140/12 mmHg
Right heart	RA pressure	<6 (mean) mmHg
	RV pressure	<25/5 mmHg
	PA pressure	25/12 (mean 22) mmHg
	PAWP	12 mmHg
	Cardiac index	2.5–4.2 l min^{-1} m^{-2}
	PVR	100 dyne s cm^{-5}
	SVR	800–1200 dyne s cm^{-5}

LV, left ventricle; RA, right atrium; RV, right ventricle; PA, pulmonary artery; PAWP, pulmonary artery wedge pressure; PVR, pulmonary vascular resistance; SVR, systemic vascular resistance.

- site and severity of coronary artery disease
- mitral and aortic valve function
- left ventricular (LV) morphology and function

The efficiency of ventricular contraction (ejection fraction) can be estimated using the formula:

$$\text{Ejection fraction (EF)} = \frac{\text{end-diastolic volume} - \text{end-systolic volume}}{\text{end-diastolic volume}}$$

Right heart catheterization allows measurement of right heart and pulmonary artery pressures. When combined with measurements of cardiac output, these can be used to determine the pulmonary and systemic vascular resistances (Table 34.2).

Echocardiography

Transthoracic echocardiography (TTE) is used frequently to define cardiac anatomy and assess ventricular and valvular function. TTE is non-invasive, and can be performed at intervals to monitor disease progression and to optimize the timing of surgical intervention before irreversible ventricular damage has occurred. It may also assist planning of the type of intervention required. Doppler techniques allow recognition of the direction and velocity of blood flow and are valuable in the diagnosis of valvular disease.

Unfortunately, TTE is of limited use in obese patients and patients with chronic lung disease (because of poor ultrasound windows caused by tissue or air). In addition, certain parts of the heart may not be visualized adequately because of their distance from the probe (such as the left atrium and interatrial septum). Therefore, transoesophageal echocardiography (TOE) may be required preoperatively (usually performed under sedation). TOE may also be indicated in mitral valve pathology to aid surgical decision-making between valve replacement and repair.

Radionuclide Imaging

By imaging the activity of an appropriate radioisotope as it passes through the heart or into the myocardium, ventricular function and myocardial perfusion can be assessed. Technetium images blood volume and can be used to demonstrate abnormal wall motion and EF. Thallium, which is taken up by the myocardium, may be used to assess regional blood flow. These techniques can be used before and after exercise or pharmacologically-induced stress, e.g. dobutamine infusion.

Computed Tomography/Magnetic Resonance Imaging

ECG-gated, multi-slice scanning, real-time motion and 3D reconstruction has led to the incorporation of CT and MRI in the preoperative assessment of many cardiac surgical patients. CT can demonstrate coronary anatomy and disease less invasively than traditional angiography, and MRI can be used to assess valvular lesions, especially in complex cases or when previous surgery has taken place. Anatomy of the aorta and pulmonary arterial system can be delineated and parameters measured accurately, facilitating surgical decision-making.

Additional Investigations

Respiratory function tests, arterial blood gas analysis, carotid ultrasonography, creatinine clearance and evaluation of a permanent pacemaker or cardio-defibrillator should be conducted as appropriate.

Preoperative Drug Therapy

Cardiac surgical patients typically take five or more prescription medicines for the control of symptoms (e.g. nitrates), cardiac risk modification (e.g. vasodilators, β-blockers) and the management of related conditions (e.g. hypoglycaemic agents, statins, bronchodilators). Care is required to balance the risks of discontinuation in the perioperative against the risk of major adverse cardiovascular events, e.g. withholding antiplatelet agents such as aspirin and clopidogrel.

β-Blocking agents. Continued administration of these drugs up to the time of surgery is desirable because discontinuation may increase the risk of perioperative myocardial infarction.

Calcium antagonists have a negative inotropic effect but, as with β-blockers, it is preferable to continue therapy throughout the perioperative period.

Nitrates should be continued to prevent rebound angina.

Digitalis. In most centres, digoxin is discontinued 24–48 h before surgery to diminish digoxin-associated arrhythmias after surgery.

Diuretics should be continued until the day before surgery.

Anticoagulants, including aspirin and clopidogrel, are usually stopped up to 1 week before surgery to permit platelet function to return towards normal. However, there is recent evidence that stopping aspirin is associated with increased morbidity, and it is continued throughout the perioperative period in many centres.

Angiotensin-converting enzyme (ACE) inhibitors are prescribed for hypertension and cardiac failure. They may produce significant vasodilatation and hypotension intraoperatively and postoperatively. Perioperative use varies from unit to unit; they may be stopped up to 1 week before surgery or continued until the day of operation.

Angiotensin receptor blockers (ARBs) are used for similar indications to ACE inhibitors and managed similarly.

Potassium-channel activators may be continued up to the day of operation.

Investigations

Blood count. Chronic anaemia (Hb <120 g L^{-1}) should be investigated because it is associated with blood transfusion and worsened outcome. Anaemia may predispose to excessive haemodilution during CPB. Iron deficiency or any other cause should be investigated and treated before surgery if detected in advance. Quantitative platelet or leucocyte abnormalities should also be excluded.

Coagulation. Clotting studies should be performed before surgery. In the absence of anticoagulant administration, the finding of a seemingly trivial prolongation of the activated partial thromboplastin time (APTT) should prompt further investigation because it may indicate the presence of a coagulopathy (e.g. factor IX or XI deficiency).

Electrolytes. Serum potassium concentration should be within normal limits; hypokalaemia is invariably associated with hypomagnesaemia. Chronic diuretic therapy may produce total body sodium depletion and uraemia. Raised serum concentrations of urea and creatinine may indicate chronic renal insufficiency and an increased risk of postoperative renal failure.

Liver function tests. Abnormal values may indicate congestive cardiac failure, alcohol abuse or metastatic malignancy.

RISK ASSESSMENT

Outcome from cardiac surgery has been the subject of intense scrutiny for the last two decades. Despite advances in surgical techniques, anaesthesia and critical care, cardiac surgery still carries a finite risk of death and serious complications. While this risk has decreased steadily over the last 10 years (<1% for isolated CABG or aortic valve replacement in young male patients), outcomes vary from centre to centre, and from surgeon to surgeon. Although helping the patient to understand the benefits (symptomatic and prognostic)

and risks of surgery during the consent process is the responsibility of the surgeon, it is essential that the anaesthetist understands how risk is assessed so that the patient is not given contradictory information.

In the late 1980s, Parsonnet and colleagues identified 14 independent risk factors for death after cardiac surgery. The so-called Parsonnet score was adopted by many centres worldwide and is still in use today. However, most present day cardiac surgeons 'out-perform' Parsonnet, reducing the usefulness of the scoring system as a measure of both risk and surgical performance. The European System for Cardiac Operative Risk Evaluation (EuroSCORE), developed in the late 1990s, provides a more robust risk assessment, which, like its predecessor, can be calculated easily at the bedside (Table 34.3). The EuroSCORE has been validated in the UK, Europe and

---

TABLE 34.3

EuroSCORE—The European System for Cardiac Operative Risk Evaluation additive risk stratification model. http://www.euroscore.org.

Factor		Points
Age	Per 5 years or part thereof >60	1
Gender	Female	1
Chronic lung disease	Bronchodilators or steroids	1
Extra cardiac arteriopathy	Claudication, carotid stenosis >50%, abdominal aortic, limb artery or carotid surgery planned or undertaken	2
Neurological dysfunction	Severe effect on ambulation or function	2
Previous cardiac surgery	Pericardium opened	3
Serum creatinine	>200 μmol L^{-1} before surgery	2
Active endocarditis	On antibiotics	3
Critical preoperative state	VT, VF, cardiac massage, invasive ventilation, inotropic support, IABP	2
Unstable angina	Angina at rest requiring intravenous nitrates	2
LV dysfunction	Moderate (LV EF 30–50%)	1
	Poor (LV EF <30%)	3
Recent myocardial infarct	<90 days	2
Pulmonary hypertension	PA systolic > 60 mmHg	2
Emergency operation	Carried out on referral, before next working day	2
Other than isolated CABG		2
Surgery on thoracic aorta		3
Post infarct septal rupture		4

VT, ventricular tachycardia; VF, ventricular fibrillation; IABP, intra-aortic balloon pump; CABG, coronary artery bypass graft; EF, ejection fraction; PA, pulmonary artery; LV, left ventricle.

North America and has been shown to be predictive of major complications, duration of critical care stay and resource utilization.

For higher risk patients, calculation of the logistic EuroSCORE provides a more accurate prediction than the simple additive score. For example, a fit 60-year-old man with asymptomatic critical left main stem coronary artery stenosis and normal LV function undergoing elective CABG surgery has a EuroSCORE predicted mortality of 1% (0.94% logistic). In contrast, a 75-year-old woman with poor LV function, chronic pulmonary disease and class IV angina undergoing emergency CABG surgery has a predicted mortality of 13% (38.74% logistic).

MONITORING

Extensive and accurate physiological monitoring is essential throughout the perioperative period for the safe practice of cardiac surgery. Instrumental monitoring should be considered an adjunct to, rather than a replacement for, routine clinical observation of the patient.

Electrocardiograph

The ECG should be monitored throughout the perioperative period. The ideal system is one which allows simultaneous multiple-lead monitoring or at least switching between leads II and V5, for accurate identification of ischaemia. Rate and rhythm should also be observed.

Systemic Arterial Pressure

Arterial cannulation is mandatory. It not only permits direct measurement of blood pressure but also facilitates sampling of arterial blood for analysis.

Central Venous Pressure

Right-sided filling pressure should be monitored by a catheter placed into a central vein. In selected cases, a flow-directed pulmonary artery catheter (PAC) may be inserted at induction to monitor left heart filling pressure.

Cardiac Output

Cardiac output (CO) can be measured by thermodilution using a PAC. This, together with the derivatives of stroke work, pulmonary and systemic vascular resistances and tissue oxygen flux, allows titration of vasoactive infusions. Modified PACs allow real-time measurement of CO and mixed venous oxygen saturation.

CO may also be measured by techniques such as oesophageal Doppler and pulse contour analysis but these have not replaced thermodilution in routine practice.

Echocardiography

Transoesophageal echocardiography (TOE) is indicated whenever valve surgery is undertaken, in cases of impaired left ventricular function or when the underlying diagnosis is uncertain. Performed immediately before surgery, it may be used to help guide the surgeon in the choice of procedure (e.g. valve repair). In addition, it may identify lesions which have not been detected or diagnosed correctly during preoperative evaluation, and may change surgical practice in up to 15% of cases. Immediately after CPB, the adequacy of surgery can be judged and the need for re-operation in case of failure identified. Abnormal motion of the ventricular wall (dyskinesia or akinesia) detected at this time but not present before surgery may indicate myocardial ischaemia, prompting further surgical revascularization or inotropic support.

Cerebral Monitoring

Despite being available for many years, monitors of cerebral function and cerebral substrate (oxygen) delivery are rarely used during routine cardiac surgery. In recent years, however cerebral near-infrared spectroscopy (NIRS) has gained popularity. This non-invasive technique allows measurement of capillary oxygen saturation in the frontal cortex throughout the perioperative period, and may prompt titration of haemodynamic and respiratory indices to improve cerebral oxygen delivery or reduce consumption (cooling). The effect of such measures on outcomes remains unproven and the subject of ongoing research.

Temperature

Core temperature should be monitored in the nasopharynx, which approximates to brain temperature, or the bladder.

Biochemistry and Haematology

Facilities should be available for immediate blood gas analysis. Many systems also measure the concentrations of sodium, potassium, calcium, lactate, haemoglobin and glucose.

Measurement of coagulation status should also be available. Activated clotting time (ACT) can be measured quickly in the operating theatre (normal = 100–120 s), but rapid access to a central laboratory is required for additional testing. Thromboelastography – the assessment of viscoelastic changes in blood during clotting – may usefully assess haemostatic function at or near the point of care.

Display

ECG, pressure waveforms and a digital output of temperature, heart rate and pressures should be clearly visible to surgeon, anaesthetist and perfusionist.

PATHOPHYSIOLOGY

The anaesthetist should have a clear understanding of the fundamental principles of cardiac and cardiovascular physiology. Accurate monitoring reveals alterations in cardiac function and permits the anaesthetist to manipulate factors which ensure adequate cardiac output and myocardial blood supply.

Preload and contractility determine the work performed by the heart (Fig. 34.3). In the failing heart, afterload determines the work expended in overcoming aortic pressure compared with that used to provide forward flow. Thus, cardiac output may be increased by increasing preload or contractility, or by reducing afterload. Any increases in heart rate, contractility, preload or afterload result in increased myocardial oxygen consumption. For this reason, augmentation of cardiac output by increasing preload or contractility may have a detrimental effect on oxygen balance. Reducing afterload may increase cardiac output while simultaneously reducing oxygen demand.

Adequate coronary perfusion demands the maintenance of an adequate diastolic aortic pressure. Oxygen supply to the myocardium occurs predominantly during diastole and is dependent on the gradient between diastolic aortic pressure and intraventricular pressure, and on the duration of diastole. The portion of myocardium most at risk of developing ischaemia is the left ventricular endocardium. Figure 34.4 illustrates how these variables affect oxygen supply and demand in the myocardium and how a satisfactory supply/demand ratio may be preserved.

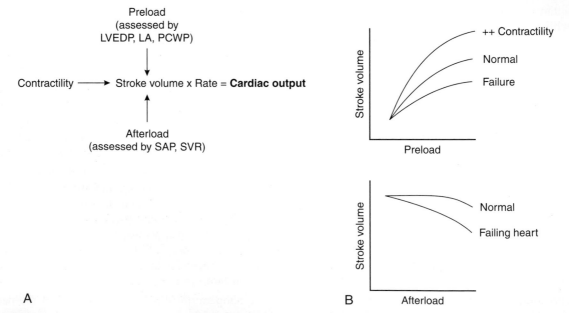

FIGURE 34.3 ■ Important aspects of mechanical function. LA, left atrium; LVEDP, left ventricular end-diastolic pressure; PCWP, pulmonary capillary wedge pressure; SAP, systolic arterial pressure; SVR, systemic vascular resistance.

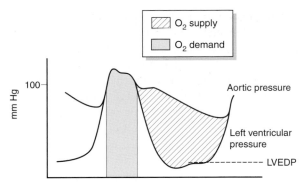

FIGURE 34.4 ■ The factors which determine myocardial oxygen supply and demand. LVEDP, left ventricular end-diastolic pressure.

Care of the patient with valvular heart disease depends on the type, severity and consequences of the valvular lesion. In general, patients with valvular heart disease are intolerant of extremes in heart rate. In patients with valvular regurgitation, reducing afterload tends to reduce the regurgitant fraction and increases forward flow. In contrast, patients with valvular stenosis often require increased preload and are intolerant of acute reductions in peripheral resistance (afterload). This is particularly true of patients with aortic stenosis, when most of the afterload to left ventricular ejection is caused by the stenosed valve itself. This afterload is fixed and cannot be reduced simply by lowering peripheral resistance. Vasodilatation in these patients produces marked hypotension and results in failure of perfusion of the hypertrophied myocardium with no increase in forward flow through the stenosed valve. Furthermore, diastolic dysfunction secondary to left ventricular hypertrophy dictates that the majority of ventricular filling occurs later in diastole as a consequence of atrial systole. For this reason, atrial fibrillation and nodal (junctional) rhythms may be tolerated poorly.

ANAESTHETIC TECHNIQUE

There is no single preferred anaesthetic technique for cardiac surgery. The choice of a specific drugs is less important than the care with which they are administered and their effects monitored. The techniques described here are suitable for standard CABG with cardiopulmonary bypass. Anaesthesia for off-pump coronary surgery may be complicated by significant

haemodynamic disturbances while the heart is positioned by the surgeon and by intraoperative myocardial ischaemia when coronary arteries are cross-clamped during anastomosis of the grafts. The reader is directed to more specialized texts for details of management.

Premedication

Most patients are sedated preoperatively with either an oral benzodiazepine (lorazepam 2–4 mg or temazepam 20–50 mg) or intramuscular opioid (morphine 10–20 mg), with or without an antisialagogue (hyoscine 0.4 mg). In the particularly anxious patient, heavy sedation may be required to prevent increases in heart rate and arterial pressure before surgery.

Induction of Anaesthesia

All drugs and equipment should be ready and the theatre and bypass circuit available for immediate use before the patient arrives in the anaesthetic room. Cross-matched blood should also be available immediately in case of rapid deterioration or surgical misadventure.

Before induction, ECG electrodes should be applied and the ECG trace displayed. Arterial and large-gauge venous cannulae should be inserted under local anaesthesia along with adequate sedation to reduce stress (e.g. midazolam 1–2 mg). The lungs should be preoxygenated.

Induction may be achieved in a variety of ways. Most often, a large dose of an opioid analgesic (e.g. fentanyl 5–15 µg kg^{-1}) is administered with a benzodiazepine (e.g. midazolam 0.05–0.1 mg kg^{-1}) to obtain unconsciousness. Alternatively, a small dose of propofol (0.5–2 mg kg^{-1}) together with opioid or benzodiazepine may be used; consciousness is obtunded by an opioid in moderate dose and hypnosis is then produced by a small dose of an intravenous induction agent. An alternative is a target-controlled infusion of propofol with the target concentration increased in small steps, accompanied by an infusion of a short-acting opioid such as alfentanil or remifentanil.

As consciousness is lost, a neuromuscular blocking drug is administered and ventilation supported when necessary. Almost all currently available relaxants have been used during cardiac surgery, although pancuronium remains a popular choice. The objective is to undertake tracheal intubation without cardiovascular stimulation and thus adequate analgesia and anaesthesia are required. A tracheal tube with a low-pressure, high-volume cuff should be used. Positive pressure ventilation is continued, usually with an oxygen/air mixture. Nitrous oxide, which may depress myocardial function and increase the volume of gaseous emboli, tends to be avoided in cardiac anaesthesia.

Percutaneous cannulation of a subclavian or internal jugular vein is performed using a multilumen catheter to allow monitoring and intravenous infusions. Ultrasound assistance should be used to facilitate central vein access, and reduces complications associated with this procedure. The nasopharyngeal temperature probe and a urinary catheter are inserted. Mechanical ventilation is continued with a breathing system containing a humidifier and bacterial filter.

Previously identified 'high-risk' patients, such as those with poor ventricular function or severe pulmonary hypertension, may require more extensive monitoring, e.g. a PA catheter. In the critical or emergency situation, the central venous catheter can be inserted under local anaesthesia, and induction of anaesthesia can be undertaken in theatre with the full team ready for immediate surgery.

Anaesthesia Pre-CPB

After the patient is prepared and draped, the sternum is opened and, if required, the left internal thoracic (mammary) artery is harvested. Many surgeons request discontinuation of mechanical ventilation during sternotomy to reduce the risk of direct injury to the lungs. The pericardium is then opened and the heart inspected. Heparin is administered (usually 300 IU kg^{-1}), to prolong the activated clotting time (ACT). The target ACT depends on local protocols, but is typically >400 s. The surgeon then places cannulae in the aorta and the vena cava. Cannulation is commonly undertaken via the right atrium into the inferior vena cava using a two-stage cannula, allowing drainage of both lower body (IVC) and upper body (right atrium). Alternatively, if the heart chambers are to be opened (for example when mitral valve surgery is scheduled), the cavae are cannulated separately.

The goals of haemodynamic management are to maintain a stable heart rate and arterial pressure during this period, particularly at moments of profound stimulation, notably skin incision, sternotomy and sternal retraction. If a technique based on opioids or volatile anaesthetics has been chosen, additional analgesia or inhalational anaesthesia should be given before stimulation. Alternatively, the opioid infusion rate can be increased temporarily as necessary, perhaps accompanied by increased target concentrations of propofol. The tendency of isoflurane to produce a 'coronary steal' (the diversion of blood away from ischaemic muscle) is considered not to be of clinical importance. There is evidence that volatile anaesthetic agents increase myocardial tolerance to ischaemia by a mechanism known as preconditioning thought to be mediated via ATP-dependent potassium channels.

If arterial pressure decreases during the period before institution of CPB, small doses of a vasoconstrictor (e.g. metaraminol or phenylephrine 250–500 µg) may be administered. A mean arterial pressure (MAP) sufficient to allow vital organ perfusion should be maintained. This will obviously depend on the individual patient, but in most patients MAP >70 mmHg is sufficient. During aortic cannulation, hypertension should be avoided to reduce the risk of aortic dissection. Many surgeons request a maximum MAP at this delicate point in the procedure (typically MAP <70 mmHg). Manipulation of the arterial pressure is required at frequent intervals to achieve a number of different goals.

Cardiopulmonary Bypass

Two factors complicate the provision of anaesthesia during CPB. First is the impact of haemodilution, hypotension, non-pulsatile blood flow and hypothermia on the pharmacokinetics of anaesthetic agents. Second is the inability to administer volatile inhalational agents via the lungs – mechanical ventilation is discontinued when full pump flow is reached and ventricular ejection ceases. Temporary loss of the lungs as a route for drug administration can be circumvented by use of total intravenous anaesthesia or the addition of a volatile agent to the CPB oxygenator 'sweep' gas.

Surgery is usually preceded by placing an aortic cross clamp proximal to the arterial cannula to isolate the coronary circulation. During CABG surgery, the distal anastomoses are usually fashioned first and the cross-clamp then removed to permit restoration of myocardial perfusion. Application of a side-biting aortic clamp then allows the proximal (aortic) anastomoses to be fashioned without interfering with perfusion of the native coronary arteries.

Myocardial Preservation

Most surgical techniques require that the heart be immobile. During CPB, the aorta is cross-clamped between the aortic cannula and the aortic valve, thus isolating the heart from the flow of oxygenated blood. Ischaemic damage to the myocardium can be reduced by hypothermia and the institution of diastolic cardiac arrest. The latter is typically achieved by instilling 500–1000 mL of crystalloid cardioplegic solution, often mixed with the patient's blood, into the coronary arteries. Many cardioplegic solutions are available; the majority contain potassium and a membrane-stabilizing agent, such as procaine.

Myocardial cooling is achieved by using ice-cold cardioplegia and by pouring cold saline (4°C) into the pericardial sac. Depending on surgical preference, the patient may also be cooled systemically. This is most often carried out when more complex or prolonged surgery is proposed, to allow better organ preservation due to reduced metabolic rate. Administration of cardioplegia is usually repeated at regular intervals, for example every 20–30 min.

Perfusion on Bypass

At normothermia, a pump flow of 2.4 L min^{-1} m^{-2} of body surface area is required to prevent inadequate perfusion of the tissues. Mean systemic (arterial) pressure is dependent on pump flow and systemic vascular resistance. Controversy exists regarding the optimum perfusion pressure because essential organs, particularly the brain, may be damaged if mean arterial pressure is <45 mmHg. Unfortunately, perfusion is difficult to assess clinically, especially in the hypothermic patient.

Following the onset of CPB, haemodilution causes marked decreases in peripheral resistance and arterial pressure, which in most instances resolve spontaneously in 5–10 min. If this does not occur, arterial pressure may be increased by raising systemic resistance with a vasoconstrictor. Frequently, peripheral resistance and arterial pressure increase during hypothermic CPB as a result of increasing concentrations of catecholamines, and then decrease during active rewarming because of profound vasodilatation.

Coagulation Control

Adequate anticoagulation must be maintained during CPB; ACT should be measured every 30 min and extra doses of anticoagulant administered as necessary.

Oxygen Delivery

Arterial blood samples should be taken at regular intervals for measurement of blood gas tensions, acid–base status and haematocrit. Continuous blood gas analysis is increasingly common. Tissue oxygen delivery is dependent on pump flow, haemoglobin concentration and oxygen tension. The haematocrit can usually be permitted to fall to 20%, but further reduction should be prevented by the addition of packed cells or blood to the bypass circuit.

Acid–Base Balance

The development of metabolic acidosis suggests that perfusion is inadequate and, if necessary (base deficit >6–8 mmol L^{-1}), sodium bicarbonate may be administered.

When systemic hypothermia is used during CPB, consideration needs to be given to the effect of hypothermia on the solubility of gases in blood, and how these affect values obtained from arterial blood gas analysis. As temperature decreases, the solubility of gases in liquids increases, and the proportion of gas in equilibrium with the gas phase (partial pressure) decreases, although the total content of each gas remains the same. The net result of this phenomenon is a metabolic acidosis secondary to reduced $PaCO_2$. There are two strategies for dealing with this issue. Not correcting arterial blood gas measurements for temperature allows a normal pH to be maintained. This is known as alpha-stat, because this maintains the degree of ionization of alpha-histidine. Alternatively, adding additional CO_2 to maintain a normal pH on the basis of corrected blood gas measurements is known as pH stat. In most centres, alpha-stat is used, but pH-stat offers a number of theoretical benefits in patients undergoing procedures requiring deep hypothermia.

Serum Potassium Concentration

Serum potassium concentration should be maintained at approximately 4.5–5.5 mmol L^{-1} by the administration of potassium chloride (10–20 mmol) into the CPB circuit as required. It should be borne in mind that repeated administration of cardioplegic solutions may cause a significant rise in serum potassium concentration.

Weaning from CPB

Following removal of the aortic cross-clamp, oxygenated blood flows into the coronary arteries again, washing out cardioplegia and repaying the oxygen debt. In many cases, the heart regains activity spontaneously. In a minority of patients, it starts to beat in sinus rhythm but reverts usually to ventricular fibrillation; internal defibrillation is required to convert fibrillation to sinus rhythm and is successful only if pH, serum potassium concentration, oxygenation and temperature are approaching normal values. The heat exchanger in the oxygenator is used to increase the temperature of blood, but peripheral temperature is often depressed for some time. If a spontaneous heartbeat cannot be maintained, external pacing via epicardial wires should be started.

When core body temperature exceeds 36°C, metabolic indices are normal and a regular heartbeat is present, the establishment of spontaneous cardiac output is attempted. By gradually restricting venous drainage to the venous reservoir, venous blood is diverted to the right atrium. When the pulmonary circulation has been restored, mechanical ventilation is restarted; 100% oxygen is given because the efficiency of pulmonary gas exchange is unknown at this stage and any gas bubbles which have not been vented may enlarge in volume if nitrous oxide or nitrogen (air) is introduced.

Left ventricular ejection produces an upward deflection on the arterial pressure trace after a QRS complex. If the myocardium is contracting satisfactorily, pump flow is reduced cautiously and the heart, now receiving all the venous return, achieves normal output.

Although arterial pressure is the most easily measured index of successful termination of CPB, it is merely the product of cardiac output and peripheral resistance. If there is doubt about efficiency of the heart, cardiac output should be measured and peripheral resistance derived.

Following successful termination of CPB, preload can be adjusted by retransfusing any blood left in the CPB circuit, by altering the patient's posture and by administering a vasodilator or vasoconstrictor.

Low Cardiac Output State

Failure to wean a patient from extracorporeal support should prompt the resumption of CPB while the cause is identified and supportive treatment initiated. TOE may be particularly helpful in this situation, permitting continuous assessment of preload, ventricular wall motion and valvular function. If causes such as failing to ventilate the lungs or an appropriate vaporizer setting have been excluded, attention should be focused on cardiac contractility and afterload.

Coronary aeroembolism, which may occur during and after separation from CPB, causes myocardial ischaemia manifest as a regional ventricular wall motion abnormality and rhythm disturbance. The problem usually resolves when arterial pressure is elevated and the heart permitted to eject on CPB.

The choice of inotrope in this setting is largely a matter of personal preference; there is little evidence to suggest that one drug is superior to another. Despite the theoretical risk of worsened myocardial reperfusion injury, calcium salts (e.g. $CaCl_2$ 250–1000 mg) are commonly used first. Other drugs commonly used – either alone or in combination – include adrenaline (0.05–0.2 µg kg^{-1} min^{-1}), dobutamine (2–20 µg kg^{-1} min^{-1}) and dopamine (2–20 µg kg^{-1} min^{-1}) by infusion; all increase myocardial oxygen demand and tend to precipitate tachyarrhythmias. Both adrenaline and dopamine cause vasoconstriction at high doses.

Phosphodiesterase III inhibitors, such as milrinone and enoximone, may be a suitable alternative or adjunct to conventional inotropes, particularly in patients with right ventricular dysfunction and pulmonary hypertension. By inhibiting the breakdown of cytosolic cyclic adenosine monophosphate, they improve myocardial performance and dilate both arterioles and veins. By reducing afterload, they reduce myocardial oxygen demand and augment ventricular ejection. Arterial hypotension, more commonly seen with milrinone, can be treated with an infusion of either noradrenaline or vasopressin.

Failure to achieve an adequate spontaneous circulation by pharmacological means alone is an indication for mechanical support such as intra-aortic balloon counterpulsation.

Intra-Aortic Balloon Pump. This device is inserted through a femoral artery and positioned in the descending aorta, just distal to the left subclavian artery. The balloon is inflated during diastole immediately after closure of the aortic valve, and deflated prior to ventricular ejection. Inflation displaces blood in the aorta, simultaneously promoting distal flow and augmenting coronary perfusion. Following deflation of the balloon, proximal aortic pressure (afterload) is reduced, favouring improved ventricular ejection and lowering left ventricular end-diastolic pressure.

Bleeding

Following decannulation of the heart, it is necessary to restore normal coagulation and achieve haemostasis. In the case of heparin anticoagulation, protamine sulphate (~1 mg for each 100 units of heparin given) is administered cautiously. Protamine typically produces a transient and occasionally profound fall in arterial pressure because of peripheral vasodilatation. Rarely, protamine may cause acute pulmonary vasoconstriction. In excessive dosage, protamine may itself act as an anticoagulant.

Excessive bleeding after cardiac surgery is associated with increased resource utilization, morbidity and mortality. Coagulopathic bleeding may be caused by residual anticoagulation or the consumption of clotting factors and platelets during CPB. Failure to achieve adequate haemostasis within 45 min of separation from CPB should prompt a full blood count, coagulation screen and, where available, thromboelastography. The results should then be used to guide the selection of blood component therapy.

While assisting the surgeon to achieve haemostasis, the anaesthetist must maintain adequate anaesthesia, maintain haemodynamic stability and correct any metabolic or biochemical abnormalities.

HAEMODYNAMICS AFTER CPB

Myocardial injury and a degree of cardiac dysfunction are inevitable consequences of cardiac surgery and CPB. Virtually all patients exhibit brief increases in serum troponin and cardiac enzyme concentrations in the early postoperative period. The net result is reduced contractility (depressed Frank–Starling curve), reduced sensitivity to adrenergic agonists (endogenous and exogenous) and increased sensitivity to myocardial depressants (e.g. β blockers). In

the normal course of events, myocardial contractility tends to improve in the week after surgery.

Peripheral vasoconstriction may persist for several hours after CPB. This may lead to hypertension in patients with preserved ventricular function (particularly after surgery for aortic stenosis) or a low cardiac output state in patients with impaired ventricular function. The treatment of hypokalaemia and hypomagnesaemia, and administration of a vasodilator such as sodium nitroprusside, decrease myocardial oxygen demand, improve peripheral perfusion and may increase cardiac output. In addition, blood pressure control reduces the stress placed on vascular anastomoses.

In some patients, however, a profound systemic inflammatory response produces excessive vasodilatation and hypotension. Having excluded hypotension secondary to low cardiac output, it may be necessary to initiate treatment with phenylephrine, noradrenaline or vasopressin.

Other Aspects

In addition to maintaining cardiac function and oxygen supply to the tissues during this period, the anaesthetist should ensure that normality is regained as soon as possible, and maintained, in respect of the following.

Temperature

The thermal gradient between body core and peripheral tissues limits both the rate and efficiency of cooling and rewarming during CPB. The rate of transfer of thermal energy is largely governed by patient weight, muscle mass, vascular tone, perfusion pressure and pump flow. The inevitable fall in core temperature secondary to redistribution after CPB (so-called 'afterdrop') can be mitigated by using external warming devices.

Biochemical Monitoring

Essential monitoring includes arterial blood gas tensions, acid–base status, serum electrolyte concentration and haematocrit.

Cardiac Rhythm

Heart Block. This may follow aortic valve surgery and operations on the ventricular septum, or as a consequence of right coronary aeroembolism.

Atrioventricular (sequential; D00, DDD) pacing using epicardial pacing wires ensures an adequate ventricular rate and maintains late diastolic ventricular filling, which is particularly important if ventricular compliance is poor.

Supraventricular Arrhythmias. Synchronized, direct current cardioversion is the most convenient treatment when the chest is open. After chest closure, options include amiodarone, β-blockade, verapamil or adenosine.

Ventricular Arrhythmias. The threshold for arrhythmias is reduced by hypokalaemia, hypomagnesaemia and hypocalcaemia. The abrupt onset of ventricular tachycardia or ventricular fibrillation after moving the patient from the operating table to the bed may herald coronary aeroembolism.

Transfer to Postoperative Care Unit

In most centres, intraoperative support and monitoring are extended into the postoperative period. The duration of this care depends on institutional practice and the patient's speed of recovery. In some centres, patients are routinely cared for in the intensive care unit (ICU). However, there may be some advantages to managing these patients on separate extended recovery units. In such instances, the interval between admission and weaning from mechanical ventilation can usually be considerably shortened. This so-called 'fast-track' approach may be associated with earlier discharge and reduced morbidity from unnecessarily prolonged sedation and mechanical ventilation of the lungs.

Transferring patients from the operating theatre is not without risk. Care must be taken to prevent inadvertent injury and avulsion of indwelling tubes, catheters and cannulae. Mechanical ventilation, drug therapy and haemodynamic monitoring should be continued throughout transfer.

POSTOPERATIVE CARE

Regardless of location, there should be a well-practised routine for the care of patients after surgery. Usually, ventilation of the lungs and full cardiovascular monitoring are recommended immediately. The principles of care in this phase are similar to those described for the period of anaesthesia after termination of bypass.

The principles underpinning the management of patients in the first few hours after cardiac surgery are the maintenance of haemodynamic stability, adequate pulmonary gas exchange, normal acid-base homeostasis, haemostasis and renal function.

In the uncomplicated patient, sedation can be discontinued 3–4 h after admission, and the patient weaned from mechanical ventilation. In a significant minority of patients however, haemodynamic instability, poor gas exchange, bleeding, hypothermia or agitation may necessitate prolonged sedation.

Bleeding

Bleeding after cardiac surgery is normal and to be expected. However, excessive bleeding (>150 mL h^{-1}) should be considered abnormal and prompt further assessment. Coagulopathic bleeding may be due to thrombocytopenia, clotting factor deficiency and residual effects of heparin, and should be treated actively on the basis of laboratory and point-of-care investigations. Temperature and acid–base balance should be normalized. In contrast, bleeding in the setting of normal coagulation should prompt consideration of early surgical re-exploration. However, it should be borne in mind that both resternotomy and massive transfusion are associated with significantly increased morbidity and mortality.

In some instances in which chest tube drainage is inadequate, the accumulation of blood within the chest may lead to haemodynamic collapse secondary to cardiac tamponade. Falling arterial blood pressure and rising central venous pressure should be considered to be due to tamponade until proved otherwise. If deterioration occurs rapidly, resternotomy must be undertaken in the ITU.

Criteria for Tracheal Extubation

- Awake, orientated, responds to commands
- Temperature >35.5C° with core-peripheral gradient <6 C°
- Chest tube drainage <100 mL h^{-1}
- Satisfactory blood gases with an inspired oxygen concentration <50%
- Haemodynamic stability

Pain Relief

Pain after sternotomy is limited because surgical wiring of the sternum during closure prevents excessive bone movement and muscle injury is not a feature. Patients tend to complain more about pain from chest drain sites and leg/arm wounds (from harvesting of the saphenous vein or radial artery). Regular paracetamol should be administered, and morphine by infusion or nurse-administered bolus is often required. Morphine can often be replaced by a strong oral analgesic such as tramadol or codeine soon after extubation of the trachea, but patient-controlled analgesia (PCA) may be required by some patients. Chest drains are usually removed on the day after surgery, and analgesia for their removal can be provided by nitrous oxide/oxygen (Entonox) inhalation.

FURTHER READING

Hensley, F.A., Martin, D.E., Gravlee, G.P., 2002. A practical approach to cardiac anesthesia, third ed. Lippincott, Williams & Wilkins, Philadelphia.

Kaplan, H.A., Reich, D.L., Konstadt, S.N. (Eds.), 2006. Cardiac anesthesia, fifth ed. WB Saunders, Philadelphia.

Klein, A.A., Vuylsteke, A., Nashef, S.A.M. (Eds.), 2008. Core topics in cardiothoracic critical care. Cambridge University Press, Cambridge.

Mackay, J.H., Arrowsmith, J.E. (Eds.), 2012. Core topics in cardiac anaesthesia, second ed. Cambridge University Press, Cambridge.

35 OBSTETRIC ANAESTHESIA AND ANALGESIA

Obstetric anaesthesia and analgesia involve caring for women during childbirth in three situations:

- provision of analgesia for labour, usually by epidural or spinal analgesic techniques
- anaesthesia for instrumental (e.g. forceps or Ventouse) or caesarean delivery
- care of the critically ill parturient.

The obstetric anaesthetist is involved in the care of the parturient as part of a multidisciplinary team, including obstetricians, midwives, health visitors, physicians and intensive care specialists. There are few other areas of anaesthetic practice where communication skills and good record-keeping are so important. Successive reports from the triennial confidential enquiries into maternal mortality currently conducted by the National Perinatal Epidemiology Unit (NPEU), and formerly by the Centre for Maternal and Child Enquiries (CMACE) have highlighted the problems of women with intercurrent medical disease and the importance of the obstetric anaesthetist in their care. This has led to the establishment of obstetric anaesthetic assessment clinics in many hospitals (an Obstetric Anaesthetists' Association (OAA) survey found that 30% of units in the UK had such clinics in 2005). The education of colleagues, patients and the public about the role of obstetric anaesthetists is essential so that patients are fully informed and hence feel more comfortable about consenting to regional anaesthetic and analgesic techniques when these may be indicated. Information leaflets produced by the OAA on analgesia in labour and caesarean section are available in up to 37 languages.

Many anaesthetists in training approach their obstetric module with trepidation for several possible reasons. All anaesthetists have heard that mothers may die, albeit rarely, as a result of general anaesthesia and that these were previously healthy young women. In addition, they may be aware of the challenge of performing a regional block under the scrutiny of a partner in patients who are awake.

The UK Royal College of Anaesthetists (RCoA) curriculum for anaesthetists in training for obstetric anaesthesia is divided into basic, intermediate, higher and advanced levels. The first three are essential in order to achieve the CCT (Certificate of Completion of Training). An initial assessment of competence in obstetric anaesthesia must also be completed to pass the basic level. Training programmes in other countries have similar objectives.

The basic obstetric module requires the trainee to gain knowledge, skills and experience of the treatment of healthy pregnant women and of the management of common obstetric emergencies. The contents of this chapter are mapped to the RCoA basic curriculum.

ANATOMY AND PHYSIOLOGY OF PREGNANCY

An understanding of the physiological changes induced by pregnancy is vital to the clinician involved in the care of pregnant women. The obstetric anaesthetist must understand maternal adaptation to pregnancy in order to manipulate physiological changes following general anaesthesia or regional analgesia and anaesthesia in such a way that the condition of the neonate at delivery is optimized.

The physiological changes of pregnancy are exaggerated in multiple pregnancy. The success of assisted conception means that obstetric anaesthetists now care for more women with twins, triplets and quadruplets.

Progesterone

The hormone progesterone may be considered the most important physiological substance in pregnancy. It is secreted initially in increasing amounts during the second half of the menstrual cycle to prepare the woman for pregnancy. Following conception, the corpus luteum ensures adequate blood concentrations until placental secretion is adequate. The most important physiological role of progesterone is its ability to relax smooth muscle. All other physiological changes stem from this pivotal function (Fig. 35.1).

Haemodynamic Changes

Blood volume increases from 65–70 to 80–85 mL kg^{-1} mainly by expansion of plasma volume, which starts shortly after conception and implantation and is maximal at 30–32 weeks (Fig. 35.2). Red cell volume increases linearly but not as much as plasma volume (Table 35.1). Thus, the haematocrit decreases, causing the 'physiological anaemia' of pregnancy.

The increase in blood volume is accompanied by an increase in cardiac output (Fig. 35.3) within the first 10–12 weeks by approximately 1.5 L min^{-1}. By the third trimester, cardiac output has increased by about 40–50% as a result of significant increases in heart rate and stroke volume (Table 35.2). In labour, cardiac output may increase by a further 45%.

In normal pregnancy, despite the increased blood volume and hyperdynamic circulation, the pulmonary capillary wedge pressure (PCWP) and central

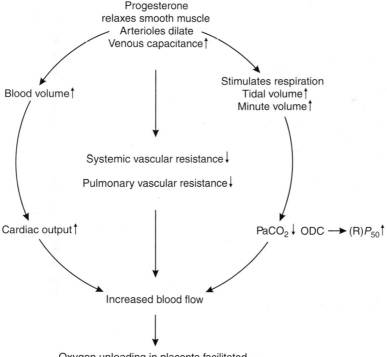

FIGURE 35.1 ■ Summary of the main actions of progesterone – it establishes the maternal physiological adaptation to pregnancy. PaCO$_2$, arterial carbon dioxide tension; ODC, oxyhaemoglobin dissociation curve; P_{50}, partial pressure of oxygen when haemoglobin is 50% saturated at pH 7.4 and temperature 37°C; HCO$_3^-$ bicarbonate.

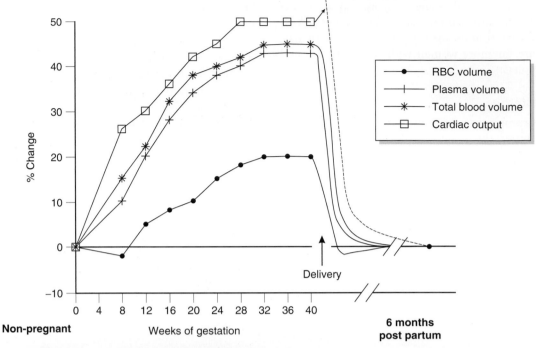

FIGURE 35.2 ■ Changes in blood, plasma and red cell volumes and cardiac output during pregnancy.

TABLE 35.1		
Haematological Changes Associated with Pregnancy		
Variable	*Non-Pregnant*	*Pregnant*
Haemoglobin	14 g dL⁻¹	12 g dL⁻¹
Haematocrit	0.40–0.42	0.31–0.34
Red cell count	4.2×10^{12} L⁻¹	3.8×10^{12} L⁻¹
White cell count	6.0×10^{9} L⁻¹	9.0×10^{9} L⁻¹
Erythrocyte sedimentation rate	10	58–68
Platelets	$150–400 \times 10^{9}$ L⁻¹	$120–400 \times 10^{9}$ L⁻¹

venous pressure do not increase, because of the relaxant effect of progesterone on the smooth muscle of arterioles and veins, and dilatation of the left ventricle. Significant decreases in systemic and pulmonary vascular resistance permit the increased blood volume to be accommodated at normal vascular pressures.

In essence, a large heart pumps a larger blood volume more quickly through an enlarged and expanding vascular bed which provides a low resistance to less viscous blood.

Despite the reductions in haemoglobin concentration and red cell mass, the physiological changes are geared to maximize oxygen transport to the placenta and eliminate carbon dioxide.

Aortocaval Compression

Pregnant women who lie supine may suffer from aortocaval compression. Arterial pressure decreases because the gravid uterus compresses the inferior vena cava to reduce venous return and therefore cardiac output. The aorta is also frequently compressed, so that femoral arterial pressure may be lower than brachial arterial pressure; this has been demonstrated to be the main cause of a reduction in uterine blood flow. Compensation for aortocaval compression occurs through sympathetic stimulation and collateral venous return via the vertebral plexus and azygous veins. The effect of aortocaval compression varies from asymptomatic mild hypotension to cardiovascular collapse and is usually prevented/relieved by left tilt/wedging although complete lateral position is required in some cases.

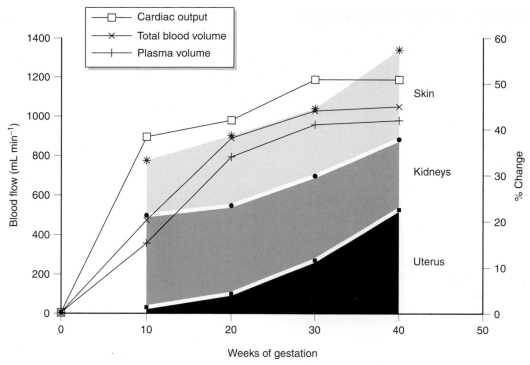

FIGURE 35.3 ■ Diagrammatic representation of changes in blood flow to various organs during pregnancy, together with percentage changes in cardiac output, and blood and plasma volumes.

TABLE 35.2
Cardiovascular Changes in Pregnancy

Variable	Change	% change
Heart rate	Increased	20–30%
Systolic blood pressure	Decreased	10–15% 2nd trimester
Diastolic blood pressure	Decreased	
Stroke volume	Increased	20–50%
Cardiac output	Increased	40–50% by 3rd trimester
Systemic vascular resistance	Decreased	20%
Central venous pressure	Unchanged	
Pulmonary vascular resistance	Decreased	30%
Pulmonary capillary wedge pressure	Unchanged	

Regional Blood Flow

There is an increased blood flow to various organs, especially the uterus and placenta, where it rises from 85 to $500\,mL\,min^{-1}$ (see Fig. 35.3). Liver blood flow is *not* increased.

Blood flow to the nasal mucosa is increased. Nasal intubation may be associated with epistaxis.

There is a considerable increase in blood flow to the skin, resulting in warm, clammy hands and feet. The purpose of this vasodilatation, together with that in the nasal mucosa, is to dissipate heat from the metabolically active fetoplacental unit.

Respiratory Changes

Respiratory function undergoes several important modifications (Table 35.3), also as a result of the actions of progesterone. The larger airways dilate and airway resistance decreases. There are increases in tidal volume (from 10 to 12 weeks' gestation) and minute volume (by up to 50%). Progesterone exerts a stimulant action on the respiratory centre and carotid body receptors.

TABLE 35.3
Changes in Respiratory Function in Pregnancy

Variable	Non-Pregnant	Term Pregnancy
Tidal volume ↑	450 mL	650 mL
Respiratory rate	16 min^{-1}	16 min^{-1}
Vital capacity	3200 mL	3200 mL
Inspiratory reserve volume	2050 mL	2050 mL
Expiratory reserve volume ↓	700 mL	500 mL
Functional residual capacity ↓	1600 mL	1300 mL
Residual volume ↓	1000 mL	800 mL
PaO$_2$ slight ↑	11.3 kPa	12.3 kPa
PaCO$_2$ ↓	4.7–5.3 kPa	4 kPa
pH slightly ↑	7.40	7.44

PaO$_2$, arterial oxygen tension; PaCO$_2$, arterial carbon dioxide tension.

Alveolar hyperventilation leads to a low arterial carbon dioxide tension (PaCO$_2$) during the second and third trimesters. By the 12th week of pregnancy, PaCO$_2$ may be as low as 4.1 kPa (PaCO$_2$ gradually decreases during the premenstrual phase of the menstrual cycle). The respiratory alkalosis is accompanied by a decrease in plasma bicarbonate concentration resulting from renal excretion (base excess decreases from 0 to −3.5 mmol L^{-1}). Arterial pH does not change significantly. The oxyhaemoglobin dissociation curve is shifted to the right because the increase in red cell 2,3-diphosphoglycerate (2,3-DPG) concentration outweighs the effects of a low PCO$_2$, which would normally shift the curve to the left. The P_{50} increases from about 3.5 to 4.0 kPa. The oxyhaemoglobin dissociation curve (ODC) of HbF is to the left of that for HbA. The loading–unloading advantages of HbF are at *low* oxygen tensions. Placental exchange of oxygen is regulated mainly by a change in oxygen affinities of HbA and HbF caused principally by altered hydrogen ion and carbon dioxide concentrations on both sides of the placenta.

Without the double Bohr and double Haldane effects, the diffusion gradients or placental blood flow would have to be increased considerably to maintain the same efficiency of gas transfer.

The functional residual capacity (FRC) and residual volume are reduced at term because of the enlarged uterus (Table 35.3). This substantial reduction, combined with the increase in tidal volume, results in large volumes of inspired air mixing with a smaller volume of air in the lungs. The composition of alveolar gas may be altered with unusual rapidity and alveolar and arterial hypoxia develop more quickly than normal during apnoea or airway obstruction. In normal pregnancy, closing volume does not intrude into tidal volume.

Oxygen consumption (Vo_2) increases gradually from 200 to 250 mL min^{-1} at term (up to 500 mL min^{-1} in labour). Carbon dioxide production parallels oxygen consumption. In the intervillous space, the diffusion gradient for oxygen is approximately 4.0 kPa, and for carbon dioxide is approximately 1.3 kPa.

The incidence of failed intubation in term parturients is approximately 1 in 300 cases, compared with 1 in 2200 in the non-pregnant population. This is caused in part by changes in pregnancy which affect the airway (Table 35.4). These factors increase the difficulty in seeing the larynx and increase the rate at which hypoxaemia develops in an apnoeic patient.

Renal Changes

These changes are shown in Table 35.5. Renal blood flow is increased (Fig. 35.3). By 10–12 weeks, glomerular filtration rate (GFR) has increased by 50% and remains at that level until delivery. Glycosuria often occurs because of decreased tubular reabsorption and the increased load. The renal pelvis, calyces and ureters dilate as a result of the action of progesterone and intermittent obstruction from the uterus, especially on the right.

TABLE 35.4
Physiological Changes of Pregnancy Which Increase the Risk of Hypoxaemia

Interstitial oedema of the upper airway, especially in pre-eclampsia

Enlarged tongue and epiglottis

Enlarged, heavy breasts which may impede laryngoscope introduction

Increased oxygen consumption

Restricted diaphragmatic movement, reducing FRC

TABLE 35.5
Renal Changes in Pregnancy

Parameter	Non-Pregnant	Pregnant
Urea (mmol L^{-1})	2.5–6.7	2.3–4.3
Creatinine (μmol L^{-1})	70–150	50–75
Urate (μmol L^{-1})	200–350	150–350
Bicarbonate (mmol L^{-1})	22–26	18–26
24 hour creatinine clearance	Increased	

Gastrointestinal Changes

These also stem from the effects of progesterone on smooth muscle.

A reduction in lower oesophageal sphincter pressure occurs before the enlarging uterus exerts its mechanical effects (an increase in intragastric pressure and a decrease in the gastro-oesophageal angle). These mechanical effects are greater when there is multiple pregnancy, hydramnios or morbid obesity. A history of heartburn denotes a lax gastro-oesophageal sphincter.

Placental gastrin increases gastric acidity. Together with the sphincter pressure changes, this makes regurgitation and inhalation of acid gastric contents more likely to cause pneumonitis in pregnancy.

Gastrointestinal motility decreases but gastric emptying is not delayed during pregnancy. However, it is delayed during labour but returns to normal by 18 h after delivery. Thus women are at risk of regurgitation of gastric contents during this time. Pain, anxiety and systemic opioids (including epidural and subarachnoid administration of opioids) aggravate gastric stasis. Small and large intestinal transit times are increased in pregnancy and may result in constipation.

Changes in liver function are summarized in Table 35.6.

TABLE 35.6
Liver Function Changes in Pregnancy

Parameter	Change in Pregnancy
Albumin	Decreased
Alkaline phosphatase	Increased (from placenta)
ALT/AST	No change
Plasma cholinesterase	Decreased

Haematological Changes

Haemoglobin concentration decreases from 14 to 12 g dL^{-1} (Table 35.1). Cell-mediated immunity is depressed. There is an increase in platelet production but the platelet count falls because of increased activity and consumption. Platelet function remains normal. Haematological changes return to normal by the sixth day after delivery.

Coagulation

Pregnancy induces a hypercoagulable state. These changes are summarized in Table 35.7.

There is an increase in the majority of clotting factors, a decrease in the quantity of natural anticoagulants and a reduction in fibrinolytic activity. Fibrinolysis decreases due to decreased tissue plasminogen activator (t-PA) activity because of inhibitors produced by the placenta.

Despite these changes, bleeding time, prothrombin time and partial thromboplastin time remain within normal limits. Thromboelastography may be useful to assess platelet function and clot stability but its use in pregnancy is unproven.

TABLE 35.7
Coagulation Changes in Late Pregnancy

Fibrinogen increased from 2.5 (non-pregnant value) to 4.6–6.0 g L^{-1}
Factor II slightly increased
Factor V slightly increased
Factor VII increased 10-fold
Factor VIII increased – twice non-pregnant state
Factor IX increased
Factor X increased
Factor XI decreased 60–70%
Factor XII increased 30–40%
Factor XIII decreased 40–50%
Antithrombin IIIa decreased slightly
Plasminogen unchanged
Plasminogen activator reduced
Plasminogen inhibitor increased
Fibrinogen-stabilizing factor falls gradually to 50% of non-pregnant value

The increase in clotting activity is greatest at the time of delivery, with placental expulsion releasing thromboplastic substances. These substances stimulate clot formation to stop maternal blood loss. Coagulation and fibrinolysis generally return to pre-pregnant levels 3–4 weeks postpartum.

The Epidural And Subarachnoid Spaces

Anatomy of the Epidural Space

The epidural space is the space between the periosteal lining of the vertebral canal and the spinal dura mater. It contains spinal nerve roots, lymphatics, blood vessels and a variable amount of fat (Figs 35.4, 35.5). Its boundaries are as follows:

- *superiorly* – the foramen magnum, where the dural layers fuse with the periosteum of the cranium; hence, local anaesthetic solution placed in the epidural space cannot extend higher than this
- *inferiorly* – the sacrococcygeal membrane
- *anteriorly* – the posterior longitudinal ligament
- *posteriorly* – the ligamentum flavum and vertebral laminae
- *laterally* – the pedicles of the vertebrae and the intervertebral foramina.

In the normal adult, the spinal cord begins at the foramen magnum and normally ends at the level of L1 or L2 (though it may end lower); here it becomes the cauda equina. The epidural space is a tube containing the spinal cord, the cerebrospinal fluid (CSF) and the meninges. It is crossed by 32 spinal nerves, each with a dural cuff. The subarachnoid space extends further than the cord, to the level of S2. Below this level, the dura blends with the periosteum of the coccyx. Between the dura and arachnoid is the subdural space, within which local anaesthetic solution may spread extensively.

The volume of the vertebral canal is finite. An increase in volume of contents of one compartment reduces the compliance of the other compartments and increases the pressures throughout.

In pregnancy, the epidural veins are dilated by the action of progesterone. These valveless veins of Batson form collaterals and become engorged as a result of aortocaval compression, during a uterine contraction or secondary to raised intrathoracic or intra-abdominal pressure, e.g. coughing, sneezing or expulsive efforts of parturition. The dose of local anaesthetic for epidural analgesia or epidural/subarachnoid anaesthesia is reduced by about one-third for the following reasons:

- Spread of local anaesthetic in either the subarachnoid or epidural space is more extensive as a result of the reduced volume.
- Progesterone-induced hyperventilation leads to a low $PaCO_2$ and a reduced buffering capacity; thus, local anaesthetic drugs remain as free salts for longer periods.
- Pregnancy itself produces antinociceptive effects. The onset of nerve block is more rapid, and human peripheral nerves have been shown to be more sensitive to lidocaine during pregnancy. Increased plasma and CSF progesterone concentrations may contribute towards the reduced excitability of the nervous system.

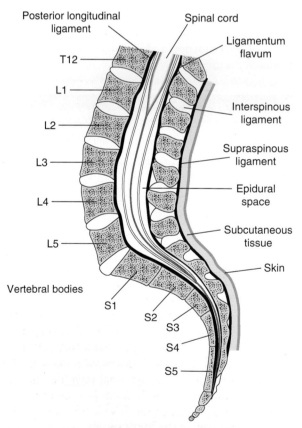

FIGURE 35.4 ■ The vertebral column. Note that the spinal cord ends at the level of L1 or L2 and that the dural sac extends to the level of the S2 vertebra.

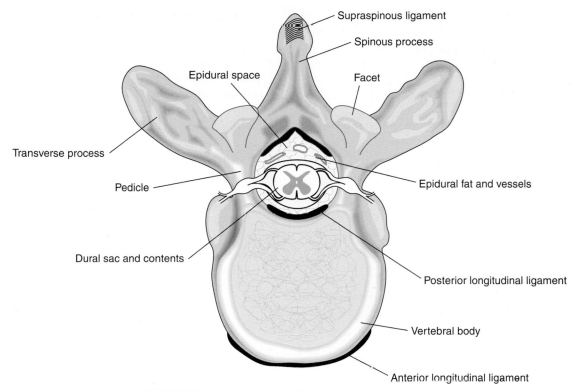

Supraspinous ligament

Spinous process

Epidural space

Facet

Transverse process

Epidural fat and vessels

Pedicle

Dural sac and contents

Posterior longitudinal ligament

Vertebral body

Anterior longitudinal ligament

FIGURE 35.5 ■ Anatomical relations of the epidural space.

- Increased pressure in the epidural space facilitates diffusion across the dura and produces higher concentrations of local anaesthetic in CSF.
- Venous congestion of the lateral foramina decreases loss of local anaesthetic along the dural sleeves.

During contractions, the pressure in the epidural space may increase by 0.2–0.8 kPa and become very high (2.0–5.9 kPa) in the second stage of labour. Because the spread of local anaesthetic is exaggerated during contractions, top-ups should not be administered at that time.

The CSF pressure increases from about 2.2 to 3.8 kPa during contractions and to 6.9 kPa in the second stage. It is therefore advised not to advance an epidural needle or insert an epidural catheter during contractions due to the increased risk of dural puncture.

Even if precautions are taken to prevent it, intermittent aortocaval compression always occurs in association with maternal movement. Consequently, the epidural veins become intermittently and unpredictably engorged.

Pain Pathways in Labour and Caesarean Section

The afferent nerve supply of the uterus and cervix is via Aδ and C fibres which accompany the thoracolumbar and sacral sympathetic outflows. The pain of the first stage of labour is referred to the spinal cord segments associated with the uterus and the cervix, namely T10–T12 and L1. Pain of distension of the birth canal and perineum is conveyed via S2–S4 nerves (Fig. 35.6). When anaesthesia is required for caesarean section, all the layers between the skin and the uterus must be anaesthetized. It is important to remember that the most sensitive layer is the peritoneum, and therefore the block should extend up to at least T4 and also include the sacral roots (S1–S5) to cold and T5 to touch.

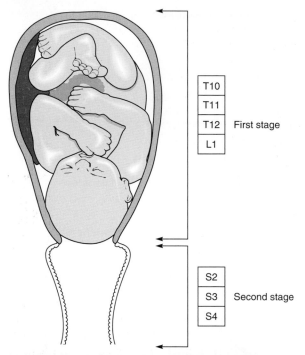

FIGURE 35.6 ■ Nerve supply to the uterus and birth canal.

The Placenta

The placenta is both a barrier and link between the fetal and maternal circulations. It consists of both maternal and fetal tissue – the basal and chorionic plates, separated by the intervillous space.

The two circulations are separated by two layers of cells – the cytotrophoblast and the syncytiotrophoblast. Fetal well-being depends on placental blood flow. Placental blood flow depends on the perfusion pressure across the intervillous space and the resistance of the spiral arteries. The spiral and uterine arteries possess α-adrenergic receptors. Placental perfusion is reduced by a reduction in cardiac output (e.g. haemorrhage) or uterine hypertonicity (e.g. overstimulation with syntocinon)

Functions of the Placenta

Transport of Respiratory Gases. This is the most important function of the placenta and is described above.

Hormone Production. Human chorionic gonadotrophin (hCG) is secreted by placental syncytiotrophoblasts and production commences very early in

pregnancy and peaks at 8–10 weeks. Its role is to stimulate the corpus luteum to secrete progesterone. hCG levels increase again near term gestation but its role in late pregnancy is unclear.

Human placental lactogen (hPL) has similar effects to growth hormone and causes maternal insulin resistance.

Oestrogens are secreted by the placenta and have a role in breast and uterus development.

Progesterone is secreted by the placenta. Its vital role in the physiology of pregnancy has been described above.

Alkaline phosphatase is secreted by the placenta but its role in pregnancy is uncertain.

Immunological. The placenta modifies the fetal and maternal immune system so that the fetus is not rejected.

IgG is transferred across the placenta and confers some passive immunity but may also produce disease.

There is a reduction in cell-mediated immunity.

Placental Transfer of Drugs. The barrier between maternal and fetal blood is a single layer of chorion united with fetal endothelium. The surface area of this is vastly increased by the presence of microvilli. Placental transfer of drugs occurs, therefore, by passive diffusion through cell membranes which are lipophilic. However, this membrane appears to be punctuated by channels which allow transfer of hydrophilic molecules at a rate that is around 100 000 times lower.

Drugs cross the placenta by simple diffusion of unionized lipophilic molecules. Fick's law of diffusion applies. The rate is directly proportional to the materno-fetal concentration gradient and the area of the placenta available for transfer, and inversely proportional to placental thickness.

Factors Determining Placental Transfer

Materno-Fetal Concentration Gradient. Drug transfer occurs down a concentration gradient in either direction. The maternal drug concentration depends on the route of administration, dose, volume of distribution, drug clearance and metabolism. The highest concentration is achieved after intravenous administration, although epidural and intramuscular administration result in similar concentrations. Fetal drug concentration depends on the usual factors of redistribution, metabolism and excretion. The fetus eliminates drugs less effectively due to immature enzyme systems. The distribution differs because of the anatomical and physiological organization of the fetal circulation; for example, drugs accumulate in the liver because of the umbilical venous flow to the liver and are metabolized before distribution. The relatively high extracellular fluid volume explains the large volumes of distribution of local anaesthetics and muscle relaxants.

Molecular Weight and Lipid Solubility. The placental membrane is freely permeable to lipid-soluble substances, which undergo flow-dependent transfer. The majority of anaesthetic drugs are small (molecular weights of less than 500 Da) and lipid-soluble and so cross the placenta readily. The main exceptions are the neuromuscular blocking drugs.

Protein Binding. A dynamic equilibrium exists between bound (unavailable) and unbound (available) drug. Reduced albumin concentration increases the proportion of unbound drug. Many basic drugs are bound to α_1-glycoprotein, which is present in much lower concentrations in the fetus than in the adult.

Degree of Ionization. The placental membrane carries an electrical charge; ionized molecules with the same charge are repelled, while those with the opposite charge are retained within the membrane. The rate of this permeability-dependent transfer is inversely proportional to molecular size. Size limitation for polar substances begins at molecular weights between 50 and 100 Da. Ions diffuse much more slowly. Factors affecting the degree of ionization alter the rate of transfer.

Maternal and Fetal pH. Changes in maternal or fetal pH alter the degree of ionization and protein binding of a drug, and thus its availability for transfer. This has most significance if the pKa is close to physiological pH (local anaesthetics), and is clinically relevant in the acidotic fetus. Fetal acidosis increases the ionization of the transferred drug, which is then unable to equilibrate with the maternal circulation, resulting in accumulation of the drug. This is known as ion trapping.

The degree of ionization of acidic drugs is greater on the maternal side and lower on the fetal side. The converse applies for basic drugs.

Placental Factors and Uteroplacental Blood Flow. Placental drug transfer depends on the area of the placenta available for transfer. Physiological shunting occurs and in pre-eclampsia the placenta itself may present an increased barrier to transfer.

Effects of Drugs on the Fetus

Drugs may have a harmful effect on the fetus at any time during pregnancy. In the early stages of pregnancy (at a stage when the woman may be unaware that she is pregnant), the conceptus is a rapidly dividing group of cells and the effect of drugs at that stage tends to be an all-or-nothing phenomenon, either slowing cell division if no harm is done or causing death of the embryo. Drugs may produce congenital malformations (teratogenesis), and the period of greatest risk is from weeks 3 to 11. In the second and third trimesters, drugs may affect the functional development of the fetus or have toxic effects on fetal tissues. Drugs given in labour or near delivery may adversely affect the neonate after delivery. Hence, drugs should be prescribed in pregnancy only if the perceived benefit of the therapy to the mother outweighs the possible detrimental effects on the fetus.

Effects of Drugs on the Neonate

In many studies, the ratio of maternal vein to umbilical vein concentration is used; this indicates the situation at delivery only and gives little information about the effects or distribution of the drug in the neonate.

Inhalational anaesthetics diffuse readily, but provided that the induction-delivery interval is short, the fetus is minimally affected. Neonatal elimination is dependent on ventilation.

Neuromuscular blocking drugs, which are quaternary ammonium compounds and ionized fully, cross the placenta very slowly. Only prolonged administration of a muscle relaxant, e.g. in the intensive care unit, might lead to neonatal paralysis. Bolus doses of succinylcholine are safe.

Thiopental is highly lipid-soluble, weakly acidic, 75% protein-bound and less than 50% ionized at physiological pH. It therefore crosses the placenta rapidly, with umbilical vein concentration closely following the relatively rapid decrease in maternal blood concentration. Fetal plasma concentration continues to increase for around 40 min after single exposure. However, because of the relatively large fetal volume of distribution, fetal and neonatal tissue concentrations are lower than maternal. The maintenance of high maternal thiopental concentration by repeated boluses maintains a high diffusion gradient, producing prolonged placental transfer and neonatal sedation. Doses of thiopental greater than 8 mg kg^{-1} produce neonatal depression, whereas doses of less than 4 mg kg^{-1} produce no significant neonatal effects provided that the induction to delivery time is less than 5 min. Thiopental in such doses does not affect Apgar score or umbilical cord gas tensions, but may produce subtle changes in the neuroadaptive capacity score (NACS), such as reduction in muscular tone, decreased excitability and a predominant sleep state in the first day of life. A dose of thiopental of 4–7 mg kg^{-1} is commonly advocated for induction of general anaesthesia because it ensures unconsciousness. Widespread clinical use testifies to the safety of thiopental.

Propofol is highly protein-bound, neutral and lipophilic. Propofol has been used for both induction and maintenance of anaesthesia for caesarean section. There is conflicting evidence concerning the effects of propofol on the neonate. Clearly, if propofol is administered by infusion and uterine blood concentrations are maintained, a high diffusion gradient is maintained across the placenta and there is persistently high transfer of propofol. Induction doses as low as 2–3 mg kg^{-1} and maintenance doses as low as 5 mg kg^{-1} h^{-1} have been shown to cause significant neonatal depression. Neonatal elimination of propofol is slower than that in adults. Unless thiopental is contraindicated, there seems little advantage in using propofol for caesarean section.

Diazepam should be avoided, if possible. It is a non-polar compound which is bound to albumin, but the feto-maternal ratio may reach 2. The neonate may suffer from respiratory depression, hypotonia, poor thermoregulation and raised bilirubin concentrations.

Opioids are mainly weak bases bound to α_1-glycoprotein. Pethidine and its metabolite norpethidine depress all aspects of neurobehaviour in the neonate. Feto-maternal ratios increase to exceed 1 after

2–4 h. Neonatal elimination is slow, resulting in prolongation of the effects. Transfer of pethidine is increased in the presence of fetal acidosis. Depressant effects are maximum if administration to delivery time is 2–3 h. Fentanyl is highly lipid-soluble and albumin-bound, and rapidly crosses the placenta. Apgar scores are low after administration of intravenous fentanyl. Epidural administration of fentanyl in doses of less than 200 µg is not associated with any adverse effect on the fetus. Alfentanil is less lipophilic but more protein-bound to α_1-glycoprotein. Feto-maternal ratios are low and at caesarean section are more related to feto-maternal α_1-glycoprotein concentration. Theoretically, Apgar and neuro-behavioural scores should be less affected.

Remifentanil crosses the placenta readily but appears to have few adverse effects on the fetus/neonate because it is rapidly metabolized. It can be used for patient-controlled analgesia (PCA) in labour (see below).

Non-steroidal anti-inflammatory drugs should be avoided in pregnancy because they can result in premature closure of the ductus arteriosus and premature birth.

Lactation and Drugs in Obstetric Anaesthesia

Women are encouraged to breastfeed. Oestrogen and progesterone stimulate mammary development during pregnancy. These hormones inhibit prolactin. This inhibition ceases at delivery. Suckling triggers lactation and stimulates the release of more prolactin and oxytocin, both of which promote production of milk.

Many women wish to suckle their infant immediately after delivery and are encouraged to do so. The anaesthetist should know, therefore, if the drugs used for obstetric anaesthesia and analgesia are secreted in the milk and, if so, whether they are likely to have an adverse effect either on the process of lactation itself or on the neonate.

The effects of a drug administered to the mother on a breastfeeding neonate are determined by peak plasma concentration of the drug, its transfer into milk, composition of milk, volume ingested, metabolism (including first-pass metabolism by the neonate), pharmacokinetics and action in the neonate. Many studies have relied on assessment of concentration of drug in milk with little consideration of resultant neonatal plasma concentration and the changing composition of breast milk. Human breast milk consists of an isosmotic emulsion of fat in water, with lactose and protein in the aqueous phase. However, its composition varies with time. Colostrum (first milk) contains abundant protein and lactose but no fat. It has a high pH and specific gravity. Over the following 7–10 days, milk has less protein, less lactose and more fat. Colostrum is more likely to be contaminated by water-soluble drugs, whereas lipid-soluble drugs are secreted into mature milk. The volume of colostrum produced is around 10–120 mL, in contrast to ingestion of mature milk by the neonate of 130–180 mL kg^{-1}day^{-1} (600–1000 mL day^{-1}). Even in mature milk, there is a significant diurnal variation in composition.

The maternal concentration of drug presented to the breast varies with dose, route of administration, volume of distribution, lipid solubility, ionization and protein binding.

The physicochemical properties of a drug which determine transfer into the milk are pK_a, the partition coefficient, degree of ionization and molecular weight. The pH of mature human milk is 7.09. Therefore, weak acids are less easily transferred than weak bases.

The total amount of drug contained in the milk depends on binding to milk protein, partition into milk lipid and the quantity which remains unbound in the aqueous phase, e.g. lipid-soluble drugs such as diazepam are concentrated in milk lipid. The dose of drug delivered to the neonate from the milk varies with the volume ingested. The higher gastric pH, different gastrointestinal flora and slow gastrointestinal transit of the neonate influence drug absorption.

The pharmacokinetics of drugs in the neonate may differ markedly from those in adults. Lipophilic and acidic drugs are bound to albumin and may displace unconjugated bilirubin. Metabolic and excretory pathways are immature so elimination may be delayed.

Opioids. Morphine appears safe with conventional administration. PCA may increase maternal plasma concentration. It is transferred readily to breast milk but does not appear to cause neonatal depression, possibly because of first-pass metabolism. Codeine and dihydrocodeine are metabolized to morphine and are not usually associated with neonatal depression. Pethidine is associated with neurobehavioural depression of the neonate. Short-acting opioids such as fentanyl and alfentanil are safe, even by continuous epidural infusion.

Non-steroidal anti-inflammatory drugs. The non-steroidal anti-inflammatory drugs (NSAIDs) ketorolac and diclofenac are safe. The neonate has immature biotransformation and excretory pathways. Aspirin should be avoided because high concentrations have been observed following a single oral dose. Neonates may be at risk of developing Reye's syndrome.

Paracetamol. Paracetamol is minimally secreted into breast milk. However, it is cleared by the liver more slowly than in adults. It is considered safe.

Thiopental and propofol. These drugs are detectable in milk and colostrum. However, the dose received by the neonate after a single induction dose is insignificant.

Diazepam. Diazepam and its metabolites are excreted in breast milk. As with placental transfer, there is the possibility of adverse effects on the neonate, especially with continuous administration.

Lidocaine and bupivacaine. The amounts excreted in breast milk are small or undetectable.

PHARMACOLOGY OF RELEVANT DRUGS

The detailed pharmacology of the drugs used during pregnancy is covered elsewhere in this textbook, but the following are of particular relevance to the obstetric anaesthetist.

Uterotonic Drugs

Syntocinon (Oxytocin)

Syntocinon is a synthetic analogue of the posterior pituitary hormone oxytocin, which is responsible for effective uterine muscle contraction. It is used during labour to augment progress, at delivery to aid placental delivery and closure of uterine vasculature and in the postpartum period to reduce postpartum haemorrhage. For augmentation or induction of labour, Syntocinon is usually administered via a syringe or volumetric pump using an increasing dose. The usual dose at delivery is 5 international units (IU), and 40 IU may be infused over 4 h to maintain myometrial contraction and reduce bleeding.

Syntocinon may cause vasodilatation and tachycardia and so should be administered cautiously in the presence of hypovolaemia and in patients with significant cardiac disease. Syntocinon also has an antidiuretic hormone effect, so care should be taken if infused in dilute dextrose solution, as hyponatraemia may occur.

Carbetocin

Carbetocin is a long-acting oxytocin analogue which can be given as a single dose to prevent postpartum haemorrhage as an alternative to an infusion of Syntocinon. The optimal dose is probably 100 μg intravenously at caesarean section. It has a plasma half-life between four and ten times that of Syntocinon.

Ergometrine

Ergometrine is also given to stimulate uterine contraction, usually in a dose of 500 μg. Ergometrine causes peripheral vasoconstriction, which may be severe, leading to hypertension and pulmonary oedema; thus it should be avoided in women with hypertensive disease. It can cause nausea and vomiting as a result of its action on other types of smooth muscle and it is usually reserved for more severe cases of uterine atony.

Syntometrine

Syntometrine is a combination of ergometrine 500 μg and Syntocinon 5 units. Until recently, it was administered routinely by intramuscular injection at the delivery of the anterior shoulder to assist in placental separation and to reduce postpartum haemorrhage; however, Syntocinon alone is now favoured because of its reduced side-effect profile.

Prostaglandins

Prostaglandins are a group of endogenous short polypeptides with a wide diversity of physiological functions. Prostaglandins are commonly used to 'ripen' the cervix on induction of labour but may cause bronchospasm and hypertension.

Carboprost

Carboprost is prostaglandin $F_2\alpha$. It has an important role in the treatment of severe uterine atony unresponsive to Syntocinon or ergometrine. It is administered intramuscularly (250 μg). It should **not** be given intravenously or intramyometrially. It may induce bronchospasm and hypertension and should be avoided in asthmatics.

Misoprostol

Misoprostol is a prostaglandin E_1 analogue. It may be used to induce labour and is given vaginally. It may be given as third or fourth line treatment of postpartum haemorrhage (600 μg p.r.). It produces pyrexia, shivering, nausea and vomiting, and diarrhoea.

Dinoprostone

Dinoprostone is prostaglandin E_2 which is given as a gel, tablets or pessary to induce labour by 'ripening the cervix' prior to rupture of membranes and intravenous infusion of Syntocinon.

Mifepristone (RU486)

Mifepristone is a prostaglandin antagonist which causes luteolysis and trophoblastic separation. It is given orally with prostaglandins to induce labour after intrauterine death of the fetus and when labour is induced for a non-viable fetus. It is associated with headache, dizziness and gastrointestinal upset.

Tocolytic Drugs

β_2-Adrenergic Receptor Agonists (Terbutaline, Salbutamol, Ritodrine)

These act on uterine β_2-receptors causing relaxation of the myometrium. They can be given orally, subcutaneously or by intravenous infusion for premature labour. The effects should be monitored carefully because severe tachycardia, hypotension, pulmonary oedema, hypokalaemia, and hyperglycaemia may occur.

The drugs may also be given by intravenous bolus injection (salbutamol or terbutaline 100–250 μg) as part of an in-utero fetal resuscitation regimen before emergency caesarean section.

Oxytocin Antagonists (Atosiban)

Atosiban is an oxytocin antagonist used to decrease uterine contractions; it has few side-effects but it is expensive.

Glyceryl Trinitrate (GTN)

GTN acts directly on uterine smooth muscle and can be given intravenously (50 μg) or sublingually (200–400 μg) to produce rapid but short-term uterine relaxation. It can be used as part of intrauterine resuscitation, or in cases of uterine hypertonicity, retained placenta and uterine inversion. It causes hypotension and headache.

Indomethacin

Indomethacin is an NSAID and a prostaglandin synthetase inhibitor. It may be given orally or rectally to inhibit contractions after cervical circlage. It can cause premature closure of the fetal ductus arteriosus and therefore should not be used after 32 weeks' gestation.

BASIC OBSTETRICS

Normal Labour

A large number of pregnant women are assessed as being 'low risk' and are predicted to have a normal labour, but the diagnosis of normal labour is retrospective. The descriptors of normal labour are:

- contractions occurring every 3 min and lasting 45 s
- progressive dilatation of the cervix (approximately 1 cm h^{-1})
- progressive descent of the presenting part
- vertex presenting with the head flexed and the occiput anterior
- labour not <4 h (precipitate) or >18 h (prolonged)
- delivery of a live healthy baby
- delivery of a complete placenta and membranes
- no complications.

The First Stage of Labour

Initially, the cervix effaces (i.e. becomes thin along its vertical axis and soft in consistency) and then cervical dilatation begins. The rate of cervical dilatation should be about 1 cm h^{-1} for a nulliparous woman and 2 cm h^{-1} for a multiparous woman. It is standard practice to examine the woman every 4 h, or more frequently if there is cause for concern. Routine observations are made as per National Institute of Clinical Excellence (NICE) guidelines and these are charted on the partogram (see Fig. 35.7):

- fetal heart rate (FHR) every 15 min
- hourly maternal pulse rate
- blood pressure and temperature 4-hourly
- frequency of emptying of the bladder
- frequency of contractions half-hourly
- vaginal examination offered 4 hourly

The fetal heart may be monitored intermittently by auscultation using a Pinard stethoscope or Doppler ultrasound. Continuous electronic fetal monitoring (EFM) can be performed using a cardiotocograph (CTG). The fetal heart rate may be recorded using either an abdominal transducer or a clip applied to the fetal head. Uterine contractions are also monitored using an abdominal transducer. Radiotelemetry is available in some units and this allows the woman to be mobile while her baby is monitored.

Indications for continuous EFM include insertion of an epidural, meconium-stained liquor, oxytocin for augmentation, abnormal FHR on auscultation, maternal pyrexia, fresh p.v. bleeding and maternal request.

The Second Stage of Labour

The second stage of labour starts at full dilatation of the cervix and ends at the delivery of the baby. At full dilatation of the cervix, the character of the contractions changes and they become associated with a strong urge to push. In normal labour, Ferguson's reflex occurs, in which there is an increase in circulating oxytocin secondary to distension of the vagina from the descending presenting part of the fetus, with consequent increased strength of uterine contractions at full dilatation. Epidural analgesia may attenuate the effect of this reflex. The second stage of labour may be classified into passive and active stages and this is particularly relevant when epidural analgesia is used. With epidural analgesia, the labouring woman does not have the normal sensation at the start of the second stage of labour produced by Ferguson's reflex, and therefore the active stage of pushing should start only when the vertex is visible or the woman has a strong urge to push. If the active second stage is prolonged, the fetus may become acidotic. A diagnosis of delay is made after 2 h in nulliparous women and 1 h in primiparous and multiparous women.

The Third Stage of Labour

The third stage of labour is the complete delivery of the placenta and membranes, and contraction of the uterus. It is usually managed 'actively' by administering an oxytocic (i.m. Syntocinon 5 IU) and early cord clamping but it may also be managed physiologically (no oxytocic and delayed cord clamping). During the third stage of labour, there is redistribution of the former placental blood flow (about 15% of cardiac output). This results in an increase in circulating blood

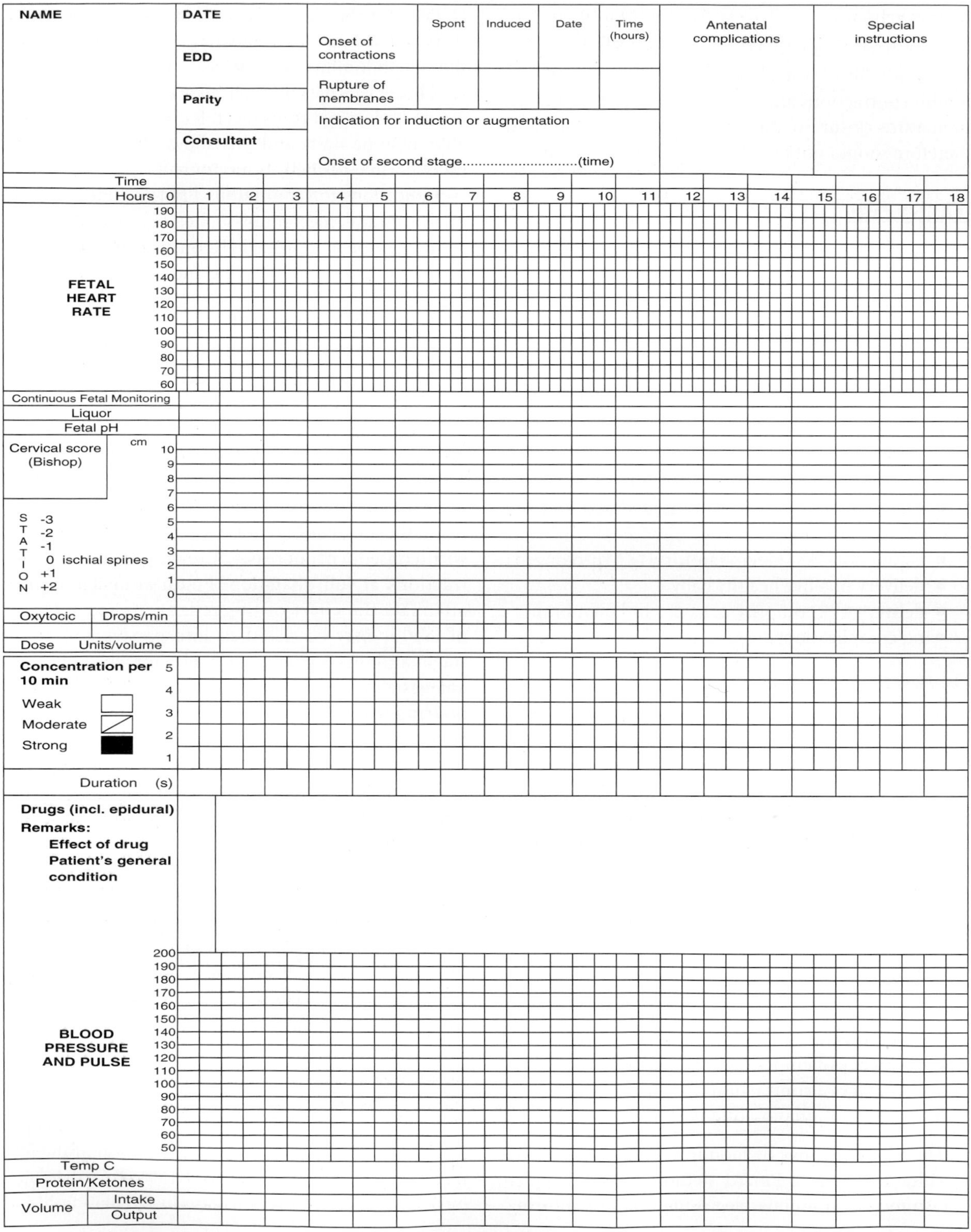

FIGURE 35.7 ■ Example of partogram.

volume which is potentially dangerous to women who have cardiac disease because it may precipitate heart failure immediately postpartum.

Fetal Monitoring

Recent developments have made it possible to assess fetal well-being in the antenatal period. An obstetric anaesthetist is often involved when a decision to deliver the baby early is made on the outcome of these assessments. The most commonly used tests are:

- serial ultrasonography
- serial umbilical artery Doppler flow studies
- cardiotocograph (CTG) monitoring.

It is important that the anaesthetist communicates with the obstetrician and understands the degree of fetal compromise when asked to give analgesia or anaesthesia to these mothers. The degree of urgency for the delivery depends on the condition of the fetus. Monitoring of the fetus is an important part of intrapartum care, as labour is a stressful event for the fetus. Fetal well-being may be monitored routinely using the following methods:

- fetal heart auscultation
- fetal heart cardiotocography
- colour of the liquor
- fetal blood sampling.

The recommended definitions and classifications of CTG monitoring are shown in Tables 35.8 and 35.9. Opioids or other sedative drugs may cause a flat trace with loss of beat-to-beat variability. Any trace which causes concern, especially in a high-risk pregnancy, is an indication for fetal blood sampling (FBS). FBS should be performed in the presence of a pathological CTG unless there is clear evidence of acute compromise (e.g. prolonged deceleration for longer than 3 min), when urgent preparations to expedite birth should be made.

The colour of the liquor may be monitored when the membranes are ruptured. The liquor colour is observed for the presence of meconium. The appearance of new meconium may indicate fetal hypoxia, because hypoxaemia may cause the fetal anal sphincter to relax. If meconium is aspirated into the lungs of the neonate, severe lung damage may ensue, and therefore a paediatrician should be present at delivery if meconium is present. When the fetus becomes hypoxic, there is an accumulation of lactic acid and a reduction in fetal pH. Fetal blood sampling allows more accurate assessment of fetal well-being than is afforded by the CTG and should be performed whenever there is anxiety about the CTG or when there is meconium in the liquor. Fetal blood sampling should be performed in the left lateral position to avoid aortocaval obstruction.

TABLE 35.8				
Classification of CTG Trace Features				
Feature	*Baseline (bpm)*	*Variability (bpm)*	*Decelerations*	*Accelerations*
Reassuring	110–160	≥5	None	Present
Non-reassuring	100–109 161–180	<5 for 40–90 min	Typical variable decelerations with over 50% of contractions, occurring for over 90 min Single prolonged deceleration for up to 3 min	The absence of accelerations with otherwise normal trace is of uncertain significance
Abnormal	<100 >180 Sinusoidal pattern≥10 min	<5 for 90 min	Either atypical variable decelerations with over 50% of contractions or late decelerations, both for over 30 min Single prolonged deceleration for more than 3 min	

TABLE 35.9
Definition of Normal, Suspicious and Pathological CTG Traces

Category	Definition
Normal	An FHR trace in which all four features are classified as reassuring
Suspicious	An FHR trace with one feature is classified as non-reassuring and the remaining features are classified as reassuring
Pathological	An FHR trace with two or more features classified as non-reassuring or one or more classified as abnormal

Values for fetal pH are as follows:

- pH >7.25: normal
- pH 7.21–7.24: borderline result and sampling should be repeated 30 min later
- pH ≤7.20: abnormal result requiring urgent delivery of the baby.

Urgency of Caesarean Section

Urgency of delivery is guided by the results of fetal monitoring and does not fall into the Confidential Enquiry into Perioperative Deaths (CEPOD) categorization for urgency.

A modification of the previous classification was proposed and adopted by the RCoA and the Royal College of Obstetricians and Gynaecologists (RCOG) in 2010 (Table 35.10).

Umbilical Cord Blood Analysis

The UK National Institute for Health and Clinical Excellence (NICE) recommends that "Paired cord

TABLE 35.10
A Classification Relating the Degree of Urgency to the Presence or Absence of Maternal or Fetal Compromise

Urgency	Definition	Category
Maternal or fetal compromise	Immediate threat to life of woman or fetus	1
	No immediate threat to life of woman or fetus	2
	Requires early delivery	3
No maternal or fetal compromise	At a time to suit the woman and maternity services	4

blood gases do not need to be taken routinely. They should be taken when there has been concern about the baby either in labour or immediately following birth". Umbilical cord blood gases may be of value in auditing outcomes of labour and predicting future development of the newborn, although opinion on their prognostic value varies. If the fetus is deprived of adequate oxygenation during labour – for example, through placental malfunction, cord compression, or excessive uterine contractions – anaerobic metabolism is activated and lactic acid is produced causing the pH to drop and base deficit to increase. Fetuses with limited metabolic reserve, such as those that are growth restricted or preterm, are less able to withstand the effects of hypoxaemia. Umbilical cord *arterial* blood normally reflects fetal acid–base balance while *venous* blood reflects a combination of maternal acid–base status and placental function. Both should be taken as it ensures that an arterial sample has definitely been obtained. The combination of results also provides further information. A large A–V difference may suggest an acute reduction in fetal blood flow whereas both venous and arterial acidaemia suggests fetal hypoxia is not acute in onset, especially in the case of metabolic acidaemia.

Physiologically significant values below which long-term sequelae are more likely are:

- Arterial pH ≤7.00 base deficit ≥12mmol L^{-1}
- Venous pH ≤7.10 base deficit ≥10mmol L^{-1}

FEEDING AND ANTACID PROPHYLAXIS IN LABOUR

Mendelson first described the syndrome of aspiration of gastric contents in 1946. He described the pathological changes seen when solid food or liquid gastric contents are inhaled during anaesthesia in pregnancy. The chemical pneumonitis which resulted from inhalation of acidic gastric contents in pregnancy prompted a number of recommendations, some of which still hold true today, such as increased use of local anaesthesia, alkalinization of stomach contents before general anaesthesia and adequate delivery room equipment including transparent masks, suction and a tilting table.

Oral intake in labour remains an area of controversy but can be managed on the basis of risk. Women at low risk of intervention are allowed to eat and drink while those at 'high risk' are allowed only clear fluids and are given regular antacids. NICE guidelines on intrapartum care produced in 2007 recommended that women may drink during established labour and be informed that isotonic drinks may be more beneficial than water. Women may eat a light diet in established labour unless they have received opioids or they develop risk factors which make a general anaesthetic more likely.

As it has been shown that acid aspiration causes chemical pneumonitis, various methods are used routinely to reduce the acidity of the stomach contents. This led to the use of non-particulate antacids such as 0.3 mol sodium citrate 30 mL administered orally less than 30 min before general anaesthesia. In addition, H_2-antagonists have now become standard gastric acid prophylaxis. NICE guidelines recommend that neither H_2-receptor antagonists nor antacids should be given routinely to low-risk women, but that H_2-receptor antagonists and antacids should be considered for women who receive opioids or who have, or develop, risk factors which make a general anaesthetic more likely; for example ranitidine 150 mg may be administered orally 6-hourly throughout labour. It is routine practice to administer oral ranitidine before elective caesarean section, e.g. in two doses – one the night before and the second on the morning of operation.

PAIN AND PAIN RELIEF IN LABOUR

It is only in the last 150 years that effective methods of pain relief have been available. Queen Victoria was given chloroform by John Snow for the birth of her eighth child and this did much to popularize the use of pain relief in labour. Many women go into labour unaware that they may need pain relief, although 75% of first-time mothers experience sufficient pain for them to request pain relief. Melzack, using the McGill pain questionnaire, found that the pain of labour is amongst the most severe in the human experience of pain, equivalent to amputation of a digit. Several studies have tried to assess the pain of labour. In nulliparous women Melzack found that 9.2% classified pain as very mild, 29.5% mild, 37.9% moderate and 23.4% severe.

The Effect of Pain and Analgesia on the Mother and Fetus

A long, painful labour may lead to an exhausted and frightened mother incapable of decision-making. Figure 35.8 summarizes the effects of pain. Pain compromises placental blood flow and renders uterine contractions less effective. Increased catecholamine secretion results in increased arterial pressure and myocardial work, and may also compromise blood flow to the placenta by peripheral vasoconstriction. Activation of the adrenocortical hormones may adversely affect electrolyte, carbohydrate and protein metabolism.

The Ideal Analgesic

The ideal analgesic for labour should provide excellent rapid-onset pain relief in both first and second stages without risk or side-effects to the mother or fetus and should also retain the mother's ability to mobilize and be independent during labour. Many women do not wish complete pain relief, and therefore the analgesic should be easy to control. There is no ideal analgesic at the present time, but it is perhaps most closely approached by low-dose central neuraxial (spinal or

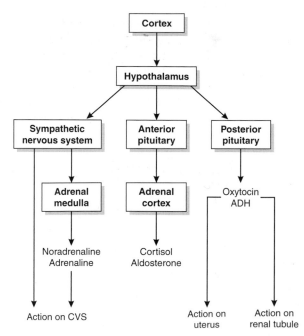

FIGURE 35.8 ■ The adverse effects of pain in labour on mother and fetus.

epidural) techniques which provide effective analgesia in over 90% of cases while preserving motor function to a large degree. Effective epidural (or spinal) analgesia reverses the adverse physiological effects of labour pain listed above by blocking the psychological and biochemical stress response, resulting in improved maternal well-being and placental perfusion.

Analgesia During Labour

Analgesia for labour may be classified broadly into the following areas:

- non-pharmacological
- parenteral
- inhalational
- regional.

Non-Pharmacological Analgesia

Birth Preparation Classes. In the 1930s, Grantly Dick-Read proposed that childbirth may be painless, as it is a normal life event, and that society had conditioned women to believe that childbirth was painful. He proposed that education of women about the process of labour and delivery and training them in relaxation therapy would obviate any need for analgesics. Active partner participation was encouraged.

The goals of childbirth preparation are to inform women fully about what to expect in labour and to enhance their ability to cope without analgesia. Fernand Lamaze popularized the technique in North America and Frederick Leboyer modified the technique to suggest birth in quiet conditions with gentle initial handling of the newborn. Although there are few controlled studies on outcome, published observations do not indicate any benefits in terms of outcome of labour and reduced maternal morbidity from childbirth preparation.

Environment and the Management of Labour. Continuous support in labour is associated with shorter labours and reduced requirement for analgesia. Traditional cultures have always had the support of experienced women to be with the woman in labour. Midwifery (literally 'with woman') has its roots in this role of emotional support. There is an increasing trend in the US and UK towards the use of professional birth partners, or doulas.

Mobility in labour is helpful in maintaining the dignity and independence of the woman, but while it is thought to be helpful, there are no randomized, controlled trials to support the view that pain is easier to cope with when ambulant.

Most would accept that a bath or shower is relaxing, and use of the birthing pool is increasing in popularity. The evidence regarding the first stage of labour suggests a reduction in labour pain and analgesic requirements with no effect on the outcome of labour or neonatal status.

Transcutaneous Electrical Nerve Stimulation. The transcutaneous electrical nerve stimulation (TENS) technique is based on Melzack and Wall's 'gate control' theory of pain. It involves passage of a small electrical current through skin to stimulate the peripheral nervous system. The TENS electrodes should be applied at the appropriate dermatomal levels involved with the transmission of pain in labour (see Fig. 35.6). The TENS machine then emits a low background stimulus which may be boosted with each contraction. There is little evidence that use of TENS reduces the need for analgesics, duration of labour or incidence of instrumental delivery; however, it is widely accepted by mothers and midwives because of its lack of side-effects on the mother and fetus.

Complementary Therapies. Hypnosis may provide reliable analgesia for a small number of women. However, they need considerable antenatal preparation and it has not proved suitable on a large scale for labour analgesia.

Acupuncture has only recently received attention for labouring women. In volunteer parturients, it was found to be ineffective in almost 80% of cases.

Aromatherapy and reflexology are also practised in labour and, although there is no evidence to support their use, many women gain emotional support and satisfaction from them.

Parenteral (Systemic) Analgesia

Many opioids have been used to provide obstetric analgesia, but the most popular have been pethidine, morphine and diamorphine. Pethidine has become established in obstetric practice without good scientific data to support its use, and in the UK two doses of 100 mg may be prescribed for a labouring woman by a midwife. Pethidine is given by intramuscular injection and the maximum effect is seen about 1 h after administration. Subcutaneous diamorphine in doses of 2.5–10 mg is used increasingly. Diamorphine has a more rapid onset of action than pethidine and, when the two were compared, diamorphine was found to be more likely to provide some pain relief and had a lower incidence of nausea and vomiting. However, the analgesic effects of the opioids are variable and they cause significant side-effects including maternal sedation, nausea and vomiting, dysphoria and inhibition of gastric emptying. They may also have adverse effects on the fetus (see above) as they freely cross the placenta, potentially causing CTG abnormalities and respiratory and neurobehavioural depression of the newborn. It is standard practice for paediatric staff to be available at delivery of an infant whose mother has received pethidine within 3h of delivery.

Several intravenous opioids have been used in patient-controlled analgesia (PCA) for labour. Remifentanil is probably the most suitable in terms of its pharmacological profile, being the most rapidly acting opioid available, with the shortest half-life. Various dosing regimens exist, for example doses of 30–50 µg with a lockout period of 2 min. However maternal side-effects still occur, necessitating close monitoring and continuous one-to-one care. In most units, remifentanil PCA is used only if there are contraindications to epidural analgesia.

Inhalational Analgesia

The ideal inhalational agent should be a good analgesic in subanaesthetic doses, have a rapid onset of action and recovery, and not accumulate. Nitrous oxide is relatively insoluble in blood and has these properties. Other anaesthetic agents have been investigated, but so far only isoflurane has shown promise and it has been used as Isonox (50% nitrous oxide and 50% oxygen with 0.2% isoflurane) but is not widely available. In the UK, nitrous oxide is supplied as Entonox, which is 50% nitrous oxide and 50% oxygen under pressure in a cylinder (see Chs 14 and 15). Entonox is administered usually via a demand valve with a face mask or mouthpiece. Administration needs to be timed for the maximum analgesic effect to coincide with the peak of the contraction. Most women tend to hyperventilate while breathing Entonox, and therefore there are often alternating phases of hyperventilation and then

hypoventilation, especially if the Entonox is administered after pethidine. Although Entonox is a reasonably effective analgesic, many women feel faint and nauseated and may vomit or become out of control.

Regional Analgesia for Labour

This is described below.

EPIDURAL AND SUBARACHNOID ANALGESIA

This is the most effective form of analgesia in labour, with up to 90% of women reporting complete or near-complete pain relief. However, it is invasive and patients require careful monitoring.

Indications for Epidural Analgesia

In addition to relief of pain and distress, there are several indications for epidural analgesia which may be helpful in securing a good outcome from labour. These are summarized in Table 35.11.

Contraindications to Epidural Analgesia in Labour

Maternal Refusal

There is a small number of women who, after a careful explanation of the risks and benefits of regional analgesia, decide against it, possibly because of medical

TABLE 35.11
Indications for Epidural Analgesia
Maternal request
Occipito-posterior presentation
Pregnancy-induced hypertension or pre-eclampsia
Prematurity or intrauterine growth retardation
Intrauterine death
Induction or oxytocin augmentation of labour
Instrumental or caesarean delivery likely
Previous caesarean delivery
Presence of significant concurrent disease (e.g. heart disease, diabetes, hypertension)
Twin pregnancy
Maternal obesity

problems, e.g. complex back surgery. Ideally, discussions should take place in the antenatal period and clear notes should be made in the medical record.

Bleeding Disorders

These may be acquired or congenital. The potential to cause bleeding in the epidural space varies widely. Epidural haematoma is a serious complication of epidural analgesia and may cause spinal cord compression with resultant paraplegia. Each patient needs careful assessment of the risks and benefits of administering the regional anaesthetic. This assessment may need team planning with haematology and obstetric staff. Most units have delivery suite guidelines for the common problems, e.g. pre-eclampsia, prophylactic heparin, etc.

Sepsis in the Lumbar Area and Systemic Sepsis

Local infection in the area adjacent to the epidural site may introduce infection into the epidural space, leading potentially to the formation of an epidural abscess. The presence of systemic infection or systemic inflammatory response syndrome (SIRS) may cause the epidural catheter to become a focus for development of a local infection. An expert assessment of the risk–benefit ratio for using epidural analgesia must be made in these circumstances.

Technique of Regional Analgesia

Preparation

Consent. Information should be given to the woman in the antenatal period about regional analgesia and anaesthesia. Leaflets, videos and parentcraft classes are important in ensuring that women are well informed before labour. It is often difficult to explain the risks and benefits of epidural analgesia to a woman who is distressed and under the effects of pethidine and Entonox. However there is a legal, ethical and professional requirement to obtain consent before performing a procedure on a patient. Women should be presumed to have capacity to make these decisions, including refusal of treatment except in very exceptional circumstances. Verbal consent should be obtained and the main elements of the discussion documented. Essential information should probably include partial or complete failure of the technique, dural puncture and headache, increased risk of instrumental delivery and neurological complications.

Other complications are listed later in this chapter and may be discussed if time allows and the patient requires.

Intravenous cannulation. A continuous infusion of crystalloid should always be started before embarking on the block.

Arterial pressure. A baseline arterial pressure value is recorded.

Bladder contents. The patient should have recently emptied her bladder.

Clothing. The patient should be wearing suitable clothing.

Positioning. The position of the patient is the same for epidural, spinal or combined spinal and epidural (CSE) block: either the lateral or the sitting position. There is no evidence that either position is superior and they are compared in Table 35.12.

TABLE 35.12	
Comparison of Sitting and Lateral Positions for Performing Spinal or Epidural Procedures	
Sitting	**Lying (Left Lateral)**
Advantages	
Midline easier to identify in obese women	Can be left unattended without risk of fainting
Obese patients may find this position more comfortable	No orthostatic hypotension
	Uteroplacental blood flow not reduced (particularly important in the stressed fetus)
Disadvantages	
Orthostatic hypotension may occur	More difficult to find the midline in obese patient
Increased risk of orthostatic hypotension if Entonox and pethidine have been administered	
Patient sitting on edge of bed may be too far away from a small anaesthetist for good manual dexterity	
Assistant (or partner) needed to support patient	
May be more difficult to monitor CTG	

Normal Labour

In either position, the knees and hips are flexed and the neck is flexed on to the chest in order to maximize the intervertebral distance.

Conduct of the Epidural

1. Epidural, spinal and CSE blocks are performed in a strictly aseptic manner. The person performing the block should scrub up properly and wear a hat, mask, and sterile gown and gloves. After cleaning the area with iodine or chlorhexidine, it is important to ensure that there is no contamination of the epidural equipment by the skin preparation fluid and that the skin is dry before the epidural is sited.
2. Cover the back with sterile drapes.
3. Identify the bony landmarks. For labour analgesia, intervertebral spaces L2–5 are the positions of choice. The intercristal line found by palpation is used to represent 'Tuffier's line' which is a radiological line joining the two iliac crests and passing through the spinous process of L4 or the L4–5 interspace (Fig. 35.9). However, studies have shown that estimation of the intervertebral space by palpation often results in the needle being inserted at a higher level than anticipated.

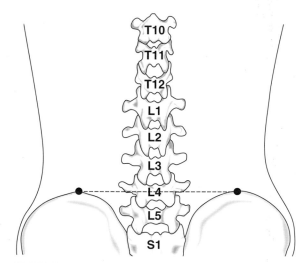

FIGURE 35.9 ■ The lumbar spine. A line drawn between the iliac crests crosses either the spinous process of the L4 vertebra or the L4–L5 intervertebral space.

Consequently, the clinically palpated intercristal line should be the upper limit for spinal (but not epidural) anaesthesia. Ultrasound can be used to identify the appropriate interspace and depth of the epidural space, with the desired point of needle insertion marked before skin preparation and scrubbing up.

4. A skin wheal of local anaesthetic (1% lidocaine) is raised at the intended point of insertion of the Tuohy needle and the superficial ligaments in the path of the epidural needle are infiltrated.
5. With the bevel cephalad, the Tuohy needle is advanced firmly through the skin and subcutaneous tissue until it becomes anchored in the superficial ligaments (supraspinous and infraspinous).
6. The epidural space is identified by loss of resistance to either air or saline. Once in the ligament, remove the stilette and attach a loss-of-resistance syringe to the Tuohy needle. As the Tuohy needle is advanced, the dorsum of the hand should be resting on the patient's back in order to control the advance of the needle using either intermittent or continuous pressure on the plunger of the loss-of-resistance syringe. This is a tactile technique, whereby there is a sudden loss of resistance to injection through the gradually advancing needle as it passes through the ligamentum flavum into the epidural space. The use of air and saline for loss of resistance are compared in Table 35.13. Loss of resistance to saline has become the standard technique.
7. When loss of resistance is confirmed, the distance from the skin at which the epidural space lies is noted.
8. The plastic catheter introducer is placed on the end of the Tuohy needle and the catheter is advanced to 15–20 cm, at the same time warning the patient that she may feel pins and needles in one of her legs or her back. The catheter should never be withdrawn back through the Tuohy needle, because part of it may be sheared off and left inside the epidural space. If withdrawal of the catheter is necessary, the needle and catheter must be removed together.

TABLE 35.13
Comparison of Air and Saline for Loss-of-Resistance Technique

Saline	Air
Advantages	*Advantages*
May give a better end-point for loss of resistance	If fluid appears during insertion it can be assumed to be CSF until proved otherwise
May push the dura away from the point of the needle, thus reducing the chances of dural puncture	No dilutional effect; the small amount of air used does not usually distort the tissues
	No possibility of confusion with other substances
Disadvantages	*Disadvantages*
May be confused with CSF	Associated with a higher incidence of dural puncture
Must be filtered to avoid introduction of minute glass particles	More likely to get a patchy block
Dilutes the local anaesthetic which is put into the epidural space	More difficult to define the point of loss of resistance with air than with saline
Another ampoule is opened, thus providing a possibility for user error	
Preservative-free saline must be used	

9. The Tuohy needle is withdrawn, ensuring that the catheter stays in position. The catheter is then withdrawn, ensuring that a length of 3–4 cm remains within the epidural space.
10. The filter is attached and the catheter is checked to ensure that no blood or CSF flows back using gravity. A test dose may now be given.
11. The epidural catheter is fixed.

Test Dose. The purpose of the test dose is to confirm or exclude intravascular or intrathecal positioning of the tip of the catheter. However, every dose injected through the epidural catheter should be considered a test dose because the tip of the catheter may migrate. The ideal test dose should allow the anaesthetist to detect abnormal positioning rapidly before endangering the patient. Hypotension, marked motor block or very rapid analgesia within 5 min of a test dose suggests intrathecal placement. If inadvertent intravascular injection occurs, the early signs are circumoral tingling and pallor and possibly a metallic taste in the mouth. The test dose of local anaesthetic should be that which could be given safely for anaesthesia if given intrathecally, e.g. 10–15 mg of levobupivacaine as a 0.1% or 0.5% solution. Common practice is to use 10 mL of levobupivacaine 0.1% with fentanyl 2 μg mL^{-1}. The addition of adrenaline 15 μg to the test dose is advocated by some for detection of an intravascular catheter. It is highly sensitive but only 65% specific.

Combined Spinal-Epidural for Labour and the 'Walking' Epidural

This was originally described in 1993 by anaesthetists in Queen Charlotte's Hospital in London. It was used to minimize motor block to the extent that a small proportion of their patients walked around the delivery suite. Some units use CSE routinely for labour analgesia, but in most it is reserved for women in whom rapid onset of analgesia is desirable.

Technique. The Tuohy needle is advanced to identify loss of resistance in the lumbar region (as for an epidural). Then, a 24–27 gauge 120-mm long pencil-point needle is advanced through the Tuohy needle to puncture the dura, and an intrathecal injection of 1 mL of bupivacaine 0.25% with fentanyl 25 μg is given. This has now been modified to use a larger volume of low-dose mixture such as 3–3.5 mL of levobupivacaine 0.1% and fentanyl 2 μg mL^{-1}. The spinal needle is withdrawn and the epidural catheter is inserted and left in place as before. The intrathecal injection usually produces a rapid onset of analgesia (<5 min) and approximately 70% of patients have normal or near-normal leg power and can walk. The intrathecal injection has an analgesic duration of the order of 90 min, after which the epidural component of the CSE is used, usually starting with a 10–15 mL bolus of bupivacaine 0.1% with fentanyl 2 μg mL^{-1}, without a test dose, as described above. Similar degrees of mobility have been achieved using epidural boluses or infusions of low-concentration bupivacaine and fentanyl mixtures without the need for the initial intrathecal injection.

Assessment. The preservation of motor function and reduced need for bladder catheterization have increased maternal satisfaction with epidural analgesia, although there have been concerns that proprioception may be affected even with this low dose of local anaesthetic, potentially making walking hazardous. The medicolegal position of the anaesthetist in the event of a fall of a parturient during a walking epidural is unclear. Nonetheless, if visual and vestibular functions are intact, proprioceptive impairment seems to have a minimal effect on walking. Many parturients do not wish to walk and, moreover, clinical trials to date have not shown that walking significantly alters outcome of labour.

Management of the Labouring Woman with Epidural Analgesia

Posture

A labouring woman who wishes to remain supine should be positioned with at least a 15° left lateral tilt to prevent aortocaval compression; alternatively, and preferably, she may sit upright at an angle of 45° or more. The weight of the gravid uterus compresses the vena cava and aorta against the vertebral bodies, thereby restricting blood flow. The reduction in systemic vascular resistance in women with epidural analgesia decreases the ability of the woman to maintain her arterial pressure, and therefore she is more likely to faint. In addition, the lumbosacral spine should be supported, as the epidural may allow unnatural positions to be adopted, which would usually produce discomfort in the back. Prolonged abnormal posture may contribute to low back pain after the epidural has worn off; in the past, this has been ascribed incorrectly to the epidural itself.

Monitoring of Mother and Baby

Routine monitoring of the mother and fetus is documented on the partogram as described previously (see Fig. 35.7). NICE guidelines recommend continuous EFM for at least 30 min during establishment of regional analgesia and after administration of each further bolus of 10 ml or more.

Analgesia for the first stage of labour requires a sensory block extending from T10 to L1, while for the second stage, a block from S2 to S5 is desirable. The aim is to provide effective analgesia with minimal side-effects. Local anaesthetics injected into the epidural space affect all nerves to some degree, in the following order: sympathetic fibres, pain fibres, proprioception fibres and finally motor fibres. The volume of local anaesthetic solution governs the spread of the block, whereas the concentration of local anaesthetic governs the density of block, with an increased risk of motor block at higher concentrations.

Maintenance of Analgesia

Epidural analgesia for labour may be maintained by the following methods.

Repeated Bolus Administration. After the first dose has been given by the anaesthetist, boluses are usually administered as required by a midwife trained in the use of epidural analgesia. The volume and concentration need to be high enough to provide adequate analgesia, but large volumes may cause too great a spread of block, with attendant toxicity and hypotension. Bupivacaine 0.25% given in 5–10 mL boluses was standard practice until relatively recently but in most units this has been replaced by the use of more dilute mixtures using 0.1% bupivacaine, levobupivacaine or ropivacaine and $2\,\mu g\,mL^{-1}$ fentanyl in 10–15 mL boluses. The lower concentration of local anaesthetic reduces the incidence of hypotension and increases the ability of the woman to mobilize. The disadvantage of boluses is the possibility of intermittent pain if top-ups are not administered at appropriate intervals and the requirement for two midwives to check and administer each top-up can cause problems on busy delivery suites.

Continuous Infusion by Syringe Pump. A mixture of local anaesthetic and fentanyl is infused epidurally at a constant rate (e.g. levobupivacaine 0.1–0.125% or ropivacaine 0.1% containing fentanyl $2\,\mu g\,mL^{-1}$ at a rate of $10\,mL\,h^{-1}$). The sensory level and the analgesia should be checked regularly to maintain good pain relief. The infusion method is indicated particularly when there is a need for cardiovascular stability (e.g. the patient with cardiac disease or pre-eclampsia). It is associated with the administration of greater amounts of local anaesthetic solution and increasing motor block as labour progresses.

Patient-Controlled Epidural Analgesia (PCEA). This involves establishing analgesia with an initial bolus dose and maintaining analgesia by allowing the patient to self-administer boluses of analgesic solution as required by depressing a button on a computer-controlled volumetric syringe. There may or may not be a low-dose background infusion, although background infusion does not improve the effectiveness of the epidural. The advantage of this method is that it gives more control to the patient.

Problems Maintaining Epidural Analgesia

Epidural is not effective. If the epidural is not providing good analgesia within 15–20 min with 15 mL of bupivacaine 0.1% and fentanyl 2 µg mL^{-1} or 10 mL of bupivacaine 0.25%, the catheter is probably not central in the epidural space and it should be partially withdrawn. If this fails, it should be re-sited.

Missed segment or unilateral block. Groin pain is the most common manifestation of a missed segment, i.e. L1, and it is important to ensure that the bladder is empty and the block is not unilateral. A bolus of dilute levobupivacaine and fentanyl or a small bolus, e.g. 5 mL of levobupivacaine 0.25%, often provides analgesia. If there is persistent groin pain between contractions, the possibility of uterine dehiscence should be excluded.

Hypotension. If the patient feels faint or her arterial blood pressure decreases, she should be turned on to her side to exclude aortocaval compression. Intravenous fluids and oxygen should be administered while extensive regional block is excluded. Catheter migration may occur and an accidental spinal may manifest itself at any stage of the epidural. If hypotension persists, ephedrine or phenylephrine should be administered.

REGIONAL ANAESTHESIA FOR THE PARTURIENT

The common indications for anaesthesia for parturients are caesarean section, forceps delivery, retained placenta and repair of trauma to the birth canal. Regional anaesthesia is the technique of choice. Anaesthesia is discussed under the following headings:

- elective caesarean section
- emergency caesarean section
- forceps and Ventouse delivery
- retained placenta
- trauma to the birth canal
- post-delivery analgesia
- complications of regional anaesthesia and analgesia in obstetrics.

Elective Caesarean Section

Regional anaesthesia is the technique of choice for elective caesarean section. Although most women presenting for elective caesarean section expect to be awake for the delivery of their baby, they still need careful preoperative explanation of the procedure with discussion of the risks. Many hospitals admit women on the day of surgery and it may be difficult to give sufficient time to the preoperative visit. Consequently, it is advisable to have an information sheet for the woman before admission to hospital. As a minimum, the woman should be informed about partial or complete failure of the regional technique, the possibility of discomfort, pain and conversion to general anaesthesia, and the risk of neurological damage. Other side-effects which should be discussed are hypotension, post-dural puncture headache, motor block, and nausea and vomiting. The techniques available are:

- spinal anaesthesia
- epidural anaesthesia
- combined spinal-epidural anaesthesia.

Spinal anaesthesia is the most popular choice for elective caesarean section, with increasing popularity of the CSE technique.

Spinal Anaesthesia

Most spinal anaesthetics are performed with the patient on the operating table because this reduces the need to move the patient after establishment of the block. The following points are mandatory:

- routine pre-anaesthetic equipment check
- monitoring of arterial pressure, ECG and oximetry
- intravenous infusion of crystalloid
- vasopressor available (phenylephrine is now the preferred choice)
- aseptic technique.

Ensure that drugs are available for the administration of general anaesthesia.

Spinal anaesthesia may be performed with the patient in either the sitting or the lateral position, curled up as for performing epidural block. The choice of needle is important to minimize the incidence of post-dural puncture headache; a pencil-point needle is preferred. It is important to remember that the spinal cord ends around L2 in a normal adult, so the spinal needle should be inserted at L3/4 or below. It has been shown that anaesthetists commonly misjudge the level at which they insert the spinal needle and are more often cephalad of the desired space. Spinal cord trauma and associated chronic neurological deficit may result from inadvertently cephalad insertion of a spinal needle. Therefore, the appropriate interspace should be chosen with care. Ultrasound can be used to guide this.

After infiltration of the skin and subcutaneous tissues with local anaesthetic, the spinal needle introducer is inserted, followed by the spinal needle, and the chosen local anaesthetic is injected when free flow of cerebrospinal fluid (CSF) is identified. If a spinal nerve is touched, the patient experiences excruciating pain radiating along the route of that nerve. The spinal needle must be removed and the patient reassured. The same applies if the patient feels pain on injection. Local anaesthetic must not be injected if there is any possibility of it being given into a nerve as this may cause permanent neurological damage.

Hyperbaric bupivacaine 0.5% is the drug of choice and 2.5 mL (12.5 mg) is usually sufficient. An opioid should be added to the local anaesthetic because this improves the quality of anaesthesia and provides postoperative analgesia. Fentanyl 25 µg, morphine 0.1 mg or diamorphine 0.25–0.4 mg may be used. NICE recommends diamorphine 0.3–0.4 mg although 0.25 mg may be an easier amount to prepare, especially in an emergency. Epidural and spinal opioids may cause delayed respiratory depression and therefore women should be monitored appropriately postoperatively. All drugs injected into the epidural space or the CSF should be in preservative-free solution. Arterial pressure should be measured at frequent intervals and the patient placed supine, ensuring that aortocaval compression is prevented by lateral tilt. The block should be tested for loss of sensation to a combination of cold and touch. It is good practice to test the block from the sacral roots to the thoracic dermatomes, even though it is unusual for a spinal block to be patchy or to miss the sacral roots. The height of the block should be T4 bilaterally to cold and T5 to touch. The level of sensory block as well as the degree of motor block should be documented.

Hypotension is treated with phenylephrine in boluses of 0.1 mg. Phenylephrine has now replaced ephedrine as the preferred vasopressor in obstetric anaesthesia because it has been shown that ephedrine causes a decrease in umbilical arterial pH and hence neonatal pH. There is increasing evidence for the benefits of a prophylactic phenylephrine infusion to prevent hypotension after spinal anaesthesia for caesarean section. A suggested regimen starts at 100 µg min^{-1} and the infusion is then titrated according to the blood pressure.

Surgery can start when the anaesthetist is happy that there is good anaesthesia. Peritoneal traction and swabbing of the paracolic gutters are the most stimulating parts of the operation and the times when pain or discomfort is most likely to be experienced. Exteriorization of the uterus is to be discouraged because this is challenging even to the most perfect block. Pain or discomfort should be treated promptly. Nitrous oxide, ketamine and/or small doses of a rapidly-acting intravenous opioid such as alfentanil are all useful to control breakthrough pain. If the pain is severe, general anaesthesia should be offered and administered if appropriate. Syntocinon 5 IU as a bolus is normally administered intravenously after the delivery of the baby to assist myometrial contraction. Routine postoperative care should take place in a well-equipped recovery area.

Epidural Anaesthesia

Epidural anaesthesia was generally the regional anaesthetic of choice until pencil-point spinal needles were introduced. The disadvantages of epidural anaesthesia are that the onset of the block is slower than that for spinal anaesthesia and that the spread of the block may be patchy, often giving poor anaesthesia of the sacral roots. The cardiovascular stability which can be achieved with an epidural anaesthetic is excellent and this implies that the technique may be considered the anaesthetic of choice in patients with heart disease or pre-eclampsia. When the epidural catheter is in place, anaesthesia can be achieved by local anaesthetic, often combined with an opioid. Epidural anaesthesia for caesarean section is most commonly used when there is already an epidural catheter *in situ* for labour analgesia and the epidural is 'topped up'.

The following are standard prescriptions for an epidural anaesthetic:

- bupivacaine or levobupivacaine 0.5% 15–20 mL with 1 in 200 000 adrenaline – this should be given in divided doses
- lidocaine 2% 15–20 mL with 1 in 200 000 adrenaline – this should be given in divided doses
- a combination of bupivacaine and lidocaine
- addition of 2 ml of sodium bicarbonate 8.4% to a 20-ml top-up mixture (lidocaine+bupivacaine) is advocated by some and may speed onset
- fentanyl 50 μg at establishment of anaesthesia or diamorphine 2.5 mg after delivery may be administered in addition to the local anaesthetic and has been shown to improve the quality of the anaesthesia
- ropivacaine 0.75% 10–15 mL

It is essential to test the block by testing each dermatome in a systematic way from the thoracic level down to the sacral roots to ensure that good anaesthesia has been produced before surgery starts.

Combined Spinal-Epidural Anaesthesia

There are various techniques for CSE, although the 'needle through needle' technique described above is probably the most popular. A full description of the other techniques is outside the remit of this chapter. The CSE allows increased flexibility by combining epidural and spinal blocks. The spinal anaesthetic is a single-shot technique and while most of the time this is no problem, delay in starting surgery or a difficult, long operation may result in failure of the block. The epidural may not achieve such profound or rapid anaesthesia, although it has the advantages of flexibility and cardiovascular stability.

In the CSE technique, the spinal is usually conducted using the same dose of drugs as listed in the spinal section and the epidural is placed as 'insurance'. The CSE may also be used as a sequential block, with a smaller intrathecal dose of local anaesthetic being given (e.g. 5–7.5 mg of bupivacaine), followed by an epidural top-up to achieve full anaesthesia. This method provides greater cardiovascular stability because the onset of the block is slower, while an

excellent sacral block is achieved with the spinal anaesthetic. This technique has extended the use of regional anaesthesia in pre-eclampsia.

Emergency Caesarean Section

Regional anaesthesia has increased in frequency for emergency caesarean section partly because of the increased use of spinal anaesthesia and the use of epidural analgesia in labour.

Topping up an Existing Epidural

A labour epidural may be topped up to achieve anaesthesia within 10–20 min using the prescriptions described previously under epidural for elective caesarean section. The epidural should be topped up incrementally while the patient is monitored continuously. Between 10 and 20 mL of local anaesthetic solution are usually needed. While the epidural is being topped up, it is important to explain what is going to happen, to ensure that the woman understands what she is likely to feel and that help is available if pain or discomfort is experienced. There is some controversy over where the top-up should be administered; if started in the labour room, the anaesthetist must stay with the patient continuously and monitor her closely.

Spinal Anaesthesia for an Emergency

Spinal anaesthesia is to be encouraged for the woman who has no epidural *in situ* and who requires an emergency caesarean section. There are times when general anaesthesia is indicated, but these decrease as experience with spinal anaesthesia increases. Spinal anaesthesia may be used in the same manner as for an elective caesarean section; however, it is important to explain the procedure to the woman as fully as possible in the time available and to be present after the caesarean section to provide a better retrospective explanation of events. Follow-up is particularly important in the emergency situation. Continuous communication with the obstetric team is vital to ensure that they are happy with the state of the fetus, and the anaesthetist must be prepared to abandon the procedure and give a general anaesthetic if the obstetric team are concerned.

'Rapid-sequence spinal anaesthesia' has been recently described; this aims to reduce some of the steps in the procedure and decrease the time taken, thereby increasing access to spinal anaesthesia in an emergency.

The technique is controversial as its proposers advocate reduced aseptic precautions. Again, continuous communication is vital.

Forceps and Ventouse Delivery

Surgical anaesthesia is required for any operative delivery, except for a simple 'lift-out' by forceps or Ventouse. For a simple lift-out, the labour epidural should be well topped up. Ideally, time to achieve good perineal anaesthesia should be allowed before the woman is placed in the lithotomy position for the assisted delivery. Bupivacaine 0.5% or lidocaine 2% with adrenaline 1 in 200 000 in a dose of around 10 mL is appropriate. If the delivery is more complex than a simple lift-out, surgical anaesthesia is required. It is preferable to deliver such patients in the operating theatre where caesarean section may be performed if there is any doubt about the ability to deliver the baby vaginally. Severe fetal distress may occur during attempted instrumental delivery, requiring immediate caesarean section. Therefore, the anaesthetist should prepare (and assess) the anaesthetic as if for caesarean section using any of the prescriptions for caesarean delivery (spinal, CSE, epidural) described above.

Retained Placenta

Regional anaesthesia may be used for manual removal of retained placenta after a careful assessment of blood loss. It is easy to underestimate the blood loss if there has been a continuous trickle of blood for some time. If the woman is not significantly hypovolaemic, the anaesthetic of choice is a spinal, unless there is an epidural *in situ*. Both techniques should provide good surgical anaesthesia with a block extending from at least T10 to the sacral roots.

Repair of Trauma to the Birth Canal

The anaesthetist is often asked to provide anaesthesia for the repair of birth trauma. The full extent of the damage may not be known as it may not be possible to examine the woman without anaesthesia. The trauma may be extensive and involve disruption of the anal sphincter, which is classified as a third-degree tear. There may be considerable blood loss and it is important to assess this before performing regional anaesthesia. If there is an epidural *in situ*, this can be topped up for the repair. If there is no epidural, then a spinal anaesthetic is the technique of choice. Hyperbaric bupivacaine 0.5% in a volume of 1.5 mL provides good sacral analgesia.

Post-Delivery Analgesia

The anaesthetist is usually involved in the continuing care of the woman after delivery and this includes the provision of pain relief for:

- normal delivery
- tears
- forceps and Ventouse
- caesarean section.

Normal Delivery

The pain experienced after a normal delivery is caused mainly by uterine contractions and also bruising of the perineum. Simple analgesia in the form of paracetamol is usually adequate, although if there is severe bruising of the perineum, NSAIDs are helpful, e.g. diclofenac suppositories.

Tears and Episiotomy

After the repair of an episiotomy or tear, there may be considerable pain which needs more than simple analgesia. NSAIDs provide excellent analgesia for most women. If the woman has had a third-degree tear repaired, she may often have had a regional anaesthetic for the repair, and the use of epidural or intrathecal opioids provides good postoperative analgesia, particularly if combined with rectal diclofenac.

Forceps and Ventouse Delivery

An episiotomy is usually performed to facilitate the forceps or Ventouse delivery and this may be extensive; therefore, pain management as above is appropriate.

Caesarean Section

The extensive use of regional anaesthesia for caesarean section has led to intrathecal and epidural opioid analgesia becoming routine practice in most units. Combined with NSAIDs, paracetamol and other simple analgesics, this enables women to mobilize early after caesarean section. It is prudent to have clear postoperative guidelines for the care of women in the postoperative period and these should include use of sedation scores. Women who are unable to have

NSAIDs do not have such good pain control. Women who have had the caesarean section under general anaesthesia may be managed with PCA using morphine in the same way as other postoperative patients. This is combined with NSAIDs where appropriate.

Transversus abdominis plane (TAP) blocks may be beneficial for women who have had a caesarean section under general anaesthesia but there is little evidence to support their use in addition to intrathecal/epidural opioids. TAP blocks are performed under ultrasound guidance using approximately 20 mL of local anaesthetic (levobupivacaine or ropivacaine) on each side.

Complications of Regional Anaesthesia and Analgesia in Obstetrics

Although regional anaesthesia is now very safe and effective, all procedures have potential complications.

Shearing of the Epidural Catheter

An epidural catheter should not be withdrawn through a needle as this may damage or shear the catheter. Any sheared portion of catheter is inert and sterile and thus unlikely to cause a problem, but a full account should be made in the medical record.

Post-Dural Puncture Headache

The incidence of post-dural puncture headache (PDPH) is 0.5–1% and is often higher in teaching hospitals. It may occur at the time of insertion of the epidural needle or be caused later by migration of the catheter into the intrathecal space (usually because of a defect in the dura caused during insertion of the needle). The clinical presentation is of an occipital headache which may radiate anteriorly, aggravated by sitting and possibly associated with nausea, distorted hearing, photophobia and, rarely, diplopia resulting from stretching of the sixth cranial nerve as it passes through the dura. The differential diagnoses of meningitis, subarachnoid haemorrhage, sagittal sinus thrombosis and cerebral space-occupying lesions should be considered and excluded by history and simple clinical examination.

Management of Dural Puncture and PDPH. Approximately 75% of women who receive a dural puncture with a 16–18G Tuohy needle will suffer from PDPH.

If dural puncture is recognized at the time (clear fluid flowing from the Tuohy needle), there are two options.

- The epidural can be performed in an adjacent interspace. After insertion, all drugs should be given cautiously because some local anaesthetic may migrate intrathecally.
- The epidural catheter can be threaded into the intrathecal space. The catheter must be clearly labelled as a spinal catheter. Analgesia is provided using intermittent intrathecal top-ups, for example bupivacaine 2.5 mg. All top-ups must be administered by an anaesthetist. Consideration should be given to leaving the catheter in place for 24 h after delivery because this may reduce the incidence of PDPH. However, the risks and benefits of this approach must be considered.

All women who have had a dural puncture must be visited by an anaesthetist following delivery and evidence of symptoms and signs of dural puncture as listed above should be sought. Prophylactic bed rest and an epidural infusion of saline are no longer recommended. Oral fluids should be encouraged to prevent dehydration, and simple analgesics should be prescribed. If conservative management fails to prevent the appearance of PDPH, then a number of other forms of treatment have been suggested.

- Caffeine produces cerebral vasoconstriction and oral intake may provide symptomatic relief. The use of intravenous caffeine is now uncommon.
- Antidiuretic hormone may relieve symptoms by an unknown mechanism.
- Corticotrophin and sumatriptan have both been used but are probably ineffective.
- Epidural blood patch (EBP) is the definitive treatment of dural puncture. A sample of the patient's own venous blood is collected under aseptic conditions and injected into the same interspace at which the dural puncture occurred, or an adjacent interspace, to seal the CSF leak. It is about 75% effective (although the quoted range is 70–98%). The procedure may be repeated. In some centres, a prophylactic blood patch is performed using the re-sited epidural catheter at the end of labour in an effort to reduce the risk and duration of PDPH, although there is limited evidence to support this.

Backache

Backache is common after childbirth, and affects 50% of women at some stage in pregnancy. An anaesthetist is often called to assess patients with backache if they have received an epidural. Insertion of an epidural catheter may contribute to short-term acute back pain if it causes:

- an epidural haematoma
- an epidural infection causing abscess or meningitis
- local bruising from poor technique.

However, long-term backache is not caused by epidural anaesthesia, and has been demonstrated clearly in two prospective studies of over 1000 obstetric patients who were followed up on the day after delivery and 3 months later. The incidence of new-onset backache was of the order of 40–50%, but there was no difference in the incidence of backache at 3 months between those who had received an epidural and those who had not. There was a trend towards a slightly higher chance of back pain on day 1, explained by minor local trauma.

Bloody Tap

Cannulation of an epidural vessel may occur with either the needle or catheter when performing an epidural. It is important because, if undetected, it can result in intravascular injection and thus local anaesthetic toxicity. If blood flows from the needle, the needle must be withdrawn. If blood is aspirated from the catheter, it should be withdrawn incrementally and flushed with saline until aspiration of blood is no longer possible, ensuring there is still sufficient epidural catheter within the epidural space. If not, it should be re-inserted.

An epidural catheter may be positioned with its tip inside a blood vessel in the absence of a bloody tap, and a test dose should always be used.

Epidural Haematoma

This is a very rare (1 in 168 000) but potentially disastrous complication. The signs of an epidural haematoma are:

- new-onset, severe back pain
- prolonged, profound motor weakness >6h after the last top-up or cessation of an infusion
- sudden onset of incontinence.

An immediate MRI scan should be undertaken to confirm the diagnosis, and neurosurgical evacuation of the haematoma within 8h of the onset of symptoms usually results in a good outcome. Delay in recognition and treatment can result in permanent paraplegia.

Epidural Abscess or Meningitis

These conditions are rare (1 in 160 000). An abscess, as with a haematoma, may give rise to a space-occupying lesion in the epidural space, resulting in compression of the spinal cord and its nutrient arteries, leading to paraplegia. Meningitis may occur as a complication of regional techniques and may be bacterial, viral or chemical. It is essential that a good aseptic technique is used when regional blocks are inserted and that meningitis is excluded in the differential diagnosis of headache.

Systemic Local Anaesthetic Toxic Reaction

This is a result of a high blood concentration of local anaesthetic, caused either by a total dose greater than the body's ability to metabolize it, by too rapid administration or by inadvertent intravascular injection. All labour suites should have Intralipid readily available for treatment of local anaesthetic toxicity. Local anaesthetic toxicity is described in Chapters 4 and 24.

Hypotension

Hypotension is usually defined as a 25% decrease in systolic or mean arterial pressure or an absolute decrease in systolic pressure of 40 mmHg. Small decreases in pressure are insignificant and may be associated with improved uteroplacental blood flow, if due to vasodilatation. Rapidly developing hypotension after spinal anaesthesia may cause unpleasant dizziness and nausea in about 50% of patients if no prophylaxis is given, and should be treated with phenylephrine until arterial pressure is restored, while at the same time maintaining normovolaemia and ensuring that there is no aortocaval compression.

Neurological Deficit

Neurological deficit may be caused by the drugs used for the procedure or by trauma from the needles or catheter. The incidence of temporary nerve damage is approximately 1 in 1000, permanent nerve damage (more than 6 months' duration) occurs with an incidence of approximately 1 in 13 000 and the incidence of severe injury including paralysis is about 1 in 250 000. When neuropraxia due to injury with the epidural needle or catheter occurs, reassurance may be given that these symptoms usually resolve over 3–6 months, but patients should be followed up on an outpatient basis. Several peripheral nerves may be injured during delivery and falsely attributed to the epidural:

- common peroneal nerve by stirrups, causing foot drop
- lateral cutaneous nerve of the thigh by groin pressure from the lithotomy position, causing anterolateral thigh numbness
- femoral nerve or sciatic nerve by the lithotomy position, causing weak quadriceps with loss of knee reflex or pain in the back of the leg with loss of ankle reflex, respectively
- sacral plexus and obturator nerves – these cross the pelvic rim and rarely may be damaged by occipital presentation or forceps delivery.

Arachnoiditis and Cauda Equina Syndrome

Inflammation of the arachnoid membrane, caused by chemical toxins (wrong substance injected) or infection, usually presents as intractable back pain, potentially leading to permanent neurological damage. It can be caused by antiseptic solutions, so extreme care must be taken when preparing for regional analgesia/ anaesthesia to ensure that there is no contamination of the equipment with antiseptic solution. It is extremely rare.

Cauda equina syndrome can occasionally be confused with arachnoiditis. It results from damage to the lumbosacral nerve roots, for example secondary to high concentrations of local anaesthetic (especially lidocaine) and presents soon after regional anaesthesia. Although rare, it can cause permanent neurological damage.

As any complications may have medicolegal implications, it is important to:

- document the problem at the time
- explain the problem to the patient and relatives
- ensure consultant involvement.

Effect on Labour and Mode of Delivery

Epidural analgesia for labour has been shown to prolong the second stage of labour by 15.5 min in a 2005 Cochrane review of epidural versus non-epidural analgesia for labour but the clinical significance of this is unclear. It also increases the rate of instrumental delivery although this risk may be reduced by low-dose epidural techniques. Epidural analgesia does not increase the incidence of caesarean section or the length of the first stage of labour.

GENERAL ANAESTHESIA FOR THE PARTURIENT

Since the 1960s, the triennial UK maternal mortality report (currently termed 'Saving Mothers Lives') has provided an audit of obstetric and anaesthetic practice. Recent reports have demonstrated decreasing numbers of deaths from anaesthesia. The increasing safety of anaesthesia in obstetrics is the result of many factors:

- increasing use of epidural analgesia in labour
- increasing use of regional anaesthesia for operative delivery
- increase in dedicated consultant obstetric anaesthetic sessions
- improved teaching of obstetric anaesthesia
- improved assistance for the anaesthetist.

Deaths caused by anaesthesia generally result from hypoxaemia and/or acid aspiration associated with a failure to intubate the trachea and difficulty in maintaining the airway during general anaesthesia (GA). Successive enquiries continue to report deaths due to general anaesthesia. In the 2006–2008 report, there was one death due to failed tracheal intubation; there were successive attempts to intubate the trachea even though the patient was being oxygenated adequately using an intubating laryngeal mask airway and then there was unrecognized oesophageal intubation. Recent surveillance of failed tracheal intubation for obstetric general anaesthesia conducted through the United Kingdom Obstetric Surveillance System (UKOSS) between April 2008 and January 2010 identified 51 women in an estimated 1.4 million maternities, giving an estimated rate of failed intubation of 36 cases per million maternities. In the 2006–2008 CMACE report, there was also a death due to aspiration of gastric contents at extubation in a patient known to have a full stomach. General anaesthesia in the parturient is more than 16 times more likely to result in death than a regional anaesthetic. The reducing use of general anaesthesia in obstetric anaesthesia further exacerbates this problem by decreasing experience of a technique that may be required in an emergency.

However, general anaesthesia continues to be required in the following situations:

- in an extreme emergency, e.g. severe fetal distress or maternal haemorrhage
- when there is a contraindication to regional anaesthesia
- when the patient refuses to have a regional anaesthetic; this may be because of a previous bad experience with regional anaesthesia
- if regional anaesthesia has failed or is inadequate

In 2001 The National Sentinel Caesarean Section Audit found that 33% of emergency and 9% of elective caesarean sections were performed under general anaesthesia in the UK. The main anaesthetic considerations are the risk of aspiration of acidic gastric contents (as little as 25 mL with pH <2.5 may lead to a 50% mortality rate) and hypoxaemia resulting from airway difficulties. The previous sections on physiology of pregnancy, anatomy and antacid therapy have highlighted many of the problems that should be considered when a pregnant woman presents for a general anaesthetic. It is essential that a thorough pre-anaesthetic check is performed, with particular attention to the difficulties that may be encountered with tracheal intubation (Table 35.14). It is mandatory that anaesthetists familiarize themselves with the operating theatre and the anaesthetic equipment, in addition to the guidelines and equipment that are available for difficult and failed intubation. Drugs and equipment should be checked at the beginning of each period of duty on the delivery suite so that an emergency can be dealt with in a calm and ordered manner.

Caesarean Section

Preparation

1. Check the equipment again. Ensure that the suction equipment is working and that the table tilts head-down.

TABLE 35.14
Clinical Methods to Assess the Airway
Mouth opening (5 cm interincisor gap, equivalent to two fingers' breadth)
Mallampati grade
Temporomandibular joint mobility (should be able to protrude lower incisors in front of upper incisors)
Neck mobility (90° flexion of head on neck)
Weight >100 kg increases risk
Risk of airway oedema (increased by pre-eclampsia, stridor, URTI)

2. Perform a pre-anaesthetic check on the patient with particular attention to the airway and gastric contents.
3. Ensure that the assistant is ready.
4. Ensure that the patient is well positioned, paying particular attention to aortocaval compression and position for tracheal intubation.
5. Insert a 16-gauge i.v. cannula and ensure that an infusion flows well.
6. Check that full routine monitoring is in use.
7. Preoxygenate the patient's lungs for 3 min or until the end-tidal oxygen partial pressure is >80 kPa using a well-applied face mask.
8. Check that the assistant knows how to apply cricoid pressure.
9. Start the anaesthetic using a rapid sequence induction.

Technique

It is standard practice to use thiopental to induce anaesthesia in a dose of at least 4 mg kg^{-1}. This should be followed rapidly by succinylcholine 1–1.5 mg kg^{-1}. There is a minority of obstetric anaesthetists who use rocuronium (1 mg kg^{-1}). Cricoid pressure should be applied as consciousness begins to be lost and continued until the tracheal tube is confirmed to be in the trachea. Anaesthesia should be continued using nitrous oxide 50% and a volatile anaesthetic agent in oxygen, using positive pressure ventilation. Isoflurane or sevoflurane are commonly used and should be administered to achieve a total end-tidal concentration (volatile and nitrous oxide) of at least 1.0 MAC. Higher concentrations cause excessive uterine relaxation, while lower concentrations predispose the patient to awareness. The historical use of techniques in which low anaesthetic concentrations were employed that caused an excessive risk of awareness is now unacceptable. When using a circle breathing system, care is needed to prime the system with an adequate fresh gas flow and concentrations of the volatile agent, so that the desired MAC level is reached quickly. If the fetus is compromised, there is evidence that the use of 100% oxygen with a volatile agent may be beneficial to the fetus by increasing oxygen transfer across the placenta (with a concomitant increase in inspired vapour concentration). There is also increasing use of conventional gas ratios of nitrous oxide and oxygen (i.e. 66:33) from the beginning of the anaesthetic. This has become more common since the introduction of oximetry and continuous analysis of expired gas concentrations. After the delivery of the baby, an opioid, e.g. morphine, may be given with oxytocin. At this stage, the concentrations of nitrous oxide and inspired volatile agent may be altered to more conventional ratios. Additional non-depolarizing muscle relaxant (e.g. atracurium 25 mg) may be administered after the effect of the succinylcholine has worn off (if used), as confirmed by a nerve stimulator. Residual neuromuscular block should be antagonized before tracheal extubation, with the patient in the lateral position and with a slight head-down tilt or sitting up. TAP blocks may be performed for postoperative analgesia before waking up. Routine postoperative care in an appropriately staffed, fully equipped recovery area is essential. At this time, postoperative pain relief should be optimized and the baby should be given to the mother whenever possible.

ASSESSMENT OF THE PREGNANT WOMAN PRESENTING FOR ANAESTHESIA AND ANALGESIA

Successive maternal mortality reports highlight the problems of women with intercurrent medical disease and the fact that they are at increased risk in pregnancy and labour. There are many more women with a coincidental significant medical problem becoming pregnant and it is important that these problems are recognized in the antenatal period. A good history should be taken. The effect of the physiological changes of pregnancy on the disease must be recognized and appropriate investigations instigated.

Women with cardiac or respiratory disease require careful assessment because the physiological changes of pregnancy and delivery may have a profound effect on the disease. Many of these women have good reserves for normal day-to-day activities but are unable to cope with the added stress of labour. Antenatal assessment often includes echocardiography, ECG and pulmonary function tests. Assessment of the medical record is particularly relevant if the woman has undergone surgery. Clear plans for labour and delivery need to be written in the record by all of the medical team, including the anaesthetist. Many obstetric units now run an anaesthetic obstetric clinic at which high-risk women can be assessed antenatally by a consultant anaesthetist.

The other more common medical conditions occurring in women of child-bearing age are neurological disease, significant back problems including major surgery, drug allergies, previous anaesthetic problems and difficulties with tracheal intubation.

Obesity, maternal age and smoking are also risk factors which should not be overlooked. Obesity is particularly important and has been highlighted in recent CMACE reports as a significant risk factor. Twenty-seven percent of women who died in the 2006–2008 report were obese. Obesity in pregnancy is associated with an increased risk of a number of serious adverse outcomes, including thromboembolism, gestational diabetes, pre-eclampsia, postpartum haemorrhage, wound infections, miscarriage, stillbirth and neonatal death. There is also a higher caesarean section rate in obese women.

EMERGENCIES IN OBSTETRIC ANAESTHESIA

Haemorrhage

Significant bleeding occurs in 3% of all pregnancies and may happen in either the antepartum or postpartum period.

Antepartum Haemorrhage

Seventy per cent of all cases of antepartum haemorrhage result from placenta praevia or abruptio placentae. Placenta praevia occurs when the placenta is inserted wholly or in part into the lower segment of the uterus. It is now classified by ultrasound imaging according to what is relevant clinically. If the placenta lies over the internal cervical os, it is considered a major praevia; if the leading edge of the placenta is in the lower uterine segment but not covering the cervical os, minor or partial praevia exists. Significant bleeding may occur which may necessitate blood transfusion or urgent delivery. There are four factors which increase the potential for significant bleeding.

- In placenta praevia, the veins on the anterior wall of the uterus are distended.
- If the placenta is anterior then the surgical incision extends through the placenta, causing significant haemorrhage.
- If the placenta covers the os then a raw area is left after its delivery. This area of the os does not have the same ability to contract as the normal myometrium, and may thus continue to bleed.
- The presence of uterine scarring, e.g. from a previous caesarean section, predisposes to pathological invasion of the uterine wall to produce a placenta accreta. In placenta accreta, the placenta grows through the endometrium to the myometrium. In placenta increta, it penetrates into the myometrium. In placenta percreta, the placenta penetrates through the myometrium and uterine serosa and into surrounding structures e.g. bladder. This may mean that separation of the placenta and uterus is impossible and profuse bleeding occurs which may require hysterectomy.

Women diagnosed with placenta praevia are delivered by elective caesarean section if it remains within 2 cm of the os on ultrasound. Because the condition may be associated with severe, potentially life-threatening haemorrhage, senior obstetric and anaesthetic staff should be involved with the delivery. Blood should always be cross-matched and equipment should be available to administer a high flow rate of warmed fluids (>1 L min^{-1}). Either general or regional anaesthesia may be used. Regional anaesthesia is associated with a reduced blood loss but may be associated with blood pressure changes which are difficult to manage, and a potentially distressed patient. These patients should be pre-optimized, for example by giving iron supplements antenatally, and cell salvage should be used if available.

The use of interventional radiology to reduce bleeding should be considered.

Abruptio placentae is defined as the premature separation of the placenta after the 20th week of gestation. It is associated with a perinatal mortality rate of up to 50%. Placental abruption may result in concealed or revealed haemorrhage. Typically, the woman presents with abdominal pain, which may be severe, together with signs indicative of acute blood loss in proportion to the amount of blood lost. A trap for the unwary is that placental abruption may be associated with pre-eclampsia; therefore, if the pre-abruption arterial pressure was markedly elevated, the post-abruption blood pressure may still appear normal, and so mask hypovolaemia. It is also important to remember that blood loss is often concealed and so may be underestimated; a coagulopathy with low platelets tends to occur early in abruption and should be corrected aggressively.

Postpartum Haemorrhage

Postpartum haemorrhage is the most frequent reason for surgery in the immediate postpartum period. Causes include:

- retained placental tissue, including placenta accreta.
- uterine atony – the failure of the uterus to contract at the site of placental separation. The risk of uterine atony may be increased by:
  - overdistension of the uterus (e.g. polyhydramnios, multiple gestation)
  - prolonged (>18 h) or precipitous (<4 h) labour
  - multiparity
  - hypotension
  - uterine infection.
- laceration of the birth canal – predisposing factors include instrumental delivery and a large infant.
- hypocoagulable states, e.g. von Willebrand's disease, HELLP syndrome.

Anaesthetic Management of Haemorrhage

Although regional anaesthesia has a role in the management of acute postpartum haemorrhage, the associated sympathetic block interferes with physiological compensatory mechanisms, potentially aggravating acute hypovolaemia. For this reason, general anaesthesia is the preferred option in this situation unless plasma volume has been fully restored.

Preoperative Assessment. Estimation of the degree of blood loss is notoriously unreliable in the obstetric setting, and hence clinical estimation of the following signs of hypovolaemia should be undertaken:

- hypotension (this is usually a late sign)
- tachycardia >120 beat min^{-1}
- urinary output <0.5 mL kg^{-1} h^{-1}
- capillary refill time >5 s
- anxiety, agitation or confusion
- transient or minimal response to 1–2 L crystalloid or 500 mL colloid fluid challenge.

Successive triennial maternal mortality reports have highlighted major obstetric haemorrhage as a significant cause of maternal mortality. The most recent triennial maternal mortality report in the UK showed a decline in the number of deaths due to haemorrhage but it still remains important. Previous reports highlight the need for all units to have clear guidelines for the management of major obstetric haemorrhage and to identify at-risk patients early. Anaesthetists should be involved in the management of such patients so that appropriate resuscitation, monitoring and planning for delivery may be developed. 'Fire drills' and regular multidisciplinary practice sessions for haemorrhage and other emergencies should be a routine in modern obstetric anaesthetic practice.

The delivery suite team, including the anaesthetist, should:

- involve senior medical staff early
- request baseline haemoglobin and haematocrit measurements
- insert two large-gauge peripheral venous cannulae
- maintain circulating fluid volume
- administer group-compatible blood if possible or O-negative blood in a life-threatening situation
- consider insertion of invasive monitoring such as CVP or arterial monitoring
- involve the haematologist early for blood products and advice
- arrange postoperative admission to the Intensive Care Unit.

Intraoperative Management. Attempts to restore circulating blood volume should precede, but not delay, definitive treatment. Rapid-sequence induction of general anaesthesia is mandatory. Care with induction agents such as thiopental and propofol is required in hypovolaemic patients, because profound hypotension may ensue, leading to cardiovascular collapse. Ketamine 1–2 mg kg^{-1} may be useful as it stimulates the sympathetic nervous system and helps to preserve arterial pressure during induction of anaesthesia.

Anaesthesia may be maintained with N_2O/O_2 mixtures and an opioid such as fentanyl 1–2 µg kg^{-1} with cautious administration of a volatile anaesthetic agent. Ultimately, hysterectomy may be a life-saving procedure and should be discussed before anaesthesia with a patient at high risk of haemorrhage. Techniques to conserve the uterus include circumferential uterine suture, intrauterine balloon, internal iliac balloon insertion or embolization of uterine vessels using interventional radiological techniques. Clotting factors (FFP, cryoprecipitate) and platelets should be administered early without awaiting results and other treatments such as Factor VIIa (Novoseven) and tranexamic acid should be considered.

Failed Intubation

Failed intubation of the trachea reflects the relatively high incidence of airway difficulties in obstetric patients (approximately 1 in 300 compared with 1 in 2220 in non-pregnant patients). The increased incidence of difficult intubation in parturients is caused by changes in the soft tissues of the airway resulting in swollen upper airway mucosa, swollen and engorged breasts and full dentition. The decreasing use of general anaesthesia in obstetrics may lead to a relative lack of experience in this technique, with increased anxiety for both junior and senior anaesthetists.

The modified failed laryngoscopy/intubation drill is an essential algorithm and should be displayed prominently in all obstetric theatres (Fig. 35.10). The essential points to take from the algorithm are to call for help when unexpected difficulty with laryngoscopy or intubation arises. Failed intubation is the inability to intubate after two attempts and repeated attempts without maintaining oxygenation should be avoided. In the presence of a poor view of the glottis at laryngoscopy, the position of the cricoid pressure should be

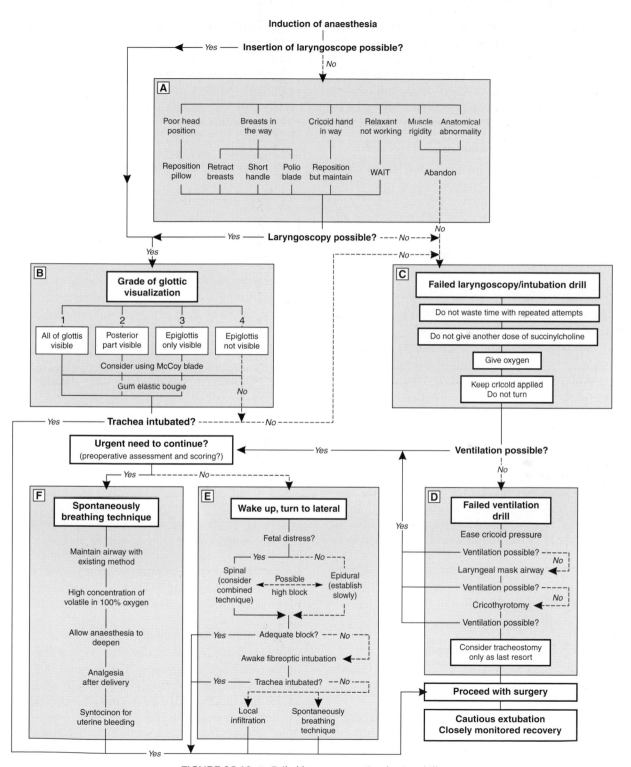

FIGURE 35.10 ■ Failed laryngoscopy/intubation drill.

checked to ensure it is central and correcting for lateral tilt of the patient. The insertion of a laryngeal mask airway (LMA) may facilitate ventilation and, if used, cricoid pressure should be applied continuously.

If rocuronium has been used for induction, then sugammadex in the appropriate dose should be given for rapid reversal of neuromuscular blockade.

Pre-Eclampsia and Eclampsia

Hypertensive disorders are among the leading causes of maternal mortality (approximately 1 in 100 000 pregnancies). Pre-eclampsia is a multisystem disorder and is defined as hypertension with proteinuria after week 20. Eclampsia is defined as the occurrence of convulsions and/or coma during pregnancy not resulting from neurological disease.

Aetiology of Eclampsia and Pre-Eclampsia

The aetiology is unknown, but current knowledge may be summarized as follows:

Immunological factors. In the normal placenta, the vascular bed is of low resistance. In pre-eclampsia, there is abnormal migration of the trophoblast into the myometrial tissue and this leads to constriction of the spiral arteries, which increases the resistance in the vascular bed. Prostacyclin and nitric oxide may be involved in this process.

Endothelial factors. Normotensive pregnant women demonstrate an increase in the activity of the renin-angiotensin-aldosterone system (RAAS) and a reduced response to exogenous angiotensin II. In pre-eclamptic women, this does not occur and this has been linked to a lack of nitric oxide production by endothelial cells.

Platelet and coagulation factors. Endothelial dysfunction may lead to a lack of nitric oxide and prostacyclin, altering the balance of platelet function in favour of platelet aggregation.

Clinical Presentation of Pre-Eclampsia

Clinically, pre-eclampsia is a multisystem disorder, and the predominant features in each system are as described below.

Cardiovascular system. Hypertension in pregnancy is defined as systolic arterial pressure >140 mmHg and/or diastolic arterial pressure >90 mmHg. There is generalized vasoconstriction leading to an increase in systemic vascular resistance and hypertension. Increased capillary permeability leads to a redistribution of plasma into the interstitial space. Blood volume is decreased by up to 30% in severe cases, but CVP and pulmonary capillary wedge pressure (PCWP) may be normal. There is a low colloid oncotic pressure (COP) and this, together with the increased capillary permeability, leads to oedema. Patients with pre-eclampsia may not have a raised arterial pressure, although it is significantly raised above baseline pressure at the beginning of pregnancy.

Central nervous system. Classically, this disease is accompanied by severe headache, visual disturbances and hyperreflexia. Seizures may occur without warning, and 40% of first fits occur in the postpartum period.

Renal system. Endothelial damage leads to protein loss and further decrease in COP. Glomerular filtration rate is reduced by 25% compared with normal pregnant women, as a result of glomerular oedema, and this can result in increases in urea and uric acid concentrations, an indicator of severity.

Haematological system. Platelet and coagulation disorders may occur as discussed above. A rapidly decreasing platelet count is indicative of a worsening of pre-eclampsia, and low platelets may be associated with HELLP syndrome (Haemolysis, Elevated Liver enzymes and Low Platelets). In general, a platelet count of $80 \times 10^9 L^{-1}$ (taken within the last 4 h) and above is safe for insertion of an epidural catheter. At levels below this, a clotting screen is advised and the risks and benefits of regional block should be assessed.

Respiratory system. Pre-eclampsia increases the risk of airway oedema, which may make tracheal intubation hazardous. Pulmonary oedema may occur at any time, including up to 24 h after delivery, as a result of increased capillary permeability and decreased COP.

Management of Pre-Eclampsia

Obstetric management is designed to stabilize the mother and deliver the baby. It is essential that the mother is assessed and monitored carefully. This includes full biochemical and haematological screening and monitoring of arterial pressure, heart rate, fluid balance and oxygen saturation. High dependency care is essential. Treatment of hypertension is essential and in the acute situation the drugs of choice are oral or intravenous labetalol, oral nifedipine and intravenous hydralazine. Aggressive treatment of severe hypertension (>170 mmHg systolic and/or >110 mmHg diastolic) is important because intracerebral haemorrhage secondary to hypertension (especially systolic) is the main cause of death in pre-eclampsia. Magnesium sulphate should be used in moderate to severe cases as prophylaxis against eclampsia. Magnesium inhibits synaptic transmission at the neuromuscular junction, causes vasodilatation, and has a central anticonvulsant effect at the NMDA receptor. A loading dose of 4 g (in 100 mL saline) is given over 30 min, followed by a maintenance dose of 1 g h^{-1}. Serum concentrations may be monitored along with hourly assessment of peripheral limb reflexes. As serum concentrations increase above 10 mmol L^{-1}, there is progressive reduction in reflexes, respiratory arrest and asystole. The therapeutic range is 4–7 mmol L^{-1}.

Pre-eclamptic patients are classically vasoconstricted and hypovolaemic, so careful fluid administration is advisable during treatment of hypertension. There is continued debate about the suitability of crystalloid or colloid in these patients; a detailed discussion of this is outside the remit of this chapter. It is important to remember that the woman may already be receiving antihypertensive therapy, e.g. methyldopa or nifedipine.

The Role of Epidural Analgesia and Anaesthesia in Pre-Eclampsia

Epidural analgesia is specifically indicated for labour analgesia in pre-eclampsia, provided that the platelet count is adequate, because:

- it provides excellent pain relief
- it attenuates the hypertensive response to pain
- it reduces circulating stress-related hormones and hence assists in controlling arterial pressure
- it improves uteroplacental blood flow
- these women have a higher incidence of caesarean section, and the presence of an epidural allows extension of the block.

If hypotension occurs, a crystalloid bolus (500 mL) may be administered, with the patient in a lateral tilt and receiving oxygen. If this is not adequate, a bolus of phenylephrine 50–100 μg may be given; however,

because of increased sensitivity of the circulation to exogenous vasopressors, caution is essential. Regional anaesthesia is the anaesthetic of choice if the woman is to be delivered by caesarean section, and although epidural anaesthesia has been the routine technique, there is increasing evidence to show that spinal anaesthesia or CSE may be the anaesthetic of choice for these women.

Eclampsia

If the woman has an eclamptic fit, the ABC of basic resuscitation should be started and it is essential that there is no compression of the aorta or vena cava during resuscitation. The treatment of eclampsia is magnesium sulphate 4 g by slow intravenous bolus as recommended in 1995 by the Eclampsia Trial Collaborative Group.

Total Spinal or Epidural Block

Too large a volume of local anaesthetic or its inadvertent deposition in the subarachnoid space may lead to profound, extensive block. The time from injection of the anaesthetic solution to onset of symptoms depends upon the exact location of the injection.

- The effects of an epidural overdose are seen 20–30 min after the bolus.
- The effects of a subarachnoid injection are seen within 2–5 min.

Local anaesthetic reaching the fourth ventricle results in respiratory arrest and may cause profound hypotension. Full resuscitation, including tracheal intubation and ventilation, external cardiac massage and vasopressors and inotropes are given as necessary. Spontaneous brainstem function returns as the excessively high block regresses over a period of 30 min to 4 h. However, when the mother has been stabilized, the baby is usually delivered by emergency caesarean section.

Thromboembolic Disease

Until the 2006–2008 Confidential Enquiry, thromboembolic disease had been the leading cause of maternal mortality for 21 years. In the latest report, the rate decreased to 19 deaths and was the lowest since the reports began in 1985; however, it remains an important cause of morbidity and mortality.

The reduction in death rate is probably due to guidelines on thromboprophylaxis for high-risk patients and these guidelines have since been refined further. All women should be risk-assessed early in pregnancy and high-risk patients should be given thromboprophylaxis antenatally and for up to 7 days postnatally. The most important risk factor is obesity but others include caesarean section, pre-eclampsia, bed rest, dehydration, multiparity, increasing age, family history, thrombophilia and long-distance travel. The dose of thromboprophylaxis should be increased appropriately for weight.

The presentation of pulmonary embolism ranges from progressive dyspnoea to sudden cardiovascular collapse. There should be a high index of suspicion in all parturients with risk factors with new-onset dyspnoea. Treatment is supportive and anticoagulation. Anticoagulation should be started immediately before investigations are completed in highly suggestive cases. This would usually be low-molecular-weight heparin (LMWH) e.g. enoxaparin 1 mg kg^{-1} 12-hourly antenatally but LMWH should be avoided if there is a possibility of imminent delivery because it may preclude the use of regional anaesthesia.

Amniotic Fluid Embolism

Amniotic fluid embolism (AFE) has been estimated to occur in 2 per 100 000 maternities and has been associated with a reported mortality approaching 100%, although the most recent maternal mortality report and UKOSS (UK Obstetric Surveillance System) reports give a combined case fatality rate of 16.5%. Amniotic fluid embolus is difficult to diagnose definitively and this may result in both under- and overreporting of cases. There were 13 deaths caused by AFE in the 2006–2008 Confidential Enquiry. Historically, amniotic fluid embolus was described as a post-mortem diagnosis dependent on the pathological finding of fetal squamous cells in the lung tissue. More recently, a clinical diagnosis has been used. Diagnosis is one of exclusion. The classic features are hypoxia, cardiovascular collapse and a coagulopathy. The mechanism of AFE is still unclear but it is suggested that the entrance into the circulation of amniotic fluid constituents is thought to cause the release of various primary or secondary endogenous mediators such as histamine, bradykinins, leukotrienes and endothelin.

The haemodynamic response has been shown to be biphasic, with initial pulmonary vasoconstriction and severe hypoxia followed by left ventricular failure. Risk factors include advancing age, multiparity and placental abruption. The woman presents with sudden collapse, usually after a rapid labour, but may present following an obstetric intervention, during labour or even during caesarean section. There may be preceding cyanosis, a confusional state, respiratory distress, left ventricular failure with hypotension and acute pulmonary oedema. This is followed rapidly by development of a consumptive coagulopathy and resultant haemorrhage. Management of this emergency involves resuscitation, with administration of oxygen and maintenance of the airway, including tracheal intubation and cardiopulmonary resuscitation, if necessary. If the fetus is undelivered, immediate caesarean section may be necessary to facilitate maternal resuscitation. Treatment is largely supportive, with early correction of coagulopathy. A protracted period of intensive care treatment may be necessary. All suspected cases of AFE in the UK should be reported to the National Amniotic Fluid Embolism Register at UKOSS.

Sepsis

In the latest triennial enquiry into maternal mortality, sepsis was the leading direct cause of death and the incidence is increasing, unlike the other direct causes. The main reason for the increase in genital tract sepsis in the latest report was the increased number of deaths caused by community-acquired β-haemolytic streptococcus Lancefield Group A (*Streptococcus pyogenes*).

It is important that all women are educated about the importance of good personal hygiene, both antenatally and postnatally. Early recognition is vital in the successful treatment of these women, so community practitioners should be aware of the clinical features and refer immediately to inpatient obstetric services. In hospital, Modified Early Obstetric Warning Scoring system (MEOWS) charts should be used to help in the more timely recognition, treatment and referral of women who have, or are developing, a critical illness. There is a 'golden hour' in the treatment of sepsis and sepsis care bundles such as the 'Surviving Sepsis' campaign should be followed. These can be summarized as early treatment (within 1 h of the recognition of severe sepsis) with broad-spectrum, appropriate intravenous antibiotics after blood cultures have been taken, fluid resuscitation and supportive measures. Critical care services should also be involved early in the management of these patients and they should be cared for in an appropriate environment with suitable monitoring.

Maternal and Neonatal Resuscitation

Severe haemorrhage, amniotic fluid embolism, pulmonary embolism or other even more uncommon causes may result in an acutely collapsed mother. In these circumstances, immediate resuscitation is required following standard resuscitation guidelines, but aortocaval compression should be avoided with tilt or wedging. Unsuccessful resuscitation is often caused by profound hypovolaemia. Perimortem caesarean section should be considered as soon as a pregnant woman has a cardiac arrest. Delivery should be completed within 5 min of cardiac arrest to maximize the chance of both maternal and fetal survival and outcome.

Neonatal Resuscitation

The condition of the infant at birth may be assessed by the following.

- Colour, tone, breathing, heart rate are used for the acute assessment. Although the Apgar score, calculated at 1 and 5 min, is of some use retrospectively, it is not used to guide resuscitation.
- Umbilical cord vein pH, which is normally 7.25–7.35.

The process of resuscitation of the infant begins with drying the baby and thus gentle physical stimulation. If, at the initial assessment after stimulation, the neonate is blue or white with irregular or inadequate respiration and the heart rate is slow (<60 beat min^{-1}), the airway should be opened and five inflation breaths of air should be given. If the heart rate remains slow despite adequate inflation breaths (chest movement seen), cardiopulmonary resuscitation should be commenced at a ratio of three compressions to one inflation breath. The newborn must be kept warm throughout.

ANAESTHESIA FOR INTERVENTIONS OTHER THAN DELIVERY OR EXTRACTION OF RETAINED PRODUCTS OF CONCEPTION

Up to 20% of all confirmed pregnancies end in spontaneous abortion within the first trimester, and extraction of retained products of conception (ERPC) is indicated if there are retained placental products. These women are often very distressed and need sympathetic care. They should be assessed for blood loss, and although there is usually no problem, there is a significant risk of severe haemorrhage which may necessitate resuscitation, including blood transfusion. In the first trimester, anaesthesia is similar to that required for cervical dilatation or hysteroscopy. Anaesthesia may be induced with an i.v. induction agent, with or without a short-acting opioid such as fentanyl (1–2 µg kg^{-1}), and maintained via a face mask or LMA (as the procedure usually lasts 5–7 min) with the patient spontaneously breathing N$_2$O/O$_2$ and 1–2 MAC of a volatile anaesthetic agent. Adequate depth of anaesthesia is required before cervical dilatation, because vagal stimulation in an inadequately anaesthetized patient may lead to bradycardia and laryngospasm. After cervical dilatation, the level of anaesthesia may be reduced to 0.5–1.0 MAC. Some practitioners avoid volatile anaesthetic agents in favour of TIVA in order to minimize uterine relaxation.

Cervical Circlage

This is a surgical procedure required occasionally for women with a history or active clinical features of an incompetent cervix, usually presenting as premature, precipitate labour. To reduce the risk of this occurring, a suture (Shirodkar suture) is placed around the cervix, in a procedure lasting 20–30 min. As this is usually performed in the second trimester or later, the anaesthetic considerations for any pregnant woman apply. Regional (spinal) anaesthesia is the technique of choice, with the required block height of T10–S5 being achieved using 1.5 mL hyperbaric bupivacaine with or without fentanyl 25 µg. If general anaesthesia must be undertaken, use of a rapid sequence induction is mandatory if the patient is at more than 12 weeks' gestation.

The Pregnant Patient with a Surgical (Non-Obstetric) Emergency

The incidence of general surgical emergencies is undiminished in pregnancy, and thus pregnant patients may require anaesthesia for laparotomy or any other procedure. If delivery is not anticipated, the anaesthetic technique should ensure good delivery of oxygen to the placenta. Use of depressant drugs such as opioids is not contraindicated. Regional techniques are recommended where possible. After the 13th week of gestation, the risk of regurgitation of gastric contents increases, so rapid sequence induction should always be performed.

ACKNOWLEDGEMENT

We would like to acknowledge C.D. Elton, A. May, D.J. Buggy.

FURTHER READING

Centre for Maternal and Child Enquiries, March 2011. Saving Mothers' Lives: Reviewing maternal deaths to make motherhood safer: 2006–2008. The Eighth Report of the Confidential Enquiries into Maternal Deaths in the United Kingdom. Royal College of Obstetricians and Gynaecologists, London.

Chestnut, D.H. (Ed.), 1999. Obstetric anesthesia, second ed. Mosby, St Louis.

Clyburn, P., Collis, R., Harries, S., Davies, S., 2008. Obstetric anaesthesia. Oxford Specialist Handbooks in Anaesthesia, Oxford University Press, Oxford.

Collis, R., Plaat, F., Urquhart, J. (Eds.), 2002. Textbook of obstetric anaesthesia. Greenwich Medical, London.

Guidelines for Obstetric Anaesthetic Services, 2005. Association of Anaesthetists of Great Britain and Ireland and Obstetric Anaesthetists' Association.

Harmer, M., 1997. Difficult and failed intubation in obstetrics. Int. J. Obstet. Anesth. 6, 25–31.

Hofmeyr, G.J., Gulmezoglu, A.M. Novikova, N., et al., 2009. Misoprostol to prevent and treat postpartum haemorrhage: a systematic review and meta-analysis of maternal deaths and dose-related effects. Bull. World Health Organ. 87(9), 666–77.

Holdcroft, A., Thomas, T., 2000. Principles and practice of obstetric anaesthesia and analgesia. Blackwell Science, Oxford.

Jones, L., Othman, M., Dowswell, T., et al., 2012. Pain management for women in labour: an overview of systematic reviews. Cochrane Database of Systematic Reviews. Issue 3. Art. No.: CD009234. http://dx.doi.org/10.1002/14651858. CD009234.pub2

MacEvilly, E., Buggy, D., 1996. Back pain and pregnancy (review). Pain 64, 405–414.

McGrady, E., Litchfield, K., 2004. Epidural analgesia in labour. Continuing Education in Anaesthesia, Critical Care and Pain 4,114–117.

National Institute of Clinical Excellence, 2007. Clinical guideline 55: Intrapartum Care.

National Institute of Clinical Excellence, 2004. Clinical guideline 13: Caesarean Section.

Reynolds, F. (Ed.), 2000. Regional anaesthesia in obstetrics. A millennium update. Springer, London.

The Royal College of Anaesthetists, 2009. NAP 3: The 3rd National Audit Project of The Royal College of Anaesthetists. Major Complications of Central Neuroaxial Blockade in the United Kingdom.

Van Zundert, A., Ostheimer, G.W., 1996. Pain relief and anesthesia in obstetrics. Churchill Livingstone, Edinburgh.

Yentis, S.M., May, A., Malhotra, S., et al., 2007. Analgesia, anaesthesia and pregnancy. A practical guide, second ed. WB Saunders, London.

http://www.oaa-anaes.ac.uk/.

36

PAEDIATRIC ANAESTHESIA

The differences in anatomy and physiology between children, especially infants, and adults have important consequences in many aspects of anaesthesia. The differences also account for the different patterns of disease seen in intensive care units (ICUs). Although major psychological differences persist throughout adolescence, a 10- to 12-year-old child may be thought of, anatomically and physiologically, as a small adult.

PHYSIOLOGY IN THE NEONATE

Respiration

Control of respiration in newborn infants, especially premature neonates, is poorly developed. The incidence of central apnoea (defined as a cessation of respiration for 15 s or longer) is not uncommon in this group. The likelihood of this increases if the patient is given a drug with a sedative effect. Potentially life-threatening apnoea may occur. The incidence is reduced by postoperative administration of xanthine derivatives such as caffeine and theophylline which act as central respiratory stimulants. Because of this problem, it is wise to admit for overnight oximetry and apnoea monitoring all children under 60 weeks' postconceptual age who have had surgical procedures, no matter how minor. Hypoxaemia in the neonate and small child appears to inhibit rather than stimulate respiration and this is contrary to what one might expect.

The newborn has between 20 and 50 million terminal air spaces. At 18 months of age, the adult level of 300 million is reached by a process of alveolar multiplication. This explains why infants who suffer with respiratory distress of the newborn improve as they grow older. Subsequent lung growth occurs by an increase in alveolar size. The lung volume in infants is disproportionately small in relation to body size. The metabolic rate is nearly twice that of the adult, and therefore ventilatory requirement per unit lung volume is increased. Thus, they have far less reserve for gas exchange.

Before the age of 8 years, the calibre of the airways is relatively narrow. Airway resistance is therefore relatively high. Small decreases in the diameter of the airways as a result of oedema or respiratory secretions significantly increase the work of breathing. Elastic tissue in the lungs of small children is poorly developed. As a result of this, compliance is decreased. This has important consequences in that airway closure may occur during normal tidal ventilation, thereby bringing about an increase in alveolar–arterial oxygen tension difference $(P_{A-a}O_2)$. This explains why PaO_2 is lower in the infant than in the child. The decreased compliance results in ventilatory units with short time constants. Consequently, the infant is able to achieve adequate alveolar ventilation whilst maintaining a high respiratory rate. However, because of the increased resistance and decreased compliance, the work of breathing may represent up to 15% of total oxygen consumption (Table 36.1). The high respiratory rate is necessary because the metabolic rate of the infant is nearly twice that of the adult. The high alveolar minute ventilation explains why induction and emergence from inhalational anaesthesia are relatively rapid in small children. The high metabolic rate also explains why desaturation occurs very rapidly in children.

TABLE 36.1
Lung Mechanics of the Neonate Compared with the Adult

	Neonate	Adult
Compliance (mL cmH$_2$O^{-1})	5	100
Resistance (cmH$_2$O L^{-1} s^{-1})	30	2
Time constant (s)	0.5	1.3
Respiratory rate (breath min^{-1})	32	15

TABLE 36.2
Respiratory Variables in the Neonate

Tidal volume (V)	7 mL kg^{-1}
Dead space (V_D)	(V_T) × 0.3 mL
Respiratory rate	32 breath min^{-1}

TABLE 36.3
Variation in Arterial Pressure (mmHg) and Heart Rate (Beat min^{-1}) with Age

Age	Systolic BP	Diastolic BP	Heart Rate
Neonate	70–80	40–50	100–180
1 year	90–100	60–80	80–130
6 years	95–100	50–80	70–120
12 years	110–120	60–70	60–100

The ratio of physiological dead space to tidal volume (V_D/V_T) is similar to that of the adult at about 0.3. However, because the volumes are smaller, modest increases in V_D produced by equipment such as humidification filters may have a disproportionately greater effect (Table 36.2).

Ventilation in small children is almost entirely diaphragmatic. Because the ribs are horizontal, there is no 'bucket handle' movement of the ribs as occurs in the adult. It is therefore important to appreciate that normal minute ventilation is respiratory rate-dependent. The infant's diaphragm is made of fast twitch fibres. This type of muscle fibre exhausts easily if it has to work against a load. This implies that in infancy, when lung compliance is low, the work of breathing is reduced by breathing rapidly. Consequently if the work of breathing is increased by an increase in airway resistance, respiratory failure may easily ensue.

It is important to appreciate that the infant's response to hypoxaemia may be bradypnoea and not tachypnoea as occurs in the adult.

Cardiovascular System

The process of growth demands a high metabolic rate. It is, therefore, not surprising that infants and children have a higher cardiac index compared with the adult, so that oxygen and nutrients may be delivered to actively growing tissues. The ventricles of neonates and infants are poorly compliant, so even though the ventricles of infants demonstrate the Frank-Starling mechanism, the main determinant of cardiac output is heart rate. Infants tolerate heart rates of 200 beat min^{-1} with ease (Table 36.3). Bradycardia may occur readily in response to hypoxaemia and vagal stimulation and it results in a decrease in cardiac output. Immediate cessation of the stimulus, and treatment with oxygen and atropine, are absolutely crucial. A heart rate of 60 beat min^{-1} in an infant is considered a cardiac arrest and requires cardiac massage. Arrhythmias are rare in the absence of cardiac disease. The usual cardiac arrest scenarios are electromechanical dissociation and asystole, not ventricular fibrillation.

Even though infants and children have a higher cardiac index, arterial pressure tends to be lower than in adults because of a reduced systemic vascular resistance associated with an abundance of vessel-rich tissues in the infant. The arterial pressure increases from approximately 80/50 mmHg at birth to the normal adult value of 120/70 mmHg by the age of 16 years. Children under the age of 8 years who are normovolaemic at the start of anaesthesia tend not to exhibit a decrease in arterial pressure when central neural blockade such as spinal anaesthesia is administered. They do not require fluid preloading as an adult would to avoid hypotension, because venous pooling tends not to occur as venous capacitance cannot increase. The reasons for this are, first, that the sympathetic nervous system is less well developed and so infants tend to be venodilated at rest. Second, they have a lower extremity:body surface ratio and as a consequence have a smaller venous capacitance.

As in all patients, the cardiovascular system must be monitored carefully. Pulse oximeter probes placed on the extremities provide a good index of peripheral perfusion. Auscultation of heart sounds, especially by an oesophageal stethoscope, is useful as the volume of heart sounds tends to be diminished as cardiac output decreases. Non-invasive measurement of arterial pressure is undertaken easily using an appropriately sized cuff. Complications preclude the use of invasive monitoring of arterial and central venous pressures for all but major cases.

Blood Volume

The stage at which the umbilical cord is clamped determines the circulating blood volume of the neonate. Variations of up to ±20% may occur. The average blood volume at birth is 90 mL kg^{-1}, and this decreases in the infant and young child to 80 mL kg^{-1}, attaining the adult level of 75 mL kg^{-1} at the age of 6–8 years. Blood losses of greater than 10% of the red cell mass should be replaced by blood, especially if additional losses are expected. However, most children who have a normal haemoglobin concentration at the start of surgery can tolerate losses of up to 20% of their red cell mass. Children may tolerate a haematocrit of 25% and the decision to transfuse blood must be balanced against the risks, which include transmitted infection and antibody formation. The latter may cause problems in later life, especially in female children during child-bearing years.

Haemoglobin

At birth, 75–80% of the neonate's haemoglobin is fetal haemoglobin (HbF). By the age of 6 months, adult haemoglobin (HbA) haematopoiesis is fully established. HbF has a higher affinity for oxygen than HbA. This is demonstrated by the leftward shift of the oxygen haemoglobin dissociation curve (Fig. 36.1). Low tissue P_{O_2} and metabolic acidosis in the tissues result in the avidity of HbF for oxygen being reduced, thereby aiding delivery of oxygen. Alkalosis produced by hyperventilation results in less oxygen being available and it is therefore sensible to maintain normocapnia.

If blood transfusion is required, it is crucial that blood is filtered and warmed – the smaller the child, the more important is this precaution. A syringe used via a tap in the intravenous giving set is probably the safest way of avoiding inadvertent overtransfusion. The circulating volume of a 1 kg neonate is of the order of 80 mL. Common sense dictates that blood loss

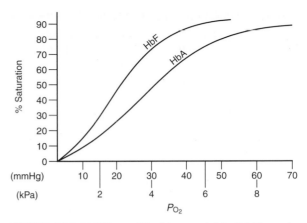

FIGURE 36.1 ■ Effects of fetal haemoglobin (HbF) on the oxygen dissociation curve. HbA, adult haemoglobin; P_{O_2}, partial pressure of oxygen.

TABLE 36.4

Distribution of Water as a Percentage of Body Weight

Compartment	Premature	Neonate	Infant	Adult
ECF	50	35	30	20
ICF	30	40	40	40
Plasma	5	5	5	5
Total	85	80	75	65

ECF, extracellular fluid; ICF, intracellular fluid.

should be monitored carefully, so swabs should be weighed and, if possible, all suction losses collected in a graduated container.

Renal Function and Fluid Balance

Body fluids constitute a greater proportion of body weight in the infant, particularly the premature infant, compared with the adult (Table 36.4). In an adult, most of the total body water is in the intracellular compartment. In a newborn infant, most of the total body water is in the extracellular compartment. With increasing age, the ratio reverses. Plasma volume remains constant throughout life at about 5% of body weight.

The kidneys are immature at birth. Both glomerular filtration rate (GFR) and subsequent reabsorption by the renal tubules are reduced. The GFR at birth is of the order of 45 mL min^{-1} 1.7 m^{-2}. This increases rapidly to about 65 mL min^{-1} 1.7 m^{-2} and then gradually approaches the adult value of $125 \, mL \, min^{-1} \, 1.7 \, m^{-2}$ by the age of 8 years. Thus, there is inability to handle excessive water and sodium loads. Overtransfusion may lead to pulmonary oedema and cardiac failure. The maturation in renal function is produced by hyperplasia in the first 6 months of life and then by a process of hypertrophy in the first year. Care must also be exercised when drugs eliminated by the renal route are used in infants; either reduced doses or an increased dosage interval should be employed. Renal maturation is not just an increase in size but also of function. The ability to modify the ultrafiltrate produced at the glomerulus increases with age. It follows that sodium bicarbonate and glucose homeostasis mechanisms are not fully developed. Medical intervention may be required to ensure that biochemical values are kept within normal ranges.

Poorly developed mechanisms exist for conserving water in the kidneys and gastrointestinal tract. Increased cutaneous water loss because of a large surface area:volume ratio through poorly keratinized skin may lead to a turnover of fluid in the infant of about 15% of total body water per day. Dehydration ensues very rapidly in an infant who is kept fasted.

Fluid Therapy

An intravenous infusion delivering maintenance fluids should be in place for all neonates requiring surgery. Maintenance fluid requirements increase over the first few days of life (Tables 36.5, 36.6). The normal infant requires of the order of $3–5 \, mmol \, kg^{-1}$ of sodium and an equivalent amount of potassium per day to maintain normal serum electrolyte concentrations. The ability of the infant's kidneys to eliminate excess sodium is limited. Exceeding this amount in the absence of loss

TABLE 36.5	
Fluid Requirements in the First Week of Life	
Day	*Rate (mL kg^{-1} Day^{-1})*
1	0
2, 3	50
4, 5	75
6	100
7	120

TABLE 36.6	
Maintenance Fluid Requirements	
Weight (kg)	*Rate (mL kg^{-1} Day^{-1})*
Up to 10 kg	100
10–20 kg	$1000 + 50 \times$ [weight (kg) – 10] mL
20–30 kg	$1500 + 25 \times$ [weight (kg) – 20] mL

results in hypernatraemia and its sequelae. Infants undergoing any procedure more than the briefest should also have their calorific needs addressed. This may be achieved by including glucose-containing fluids in the regimen; failure to do so results in hypoglycaemia and ketosis. This may occur rapidly because of the limited glycogen stores and high metabolic rate of the infant.

It is imperative that the anaesthetist recognizes and resuscitates the dehydrated infant appropriately before surgery. Clinical examination of skin turgor, capillary refill, tension of fontanelles, arterial pressure and venous filling may aid estimation of hydration, but electrolyte and haemoglobin concentrations and haematocrit, urine volumes and plasma and urine osmolalities should be monitored if problems of fluid balance exist (Table 36.7).

TABLE 36.7			
Effects of Dehydration in the Young Infant			
	Mild	*Moderate*	*Severe*
Percentage loss of body weight	5	10	15
Clinical signs	Dry skin and mucous membranes	Mottled cold periphery Depressed fontanelles Oliguria++	Shocked Moribund Unresponsive to pain
Replacement	50 mL kg^{-1}	100 mL kg^{-1}	150 mL kg^{-1}

Intravenous fluids should be administered using a system that allows small volumes to be given accurately. This may vary from the anaesthetist injecting fluid using a syringe to microprocessor-controlled syringe driver pumps. The latter are preferable, as fluid is given at a steady rate and the anaesthetist's hands are free to attend to other tasks. During surgery, fluid administration should be increased to account for increased losses occurring through evaporation from exposed viscera and third-space losses.

The intraosseous route may be used to carry out fluid resuscitation and drug therapy in shocked children. The needle should be inserted in an aseptic fashion to minimize the risk of osteomyelitis. Although various sites have been described for needle insertion, the proximal end of the tibia below the tuberosity is probably the easiest to perform. The intraosseous route is safer than attempting central venous cannulation in the shocked child in whom veins are difficult to discern. The usual fluid administered in this situation is a colloid solution. This is given as a 10 mL kg^{-1} bolus and repeated until clinical improvement occurs.

Temperature Regulation and Maintenance

Homeothermic animals possess the ability to produce and dissipate heat. Heat loss occurs by one of four processes: radiation, convection, evaporation and conduction. The environment in which the patient is situated governs the relative contribution of each. The neutral thermal environment is defined as the range of ambient temperatures at which temperature regulation is achieved by non-evaporative physical processes alone.

The metabolic rate at this temperature is minimal. The temperature of such an environment is 34°C for the premature neonate, 32°C for the neonate at term and 28°C for the adult.

Heat may be produced by one of three processes: voluntary muscle activity, involuntary muscle activity and non-shivering thermogenesis. Infants under the age of 3 months do not shiver. The only method available to increase their temperature in the perioperative period is non-shivering thermogenesis. The process is mediated by specialized tissue termed brown fat. It differentiates in the human fetus between 26 and 30 weeks of gestation. It comprises between 2% and 6% of total body weight in the human fetus and is located mainly between the scapulae and in the axillae. It is also found around blood vessels in the neck, in the mediastinum and in the loins. Brown fat is made of multinucleated cells with numerous mitochondria and has an abundant blood and nerve supply. Its metabolism is mediated by catecholamines. The substrate used for heat production is mainly fatty acids.

Radiation accounts for about 60% of the heat loss from a neonate in a 34°C incubator placed in a room at 21°C. If the infant was in a thermoneutral environment of 34°C, the percentage loss by radiation would decrease to about 40% of the total heat loss, and, in addition, the total heat loss in this environment would be lower. The reason for this is that heat loss by radiation is a function of skin surface area and the difference in temperature between the skin and the room. The second major source of heat loss in the neonate is convection. This is a function of skin temperature and ambient temperature. The neonate possesses minimal subcutaneous fat that may act as thermal insulation and as a barrier to evaporative loss. A neonate has a body surface area:volume ratio about 2.5 times greater than the adult; thus, a neonate may become hypothermic very rapidly.

If neonates are allowed to become hypothermic during anaesthesia, unlike adults they attempt to correct this by non-shivering thermogenesis. Metabolic rate increases and oxygen consumption may double. The increase in metabolic rate puts an additional burden on the cardiorespiratory system and this may be critical in neonates with limited reserves. The release of noradrenaline in response to hypothermia causes vasoconstriction, which in turn causes a lactic acidosis. The acidosis favours an increase in right-to-left shunt, which causes hypoxaemia. As a result, a vicious positive feedback loop of hypoxaemia and acidosis is set up. The protective airway reflexes of a hypothermic neonate are obtunded, thereby increasing the risks of regurgitation and aspiration of gastric contents. The action of most anaesthetic drugs is potentiated by hypothermia. This effect is particularly important with regard to neuromuscular blocking drugs. The combination of hypothermia and prolonged action of these drugs increases the chances of the neonate hypoventilating after surgery.

Many precautions should be taken to ensure that the neonate's body temperature is maintained. First, the child must be transported to theatre wrapped up and in an incubator set at the thermoneutral temperature. The theatre should be warmed up to the thermoneutral temperature, ideally a few hours before the planned start of surgery. This interval allows the walls of the theatre to warm up and this reduces the net heat loss by radiation. Heat loss by radiation is a two-way process. The child loses heat by radiation to the walls and also gains heat from the walls. All body parts which are not needed for insertion of cannulae and for monitoring should remain covered until the child has been draped with surgical towels. If the child has to be exposed, overhead radiant heaters may be used. During surgery, the child should lie on a thermostatically controlled heated blanket. Forced air warming systems are effective in maintaining the child's temperature during surgery; these work on the principle of blowing filtered, warmed air into quilted blankets with perforations. This allows warmed air to come into direct contact with the patient. Simple measures such as using a bonnet to reduce heat loss from the head are very effective. Intravenous fluids and fluids used to perform lavage of body cavities must be warmed. Anaesthetic gases should be humidified and warmed in order to preserve ciliary function and to reduce heat loss from the respiratory tract.

Monitoring

It is important in all procedures to measure temperature. For short procedures, an axillary temperature probe may be sufficient. In longer operations, core temperature should be measured at one of a variety of sites, such as rectal, bladder, nasopharyngeal or oesophageal. The oesophageal probe is often the preferred method, as most modern oesophageal probes may be connected to a stethoscope. The anaesthetist is therefore able to listen to heart sounds in addition to recording the patient's temperature. When active heating methods such as cascade humidifiers and heated blankets are used, it is important that temperature gradients between the patient and the warming device are kept to less than 10°C. Failure to observe this may result in burns to the skin and the respiratory tract. In the ICU, simultaneous measurement of core and peripheral temperatures, though not often used in theatre, may serve as a useful guide to adequacy of the cardiac output. Decreases in cardiac output result in a reduction of blood flow to the peripheries and this is reflected in a core-peripheral temperature gradient greater than 3–4°C.

PHARMACOLOGY IN THE NEONATE

Developmental Pharmacology

Drugs given via the oral or rectal route are absorbed by a process of passive absorption. This process is dependent on the physicochemical properties of the drug and the surface area available for absorption. Most drugs are either weak bases or weak acids. The un-ionized portion of the drug therefore depends on the pH of the fluid in the gut. The gastric pH of the neonate is higher than that of the older child and adult. The consequence is that drugs inactivated by a low pH undergo greater absorption. Examples of these include antibiotics such as penicillin G.

Factors which determine the distribution of intravenously administered drugs include protein and red cell binding, tissue volumes, tissue solubility coefficients and blood flow to tissues. Neonates, in particular preterm infants, have lower plasma concentrations of albumin. In addition, the albumin is qualitatively different in that its ability to bind drugs is lower than that of adult albumin. The concentration of α_1-acid glycoprotein is also lower in this group of patients; this protein is the major binding protein for alkaline drugs, which include opioid analgesics and local anaesthetics.

The blood–brain barrier is immature at birth; thus, it is more permeable to drugs. In addition, the neonate's brain receives a larger proportion of the cardiac output than does the adult brain. Consequently, brain concentrations of drugs are higher in neonates than in adults. For example, administration of morphine, which has low lipid solubility, results in high concentrations in the neonate's brain and therefore it should be used with caution and in reduced amounts.

In a neonate, total body water, extracellular fluid and blood volume are proportionally larger in comparison with an adult. This results in a larger apparent volume of distribution for a parenterally administered drug. This explains in part why neonates appear to require larger amounts of some drugs on a weight basis to produce a given effect. However, plasma concentrations tend to remain high for longer because they have smaller muscle mass and fat stores to which drugs redistribute.

The action of most drugs is terminated by metabolism or excretion through the liver and kidneys. In the liver, phase I reactions convert the original drug to a more polar metabolite by the addition or unmasking of a functional group such as -OH, $-NH_2$ or -SH. These reduction/oxidation reactions are a function of liver size and the metabolizing ability of the appropriate microsomal enzyme system. The volume of the liver relative to body weight is largest in the first year of life. The enzyme systems in the liver responsible for the metabolism of drugs are incompletely developed in the neonate. Their activity appears to be a function of postnatal rather than post-conceptual age, because premature and full-term infants develop the ability to metabolize drugs to the same degree in the same period after birth. Adult levels of activity are achieved within a few days of birth. Phase II reactions which involve conjugation with moieties such as sulphate, acetate, glucuronic acid, etc., are severely limited at birth. Most of these conjugation reactions are in place by the age of 3 months. The kidneys ultimately eliminate most drugs. As mentioned above, GFR is lower in young children than in adults. However, by the age of 3 months, the clearance of most drugs approaches adult values.

Specific Drugs in Paediatric Anaesthesia

Inhalational Agents

Alveolar and brain concentrations of inhalational anaesthetic agents increase rapidly in children, because they have a greater alveolar ventilation rate in relation to functional residual capacity (FRC) and because of the preponderance of vessel-rich tissues. Induction and excretion of the agent at the termination of anaesthesia are more rapid.

The minimum alveolar concentration (MAC) of anaesthetic agents changes with age, because of age-related differences in blood/gas solubility coefficients. From birth, MAC increases to a peak at the age of 6 months and then declines gradually until the adult value is reached. It is worth stating at this juncture that malignant hyperthermia has been reported or is possible with all the presently available volatile anaesthetic agents and that all potentiate the duration of neuromuscular blocking drugs.

Nitrous Oxide. Nitrous oxide is used as a carrier gas for most inhalational anaesthetic agents. It is also used for its MAC-sparing effect. The effect is most marked with halothane, with which a 60% reduction can be achieved. However, with the newer agents such as sevoflurane, only a 25% reduction may be produced. Thus, there would appear to be little to be gained by adding nitrous oxide to a sevoflurane anaesthetic. A major problem with nitrous oxide is its greater solubility compared with nitrogen. It diffuses into closed nitrogen-containing spaces at a greater rate than nitrogen leaves, thereby causing expansion. This effect is particularly important in lung lesions such as pneumothorax and congenital lobar emphysema. Expansion of the bowel in exomphalos or gastroschisis may make surgical reduction into the peritoneal cavity difficult.

Halothane. This agent has been the gold standard for induction of anaesthesia in children, because until recently its odour was one of the least pungent. It shares with all anaesthetic agents the ability to depress the myocardium. However, it also slows heart rate, causing a decrease in cardiac output. It is therefore prudent to give an anticholinergic before its administration. Induction with halothane is smooth, and because most vaporizers allow $5 \times MAC$ to be administered, it may be given in almost 100% oxygen. This is a useful feature when anaesthetizing a child with an airway problem. Another property which makes halothane useful in this situation is its prolonged action compared with the newer volatile agents, as it is undesirable that anaesthesia 'lightens' during instrumentation of the airway. In adult anaesthetic practice, repeat administrations of halothane within a period of less than 3 months may be associated with hepatic dysfunction and occasionally with fulminant hepatic failure. The exact mechanism of this toxic effect is not clear, but some have speculated that a reductive metabolite of halothane is responsible. Reductive hepatic metabolism of drugs is developed poorly in children and this may explain why this problem is extremely rare in children. However, if a child needs a second anaesthetic within 3 months of a first halothane anaesthetic, a risk–benefit assessment has to be undertaken. Economic considerations dictate that this is the most widely used inhalational agent for induction and maintenance of anaesthesia in children worldwide. As one might predict from its physical characteristics, emergence from halothane anaesthesia tends to take longer compared with the newer agents.

It is acceptable to induce anaesthesia with halothane and then to use a less lipid-soluble agent for maintenance.

Isoflurane. Cardiac output tends to be well maintained when less than 1 MAC of this agent is used for maintenance of anaesthesia. However, because of its pungency, it is not a suitable agent for induction. In spite of the fact that it has a low blood/gas partition coefficient, induction tends to be slow because of breath-holding. It may be used for maintenance of anaesthesia after sevoflurane or intravenous induction.

Sevoflurane. The blood/gas partition coefficient of 0.68 results in rapid induction of anaesthesia with this agent and also a quick recovery. It is the least pungent of the currently available agents. It is possible to turn the vaporizer to its maximum output of 8% without experiencing significant problems of coughing, breath-holding or laryngeal spasm. There is little to be gained by including nitrous oxide during induction, as the MAC-sparing effect on sevoflurane is not as great as with other agents. It is not unusual to observe slowing of the heart rate during induction, but it is not usually necessary to give an anticholinergic. Cardiac arrhythmias do not commonly occur during induction or maintenance with sevoflurane. Economic considerations dictate that the agent is used mainly for induction, followed by a cheaper agent such as isoflurane for maintenance. Sevoflurane is an excellent choice for induction in children with upper airway obstruction. The agent is partly degraded by soda lime to compound A, which is nephrotoxic in rats because they possess the enzyme β-lyase. This hazard would appear to be theoretical in humans.

Desflurane. The blood/gas partition coefficient of 0.42 suggests that induction should be rapid, but this is not so because desflurane is very irritant to the upper airway. It may be used for maintenance of anaesthesia with the benefit that emergence is very rapid. This may be particularly desirable in the ex-premature infant. Cost and the fact that the agent has to be delivered using a special vaporizer limit the use of desflurane in paediatric practice.

Intravenous Agents

The availability of topical local anaesthetic creams has resulted in venepuncture and cannulation being relatively atraumatic for children. As a consequence, intravenous induction has become more common.

Barbiturates. Thiopental is the most widely used in this class of agents. A dose of 5–6 mg kg^{-1} of a 2.5% solution is required in the healthy child. The main advantage is that injection into a small vein is pain-free. The agent can be given rectally using a 10% solution at a dose of 30 mg kg^{-1}, but induction and recovery tend to be slow with this technique.

Propofol. Propofol may be used for both induction and maintenance of anaesthesia as part of a total intravenous technique. Although not common in paediatric anaesthetic practice, the technique of total intravenous anaesthesia using propofol is very useful in the child prone to malignant hyperthermia or the child with porphyria. Induction and maintenance doses tend to be larger in the younger healthy patient. The reasons for this are because of a larger central volume of distribution and because the clearance of the agent is higher compared with the adult. Pain on injection is a problem and this may be lessened by the addition of 0.2 mg kg^{-1} of lidocaine. Propofol stabilized in a medium-chain triglyceride emulsion appears to cause less pain on injection.

Ketamine. The current formulation of this drug is a racemic mixture of the S(+) and R(−) enantiomers. It is possible to separate the two enantiomers, although at present this does not appear to be a commercially viable proposition. The reason for doing this is that the S(+) enantiomer is twice as potent, recovery is quicker and the incidence of emergence reactions is lower. One of the major advantages of ketamine is the intense analgesia it provides. The analgesia has both spinal and supraspinal components. Epidural administration of the drug in combination with local anaesthetic significantly prolongs the duration of analgesia compared with local anaesthetic alone. The lack of cardiovascular depression *in vivo* is a feature which allows the drug to be used for inducing anaesthesia in children with congenital heart disease. Occasionally, pulmonary vascular resistance may increase, and as a consequence pulmonary pressures also increase. Even though upper airway reflexes are relatively well preserved, aspiration of gastric contents may still occur. The drug has bronchodilator properties and may be used for sedating the child with status asthmaticus to allow artificial ventilation in the ICU. It is prudent to administer an anti-cholinergic when the drug is used for maintenance of anaesthesia, because increased salivation and bronchial secretions are potential problems. Emergence from ketamine anaesthesia is slower than with other agents. It may be accompanied by emergence phenomena such as hallucinations and unpleasant dreams. The incidence of these can be reduced by concurrent administration of a benzodiazepine.

Opioids. These may be used in large doses as the sole agent to provide stable haemodynamic conditions for children with cardiac disease. The major disadvantage of using this technique is that drug effects persist into the postoperative period, causing respiratory depression. As a result, postoperative mechanical ventilation is mandatory. Morphine is the drug used most commonly for the management of severe pain in children. Hepatic glucuronidation is the process by which it is eliminated. Morphine is converted to morphine-3- and morphine-6-glucuronide. These metabolites are active. Morphine-3-glucuronide antagonizes the analgesic effects of morphine-6-glucuronide. The very young suffer from respiratory depression at lower morphine infusion rates. This is probably because of sensitivity of the brainstem and also because the ratio of morphine-3- to morphine-6-glucuronide is lower. Remifentanil is the newest of the synthetic opioids. This drug is unique in that its metabolism to a virtually inactive metabolite is by non-specific esterases in blood and tissue. The half-life of the drug is independent of the duration of infusion. There are few data on the use of this drug in infants and children, and at present it is unlicensed for use in children under the age of 2 years. However, it is likely to be valuable in infants because of its lack of accumulation and short half-life. Opioid-induced respiratory depression may be reversed by naloxone. The reversal is short-lived and it is probably wise to mechanically ventilate the lungs of children in this state.

Neuromuscular Blocking Drugs and their Antagonists

The neuromuscular junction in infants is not mature. Electrophysiological studies demonstrate that the response of the junction is similar to what one might observe in a patient with myasthenia gravis. In other words, the junction is very sensitive to the effects of neuromuscular blockers. These drugs are polar and as a result distribute mainly to the extracellular space. Because this space is larger in the infant, the dose of drug required to depress twitch tension is similar or slightly larger than that required for adults on a dose/unit weight basis. The larger volume of distribution explains why drugs that depend on the kidneys or liver for elimination have a longer duration of action. Conversely, drugs such as atracurium, which is degraded by a combination of ester hydrolysis and Hoffman elimination, act for a shorter time because of the larger extracellular space.

Anticholinesterases are used to antagonize residual neuromuscular blockade. The appropriate anticholinergic to match the duration and onset should be combined with the anticholinesterase in order to minimize muscarinic side-effects. Atropine with edrophonium and glycopyrronium with neostigmine are the recommended combinations. The dose requirements are similar to those of adults and reversal should not be attempted in the presence of profound blockade. The edrophonium/atropine combination has a quicker onset of action and a shorter duration of action. This combination, although not readily available, might be more appropriate for reversing the currently widely used intermediate-duration drugs.

Succinylcholine. This depolarizing neuromuscular blocking drug has the most rapid onset of action of any currently readily available agent. It is therefore the drug of choice for the patient with a full stomach and also for the treatment of laryngeal spasm. In the infant, it has the ability to cause bradycardia after only a single dose. It is wise to administer an anticholinergic before administration. A hyperkalaemic response is not seen after administration to children with myelomeningocoele or cerebral palsy. It is one of the most potent triggers for malignant hyperthermia. The incidence of this increases if succinylcholine is preceded by induction of anaesthesia with halothane. Fatal cardiac arrest has occurred in a small number of patients. It is presumed that these patients had unsuspected muscular dystrophies and that the drug caused massive muscle breakdown. As it is not possible to predict which patients might exhibit this response, it is wise to limit the use of the drug to patients with a full stomach and for the relief of laryngospasm.

Non-Depolarizing Agents. Onset and duration of action and the response in patients with renal and hepatic disease are probably the most important considerations when choosing one of these agents. Rocuronium has the most rapid onset of all the currently available agents. The onset of all these drugs may be increased by giving larger doses, but this is counterbalanced by a correspondingly longer duration of action. Recently, a new amino-steroid, rapacuronium, was evaluated in paediatric practice. Data suggested that its onset of action was similar to that of succinylcholine and that its duration of action was comparable to that of mivacurium. However, there were several reports of bronchospasm and hypoxaemia, especially in small children, and the drug was withdrawn. Mivacurium has the shortest duration of action of the currently available drugs. Mivacurium is best suited for the short surgical procedure, which usually matches its duration of action. Very occasionally, a patient may be cholinesterase-deficient, in which case its duration is long. Atracurium, rocuronium and vecuronium have an intermediate duration of action, making them the most commonly used, as the duration of most paediatric operations falls into this category. Cisatracurium and pancuronium are best reserved for longer procedures. Pancuronium is excreted renally and should be used with caution in the patient with renal failure. In spite of the fact that vecuronium and rocuronium are excreted by the liver, their duration of action is minimally affected by hepatic disease. Atracurium or cisatracurium are the most obvious choices for patients with renal or hepatic disease because elimination is altered minimally by organ failure.

ANAESTHETIC MANAGEMENT

Preoperative Preparation

For all elective surgery, it should be possible to prepare the child and family for what is to be expected in the perioperative period. This may be done in a wide variety of ways, including hospital tours, educational videotapes and pamphlets. The optimum choice depends on the age and intellectual ability of the child. Children possess great insight, and to attempt to keep forthcoming events secret is only likely to lead to mistrust and fear. All children should be visited preoperatively by the anaesthetist responsible for caring for them in the perioperative period. This is the opportunity not only to assess fitness for anaesthesia and surgery but also, when appropriate, to allay anxiety, answer questions and to find out what the child's preferences are for mode of induction, pain relief, etc.

Children who are systemically unwell should not have elective surgery. It is not unusual for a child to present with coryzal symptoms alone. There is an increased incidence of airway problems during anaesthesia; these children are more at risk of laryngeal spasm, breath-holding and bronchospasm, and in the postoperative period the chance of post-intubation croup is increased. The decision to proceed should be made only by a senior anaesthetist. Occasionally, these symptoms precede a more serious upper or lower respiratory tract infection. In very rare cases, the viraemic phase of the illness may be associated with a myocarditis. Each case should be dealt with on its merits. Children who have active viral illnesses such as chickenpox should not have elective surgery, nor should children who have recently been immunized using live vaccines, for two reasons: first, there is an associated myocarditis or pneumonitis; and, secondly, to protect others on the ward who may be immunocompromised.

It is extremely important that the child is weighed before arrival in theatre, because body weight is the simplest and most reliable guide to drug dosage. Veins suitable for insertion of a cannula should be identified and, if possible, local anaesthetic cream applied and covered with an occlusive dressing. If it has not been possible to weigh the child, the weight may be estimated from the child's age (Table 36.8).

Preoperative Fasting

Morbidity and mortality caused by aspiration of gastric contents are extremely rare in children undergoing elective surgery. What is becoming increasingly clear is that prolonged periods of starvation in children, especially the very young infant, are harmful. These children, who have a rapid turnover of fluids

TABLE 36.8
Estimates of Children's Weight

Age	Approximate Body Weight (kg)
Neonate	3
4 months	(Age in months × 0.5) + 4 = 6
1–8 years	(age in years × 2) + 8
9–13 years	(age in years × 3) + 7

and a high metabolic rate, are at risk of developing hypoglycaemia and hypovolaemia. Research has shown that children allowed unrestricted clear fluids up to 2 h before elective surgery have a gastric residual volume equal to or less than that of children who have been fasted overnight. The essential message is that children should, rather than could, be given clear fluids up to 2 h before induction. Solids (including breast and formula milk) should not be given for at least 6 h before the anticipated start of induction. In the emergency setting, e.g. the child who has sustained trauma shortly after ingesting food, it is probably best (if possible) to wait 4 h before inducing anaesthesia. Clearly, in this situation risk–benefit judgements have to be made. If it is surgically possible to wait 4 h, an i.v. infusion of a glucose-containing solution such as 5% dextrose with 0.9% NaCl, must be commenced and, if necessary, appropriate fluid resuscitation undertaken.

Premedication

The advent of local anaesthetic creams has reduced the necessity for sedative premedication. Currently, two formulations are available:

- *EMLA* (eutectic mixture of local anaesthetics) has been available for nearly two decades. Venepuncuture is usually painless if it has been applied and an occlusive dressing placed over the site at least 1 h before the planned procedure. It is wise to apply it over at least two locations marked by the anaesthetist in case the first attempt fails. It should not be used in the very small child or on mucous membranes because of the danger of systemic absorption of prilocaine that results in methaemoglobinaemia. It should not be left on the skin for more than 5 h. A major disadvantage of EMLA is that it causes some venoconstriction and this may obscure the vein.

- *Tetracaine gel* is the other agent available for this purpose. It has the advantage of a quicker onset of action and also provides analgesia for a considerable period of time after the occlusive dressing has been removed (4 h). This is an advantage in the day-care unit, because it may be applied as part of the admission procedure for all the children, left on for about 45 min and then removed, as small children often object to the presence of the occlusive dressing.

Occasionally, a sedative premedicant drug is required. This is particularly useful for the child who, in spite of good preoperative preparation, remains apprehensive. Currently, the injectable form of midazolam given orally is gaining widespread popularity. The dose used is $0.5 \, \text{mg kg}^{-1}$. An effect occurs within 10 min, with the peak at 20–30 min after administration. It may be used for day-case patients without a significant effect on discharge time. The bitter taste is a disadvantage. This should be eliminated when an oral formulation becomes available. One should err on reducing the dose if the patient is concurrently taking drugs which inhibit hepatic enzymes, because the duration of action of midazolam may be significantly prolonged.

An alternative to midazolam is oral ketamine in a dose $3–10 \, \text{mg kg}^{-1}$. An antisialagogue (e.g. atropine $0.02 \, \text{mg kg}^{-1}$) should be added to prevent excess salivation. The larger the dose, the more likely it is that the child may experience postoperative nausea and vomiting. If profound degrees of sedation are required, it is possible to combine midazolam and ketamine. The incidences of nausea and vomiting and of excess sedation in the postoperative period are increased.

Intramuscular premedication is generally not tolerated well by children. Often, it is the event in their hospital stay which they dislike the most. Rectal administration of induction agents has been used, such as thiopental in doses of $25–30 \, \text{mg kg}^{-1}$. This form of premedication should be used only under the direct supervision of the anaesthetist, as respiratory depression is a distinct possibility. A relatively new route for premedication administration is the intranasal route. This is particularly useful for the child who refuses to swallow an oral premedication. Drugs which have been used by this route include ketamine and midazolam in the doses mentioned above. At this stage, it is not known how much of the drug goes through the cribriform plate directly into the central nervous system. Until this issue is clarified, it is best not to use this route routinely, because midazolam or its preservative and the preservative used with ketamine are neurotoxic when applied directly to neural tissue.

Induction

It is important that children are accompanied into the anaesthetic room by someone with whom they are familiar. This person is usually a parent but may be a ward play specialist with whom the child feels comfortable. It is equally important that whoever accompanies the child is not coerced into doing so. Children usually detect anxiety in their parents and this tends to have an adverse effect on their behaviour.

The person accompanying the child should be informed on the ward of what to expect in the anaesthetic room. For example, if an inhalational induction is planned, he or she should be made aware of some of the signs of the excitation phase that the child might exhibit. If an i.v. induction is planned, the person should be made aware of how to assist the anaesthetist by distracting the child.

Unlike adult practice, it is not possible to have all the necessary monitoring devices placed on the child before induction. In most cases, it should be possible to place an appropriately sized pulse oximeter probe on a digit. Most children also allow the placement of a precordial stethoscope. The appropriate monitoring should be applied as soon as possible after the start of anaesthesia. The anaesthetist must always have present an assistant who is used to paediatric anaesthesia.

When inhalational induction is planned, clear, scented plastic masks are much more acceptable to small children than the traditional Rendell–Baker rubber masks. Clear masks allow respiration and the presence of vomitus to be observed. An alternative to using a mask is cupping the hands over the face of the child while holding the T-piece. It is important to ensure that the flow of fresh gas is directed away from the child's eyes because anaesthetic gases may be irritant.

Airway Management

The ratio of dead space to tidal volume tends to remain constant at about 0.3 throughout life in the healthy person. Anaesthetic apparatus such as connectors and humidification devices significantly increase dead space and should be kept to the minimum. This is especially important if the child breathes spontaneously during anaesthesia.

The Rendell–Baker masks were developed to fit around the facial anatomy of the child in an attempt to minimize equipment dead space. However, the flow of gas in a clear mask is such that the advantage of using Rendell-Baker masks is minimal. These masks are much more difficult to use than the clear ones with a pneumatic cushion. When using a face mask, it is important that the soft tissue behind the chin is not pushed backwards by the fingers, thereby obstructing the airway. The anaesthetist's fingers should rest only on the mandible.

The Jackson–Rees modification of the Ayre's T-piece is the breathing system used traditionally for children under 20 kg in weight. It has been designed to be lightweight with a minimal apparatus dead space. The apparatus may be used for both spontaneous and controlled ventilation. The open-ended reservoir bag is used for manually controlled ventilation. This mode of ventilation is especially useful in the neonate and infant, as the anaesthetist is able to detect changes in compliance produced by tube displacement. The reservoir bag also allows the application of continuous positive airway pressure for both the spontaneously breathing child and one undergoing artificial ventilation. This may be helpful in improving oxygenation. The bag may be removed and an appropriate ventilator such as the Penlon 200 attached to the expiratory limb. A minimum gas flow rate of 3 L min^{-1} is required to operate this apparatus satisfactorily. Fresh gas flows of 300 mL kg^{-1} for spontaneous respiration and flows of 1000 mL plus 100 mL kg^{-1} for controlled ventilation usually result in normocapnia. It is difficult to scavenge the T-piece system. For the older child, it is satisfactory to use a Bain, Humphrey ADE or circle absorber system. It is easy to scavenge the waste gases from these systems with the resultant benefit of reducing pollution of the theatre environment. In addition, the circle system offers economic advantages because of the low fresh gas flows required.

The Guedel airway is a useful adjunct in maintaining the airway of a child undergoing anaesthesia. It is important that the appropriate size of airway is used. If an airway is too small or too large, it may obstruct the child's airway completely. A reliable way of selecting the correct size is to place the flange of the airway at the angle of the mouth. The correctly sized airway should reach the angle of the mandible. The tongue should be depressed using a depressor or even the blade of the laryngoscope and the airway inserted. The method used in adults of rotating the airway through 180° during insertion is not recommended for small children because of the possibility of damaging the pharynx and subsequently compromising the airway. It is important that all procedures involving the airway of a child, including suction of the pharynx, are performed under direct vision.

The laryngeal mask airway is a major advance in anaesthetic airway management. It does not protect the airway against aspiration of refluxed gastric contents. It should be used only when it is planned that the child is to breathe spontaneously during surgery. It follows that it is unwise to use the device when neuromuscular blocking drugs are used. The mask may be displaced easily, which may result in airway obstruction and gastric insufflation. With these provisos, it may be used for a variety of operations where in the past tracheal intubation would have been mandatory, such as squint correction and tonsillectomy. Because of the large cross-sectional area of the mask tube, airway resistance increases only a small amount, if at all. Masks are available to fit all children, including neonates. The neonatal (size 1) mask is not popular for several reasons: it is relatively difficult to insert; it may be displaced very easily; and it increases apparatus dead space, resulting in rebreathing and hypercapnia.

It is mandatory to intubate the trachea during artificial ventilation. Intubation of the trachea confers many advantages. The lungs are protected against aspiration of gastric contents, ventilation is controlled and bronchoalveolar toilet may be performed. Operations in the oral cavity of a small child are not possible without tracheal intubation. It is very difficult to maintain the airway of a neonate using an airway and a face mask for any but the shortest surgical procedure requiring general anaesthesia. It is usually wise to intubate the trachea electively in most situations. Insertion of a tracheal tube results in a reduction of the cross-sectional area of the airway. A 3.5 mm tube in a neonate causes an increase in resistance by a factor of 16. Neonates with a tracheal tube must undergo artificial ventilation in order to reduce the work of breathing.

The vocal cords should be visible in order to be certain of intubating the trachea. In order to be able to do this, the anaesthetist has to align three imaginary axes: one through the trachea, one through the pharynx and one through the mouth. In the older child and adult, this is usually achieved by placing a pillow under the head – the familiar 'sniffing the morning air' position. A laryngoscope blade is then put into the vallecula in front of the epiglottis and the laryngeal structures lifted. Because of anatomical differences, the technique needs to be modified for the infant. Infants have a head which is large and a neck which is short relative to the size of the body. Instead of placing a pillow under the head, it is usually necessary to place a small pad or pillow under the torso. An alternative is to ask the assistant to gently raise the torso off the surface on which the child is lying. The larynx of a child under the age of 2 years tends to sit higher in the neck opposite the vertebral bodies of C3–4, whereas in the older child it is opposite C5–6. This results in the larynx being more anterior during laryngoscopy. The epiglottis of the infant is relatively large and, because the cartilaginous support is not fully developed, tends to be floppy. The anaesthetist cannot usually elevate the epiglottis sufficiently in order to be able to see the vocal cords if a curved blade such as the Macintosh is used. Instead, the anaesthetist has to use a straight blade and place it on the posterior surface of the epiglottis whilst lifting. In addition to the above, gentle cricoid pressure helps to bring the three axes into alignment. This may be performed with the little finger of the left hand.

In the adult, the narrowest part of the airway is the glottic opening. In the child, the narrowest part is the cricoid ring, which cannot be seen during laryngoscopy. It is very important that the correct size of tube is selected. If too large a tube is selected, the tracheal mucosa is damaged and the child may develop post-intubation croup; if it is too small, excessive leak makes effective positive pressure ventilation impossible. The ring forms a natural cuff around the tube, thereby eliminating the need for a pneumatic cuff. Generally, cuffed tubes are used only in children above the age of 8 years. The reason for this is that the pressure may render the underlying trachea ischaemic and subsequently lead to post-intubation croup. If possible, tracheal intubation should not be performed in children having day-case procedures. The laryngeal mask has eliminated the need for this.

The following formulae are used to calculate the internal diameter of the appropriate size of tube for children greater than one year:

$$(age/4) + 4.5 \text{ mm (uncuffed)}$$
$$(age/4) = 3.5 \text{ mm (cuffed)}$$

An alternative is to use a tube with an external diameter similar to that of the child's little finger. It is important that tubes with internal diameters 0.5 mm larger and smaller than the predicted size are readily available.

The tip of the tracheal tube should lie at the mid-trachea. For oral intubation, the measurement from the alveolar ridge to the mid-trachea is about (age/2)+12 cm. An alternative is three times the internal diameter of the tube. For nasal intubation, the measurement is (age/2)+15 cm.

For neonates, the best guide is related to weight (Table 36.9).

After tracheal intubation has been performed, the lung fields and epigastrium should be auscultated to confirm correct placement. Additional confirmation of correct placement using a capnograph is essential. If intubation has been preceded by a period of difficult mask ventilation, it is not unusual for the stomach to become inflated. The inflated stomach decreases excursion of the lungs and results in arterial desaturation. If this has occurred, the stomach should be deflated by passing an orogastric tube, which is removed as soon as the task is complete.

Because children have a relatively short trachea, it is easy for the tube to become displaced and enter a main bronchus or for the trachea to become extubated. It is vital that the tube is well secured. It is best to use adhesive tape and secure the tube to the immobile maxilla rather than to the mandible. Preformed tubes such as the RAE are not recommended for the infant because inadvertent bronchial intubation easily occurs.

Monitoring

There is no substitute for an experienced, vigilant anaesthetist directly observing the child. Changes in colour, inappropriate movement, respiratory obstruction and changes in respiratory pattern may be observed quickly and treated. Temperature should be monitored at an appropriate site for all but the shortest procedures. It is unwise even to consider extubating the trachea of a hypothermic infant. Ideally, ECG and arterial pressure monitoring should be in place before induction. In practice, this is not always possible. Usually, these devices are put in place as soon as the child is asleep. Capnography is mandatory for the child who has a tracheal tube or laryngeal mask.

Day Surgery

Day-case surgery confers many advantages in children. Children who are admitted to hospital often develop behavioural problems, perhaps as a result of separation from parents and disruption of family life. These problems may manifest as an alteration of sleep pattern, bedwetting and regression of developmental milestones.

Most children make excellent candidates for day-case surgery. They are usually healthy and the procedures performed are usually of short to intermediate duration. Only experienced surgeons and anaesthetists should undertake day-case surgery. Because this form of surgery is performed by experienced personnel, even ASA III patients may be considered. Children who are under 60 weeks' postconceptual age, those who have diseases that are not well controlled (e.g. poorly controlled epilepsy) and those with metabolic disease (e.g. insulin-dependent diabetes) which may result in hypoglycaemia should always be admitted electively for overnight stay.

Parents must be given clear written instructions well before the planned date of surgery. They should be told how long their child should be fasted before surgery. They should also be asked to make

TABLE 36.9
Estimates of Tracheal Tube Size in Neonates

Weight (kg)	Internal Diameter (mm)	Length from Alveolar Ridge (cm)
1	2.5	7
2	3	8
3	3.5	9

arrangements so that two responsible adults with their own transport accompany the child home.

Sedative premedication is rarely required for a child who has been well prepared. Children accompanied to the anaesthetic room by their parents usually remain calm. It makes sense to use agents with the shortest half-life. Regional anaesthesia performed after induction is useful in reducing the amount of anaesthetic needed intraoperatively and also provides excellent postoperative analgesia, especially when long-acting agents such as bupivacaine or ropivacaine are used. Paracetamol or diclofenac given as suppositories at the end of surgery ensure that the child remains comfortable when the local anaesthetic has regressed. It is essential to seek the parent's informed consent for regional anaesthesia and rectal analgesics.

After surgery, the child should be allowed to recover in a fully equipped and staffed recovery ward. The child is returned to the day ward only when protective reflexes have returned. The child is discharged home when oral fluids are tolerated, but if the child has received intraoperative hydration, it is possible to ignore this criterion. Another yardstick used is whether the child has passed urine or not; this is particularly important if the child has been given a caudal block. Occasionally, caudal blocks and inguinal blocks result in weakness of the leg. In this case, it is advisable to wait for the block to regress before discharging the child; clearly, this applies only to children who are walking. Ondansetron is useful in the treatment of postoperative nausea and vomiting, as the lack of any sedative effect is conducive to an early discharge. Children who have undergone tracheal intubation should remain on the day ward for at least 2 h to ensure that post-intubation croup does not occur.

Parents should be given an adequate supply of postoperative analgesics. It is crucial to emphasize the importance of giving analgesics pre-emptively 'by the clock' instead of waiting for the child to complain of pain.

Paediatric Regional Anaesthesia

Most children admitted to hospital experience regional anaesthesia. The commonest use is probably the application of topical preparations of lidocaine/prilocaine or tetracaine before venesection or intravenous cannulation. Topical anaesthesia is not limited to these uses. It may be used as the sole anaesthetic, in suitable children, for procedures such as division of preputial adhesions and removal of simple skin lesions. Procedures performed in this way often do not involve an anaesthetist.

Whenever possible, regional anaesthesia is combined with general anaesthesia. Children who are anaesthetized in this way wake up quickly and appear to be less troubled by nausea and vomiting than when general anaesthesia is used without a regional block. In the day-case surgery setting, this leads to earlier discharge and a more pleasant experience for the child and the family.

Wound infiltration is a technique which is not usually performed by, but which is supervised by, the anaesthetist. Examples include wound infiltration after pyloromyotomy or herniotomy. The anaesthetist advises the surgeon as to the volume of anaesthetic that may be used safely. This technique is mostly used at the end of surgery because of the distortion of anatomy that the infiltration of local anaesthetic might cause. Occasionally, the surgeon may be persuaded to inject at the beginning, especially if local anaesthetic with a vasoconstrictor is used, as this provides the surgeon with a 'dry' field. A good example of this would be for removal of accessory auricles or encapsulated subcutaneous lesions.

Central neuraxial and peripheral nerve blocks are almost always performed on anaesthetized children. The anaesthetist must therefore be experienced in identifying fascial planes with needles and must also be confident with the use of the nerve stimulator. A peripheral block is usually preferred to a neuraxial block because of a lower complication rate. Complications associated with neuraxial blocks include inadvertent intravascular or intrathecal injection and permanent nerve injury. The risk:benefit ratio and surgical/patient considerations have to be taken into account before selecting a block. For example, a penile ring block, while safe and simple, might make it difficult for the surgeon to perform a circumcision.

The ilioinguinal/iliohypogastric block is used for surgery in the groin area. It provides excellent analgesia for inguinal herniotomy. This block may be combined with infiltration anaesthesia if the child needs orchidopexy. Local anaesthetic is deposited under the aponeurosis of the external oblique muscle at a point a finger's breadth medial to the anterior superior iliac spine. Very occasionally, the local anaesthetic may block the femoral nerve. The parents should be warned about this beforehand so that they can assist their child when taking the first steps after anaesthesia.

The dorsal nerves of the penis are blocked by injection of local anaesthetic, each side of the midline, into the subpubic space. If more than 0.1 mL kg^{-1} is injected, the anatomy may be distorted. The block is appropriate for circumcision but for hypospadias surgery a caudal epidural is probably a better choice. The dorsal penile arteries, which run alongside the nerves, are end arteries. The local anaesthetic solution should not contain vasoconstrictor.

The paediatric equivalent of the 3-in-1 femoral nerve block is the fascia iliaca block. The femoral, obturator and lateral cutaneous nerves of the thigh are blocked reliably using this approach. The block has the advantage of being distant from neurovascular structures, thereby reducing the opportunity for complications. The injection point is as follows. A line is drawn from the anterior superior iliac spine to the pubic tubercle. The needle is inserted 0.5 cm below this line at the junction of the medial two-thirds and lateral one-third. The regional block needle is advanced until two 'pops' have been felt and the local anaesthetic is then deposited. The two 'pops' represent the needle traversing the fascia lata and fascia iliaca, respectively. The block may be used to reduce femoral fractures in the Accident and Emergency department. An elegant technique is to apply topical local anaesthetic to the injection site before performing the block. The block may also be used to obtain muscle biopsies. Metatarsal and metacarpal blocks are usually the only blocks required for surgery on the extremities. It is unusual to require a brachial plexus block.

The combination of auriculotemporal and great auricular nerve blocks is useful for pinnaplasty. Operation on the ears is associated with nausea and vomiting and it is probable that these blocks help to reduce the incidence of these side-effects. The great auricular nerve is a branch of the superficial cervical plexus. It is blocked by infiltrating about 3 mL of local anaesthetic anterior to the tip of the mastoid process. This anaesthetizes the posterior aspect and the lower third of the anterior surface of the ear. The auriculotemporal nerve is a branch of the mandibular division of the trigeminal nerve and it supplies the superior two-thirds of the anterior surface of the ear. An additional 1–2 mL of local anaesthetic deposited subcutaneously immediately anterior to the external auditory meatus blocks this nerve.

Caudal epidural blockade is probably the most commonly used block in children. The sacrococcygeal membrane (otherwise known as the sacral hiatus) represents the unfused laminae of the S5 vertebral body. The sacral hiatus is at the apex of an equilateral triangle, the base of which is a line joining the posterior iliac spines. In children, this point is higher than might be expected and it is always above the natal cleft. The epidural space in children is devoid of fat. This implies that by increasing the volume of solution injected, a predictably higher dermatomal level may be reached. The Armitage formula is the most commonly used to calculate the volume of local anaesthetic. Analgesia over the sacral dermatomes is achieved by injecting 0.5 mL kg^{-1} volume of solution. It is necessary to inject 1 mL kg^{-1} to reach the lower thoracic dermatomes and 1.25 mL kg^{-1} to reach the mid-thoracic dermatomes. Another benefit derived from the absence of epidural fat is that it is possible to advance a catheter from the sacral region to the mid-thoracic region. This is used to provide analgesia after laparotomy in neonates. In small babies, the epidural space may be found at a depth of approximately 1 mm kg^{-1} from skin. In older children, the thoracic dermatomes may be blocked by threading the catheter from the lumbar epidural space to the thoracic. It is safer to avoid a direct thoracic approach because the tributaries to the anterior spinal artery may be damaged easily. Sometimes, preservative-free clonidine or ketamine is added to the local anaesthetic mixture to prolong the duration of a single-shot caudal. The dural sac in babies usually ends opposite the S3–S4 intervertebral space and, because of differential growth, rises to end opposite the S1–S2 intervertebral space. Therefore, there is a potential for a total spinal block after caudal injection. The chances of this complication occurring may be reduced significantly by careful attention to how far the needle or cannula is inserted into the space. After insertion of the needle or cannula, the anaesthetist should wait a short while with the hub open to air so that blood or CSF may drip out; if this happens, the technique has to be abandoned.

In babies, the spinal cord ends opposite the body of L3. Because of differential growth, the spinal cord 'ascends' in the spinal canal so that by the time the child is 1 year old it is at the adult level opposite the L1–2 intervertebral space. In the UK, spinal anaesthesia may be used to provide anaesthesia for infraumbilical surgery in the ex-premature infant who is less than 60 weeks' postconceptual age. At any age, damage to the spinal cord is avoided by injecting below an imaginary line joining the iliac crests.

The introduction of portable ultrasound to the theatre environment has greatly facilitated the provision of regional anaesthesia for children. The fact that neural structures and the anatomical planes through which they traverse are quite superficial means that high resolution ultrasound can be used. Consequently, local anaesthetic can be deposited very precisely in patients who are under general anaesthetic. Smaller volumes of local anaesthetic can be used and the quality of analgesia is generally excellent. When ultrasound is used, peripheral blocks can be a reliable alternative to central neuraxial blockade. In the very young, ultrasound can aid the performance of central neuraxial blocks both for the definition of anatomy and visualization of the catheter.

SPECIFIC OPERATIONS IN THE NEONATE

Inguinal Hernia Repair

This is one of the commonest operations in the neonatal period. The incidence in this age group is highest amongst preterm infants. There is debate about the most appropriate method of anaesthesia; the choice is based on individual patient factors and the particular skills and experience of the surgeon and anaesthetist. Spinal anaesthesia offers the advantage of a quick onset with profound muscle relaxation in less than 2 min. Unfortunately, the duration of action is very short – of the order of about 40 min; the reason for this is probably a higher cardiac index than in adults. Addition of an α_1-agonist such as phenylephrine or adrenaline may prolong the block to about 1 h. Caudal anaesthesia is also possible in this situation, the main disadvantages being a slower onset time and the potential complications of injecting large quantities of local anaesthetic.

However, the block lasts a long time so that bilateral hernia repair is easily possible. The child should have an intravenous cannula *in situ*, but unlike adult practice, there is no need for volume preloading, nor is there a need to administer vasoactive drugs such as ephedrine.

Pyloromyotomy

Pyloric stenosis usually presents in weeks 4–8 of life. A previously well male child develops projectile vomiting. Untreated, the child becomes severely dehydrated with a hypokalaemic, hypochloraemic metabolic alkalosis. Because the obstruction is at the level of the pylorus, the body loses hydrogen and chloride ions but none of the alkaline small bowel secretions. The kidney is thus presented with a large bicarbonate load, which exceeds its absorptive threshold and this results initially in alkaline urine. As further fluid depletion occurs, the renin-angiotensin-aldosterone axis is activated in an attempt to preserve circulating volume. This results in an exchange of sodium ions for hydrogen and potassium ions, which leads to a paradoxical aciduria with a worsening hypokalaemia and metabolic alkalosis.

The initial management is insertion of a nasogastric tube and an intravenous cannula. A solution of 5% glucose in 0.45% saline to which 40 mmol L^{-1} of potassium chloride has been added is given at a rate of 6 mL kg^{-1} h^{-1}. The nasogastric tube is aspirated and the aspirate replaced with 0.9% saline. The child is ready for surgery between 24 and 48 h after this regimen is started. A normal serum potassium concentration and a bicarbonate concentration of 25 mmol L^{-1} are used to indicate that sufficient volume replacement has taken place.

In theatre, the child's stomach should be washed with warm saline until the aspirated fluid is clear. Induction should be smooth, by either the inhalational or intravenous route according to the experience of the anaesthetist. Postoperative analgesia is provided by wound infiltration followed by either rectal or oral paracetamol, depending on when the surgeon decides that the child may be fed.

Tracheo-Oesophageal Fistula and Oesophageal Atresia

Six types of this condition (A–F) have been described. The commonest is C in which the proximal oesophagus ends as a diverticulum and the lower part exists as a fistula off the trachea just above the carina. Cardiovascular anomalies such as a septal defect or coarctation of the aorta often coexist with this condition. An echocardiogram should always be performed before surgery. The corrective surgery should be performed as a matter of urgency as a one-stage repair because delay results in soiling of the lungs and pneumonitis. Preoperatively, the child should be nursed in an upright position to prevent soiling of the lungs by gastric fluid. It is important that a tube is placed in the diverticulum and continuous suction applied to aspirate the saliva that the child cannot swallow. If the lungs become soiled, then antibiotics and physiotherapy are required and the operation should be performed as soon as the child's condition has been optimized.

An inhalational induction is the preferred method for induction. Positive-pressure ventilation results in distension of the stomach and subsequent impairment of oxygenation. The tracheal tube should be inserted with the bevel facing up so that the posterior wall of the tube occludes the fistula. Initially, the tube should be inserted further than predicted and then withdrawn gently until both lungs are being ventilated. Manual ventilation is recommended because surgical traction may easily occlude the neonate's soft trachea.

Postoperatively, the lungs should be ventilated artificially so that adequate amounts of analgesia may be given and also to prevent traction on the oesophageal anastomosis by movement of the head.

Diaphragmatic Hernia

In this condition, the abdominal contents herniate through a defect in the diaphragm, usually on the left side. The abdominal contents exert pressure on the developing lung and, if the defect is large enough, the mediastinum is shifted to the right and the growth of the contralateral lung is also impaired. Repair of the hernia is not an emergency and the child should be managed medically. Problems which have to be managed include ventilation, acidosis and pulmonary hypertension. Surgery is considered when the child's condition has been optimized medically. Positive-pressure ventilation by bag and mask may expand the abdominal viscera and should be avoided. Nitrous oxide should also be avoided for the same reason.

The defect is usually repaired through an abdominal incision. It is not always possible to fit the viscera in the peritoneal cavity, in which case a silastic silo may be used and the contents introduced gradually. It is wise to avoid cannulation of veins in the lower extremity because the return of abdominal viscera increases the pressure in the inferior vena cava. Infants who present soon after birth with severe symptoms do not usually survive because they have inadequate amounts of lung tissue to sustain life.

Exomphalos and Gastroschisis

Embryologically, these are two separate conditions. However, both present similar challenges to the anaesthetist. The abdominal contents, which have herniated through the abdominal wall, offer a large surface area from which heat and fluid may be lost. It is imperative that the abdominal contents are placed into a clear sterile polythene bag as soon as possible after birth. The defects should be corrected as a matter of urgency. Nitrous oxide should be avoided to facilitate surgery and a nasogastric tube must be in place to decompress the stomach. If it is not possible to return all the viscera into the peritoneal cavity a silastic silo may be used. It is usual to ventilate the child's lungs postoperatively because of the reduction in compliance caused by return of the viscera to the peritoneum. As with all congenital anomalies, associated abnormalities are described with these conditions, particularly with exomphalos.

Postoperative Care

Unless they are to be admitted to an ICU, all children should be nursed in a properly equipped and staffed recovery unit. Oxygen should be administered until the child has a good oxygen saturation breathing room air. The cardiovascular and respiratory systems should be monitored and interventions carried out appropriately. It is becoming increasingly popular to have a step-down area attached to the recovery unit. This is an area where the child may be accompanied by the parents but may still be monitored closely. The child is returned to the ward when warm, pain-free and haemodynamically stable. It is the anaesthetist's responsibility to ensure that appropriate analgesia and intravenous fluids have been prescribed.

Useful information for dealing with paediatric emergencies is shown in Table 36.10.

TABLE 36.10
Paediatric Resuscitation Chart

AGE AND WEIGHT

	Neonate 3.5 kg	3 Months 5 kg	1 Year 10 kg	3 Years 15 kg	6 Years 20 kg	8 years 25 kg	12 years 40 kg
Tracheal Tube							
Size; mm	3.0–3.5	3.5–4.0	4.5	5.0	6.0	5.5 (cuffed)	6.5 (cuffed)
Length (oral); cm	9	10	11	13	14	15	17
Length (nasal); cm	11	13	14	16	19	20	22
Adrenaline 1:10 000							
i.v./i.o./t.0.1 mL kg⁻¹ repeated as necessary	0.5 mL	0.5 mL	1 mL	1.5 mL	2 mL	2.5 mL	4 mL
Sodium Bicarbonate 8.4%							
1 mL kg⁻¹ i.v.	3 mL	5 mL	10 mL	15 mL	20 mL	25 mL	40 mL
Atropine 500 µg in 5 mL							
0.2 mL kg⁻¹ i.v./t.	1 mL	1 mL	2 mL	3 mL	4 mL	5 mL	8 mL
Calcium Chloride 10%							
0.1 mL kg⁻¹ i.v.	0.5 mL	0.5 mL	1 mL	1.5 mL	2 mL	2.5 mL	4 mL
Defibrillation (J)							
4 J kg⁻¹	10	20	40	60	80	100	160
Colloid Volume (mL)							
10 mL kg⁻¹ × 2–3 as necessary	35	50	100	150	200	250	400

i.v., intravenous; i.o., intraosseous; t., tracheal.
N.B. All drugs and fluids may be administered via the intraosseous route.
Drug infusions
Adrenaline: 0.03 mg kg⁻¹ in 50 mL glucose 5%; start at 2 mL h⁻¹.
Dopamine: 3 mg kg⁻¹ in 50 mL glucose 5%; 3–20 mL h⁻¹.
Dobutamine: 3 mg kg⁻¹ in 50 mL glucose 5%; 5–20 mL h⁻¹.

FURTHER READING

Anon, 1999. Postgraduate educational issue: the paediatric patient. Br. J. Anaesth. 83, 16–129.

Arthurs, G., Nicholls, B., 2009. Ultrasound in anaesthetic practice. Cambridge University Press, Cambridge.

Baum, V., O'Flaherty, J., 2006. Anesthesia for genetic, metabolic and dysmorphic syndromes of childhood. Lippincott Williams & Wilkins, Baltimore.

Dalens, B., 2001. Regional anesthesia for infants, children and adolescents, second ed. Williams & Wilkins, Baltimore.

In: McKenzie, I., Gaukroger, P.B., Ragg, P., Brown, T.C.K., (eds), 1997. Manual of acute pain management in children. Churchill Livingstone, Edinburgh.

Motoyama, E.K., Davis, P.J., 2006. Smith's anesthesia for infants and children. Mosby, St Louis.

Peutrell, J.M., Mather, S.J., 1997. Regional anaesthesia for babies and children. Oxford University Press, Oxford.

Rowney, D.A., Doyle, E., 1998. Epidural and subarachnoid blockade in children. Anaesthesia 53, 980–1001.

37

EMERGENCY ANAESTHESIA

P atients scheduled for elective surgery are usually in optimal physical and mental condition, with a definitive surgical diagnosis; any coexisting medical disease is defined and well controlled. In contrast, the patient with a surgical emergency may have an uncertain diagnosis and uncontrolled coexisting medical disease, in addition to any physiological derangements resulting from their surgical pathology. Thus, a major principle governing the practice of emergency anaesthesia is to identify and, if time permits, correct any major physiological abnormalities preoperatively. In addition, the anaesthetist must be prepared for potential complications arising as a consequence of anaesthetizing a patient in sub-optimal condition. These include vomiting and regurgitation, hypovolaemia and haemorrhage, and abnormal reactions to drugs in the presence of electrolyte disturbances and renal impairment.

PREOPERATIVE ASSESSMENT

The objective of emergency anaesthesia is to permit correction of the surgical pathology with the minimum risk to the patient. This requires adequate and accurate preoperative evaluation of the patient's general condition, with particular attention to specific problems that may influence anaesthetic management.

The likely surgical diagnosis, and the extent and urgency of the proposed surgery must be discussed with surgical and medical colleagues preoperatively. The urgency for surgery is most helpfully conveyed using a recognized classification system, such as the one created by the National Confidential Enquiry into Patient Outcome and Death (NCEPOD) (Table 37.1).

The nature and urgency of the planned surgery dictate the extent of preoperative preparation and anaesthetic technique. They also influence plans for postoperative care, which may include transfer to a HDU/ICU facility.

During the preoperative visit a past medical and drug history is elicited. In particular, the patient's degree of cardiorespiratory reserve should be established, even if there is no formal diagnosis of cardiovascular or respiratory disease. The presence and severity of symptoms suggestive of reduced reserve such as angina, productive cough, orthopnoea or paroxysmal nocturnal dyspnoea should be sought. The patient's functional capacity is of useful prognostic value and can be simply quantified in terms of *metabolic equivalents (METs)*. 1 MET is a unit of resting oxygen consumption and appropriate questioning can allow an estimate of the patient's maximal oxygen consumption capacity (VO_2 max) (Table 37.2 and Ch 18 [Table 18.1]). A patient who is unable to perform activity at 4 METs or more is at increased risk of perioperative cardiac complications.

Depending upon the urgency of surgery, the physical examination may be targeted to identify significant cardiorespiratory dysfunction or any abnormalities that might lead to technical difficulties during anaesthesia. Basal crepitations, pitting oedema and raised jugular venous pulse signify impaired ventricular function and limited cardiac reserve, which significantly increase the risk of anaesthesia. It is also important to exclude arrhythmias and heart sounds indicative of valvular heart disease, as these influence the patient's response to physiological challenges and

TABLE 37.1

NCEPOD Classification of Intervention

Code	Category	Description	Target Time to Theatre	Expected Location	Examples	Typical Procedures
1	Immediate	Immediate (A) life-saving or (B) limb or organ saving intervention. Resuscitation simultaneous with surgical intervention	Within minutes of decision to operate	Next available operating theatre – "break in" to existing lists, if required	-Ruptured aortic aneurysm -Major trauma to abdomen or thorax -Fracture with major neurovascular deficit	-Repair of ruptured aortic aneurysm -Laparotomy/ thoracotomy for control of haemorrhage
2	Urgent	Acute onset or deterioration of conditions that threaten life, limb or organ survival; fixation of fractures; relief of distressing symptoms	Within hours of decision to operate and normally once resuscitation complete	Day time "emergency list" Or Out-of-hours emergency theatre (including at night)	-Compound fracture -Perforated bowel with peritonitis -Critical organ or limb ischaemia -Penetrating eye injury	-Debridement plus fixation of fracture -Laparotomy for perforation
3	Expedited	Stable patient requiring early intervention for a condition that is not an immediate threat to life, limb or organ survival	Within days of decision to operate	Elective list which has "spare" capacity Or Day time emergency list (not at night)	-Tendon and nerve injuries -Stable & non-septic patients for wide range of surgical procedures -Penetrating eye injuries	-Repair of tendon and nerve injuries -Excision of tumour with potential to bleed or obstruct
4	Elective	Surgical procedure planned or booked in advance of routine admission to hospital	Planned	Elective theatre list booked & planned before admission	-Encompasses all conditions not classified as immediate, urgent or expedited	-Elective AAA repair -Laparoscopic cholecystectomy

TABLE 37.2	
Metabolic Equivalents	
MET Score	Approximate Level of Activity
1	Dress, walk indoors
2	Light housework, slow walk
4	Climb one flight of stairs
6	Moderate sport eg golf or dancing
10	Strenuous sport or exercise

thus anaesthetic management. Assessment of respiratory function is particularly difficult, as the patient in pain (with or without peritoneal irritation) may be unable to cooperate with pulmonary function testing.

Valuable information about the patient's condition can also be obtained from the bedside observations chart. In particular, trends in physiological variables such as arterial pressure, heart rate and respiratory rate may signal a deteriorating condition, and even impending decompensation.

Preoperative evaluation of the airway is always important. The standard clinical tests of airway assessment should be used (see Ch 21: The practical conduct of anaesthesia) and any previous anaesthetic charts consulted if available. A history of difficult intubation is of considerable significance; however, a past record of easy tracheal intubation does not guarantee future success. In emergency anaesthesia, airway difficulties may be caused by the patient's usual anatomy, but also surgical pathology such as dental abscesses, trauma and bleeding or haematoma. If a rapid-sequence induction is contemplated, then contingency plans are required for management of the patient in the event of failure to intubate the trachea. If a high degree of difficulty in tracheal intubation is anticipated then an awake technique may be necessary.

The final stage of the preoperative assessment is to review any laboratory investigations, including ECGs, radiological imaging and arterial blood gases where appropriate. The availability of blood products should be checked if necessary and urgent requests should be made for any additional tests which may influence patient management.

Assessment of Circulating Volume

Assessment of intravascular volume is essential, as underestimated or unrecognized hypovolaemia may lead to circulatory collapse during induction of anaesthesia, which attenuates the sympathetically mediated increases in arteriolar and venous constriction as well as reducing cardiac output. In any patient in whom fluid is sequestered or lost (e.g. peritonitis, bowel obstruction) or in whom haemorrhage has occurred (e.g. trauma), the anaesthetist should try to quantify the circulating/intravascular blood volume or extracellular fluid volume, and correct any deficit.

Intravascular Volume Deficit

Blood loss may be assessed using the patient's history and any measured losses, but more commonly the anaesthetist has to rely on clinical evaluation of the patient's current cardiovascular status. Profound circulatory shock with hypotension, poor peripheral perfusion, oliguria and altered cerebration is easy to recognize. However, a more careful assessment is needed to recognise the early manifestations of haemorrhage, such as tachycardia and cutaneous vasoconstriction. Useful indices include heart rate, arterial pressure (especially pulse pressure), the state of the peripheral circulation, central venous pressure and urine output. Table 37.3 describes approximate correlations among these clinical indices and the extent of haemorrhage, but it should be stressed that these refer to the 'ideal' patient. In young, healthy adults, arterial pressure may be an unreliable guide to volume status because compensatory mechanisms can prevent a measurable decrease in arterial pressure until more than 30% of the patient's blood volume has been lost. In such patients, attention should be directed to pulse rate, skin circulation and a narrowing pulse pressure. Tachycardia in the presence of a normal arterial pressure should never automatically be attributed to pain or anxiety if there is a clinical history consistent with the potential for intravascular volume loss. In elderly patients with widespread arterial disease, limited cardiac reserve and a rigid vascular tree (fixed total peripheral resistance), signs of severe hypovolaemia may become evident when blood volume has been reduced by as little as 15%. However, as baroreceptor sensitivity decreases with age, elderly patients may exhibit less tachycardia for any degree of volume depletion.

TABLE 37.3
Clinical Indices of Extent of Blood Loss

Class of Hypovolaemia	1 Minimal	2 Mild	3 Moderate	4 Severe
Percentage blood volume lost	10	20	30	Over 40
Volume lost (mL)	500	1000	1500	2000+
Heart rate (beat min^{-1})	Normal	100–120	120–140	Over 140
Arterial pressure (mmHg)	Normal	Orthostatic hypotension	Systolic below 100	Systolic below 80
Urinary output (mL h^{-1})	Normal (1 mL kg^{-1} h^{-1})	20–30	10–20	Nil
Sensorium	Normal	Normal	Restless	Impaired consciousness
State of peripheral circulation	Normal	Cool and pale	Cold and pale, slow capillary refill	Cold and clammy Peripheral cyanosis

In general, hypovolaemia does not become apparent clinically until circulating blood volume has been reduced by at least 20% (approximately 1000 mL). A reduction by more than 30% of blood volume occurs before the classic 'shock syndrome' is produced, with hypotension, tachycardia, oliguria and cold, clammy extremities. Haemorrhage greater than 40% of blood volume may be associated with loss of the compensatory mechanisms that maintain cerebral and coronary blood flow, and the patient becomes restless, agitated and eventually comatose. In patients with major trauma, it is valuable to compare the clinical assessment of the extent of haemorrhage with the measured or assumed loss. A marked disparity between these two estimates often leads to a diagnosis of a further concealed source of haemorrhage.

Whilst clinical evaluation remains the most important and most frequently used guide to the management of intravascular volume deficit, the use of non-invasive and minimally-invasive methods of cardiac output measurement in this setting is growing. These techniques may be of particular benefit in guiding the immediate resuscitation of frail or critically ill patients.

Extracellular Volume Deficit

Assessment of extracellular fluid volume deficit is difficult. Guidance may be obtained from the nature of the surgical condition, the duration of impaired fluid intake and the presence and severity of symptoms associated with abnormal losses (e.g. vomiting). At the time of the earliest radiological evidence of intestinal obstruction, there may be 1500 mL of fluid sequestered in the bowel lumen. If the obstruction is well established and vomiting has occurred, the extracellular fluid deficit may exceed 3000 mL. Table 37.4 describes some of the clinical features seen with varying degrees of severity of extracellular fluid losses. It is clear that considerable losses must occur before clinical signs are apparent, and that these signs are often subjective in more minor degrees of extracellular fluid deficit.

In addition to clinical signs, laboratory investigations may also indicate extracellular fluid volume deficit. Haemoconcentration results in an increased haemoglobin concentration and an increased packed cell volume. As dehydration becomes more marked, renal blood flow diminishes, reducing renal clearance of urea and consequently increasing the blood urea concentration. Patients with moderate volume contraction exhibit a 'pre-renal' pattern of uraemia characterized by an increase in blood urea out of proportion to any increase in serum creatinine concentration. Under maximal stimulation from ADH and aldosterone, conservation of sodium and water by the kidneys results in excretion of urine of low sodium concentration (0–15 mmol L^{-1}) and high osmolality (800–1400 mosmol kg^{-1}).

TABLE 37.4
Indices of Extent of Loss of Extracellular Fluid

Percentage Body Weight Lost as Water	mL of Fluid Lost per 70 kg	Signs and Symptoms
Over 4% (mild)	Over 2500	Thirst, reduced skin elasticity, decreased intraocular pressure, dry tongue, reduced sweating
Over 6% (mild)	Over 4200	As above, plus orthostatic hypotension, reduced filling of peripheral veins, oliguria, low CVP, apathy, haemoconcentration
Over 8% (moderate)	Over 5600	As above, plus hypotension, thready pulse with cool peripheries
10–15% (severe)	7000–10 500	Coma, shock followed by death

Once the extent of blood volume or extracellular fluid volume deficit has been estimated, deficits should be corrected with the appropriate intravenous fluid. The overall priority is to maintain adequate tissue perfusion and oxygenation, therefore correction of intravascular deficit takes precedence – hypovolaemia due to blood loss should be treated with either a balanced crystalloid solution (such as Hartmann's solution) or a suitable colloid until packed red cells are available (see Ch 12: Fluid, electrolyte and acid–base balance). Resuscitation is usually guided by clinical indices of circulating volume status and organ perfusion. Central venous pressure (CVP) measurement has often been used to guide fluid therapy but CVP has limitations when used to predict intravascular volume status and responsiveness to infused fluids. High-risk surgical patients may benefit from the use of (non-invasive) cardiac output measuring devices to direct fluid resuscitation towards predetermined goals for cardiac output and systemic oxygen delivery.

Extracellular fluid deficit is usually corrected after the correction of any intravascular deficit, by adjusting maintenance fluid infusion rates. Losses from vomiting or gastric aspirates are best replaced by crystalloid solutions containing an appropriate potassium supplement. Hartmann's solution is often used, although hypochloraemia is an indication for saline 0.9% (with additional potassium). Lower GI losses, such as those due to diarrhoea or intestinal obstruction, are normally replaced volume-for-volume with Hartmann's solution.

THE FULL STOMACH

Vomiting or regurgitation of gastric contents, followed by aspiration into the tracheobronchial tree whilst protective laryngeal reflexes are obtunded, is one of the commonest and most devastating hazards of emergency anaesthesia.

Vomiting is an active process that occurs in the lighter planes of anaesthesia. Consequently, it is a potential problem during induction of, or emergence from, anaesthesia, but should not occur during maintenance if anaesthesia is sufficiently deep. In light planes of anaesthesia, the presence of vomited material above the vocal cords stimulates spasm of the cords. This reflex provides a degree of protection against material entering the larynx and tracheobronchial tree. However, apnoea occurs as a consequence and may persist until severe hypoxaemia or even cardiac arrest occurs. If the spasm does resolve then aspiration may occur unless the supraglottic debris has been cleared by the anaesthetist before the resumption of ventilation.

In contrast to vomiting, regurgitation is a passive process that may occur at any time, is often 'silent' (i.e. not apparent to the anaesthetist) and, if aspiration occurs, may have clinical consequences ranging from minor pulmonary sequelae to fulminating aspiration pneumonitis and acute respiratory distress syndrome (ARDS). Regurgitation usually occurs in the presence of deep anaesthesia or at the onset of action of neuromuscular blocking drugs, when laryngeal protective reflexes are absent and so the risk of aspiration is increased.

The most important factors determining the risk and degree of gastric regurgitation are lower oesophageal sphincter function and residual gastric volume, which itself is largely determined by the duration of fasting and rate of gastric emptying.

The Lower Oesophageal Sphincter

The lower oesophageal sphincter (LOS) is a 2–5 cm length of oesophagus with higher resting intraluminal pressure situated just proximal to the cardia of the stomach. The sphincter relaxes during oesophageal peristalsis to allow food into the stomach, but remains contracted at other times. The structure cannot be defined anatomically but may be detected using intraluminal pressure manometry.

The LOS is the main barrier preventing reflux of gastric contents into the oesophagus. Many drugs used in anaesthetic practice affect the resting tone of the LOS. Reflux is related not to the LOS tone per se, but to the difference between gastric and LOS pressures; this is termed the *barrier pressure*. Drugs that increase the barrier pressure (e.g. cyclizine, anticholinesterases, α-adrenergic agonists and metoclopramide) decrease the risk of reflux. For many years it was thought that the increase in intragastric pressure during succinylcholine-induced fasciculations predisposed to reflux. However, LOS tone is also increased by succinylcholine and so barrier pressure is maintained.

Anticholinergic drugs, ethanol, tricyclic antidepressants, opioids and thiopental reduce LOS pressure and it is reasonable to assume that these drugs increase the tendency to gastro-oesophageal reflux.

Gastric Emptying

Gastric emptying results from peristaltic waves sweeping from cardia to pylorus at a rate of approximately three per minute, although temporary inhibition of gastric motility follows recent ingestion of a meal. The gastric emptying of clear fluids is an exponential process, i.e. the rate of emptying at any given time is proportional to the volume of liquid in the stomach. The half-time for this process is about 20 min, so less than 2% of ingested clear fluid remains in the stomach at 2 h. The gastric emptying of solids is roughly linear, i.e. occurs at a constant rate, and usually begins about 30 min after ingestion of a meal. The rate of emptying varies depending on the composition of food ingested. Typically, about 50% of food reaches the duodenum within 2 h although meals high in fat content may take considerably longer. The rate of gastric emptying is also significantly delayed if the mixture reaching the duodenum is very acidic or hypertonic (the inhibitory enterogastric reflex), but both the nervous and

humoral elements of this regulating mechanism are still poorly understood. Many pathological conditions reduce gastric emptying (Table 37.5). In the absence of any of these factors, it is reasonably safe to assume that the stomach is empty provided that solids have not been ingested within the preceding 6 h, or clear fluids consumed in the preceding 2 h, and provided that normal peristalsis is occurring. This is the usual case for elective surgical patients. However, in emergency surgery it may be necessary to induce anaesthesia urgently before an adequate period of starvation occurs. In addition, the patient's surgical condition is often accompanied by delayed gastric emptying or abnormalities of peristalsis. In these circumstances, even if the usual period of fasting has been observed it cannot be assumed that the patient's stomach is empty.

In patients who have sustained a significant trauma injury, gastric emptying virtually ceases as a result of the combined effects of fear, pain, shock and treatment with opioid analgesics. In these patients, the interval between ingestion of food and the injury is a

TABLE 37.5
Situations in Which Vomiting or Regurgitation May Occur

Full stomach

With absent or abnormal peristalsis
    Peritonitis of any cause
    Postoperative ileus
    Metabolic ileus: hypokalaemia, uraemia, diabetic ketoacidosis
    Drug-induced ileus: anticholinergics, those with anticholinergic side-effects

With obstructed peristalsis
    Small or large bowel obstruction
    Gastric carcinoma
    Pyloric stenosis

With delayed gastric emptying
    Diabetic autonomic neuropathy
    Fear, pain or anxiety
    Late pregnancy
    Opioids
    Head injury

Other causes

Hiatus hernia

Oesophageal strictures – benign or malignant

Pharyngeal pouch

more reliable index of residual stomach volume than the period of fasting observed since injury. It is not uncommon to encounter vomiting 24 h or longer after ingestion of food when trauma has occurred very shortly after a meal. In these patients, a patient's sensation of hunger should not be used to indicate an empty stomach: sensations of hunger and satiety are complex and are unreliable indicators of stomach volume. Bedside ultrasonography is a more objective tool for determining gastric content and its use may become more widespread.

Injury from aspiration of gastric contents results from three different mechanisms: chemical pneumonitis (from acid material), mechanical obstruction from particulate material and bacterial contamination. Aspiration of liquid with a pH <2.5 is associated with a chemical burn of the bronchial, bronchiolar and alveolar mucosa, leading to atelectasis, pulmonary oedema and reduced pulmonary compliance. Bronchospasm may also be present. The claim that patients are at risk if they have more than 25 mL of gastric residue with a pH <2.5 is based on data from animal studies extrapolated to humans and should not be regarded as indisputable fact. Day-case patients often have residual gastric volumes greater than 25 mL.

If aspiration of gastric contents occurs, the first manoeuvre after the airway is secured is to suction the trachea to remove as much foreign material as possible. If particulate matter is obstructing proximal bronchi, bronchoscopy may be necessary. Hypoxaemia is managed with O_2, IPPV and PEEP. Steroids are not recommended and antibiotics are not given routinely unless the aspirated material is considered unsterile.

TECHNIQUES OF ANAESTHESIA

It is important to recognize any patient who may have significant gastric residue and who is in danger of aspiration. The anaesthetic management of such a patient may be described in five phases: preparation, induction, maintenance, emergence and postoperative management.

Phase I – Preparation

Whilst it may be necessary to postpone surgery in the emergency patient to obtain investigations and resuscitate with i.v. fluids, there is usually little benefit in terms of reducing the risk of aspiration of gastric contents; the risk of aspiration must be weighed against the risk of delaying an urgent procedure. However, two manoeuvres are available:

- Although not completely effective, insertion of a nasogastric tube to decompress the stomach and to provide a low-pressure vent for regurgitation may be helpful. Aspiration through the tube may be useful if gastric contents are liquid, as in bowel obstruction, but is less effective when contents are solid. Cricoid pressure is still effective at reducing regurgitation even with a nasogastric tube *in situ*.

- Clear oral antacids (e.g. sodium citrate) may be used to raise the pH of gastric contents immediately before induction. However, this also increases gastric volume. Particulate antacids should not be used, as they may be very damaging to the airway if aspirated. The preoperative administration of H_2-receptor antagonists consistently raises gastric pH and may reduce the chance of chemical pulmonary injury occurring in the event of inhalation. Although this is standard practice in obstetric anaesthesia, few anaesthetists employ these measures for emergency general surgery. The regimens available are described in Chapter 35.

Phase II – Induction

Rapid-Sequence Induction

This is the technique used most frequently for the patient with a full stomach. The phrase 'rapid-sequence' hints at one of the fundamental goals of this technique, which is to minimize as much as possible the duration of time between loss of consciousness and tracheal intubation, during which the patient is at greatest risk of aspiration of gastric contents. In achieving this goal, this technique contravenes one of the fundamental rules of anaesthesia, namely that neuromuscular blockers are not injected until control of the airway is assured. The decision to employ the rapid-sequence induction technique balances the risk of losing control of the airway against the risk of aspiration. Therefore it is vital to assess carefully the likelihood of difficult laryngoscopy or tracheal intubation. The anaesthetist must have a contingency plan prepared for patient management should intubation fail. If preoperative evaluation indicates a particularly difficult airway, alternative methods should be considered, e.g. local anaesthetic techniques or 'awake intubation' under local anaesthesia.

For rapid-sequence induction to be consistently safe and successful, it should be performed with meticulous attention to detail and preparation is necessary. The patient *must* be on a tipping trolley or table, preferably with an adjustable headpiece so that the degree of neck extension/flexion may be altered quickly. Ideally the patient's head should be in the classic 'sniffing position' with the neck flexed on the shoulders and the head extended on the neck. Failure to appreciate this point increases the likelihood of difficult intubation. The optimal incline of the operating table is debatable: some authorities recommend the reverse Trendelenburg (head-up) position (to prevent regurgitation) and others the classic Trendelenburg position (to prevent aspiration of any regurgitated or vomited material). In general, the optimum position is that in which the trainee anaesthetist has gained greatest experience in performing intubation.

The anaesthetist *must* be aided by at least one skilled assistant to perform cricoid pressure, assist in turning the patient, obtain smaller tracheal tubes, supply stylets for tubes, etc. High-volume suction apparatus *must* be functioning and the suction catheter should be within easy reach of the anaesthetist's hand (commonly placed under the patient's pillow). As with any anaesthetic, the machine should have been checked before starting, the ventilator adjusted to appropriate settings and all drugs drawn up into labelled syringes before induction. An i.v. cannula should be sited and connected to running fluid, to aid circulation of drugs to the brain. Appropriate monitoring devices should be attached.

Before inducing anaesthesia, it is essential to preoxygenate the patient's lungs with 100% oxygen. The aim is to denitrogenate the lungs and maximize the oxygen reservoir available to the patient from their functional residual capacity, which will delay the onset of hypoxia if difficulty is encountered whilst securing the airway. The patient should breathe 100% O_2 for 3–5 min, or until the end-tidal oxygen concentration is >85%. In extreme emergencies this process can be quickened by asking the patient to make 8 vital capacity breaths.

Heart rate, arterial pressure (and, when appropriate, central venous pressure) and ECG are monitored before induction of anaesthesia, and a skilled assistant is in position at the patient's side to perform Sellick's manoeuvre (cricoid pressure). It is important that the assistant can identify the cricoid cartilage, as compression of the thyroid cartilage distorts laryngeal anatomy and may render tracheal intubation very difficult. To perform Sellick's manoeuvre correctly, the thumb and forefinger press the cricoid cartilage firmly in a posterior direction with a force of 20–40 N, thus compressing the oesophagus between the cricoid cartilage and the vertebral column. Because the cricoid cartilage forms a complete ring, the tracheal lumen is not distorted (Fig. 37.1).

Opinions differ with regard to the time at which cricoid pressure should be applied. Some prefer to inform the patient and apply it just before administration of the i.v. induction agent; others apply it as soon as consciousness is lost.

With the assistant in position, a predetermined sleep dose of i.v. anaesthetic induction agent is injected. This is followed immediately by the administration of a paralysing dose of succinylcholine (1.5 mg kg^{-1}) without waiting to assess the effect of the induction agent. Manually ventilating the patient's lungs whilst waiting for muscle paralysis is sometimes avoided for

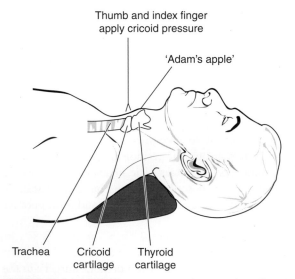

FIGURE 37.1 ■ Sellick's manoeuvre. The cricoid cartilage is palpated immediately below the thyroid cartilage.

fear of causing gastric insufflations and increasing the risk of aspiration. As soon as the jaw begins to relax or fasciculations have ceased, laryngoscopy is performed and the trachea intubated. Cricoid pressure is maintained until the cuff of the tracheal tube is inflated and correct placement of the tube has been confirmed, by auscultation of both lungs and the presence of end-tidal carbon dioxide. The exception to this rule is in instances of vomiting after induction, where maintenance of cricoid pressure could lead to oesophageal rupture.

After successful intubation, the lungs are gently ventilated by hand, as excessive increases in intrathoracic pressure may have harmful effects on circulatory dynamics. One of the main disadvantages of the rapid-sequence induction technique is the haemodynamic instability that may result if the dose of induction agent is excessive (hypotension, circulatory collapse) or inadequate (hypertension, tachycardia).

Thiopental has long been regarded as the i.v. induction agent of choice for RSI. It provides a rapid loss of consciousness with a clearly defined end-point. A dose of 4–$5\,mg\,kg^{-1}$ can reliably be predicted to be sufficient for healthy young patients, but much less (1.5–$2\,mg\,kg^{-1}$) is required in the elderly and frail or hypovolaemic patient. In the critically ill patient with a metabolic acidosis, the unbound fraction of the drug is increased and this will also reduce dose requirements. In comparison to thiopental, propofol 1.5–$2\,mg\,kg^{-1}$ causes greater suppression of laryngeal reflexes and may be more familiar to junior anaesthetists, owing to its everyday use in anaesthesia for elective procedures. However, propofol causes more cardiovascular depression than thiopental and should be used with caution. Another alternative is etomidate 0.1–$0.3\,mg\,kg^{-1}$ which has the advantage of less cardiodepressant effects but its use is limited by adverse effects of adrenal suppression. Ketamine $1.5\,mg\,kg^{-1}$ has a slower speed of onset and poorly defined end-point compared to thiopental. However, it causes the least cardiovascular depression of any induction agent and is often used in severely shocked patients.

It is sometimes inferred from the term RSI that the i.v. anaesthetic should be injected rapidly. This is not the case: RSI means that a predetermined dose of i.v. anaesthetic drug is immediately followed by injection of the neuromuscular blocking drug, and before waiting for signs of unconsciousness. Too rapid an injection of i.v. agent may exaggerate cardiovascular depression in the compromised patient, and bolus doses of all intravenous anaesthetics during RSI should be given over several seconds. Opioids are often injected along with intravenous anaesthetics at induction of anaesthesia for elective surgery, but 'classical' teaching suggests they should be omitted during RSI despite their potential benefits – for example attenuating the sympathetic response to intubation. This is largely because of concerns about delaying the onset of spontaneous respiration in the event of failed intubation. However, shorter acting drugs such as alfentanil are increasingly used as part of an RSI and may allow reduced doses of i.v. anaesthetic induction agents.

Succinylcholine is used as the neuromuscular blocker for RSI because it has two very desirable properties: a rapid onset of action facilitates speedy intubation and therefore minimizes the risk of aspiration, whilst a short duration of action allows for a quicker onset of spontaneous ventilation in the event of failed intubation. However, it also causes a number of undesirable effects including increased serum potassium concentrations, muscle pains and, rarely, malignant hyperthermia. The incidence of anaphylaxis is also higher than that of other neuromuscular blocking drugs. High-dose rocuronium (0.9–$1.2\,mg\,kg^{-1}$) achieves intubating conditions in a comparable time to succinylcholine but its use in RSI has been limited by a more prolonged duration of action. However, su gammadex allows rapid reversal of the effects of rocuronium through encapsulation of the rocuronium molecule. The availability of sugammadex may therefore enable high-dose rocuronium to be used as an alternative to succinylcholine in RSI.

Inhalational Induction

If there is reasonable doubt about the ability to perform intubation or to maintain a patent airway in a patient with a full stomach (e.g. the patient with facial trauma, epiglottitis or bleeding tonsil), an inhalational induction may be used with oxygen and halothane or sevoflurane. When the patient has reached a deep plane of anaesthesia, laryngoscopy is performed followed by an attempt at tracheal intubation during spontaneous ventilation. Normally, the patient should be placed in the left lateral, head-down position, but if circumstances do not allow the lateral position then the supine posture with cricoid pressure may have to be accepted. Indeed a modification of this technique may be used in any elderly, frail patient who may not tolerate i.v. induction agents. Anaesthesia may be induced by inhalational induction with the maintenance of cricoid pressure and, when the patient is sufficiently anaesthetized, succinylcholine injected and the trachea intubated.

Awake Intubation

Although blind nasal intubation is a valuable skill, the introduction of the narrow-gauge fibreoptic intubating laryngoscope has replaced it as the technique of choice in those patients who are likely to develop unrelievable airway obstruction when loss of consciousness occurs (e.g. trismus from dental abscess) or who are known or suspected to pose difficulties with intubation. Such endoscopic tracheal intubations may be performed via either the nasal route (more commonly used) or the oral route (see Ch 22: Management of the difficult airway). Before embarking on awake fibreoptic nasal intubation, the nasopharynx and, to a greater or lesser extent, the upper airway must be rendered insensitive, so that the patient can tolerate the introduction of a tracheal tube (see Ch 43: Complications during anaesthesia).

Regional Anaesthesia

The use of regional anaesthesia is increasing in the UK, partly because of the growth in the practice of ultrasound-guided regional anaesthetic techniques. Many regional techniques are eminently suitable for emergency procedures on the extremities (e.g. to reduce fractures or dislocations).

Brachial plexus block by the axillary, supraclavicular or interscalene approach is satisfactory for orthopaedic manipulations or surgical procedures involving the upper extremity. It satisfies surgical requirements for analgesia, muscle relaxation and immobility. There are minimal effects on the cardiovascular system and there is a prolonged period of analgesia postoperatively. Similarly, i.v. regional anaesthesia is useful for the manipulation or reduction of a fractured wrist; prilocaine 0.5% plain is the drug of choice as it is the least toxic local anaesthetic drug and has the largest therapeutic index. If prilocaine is not available, then lidocaine 0.5% plain is acceptable.

For regional anaesthesia of the lower extremity, available techniques include subarachnoid, epidural and sciatic/femoral blocks. Spinal and epidural blocks are contraindicated if there is doubt about the adequacy of extracellular fluid or vascular volumes, as large decreases in arterial pressure may result from the associated pharmacological sympathectomy.

It is a common surgical misconception that subarachnoid or epidural anaesthetic techniques are safer than general anaesthesia for patients in poor physical condition. It must be emphasized that for the *inexperienced* anaesthetist, these techniques are invariably more dangerous than general anaesthesia for the patient with moderate/major trauma or any intraabdominal emergency condition.

Phase III – Maintenance of Anaesthesia

If a rapid-sequence induction has been performed, the patient's lungs are gently ventilated manually whilst heart rate and arterial pressure measurements are repeated to assess the cardiovascular effects of the drugs used and of the stimulus of tracheal intubation. Capnography is essential throughout anaesthesia and gives valuable information about perfusion and ventilation of the lungs.

When there is evidence of return of neuromuscular transmission (by clinical signs or from a nerve stimulator) as succinylcholine is degraded, a nondepolarizing neuromuscular blocker is administered. The choice depends on the patient's condition, and the effect of the induction of anaesthesia on the patient's cardiovascular status. Both rocuronium and atracurium are appropriate drugs for routine use, although the pharmacokinetics of atracurium make it the logical choice for the older patient. Atracurium has virtually no cardiovascular effects in clinical doses and is useful if there is any doubt about renal function.

When the neuromuscular blocker has been injected, the tracheal tube is connected to a mechanical ventilator and minute volume adjusted to produce normocapnia. Ventilators are now increasingly sophisticated and incorporate a choice of ventilation modes. The choice is usually between pressure controlled or volume controlled ventilation. It can be difficult to predict ventilator requirements, but initial settings should aim to produce a minute volume of $75-100\,mL\,kg^{-1}\,min^{-1}$ with a tidal volume of $6-8\,mL\,kg^{-1}$. The inspiratory flow rate should be adjusted to minimize peak airway pressure, and the capnograph waveform and pressure volume loops should be inspected regularly to guide the further adjustment of ventilator settings. Maintenance of core temperature is a very important aspect of intraoperative management – core temperature should be monitored throughout the procedure and hypothermia avoided whenever possible (see Ch 43: Complications during anaesthesia).

Before the initial surgical incision is made, analgesia may be supplemented by incremental i.v. doses of morphine 1–5 mg or fentanyl 25–100 μg. Morphine is probably the analgesic of choice for emergency surgery. With repeated doses, fentanyl can accumulate and may have an even longer elimination half life than morphine. Other drugs are often used to augment analgesia in emergency surgery, including low dose ketamine (0.15 mg kg^{-1}) and paracetamol i.v. Non-steroidal anti-inflammatory agents are sometimes used but with caution in those with, or at risk of, acute kidney injury or postoperative bleeding. They should be reserved for young ASA 1 & 2 patients.

The use of supplemental doses of analgesic and neuromuscular blocking drugs is described in Chapters 5 (Analgesic drugs) and 6 (Muscle function and neuromuscular blockade). The trainee should be familiar with the pharmacokinetics and pharmacodynamics of all drugs used and be aware that these may change during emergency anaesthesia, when acute circulatory changes or impaired organ function often occur.

Fluid Management

During emergency intra-abdominal surgery, there may be large blood and fluid losses, which exceed the patient's maintenance fluid replacement. Hartmann's solution (compound sodium lactate) is still the preferred i.v. fluid during surgery. More sophisticated methods of determining intravascular volume status and cardiac output are increasingly used. Although much of the work in this field has been performed in patients undergoing elective surgery, there are a few examples of fluid optimization using cardiac output monitoring proving beneficial in emergency patients (Sinclair et al 1997). Methods of determining cardiac output are covered in Chapter 16 (Clinical measurement and monitoring).

The requirement for blood transfusion varies in different groups of patients. In general the threshold for transfusion of blood (or more commonly packed red blood cells), the 'transfusion trigger', is a haemoglobin concentration 8 g dL^{-1} (Carless et al 2010). A higher transfusion trigger is often used for certain patient populations, for example 10 g dL^{-1} in patients with ischaemic heart disease, though the evidence for this is not established. Near-patient-testing devices, sampling from arterial or venous catheters are invaluable aids to guide transfusion during surgery.

Phase IV – Reversal and Emergence

After insertion of the last skin suture, anaesthetic drugs can be discontinued, if the patient is deemed stable enough for tracheal extubation. Direct pharyngoscopy is performed and secretions/debris removed from the pharynx; if a nasogastric tube is *in situ*, it is aspirated and left unspigoted. Glycopyrrolate 20 μg kg^{-1} and neostigmine 50 μg kg^{-1} are given as a bolus and ventilation continued to eliminate volatile agents until signs of awakening appear. The end-tidal concentration of volatile anaesthetic is usually below 0.1 MAC before eye opening occurs. Because the risk of aspiration of gastric contents is as great on recovery as at induction, tracheal extubation should not be performed until protective airway reflexes have returned fully and the patient responds to commands such as 'open your eyes' or 'lift your hand up'. Both the level of consciousness and neuromuscular transmission should be assessed to demonstrate the adequacy of reflexes.

The adequacy of reversal of paralysis may be determined by observing the patient's ability to sustain a head lift for 5 s and sustain a firm grip without fade, although clinical signs can be misleading. Preferably, a nerve stimulator is used to define reversal of neuromuscular transmission (see Ch 6: Muscle function and neuromuscular blockade).

Tracheal Extubation

If extubation is planned after emergency anaesthesia, this should take place in the operating room with the presence of a trained anaesthetic assistant. Immediately before tracheal extubation, the patient is turned to the lateral position (if possible) and asked to take a deep inspiration while gentle positive pressure is applied to the airway. At the peak of inspiration, the cuff is deflated and the tracheal tube removed as the patient exhales, thus assisting removal of any secretions which may have accumulated above the cuff. Oxygen 100% is administered until a regular respiratory rhythm is re-established and the patient has demonstrated an ability to cough and maintain a patent airway. Breathing 40% O_2, the patient is transported in the lateral position to the recovery room and remains there until all vital signs are stable.

Phase V – Postoperative Management

Appropriate analgesia and fluids should be prescribed before the patient is discharged to the ward. There may be a need for Level 2 or 3 care in some circumstances and good documentation and clear patient handovers between staff are essential.

The need for further blood replacement is assessed by regular observation of vital signs and drainage measurements and postoperative Hb or haematocrit measurements, which can be performed at the bedside.

Prophylactic Postoperative IPPV

Continuation of IPPV should be considered electively in several circumstances, some of which are listed in Table 37.6. There should be close cooperation between intensive care colleagues, surgeons and anaesthetists when the decision is made to continue ventilation.

Emergency Laparotomy in the Older Patient

Elderly patients undergoing emergency laparotomy are at particularly high risk of complications or death, as highlighted by the UK NCEPOD (National Confidential Enquiry into Patient Outcome and Death) report of 2010 (see further reading). The decision to perform emergency surgery on older patients requires the input of senior surgical, anaesthetic, medicine for the elderly and critical care clinicians.

TABLE 37.6
Indications for Postoperative Ventilation

Prolonged shock/hypoperfusion state of any cause

Massive sepsis (faecal peritonitis, cholangitis, septicaemia)

Severe ischaemic heart disease

Extreme obesity

Overt gastric acid aspiration

Severe pulmonary disease

The risks and potential benefits should be carefully assessed and frail, older patients should not necessarily undergo major surgery followed by prolonged intensive care treatments if it is considered that the burden of surgical treatment and poor prognosis outweigh the likely benefit of surgery. This is a very difficult decision and should only be made by senior clinicians. It is emphasized that such decisions must be individualized and the views of the patient are paramount.

Before embarking on emergency, potentially major surgery in frail, elderly patients with an acute abdomen, some questions must be answered:

- Is it likely that the patient will die *with* or *without surgery*? If the answer is yes, then surgery is *not* indicated unless it is likely that it will contribute to the physical comfort of the patient during the dying process, i.e. contribute to a 'good death'.
- Is it likely that the patient would survive a laparotomy if the underlying cause were found to be curable/treatable (e.g. perforated duodenal ulcer, appendicitis)? If the answer is yes, then surgery is indicated and agreement on the appropriate level and duration of postoperative organ support must be reached.
- If, having embarked on surgery, the underlying cause is found to be treatable but not curable (e.g. perforated carcinoma with metastases, gangrenous bowel), would radical surgery be appropriate, given the patients overall state? If not, aggressive postoperative intensive care is not indicated. If yes, then what would be an appropriate level and duration of postoperative support? These questions need to be answered by experienced clinicians.

The concept of 'damage control surgery', which has developed from military situations in young patients with severe injuries, may be appropriate for the older person requiring emergency surgery. There are no randomized studies looking at this age group but in theory several staged interventions of a shorter duration, with the aim of restoring physiology (or at least preventing further deterioration), may be better than a single prolonged, definitive operation. Time is valuable when physiological reserve is diminished. There should be rapid access to radiology and other investigations and these patients should be treated as a priority.

THE ANAESTHETIST AND MAJOR TRAUMA

The management of the patient with major trauma requires a multidisciplinary team effort. The UK National Audit Office (2010) estimated there were 20 000 cases of major trauma in England per year, resulting in 5400 deaths. Perceived deficiencies in care have resulted in the formation of regional trauma networks with resources being concentrated at major centres. One consequence of this is that the numbers of patient transfers between hospitals is likely to increase, and most will involve an anaesthetist. A successful outcome depends on the quality of the initial resuscitation and correct prioritisation of treatment. The anaesthetic/ICU trainee should be an integral member of the 'trauma team' called to manage a patient with multiple injuries. Trauma management is based on major trauma protocols which have evolved from ATLS® and experience from military and civilian trauma. The anaesthetist must be familiar with these. All major trauma networks have an education function and trainee anaesthetists should avail themselves of the education and training provided. Major trauma is a dynamic, high-stakes environment with difficult decision making. Excellent team working, communication and non-technical skills are fundamental to successful trauma management and the anaesthetist should spend time and effort to learn and practice these.

Effective management of major trauma requires:

1. *Rapid primary survey*. Recognition and treatment of any immediately life-threatening injuries, such as airway obstruction, tension/open pneumothorax, massive bleeding (chest, abdomen, pelvis, long bones or external), cardiac tamponade or intracranial injury.
2. *Damage control resuscitation*. Control of haemorrhage, achieving adequate tissue perfusion, haemostatic resuscitation and damage control surgery.
3. *On-going, repeated examination* to identify threats to life or limb and all associated injuries.
4. *Definitive care*.

Although these processes are described sequentially, a well-run trauma team will prioritise, communicate and assess and treat in parallel. The anaesthetic trainee may be involved in any or all of the above areas of management.

Primary Survey/Damage Control Resuscitation

As soon as the patient arrives in the emergency department, rapid primary survey is performed at the same time as resuscitation. A cABC approach is taken:

- **C**atastrophic haemorrhage control: less common in civilian than military trauma but does occur.
- **A**irway
- **B**reathing
- **C**irculation: haemorrhagic and non-haemorrhagic causes may co-exist. There is a strong emphasis on haemorrhage control.

Control of exsanguinating haemorrhage

- In the limbs apply direct pressure and elevate
- For continued bleeding use indirect pressure and apply a military tourniquet
- Pelvic binder – should have been applied pre-hospital; ensure correctly positioned

Airway/Breathing

In general, airway assessment reveals one of three clinical scenarios:

- *Patient is conscious, alert, talking.* Give high-flow oxygen via face mask. There is no need for immediate airway intervention and a full clinical evaluation can be done. Persisting signs of shock and/or the diagnosis of serious underlying injuries might be an indication for planned endotracheal intubation and mechanical ventilation
- *Patient has a reduced conscious level but some degree of airway control and gag reflex still present.* If the patient is maintaining the airway and breathing adequately then there is no need for immediate intervention. Endotracheal intubation will be necessary but a clinical evaluation can be done whilst equipment is being readied.
- *Patient has a reduced conscious level, gag reflex absent.* If the patient is unable to maintain the airway or is breathing poorly tracheal intubation and artificial ventilation should be carried out at once.

When confronted with an unconscious trauma victim the anaesthetist must establish the patency of the patient's airway whilst assuring immobilization of the cervical spine. Unstable cervical spine injuries are relatively uncommon, however, *all* patients should be assumed to be at risk until proven otherwise. If upper airway obstruction is present, the pharynx is cleared of any debris and the jaw displaced forward (jaw thrust). Avoid neck tilt.

If the patient is apnoeic, bag-mask ventilation with 100% oxygen must be started immediately to control oxygenation and $PaCO_2$. Orotracheal intubation should be performed with care. Do not try to intubate the patient with a collar in place. The C-spine should be protected by manual in line immobilisation during intubation, and the collar subsequently replaced. Have a very low threshold for the use of a bougie and McCoy laryngoscope to facilitate intubation, and do not necessarily try to obtain the 'best possible' view of the glottic opening. Achieve a good enough view to facilitate easy passage of the bougie. This will minimise potential neck movement. There is a higher incidence of failed intubation in the emergent trauma setting, partly attributable to cervical immobility. A genuinely deliverable airway strategy must be planned and communicated with the trauma team, up to and including a surgical airway. There is rarely a 'wake-up' option in the polytrauma setting.

Patients with severe facial trauma who are cooperative and awake despite their injuries may not require immediate tracheal intubation, but do need frequent and regular upper airway evaluation to assess the rate of progress of pharyngeal or laryngeal oedema, which may proceed to complete airway obstruction with alarming speed.

If there are clinical signs suggesting a pneumothorax or surgical emphysema and/or a flail segment is apparent, then a chest drain should be inserted simultaneously or before mechanical ventilation is commenced. Persistence of hypoxaemia after institution of mechanical ventilation suggests unrecognized pneumothorax, haemothorax, pulmonary contusion or poor cardiac output caused by hypovolaemia, cardiac tamponade, or other causes.

Damage Control Resuscitation

There has been a significant shift in management of major trauma away from 'full' resuscitation and 'definitive' surgery towards a concept of damage control resuscitation. This approach combines *time-limited* permissive hypotension, haemostatic resuscitation and *damage control surgery*. It is important to understand that permissive hypotension is not an end in itself. The presence of a peripheral pulse is deemed to be evidence of adequate perfusion only until the source of bleeding is controlled. The emphasis is on rapid and effective control of bleeding.

Circulation

Haemorrhage is the most common cause of shock in the injured patient and virtually all patients with multiple injuries have an element of hypovolaemia. Patients with major trauma often require urgent restoration of sufficient circulating blood volume to ensure:

- Adequate oxygen delivery to the tissues;
- Stabilisation and/or correction of metabolic derangements;
- Correction of acute coagulopathy of trauma and prevention of iatrogenic coagulopathy.

Initial response to adequate boluses of warmed isotonic fluids may give some guide as to degree of hypovolaemia. However, if a patient has clear signs or a strong history suggestive of significant blood loss, there is nothing to be gained by administration of crystalloids. Blood should be given at the earliest opportunity.

All fluids given must be warmed as the triad of hypothermia, acidosis and clotting derangement can be lethal. At least two large (14-gauge) i.v. cannulae are inserted into peripheral veins in one or two limbs and both attached to infusions running through blood-warming coils.

Concurrently with administration of fluid replacement the team should be instituting measures to reduce further blood loss. The most important of these are:

- Application of a pelvic binder
  - The binder should be placed around the trochanters not the iliac crests. The aim is to close the pelvis, not compress it.
  - If the binder was applied pre-hospital leave it in place, check it is positioned correctly, and x-ray.
- Administration of tranexamic acid
  - The CRASH-2 study reported a significant reduction in mortality following major trauma with few adverse events.
  - 1g IV stat followed by 1g infusion over 8 hours.

- Avoidance of over-resuscitation
  - Fluid should be given to achieve restoration of a palpable peripheral pulse.
  - Excessive fluid risks disruption of early clots and may worsen coagulopathy and overall blood loss.

Transfusion protocols have changed over the last few years, largely as a result of experience gained in conflict zones. Hospitals will have their own protocols for massive haemorrhage; these vary in their ratios of packed red cells: FFP: cryoprecipitate: platelets. However, the overall aim is the same: correction/avoidance of coagulopathy (*haemostatic resuscitation*) and adequate tissue oxygen delivery and perfusion. Good transfusion practice requires the use of near patient testing and close co-operation with haematology services. Further detail is given below (p 767).

Pump Function

Pump failure in major trauma is commonly due to the presence of a tension pneumothorax, but other possibilities include severe myocardial contusion and traumatic pericardial tamponade. Tension pneumothorax causes compression of the mediastinum (heart and great vessels) and presents with extreme respiratory distress, shock, unilateral air entry, a shift of the trachea towards the normal side and distension of the veins in the neck, although the last sign may not be seen in hypovolaemic shock. Tension pneumothorax is a clinical diagnosis, and should be treated if suspected. X-ray simply delays treatment. It may be relieved immediately by insertion of a 14-gauge cannula through the second intercostal space in the midclavicular line. This should be followed by standard chest drainage. Patients with blunt chest trauma and fractured ribs may develop a tension pneumothorax rapidly when positive-pressure ventilation is commenced, and the prophylactic insertion of a chest drain should be considered in such patients.

Damage Control Surgery

An early decision by the team is needed regarding the most appropriate pathway for the patient. Urgent trauma CT provides important anatomical information about actual or potential threat to life and is indicated in patients with adequate perfusion. Patients with inadequate perfusion and not responding to resuscitation should go straight to the operating theatre. Patients intermediate between these two groups require a more complex decision. The most important action is to **make a decision**. Waiting in ED is not going to further the patient's care. Well-run trauma units expect to have major trauma patients through CT and with initial reporting of major findings within 30 minutes of ED arrival.

- Systolic blood pressure >90 mmHg: urgent trauma CT
- Systolic blood pressure 70-90 mmHg: senior decision making; if choose CT **MUST** be accompanied by trauma team
- Systolic blood pressure <70 mmHg and not responding: operating theatre

A FAST (Focused Abdominal Sonography for Trauma) scan by a skilled operator may provide helpful information if positive. A negative FAST scan does not rule out significant injury. Based on the CT findings and clinical picture, senior members of the trauma team will make a prompt decision regarding intervention: operating theatre for damage control surgery; embolization; non-operative continued resuscitation (critical care).

The anaesthetist must be involved in ongoing discussions with the surgical teams about the extent and intent of surgery.

The aims of Damage Control Surgery are:

- control haemorrhage: packs, clamps, ligation, splinting of fractures
- decompression of at risk compartments: head, heart, limbs, abdomen
- minimise contamination: debridement of fractures and wounds, closure or resection of hollow viscus injuries.

The duration of surgery is limited, and additional surgical trauma is minimised. During this time, particularly once haemorrhage has been controlled, the anaesthetist should be aiming to correct metabolic, fluid and haemostatic derangements. In particular:

- Normothermia
- Normal pH
- Normal coagulation: fibrinogen >1.5 g dL^{-1}; normal APTT and PT.

- Normal or improving lactate – a marker of adequacy of resuscitation
- Haemoglobin – generally around 10-11 g dL^{-1} is accepted

For patients who do not require immediate surgery for haemorrhage, decontamination or decompression, a team decision may need to be made whether to proceed to Early Total Care (ETC: definitive treatment of all long-bone fractures) or Damage Control Orthopaedic Surgery. These decisions should be based on an overall assessment of patient condition, particularly the trend in arterial lactate. If lactate is <2.0 mmol L^{-1} then ETC can be considered; if >2.5 mmol L^{-1} then continued resuscitation is required.

It is often necessary to induce anaesthesia in a hypovolaemic patient; this requires meticulous attention to fluid and drug management. A controlled rapid-sequence induction using thiopental, propofol or ketamine should be performed, but with extreme care over the dose of induction agent. Often very small doses of ketamine (0.3–0.7 mg kg^{-1}) suffice. The use of etomidate in trauma is still contentious due to its metabolic effects. The depressant effects of i.v. induction agents are exaggerated because the proportion of the cardiac output going to the heart and brain is increased. In addition, the rate of redistribution and/or metabolism is decreased as a result of reduced blood flow to muscle, liver and kidneys and thus blood concentrations remain increased for longer periods in comparison with healthy patients. Ketamine can be used in patients with a significant head injury as the benefits of maintained arterial blood pressure outweigh any concerns about cerebrometabolic effects. Figure 37.2 illustrates monitoring often used for the

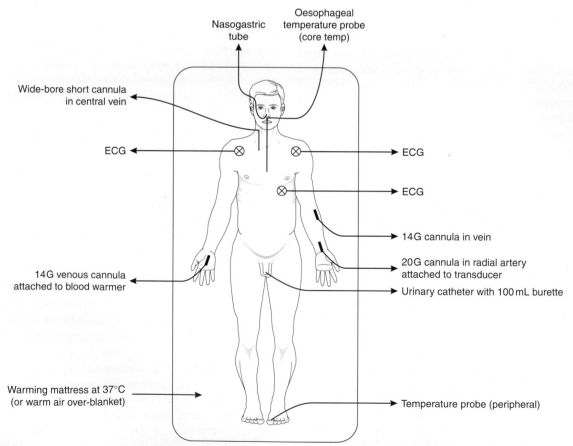

FIGURE 37.2 ■ Commonly used monitoring and resuscitation attachments in management of a patient with multiple injuries. Pulse oximetry and capnography are also used during anaesthesia.

management of major trauma. Particular care needs to be taken in the presence of hypovolaemia and severe traumatic brain injury as hypotension is associated with a doubling of mortality.

After tracheal intubation, the lungs are ventilated at the lowest peak airway pressure consistent with an acceptable tidal volume. Judicious doses of muscle relaxant and analgesia (usually fentanyl) are given as necessary. As the cardiovascular status normalises and systolic pressure exceeds 90 mmHg, anaesthesia should be deepened as tolerated. This should be undertaken cautiously and, in principle, agents which are rapidly reversible or rapidly excreted should be used. In the shock state, there is very rapid uptake of inhalational agents. Reduced cardiac output and pulmonary blood flow decrease the rate of removal of anaesthetic agent from the alveoli, producing a rapid increase in alveolar concentration. Thus, the MAC value is approached more rapidly than in normovolaemic patients.

Basic monitoring will have been instituted in the emergency department. Insertion of arterial lines should not delay time to CT or surgical control of haemorrhage. However, blood may be sampled from an arterial cannula to monitor changes in acid-base state, haemoglobin concentration, coagulation and electrolyte concentrations. Central venous access is not usually a high priority in trauma resuscitation, but may be essential for i.v. access in the presence of four limb trauma. Short wide cannulae (e.g. 'Swan sheaths') should be used. Urine output is a useful guide to adequacy of resuscitation.

When surgical bleeding has been controlled, the patient's cardiovascular status should improve, but if hypotension persists despite apparently adequate fluid administration, other causes of haemorrhage should be sought (Table 37.7). It is important that the anaesthetist assesses the patient regularly during prolonged anaesthesia to exclude these latent complications of major trauma.

Massive Transfusion

This is defined arbitrarily as either replacement of >50% of a patient's blood volume within 1 hour, or replacement of 1–1.5 blood volumes within a 24-hour period. These are life-threatening situations and good management requires an appreciation of both the clinical and logistical issues surrounding large-scale blood component replacement. Massive haemorrhage protocols, developed in collaboration between the emergency department, anaesthesia, blood bank and other key support services are a fundamental component of good clinical care. If possible, a named individual should be given responsibility for liaising directly with colleagues in blood bank and ensuring timely request and collection of blood products.

The shocked polytrauma patient is very likely to be coagulopathic on arrival: acute coagulopathy of trauma (ACOT). The UK transfusion service now provides almost all stored blood as red cells in optimal additive solution, containing no plasma, platelets, coagulation factors or leucocytes. Therefore, the treatment of massive haemorrhage by volume replacement solely with red cells will not correct ACOT and places the patient at high risk of further dilutional coagulopathy. Early infusion of fresh frozen plasma (FFP) 15 mL kg^{-1} is required and it is increasingly common to transfuse red cells and FFP in set ratios of 4:1 or 3:1 to prevent disorders of haemostasis. In military trauma settings red cell:FFP:platelet ratios as high as 1:1:1 are sometimes used. Transfusing according to set ratios is particularly useful if blood loss is rapid and laboratory turnaround time is excessive. The anaesthetist should not be waiting for coagulation test results to treat coagulopathy. Near-patient tests of clotting such as thromboelastography (TEG) may have a role.

FFP alone corrects fibrinogen and most coagulation factor deficiencies. However, if fibrinogen concentration remains <1.5 g L^{-1}, cryoprecipitate or fibrinogen concentrate therapy should be considered. It is necessary to give platelet concentrate for all instances of severe thrombocytopenia (platelet count less than $50 \times 10\ 9\ L^{-1}$) or milder thrombocytopenia

---

TABLE 37.7
Causes of Persistent Hypotension

Surgical or medical (check platelets and clotting screen)
    Continued overt bleeding
    Continued concealed bleeding – chest, abdomen, retroperitoneal space, pelvis, soft tissues of each thigh

Pump failure – haemothorax, pneumothorax, tamponade, myocardial contusion

Metabolic problem – acidaemia (only correct pH less than 7.1), hypothermia (largely preventable), hypocalcaemia (platelet count less than $75 \times 10\ 9\ L^{-1}$) in patients with high-energy trauma, central nervous system injury or ongoing haemorrhage. In assessing the requirement for platelets, frequent measurements are needed, as it may be necessary to request platelets at levels above the desired target in order to ensure their availability when needed. Requests for blood products should be made early as there is often delay in obtaining them and it is better to prevent the development of coagulation failure. Although diffuse pathological bleeding may be secondary to dilutional effects, it is also a manifestation of tissue hypoperfusion resulting from shock and inadequate or delayed resuscitation. Clinically, this microvascular bleeding produces oozing from mucosal or raw surfaces and puncture sites and may increase the extent of soft tissue and pulmonary contusions. It is difficult to treat and this underscores the importance of rapid and adequate resuscitation. Frequent estimation of platelet count, fibrinogen, PT and APTT is required.

Inadequate volume replacement is the most common complication of haemorrhagic shock. Mortality increases with increasing duration and severity of shock and so rapid and effective restoration of an adequate circulating blood volume is crucial in the management of major haemorrhage once the source has been controlled. The importance of the prevention of hypothermia during massive transfusion cannot be overstated. Hypothermia causes platelet dysfunction, an increased tendency to cardiac arrhythmias and a left-shift of the oxyhaemoglobin dissociation curve thereby decreasing oxygen delivery to the tissues. Hypothermia also decreases the metabolism of citrate and lactate, both of which are usually present in stored blood. If the normally rapid metabolism of these substances is slowed then a profound metabolic acidosis can develop. Core temperature should be measured continuously during massive transfusion and every effort must be made to prevent heat loss. Warm air over-blankets (e.g. Bair Hugger™) are usually helpful. Efficient systems for heating stored blood and allowing rapid infusion are available, but all fluids should be warmed to body temperature if possible. In addition, calcium chelation by citrate can lead to clinically significant hypocalcaemia, which should be treated and monitored.

ACKNOWLEDGEMENT

The editors acknowledge the significant input of Jo Haycock, Chris Moran, Jo Ollerton, Daren Forward and members of the East Midlands Trauma Centre steering group into the section on Major Trauma.

FURTHER READING

American College of Surgeons, 1997. Advanced trauma life support program for doctors, sixth ed. American College of Surgeons, Chicago.

Carless, P.A., Henry, D.A., Carson, J.L., 2010. Transfusion thresholds and other strategies for guiding allogenic red blood cell transfusion (Review). The Cochrane Collaboration 2010. Cochrane Database Syst. Rev. CD002042.

Funk, D.J., Moretti, E.W., Gan, T.J., 2009. Minimally invasive cardiac output monitoring in the perioperative setting. Anesth. Analg. 108, 887–897.

Marik, P.E., Baram, M., Vahid, B., 2008. Does central venous pressure predict fluid responsiveness?; a systematic review of the literature and the tale of seven mares. Chest 134, 172–178.

Moran, C.G., Forward, D., 2012. The early management of patients with multiple injuries : an evidence-based, practical guide for the orthopaedic surgeon. J. Bone Joint Surg. Br. 94-B, 446–453.

National Confidential Enquiry into Patient Outcome, Death (NCEPOD), 2010. An age old problem: 'A review of the care received by elderly patients undergoing surgery'. Available from http://www.ncepod.org.uk/2010report3/downloads/EESE_fullReport.pdf.

Sinclair, S., James, S., Singer, M., 1997. Intraoperative intravascular volume optimisation and length of hospital stay after repair of proximal femoral fracture: randomised controlled trial. BMJ 315, 909–912.

Stainsby, D., MacLennan, S., Hamilton, P.J., 1997. Management of massive blood loss: a template guideline. Br. J. Anaesth. 85, 487–496.

www.ncepod.org.uk/2007report2/Downloads/SIP_report.pdf.

www.nao.org.uk/publications/0910/major_trauma_care.aspx.

ANAESTHESIA OUTSIDE THE OPERATING THEATRE

General anaesthesia outside the operating theatre suite is often challenging for the anaesthetist, because specialized environments pose unique problems. In hospital, the anaesthetist must provide a service for patients with standards of safety and comfort which are equal to those in the main operating department. Outside the hospital, this level of service is more dependent on location and available resources.

ANAESTHESIA IN REMOTE HOSPITAL LOCATIONS

In-hospital remote locations include radiology, radiotherapy, the Accident and Emergency (A & E) department and wards with areas designated for procedures such as ECT, assisted conception, cardioversion and intrathecal chemotherapy administration.

General Considerations and Principles

Anaesthetists are frequently required to use their skills (e.g. administer anaesthesia, analgesia, sedation, resuscitate, cannulate, etc.) outside the familiar operating theatre environment. When requests are made for anaesthetic intervention in remote locations, there are multiple considerations which the anaesthetist must be aware of. These include the following.

1. *Appropriate personnel.* Only senior experienced anaesthetists who are also familiar with the particular environment and its challenges should normally administer anaesthesia in remote locations. Additional skilled anaesthetic help may not be readily available compared with an operating theatre suite and patients are often challenging, e.g. paediatric or critically ill.

2. *Equipment.* The remote clinical area may not have been designed with anaesthetic requirements in mind. Anaesthetic apparatus often competes for space with bulky equipment (e.g. scanners) and, in general, conditions are less than optimal. Monitoring capabilities and anaesthetic equipment should be of the same standard as those used in the operating department. In reality, such equipment may not be readily available and the equipment used is often the oldest in the hospital. Nevertheless, the monitoring equipment should meet the minimum standards set by the Association of Anaesthetists of Great Britain and Ireland (AAGBI, 2006). The anaesthetist who is unfamiliar with the environment should spend time becoming accustomed to the layout and equipment. Compromised access to the patient and the type of monitors used during the procedure require careful consideration. Advanced planning helps to prepare for unanticipated scenarios. Clinical observation may be limited by poor lighting.

3. *Patient preparation.* Preparation of the patient may be inadequate because the patient is from a ward where staff are unfamiliar with preoperative protocols, or patients may be unreliable, e.g. those presenting for ECT.

4. *Assistance.* An anaesthetic assistant (e.g. operating department practitioner) should be present, although this person may be unfamiliar with the environment. Maintenance of anaesthetic equipment may be less than ideal. Consequently, the anaesthetist must be particularly vigilant in

checking the anaesthetic machine, particularly because it may be disconnected and moved when not in use. Empty gas cylinders need to be replaced in older suites without piped gases, and also the anaesthetist must ensure the presence of drugs, spare laryngoscope and batteries, suction and other routine equipment.

5. *Communication.* Communication between staff of other specialities and the anaesthetist may be poor. This may lead to failure in recognizing each other's requirements. Education programmes for non-anaesthesia personnel regarding the care of anaesthetized patients may be of benefit.

6. *Recovery.* Recovery facilities are often non-existent. Anaesthetists may have to recover their own patients in the suite. Consequently, they must be familiar with the location of recovery equipment including suction, supplementary oxygen and resuscitation equipment. Alternatively, patients may be transferred to the main hospital recovery area. This requires the use of routine transfer equipment which should ideally be available as a 'pack' kept alongside monitoring equipment and a portable oxygen supply. This avoids searching for various pieces of equipment which may delay transfer, and ensures that nothing is forgotten. The pack should be regularly checked and maintained.

There should be a nominated lead anaesthetist responsible for remote locations in which anaesthesia is administered in a hospital. This individual should liaise with the relevant specialities, e.g. radiologists, psychiatrists, to ensure that the environment, equipment and guidelines are suitable for safe, appropriate and efficient patient care.

Anaesthesia in the Radiology Department

In most hospitals, members of the anaesthetic department are called upon to anaesthetize or sedate patients for diagnostic and therapeutic radiological procedures. These procedures include ultrasound, angiography, computed tomography (CT) scanning and magnetic resonance imaging (MRI). The major requirement of all these imaging techniques is that the patient remains almost motionless. Thus, general anaesthesia may be necessary when these investigations and interventions are performed in children, the critically ill

or the uncooperative patient. The presence of pain or prolonged procedures may also be an indication for anaesthesia.

Radiological studies may require administration of conscious sedation. This term describes the use of medication, often given by a non-anaesthetist, to alter perception of painful and anxiety-provoking stimuli while maintaining protective airway responses and the ability to respond appropriately to verbal command. Medical personnel responsible for the sedation should be familiar with the effects of the medication and skilled in resuscitation (including airway management). All the equipment and drugs required for resuscitation should be readily available and checked regularly. It is undesirable for a single operator to be responsible for both the radiological procedure and administration of sedation because there is the potential to be distracted from one responsibility and to allow side-effects to go untreated. Ideally, different individuals should be responsible for each of these tasks. Guidelines for prescribing, evaluating and monitoring sedation should be readily available. Chloral hydrate may be used in young children and benzodiazepines, opioids or propofol in adults. Patients should be starved before sedation and vital signs monitored and documented.

Iodine-containing intravascular contrast agents are used routinely during angiographic and other radiological investigations. The anaesthetist must always be aware of the risk of adverse reactions to contrast dyes. In recent years, low-osmolarity contrast media have been introduced; these cause less pain and have fewer toxic effects than the older contrast agents, but are more expensive. Factors contributing to the development of adverse reactions include speed of injection, type and dose of contrast used and patient susceptibility.

Coronary and cerebral angiography are associated with a high risk of reaction. Other major risk factors include allergies, asthma, extremes of age (under 1 and over 60 years), cardiovascular disease and a history of previous contrast medium reaction. Fatal reactions are rare, occurring in about 1 in 100 000 procedures. Nausea and vomiting are common and reactions may progress to urticaria, hypotension, arrhythmias, bronchospasm and cardiac arrest. Treatment of allergic reactions depends on the severity of the reaction.

This usually consists of fluids, oxygen and careful monitoring. An anaphylaxis protocol should be readily available along with adrenaline, antihistamines, steroids and fluids, preferably as an 'anaphylaxis kit'. Adequate hydration is important, because patients undergoing contrast dye procedures usually have an induced osmotic diuresis, which may exacerbate preexisting renal dysfunction. Patients at particular risk are dehydrated patients, those with chronic renal dysfunction and patients in the recovery phase of acute renal failure for which renal replacement therapy has been required. In these patients, even small doses of contrast may cause sufficient deterioration to necessitate further haemofiltration. Some intensive care units have a policy of giving acetylcysteine with a fluid load up to 1 h before the scan, with a further dose after the scan to protect against contrast-induced nephropathy. A urinary catheter may be useful for patients undergoing long procedures.

Healthcare workers are exposed to X-rays in the radiology and imaging suites. The greatest source is usually from fluoroscopy and digital subtraction angiography. Although the patient dose is high, ionizing radiation from a CT scanner is relatively low because the X-rays are highly focused. Radiation intensity and exposure decrease with the square of the distance from the emitting source. The recommended distance is 2–3 m. This precaution, together with lead aprons, thyroid shields and movable lead-lined glass screens, keeps exposure at a safe level. A personal-dose monitor should be worn by personnel who work frequently in an X-ray environment.

Computed Tomography

General Principles. A CT scan provides a series of tomographic axial 'slices' of the body. It is used most frequently for intracranial imaging and for studies of the thorax and abdomen and is the investigation of choice in the evaluation of major trauma when whole body CT may be used in place of plain X-rays. Each image is produced by computer integration of the differences in the radiation absorption coefficients between different normal tissues and between normal and abnormal tissues. The image of the structure under investigation is generated by a cathode ray tube and the brightness of each area is proportional to the absorption value.

One rotation of the gantry produces an axial slice or 'cut'. A series of cuts is made, usually at intervals of 7 mm, but this may be larger or smaller depending on the diagnostic information sought. The first-generation scanners took 4.5 min per cut, but the newest scanners take only 2–4 s.

The circular scanning tunnel contains the X-ray tube and detectors, with the patient lying stationary in the centre during the study. The procedure is noisy and patients are occasionally frightened or claustrophobic.

Anaesthetic Management. Computed tomography is non-invasive and painless, requiring neither sedation nor anaesthesia for most adult patients. A few patients may require conscious sedation to relieve fears or anxieties. However, patients who cannot cooperate (most frequently paediatric and head trauma patients or those who are under the influence of alcohol or drugs) or those whose airway is at risk may need general anaesthesia to prevent movement, which degrades the image. Anaesthetists may also be asked to assist in the transfer from the ICU and in the care of critically ill patients who require CT scans.

General anaesthesia is preferable to sedation when there are potential airway problems or when control of intracranial pressure (ICP) is critical. Because the patient's head is inaccessible during the CT scan, the airway needs to be secured. In the majority of situations, tracheal intubation is more appropriate than the use of a laryngeal mask airway (e.g. full stomach). The scan itself requires only that the patient remains motionless and tolerates the tracheal tube. If ICP is high, controlled ventilation is essential to maintain normo- or hypocapnia.

Because these patients are often in transit to or from critical care areas or A & E, a total intravenous technique with neuromuscular blockade is usually the technique of choice with tracheal intubation and controlled ventilation. Use of volatile anaesthetic agents during the scan is also acceptable but may involve changing from one technique to another for transfer. In addition, the anaesthetic machine may be left unplugged when not in use in the scanner and reconnecting and checking it may be distracting and time-consuming. A portable ventilator with CO_2 monitoring removes the need to change breathing systems. If the scan is likely to take a long time, it may be advisable to change from cylinder to piped oxygen supply to conserve supplies for transfer. Anaesthetic complications while in the scanner include kinking of the tracheal tube or disconnection of the breathing system, particularly during positioning and movement of the gantry, hypothermia in paediatric patients and disconnection of drips and lines during transfer. In addition, in the trauma setting, patients may become markedly unstable during movement on to the scanning table, and emergency drugs and fluids should be readily available. If, during the scan, the anaesthetist is observing the patient from inside the control room, it is imperative that alarms/monitors have visual signals which may be seen easily.

Stereotactic-guided surgery is possible using CT scanners although this has largely been replaced by frameless image guidance systems which allow tumour localization in the theatre suite from an existing scan. Most procedures involve aspiration or biopsy of intracranial masses in eloquent or important motor areas to give a tissue diagnosis with minimal risk to surrounding structures. The patient may either be anaesthetized in the theatre suite and then transferred to the CT scanner or anaesthetized in the scanner itself. Advantages of the former are induction of anaesthesia in a familiar environment with assistance and equipment readily available; the disadvantage is that the patient then must be transferred to the CT scanner and back again to theatre. The advantage of inducing anaesthesia in the CT scanner is that the need for initial transfer is removed, but there are the risks already outlined of anaesthesia in a remote location. Pins are used to hold a radiolucent frame around the head and then coordinates are mapped onto the frame from the scan to allow precise location of the tumour. Application of the frame via the pins is painful and access to the patient and airway with the frame attached inside the scanner is difficult.

Magnetic Resonance Imaging

General Principles. Magnetic resonance imaging (MRI) is an imaging modality which depends on magnetic fields and radiofrequency pulses for the production of its images. The imaging capabilities of MRI are superior to those of CT for examining intracranial, spinal and soft tissue lesions. MRI differentiates clearly between white and grey matter in the brain, thus making possible, for example, the *in vivo* diagnosis of demyelination. It may display images in the sagittal, coronal, transverse or oblique planes and has the advantage that no ionizing radiation is produced.

An MRI imaging system requires a large magnet in the form of a tube which is capable of accepting the entire length of the human body. A radiofrequency transmitter coil is incorporated in the tube which surrounds the patient; the coil also acts as a receiver to detect the energy waves from which the image is constructed. In the presence of the magnetic field, protons in the body align with the magnetic field in the longitudinal axis of the patient. Additional perpendicular magnetic pulses are applied by the radiofrequency coil; these cause the protons to rotate into the transverse plane. When the pulse is discontinued, the nuclei relax back to their original orientation and emit energy waves which are detected by the coil. The magnet is over 2 m in length and weighs approximately 500 kg. The magnetic field is applied constantly even in the absence of a patient. It may take several days to establish the magnetic field if it is removed and this is only done in an emergency because it is very expensive to shut down the field. The magnetic field strength is measured in tesla units (T). One tesla is the field intensity generating 1 Newton of force per 1 ampere of current per 1 metre of conductor. One tesla equals 10 000 gauss; the earth's surface strength is between 0.5 and 1.0 gauss. MRI strengths usually vary from 1 to 3 T although some research facilities have scanners which may produce fields up to 9.4 T. The force of the magnetic field decreases exponentially with distance from the magnet and a safety line at a level of 5 gauss is usually specified. Higher exposure may result in pacemaker malfunction and unscreened personnel should not cross this level. At 50 gauss, ferromagnetic objects become dangerous projectiles. The magnetic fields present are strong static fields which are present all around the magnet area, and fast-switching and pulsed radiofrequency fields in the immediate vicinity of the magnet.

The final MR image is made from very weak electromagnetic signals, which are subject to interference from other modulated radio signals. Therefore, the scanner is contained in a radiofrequency shield (Faraday cage). A hollow tube of brass is built into this cage to allow monitoring cables and infusion lines to pass into the control room. This is termed the waveguide.

Anaesthetic Management

STAFF SAFETY. Staff safety precautions are essential. The supervising MR radiographer is operationally responsible for safety in the scanner and anaesthetic staff should defer to him or her in matters of MR safety. Screening questionnaires identify those at risk and training should be given in MR safety, electrical safety, emergency procedures arising from equipment failure and evacuation of the patient. Anaesthetists should also understand the consequences of quenching the magnet and be aware of recommendations on exposure and the need for ear protection. Long-term effects of repeated exposure to MRI fields are unknown, and pregnant staff should be offered the option not to work in the scanner. All potentially hazardous articles should be removed, e.g. watches, bleeps and stethoscopes. Bank cards, credit cards and other belongings containing electromagnetic strips become demagnetized within the vicinity of the scanner and personal computers, pagers, phones and calculators may also be damaged.

PATIENT SAFETY. Metal objects within or attached to the patient pose a risk. Jewellery, hearing aids or drug patches should be removed. Absolute contraindications include implanted surgical devices, e.g. cochlear implants, intraocular metallic objects and metal vascular clips. Pacemakers remain an absolute contraindication in most settings although some patients with a pacemaker have undergone scanning under tightly controlled conditions when the benefit has been deemed to outweigh the risk. Metallic implants, e.g. intracranial vascular clips, may be dislodged from blood vessels. Programmable shunts for hydrocephalus may malfunction because the pressure setting may be changed by the magnetic field, leading to over- or underdrainage. The use of neurostimulators such as spinal cord stimulators for chronic pain is increasing. These devices may potentially fail or cause thermal injury on exposure to the magnetic field. Each must be considered individually, some may be safe if strict guidelines are adhered to. Joint prostheses, artificial heart valves and sternal wires are safe because of fibrous tissue fixation. Patients with large metal implants should be monitored for implant heating. A description of the safety of various devices is available on dedicated websites. All patients should wear ear protection because noise levels may exceed 85 dB.

Other unique problems presented by MRI include relative inaccessibility of the patient. In most scanners, the body cylinder of the scanner surrounds the patient totally; manual control of the airway is impossible and tracheal intubation or use of a laryngeal mask airway is essential when general anaesthesia is necessary. The patient may be observed from both ends of the tunnel and may be extracted quickly if necessary. Because there is no hazard from ionizing radiation, the anaesthetist may approach the patient in safety.

EQUIPMENT. The magnetic effects of MRI impose restrictions on the selection of anaesthetic equipment. Any ferromagnetic object distorts the magnetic field sufficiently to degrade the image. It is also likely to be propelled towards the scanner and may cause a significant accident if it makes contact with the patient or with staff. Terminology regarding equipment used in the MRI scanner has now changed from 'MR compatible' or 'MR incompatible' to 'MR conditional', 'MR safe' or 'MR unsafe'. MR conditional equipment is that which poses no hazards in a specified MR environment with specified conditions of use. The conditions in which it may be used must accompany the device and it may not be safe to use it outside these conditions, e.g. higher field strength or rate of change of the field. MR safe equipment is that which poses no safety hazard in the MR room but it may not function normally or may degrade the image quality. Consideration needs to be given to replacing equipment if a scanner is replaced by one of higher field strength.

The layout of the MRI room/suite determines whether the majority of equipment needs to be inside the room (and therefore MR conditional or safe), or outside the room with suitable long circuits, leads and tubing to the patient. Suitable anaesthetic machines and ventilators are manufactured and may be positioned next to the magnetic bore to minimize the length of the breathing system. They require piped gases or special aluminium oxygen and nitrous oxide cylinders. Consideration also needs to be given to intravenous fluid stands, infusion pumps and monitoring equipment, including stethoscopes and nerve stimulators. Laryngoscopes may be non-magnetic, but standard batteries should be replaced with non-magnetic lithium batteries. Laryngeal mask airways without a metal spring in the pilot tube valve should be available.

All monitoring equipment must be appropriate for the environment. Technical problems with non-compatible monitors include interference with imaging signals, resulting in distorted MRI pictures, and radiofrequency signals from the scanner inducing currents in the monitor which may give unreliable monitor readings. Special monitors are available or unshielded ferromagnetic monitors may be installed just outside the MRI room and used with long shielded or non-ferromagnetic cables (e.g. leads may be fibreoptic or carbon fibre cable). Ambient noise levels are such that visual alarms are essential. The 2010 AAGBI guidelines on services for MRI suggest that monitoring equipment should be placed in the control room outside the magnetic area. A non-invasive automated arterial pressure monitor, in which metallic tubing connectors are replaced by nylon connectors, should be used. Distortion of the ECG may occur, which interferes with arrhythmia and ischaemia monitoring. Interference may be reduced by using short braided leads connected to compatible electrodes placed in a narrow triangle on the chest. There should be no loops in cables because these may induce heat generation and lead to burns. Side-stream capnography and anaesthetic gas concentration monitoring require a long sampling tube, which leads to a time delay of the monitored variables. The use of 100% oxygen during the scan should be indicated to the radiologist reporting the images because this may produce artefactually abnormal high signal in CSF spaces in some scanning sequences.

CONDUCT OF ANAESTHESIA. The indications for general anaesthesia during MRI are similar to those for CT. In addition, the scanner is very noisy and, in general, the patient lies on a long thin table in a dark, confined space within the tube (typical diameter 50–65 cm). This may cause claustrophobia or anxiety-related problems which may require sedation or anaesthesia. Obese patients cannot be examined in this small magnetic bore. A complex scan may take up to 20 min and an entire examination more than 1 h. Open scanners have been developed and some are available which allow the patient to stand up, allowing a greater range of patients to be scanned. Outside normal working hours, only neuraxial scanning is usually performed, for acute brain or spinal cord evaluation.

Anaesthesia is induced usually outside the MRI room in an adjacent dedicated anaesthetic area where it is safe to use ferromagnetic equipment (distal to the 5 gauss line). Most patients benefit from the use of short-acting drugs because these are associated with rapid recovery and minimal side-effects. Sedation of children by organized, dedicated and multidisciplinary teams for MRI has been shown to be safe and successful. However, general anaesthesia allows more rapid and controlled onset, with immobility guaranteed. All patients must be transported into the magnet area on MRI-appropriate trolleys. During the scan, the anaesthetist should ideally be in the control room but may remain in the scanning room in exceptional circumstances if wearing suitable ear protection. If an emergency arises, the anaesthetist needs to be aware of the procedure for rapid removal of the patient to a safe area.

Occasionally, ICU patients may require scanning. Careful planning is required and screening checklists should be used. Non-essential infusions should be discontinued and essential infusions may need to be transferred to MR safe pumps. This may induce a period of instability in the patient while the infusions are being moved and high requirements for drugs such as vasopressors may be a relative contraindication to scanning. The tracheal tube pilot balloon valve spring should be secured away from the scan area. Pulmonary artery catheters with conductive wires and epicardial pacing catheters should be removed to prevent microshocks. Simple central venous catheters appear safe if disconnected from electrical connections, etc. All anaesthetized patients, especially infants, are at risk from hypothermia because the MRI room may be cold.

Gadolinium-based contrast agents are used in MR and are generally safe, with a high therapeutic ratio. However, the use of these contrast agents in patients with renal failure may precipitate a life-threatening condition called nephrogenic systemic fibrosis. If the GFR is less than 30 mL min^{-1} per 1.73 m^2, only minimal amounts of contrast should be given (if deemed absolutely necessary). No more should be given for at least 7 days.

MRI-guided surgery is a new, highly specialized form of surgery which may continue to be developed. It offers surgeons radiological images of the tissues immediately beyond their operative field. This makes use of an open-configuration scanner rather than the traditional closed tubular scanner. The absence of ionizing radiation places less restriction on the duration of staff presence, but the anaesthetic considerations are similar to those of the traditional MRI scanner and the anaesthetist and all the related equipment including surgical instruments are required to be in the vicinity of the scanner and therefore compatible with a magnetic field. Surgery which has been performed in this environment includes endoscopic sinus surgery and neurosurgery.

Diagnostic and Interventional Angiography

General Principles. Direct arteriography using percutaneous arterial catheters is used widely for the diagnosis of vascular lesions. Catheters are usually inserted by the Seldinger technique via the femoral artery in the groin and injection of contrast medium provides images which are viewed by conventional or digital subtraction angiography. In addition, it is becoming increasingly common to consider vessel embolization both in the elective preoperative setting (e.g. vascular tumours or malformations) and in the emergency management of major haemorrhage (e.g. major trauma or massive obstetric or gastrointestinal haemorrhage). The procedure involves the injection of an embolic material to stimulate intravascular thrombosis, resulting in occlusion of the vessel. There is a risk of distal organ damage if the blood supply is completely occluded. Non-invasive angiographic techniques used with CT or MRI have reduced the need for direct arteriography for diagnosis of some vascular lesions. The advent of spiral and double helical CT scanners allows whole vascular territories to be mapped within 30 s and produces superior images, including three-dimensional pictures. MRI is sensitive to the detection of flow and, together with more sophisticated scanning and data collection techniques, is used increasingly for assessment of vascular structures.

Anaesthetic Management. Most angiographic procedures may be carried out under local anaesthesia, with sedation if necessary during more complex investigation. If the procedure is likely to be prolonged, general anaesthesia may be more appropriate; the same applies to nervous patients, those unable to cooperate and children. Complete immobility is required during the investigation and particularly if any interventional procedures are to be performed. Sedation to augment

local anaesthesia must be avoided in the presence of intracranial hypertension, because the increased $PaCO_2$ leads to vasodilatation and a further increase in ICP; in addition, vasodilatation results in poor-quality angiography. Major trauma patients and those with life-threatening haemorrhage are nearly always sedated, with ventilation controlled, before arrival in the angiography suite. The drawbacks of general anaesthesia include prolonging the time taken for the investigation and increasing the cost and risks associated with anaesthesia. Moreover, the patient is unable to react to misplaced injections and alert staff to untoward reactions.

Adequate hydration is essential for patients undergoing angiography because they are often fasted and the contrast medium causes an osmotic diuresis. Intravenous cannulae and monitor leads may require extensions to enable the anaesthetist to remain at an acceptable distance from the patient, to minimize exposure. This also allows the anaesthetist to remain outside the range of movement of the imaging machine.

Complications of Angiography

- *Local* – haematoma and haemorrhage, vessel wall dissection, thrombosis, perivascular contrast injection, adjacent nerve damage, loss and knotting of guide wires and catheters.
- *General* – contrast reactions of varying severity; emboli from catheter clots, intimal damage and air; sepsis and vagal inhibition.

Interventional Neuroradiology. Cerebral angiography may be used to demonstrate tumours, arteriovenous malformations, aneurysms, subarachnoid haemorrhage and cerebrovascular disease. Since the ISAT (International Subarachnoid Aneurysm Trial) in 2002 (which compared coiling in patients with a ruptured aneurysm of good clinical grade with surgical clipping) showed a favourable initial outcome, endovascular treatment has become the technique of choice for most patients. Detachable coils are used to pack the aneurysm to prevent rebleeding. These patients are often systemically unwell as a result of subarachnoid haemorrhage and may be profoundly cardiovascularly unstable during induction of anaesthesia. A thorough preoperative assessment should be made, including cardiovascular, respiratory, neurological and metabolic status. The risk of complications is generally increased in the elderly and those with pre-existing vascular disease, diabetes, stroke or transient ischaemic attacks. Many of these patients have intracranial hypertension and cerebral vasospasm; consequently, control of arterial pressure and carbon dioxide tension is essential. Obtunding the pressor response to tracheal intubation and careful positioning to avoid increasing central venous pressure are necessary to prevent elevation of intracranial pressure. A relaxant/IPPV technique with ventilation to mild hypocapnia ($PaCO_2$=4.5–5.0 kPa) is usually used. A moderate reduction in $PaCO_2$ causes vasoconstriction of normal vessels, slows cerebral circulation and contrast medium transit times and improves delineation of small vascular lesions.

Transient hypotension and bradycardia or asystole may occur during cerebral angiography with contrast dye injection. This usually responds to volume replacement and atropine. Complications during interventional neuroradiology include haemorrhage from rupture of the vessel, which may necessitate reversal of anticoagulation with protamine, and ischaemia as a result of thromboembolism (e.g. clot forming around the catheter tip), vasospasm, embolic material or hypoperfusion. Heparin and glycoprotein IIb/IIIa inhibitors (e.g. abciximab) may be required if an occlusive clot forms. All complications may occur rapidly and with devastating results. Occasionally, urgent craniotomy may be required.

Cardiac Catheterization.
General anaesthesia is required mainly for children (rarely in adults because sedation is usually adequate). In children (premature neonates to teenagers), congenital heart disease may cause abnormal circulations and intracardiac shunts, which often present with cyanosis, dyspnoea, failure to thrive and congestive heart failure. Patients may also have coexisting non-cardiac congenital abnormalities. Neonatal patients may be deeply cyanotic and critically ill. Initial echocardiography often gives a diagnosis but catheterization is required for treatment or determining the possibility of surgery. These radiological procedures include pressure and oxygen saturation measurements, balloon dilatation of stenotic lesions (e.g. pulmonary valve), balloon septostomy for transposition of the great arteries and ductal closure.

The ideal anaesthetic technique would not produce myocardial depression, would avoid hypertension and tachycardia, preserve normocapnia and maintain spontaneous respiration of air. All techniques have their limitations. Positive-pressure ventilation causes changes in pulmonary haemodynamics and therefore influences measurements of flow and pressure. Spontaneous respiration with volatile agents may not be suitable for patients with significant myocardial disease. The onset of action of anaesthetic drugs is affected by cardiac shunts and congestive failure. Contrast medium in the coronary circulation may cause profound transient changes in the ECG. Therefore, ECG and invasive arterial pressure monitoring should be used to allow rapid assessment of arrhythmias and hypotension. Children with cyanotic heart disease may be polycythaemic, thereby predisposing to thrombosis.

Pacemaker and Cardioverter/Defibrillator Implantation.
These devices may be inserted in the cardiac catheter laboratory. These procedures may be performed under local or general anaesthesia depending on the circumstances. Implantation requires placing transvenous leads in the cardiac chambers and subcutaneous tunnelling to the device pocket. Testing of cardioverter/defibrillator units should be performed under general anaesthesia and the benefit of using direct arterial monitoring considered.

TIPS Procedures.
Transjugular intrahepatic portosystemic shunt (TIPS) procedures are increasingly being carried out in the management of refractory portal hypertension, often secondary to cirrhosis. This decreases the risk of developing complications such as variceal bleeding or ascites. A shunt is created between the portal and hepatic veins to decrease vascular resistance. Complications include bleeding and liver injury (usually rare), hepatic encephalopathy as a result of increased nitrogen load from the gut and hepatic ischaemia. Patients are often acutely unwell with ascites, poor cardiovascular reserve and disordered fluid balance. General anaesthesia is usually required for comfort but may be challenging.

Anaesthesia for Radiotherapy
Adults may require general anaesthesia for insertion of intracavity radioactive sources to treat some types of tumour. The commonest tumours to be treated in this way are carcinoma of the cervix, breast or tongue. These

procedures are undertaken in the operating theatre and the anaesthetic management is similar to that for any type of surgery in these anatomical sites. These patients may require more than one anaesthetic for radiotherapy treatment. The anaesthetist may be exposed to radiation and appropriate precautions should be taken.

Radiotherapy is used increasingly in the management of a variety of malignant diseases which occur in childhood. These include the acute leukaemias, Wilms' tumour, retinoblastoma and central nervous system tumours. High-dose X-rays are administered by a linear accelerator and all staff must remain outside the room to be protected from radiation.

Anaesthesia in paediatric radiotherapy presents several problems.

1. Treatment is administered daily over a 4–6 week period and necessitates repeated doses of sedation or general anaesthesia.
2. The patient must remain alone and motionless for short periods during treatment, but immediate access to the patient is required in an emergency.
3. Monitoring is difficult because the child may be observed only on a closed-circuit television screen during treatment.
4. Recovery from anaesthesia must be rapid, because treatment is organized usually on an outpatient basis and disruption of normal activities should be minimized.

Before treatment begins, the fields to be irradiated are plotted and marked so that the X-rays may be focused on the tumour to avoid damaging the surrounding structures. This procedure requires the child to remain still for 20–40 min and takes place in semi-darkness. Radiotherapy treatment is of much shorter duration; two or three fields are irradiated for 30–90 s each. Anaesthesia or sedation may be required for both the focusing and the administration of radiation.

Anaesthetic Management

Frequently, these children have a Hickman line *in situ* to ensure reliable intravenous access for a range of medications and blood sampling. This makes induction of anaesthesia far simpler and avoids repeated i.v. cannulation, which may become technically difficult and also increasingly distressing for the patient, parent and anaesthetist. The dead space volume of Hickman lines must always be remembered and an attempt made to keep them clean. Failure to flush these lines immediately after administering drugs may lead to disastrous consequences when the anaesthetic drugs are flushed into the bloodstream at a later time. Inhalational induction with the child sitting on the parent's knee is an alternative technique. Agents such as ketamine are unsatisfactory because sudden movements may occur and excessive salivation may risk airway compromise.

When anaesthesia has been induced, the child is placed on a trolley and anaesthesia maintained with nitrous oxide, oxygen and volatile agent delivered via a laryngeal mask. No analgesia is required and tracheal intubation is generally not necessary. There is virtually no surgical stimulation and patients may be maintained at relatively light anaesthetic levels, allowing for rapid emergence and recovery. Monitoring during radiotherapy requires the patient, anaesthetic monitors and equipment to be observed continuously by closed-circuit television.

The same principles apply when anaesthetizing children for other oncology procedures such as bone marrow aspiration, lumbar puncture and administration of intrathecal chemotherapy. This often takes place in a dedicated suite on the oncology ward and patients attend as day cases to avoid the need to come to operating theatre. It is helpful to keep records of how best to manage these children both physically and emotionally to allow continuity and minimize the impact on the child and its family.

Anaesthesia for Electroconvulsive Therapy

Electroconvulsive therapy (ECT) is controlled electrical stimulation of the central nervous system to cause seizures. It is often administered in a dedicated ward area within a psychiatric hospital. Indications include severe depression, including postnatal depression and certain psychoses. The mechanism of the therapy remains unknown. The electrical stimulus applied transcutaneously to the brain results in generalized tonic activity for about 10 s followed by a generalized clonic episode lasting up to 1 min or more. The hand-held electrodes are placed in the bifrontotemporal region for bilateral ECT, or with both electrodes over the non-dominant hemisphere for unilateral therapy. The duration of the seizure may be important for outcome and depends on age, stimulus site, stimulus energy and drugs, including anaesthetics. Seizure activity lasting 25–50 s is optimal for the antidepressant effect. Treatment may initially be 2 or 3 times per week for 3 weeks. Contraindications include increased intracranial pressure, recent cerebrovascular accident, phaeochromocytoma, cardiac conduction defects, and cerebral or aortic aneurysms. The risks from ECT and anaesthesia need to be balanced against potential benefits. Drug interactions with tricyclic antidepressants, monoamine oxidase inhibitors and lithium should be considered and managed appropriately. Seizures cause parasympathetic followed by sympathetic discharge, producing bradycardia followed by tachycardia and hypertension. Myocardial and cerebral oxygen demands increase and cardiac arrhythmias and changes in blood pressure of variable magnitude and significance, depending on any underlying medical conditions (e.g. hypertension, coronary artery disease, peripheral vascular disease), may be precipitated. Emergence agitation, nausea, headache and fracture dislocations are other described complications.

Anaesthesia

The patient may be a poor historian because of the psychiatric condition, so a careful preoperative evaluation is essential, including dentition, reflux and fasting status. Anaesthesia with neuromuscular blockade is necessary to reduce physical and psychological trauma. The anaesthetic technique should allow a rapid recovery. Routine anaesthetic equipment and minimum standards of monitoring should be available. Pretreatment with glycopyrrolate may be useful to reduce bradycardia and oral secretions. After preoxygenation, an intravenous induction agent and a neuromuscular blocker are administered. A bite block is inserted when mask ventilation with oxygen is achieved and then the stimulus is applied to produce a seizure. Intubation of the trachea would be required in late pregnancy or other full-stomach situations. Ventilation should continue until the patient is breathing, because hypoxia and hypercapnia may shorten the seizure.

Propofol is the most commonly used intravenous anaesthetic agent, replacing methohexital in this role. If seizure activity is deemed inadequate, etomidate is sometimes used, although consideration must be given to the potential effect of adrenal suppression with repeated administration. Recovery is also likely to be less rapid. Thiopental is used occasionally but may

shorten the duration of the seizure. Sevoflurane has no advantages when compared with intravenous agents and is generally more time-consuming to administer.

Partial neuromuscular blockade is required to allow monitoring of the duration of the peripheral seizure and to reduce physical symptoms in an attempt to help to avoid trauma and minimize post-seizure muscle pain. Succinylcholine is often used in a dose of 0.5 mg kg^{-1} because it has a short duration. Subsequent doses for ECT may be modified as appropriate. Use of other neuromuscular blockers (e.g. mivacurium) may necessitate short post-procedural artificial ventilation and may not be as effective in preventing muscle contractions.

Cardiovascular drugs such as esmolol or labetalol may be required to minimize the acute haemodynamic changes of ECT in high-risk patients.

Anaesthetic drug administration and the patient's response should be accurately recorded, as in other anaesthetic situations. This is particularly important with ECT because the therapy is repeated frequently over several weeks. Each individual responds differently to the drugs used and consistent conditions are required to obtain the best ECT stimulus response.

Anaesthesia in the Accident and Emergency Department

Anaesthetists' involvement in the Accident and Emergency (A & E) department varies among hospitals, depending on the skills of the resident A & E medical staff. The following clinical conditions usually require an anaesthetist to attend the A & E department.

■ Preoperative assessment and resuscitation before emergency surgery, e.g. ruptured ectopic pregnancy.
■ Specialist airway management for a patient with respiratory failure or acute airway compromise.
■ Intensive care admission for a patient needing ventilatory and/or other organ support.
■ Resuscitation as part of the cardiac arrest or trauma team.
■ Patients requiring specialist cannulation skills.
■ Anaesthesia for patients requiring procedures such as cardioversion or gastric lavage.
■ Anaesthesia for patients requiring CT scan, e.g. suspected intracranial haemorrhage.

The anaesthetist attending A & E should be trained and experienced enough to manage these seriously ill patients. As in other remote locations, trained anaesthetic assistance is mandatory. Equipment and monitoring should match the minimum standard agreed for the main operating theatres. Although the anaesthetist should ideally be available continuously (assuming the A & E department is admitting patients), there may be a delay if he or she is busy in theatre or ICU. Therefore, the emergency physician or A & E doctor may sometimes have provided the initial care of the patient. In these situations, it is essential for the anaesthetist to obtain appropriate handover information and to check the patient/equipment carefully before accepting responsibility, e.g. before transferring the patient for CT scan or to the ICU.

ANAESTHESIA IN THE PRE-HOSPITAL ENVIRONMENT

The difficulties described in giving anaesthesia outside the operating theatre are compounded when working outside the hospital and the AAGBI has produced a safety guideline for pre-hospital anaesthesia. Anaesthetic intervention may be life-saving in specific situations. However, these situations are relatively infrequent and it can result in harm if performed poorly. It should only be performed by appropriately trained personnel with similar standards as those expected in hospital. There should also be a robust clinical governance structure integral to every pre-hospital service including audit, appraisal, case review, standard algorithms and a clearly defined lead clinician. Hospital staff may find themselves providing care in several situations:

- as a member of a hospital flying squad
- as an immediate care practitioner
- on duty (either paid or with the voluntary services) at an event such as a football match or festival
- Armed Forces medical staff in an incident response team.

Each of these situations has different clinical and logistical issues but there are some common areas. For this chapter, the main example used is that of hospital staff attending a road accident. Working safely in the pre-hospital environment demands consideration of hazards at the scene and of the roles of the other emergency services.

For example, at a road accident, potential hazards include:

- broken glass
- spilt fuel
- fire and smoke
- jagged metal edges in damaged vehicles
- other traffic moving around the incident
- cutting and lifting equipment being used by the fire brigade.

Personal Preparation for Working in the Pre-Hospital Environment

It is unreasonable to expect hospital staff to get into an ambulance and attend a road accident and function effectively without training and preparation. The road accident is also a remote and unsupervised location and hospitals should deploy only staff with the correct clinical background to work in these situations.

Preparation includes having appropriate safety clothing and equipment such as:

- coveralls
- high-visibility jackets
- helmets
- eye and ear protection
- safety boots
- gloves.

For people attending ballistic incidents, this needs to include ballistic helmets and body armour.

Staff also need insurance to cover travelling to and from the incident, and working at the incident. Advice on suitable equipment may be found on the British Association for Immediate Care (BASICS) website: *http://www.basics.org.uk*

Training in Pre-Hospital Care

Several organizations provide training in pre-hospital care. These include the following:

- BASICS runs courses in casualty extrication from vehicles and a pre-hospital emergency care certificate (PHEC, awarded jointly with the Royal College of Surgeons of Edinburgh). Information may be obtained from its website (see above).

- The Royal College of Surgeons (RCS) of Edinburgh examines for a Diploma and Fellowship in Immediate Medical Care. Information may be obtained from the Faculty of Pre-hospital Care at the RCS, Edinburgh.
- The Royal College of Surgeons of England oversees the Pre-hospital Trauma Life Support Course, PHTLS.

Team Working

Hospital personnel at an incident are there to support the Ambulance Service and they need to know whom to report to and how to work with ambulance staff and police. In addition, the Fire Service may be present to manage hazards and provide cutting equipment if needed for extrication. The police are present to coordinate the incident and the area around it, managing traffic flow and protecting evidence at the scene.

While everyone is concentrating their efforts on saving and treating the casualties, hospital staff need to understand that the other emergency services have their own roles, and the management of the incident continues after they and the casualties have left the scene.

Interservice working is addressed by the Major Incident Medical Management and Support (MIMMS) Course run by the Advanced Life Support Group: *http://www.alsg.org* and described in the MIMMS manual.

Working at the Scene

On arriving at an incident, the anaesthetist should report to the senior ambulance person, who has called the hospital flying squad or immediate care practitioner for a reason, such as:

- multiple casualties
- trapped casualties.

They may also provide an explanation of what has happened, from which the mechanism of injury may be inferred and likely injuries anticipated.

Problems likely to be encountered are:

- *Access to the casualty.* The vehicle compartment around the casualty may be deformed and intruded. The vehicle may be on its side, upside down or in a ditch, making access to the casualty difficult.

- *Lighting.* The emergency services may provide portable lights, but in pre-hospital care, the anaesthetist is often trying to assess and manage a casualty in poor light.
- *Noise.* Noise from generators and vehicles makes auscultation very difficult and interferes with communication with other team members and the other emergency services.
- *Environment.* Wet weather and cold conditions imply that casualties (and staff not wearing appropriate clothing) become hypothermic quickly.

Logistical Considerations

The aim is to move the patient in the best clinical condition possible to the most appropriate hospital in the shortest time possible. In reality, a series of compromises is needed. Before carrying out any procedure, the clinician on the scene needs to ask:

- Is this essential?
- Should it be carried out now, during the move to hospital or at the hospital?
- Am I helping the patient and the situation or causing undue delay? For example, is it appropriate to struggle for 15 min to set up an intravenous infusion when the hospital is only 5 min travel time away?
- If the casualty is trapped and needs intravenous analgesia or anaesthesia to facilitate release, then probably yes, unless there are alternatives.
- If the casualty is ready to leave the scene except for this intervention, then probably no (unless there is no vehicle available to move the casualty).

Decisions such as these depend on many factors, including the overall situation, travel time to hospital, availability of ambulances and the needs of other casualties.

Clinical Considerations

Airway. The main issue is oxygenation. As in hospital practice, simple methods should be tried first, such as chin lift, jaw thrust, oral airway, nasopharyngeal airway and laryngeal mask.

Tracheal intubation may be desirable in a casualty at risk of aspiration or with a severe head injury but this may not be practical if access to the casualty is restricted. Simple methods should be used first and the situation reassessed because access to the casualty may be improved (e.g. when the roof of the car has been cut off or when the casualty has been released from the vehicle). The NCEPOD Report from 2007 highlighted the deficiencies in airway management in trauma and emphasized the need for pre-hospital anaesthesia when appropriate. Rapid-sequence induction (RSI) with oral intubation is usually the technique of choice but this should be performed only by appropriately trained individuals with adequate resources. A surgical cricothyroidotomy is an alternative definitive airway if tracheal intubation is not possible.

Children are a separate group in whom the threshold for RSI and tracheal intubation should be high (i.e. tracheal intubation should generally be used only if other techniques have failed) because not all anaesthetists are familiar with the management of small children. The risk:benefit ratio should be considered and most can be treated with simple airway interventions.

Cervical Spine Control. Many road accident casualties are at risk of cervical spine injury. Neck collars and other immobilization devices limit mouth opening and make airway management difficult. The front of the collar may be removed and paramedics may be asked to substitute manual in-line immobilization if the anaesthetist is having difficulty establishing a clear airway.

Breathing. As in hospital, inadequate ventilation is supported if necessary using a bag/valve mask. Life-threatening injuries such as tension pneumothorax may be difficult to diagnose. Some clinical signs, such as tracheal deviation, present late. Breath sounds may be difficult to hear because of the noisy environment. Clinical signs such as the presence of subcutaneous emphysema, indicating an air leak, should be sought. The decision to decompress a chest may have to be made on the basis of deteriorating ventilation and 'most likely' diagnosis.

Circulation. Control of bleeding with pressure dressings or tourniquet should be achieved before attempting intravenous access. Intravenous fluid resuscitation should be targeted at the injury being managed. Some injuries require hypotensive resuscitation until surgical control is achieved; others require normotension

(for example, head injury to maintain cerebral perfusion). Blood loss may be very difficult to assess in the field. Blood can be difficult to see on soft muddy ground and may pool out of sight on the floor of vehicles.

Deficit. Casualties with a reduced Glasgow Coma Score (GCS) and at risk of pulmonary aspiration require airway protection (but see above).

Extremity. Fractures and dislocations may need to be reduced at the site of the accident, especially if this reduces bleeding or restores circulation to the distal limb. Analgesia is often needed (see below).

Anaesthetic and Analgesic Techniques

The principles of emergency anaesthesia are discussed in Chapter 37. In the pre-hospital environment, the same principles apply. Techniques which are familiar to the anaesthetist should be used. If the technique causes problems (e.g. apnoea or airway obstruction), the anaesthetist should have adequate access to the patient for appropriate management.

Local/Regional Anaesthesia. Ring blocks are effective for fingers trapped in machinery. Femoral block may help in the management of pain from a fractured femur.

Intravenous Analgesia. The anaesthetist is limited to those drugs carried by the ambulance service and deployed by the flying squad. Intravenous morphine, nalbuphine and tramadol have all been used pre-hospital; they should be titrated to effect, and any complications arising from their use should be managed.

Low-dose intravenous ketamine is an effective analgesic. Small bolus doses of 10–20 mg, titrated to effect, are adequate in some casualties to allow fracture alignment or release of a trapped limb.

Inhalational Analgesia. Many ambulances carry Entonox, which may be used alone or in combination with other drugs. The main concern with the nitrous oxide in Entonox is enlargement of a pneumothorax or other air-filled cavity.

Intravenous Anaesthesia. Rapid-sequence induction using an i.v. anaesthetic agent may be the technique of choice to allow airway protection and control of ventilation in the injured casualty. Appropriate agents include ketamine, etomidate and propofol but with the dose moderated according to the casualty's haemodynamic status. Before embarking on general anaesthesia, the anaesthetist should consider such issues as:

- Is there suitable access to the casualty?
- Who is available to provide assistance?
- Is there appropriate monitoring?
- Is appropriate equipment available? Unlike the anaesthetic room where equipment is easily to hand, the pre-hospital practitioner works using a rucksack or other bag containing a very limited range of equipment.

Ideally, there should be four people available to perform intubation, assist the anaesthetist, provide manual in-line stabilization and perform cricoid pressure.

Pre-oxygenation should be performed as in the standard hospital setting. If the casualty is combative and aggressive as a result of low GCS or the effects of drugs or alcohol, consideration may be given to carefully titrated sedation to allow adequate preoxygenation to take place rather than a 'smash and grab' approach which may result in significant hypoxaemia.

Even with a supine casualty on the roadside, laryngoscopy and successful tracheal intubation are often more difficult than in the anaesthetic room. A bougie or introducer should always be immediately to hand. In bright sunlight, it is difficult to see the light from the laryngoscope bulb in a casualty's airway and an assistant may be posted between the sunlight and the casualty. There should be a well rehearsed failed intubation plan. Tracheal tube placement should be confirmed using capnography and the tube should be secured so as not to impair venous drainage of the head and neck. Anaesthesia should be maintained with midazolam or propofol either as intermittent boluses or infusions, although infusion pumps are rarely to hand. Ventilation should aim to produce normocapnia and consideration should be given to the adequacy of the oxygen supply. Clinical assessment and monitoring should be employed continuously and recorded as fully as practicable. Observations should include:

- Pulse rate and rhythm
- Respiratory rate
- Pupil size and reactivity
- Lacrimation
- Presence or absence of muscular activity
- Non-invasive blood pressure (invasive monitoring is rarely used)
- Oxygen saturation
- Capnography
- ECG.

Transfer to Hospital

The choice of hospital is decided usually by the medical and ambulance staff on scene and relayed to ambulance control. Ambulance control or the personnel on scene should contact the hospital so that the receiving team is placed on standby and receives as much information about the casualty (or casualties) as possible in advance.

A checklist for transfer includes the following:

- Is the airway secured for transport? A tracheal tube or laryngeal mask should to be tied or taped in place.
- Is oxygen being provided in adequate quantities?
- Is breathing adequate or is assistance required? If the patient's lungs are being ventilated using a mechanical ventilator, is the power capacity (gas, electricity or battery) adequate for the journey? Is there a back-up such as a self-inflating bag?
- Is external bleeding controlled? Are i.v cannulae/catheters taped securely in place? What variables have been selected (arterial pressure and/or pulse) as indicators of resuscitation requirements?
- If the patient has a reduced GCS, have remediable causes such as hypovolaemia or hypoglycaemia been considered?
- Are splints secured? Is spinal immobilization in place (where indicated)? Has a check been made that straps from splints and spinal immobilization devices are not interfering with respiration?
- Is the patient being kept warm with blankets?
- Is appropriate monitoring in place?

In some situations, it is necessary to ignore much of this preparation and 'load and go' as fast as possible, e.g. some stabbing or gunshot incidents in which the overriding need is surgical intervention.

Civilian helicopter ambulances provide a fast method of transporting a patient to hospital but these have some limitations. The attending staff may be unfamiliar with working in a helicopter, the space around the casualty is restricted compared with a ground ambulance and the environment is noisy; also, a second ambulance journey is often required at many UK hospitals to transport the patient from the helicopter landing site to the A & E department.

FURTHER READING

AAGBI, 2006. Recommendations for standards of monitoring during anaesthesia and recovery. The Association of Anaesthetists of Great Britain and Ireland.

AAGBI, 2009. Pre-hospital Anaesthesia. The Association of Anaesthetists of Great Britain and Ireland.

AAGBI, 2010. Provision of anaesthetic services in MRI units. Anaesthesia 65, 766–770.

Advanced Life Support Group, 2002. Major incident medical management and support. second ed. BMJ Books, London.

Ding, Z., White, P.F., 2002. Anesthesia for electroconvulsive therapy. Anesth. Analg. 94, 1351–1364.

Greaves, I., Porter, K. (Eds.), 1999. Pre-hospital medicine: the principles and practice of immediate care. Arnold, London.

Hashimoto, T., Gupta, D.K., Young, W.L., 2002. Interventional neuroradiology – anesthetic considerations. Anesthesiol. Clin. North America 20, 347–359.

Holleran, R.S. (Ed.), 2003. Air and surface patient transport: principles and practice, third ed. Mosby, St Louis.

Trauma: Who Cares? 2007. National Confidential Enquiry into Patient Outcome and Death.

39

ANAESTHESIA FOR THE PATIENT WITH A TRANSPLANTED ORGAN

INTRODUCTION

There have been several advances in surgical techniques, perioperative management and immunosuppressive regimens to prevent early and late organ rejection. These have led to improvements in short and long-term outcomes after transplantation, with most patients now able to lead a relatively normal life (see Table 39.1). Furthermore, outcomes following patient re-transplantation after rejection or graft failure have improved. As a result, it is likely that non-transplant anaesthetists are more likely to encounter transplant recipients presenting for elective surgery in the future. Transplant recipients are more likely than the general population to require surgery for malignancy or emergency procedures especially for acute gastrointestinal pathology. In addition, the increased success of solid organ transplantation has led to the recipient population being older and having more comorbidities than previously. Furthermore, the use of 'marginal' donor organs, secondary to the relative shortage of organs, is likely to make the management of these patients more complex. In general, wherever recipients present for non-transplant surgery, the patient is likely to have both residual evidence of chronic disease, be immunocompromised and have reduced organ function. In the emergency situation, the effect of acute illness may also complicate further anaesthetic management.

Careful attention to detail in the anaesthetic management of these patients will allow a smooth transition through the current surgical problem and perioperative process without disruption of the complex immunosuppressive regimens and without the risk of rejection.

TABLE 39.1

Patient Survival After First Organ Transplantation (UK Figures: Year of Transplant 2001–2003)

	1 Year Survival (%)	2 Year Survival (%)	5 Year Survival (%) (3 Year*)
Kidney (live related)	98	97	95
Kidney (heart beating donation)	95	93	88
Kidney (non heart beating donation)	95	94	86
Liver	88	85	76
Heart	82	79	71
Lung	68	60	54*
Pancreas (including SPK)	95	-	-

GENERAL CONSIDERATIONS

Immunosuppression

Immunosuppressive regimens are an absolute necessity in promoting long-term benefit from transplantation. The use of mainly steroid-based immunosuppressive regimens is gradually being substituted with the development of newer agents which have fewer generalized adverse effects. As a result, the complications of steroid overdose are seen less commonly and iatrogenic

Cushing's syndrome is rare. However, even newer regimens have significant adverse effects and require careful monitoring. The greatest risk of graft rejection is within the first year after transplantation, especially in the first few months. Immunosuppressive regimens may be classified as:

- induction therapies – to reduce both early rejection episodes and complications associated with long-term treatments using either high dose conventional immunosuppressive agents or polyclonal/monoclonal antibodies.
- maintenance treatments – to prevent chronic rejection episodes with reduced dose therapies.

The characteristics, side effects and drug interactions of the main immunosuppressive agents are shown in Table 39.2.

Plasma drug monitoring is usually performed by transplant physicians and most patients presenting for elective surgery are on a stable regimen of immunosuppressive drugs. Even with stable chronic treatment these patients remain at risk of:

- increased risk of infection (see Table 39.3) – all staff should be aware of the risks of opportunistic infections and take appropriate precautions, including aseptic techniques and microbiological monitoring.
- reduced wound healing – long-term immunosuppression also reduces the tensile strength of tissues and therefore may impair wound healing.
- major drug interactions – immunosuppressive drugs can cause interactions with a number of medications used for anaesthesia or postoperative pain relief.
- damage to other organ systems.

The presence of acute illness in combination with surgical stress is likely to create a period of instability. Early communication with the transplant team regarding immunosuppressive therapy is important to prevent large alterations of plasma drug concentrations. These may cause:

- drug toxicity – caused by reduced drug elimination or metabolism.
- risk of rejection – inadequate plasma levels lead to risk of rejection. This risk is greater in the early period after transplantation and during periods of acute rejection.

Residual Comorbidity

It is important to consider the nature of the disease process leading to the initial requirement for transplantation. Although some systemic manifestations are reduced by successful transplantation, residual disease in other organs associated with pre-transplant disease may remain (e.g. lung disease secondary to impaired liver function, cardiac disease secondary to renal failure).

The interval between organ transplantation and subsequent elective surgery determines the likelihood, nature and complexity of anaesthetic problems. Within the first 6 months after transplantation, the major considerations for the anaesthetist are those of graft rejection and acute changes in physiology. One year after successful transplantation, the likelihood of significant physiological changes is lower although the risk of chronic rejection always remains.

ANAESTHETIC CONSIDERATIONS

Preoperative

Immunosuppressive Regimens

It is important to understand the status and stability of the patient's immunosuppressive regimen and it is appropriate to communicate with the transplant team at an early stage. As a general rule, all current immunosuppressive therapy should be continued throughout the perioperative period. However, if gastrointestinal absorption is likely to be compromised after surgery, oral immunosuppressive drugs should be converted to intravenous preparations; drug doses must be guided by drug bioavailability. Complete omission of immunosuppressive regimens must be limited to the most extreme cases, where sepsis is potentially life threatening and where the risk of graft rejection becomes a secondary issue.

Transplanted Organ Status

Although many standard biochemical tests of renal, liver and cardiac function are normal in transplant recipients, the functional reserve of most transplanted organs is reduced. Any degree of surgical stress can potentially reduce organ function further and may lead to organ failure. Therefore, any measure available to reduce surgical stress (e.g. by changes in anaesthetic

TABLE 39.2

Immunosuppressive Drugs: Mechanisms of Action, Side Effects and Interactions

Drug Type	Mechanism of Action	Side Effects	Interactions
Maintenance Regimens			
Steroids	Block T and B cell activation via inhibition of IL and cytokine gene transcription	Hypertension, hyperlipidaemia, diabetes, osteoporosis	
Calcineurin inhibitors (e.g. Cyclosporin A, Tacrolimus)	Inhibit IL-2 T cell activation: relies on CYP450 metabolism	CyA - Hypertension, nephrotoxicity, hyperkalaemia, neurological Tacrolimus – diabetes, nephrotoxicity, neurological	Macrolides
Antiproliferatives (Mycophenolate mofetil (MMF), Azathioprine)	MMF - Inhibitor of T and B cell inosine monophosphate dehydrogenase AZA – Inhibits purine nucleotide synthesis	GI upset, marrow suppression (anaemia, leucopaenia, thrombocytopaenia)	Metronidazole, norfloxacin
mTOR inhibitor (e.g. Sirolimus)	Combines with mTOR via FK-binding resulting in cell cycle arrest	Marrow suppression (anaemia, leucopaenia), hypercholesterolaemia	Antifungals, some antimicrobials
Induction Therapy			
Polyclonal antibodies (e.g. Anti-thymocyte globulin (ATG))	Polyclonal antibodies: act against most T cell antigens	Cytokine response (fever, anaphylaxis)	
Monoclonal antibodies (e.g. OKT3, Daclizumab, basiliximab, alemtuzumab)	Monoclonal antibodies: (1) OKT3 – Act against CD3 on T cells (2) Daclizumab, basiliximab - Block IL-2 T-cell activation (3) Alemtuzumab (Campath) – Specific action against common lymphocyte and monocyte CD52 antigen: depletes lymphocytes without reducing neutrophils, etc	Haematological suppression, fever, nausea, pulmonary oedema (ARDS) Alemtuzumab – hypotension, bleeding, allergic reaction	

TABLE 39.3

Organisms Causing Common Opportunistic Infections in Transplant Recipients

CMV (cytomegalovirus)

Fungi – *Aspergillus* sp, *Candida* sp

Pneumocystis sp

Legionella sp

Toxoplasma sp

Listeria sp

management or minimally invasive surgery) should be used where appropriate. Where either biochemical or clinical evidence of rejection is present, further investigation and graft optimization is mandatory before any surgical procedure.

Presence of Infection

In addition to the presence of infection causing the initial requirement for transplantation (e.g hepatitis or CMV), the development of *de novo* infection must be investigated. However, the diagnosis may be difficult in these patients because typical presenting features may be absent. Fever may not be present and given that some drug regimens cause leucopoenia, an increased white cell count for a particular patient may lie within the 'normal' range. In elective situations, a recent culture screen for infection should have been performed before surgery and will guide further management. Early discussion with microbiology colleagues should take place to assess the correct regimen for surgical prophylaxis. There is no evidence to support an increase in the use or duration of prophylactic perioperative antibiotics in the transplant recipient.

Function of Other Organ Systems

Although the status of the transplanted organ and associated system is important, the systemic effect of the disease process that created the need for transplant must also be considered. Although transplantation may reduce the effects of this disease, full reversal of major systemic disease is unlikely.

Cardiovascular issues are common to many multisystem diseases requiring transplantation especially renal, pancreatic, and liver disease and are a common cause of mortality after transplantation. Paradoxically, the presence of coronary artery disease in cardiac transplant recipients is less likely unless rejection is present. Although most patients undergoing these transplants will have had a full investigation of their cardiac status before transplantation, presentation for surgical procedures may occur sometime after the transplantation. Therefore, depending on the complexity of the surgery contemplated, more up to date investigation may be warranted. The presence and stability of diabetes must be known. As previously mentioned, systemic toxicity caused by immunosuppressive regimens, must also be considered before surgery.

Intraoperative

The overriding principles for anaesthetic management of transplant recipients are to reduce the degree of surgical stress, avoid injury to the transplanted organ and to protect against infection.

Avoidance of Surgical Stress

Laparoscopic surgical techniques have the advantage of reducing surgical stress. However, especially in the case of abdominal solid organ transplants (i.e. liver,

pancreas, intestinal) this must be balanced with the increased intra-abdominal pressures during laparoscopy and the potential to reduce organ perfusion. Regional analgesic techniques also reduce surgical stress but may have relative contraindications if coagulation (liver), haemodynamic (cardiac) or autonomic (e.g. renal, pancreatic) dysfunction are present.

Reduce Injury to Transplanted Organ

It is vital to maintain adequate perfusion of the transplanted organ, and hypovolaemia must be avoided. Minimally invasive techniques are now available to optimize fluid balance and cardiac output and these are recommended in major surgery, where blood loss and fluid shifts are most likely. Perfusion pressures must be maintained for renal transplant recipients and direct arterial monitoring is indicated in these patients for all but the most minor procedures, especially where preoperative hypertension exists. Other measures should be used to maintain organ perfusion in addition to maintaining circulating volume, particularly in liver transplant recipients. These include the avoidance of high central venous pressures, high levels of PEEP and excessive doses of volatile anaesthetic agents. It is important to avoid high airway pressures and excessive airway manipulation to prevent organ injury in lung transplant recipients. Direct injury to cardiac function in heart transplant recipients is less likely during noncardiac surgery.

The use of anaesthetic agents that are non-toxic to the transplanted organ is important, given reduced organ reserve. Large volumes of radiological contrast agents, aminoglycosides and non-steroidal anti-inflammatory drugs are best avoided in renal transplant recipients. Liver transplant function is rarely affected by anaesthetic drugs and, importantly, paracetamol in analgesic doses is not contraindicated.

Infection

Strict asepsis must be adhered to at all times especially when inserting central venous access lines or performing regional anaesthetic techniques. It is best to avoid using dedicated *in situ* TPN lines for the administration of anaesthetic drugs. Although predominantly determined by the type of surgery, some advocate minimal airway manipulation and the avoidance of nasal intubation.

Postoperative

Postoperative management of transplant recipients must be carefully planned and the requirement for enhanced postoperative care facilities must be considered; this depends on the preoperative status of the patients and the type of surgery. If admission to critical care is contemplated, the risk of infection must be considered and a separate cubicle may be required.

Analgesia is best provided with regional techniques, thereby preventing the administration of intravenous or oral agents that have the potential for transplanted organ toxicity. Reduced metabolism and excretion of analgesic agents, especially opioids, may require alteration in drug type dose or interval and more rapid acting agents are commonly used in liver and renal transplant recipients.

The administration of additional steroid doses to prevent the possibility of adrenal unresponsiveness is controversial. Although hypothalamic-pituitary axis suppression is common, the incidence of severe perioperative events including hypotension and adrenal crisis is rare. Some authors suggest that supplementation is not required unless the maintenance steroid dose is >20 mg prednisolone per day. In the absence of clear evidence, the use of prolonged supraphysiological doses of steroids is best avoided and the continuation of chronic steroid doses with short term steroid augmentation is recommended. A dose of 25–75 mg day^{-1} hydrocortisone for 24–48 h is adequate for all but the most major procedures.

SPECIFIC ISSUES

Renal

The kidney is the most commonly transplanted organ and renal transplantation has the most successful patient outcome. The success of the live-related kidney program has further increased the number of transplants being performed and allowed patients with more severe comorbidities to undergo transplantation. For these reasons, the non-transplant anaesthetist is most likely to encounter patients with a renal transplant.

Indications for Renal Transplantation

Typical indications for renal transplantation include:

- diabetic nephropathy (often combined as simultaneous kidney–pancreas transplant)
- hypertensive nephrosclerosis
- acute and chronic glomerulonephritis
- polycystic kidney.

The effects of renal transplantation on quality of life issues are profound: most recipients are rendered dialysis-free. However, any systemic complications already present as a component of renal disease may continue to pose problems. Patients presenting for surgery may retain diabetic-related illnesses, ischaemic heart disease, hypertension and pulmonary disease. They are also maintained on relatively severe immunosuppressive regimens with the risk of adverse effects (Table 39.2).

Preoperative Status

Serum creatinine concentrations are often normal, but in most cases, glomerular filtration rate and renal plasma flow are reduced. This may have a covert effect on drug metabolism and excretion. Nephrotoxic drugs (e.g. contrast agents, aminoglycosides) should be given in reduced doses, whereas non-steroidal anti-inflammatory drugs are relatively contraindicated. Hypertension, often induced by Cyclosporin A, is a common problem after transplantation, with 50% of renal recipients requiring therapy at one year after transplant.

Surgical Presentation

Renal recipients present early after transplantation for bleeding problems or inadequate urine output. Later presentation for non-transplant surgical intervention is often due to urological complications or the need for further fistula formation where transplantation has been unsuccessful. Systemic complications of renal disease including osteoporosis may require orthopaedic intervention. Gastrointestinal and cardiac diseases are also more common in these patients and may require surgical intervention.

Anaesthetic Considerations

Regional anaesthesia is safe in renal transplant recipients and should be considered in the first instance. However, general anaesthesia is often required and is best performed using rapid acting agents, which do not rely on renal excretion. Desflurane or isoflurane are the volatile agents of choice. Sevoflurane is also safe and early reports of high doses of fluoride ions after prolonged surgical procedures have not been shown to be harmful in humans. Scrum potassium concentrations must be determined where suxamethonium is being used. All non-depolarizing neuromuscular blockers may be used but atracurium or cisatracurium have theoretical advantages, given the likelihood of reduced renal reserve. All drugs that have active intermediate metabolites (e.g. morphine) may have a prolonged action and should be used with caution. Alternatively, analgesia may be provided by regional or central neuraxial blockade. Since the transplanted kidney has no autoregulatory mechanisms, it is particularly susceptible to damage if perfusion pressure is reduced. Therefore, an appropriate blood pressure must be maintained by both the judicious use of vasopressor therapy and the assiduous avoidance of hypovolaemia, especially where dialysis has been performed before surgery. In this regard, a non-invasive monitor of fluid status with or without invasive arterial pressure monitoring is appropriate.

Liver

Liver transplantation is now the second commonest transplant surgery performed in the UK. The requirement for liver transplantation is likely to increase given the recent trend for an increased incidence of fatty liver and alcohol-related illnesses in younger individuals. The limiting factor to liver transplantation is the paucity of donor organs although live-related transplantation is now being performed in some centres in the UK. The survival rates for liver transplantation are high: 85–90% of patients survive to 1 year and 75% survive for 5 years.

Indications for Transplantation

Common indications for orthoptic liver transplantation include:

- alcoholic liver disease (abstinent/reformed patients)
- viral hepatitis (e.g. hepatitis C, B)
- primary biliary cirrhosis
- drug-induced hepatitis
- paracetamol-induced liver failure – acute transplantation.

Preoperative Status

Successful transplantation leads to an early return to normal hepatic function and coagulation. Drug metabolism starts earlier within hours of reperfusion in a well functioning graft. Many of the systemic manifestations of liver disease including pulmonary abnormalities return to normal postoperatively. Resolution of pleural effusions, ascites and pulmonary shunting occurs within the first few weeks. Hepatopulmonary syndrome usually resolves and oxygenation is rarely a problem in patients after transplant. Porto-pulmonary hypertension, secondary to chronic liver disease, was previously a contraindication to transplantation. However, preoperative therapy with pulmonary vasodilator therapy has allowed successful transplantation in these patients. However, complete resolution of this problem is uncommon and many patients remain on therapy. These drugs must be continued throughout the perioperative period and any factors leading to pulmonary vasoconstriction must be eliminated. The haemodynamic stigmata of chronic liver disease (systemic vasodilatation and high cardiac output) usually return to a normal level within months of transplantation but tolerance of a low systemic vascular resistance in the early postoperative period is important as long as adequate blood pressure allows. Similar to the renal allograft, lack of autoregulation makes the organ susceptible to ischaemia-reperfusion injury. Hypovolaemia, high levels of PEEP, and increased central venous pressures, may lead to worsening of liver function.

Surgical Presentation

Liver transplantation has a high incidence (15–20%) of needing early re-operation and this may not always be dealt with by the transplant team. Indications include surgical bleeding from the gallbladder bed, posterior to the liver, from any vascular anastamosis or from portal varices. Surgical bleeding may be difficult to differentiate from coagulopathy and may lead to a 'negative' laparotomy. However, removal of surgical packs may also necessitate intervention. Where there has been delayed normalization of coagulation, haematoma formation may lead to abdominal tamponade which must be released to avoid renal and liver compromise. There is a risk of cardiovascular collapse caused by release of tamponade and reduction of venous return and it is important to have methods available to perform rapid transfusion including adequate venous access, although many of the access lines will still be in position from the original transplant.

Hepatic artery or portal vein thrombosis may lead to graft failure and are surgical emergencies. Most centres use ultrasound investigation of the graft postoperatively to ensure vessel patency. However, a worsening metabolic acidosis and coagulopathy are signs of impending thrombosis. Early diagnosis will allow return to theatre with a chance of rescuing the threatened graft. Complete thrombosis of vessels is difficult to rectify and may need urgent re-transplantation.

Biliary tract drainage procedures (including Roux en Y formation) are often required after transplantation and especially where there has been a hepatic artery complication. Incisional hernia repair is also a common surgical intervention.

Anaesthesia

After successful liver transplantation, many of the sequelae of chronic liver disease will have resolved and functional reserve will have improved. However, ischaemic heart disease may still be present and must be investigated. Similarly, pretransplant evidence of pulmonary hypertension should be noted and current therapy optimized if necessary. Clinical evidence of sepsis may suggest active cholangitis and this should be treated before biliary drainage procedures are performed. Recidivism after a transplant for alcoholic liver disease is common and assessment of alcohol intake must be ascertained. Preoperative investigations should include full clotting studies, liver function tests and electrolytes. The presence of ongoing viral illness is important for both theatre safety and blood cross-matching.

Further abdominal surgery may be complex and haemorrhage is a real possibility. Good venous access is mandatory. Regional anaesthesia is not contraindicated unless clotting dysfunction remains an issue. Unpredictable drug metabolism is important within the first few months after liver transplantation. However, if liver function tests have returned to baseline, it can be assumed that the response to anaesthetic drugs will be normal. Vecuronium is not contraindicated in this population, although it is probably prudent to use atracurium wherever coexisting renal disease is present. Paracetamol in standard analgesic doses is not contraindicated.

Cardiac

Indication for Transplantation

The main indications for heart transplantation are:

- severe heart failure (e.g. viral cardiomyopathy, hypertension, ischaemic heart disease)
- pulmonary hypertension
- congenital heart disease.

Preoperative Status

In contrast to renal and liver transplant recipients, the diseases that lead to the requirement for cardiac transplantation are less likely to be systemic in nature. However, the transplanted organ must not be considered normal in terms of its innervation and haemodynamic responses. Autonomic denervation leads to a loss in vagal control of the sinoatrial node and a persistent tachycardia. The ECG may show two 'p' waves due to remnants of the explanted organ conduction system. There may also be minor arrhythmias, bundle branch blocks and in some cases pacemaker fitting may have been necessary. Cardiac functional capacity is usually normal or minimally reduced. Early preload dependency is followed by a steady improvement in function due to an appropriate cardiac response to increased catecholamine concentrations. Indeed, most successfully transplanted patients eventually return to having a normal cardiac output, stroke volume and ejection fraction. The highest risk of rejection occurs within the first six months after transplantation and is diagnosed by myocardial biopsy. Increased troponin levels may also be associated with rejection. Chronic rejection often presents as progression of coronary artery disease without angina, due to reduction in sympathetic innervation and is angiographically present in 20% of patients, 5 years after transplantation.

Surgical Presentation

Early reoperation may be required due to surgical bleeding and the inherent risk of cardiac tamponade, although these complications are commonly dealt with by the transplant team. Cardiac recipients are more likely to present to the non-transplant anaesthetist for abdominal surgery. Cardiopulmonary bypass in conjunction with a debilitated immune system and high dose immunosuppression makes these patients more susceptible to intra-abdominal complications and mucosal perforation. Furthermore, sternal wound breakdown may require multiple surgical operations with complex tissue grafting procedures.

Anaesthetic Considerations

Preoperatively, hypertension (often induced by Cyclosporin A) is present in two third of patients and may require adjustment of drug therapy or treatment. Permanent pacemakers must be checked before the procedure and appropriate measures taken for intra-operative management. Persistent atrial arrhythmias may suggest rejection and require further investigation.

Intraoperatively, the use of regional anaesthesia is somewhat controversial but where there is normal cardiac function, it is unlikely to cause major complications. Right internal jugular vein cannulation is best avoided since it provides venous access for frequent myocardial biopsies. Drugs affecting the autonomic system are of minimal use in these patients due to the denervation occurring after heart transplantation. A requirement for an increased chronotropic or inotropic effect requires the use of direct-acting drugs including dobutamine, ephedrine and noradrenaline. Drugs that have direct action on heart allografts are shown in Table 39.4.

In the early stages after transplantation, cardiac output relies on an adequate preload. Fluid therapy should be optimized, guided by appropriate monitoring techniques (e.g. TOE, non-invasive cardiac output devices)

TABLE 39.4
Drugs that have Direct Action on Heart Allografts

Direct-Acting Drugs – Retained Action on Denervated Heart	No Activity on Denervated Heart
Dobutamine	Atropine, Glycopyrrolate
Ephedrine	Neostigmine
Dopamine	Pancuronium
Glugacon	Pyridostigmine
Digoxin	
Adrenaline	
Noradrenaline	
Beta-blockers	
Phosphodiesterase inhibitors	

and avoiding reductions in afterload. All current volatile and analgesic agents in judicious doses are suitable.

Pulmonary
Indications for Transplantation

The common indications for lung transplantation are:

- COPD and emphysema (45%)
- cystic fibrosis
- pulmonary fibrosis
- pulmonary hypertension
- others: including Eisenmenger's complex.

Transplantation may be either single (SLT) or double lung (DLT) or may occur in combination with a heart transplant (en bloc).

Preoperative Status

Pulmonary function after both single and double lung transplantation improves over the first six months. Persistent hypercapnia suggests allograft dysfunction. Lung volumes are reduced in the first month after both SLT or DLT. Successful DLT results in return of full lung function and at 3 months after transplant, PO_2, PCO_2 and exercise tolerance are likely to be close to normal. SLT has a more variable return of function depending on the underlying disease process. The commonest complications of both forms of lung transplantation are infection and rejection. Rejection often presents as an obliterative bronchiolitis which occurs around 8–12 months post-transplant and is present in up to 70% of patients who survive for 5 years.

Surgical Presentation

Early re-exploration is required for surgical bleeding and repair of anastomotic leaks. The anaesthetist is likely to encounter these patients for investigation of airway stenosis, drainage of infection and diagnostic bronchoscopy. There is also an increased risk of intra-abdominal lymphoproliferative disease and this may require surgery.

Anaesthetic Considerations

Many of these patients will have recent pulmonary function tests available. However, a worsening of functional symptoms since previous testing requires further testing. In some cases, an echocardiogram may be appropriate to rule out concomitant cardiac disease. Baseline blood gases are useful where supplemental oxygen is required, especially in SLT recipients. Recent chest infection should trigger preoperative sputum culture with appropriate therapy and awareness for a requirement for physiotherapy.

Intraoperatively, the anaesthetist should always be aware of possible altered upper airway anatomy and airway responses in both SLT and DLT recipients. DLT (or combined heart–lung) recipients have no airway reflexes. Postoperative sputum retention and chest infection are common and extubation under deep anaesthesia is not appropriate. In addition, fluid overload may lead to pulmonary oedema due to the disruption of pulmonary lymphatics.

SLT patients retain airway and carinal responses. However, the presence of an allograft with normal structure in combination with a lung retaining the original disease process may cause specific ventilatory problems. Pulmonary blood flow preferentially diverts to the allograft and during lateral positioning, especially where the diseased lung is dependent, difficult oxygenation and overt hypoxia may occur. Different lung compliances may lead to volutrauma or barotrauma; differential lung ventilation must be considered in this situation. However, given altered airway anatomy, the siting of a double lumen tube may be very difficult and other methods of lung isolation may be required.

Pancreas

Isolated pancreas transplant alone is less common than simultaneous kidney–pancreas transplantation (SPK; the latter potentially prolongs the survival of both grafts).

Indications for Transplantation

The indication for transplantation is almost exclusively for longstanding poorly controlled diabetes. Although patients have the ability to be free from insulin administration there is a compromise trade-off in that patients remain on immunosuppressive therapy thereafter, with the inherent risk of infection.

Preoperative Status

Early graft function allows rapid discontinuation of exogenous insulin therapy. However, even when this occurs, stabilization of the patient on an appropriate immunosuppressive regimen may delay recovery for some weeks. Where recovery of insulin secretion is not rapid, a more prolonged period of instability is expected. Drainage of pancreatic secretions is an important component of the initial transplant procedure since exocrine secretions may cause major injury to internal organs. Drainage procedures have included enteric or urinary drainage procedures. The latter allows for measurement of urinary pancreatic amylase but where SPK has been performed, this monitoring is rarely needed as renal failure often precedes pancreatic graft failure. Furthermore, bicarbonate losses are considerable requiring intravenous replacement in the early phase. Enteric drainage allows bicarbonate reabsorption, and acidosis and dehydration are uncommon.

Surgical Presentation

There is a high incidence of early postoperative return to theatre due to surgical bleeding. This may be either a major (mesenteric axis or splenic vein) or more insidious haemorrhage (pancreas surface). Timely surgery may allow recovery from graft thrombosis which occurs in 10–15% of transplants, although this is rarely successful and more often graft loss occurs.

Anaesthetic Considerations

Preoperative blood tests must include electrolytes and especially bicarbonate where urinary drainage has been performed. Residual requirement for insulin must be noted and a similar insulin regimen to those for other diabetics presenting for surgery should be used. The systemic effects of long-term, uncontrolled diabetes may remain even after successful pancreas transplantation. Patients may have persistent ischaemic heart disease, often silent, that must be investigated where there has been recent functional deterioration. Discontinuation of anti-thrombotic agents prescribed after previous coronary intervention must be considered. Autonomic neuropathy is common and leads to a delay in gastric emptying, hypotension and a vagolytic response to surgery. Wherever there is a combination of anti-thrombotic medication and autonomic dysfunction, the use of regional anaesthetic must be carefully considered.

Intestinal (Including Multivisceral) Transplants

Intestinal transplants are performed in a limited number of UK centres and are indicated mainly for loss of intestinal function (surgical or non-surgical reasons). These patients have significant problems after the initial transplantation but these are commonly dealt with in specialist units. However, patients may present for incidental elective and emergency procedures in other hospitals and may pose significant practical anaesthetic problems. Parenteral nutritional support is needed in the early postoperative period and this may lead to later difficulties with venous access. Indeed, the patient's nutritional state may remain poor for some time after transplantation. The initial transplantation makes further surgical access difficult with the risk of haemorrhage and prolonged procedures. Postoperative care in a critical care environment is advisable, given the degree of debility, ongoing nutritional requirements and the need for multidisciplinary care.

Bone Marrow Transplantation

The indications for bone marrow transplantation continue to increase and include many forms of haematological malignancy. The initial procedures rarely concern anaesthetic services. However, the complications caused by infection, chemotherapy and the requirement for multiple radiological procedures and investigations often require anaesthetic input. Many of these occur in remote locations and children make up a significant proportion of patients.

SUMMARY

The increasing number of patients obtaining long-term survival benefits after various forms of transplantation means that more will present for alternative elective and emergency surgery. General issues relate to alterations in immunosuppressive regimens, the risk of infection and rejection and the presence of systemic diseases related to the original disease process. In most circumstances, where the initial transplant has been successful, the patient will have made an appropriate return to normal capacity. Even so, the functional reserve of the transplanted organ remains limited, even where simple biochemical markers of organ function are within normal range. The transplanted organ therefore remains at serious risk of further damage wherever the stress of a major surgical procedure is applied. In addition, the issues related to specific organ disease must also be considered.

FURTHER READING

Keegan, M.T., Plevak, D.J., 2004. The transplant recipient for non-transplant surgery. Anesthesiol. Clin. North America 22, 827–861.
UK Transplantation Website. http://www.organdonation.nhs.uk/.

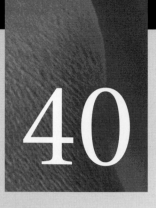

POSTOPERATIVE CARE

In modern anaesthetic practice, the patient is monitored and supervised closely and continuously during induction and throughout the operative procedure. However, many problems associated with anaesthesia and surgery may occur in the immediate postoperative period, and it is essential that supervision by adequately trained and experienced personnel is continued during the recovery period. In addition, some major and minor complications of anaesthesia and surgery may occur at any time in the first few days after operation.

THE EARLY RECOVERY PERIOD

Most hospitals have a recovery ward (or postanaesthesia care unit, PACU) within, or in close proximity to, the operating theatre suite (see Ch 20). The Association of Anaesthetists of Great Britain and Ireland (AAGBI) recommends that fully staffed recovery facilities must be available at all times in hospitals with an emergency surgical service. Some locations where anaesthesia is provided (e.g. the X-ray department) may not have a recovery ward. This section describes common problems which occur in the immediate postoperative period and refers specifically to their management in a recovery ward; however, the same principles are applicable to recovery in other locations.

The recovery period starts as soon as the patient leaves the operating table and the direct supervision of the anaesthetist. All the complications described below may occur at any time, including the period of transfer from operating theatre to recovery ward; in some operating theatre suites, the transfer to the recovery ward may last for several minutes, and it is essential that the standard of observation does not diminish during the journey. The patient must be supervised and monitored closely *at all times.*

Systems Affected

Central Nervous System

Consciousness may not return for several minutes after the end of general anaesthesia and may be impaired for a longer period of time. During this period, a patent airway must be maintained. There is a risk of aspiration into the lungs of any material, e.g. gastric content or blood, which is present in the pharynx. Consciousness may also be depressed in patients who have received sedation to facilitate endoscopy or regional anaesthesia.

Excitement and confusion may occur during recovery and may result in injury. Pain may be severe if long-acting analgesics or a nerve block have not been provided during surgery.

Cardiovascular System

Peripheral vascular resistance and cardiac output may be reduced because of residual effects of anaesthetic drugs in the absence of surgical stimulation. Hypovolaemia may be present because of inadequate fluid replacement during surgery, continued bleeding postoperatively or expansion of capacitance of the vascular system as a result of rewarming. Cardiac output may also be reduced as a result of arrhythmias or pre-existing disease. Hypertension may occur as a result of increased sympathoadrenal activity after restoration of consciousness, especially if analgesia is inadequate.

Respiratory System

Hypoventilation occurs commonly, usually as a result of residual effects of anaesthetic drugs or incomplete antagonism of neuromuscular blocking drugs. Hypoxaemia may result from hypoventilation, ventilation/perfusion imbalance or increased oxygen consumption produced by restlessness or shivering.

Gastrointestinal System

Nausea and vomiting are common in the immediate postoperative period.

Staff, Equipment and Monitoring

The recovery ward should be staffed by trained and experienced nurses. One nurse must remain with each patient at all times until consciousness and airway reflexes return. The responsibility for the patient's welfare remains with the anaesthetist. Ideally, an anaesthetist should be available immediately to treat complications detected by the nursing staff in the recovery ward.

The patient is nursed in a bed if available or if a prolonged stay is anticipated, but sometimes on a trolley (Fig. 40.1). All beds and trolleys must have the facility to be tipped head-down. Suction apparatus, including catheters, an oxygen supply with appropriate face mask, a self-inflating resuscitation bag and anaesthetic mask, a pulse oximeter and an automated non-invasive blood pressure monitor must be available for each

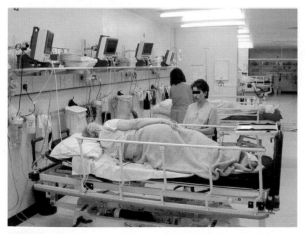

FIGURE 40.1 ■ Part of a recovery ward. Many patients are nursed on a trolley, but a bed is used if available, and particularly for those who have undergone major surgery and those who need to stay for several hours.

patient. In addition, there should be a complete range of resuscitation equipment within the recovery area; this includes an anaesthetic machine, a range of laryngoscopes, tracheal tubes, bougies, intravenous (i.v.) cannulae, fluids, emergency drugs, electrocardiogram (ECG) monitor and defibrillator. Facilities for emergency airway management including surgical airways should also be available (see Ch 22).

A wide range of drugs should be stored in the recovery area for the treatment of common complications and also emergency events (Table 40.1).

On arrival in the recovery ward, the anaesthetist should give the nurse full details of pre-existing medical problems, surgical procedure, anaesthetic technique, drugs, regional blocks, fluids, blood loss/replacement, any untoward events and any anticipated problems during recovery. All patients should be monitored by measurement of pulse rate, arterial pressure, arterial oxygen saturation and respiratory rate, and by assessment of level of consciousness, peripheral circulation and adequacy of ventilation. Depending on the nature of work undertaken in the theatre suite, a proportion of bed stations should have the facility for monitoring ECG, systemic and pulmonary arterial pressures and central venous pressure (CVP) continuously; this may be required in high-risk patients or those who have undergone major surgery. Capnography should be available for use in patients who require tracheal intubation. At least one mechanical ventilator should be available, although more may be required depending on the workload. Urine output should be measured routinely in patients who have undergone major surgery. Wounds and surgical drains should be inspected regularly for signs of bleeding.

It is important that the handover from anaesthetist to recovery nurse is systematic and undertaken in an unhurried way when both anaesthetist and nurse can concentrate on the handover. In general this will be after essential monitoring, such as pulse oximetry and blood pressure, has been reapplied and checked. The anaesthetist should not leave the patient until he or she is satisfied that there are no immediate problems, particularly with regard to the airway, and respiratory and cardiovascular systems.

A record should be made of pulse rate, arterial pressure and arterial oxygen saturation, respiratory rate, level of consciousness, pain score, sensory level (if

TABLE 40.1
Drugs Which Should be Available in the Recovery Room

Adenosine	Digoxin	Isoprenaline (isoproterenol)	Pethidine
Alfentanil	Dobutamine	Ketamine	Phentolamine
Aminophylline	Dopamine	Ketorolac	Phenytoin
Antibiotics	Doxapram	Labetalol	Phytomenadione
Aprotinin	Edrophonium	Lidocaine	Potassium chloride
Aspirin	Ephedrine	Metaraminol	Procainamide
Atracurium	Adrenaline	Methoxamine	Prochlorperazine
Atropine	Fentanyl	Methylprednisolone	Propranolol
Bupivacaine	Flumazenil	Metoclopramide	Protamine
Calcium chloride	Furosemide	Midazolam	Ranitidine
Calcium gluconate	Glucose	Morphine	Salbutamol
Calcium heparin	Glyceryl trinitrate	Naloxone	Sodium citrate
Chlorphenamine (chlorpheniramine)	Glycopyrronium	Neostigmine	Sodium nitroprusside
Co-proxamol	Hyaluronidase	Nifedipine	Succinylcholine
Cyclizine	Hydralazine	Noradrenaline	Tranexamic acid
Dexamethasone	Hydrocortisone	Ondansetron	Verapamil
Diazepam	Hyoscine	Papaverine	
Diclofenac	Insulin	Paracetamol	

regional anaesthesia has been used), and any other relevant information (such as complications, and drug and fluid administration) obtained while the patient is in the recovery area. In most units, recordings of physiological measurements are made every 5 min until consciousness has returned and then at intervals of 10–15 min.

The patient should not be discharged to the surgical ward until the following criteria have been met.

■ Consciousness has returned fully, a patent airway can be maintained and protective reflexes are present.
■ Ventilation and oxygenation are satisfactory.
■ The cardiovascular system is stable with no unexplained cardiac irregularity or persistent bleeding. Consecutive measurements of pulse rate and arterial pressure should approximate to the patient's normal preoperative values or be at an acceptable level commensurate with the planned postoperative care. Peripheral perfusion should be adequate.

■ Pain and nausea are controlled.
■ Temperature is within acceptable limits.

High-risk patients or those who have undergone major surgery may stay in the recovery ward for up to 24 h. If this is not feasible, or if instability persists for longer than 24 h, the patient should be transferred to a high-dependency or intensive care unit. The level of monitoring and care during transfer should be the same as that in the recovery room.

Although the recovery room nurse undertakes the direct care of the patient, the responsibility for the patient remains with the anaesthetist. Patients must only be discharged to the ward with the anaesthetist's consent.

The remainder of this chapter is devoted to the diagnosis and management of common problems which occur in the postoperative period. Some of these occur most frequently in the immediate recovery period, while others may occur at any time during the patient's convalescence from surgery. Some surgical procedures are associated with specific complications.

CENTRAL NERVOUS SYSTEM

Conscious Level

Many patients are unconscious on arrival in the recovery ward because of residual effects of anaesthetic drugs. The duration of impaired consciousness depends on:

- *The drugs used.* Recovery of consciousness may be delayed if the following agents have been used:
  - volatile anaesthetics with a high blood/gas solubility coefficient
  - barbiturates, particularly if large total doses have been given
  - benzodiazepines
  - opioids with a long duration of action, including large doses of fentanyl.
- *The timing of drug use.* Delayed recovery may occur if a long-acting i.v. anaesthetic or analgesic drug has been given towards the end of the procedure, or if the more soluble volatile agents have been continued until the end of surgery.
- *Pain.* The presence of pain speeds recovery of consciousness. Recovery may be delayed after minor procedures or if potent analgesia has been provided by administration of opioids or by regional anaesthesia.

Undue prolongation of unconsciousness should not be attributed to these factors alone. Other causes should be considered, as their early recognition may prevent serious sequelae. These are:

- hypoxaemia – in the presence of an adequate circulation, coma occurs only if profound hypoxaemia is present; agitation is a more common sign of hypoxia
- hypercapnia – unconsciousness may occur if arterial carbon dioxide tension ($PaCO_2$) exceeds 9–10 kPa
- hypotension
- hypothermia.

Hypoglycaemia

This occurs most commonly in diabetic patients treated with oral hypoglycaemic agents or insulin and an inadequate intake of glucose. The perioperative management of the diabetic patient is discussed in Chapter 18.

Hyperglycaemia

Hyperglycaemia in known diabetics may occur as a result of inadequate provision of insulin or injudicious infusion of glucose. However, coma is unusual in acute hyperglycaemia. Undiagnosed diabetics with hyperglycaemia and ketosis may present for surgery because of abdominal pain, and prolonged postoperative coma may occur unless the metabolic defect is diagnosed and treated.

Cerebral Pathology

Consciousness may be impaired by functional or structural cerebral damage. Possible causes include:

- episodes of cerebral ischaemia (e.g. carotid artery surgery, profound hypotension) or cerebral hypoxia during anaesthesia
- intracranial haemorrhage, thrombosis or infarction – these may occur coincidentally or may have been associated with intraoperative hypertension, hypotension or arrhythmias
- pre-existing cerebral lesions, e.g. tumour, trauma – anaesthetic techniques which increase intracranial pressure are likely to impair cerebral function
- epilepsy – convulsions may have been masked by anaesthesia or neuromuscular blocking drugs
- air embolism
- intracranial spread of local anaesthetic solution after subarachnoid injection – introduction into the subarachnoid space may be accidental, e.g. during epidural block or, rarely, interscalene brachial plexus block; unconsciousness is almost always accompanied by apnoea.

Other Causes

- *Hypo-osmolar or TURP syndrome.* This results most commonly from absorption of water from the bladder during transurethral resection of the prostate (TURP). The investigation and management of this condition are described on page 570.
- *Hypothyroidism.*
- *Hepatic or renal failure.*

Confusion and Agitation

These occur occasionally during emergence from an otherwise uncomplicated anaesthetic.

Various drugs are associated with postoperative confusion, including:

- opioids
- benzodiazepines
- anticholinergics including atropine and cyclizine.

Atropine crosses the blood–brain barrier and may result in the central anticholinergic syndrome, characterized by restlessness and confusion, together with obvious antimuscarinic effects. Glycopyrronium does not cross the blood–brain barrier and is preferable to atropine for antagonism of the muscarinic effects of neostigmine in elderly patients; in addition to its lack of central effects, it produces less tachycardia and antagonizes the effects of neostigmine for a longer period.

All the factors listed above as causes of prolonged coma may also result in confusion and agitation. Pain may also contribute, although it is seldom responsible alone. Emergence delirium is associated particularly with the use of ketamine and may occur after the administration of etomidate. Septicaemia may result in confusion, as may distension of the stomach or bladder.

A lightly sedated, conscious patient with inadequate antagonism of neuromuscular blocking drugs may appear to the inexperienced observer to be agitated and confused. Movements are uncoordinated.

The condition is distressing to the patient and is an indication of a poor anaesthetic technique. It should never be allowed to develop.

Pain

This subject is discussed fully in Chapter 41. The effects of pain should be differentiated from those of hypercapnia and hypovolaemia (Table 40.2).

RESPIRATORY SYSTEM

Hypoventilation

Common causes of hypoventilation in the immediate postoperative period are listed in Table 40.3. Hypoventilation results in an increase in $PaCO_2$ (Fig. 40.2) and a decrease in alveolar oxygen tension (PaO_2), and thus hypoxaemia, which may be corrected by increasing the inspired concentration of oxygen. The risk factors for developing hypoventilation include:

- old age
- obesity
- prolonged surgical operations
- opioids
- upper abdominal or thoracic surgery.

Airway Obstruction

Airway obstruction caused by the tongue, by indrawing of the pharyngeal muscles or by blood or secretions in the pharynx may be ameliorated by placing the patient

	TABLE 40.2		
	Common Problems in the Recovery Room: Symptoms and Signs		
	Pain	*Hypercapnia*	*Hypovolaemia*
Conscious level	May be restless. May be quiescent if severe pain	Comatose	Restless or quiescent depending on extent of analgesia and residual anaesthesia
Periphery	Vasoconstriction, pallor ± sweating	Warm, flushed with bounding pulse (if normovolaemic)	Vasoconstriction, pallor ± sweating
Heart rate	Tachycardia	Tachycardia	Tachycardia
Arterial pressure	Systolic ↑. Diastolic ↑. Pulse pressure normal	Systolic ↑. Diastolic ↑ ↓. Pulse pressure ↑	Systolic and diastolic may be normal until marked reduction in stroke volume, then ↓. Pulse pressure ↓

TABLE 40.3
Causes of Postoperative Hypoventilation

Factors Affecting Airway	Factors Affecting Ventilatory Drive	Peripheral Factors
Upper airway obstruction	Respiratory depressant drugs	Muscle weakness
Tongue	Preoperative CNS pathology	Residual neuromuscular block
Laryngospasm	Intra- or postoperative cerebrovascular accident	Preoperative neuromuscular disease
Oedema	Hypothermia	Electrolyte abnormalities
Foreign body	Recent hyperventilation (PaCO$_2$ low)	Pain
Tumour		Abdominal distension
Bronchospasm		Obesity
		Tight dressings
		Pneumo-/haemothorax

CNS, central nervous system; PaCO$_2$, arterial carbon dioxide tension.

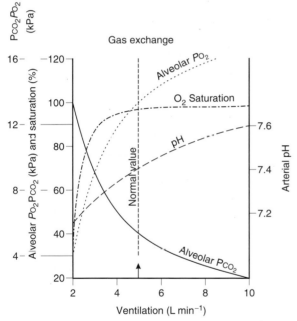

FIGURE 40.2 ■ Gas exchange during hypoventilation. Note the relatively rapid increase in alveolar partial pressure of carbon dioxide (PCO$_2$) compared with the slow decrease in arterial oxygen saturation. PO$_2$, partial pressure of oxygen.

by absent sounds of breathing and paradoxical movement of the chest wall and abdomen.

In many patients, a clear airway is maintained only by displacing the mandible anteriorly and extending the head. In some, it is necessary also to insert an oropharyngeal airway, although this may stimulate coughing, gagging and laryngospasm during recovery of consciousness. A nasopharyngeal airway is often tolerated better, but there is a risk of causing haemorrhage from the nasopharyngeal mucosa. Occasionally, insertion of a laryngeal mask airway is necessary to maintain the airway until consciousness has returned fully; very occasionally, tracheal intubation is required.

Blood, oral secretions or regurgitated gastric fluid which have accumulated in the pharynx should be aspirated and the patient placed in the recovery position to allow any further fluid to drain anteriorly.

Foreign bodies, such as dentures (particularly partial dentures) or throat packs, may cause airway obstruction. It may be difficult to maintain a patent airway in an unconscious patient with an oral, pharyngeal or laryngeal tumour.

Obstruction of the upper airway occurs intermittently after recovery from anaesthesia. Obstructive sleep apnoea is common in the postoperative period and may result in decreases of arterial oxyhaemoglobin saturation (SaO$_2$) to less than 75%. Episodes occur with the greatest frequency in the first 4 h after anaesthesia and are more common and severe in patients who receive opioids for postoperative analgesia than in those in whom analgesia is provided by a regional technique. However, the use of regional techniques does not reduce the risk to zero.

in the lateral or recovery position (see Fig. 21.7). This position should be used for all unconscious patients who have undergone oral or ear, nose and throat surgery, and for patients at risk of gastric aspiration.

Partial obstruction of the airway is characterized by noisy ventilation. As the obstruction increases, tracheal tug and indrawing of the supraclavicular area occur during inspiration. Total obstruction is signalled

Airway obstruction may result from haemorrhage after surgery to the neck, including thyroid, carotid and spinal surgery; the wound should be opened urgently and the haematoma drained. This may not relieve the obstruction if venous engorgement or tissue oedema are marked. Occasionally, tracheal collapse occurs after thyroidectomy in patients who have developed chondromalacia of the cartilaginous rings of the trachea caused by pressure from a large goitre. Inspiratory stridor may be present or there may be total obstruction during inspiration; the trachea must be reintubated immediately.

Laryngeal Spasm

This complication is relatively common after general anaesthesia. In particular, children undergoing oropharyngeal surgery are more at risk. It may be partial or complete and is caused usually by direct stimulation of the cords by secretions or blood, or of the epiglottis by an oropharyngeal airway or laryngeal mask. It may follow extubation of the trachea in the semiconscious patient. It may be difficult to differentiate this condition from airway obstruction caused by the pharyngeal wall; if airway obstruction persists despite implementation of the measures described above, laryngoscopy should be undertaken.

Any obvious foreign material causing laryngospasm should be removed by aspiration, and oxygen 100% administered. If obstruction is complete, positive-pressure ventilation by mask may force some oxygen through the cords to maintain arterial oxygenation until the spasm has subsided; there is a significant risk of inflating the stomach with oxygen during this procedure. If attempts to oxygenate the lungs fail, a small dose of succinylcholine should be administered, and the lungs ventilated with oxygen when the spasm is relieved. When satisfactory oxygenation has been achieved, it may be advisable to intubate the trachea to reduce the risk of regurgitation of gastric contents, as the stomach may have been inflated with oxygen. Appropriate methods to avoid awareness should be instituted. When the effects of succinylcholine have terminated, oxygen 100% is administered and the trachea is extubated when the patient regains consciousness.

Rarely, laryngeal obstruction occurs after thyroid surgery if both recurrent laryngeal nerves have been traumatized.

Laryngeal Oedema

This occurs occasionally after tracheal intubation and may result in severe obstruction, particularly in a child. Treatment depends on the severity of the obstruction; immediate reintubation may be required if obstruction is complete, but partial obstruction may subside if the patient is treated with heated humidified gases. Dexamethasone may hasten resolution of the oedema.

Bronchospasm

This may result from stimulation of the airway by inhaled material. It is commoner in asthmatic or bronchitic patients and in smokers. It may result directly from intrinsic asthma or may be part of an anaphylactic reaction. Several drugs used in anaesthetic practice may precipitate bronchospasm either by a direct effect on bronchial muscle or by releasing histamine; these include barbiturates, morphine, mivacurium and atracurium. Treatment comprises the removal of any predisposing factor and the administration of oxygen and bronchodilators.

Ventilatory Drive

There are several possible causes of reduced ventilatory drive during recovery from anaesthesia (see Table 40.3). The presence of intracranial pathology, e.g. tumour, trauma or haemorrhage, may affect ventilatory drive in the postoperative period. Ventilation is reduced in the presence of hypothermia, although it is usually appropriate for the metabolic needs of the body. Hypoventilation occurs in the hypocapnic patient, e.g. after a period of hyperventilation until $PaCO_2$ is restored to normal, and in the presence of primary metabolic alkalosis.

The most important cause of reduced ventilatory drive during recovery is the effect of drugs administered by the anaesthetist in the perioperative period. All the volatile and i.v. anaesthetic agents – with the exception of ketamine – depress the respiratory centre; significant concentrations of these drugs remain in the brainstem during the early postoperative period.

All opioid analgesics depress ventilation. With most opioids, the effect is dose-dependent, although the agonist-antagonist agents are claimed to have a ceiling effect. In the majority of patients, opioids do not produce apnoea, but result in decreased ventilatory drive and an increase in $PaCO_2$, which plateaus at an elevated value. The elderly are particularly sensitive to drug-induced ventilatory depression. The treatment of postoperative pain begins in the recovery area, often by administration of i.v. opioids by the medical or nursing staff, and ventilation must be monitored carefully after each dose.

Spinal (intrathecal or epidural) opioids, particularly lipid-insoluble agents such as morphine, may produce ventilatory depression some hours after administration. Patients who have received subarachnoid or epidural opioids should be cared for in areas where protocols and training programmes for surgical ward nurses have been implemented.

Reduced ventilatory drive is easy to diagnose if the ventilatory rate or tidal volume is clearly reduced. However, lesser degrees of hypoventilation may be difficult to detect, and the signs of moderate hypercapnia, e.g. hypertension and tachycardia, may be masked by the residual effects of anaesthetic agents, or misdiagnosed as pain-induced (see Table 40.2).

Mild hypoventilation is acceptable provided that oxygenation remains adequate; this may easily be achieved by a modest increase in the inspired fractional concentration of oxygen (FiO_2; see below). If ventilatory drive is reduced excessively by opioids, resulting in an increasing $PaCO_2$ or delayed recovery of consciousness, naloxone in increments of 1.5–$3\,\mu g\,kg^{-1}$ should be administered every 2–3 min until improvement occurs. Administration of excessive doses of naloxone reverses the analgesia induced by systemic (but not to the same extent by spinal) opioids; large doses may cause severe hypertension and have been associated with cardiac arrest on rare occasions. The effects of i.v. naloxone last only for 20–30 min; in order to prevent recurrence of reduced ventilation after long-acting opioids, an additional dose (50% of the effective i.v. dose) may be administered intramuscularly or an i.v. infusion commenced.

Peripheral Factors

The commonest peripheral factor associated with hypoventilation is residual neuromuscular blockade. This may be exaggerated by disease of the neuromuscular junction, e.g. myasthenia gravis, or by electrolyte disturbances. Inadequate reversal of neuromuscular blockade is usually associated with uncoordinated, jerky movements, although these may

TABLE 40.4
Clinical Assessment of the Adequacy of Antagonism of Neuromuscular Block
Subjective
Grip strength
Adequate cough
Objective
Ability to sustain head lift for at least 5 s
Ability to produce vital capacity of at least $10\,mL\,kg^{-1}$

occur occasionally during recovery of consciousness in patients with normal neuromuscular function. Measurement of tidal volume is not a reliable guide to adequacy of reversal of neuromuscular blockade; a normal tidal volume may be achieved with only 20% return of diaphragmatic power, but the ability to cough remains severely impaired. Traditional clinical signs of adequacy of reversal of neuromuscular blockade (such as if the patient is able to lift the head from the trolley for 5 s or maintain a good hand grip) correlate poorly with objective signs of neuromuscular function. Some more objective means of assessment are listed in Table 40.4, but these require the cooperation of the patient. In the unconscious or uncooperative patient, nerve stimulation (see Ch 6) provides the best means of assessing neuromuscular function, although there are differences among the non-depolarizing relaxants in the relationship between their actions in the forearm and diaphragm.

If residual non-depolarizing blockade is confirmed, further doses of neostigmine may be administered (with glycopyrronium) up to a total of 5 mg; in higher doses, neostigmine can worsen neuromuscular function. Patients who have received rocuronium or vecuronium can be given sugammadex ($2\,mg\,kg^{-1}$ if there are signs of reversal of neuromuscular blockade; or $4\,mg\,kg^{-1}$ if there are no twitches present using train-of-four stimulation). If the block persists, artificial ventilation must be maintained while the cause is sought.

Factors responsible most commonly for difficulty in antagonism of neuromuscular block include overdosage with muscle relaxant, too short an interval between administration of the drug and the antagonist, hypokalaemia, respiratory or metabolic acidosis, administration of aminoglycoside antibiotics, local anaesthetic agents, diseases affecting neuromuscular transmission and muscle disease.

Delayed elimination of all of the non-depolarizing muscle relaxants (except atracurium and cisatracurium) has been reported, and causes prolonged neuromuscular block. Delayed elimination occurs most frequently in the presence of renal or hepatic insufficiency, or in dehydrated patients with low urine output. Muscle paralysis may recur 30–60 min after administration of neostigmine if elimination of the relaxant is inadequate, even if antagonism appears to be satisfactory initially. A similar phenomenon may occur if acidosis develops, or when patients who have been hypothermic are rewarmed.

Prolonged neuromuscular block after succinylcholine or mivacurium occurs in the presence of atypical plasma cholinesterase or a low concentration of normal plasma cholinesterase. Paralysis after succinylcholine may persist for up to 8 h, although in most instances recovery occurs within 20–120 min. Neostigmine should not be administered if prolonged neuromuscular block occurs after administration of succinylcholine.

Artificial ventilation of the lungs must be maintained or resumed in any patient who has inadequate neuromuscular function. Anaesthesia should be provided to prevent awareness.

Hypoventilation may be caused also by restriction of diaphragmatic movement resulting from abdominal distension, obesity, tight dressings or abdominal binders. Pain, particularly from thoracic or upper abdominal wounds, may cause reduced ventilation.

The presence of air or fluid in the pleural cavity may result in hypoventilation. Pneumothorax may occur during intermittent positive-pressure ventilation (IPPV). It is an occasional complication in healthy patients, but is a particular risk in those with chronic obstructive airways disease, especially if bullae are present, and after chest trauma. It may complicate brachial plexus nerve block, central venous cannulation or surgery involving the kidney or neck. Haemothorax may result from chest trauma or central venous cannulation. Hydrothorax may be caused by pleural effusions or inadvertent infusion of fluids through a misplaced central venous catheter. These rapidly remediable causes of hypoventilation are often overlooked.

TABLE 40.5
Functional Classification of the Causes of Hypoxaemia in the Postoperative Period
Reduced inspired oxygen concentration
Ventilation–perfusion abnormalities
Shunting
Hypoventilation
Diffusion deficits
Diffusion hypoxia after nitrous oxide anaesthesia

Treatment

This consists primarily of treatment of the cause. Mild or moderate hypoventilation resulting from residual effects of anaesthetic drugs may respond to a bolus dose or infusion of doxapram. Artificial ventilation should be started if severe hypercapnia is present or $PaCO_2$ continues to increase, or if the clinical condition of the patient is deteriorating.

Hypoxaemia

A functional classification of causes of hypoxaemia in the early recovery period is shown in Table 40.5. An inspired oxygen concentration of less than 21% should never occur, although PaO_2 is decreased when air is breathed at high altitudes.

Ventilation–Perfusion Abnormalities

These are the commonest cause of hypoxaemia in the recovery room. Cardiac output and pulmonary arterial pressure may be reduced after general or regional anaesthesia, causing impaired perfusion of some areas of the lungs. Functional residual capacity (FRC) is reduced during and immediately after anaesthesia. Patients who are elderly, obese or those undergoing thoracic or upper abdominal surgery are particularly at risk. The closing capacity may encroach on the tidal breathing range, resulting in reduced ventilation of some lung units, particularly those in dependent alveoli. Thus, the scatter of ventilation/perfusion ($\dot{V}/\dot{Q}$) ratios is increased. Areas of lung with increased ratios constitute physiological dead space. Areas of lung with low $\dot{V}/\dot{Q}$ ratios increase venous admixture which results in hypoxaemia unless the inspired oxygen concentration is increased.

Shunt

Physiological shunt may be increased in the immediate postoperative period if small airways closure has been extreme. Shunting may be present also in patients with pulmonary oedema of any aetiology, or if there is consolidation in the lung. Shunt may be increased in the later postoperative period as a result of retention of secretions and underventilation of the lung bases because of pain; these changes lead to alveolar consolidation and collapse.

Hypoventilation

This has been discussed in detail above. Moderate hypoventilation, with some elevation of $PaCO_2$, leads to a modest reduction in PaO_2 (Fig. 40.2). Obstructive sleep apnoea may produce profound transient but repeated decreases in arterial oxygenation. SaO_2 may decrease to less than 75%, corresponding to a PaO_2 of less than 5 kPa (40 mmHg). These repeated episodes of hypoxaemia cause temporary, and possibly permanent, defects in cognitive function in elderly patients and may contribute to perioperative myocardial infarction. Obstructive sleep apnoea is exacerbated by opioid analgesics, and patients who are known to suffer from this condition should be monitored carefully in the postoperative period, preferably in a high-dependency unit. Patients who normally use a continuous positive airways pressure (CPAP) mask to reduce obstructive sleep apnoeic episodes should use the mask at night throughout the postoperative period.

Diffusion Defects

Interstitial oedema produced by overtransfusion of fluids or by left ventricular dysfunction may cause hypoxaemia by impairment of oxygen transfer across the alveolar–capillary membrane.

Diffusion Hypoxia

Nitrous oxide is 40 times more soluble than nitrogen in blood. When administration of nitrous oxide is discontinued at the end of anaesthesia, nitrous oxide diffuses out of blood into the alveoli in larger volumes than nitrogen diffuses in the opposite direction. Consequently, the alveolar concentrations of other gases are diluted. PaO_2 is reduced and arterial oxygenation impaired if the patient breathes air; $PaCO_2$ decreases as a result of effective alveolar hyperventilation. SaO_2 is reduced to values as low as 90% for several minutes in normal individuals after breathing 50% nitrous oxide in oxygen. Arterial desaturation is greater in elderly patients, if higher concentrations of nitrous oxide have been used, or if $PaCO_2$ is initially low because of hyperventilation during anaesthesia.

Diffusion hypoxia is avoided by the administration of oxygen for 10 min after discontinuation of nitrous oxide anaesthesia.

Reduced Venous Oxygen Content

Assuming that oxygen consumption remains unchanged, anaemia or reduced cardiac output result in increased oxygen extraction from circulating arterial blood, and consequently in a reduction in mixed venous oxygen content. In the presence of increased $\dot{V}/\dot{Q}$ scatter or intrapulmonary shunt, this causes a variable degree of arterial hypoxaemia. Similarly, if cardiac output remains constant, increased oxygen utilization by the tissues (as may occur during shivering, restlessness or malignant hyperthermia) causes a reduction in mixed venous oxygen content and a worsening of arterial hypoxaemia if any shunt is present.

Tissue Hypoxia

Oxygenation of the tissues is a function of arterial oxygenation, oxygen carriage in blood, delivery of blood to the tissues and transfer of oxygen from the blood. It may be impaired by respiratory or cardiovascular dysfunction, by severe anaemia or by a leftward shift of the oxyhaemoglobin dissociation curve (reduced P_{50}).

Pulmonary Changes after Abdominal Surgery

Patients with previously normal lungs suffer impairment of oxygenation for at least 48 h after abdominal surgery. The extent of this impairment is related to the site of operation. It is less marked after lower abdominal surgery, more severe if there has been a large incision in the upper abdomen and worst after thoracoabdominal procedures. In these circumstances, the differences between pre- and postoperative PaO_2 may be as much as 4 kPa.

Impairment of oxygenation in the postoperative period is related to a reduction in FRC. After induction of anaesthesia, there is an abrupt decrease in FRC. The magnitude of the decrease is similar for anaesthetic techniques in which the patient breathes spontaneously and those in which IPPV is employed. Postoperatively, this decrease is maintained by wound pain, which causes spasm of the expiratory muscles, and abdominal distension, which leads to diaphragmatic splinting. This is also influenced by the site of surgical incision; the greatest reduction follows thoracic or upper abdominal surgery. The supine position also reduces FRC.

The reduction in FRC may lead to closing capacity impinging upon the tidal breathing range. This results in small airways closure during normal tidal ventilation. Gas trapping occurs in the affected airways and subsequent absorption of air may lead to the development of small, discrete areas of atelectasis which are not visible on chest X-ray. This occurs mainly in the dependent parts of the lung and may be demonstrated by CT scan very soon after induction of anaesthesia. The result is an increase in the number of areas of low $\dot{V}/\dot{Q}$ ratio within the lungs. The relationship between changes in FRC and PaO_2 postoperatively is shown in Figure 40.3.

In most patients, these abnormalities return towards normal by the fifth or sixth postoperative day. However, if the changes have been marked, the areas of low $\dot{V}/\dot{Q}$ ratio may become a focus for infection, particularly in the presence of retained secretions. The following factors contribute to retention of secretions after surgery.

- *Inability to cough.* This results mostly from wound pain. However, excessive sedation may also contribute. Postoperative electrolyte imbalance, especially hypokalaemia or hypophosphataemia, may compound the situation by interfering with muscle function.
- *Suppression of bronchial mucosal ciliary activity.* This results from the use of unhumidified anaesthetic gases.
- *Antisialagogue drugs.* When antisialagogue premedicants have been used, the secretions become more viscid. The dry mucosa itself is more prone to inflammatory reaction. If this occurs, the exudate produced increases the problem still further.
- *Infection.* If pulmonary infection supervenes, impairment of oxygenation may contribute to a lack of cooperation in clearing secretions.

A combination of these factors may result in retention of secretions, leading to areas of visible pulmonary collapse on chest X-ray and an increase in the work of breathing. Ultimately, oxygenation of the blood may become inadequate despite oxygen therapy, or carbon dioxide retention may occur. The sequence of events that culminate in ventilatory failure is shown in Figure 40.4.

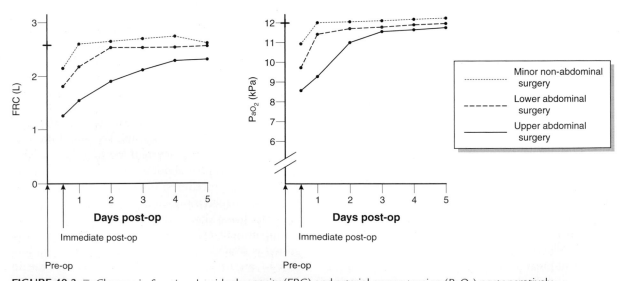

FIGURE 40.3 ■ Changes in functional residual capacity (FRC) and arterial oxygen tension (PaO_2) postoperatively.

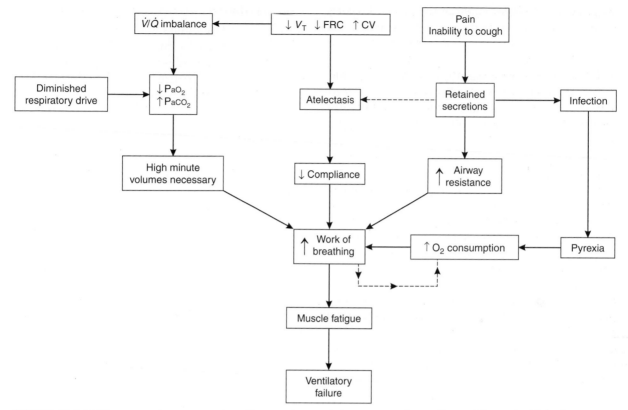

FIGURE 40.4 ■ Diagrammatic representation of events that result in postoperative ventilatory failure. V_T, tidal volume; FRC, functional residual capacity; CV, closing volume; $\dot{V}/\dot{Q}$, ventilation/perfusion; PaO_2, arterial oxygen tension; $PaCO_2$, arterial carbon dioxide tension.

Predisposing Factors

- *Site of surgery.* Pulmonary complications occur more commonly after upper abdominal or thoracic surgery than after lower abdominal operations.
- *Pre-existing respiratory disease* increases the complication rate. This is particularly so in the presence of concurrent infection or excessive secretions.
- *Smokers* have an increased incidence of pulmonary complications compared with non-smokers.
- *Obesity* is associated with a high incidence of pulmonary complications. Obese patients have a low FRC and increased work of breathing postoperatively.

The anaesthetic technique has little effect on the incidence of postoperative pulmonary complications.

Clinical Findings

Collapse of Lung Units. In patients who develop clinical symptoms, the first signs of atelectasis are usually seen within 24 h of operation. The triad of pyrexia, tachycardia and tachypnoea is often present. Temperature is usually in the range of 38–39 °C. There is often a productive cough. If atelectasis is extensive, the patient is cyanosed. On physical examination, localizing signs are uncommon unless the area of involvement is large. Chest X-ray reveals patchy areas of atelectasis.

Pneumonia. Lobar pneumonia is rarely seen postoperatively. Bronchopneumonia is more common, especially in the elderly. The onset of symptoms is not as rapid as in atelectasis. There is usually fever and associated tachycardia, with an increase in the ventilatory rate. Physical examination usually reveals areas of consolidation, predominantly at the lung bases, which are evident on chest X-ray.

Treatment

If a pulmonary complication is suspected, a sputum sample should be sent to the laboratory for bacteriological analysis. Appropriate antibiotic therapy may then be started. Intensive physiotherapy should be prescribed in an attempt to remove secretions and re-expand atelectatic areas of the lung.

Patients with pulmonary collapse are usually hypoxaemic, but $PaCO_2$ remains normal or may be low as a result of tachypnoea, at least in the early stages. Usually, oxygen in moderate concentrations (30–40%) is sufficient to correct hypoxaemia, but this should be confirmed by blood gas analysis; CPAP given via a tightly fitting face mask is effective in re-expanding the collapsed alveoli and improving the mechanics of breathing. If the patient fails to respond to these measures, signs of respiratory distress develop. The patient becomes drowsy and ventilation is laboured, with rapid shallow breathing involving the accessory muscles. $PaCO_2$ increases and arterial oxygenation deteriorates despite oxygen therapy. The presence of continued deterioration in blood gases is an indication for ventilatory support.

Reducing Pulmonary Complications

Preoperative

Measures to reduce pulmonary complications should begin preoperatively. Ideally, patients should be free from ongoing upper or lower respiratory tract infections but this may not always be possible, for instance in young children, adults with recurrent infective complications (such as COPD or bronchiectasis) or patients presenting for urgent or emergency surgery.

Pre-existing chronic respiratory disorders should be treated so that the patient is in optimal condition before surgery. Spirometry may be useful to monitor the effects of such treatment, but arterial blood gas analysis is the only assessment which has been demonstrated to correlate well with the need for postoperative ventilatory support. Smoking should be discouraged and weight loss encouraged where indicated. In patients with increased risk factors, heavy premedication should be avoided to ensure minimal ventilatory depression at the end of the procedure.

Intraoperative

At induction, care should be taken not to introduce infection by contaminated equipment. Anaesthetic gases should be humidified. If neuromuscular blocking agents are used, particular care should be taken to ensure that antagonism is adequate.

Postoperative

Analgesia should be optimal to ensure adequate coughing and cooperation during physiotherapy, which should be started as soon as possible after operation. Early mobilization should be encouraged.

Oxygen Therapy

Hypoxaemia may occur to some degree in any patient during the early recovery period as a result of one or more of the mechanisms described above. Consequently, *all* patients should receive additional oxygen for the first 10 min after general anaesthesia has been discontinued. Oxygen therapy should be continued for a longer period in the presence of any of the conditions listed in Table 40.6.

Oxygen therapy is particularly beneficial in treating hypoxaemia caused by hypoventilation; PaO_2 is substantially increased by a modest increase in FiO_2. In contrast, higher concentrations are required in the presence of a shunt fraction in excess of 0.1–0.15 (Fig. 40.5). Known concentrations of oxygen may be

TABLE 40.6
Conditions in Which Prolonged Oxygen Therapy is Required After Operation
Hypotension
Ischaemic heart disease
Reduced cardiac output
Anaemia
Obesity
Shivering
Hypothermia
Hyperthermia
Pulmonary oedema
Airway obstruction
After major surgery

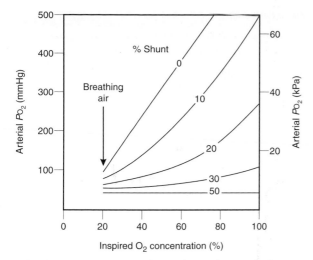

FIGURE 40.5 ■ Response of arterial partial pressure of oxygen (PO_2) to increased inspired oxygen concentrations in the presence of various degrees of shunt. Note that, in the presence of shunt, arterial PO_2 remains well below the normal value when 100% oxygen is breathed. Nevertheless, useful increases in arterial oxygenation occur with a shunt of up to 30%.

administered by a tightly fitting mask supplied with metered flows of air and oxygen via either an anaesthetic breathing system or a CPAP system. In small children, an oxygen tent or headbox may be used. However, oxygen is usually administered by less cumbersome disposable equipment.

Oxygen Therapy Devices

The characteristics of oxygen face masks depend predominantly on their volume, the flow rate of gas supplied and the presence of holes in the side of the mask. If no gas is supplied, face masks act as increased dead space and result in hypercapnia unless minute volume is increased; the increase in dead space is proportional to the volume of the mask. If the mask contains holes, air is entrained readily during inspiration.

When oxygen is supplied, the inspired oxygen concentration increases, but to an extent which depends upon the relationship between the oxygen flow rate and the ventilatory pattern. If there is a pause between expiration and inspiration, the mask fills with oxygen and a high concentration is available at the start of inspiration; during inspiration, the inspired oxygen is diluted by air drawn in through the holes when the inspiratory flow rate exceeds the flow rate of oxygen.

During normal tidal ventilation, the peak inspiratory flow rate (PIFR) is 20–30 L min^{-1}, but is considerably higher during deep inspiration or in the hyperventilating patient. If there is no expiratory pause, alveolar gas may be rebreathed from the mask at the start of inspiration; this occurs especially when the oxygen flow rate is low or when no holes are present in the mask. A predictable and constant inspired oxygen concentration may be achieved only if the total gas flow to the mask exceeds the patient's peak inspiratory flow rate (PIFR).

Fixed-Performance Devices. These masks, also termed high air flow oxygen enrichment (HAFOE) devices, provide a constant and predictable inspired oxygen concentration irrespective of the patient's ventilatory pattern. This is achieved by supplying the mask with oxygen and air at a high total flow rate. Oxygen is passed through a jet which entrains air (Fig. 40.6). The mask is designed in such a way that the total flow rate of gas to the mask exceeds the expected PIFR of most patients who require oxygen therapy. For example, if a jet designed to supply 28% oxygen is supplied with an oxygen flow rate of 4 L min^{-1}, approximately 41 L min^{-1} of air is entrained and a total flow of 45 L min^{-1} passes to the patient's face.

Various types of HAFOE device are available; an example is shown in Figure 40.7. Ventimasks are the most accurate, but a different mask is required for each of the range of oxygen concentrations available. Some manufacturers produce masks in which the jet device can be changed by the user, so that the oxygen concentration may be adjusted as appropriate.

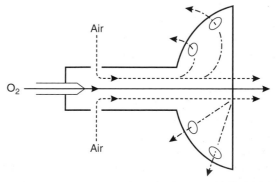

FIGURE 40.6 ■ Diagram of high air flow oxygen enrichment (HAFOE) mask (see text for details).

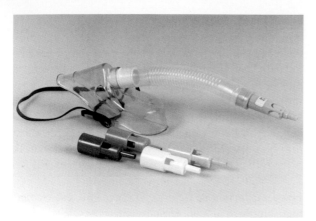

FIGURE 40.7 ■ A high air flow oxygen enrichment (HAFOE) face mask.

TABLE 40.7
Oxygen Masks, Flow Rates and Approximate Oxygen Concentration Delivered

Type of mask	Oxygen flow ($L\,min^{-1}$)	Oxygen concentration (%)
Edinburgh	1	24–29
	2	29–36
	4	33–39
Nasal cannulae	1	25–29
	2	29–35
	4	32–39
Hudson	2	24–38
	4	35–45
	6	51–61
	8	57–67
	10	61–73
MC	2	28–50
	4	41–70
	6	53–74
	8	60–77
	10	67–81

The air-entraining jets of HAFOE devices provide a relatively constant oxygen concentration irrespective of the flow rate of oxygen. The recommended oxygen flow rates are larger when jets providing a high concentration are used (e.g. $8\,L\,min^{-1}$ for 40%, $15\,L\,min^{-1}$ for 60%) so that the total flow rate supplied to the mask remains adequate despite the smaller proportion of air entrained. The total flow rates through masks which deliver more than 28% oxygen are between 20 and $30\,L\,min^{-1}$ when the recommended oxygen flow rates are provided; higher flow rates of oxygen may be used in patients who are thought to have an increased PIFR.

Because of the high fresh gas flow rate, expired gas is rapidly flushed from the mask. Thus, rebreathing does not occur, i.e. fixed-performance devices do not act as an additional dead space.

Variable-Performance Devices. All other disposable oxygen masks and nasal cannulae provide an oxygen concentration which varies with the oxygen flow rate and the patient's ventilatory pattern. Although there is no increase in dead space when nasal cannulae are used, all variable-performance disposable face masks add dead space, the magnitude of which depends on the patient's pattern of ventilation. Table 40.7 gives an indication of the range of oxygen concentrations achieved with a number of commonly used variable-performance devices; an example is shown in Figure 40.8.

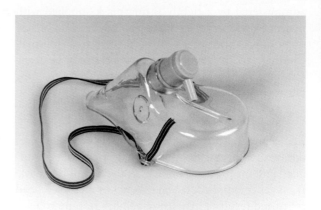

FIGURE 40.8 ■ A variable-performance oxygen face mask.

Oxygen Therapy in the Recovery Ward

The large majority of patients recovering after anaesthesia require only a modest increase in FiO_2 to overcome the combined effects of mild hypoventilation, diffusion hypoxia and some degree of increased $\dot{V}/\dot{Q}$ scatter. Usually, an inspired concentration of 30% is adequate and this may be achieved in most instances by supplying an oxygen flow rate of $4\,L\,min^{-1}$ to any of the variable-performance devices (see Table 40.7).

However, in a small proportion of patients, it is necessary to control the FiO_2 more strictly.

Controlled Oxygen Therapy. This is required in two categories of patient:

- Some patients with chronic bronchitis develop chronic hypercapnia, and ventilatory drive is produced largely by hypoxaemia. If PaO_2 increases above the level which stimulates breathing, ventilatory depression may occur. However, these patients may become dangerously hypoxaemic after anaesthesia, and oxygen therapy is required so that adequate oxygenation of the tissues is maintained. The aim of oxygen therapy in these circumstances is to increase arterial oxygen content without an excessive increase in PaO_2. This is achieved by a modest increase in FiO_2. In the hypoxaemic patient, the relationship between arterial oxygen tension and saturation (and therefore oxygen content) is represented by the steep portion of the oxyhaemoglobin dissociation curve, and a small increase in oxygen tension results in significant increases in saturation and oxygen content (Fig. 40.9). The use of a variable-performance device in these patients is unsatisfactory, as an unacceptably high FiO_2 may be delivered. A fixed-performance device delivering 24% oxygen should be used initially, and the response assessed. If the patient remains clinically well, and the $PaCO_2$ does not increase by more than 1–1.5 kPa, 28% oxygen – and subsequently higher concentrations – may be administered if further increases in PaO_2 are desirable. The aim is not to achieve 'normal' PaO_2 or SaO_2 but to provide acceptable oxygenation for that patient. Patients whose normal SaO_2 is in the low 90s do not need postoperative SaO_2 in the high 90s. Most patients with chronic bronchitis do not depend on hypoxaemia for respiratory drive and should not be denied adequate inspired concentrations of oxygen.

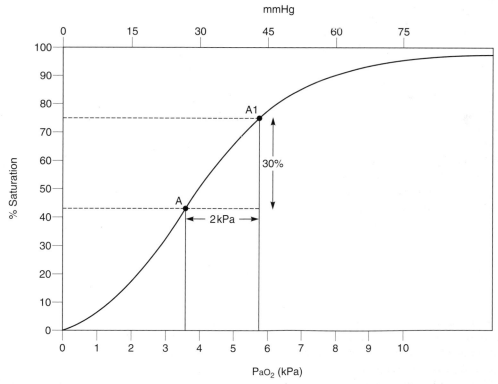

FIGURE 40.9 ■ Effect of controlled oxygen therapy on oxygen saturation in a hypoxaemic chronic bronchitic patient. A small increase in inspired oxygen concentration produces a modest increase in arterial oxygen tension (PaO_2) but a substantial increase in arterial oxygen saturation.

■ Patients with increased shunt, e.g. those with acute respiratory distress syndrome (ARDS), pulmonary oedema or pulmonary consolidation, may require a high inspired oxygen concentration (see Fig. 40.5), which cannot be guaranteed if a variable-performance device is used. In addition, serial blood gas analysis is normally used to assess improvement or deterioration in their condition. Changes in PaO_2 and the degree of shunt may be interpreted accurately only if the FiO_2 is known. Thus, controlled oxygen therapy should be employed, using a fixed-performance device which delivers 40% oxygen *or more*.

CARDIOVASCULAR SYSTEM

Hypotension

Residual Effects of Anaesthetic Drugs

Hypotension may result from the residual vasodilator effect of i.v. or inhalational anaesthetic drugs, particularly in patients who are experiencing little pain. Subarachnoid or epidural nerve block may also cause hypotension which persists into the postoperative period. Heart rate is seldom elevated, and the peripheries are warm if anaesthetic drugs or regional anaesthesia are the cause of hypotension. Up to 20% decrease in the mean arterial pressure is tolerated well except by the elderly or patients with myocardial disease. No treatment is required in most patients. Elevation of the legs often increases arterial pressure by increasing venous return. Intravenous infusion of $7–10\,mL\,kg^{-1}$ of colloid solution is usually effective in restoring normotension if there is concern; infusion should be undertaken cautiously in elderly patients and in those with cardiovascular disease.

Other causes of hypotension in the recovery period are more sinister and must be excluded before it may be assumed that residual anaesthesia is responsible.

Hypovolaemia

This may result from inadequate or inappropriate replacement of preoperative or intraoperative fluid and blood losses, or from postoperative haemorrhage. Surgical bleeding may be obvious from inspection of wounds and drains, but may be concealed, particularly in the abdomen, retroperitoneal space or thorax, even when drains are present.

Inadequate surgical haemostasis is the usual cause of postoperative bleeding, but coagulation disorders may be present in the following circumstances:

■ after massive blood transfusion, which results in decreased concentrations of clotting factors and reduced platelet numbers
■ pre-existing bleeding tendency, e.g. haemophilia
■ disseminated intravascular coagulation produced by sepsis, amniotic fluid embolism, etc.
■ if anticoagulant drugs have been administered.

A coagulation disorder is frequently associated with prolonged bleeding after venepuncture, oozing from the wound and the development of petechiae or bruises. The investigation and management of coagulation disorders are discussed in Chapter 13.

Hypotension caused by hypovolaemia may be accompanied by signs of poor peripheral perfusion, e.g. cold, clammy extremities and pallor. Tachycardia may be present but is masked, not infrequently, by the effects of drugs (e.g. anticholinesterases, β-blockers). Central venous pressure is a poor guide to volaemic status. Urine output is reduced ($<30\,mL\,h^{-1}$). The effects of hypovolaemia on arterial pressure are more pronounced in the presence of vasodilatation or reduced myocardial contractility resulting from the effects of residual anaesthetic drugs, or antihypertensive, calcium channel or β-blocker therapy. In patients who have undergone prolonged surgery, and particularly if the core temperature is below normal, vasoconstriction may be profound and hypovolaemia may be unmasked at a relatively late stage, as normal vasomotor tone returns with rewarming.

Treatment comprises elevation of the legs and administration of appropriate crystalloid or colloid solutions; in elderly or high-risk patients, or if hypovolaemia is profound, administration of fluids should be monitored with the assistance of invasive arterial blood pressure and often some form of cardiac output monitoring. Red cells, clotting factors or platelets should be administered if appropriate, and surgical bleeding treated by re-operation if necessary.

Arrhythmias

These are discussed below.

Ventricular Failure

Left or right ventricular failure may cause hypotension. Right ventricular failure is uncommon in the postoperative period and is secondary usually to acute pulmonary disease, e.g. ARDS.

Left ventricular failure in the postoperative period is associated most commonly with perioperative myocardial infarction or ischaemia, or sometimes with fluid overload. The peripheral circulation is poor. Usually, tachycardia is present and there is clinical and radiological evidence of pulmonary oedema. Jugular venous pulse and CVP are usually elevated, but they may remain normal despite a substantial increase in left atrial pressure, particularly if right ventricular hypertrophy is present. Thus, left ventricular failure may be misdiagnosed as hypovolaemia in some patients, and in some instances the two conditions coexist. If there is doubt about the diagnosis, a small intravenous fluid bolus may be administered (no more than 200 mL) and the response of arterial pressure and CVP monitored; if the diagnosis remains uncertain, more involved testing may include echocardiography or rarely the insertion of a pulmonary artery catheter.

Treatment comprises administration of oxygen, fluid restriction, diuretics and, if necessary, inotropic support or vasodilator therapy. ECG, arterial pressure and CVP should be monitored. The possibility of myocardial infarction should be investigated.

Sepsis with Shock

In this condition, hypotension is accompanied by elevated cardiac output and peripheral vasodilatation in the early stages, followed by vasoconstriction and reduced cardiac output caused partly by loss of fluid from the circulation. Treatment should be according to local guidelines ('Sepsis Bundles') and includes infusion of appropriate volumes of colloid solutions, early antibiotic therapy, surgical treatment of the source if necessary, monitoring of response (e.g. blood lactate concentration) and inotropic support.

Hypertension

Arterial hypertension is a common complication in the early postoperative period. The causes include the following:

- pain
- pre-existing hypertension, particularly if controlled inadequately
- hypoxaemia
- hypercapnia
- administration of vasopressor drugs
- after aortic surgery, as a result partly of increased plasma concentration of renin.

A combination of these causes may be present. Hypertension results in increased cardiac work and myocardial oxygen consumption, and may result in myocardial ischaemia or infarction, left ventricular failure or cerebral haemorrhage. The cause should be elicited rapidly and treated if possible. Oxygen should be administered. If no remediable cause is found and the hypertension is felt to be a risk to the patient, careful antihypertensive treatment can be started using vasodilators such as hydralazine (i.v.), nifedipine (sublingual) or glyceryl trinitrate (sublingual or i.v.), or beta-blockade (labetalol has combined α- and β-antagonism, esmolol is short-acting). Such treatment may unmask hypovolaemia (see above) and additional i.v. fluids may be required.

Arrhythmias

These are common during and immediately after anaesthesia (see also Ch 8). The majority are benign and require no treatment. However, the cause should be sought and its effect on the circulation assessed. Common causes include the following:

- residual anaesthetic agents
- hypercapnia
- hypoxaemia
- electrolyte or acid–base disturbance
- vagal stimulation, e.g. by tracheal tube or suction catheters
- myocardial ischaemia or infarction
- pain.

Sinus tachycardia is common and may be a reflex response to hypovolaemia or hypotension. It also occurs in the presence of hypercapnia, anaemia or hypoxaemia, and if the metabolic rate is elevated by fever, shivering, restlessness or malignant hyperthermia. The commonest cause is pain. Tachycardia increases myocardial oxygen consumption and decreases coronary artery perfusion by reducing diastolic time. The combination of arterial hypertension and tachycardia is dangerous in the presence of ischaemic heart disease and should *not* be allowed to persist, as it may result in myocardial infarction. Sinus tachycardia should be treated specifically only if it persists after therapy for underlying causes has been given; a small i.v. dose of a short-acting β-blocker (esmolol) should be administered, followed by a continuous intravenous infusion. The ECG must be monitored.

Sinus bradycardia may result from inadequate antagonism by glycopyrronium of vagal stimulation by neostigmine, pharyngeal stimulation during suction or the residual effects of volatile anaesthetic agents. Other causes include hypoxaemia (especially in neonates and infants), raised intracranial pressure, myocardial infarction and some cardiac drugs, e.g. β-blockers, digoxin. Oxygen should be administered. Intravenous atropine or glycopyrronium is usually effective if there is associated hypotension or evidence of inadequate cardiac output. In the presence of severe bradycardia, external cardiac massage is necessary to increase cardiac output.

Bradycardia may also occur as a result of complete heart block; this may require electrical pacing.

Bradycardia may also be normal for certain individuals in which case treatment is likely to cause more problems than it solves.

Supraventricular arrhythmias, including atrial fibrillation, flutter or supraventricular tachycardia, are treated as in other circumstances. Rapid arrhythmias are best treated by cardioversion, but may require pharmacological therapy to prevent recurrence. Nodal rhythm with a normal heart rate is common in the perioperative period, particularly when volatile anaesthetic agents have been used. Supraventricular arrhythmias may cause moderate hypotension because of the loss of synchronization between atrial and ventricular contractions.

Ventricular arrhythmias. Ectopic beats usually require no treatment. Ventricular tachycardia should be treated according to current Resuscitation Council (or equivalent) guidelines.

Conduction Defects

In the perioperative period, these usually occur in patients with pre-existing heart disease. Patients who develop complete heart block and who have cardiovascular compromise will usually require temporary (external or internal) cardiac pacing and cardiological advice should be sought. Patients who develop second-degree heart block during anaesthesia or in the recovery ward should be transferred to a coronary care or intensive therapy unit for an appropriate period of observation.

Myocardial Ischaemia

This occurs most commonly in patients with pre-existing coronary artery disease, and most often in the presence of hypoxaemia, hypotension, hypertension or tachycardia. The ECG should be monitored throughout the recovery period in patients known to be at risk, and precipitating factors should be avoided. Angina occurring during the recovery period should be treated by elimination of any predisposing factor (particularly pain) and administration of glyceryl trinitrate sublingually or intravenously.

Acute Coronary Syndrome

Myocardial infarction (MI) occurs in 1–2% of unselected patients over 40 years of age undergoing major non-cardiac surgery. Pre-existing coronary artery disease and, in particular, evidence of a previous MI, result in a higher risk. Mortality in patients who suffer a perioperative MI used to be as high as 60% but is somewhat lower now. Perioperative MI occurs most commonly on the second or third postoperative day, but may happen at any time during or after surgery. Acute coronary syndromes in the perioperative period are most commonly caused by atheromatous plaque rupture, in the same way as non-operative events. Non-thrombotic acute coronary syndrome (ACS) may also occur when myocardial oxygen delivery is insufficient for demand.

Several factors which may be detected during preoperative assessment are known to increase the likelihood of perioperative MI (see Ch 17). The most important of these is the time interval between surgery and a previous MI. One extensive study of risk factors which might predict major cardiac complications (including, but not exclusively, MI) showed that preoperative evidence of cardiac failure, arrhythmias (of any type) or aortic stenosis, and age were also associated with a high risk. In addition, there is evidence that pre-existing uncontrolled hypertension is associated with increased risk. These problems are discussed more fully in Chapter 18.

The incidence of perioperative MI is related also to intraoperative and postoperative factors. The magnitude and type of surgery are important determinants; in patients with a history of previous MI, the incidence of perioperative reinfarction associated with major vascular surgery is considerably higher than when surgery is performed outside the thorax and abdomen. In patients with ischaemic heart disease, postoperative MI is more likely if there is evidence of ischaemic changes on ECG during operation. Such changes are associated most commonly with episodes of intraoperative hypotension, hypertension or tachycardia; the last two occur most frequently in response to noxious stimuli, e.g. tracheal intubation, surgical incision. The drugs used and the manner in which they are employed by the anaesthetist influence the incidences of both intraoperative ischaemia and perioperative MI. There is ongoing debate as to whether regional anaesthesia reduces risk when major surgery is undertaken.

Reduction of Risk

The incidence of perioperative MI may be reduced by the following.

- *Identification of patients at risk.* Elective surgery should be postponed if possible until at least 3 months after a previous MI.
- *Treatment of risk factors.* Cardiac failure, hypertension and arrhythmias should be controlled before surgery. If necessary, the operation should be postponed until control is achieved. Coronary artery bypass grafting or aortic valve replacement may be required in patients with severe coronary artery disease or aortic stenosis, respectively, before other major abdominal or thoracic surgery is undertaken.
- *Avoidance of ischaemia.* The anaesthetic technique and postoperative management should ensure adequate oxygenation of the myocardium and should minimize myocardial oxygen demand (see Ch 18).
- *Monitoring.* ECG must be monitored throughout anaesthesia, including induction, in all patients at risk; the CM5 electrode configuration (see Fig. 16.2) is suitable for detection of ischaemic

changes. Arterial pressure should be monitored regularly, and continuously in patients undergoing major surgery.

Diagnosis

Perioperative MI may be difficult to diagnose. It occurs most commonly on the second or third postoperative days. The classic distribution of pain is present in only 25% of patients.

The diagnosis should be considered in any patient at risk who develops an arrhythmia or becomes hypotensive in the postoperative period. Premature ventricular contractions occur in 90% of patients who experience an MI; sinus bradycardia and the development of any degree of atrioventricular conduction defect are also common. The diagnosis is confirmed by changes in serial ECG recordings and serum troponin concentrations.

OTHER MAJOR POSTOPERATIVE COMPLICATIONS

Deep Venous Thrombosis

The main factors postulated by Virchow as contributing to the formation of venous thrombi are:

- changes in the composition of blood
- damage to walls of blood vessels
- decreased blood flow.

However, the exact trigger mechanism which initiates venous thromboembolic disease in some patients but not others remains unknown. Most DVTs are subclinical and peak occurrence is around 7 days after surgery. The degree of association between subclinical distal (calf) DVT and fatal pulmonary embolism (PE) is unclear. There remains a degree of controversy over the optimal approach to management.

Risk Factors

A higher incidence of deep venous thrombosis (DVT) has been reported in patients with:

- extensive trauma
- infection
- heart failure
- blood dyscrasias
- malignancy
- metabolic disorders.

DVT is commoner after hip, pelvic and abdominal surgery than after other types of surgery; regional anaesthetic techniques, with general anaesthesia or in isolation, may reduce the risk. There is a well-established association between spontaneous DVT and oestrogen, and DVT may occur in women who take some types of oral contraceptive pill. The number of women who develop this complication is small. However, the incidence increases if surgery is performed while the patient is currently taking the drug. The risk is reduced but not abolished if a low-oestrogen (50 μg or less) preparation is used. Women who take hormone replacement therapy are also at increased risk.

Diagnosis

Approximately 70% of patients with a DVT have neither symptoms nor signs. Fifty per cent of patients with calf pain and tenderness on dorsiflexion of the foot do not have a DVT. Often there is mild pyrexia.

Investigations

Ultrasonography. This is non-invasive and simple to perform. However, it is relatively insensitive and is useful only for confirming the diagnosis of a major thrombus.

CT/MR Venography. These may be of use for selected patients.

D-Dimers. These are degradation products from the action of plasmin on fibrin. Although they are useful as a screening test in outpatients, they are of little value in postoperative patients due to the frequency of elevated concentrations in surgical patients.

Prophylaxis

As with most complications, appropriate assessment is a key step in reduction of events. Prophylactic measures to minimize the risk of DVT and PE are detailed in Chapter 13.

Elimination of Stasis. Early ambulation after operation is widely promoted as a method to reduce the incidence of DVT, although the degree of benefit is not clear. Attempts directed at preventing stasis, including physiotherapy, elastic stockings and elevation of the feet, may reduce the incidence of DVT but have not been shown to influence the incidence of pulmonary embolism.

Two methods are currently used for increasing venous return from the lower limbs during surgery.

■ *Pneumatic compression of the calves.* The legs are encased in an envelope of plastic material, which is inflated and deflated rhythmically, thus squeezing the calves intermittently. These devices mimic the effect of the calf muscle pump, promoting venous return, and also stimulate fibrinolytic activity. This technique may be continued postoperatively.

■ *Anti-embolism stockings.* It is important that these are fitted properly because ill-fitting stockings are at best useless and at worst may cause injury due to local constrictions. There is no good evidence that thigh-length stockings confer benefit over knee-length stockings. They are contraindicated in patients with:
  - suspected or proven peripheral arterial disease
  - peripheral arterial bypass grafting
  - peripheral neuropathy or other causes of sensory impairment
  - any local conditions in which stockings may cause damage, e.g. fragile 'tissue paper' skin, dermatitis, gangrene or recent skin graft
  - known allergy to material of manufacture
  - cardiac failure
  - severe leg oedema or pulmonary oedema from congestive heart failure
  - unusual leg size or shape
  - major limb deformity preventing correct fit.

Although the incidence of DVT is reduced substantially by these techniques, there is no reduction in the incidence of, or mortality from, PE. However, there is no increased risk of bleeding, and if fitted appropriately, few complications.

Alteration of Blood Coagulability

Platelet Aggregation. Various drugs which interfere with different aspects of platelet function have been investigated. These include dextran 70, dipyridamole, aspirin and chloroquine. High dose, but not low dose, aspirin reduces the incidence of DVT and PE. Infusion of dextran during and after surgery may reduce the incidence of fatal postoperative pulmonary embolism but its role in the prevention of peripheral venous thrombosis is undetermined.

The Coagulation Mechanism. Low-molecular-weight heparins reduce the rate of DVT and PE, but at the expense of an increase in major bleeding. Pharmacological methods should therefore be used only in patients at risk of major bleeding if the risk of venous thromboembolism (VTE) is felt to outweigh the risk of bleeding. This is described more fully in Chapter 13. Pharmacological prophylaxis is usually with low-molecular-weight heparin. The anaesthetist should be aware of when this is given as it may impact on the use of neuraxial blockade and removal of epidural catheters.

Temporary inferior vena caval filters should be considered for patients at high risk of VTE where mechanical or pharmacological methods are contraindicated or likely to be insufficient.

Pulmonary Embolism

This term covers a range of events from sudden circulatory collapse and death, through minor episodes of pleurisy and haemoptysis, to the long-standing disability of patients with chronic thromboembolic pulmonary hypertension. The acute forms of pulmonary embolism are encountered after anaesthesia and surgery. In the elderly, multiple small pulmonary emboli may be misdiagnosed as bronchopneumonia.

The common sites of origin for thrombi which result in pulmonary embolus are the veins of the pelvis and lower extremities. The most common time for presentation of a postoperative pulmonary embolism is during the second week. In some patients, predisposing factors may have existed preoperatively for some time, and the whole time-scale of events may be shifted; the embolus may occur at the time of, or shortly after, surgery.

Diagnosis

Presenting features. The principal features are circulatory collapse and sudden dyspnoea, often associated with chest pain. If the embolus is large, the pulmonary artery outflow is blocked and sudden death results. If the embolus involves more than 50% of the main pulmonary arteries, or is associated with arterial hypotension or shock, it is termed massive.

Physical Signs. A low cardiac output state develops. Tachypnoea and central cyanosis are usual. There is arterial hypotension, sinus tachycardia and a constricted peripheral circulation. The jugular venous pressure is elevated.

Investigations

- ***ECG*** (Fig. 40.10). This reflects acute right ventricular strain, with features that often include right axis deviation, T-wave inversion in leads V_1–V_4 and sometimes right bundle branch block. The classic S1–Q3–T3 pattern is less common.
- ***Chest X-ray.*** This is often unremarkable but may show areas of oligaemia reflecting pulmonary vascular obstruction.

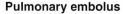

Pulmonary embolus

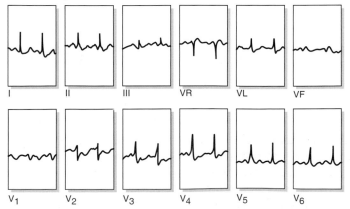

FIGURE 40.10 ■ Typical electrocardiogram changes in pulmonary embolism.

- *Arterial blood gases.* There is usually hypoxaemia because of ventilation–perfusion imbalance, and hypocapnia resulting from hyperventilation.
- *Pulmonary angiography.* This provides a definitive diagnosis of major obstruction in the pulmonary circulation, and is now performed usually by CT scan. This investigation is particularly useful if the patient is critically ill and the diagnosis is in doubt, and is essential if pulmonary embolectomy is planned. However, it requires transfer of the patient to the X-ray department.

Treatment

Deep Venous Thrombosis. The mainstay of therapy is anticoagulation. Low molecular weight heparin is started at a therapeutic dose. At the same time, oral anticoagulant therapy is started. Warfarin is used most commonly. Heparin is continued until adequate anticoagulation is in place with oral agents (warfarin). Oral anticoagulants are usually continued for at least 3 months depending on the underlying cause.

Pulmonary Embolism. Immediate treatment consists of administration of oxygen in a high concentration and therapeutic doses of low-molecular-weight heparin. Sometimes it is necessary to use additional inotropic support for the circulation. Heparin is continued until adequate anticoagulation is in place with oral agents (warfarin). Oral anticoagulant therapy is started as soon as possible and is continued for several months in consultation with the haematologists.

Massive pulmonary embolus which does not respond to the above measures may warrant the use of thrombolytic agents (e.g. TPA), surgical embolectomy (under cardiopulmonary bypass) or interventional radiological procedures.

Postoperative Renal Dysfunction

The kidney is vulnerable to a wide range of drugs (see Ch 10), chemicals and pathological insults. It is particularly susceptible to toxic substances for the following reasons:

- large blood flow per unit mass
- high oxygen consumption
- non-resorbable substances concentrated by tubules
- permeability of tubular cells.

Acute kidney injury (AKI) following surgery is relatively common; almost 25% of elderly patients who died following emergency surgery were found to have evidence of acute kidney injury on admission. There is no single diagnostic criterion for defining acute kidney injury, but a consensus clinical tool is the 'RIFLE' criteria (Table 40.8).

Unfortunately, the RIFLE criteria essentially give information about what has happened already, rather than providing information about current injury at a time when preventative action may be possible. There is ongoing research into biomarkers of early/ongoing renal injury but there is no reliable and practical test available yet.

Acute kidney injury in the surgical patient is often multifactorial. Key factors are:

- increased age
- sepsis/systemic inflammatory response syndrome
- intravascular volume depletion
- nephrotoxic drugs:
  - aminoglycosides
  - radiocontrast

TABLE 40.8		
RIFLE (Risk, Injury, Failure, Loss, End-Stage) Criteria for Acute Kidney Injury		
	GFR Criteria	*Urine Output (UO) Criteria*
Risk	GFR decreased >25% or [Creatinine] x 1.5	UO<0.5 mL h^{-1} for 6 h
Injury	GFR decreased >50% or [Creatinine] x 2	UO<0.5 mL h^{-1} for 12 h
Failure	GFR decreased >75% or [Creatinine] x 3 or [Creatinine] >355 μmol L^{-1} (with a rise of >44 μmol L^{-1})	UO<0.3 mL h^{-1} for 24 or anuria for >12 h
Loss	Persistent acute renal failure – complete loss of kidney function >4 weeks	
End-stage	End-stage kidney disease	

- comorbidities:
    - diabetes
    - vascular disease
- abdominal compartment syndrome.

Outcome following illness and surgery is worse when complicated by AKI, with increased length of stay and increased mortality.

Postoperative care should therefore focus on:

- identifying patients at high risk of developing AKI
- avoiding factors which may increase risk of or from AKI
- close monitoring and intervention in those patients who develop signs of AKI.

Effects of Anaesthesia

All anaesthetic techniques depress renal blood flow and, secondary to this, interfere with renal function. Provided that prolonged hypotension is avoided, the effects are temporary. However, there is the potential for some anaesthetic agents to produce permanent renal damage.

The administration of the volatile anaesthetic agent methoxyflurane was associated with a relatively high incidence of renal dysfunction. Clinically, the defect was characterized by failure of the concentrating ability of the kidney. In certain instances, this progressed to high-output renal failure. The nephrotoxicity of methoxyflurane was dose-dependent and was caused by inorganic fluoride ions produced during its metabolism. Administration of methoxyflurane in combination with other nephrotoxic drugs, e.g. aminoglycosides, was particularly hazardous.

Large quantities of fluoride ion are also produced during metabolism of enflurane and sevoflurane, although a much smaller proportion of these drugs (2–3%) is metabolized in comparison with methoxyflurane (45%). Concentrations of fluoride ion in blood following administration of sevoflurane may exceed the value associated with renal impairment after anaesthesia with methoxyflurane. However, there has been no evidence to suggest that either enflurane or sevoflurane is associated with renal impairment related to the production of fluoride ions. The reason is probably related to the fact that the very soluble methoxyflurane continues to be metabolized for some days, resulting in prolonged production of fluoride ions, whereas the peak concentrations associated with the use of enflurane and sevoflurane are of short duration because of their relative insolubility in tissues.

Postoperative Hepatic Dysfunction

There are many causes of postoperative hepatic dysfunction (Table 40.9). Most patients show no evidence of hepatic damage after anaesthesia and surgery. If it occurs, it is usually attributable to one of the causes shown in Table 40.9. However, if other causes are excluded, consideration should be given to the possibility of hepatotoxicity from anaesthetic drugs.

Chloroform was the first anaesthetic agent to be suspected of causing hepatic damage. In large doses, chloroform is a direct hepatotoxin, and after anaesthesia a hepatitis-like syndrome, with histological evidence of centrilobular hepatic necrosis, occurred occasionally. Methoxyflurane was also associated with hepatic damage, causing a syndrome clinically similar to viral hepatitis. Two of the volatile agents in current use have been implicated in cases of postoperative hepatic dysfunction.

Halothane

Attention was first focused on halothane-associated hepatitis in the early 1960s. Numerous case reports prompted institution in 1969 of the largest retrospective anaesthetic study ever undertaken (United States National Halothane Study). The incidence and causes of fatal hepatic necrosis occurring within

TABLE 40.9

Causes of Postoperative Hepatic Dysfunction

Increased Bilirubin Load	Hepatocellular Damage	Extrahepatic Biliary Obstruction
Blood transfusion	Pre-existing	Gallstones
Haemolysis and	liver disease	Ascending
haemolytic disease	Viral hepatitis	cholangitis
Abnormalities	Sepsis	Pancreatitis
of bilirubin	Hypotension/	Surgical
metabolism	hypoxia	misadventure
	Drug-induced	
	hepatitis	
	Congestive	
	heart failure	

6 days of anaesthesia were reviewed. The overall incidence was 1 in 10 000; that associated with halothane was 1 in 35 000 and was no greater than the incidence associated with other anaesthetic agents. However, it is believed at present that there is a small number of patients who develop postanaesthetic jaundice in which halothane is the aetiological agent.

There are two categories of halothane hepatotoxicity. *Type 1* is common and self-limiting. It is characterized by modest increases in liver transaminases and changes in drug metabolism. There is no jaundice and there are no signs of liver disease. It appears to be essentially halothane-specific and is probably due to reductive rather than oxidative metabolism of halothane. *Type 2* is associated with centrilobular necrosis and acute liver failure. It is clinically similar to viral hepatitis with fever, jaundice and markedly elevated transaminases. The exact mechanism of liver damage is not known. At present, there are two main hypotheses.

■ Metabolites of reductive halothane metabolism bind covalently to hepatocyte macromolecules, causing hepatocellular damage.
■ Halothane or more likely its trifluoroacetyl metabolites react with hepatocyte proteins to form antigenic compounds, against which the body mounts an immune response which results in hepatocellular damage. There may be a genetic predisposition to this response.

Antibodies to halothane have been demonstrated in patients who have suffered hepatic damage after administration of the drug. At present, this is the most promising method for evaluating the aetiology of a condition which has been a source of great controversy.

The following groups of patients are believed to be at the greatest risk of developing hepatic dysfunction after halothane anaesthesia:

■ patients subjected to repeated halothane anaesthetics, especially within a 3-month period
■ patients who have developed unexplained pyrexia or jaundice after a previous halothane anaesthetic
■ obese patients, particularly women.

Pre-existing liver disease is not a risk factor for developing hepatotoxicity. Type 2 hepatotoxicity has been reported rarely with other volatile anaesthetics and appears to be related to the degree of hepatic metabolism.

OTHER COMPLICATIONS
(TABLE 40.10)

Serious complications are described in detail in Chapter 43.

TABLE 40.10
Minor Morbidity Resulting from Anaesthesia
Nausea and vomiting (see Chapter 42)
Related to nature of operation
Females>males
Sore throat
Around 12% of all general anaesthesia
Around 45% of those with tracheal tubes
Hoarseness
Around 50%
Laryngeal granulomata
Headache
Up to 60% of patients
Backache
Discomfort from catheters, drains, nasogastric tubes
Anxiety
Muscle pains
Up to 100% of those who receive succinylcholine
Shivering
Drowsiness
Anorexia
Disorientation
Thrombophlebitis at injection site
Oral trauma
Around 5%
Dental injury
Around 1%; 0.02% require surgical treatment
Corneal abrasions
Around 0.05–0.1%

Nausea and Vomiting

Although often regarded by medical and nursing staff as only a minor complication of anaesthesia and surgery, nausea and vomiting are frequently the cause of great distress to patients. Many studies have been undertaken to investigate nausea and vomiting after anaesthesia and surgery. The incidence varies from 14% to 82%, the wide range resulting partly from differences in design of studies. Many factors contribute to the aetiology of postoperative nausea and vomiting and these are discussed in detail in Chapter 42.

Prevention and Treatment

The incidence of postoperative vomiting may be reduced by careful selection of drugs in the perioperative period, and the prophylactic use of antiemetic agents (see Ch 42).

Headache

The reported incidence of severe headache after anaesthesia and surgery ranges from 12% to 35%, but up to 60% of patients complain of some headache. Individuals who are susceptible to headaches caused by stress, etc., are more likely to complain of postoperative headache. Most investigations have failed to identify any single agent as being responsible for postoperative headache after general anaesthesia. Severe postural headache may occur after dural puncture (see p. 529).

Sore Throat

Around 12% of patients complain of sore throat after anaesthesia and surgery. Some of the common causes include the following.

- *Trauma during tracheal intubation.* Damage to the pharynx and tonsillar fauces may be caused by the laryngoscope blade.
- *Trauma to the larynx.* This is more likely if the tube has been forced through the vocal cords. A poorly stabilized tube causes more frictional damage to the larynx than one which is securely stabilized.
- *Trauma to the pharynx.* This may occur during passage of a nasogastric tube or insertion of an oropharyngeal or laryngeal mask airway, and is particularly common when a throat pack has been used. Occasionally, the pharynx or upper oesophagus may be perforated during insertion of a nasogastric tube, or during difficult tracheal intubation, and severe pain in the throat is often the first symptom. Sore throat is likely if a nasogastric tube remains *in situ* during the postoperative period.
- *Other factors.* The mucous membranes of the mouth, pharynx and upper airway are sensitive to the effects of unhumidified gases; the drying effect of anaesthetic gases may cause postoperative sore throat. The antisialagogue effect of anticholinergic drugs may also contribute to this symptom.

The use of topical local anaesthetics does not reduce the incidence of sore throat. Lubrication of the tracheal tube is effective in reducing the incidence, although there is no difference in this respect between plain or local anaesthetic jellies. Sore throat is less common, but not completely avoided, when a face mask or supraglottic airway is used for airway management.

In the absence of a nasogastric tube, postoperative sore throat is usually of short duration; most patients are symptom-free within 48 h.

Hoarseness

This should not be confused with sore throat. It is almost always associated with tracheal intubation and is caused predominantly by prolonged abduction of, and pressure on, the vocal cords. However, traumatic tracheal intubation can cause direct trauma to the vocal cords, resulting in prolonged hoarseness.

Laryngeal Granulomata

These may occur after tracheal intubation, and arise from areas of ulceration, usually on the posterior aspect of the vocal cords. The ulcers are caused by pressure and consequent ischaemia. Granulomata are reported most frequently after thyroidectomy.

If hoarseness persists for longer than 1 week, indirect laryngoscopy should be performed. If ulceration is present, complete voice rest is indicated. Any granulomata present should be excised; untreated granulomata may grow to such a size as to obstruct the airway.

Dental Trauma

This is the commonest cause of litigation against anaesthetists. Damage usually occurs during laryngoscopy, especially if tracheal intubation is difficult, or in association with removal of a supraglottic airway. Loose teeth, crowns, caps and bridges are particularly susceptible to damage. Preoperative enquiry and examination should alert the anaesthetist to the possibility of damage.

Ocular Complications

Carelessness is the commonest cause of damage to the eyes; corneal abrasion is the most frequent lesion. The eyes should not remain open during anaesthesia. The cornea is then exposed and vulnerable to the irritant effects of skin preparations, dust and surgical drapes. This type of damage is easily prevented by securing the eyelids in a closed position with adhesive tape.

Retinal infarction has occurred on rare occasions as a result of pressure on the eyeball from a face mask. It can also occur if patients are placed in the prone position in such a way that pressure is exerted on the eye, e.g. by a horseshoe head rest.

Muscles

Problems associated with inadequate reversal of neuromuscular blocking drugs are discussed above. The detection and treatment of malignant hyperthermia are described on page 879; it is important to appreciate that this condition may present during recovery.

Shivering

This is a common complication in the recovery room. It may occur in patients who are hypothermic as a result of prolonged surgery, or during injection of local anaesthetic solution into the epidural space. However, in most patients, the onset of shivering is not related to body temperature, and there is evidence from electromyography that the characteristics of postoperative (or postanaesthetic) shivering differ from those of thermoregulatory shivering. The incidence and severity of shivering are increased in patients who have received an anticholinergic premedication, and women are more likely to shiver in the luteal than in the follicular phase of the menstrual cycle.

Shivering increases oxygen consumption and carbon dioxide production and may result in hypoxaemia and hypercapnia if the response of the respiratory centre to carbon dioxide is impaired by drugs. Oxygen should be administered. A small dose of pethidine (20 mg i.v.) is frequently effective in aborting postoperative shivering.

Succinylcholine Pains

Muscle pains after succinylcholine are very common, occurring in at least 50% of patients who receive the drug. The muscles involved most frequently are those of the shoulder girdle, neck and thorax. The pain is similar in nature to that caused by viral-related myositis. The incidence is influenced by the following factors.

- *Age.* Succinylcholine pains are unusual in young children and the elderly.
- *Gender.* Women are more susceptible than men. The incidence is reduced during pregnancy.
- *Type of surgery.* There is an increased incidence after minor procedures, when early ambulation is likely.
- *Physical fitness.* The incidence is higher in individuals who are physically fit.
- *Repeated doses.* The incidence is increased if repeated doses of succinylcholine are administered.

The exact cause of muscle pains after succinylcholine is unknown, although it is thought that fasciculations produced by depolarization of the motor nerve end-plate are involved in the pathogenesis. However, the visible extent of fasciculations does not correlate with the severity of subsequent pain. Myoglobinuria occurs after administration of succinylcholine, demonstrating that muscle cell injury does occur.

After minor surgery, the patient may be disturbed by the muscle pains to a greater extent than the discomfort caused by the operative procedure. Analgesics such as paracetamol or NSAIDs may be required for 2–3 days to relieve the pain.

It is possible to reduce, but not to eliminate, the incidence of succinylcholine pains by pretreatment with one of the following agents:

- a small dose of non-depolarizing muscle relaxant (usually 10% of the normal dose) 2–3 min before induction of anaesthesia

- lidocaine $1\,mg\,kg^{-1}$
- diazepam $0.15\,mg\,kg^{-1}$ i.v. before induction of anaesthesia.

Surgical Considerations

During the recovery period, several surgical complications may occur. These include haemorrhage, blockage of drains or catheters and soiling of dressings. Prosthetic arterial grafts may block, resulting in ischaemia of the limbs. Recovery ward nurses and anaesthetists must be aware of potential surgical complications, as rapid surgical intervention may be required.

The recovery period may also be used to commence orthopaedic traction before the patient returns to the ward.

FURTHER READING

Association of Anaesthetists of Great Britain and Ireland, 2013. Immediate postanaesthetic recovery 2013. AAGBI, London.

Mecca, R.S., 2002. Postanesthesia recovery. In: Kirby, R.R., Gravenstein, N., Lobato, B., Gravenstein, N. (Eds.), Clinical anesthesia practice. WB Saunders, Philadelphia, pp. 83–127.

Venkataraman, R., Kellum, J.A., 2007. Defining acute renal failure: the RIFLE criteria. J. Intensive Care Med. 22, 187–193.

POSTOPERATIVE PAIN

Pain is an extraordinarily complex and emotive sensation which is difficult to define and equally difficult to measure in an accurate, objective manner. It has been defined as the sensory appreciation of afferent nociceptive stimulation, which elicits an affective (or autonomic) component; both are subjected to rational interpretation by the patient. It may be represented as a Venn diagram (Fig. 41.1), the shaded area of which represents the quantum of suffering experienced by the patient. The Venn diagram illustrates easily and effectively that the sensation of pain differs among individual patients; the emotional component may vary according to the patient's current psychological state and pre-existing psychological composition and the rational component varies with the patient's previous experience, insight and motivation.

Postoperative pain differs from other types of pain in that it is usually, but by no means always, transitory, with progressive improvement over a relatively short time-course. Typically, the affective component tends towards an anxiety state associated with diagnosis of the condition, concern regarding the effectiveness of surgery to provide a cure and/or relief of existing pain, and fear of delay in provision of adequate analgesic therapy by attendants. In contrast, chronic pain is persistent, frequently with fluctuating intensity, may remain without an acceptable diagnosis and the affective component contains a greater depressive element, with the patient needing and potentially actively searching for adequate pain relief. Thus, postoperative pain is more easily amenable to therapy than chronic pain. Despite this, a recent survey showed that most adults still expect to have significant postoperative pain after surgery, and that this is their primary concern before surgery. Such concern may be justified, because traditional management of postoperative pain, using intramuscular opioid administration given on demand, often failed to produce good analgesia. This was highlighted by the Royal College of Surgeons' report on postoperative pain in 1990, which paved the way to the national development of Acute Pain Services and improved methods of administering pain relief.

The traditional management of postoperative pain comprised the prescription of a standard dose of an opioid, to be given on demand by a nurse when the patient's pain threshold had been exceeded. This leads to poor control of postoperative pain for the following reasons:

- Responsibility for management of pain is delegated to the nursing staff, who err on the side of caution in the administration of opioids. They tend to give too small a dose of drug too infrequently because of exaggerated fears of producing ventilatory depression or addiction.
- The roles and availability of nurses have changed in line with an evolving healthcare system. This has reduced the number of nurses available to administer opioid analgesia in an effective and safe manner. The statutory regulations on the prescribing and administration of opioid medication remains unchanged, but with reduced staffing levels, this can impact on the time delay between the request for analgesia and the administration of the medication. This is often most noticeable at night.

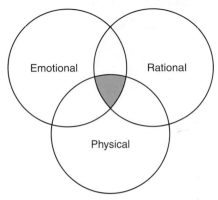

FIGURE 41.1 ■ The interrelationship between emotional, rational and physical components of pain. Perceived pain is represented by the area of intersection of all three components.

- Because the administration of drugs is left entirely to the discretion of the nursing staff, the degree of empathy between nurse and patient affects analgesic administration. This may be part of the explanation for the common observation that the mean dose of morphine given for a standard operation varies among hospitals and even among wards in the same hospital.
- Because the measurement of pain is difficult, it is seldom possible to adjust the dose of drug to match the extent of pain.
- There are enormous variations in the extent of analgesic requirements depending upon the type of surgery, pharmacokinetic variability, pharmacodynamic variability, etc.

These inadequacies in the traditional management of postoperative pain have been confirmed by a survey of ethical problems faced by nurses, which showed that they regard pain management to be a significant problem in their clinical practice.

PHYSIOLOGY

The physiology of acute pain is no longer considered to be a simple 'hard-wired' system with a pure 'stimulus-response' relationship. Rather, tissue damage or disease sets up a process involving tissue receptors, the peripheral, central and autonomic nervous systems, and higher centres in the brain which produce the perception of pain.

Nociceptors

Nociceptors are receptors which require a strong (high threshold) stimulus for activation. Most are polymodal, i.e. respond to a variety of noxious stimuli (heat, mechanical, chemical). The usual stimulus for activation is mechanical distortion of the receptor, followed by local increases in K^+ and H^+ ions. Inflammation leads to a reduction in the threshold for stimulation, and activation of dormant or 'silent' nociceptors. This is termed 'peripheral sensitization'.

Primary Afferent Fibres

Primary afferent fibres conduct impulses from the nociceptor to the spinal cord, and have their cell bodies in the dorsal root ganglion. There are two types of primary afferent fibres from nociceptors, and they are distinguished mainly by their speed of conduction. Aδ fibres have a high speed of conduction, and are responsible for 'immediate', sharp pain and reflex withdrawal. C fibres conduct at a lower speed, and are responsible for persistent pain and central sensitization in the spinal cord (Table 41.1). Most primary afferent fibres terminate by synapsing with dorsal horn neurones (Fig. 41.2).

TABLE 41.1			
Characteristics of Primary Afferent Fibre (Aβ is Included for Comparison)			
	C	*Aδ*	*Aβ*
Conductive velocity	IV (<2 m s⁻¹)	III (10–40 m s⁻¹)	II (>40 m s⁻¹)
Myelination	No	Yes	Yes
Receptors	High threshold	High and low threshold	Low threshold

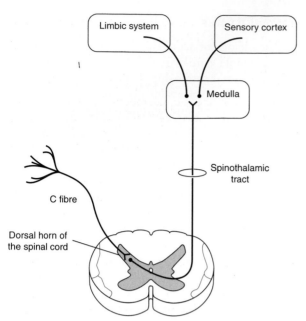

FIGURE 41.2 ■ Basic anatomy of the pain pathway.

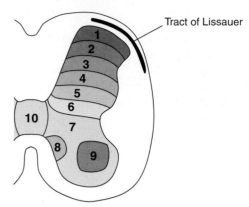

FIGURE 41.3 ■ Rexed laminae.

Dorsal Horn Neurones

A cross-section of the spinal cord shows 10 anatomically and physiologically distinct layers called Rexed laminae (Fig. 41.3). Laminae 1–6 and lamina 10 are sites at which sensory afferents synapse with dorsal horn cells. Laminae 7, 8 and 9 represent the motor horn. Aδ and C fibres terminate in several layers, including the outer (marginal) zone and in particular lamina 2 (substantia gelatinosa).

Some dorsal horn cells respond to painful and non-painful stimuli, and are called 'wide dynamic range' (WDR) neurones. They exhibit 'wind up' in which their output increases in the presence of a continuous, low frequency, C fibre (i.e. painful) input. In this case, the C-fibre input has 'sensitized' the dorsal horn cell, and animal models have demonstrated that NMDA (N-methyl-D-aspartate) receptor activation is a key feature. This process is termed 'central sensitization'.

Allodynia and Hyperalgesia

Allodynia is the term for pain induced by a previously non-painful stimulus. Hyperalgesia is increased pain from a previous painful stimulus. Both occur following peripheral and central sensitization, and they should be regarded as normal physiological processes following tissue injury, designed to encourage the organism to protect the injury.

The receptive field of a dorsal horn neurone refers to the area in the periphery where stimulation triggers action potentials in that dorsal horn neurone. Following tissue injury, the receptive field expands, and minor changes in excitability cause major changes in the size of the receptive field.

Ascending Tracts and Supraspinal Systems

Most dorsal horn neurones project to the brain by ascending several segments in the spinal cord before crossing over to the opposite ventrolateral side, and joining one of three major spinal systems:

- Spinothalamic tract: probably the most important tract for pain transmission, this tract projects to several nuclei in the thalamus. It is the target for treating intractable cancer pain with cordotomy.
- Spinoreticular tract: terminates in the reticular nuclei in the brainstem.
- Spinomesencephalic tract: terminates in the mesencephalic reticular formation and periaqueductal grey.

All the terminal sites of spinal tracts project to the somatosensory cortex, associated with the sensory aspect of pain. The limbic system is associated with the affective aspect of pain.

Descending Systems

Descending inhibitory pathways, originating in particular from the periaqueductal grey matter in the midbrain and the rostral ventromedial medulla, may modulate transmission across spinal cord synapses. Both these areas contain high concentrations of endogenous opioids and opioid receptors. Activation of these receptors increases activity in descending monoamine (serotonin and noradrenaline) pathways (indirectly, by reducing stimulation of inhibitory interneurones), and reduces transmission across dorsal horn synapses.

Visceral Pain

Afferent C fibres from abdominal viscera travel with autonomic nerves, particularly sympathetic, and synapse with dorsal horn cells. Thus, sympathetic denervation may be useful for intractable visceral pain (e.g. coeliac plexus block for pancreatic cancer). There is no distinct spinothalamic tract for visceral afferents.

Neuropathic Pain

This is pain arising from an abnormality or change in either the peripheral or central nervous systems. It is usually accompanied by other sensory (numbness, paraesthesiae), motor (weakness) or autonomic dysfunction, and so may be distinguished from referred pain. Radicular pain is pain arising in the distribution of a spinal nerve, and may be caused by compression of the spinal cord, nerve root, or plexus.

Referred Pain

Referred pain is experienced at a site distant from the pain source, and occurs because of convergence of different pain afferents on to common dorsal horn neurones. Segmental embryonic innervation remains throughout growth and accounts for the distance between the source of pain and referred site. Referred pain is often described as an ache, and is not accompanied by any other sensory abnormality.

EFFECTS OF NOXIOUS SURGICAL STIMULATION

Changes occur within the nervous system following any prolonged, noxious stimulus, as in the postoperative period where the surgical wound sends afferent neuronal information to the central nervous system for some time. Both 'peripheral' and 'central' sensitization occurs and alters the body's response to further peripheral sensory input.

Moreover, surgery generates a catabolic state by changes in endocrine hormonal control, with increased secretion of catabolic hormones and decreased secretion of anabolic hormones. The results include: pain; nausea, vomiting and intestinal stasis; alterations in blood flow, coagulation and fibrinolysis; alterations in substrate metabolism; alterations in water and electrolyte handling by the body; and increased demands on the cardiovascular and respiratory systems.

New principles of pain management have been developed to improve analgesia after surgery in the light of our improved understanding of the processes involved. These include the recognition of the adverse effects of unrelieved pain, the need for an experienced and flexible approach to the problem by medical and nursing staff, and the necessity of informing the patient about the pain relief process. It is best to make plans for analgesia before surgery takes place, and this is especially important in short-stay surgery, when the patient is discharged home soon after the operation. The safety and efficacy of postoperative pain management may be improved by frequent assessment of the patient, good education of the staff and patients about the techniques and drugs used, preparation of protocols and guidelines for staff to follow, and regular evaluation by quality assurance programmes. These principles have been developed and incorporated into Acute or more recently Inpatient Pain Teams. Whilst acute postoperative pain normally settles over a relatively short time period, it is recognized that there is a significant incidence of chronic, severe pain after surgery including thoracotomy, mastectomy, limb amputation, and the less invasive operation of vasectomy. The aetiology of ongoing severe pain after surgery must lie in the pathophysiological changes, described above, which occur after tissue damage.

INPATIENT PAIN TEAMS

Since the publication of the Royal College of Surgeons' and College of Anaesthetists' report on postoperative pain in 1990, there has been a gradual and effective formation of Acute Pain Teams; more recently, these have become Inpatient Pain Teams. Their role is multi-dimensional, multidisciplinary and aimed at improving analgesia, maintaining safety, education and, in the long term, reducing morbidity, mortality and potentially bed days.

In broad terms, these teams have the following functions:

- Assessment of pain
- Standardization of orders of analgesic prescription and monitoring of patients
- Education of nurses, doctors and staff allied to medicine who deal with patients in acute pain
- Provision and monitoring of new or specialist analgesic methods
- Advice to staff on managing acute pain
- Constant evaluation of analgesic regimens e.g. efficacy, side-effects and safety
- Audit
- Adherence to national standards

The teams are usually multidisciplinary but managed by senior nursing staff trained in Pain Management, who often have postgraduate qualifications in the management of pain. Guidance and assistance, which is both practical and educational, is provided by consultant anaesthetists trained in Pain Management, and usually anaesthetists in training. Further assistance at ward level is provided by a system of link nurses who have a special interest in Pain Management on their ward.

The whole team requires administrative and audit support. Specific resources include specialist equipment and computers.

These Pain Teams now deal with a wide variety of acute pain problems, not only postoperative, which are categorized below.

- Acute postoperative
  - Major surgery
  - Intermediate surgery
  - Minor surgery
  - Ambulatory and day surgery
  - Specialist surgery e.g. bariatric, emergency, fractured neck of femur in the elderly
- Secondary to trauma
  - Skeletal
  - Blunt trauma
  - Penetrating trauma
  - Accidental/deliberate

- Secondary to a disease process
  - Infection
  - Inflammation
  - Ischaemia
  - Burns
  - Infiltration/Cancer
  - Compression

A patient's experience of pain as illustrated in the previous Venn diagram (Fig. 41.1) is multidimensional, requiring input from a wide variety of professionals experienced in pain management.

CAUSES OF VARIATION IN ANALGESIC REQUIREMENTS

Using patient-controlled analgesic apparatus (see below), it has been shown that there is marked interindividual variation in analgesic requirements. Thus, after open cholecystectomy, some patients may require no morphine within the first 24 h, whereas others may require as much as 120 mg. Unfortunately, there is no way of predicting in advance the extent of opioid requirements of an individual patient. In clinical practice, requirements are assessed on a trial-and-error basis; anaesthetists are therefore in an ideal position to be involved in prescribing postoperative analgesia, as they obtain a 'feel' for dose requirements during the management of anaesthesia.

Site and Type of Surgery

In general, upper abdominal surgery produces greater pain than lower abdominal surgery, which in turn is associated with greater pain than peripheral surgery. This generalization is not entirely accurate; operations on the richly innervated digits may be associated with quite severe pain.

The type of pain may differ with different types of surgery. Operations on joints are associated with sharp pain. In contrast, abdominal surgery is associated with three types of pain: a continuous dull nauseating ache (which responds well to morphine); a spasmodic, intermittent cramping pain originating from motile viscera, which may respond to hyoscine (Buscopan); and a sharper pain induced by coughing and movement (which responds poorly to morphine). Pain associated with surgery on the digits may respond relatively poorly to opioids but well to non-steroidal

TABLE 41.2
Duration and Severity of Postoperative Pain

Site of Operation	Duration of Opioid Use (h)	Severity of Pain (0–4)
Abdominal		
Upper	48–72	3
Lower	Up to 48	2
Inguinal	Up to 36	1
Thoracotomy	72–96	4
Limbs	24–36	2
Faciomaxillary	Up to 48	2
Body wall	Up to 24	1
Perineal	24–48	2
Hip surgery	Up to 48	2

TABLE 41.3
Psychological Factors Which Influence Postoperative Analgesic Requirements

Personality – more pain if high neuroticism/extroversion

Social background

Culture

Motivation

Preoperative psychotherapy

anti-inflammatory drugs. There is increasing evidence that minimally invasive, laparoscopic surgery produces less-prolonged postoperative pain than do traditional techniques, but the pain may still be severe, especially in the immediate postoperative period.

Table 41.2 provides an approximate guide to the duration and severity of postoperative pain.

Age, Gender and Body Weight

The analgesic requirements of males and females are identical for similar types of surgery, but variations in opioid receptor type (more OPRK1 [κ] receptors in females) may influence gender response to different opiates. However, there is a reduction in analgesic requirements with advancing age. Consequently, it is essential that the anaesthetist reduces the dosage of opioid drugs in elderly patients. For example, reasonable starting doses for intramuscular (or subcutaneous) postoperative morphine administration would be 7.5–12.5 mg for patients aged 20–39 years, but the dose should be reduced to only 2.5–5.0 mg for patients of 70–85 years of age.

The established anaesthetic practice of prescribing the potent opioid drugs on a milligram or microgram per body weight basis lacks scientific validity. There is no evidence to suggest that variations in body weight in the adult population affect opioid requirements significantly.

Psychological Factors

The patient's personality affects pain perception and response to analgesic drugs. Thus, patients with low anxiety and low neuroticism scores on a personality scale exhibit less postoperative pain and require smaller doses of opioid than patients who rate highly on these scales. Patients with high scores may exhibit a higher incidence of postoperative chest complications (Table 41.3).

The extent of a patient's anxiety also affects pain perception; increased anxiety results in a greater degree of perceived postoperative pain and increased opioid requirements.

These psychological factors help to explain the efficacy of preoperative psychotherapy. Anxiety and postoperative analgesic requirements are reduced if the preoperative assessment by the anaesthetist includes an explanation of forthcoming perioperative events and details regarding the provision of pain relief.

Pharmacokinetic Variability

After the intramuscular injection of an opioid, there is a three- to sevenfold difference among patients in the rate at which peak plasma concentration of the drug occurs and a two- to fivefold difference in the peak plasma concentration achieved. This is illustrated in Figure 41.4, which shows the mean change in plasma concentration after the first and second, and seventh and eighth injections. The variability in the plasma concentration is reflected by the large standard deviation of the mean. In addition, average concentrations increase after each of the first few injections; oscillation around a steady mean concentration does not occur until after approximately the fourth injection.

This pharmacokinetic variability helps to explain the relatively poor response to a single intramuscular injection given in the postoperative period.

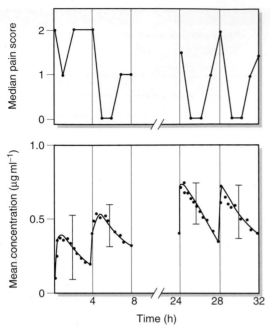

FIGURE 41.4 ■ Blood concentrations of pethidine and pain score after surgery; a pain score of 0 indicates no pain. Doses of pethidine 100 mg have been given 4-hourly. Mean blood concentration of pethidine continues to rise for 24 h before a plateau is reached. Little pain relief is provided by the first dose. Even after 24 h, significant pain is present 3 and 4 h after each injection, as blood concentrations decline.

TABLE 41.4	
Minimum Effective Analgesic Concentration (MEAC) in Blood for a Number of Analgesic Drugs. (Note the Wide Range of Values for Each Agent)	
Drug	*MEAC (ng mL^{-1})*
Fentanyl	1–3
Alfentanil	100–300
Pethidine	300–650
Morphine	12–24
Methadone	30–70

MEASUREMENT OF PAIN

Although pain measurement is subjective, it is a useful tool to aid assessment of the patient and the effect of treatment. Patient and doctor recall of the effectiveness of previous treatment is an unreliable way of monitoring response to therapy, and it is much better to record some type of repeatable measure. Recently, pain it has been named as the fifth vital sign and many hospitals encourage/require nursing and medical staff to record a 'Pain Score' along with temperature, respiratory rate, pulse rate and blood pressure. Some simple ways of measuring pain are listed below. It is important to involve the patient in the assessment process because individual responses to treatment are so variable. Pain should be assessed on movement, not simply when the patient is lying perfectly still in an attempt to minimize discomfort. A typical standard movement is to ask the patient to reach over to the other side of the bed while in a lying or semirecumbent position.

- Verbal rating scales tend to be short, easy to administer and easy to understand (e.g. 'none, mild, moderate or severe'), but not as accurate as the methods below.
- The Visual Analogue Scale (VAS) and the numeric rating scale (NRS) are validated in clinical use, but some patients find them more difficult to understand than scales using word descriptors. These scales are often understood better as a vertical score with increasing pain at the top and less pain at the bottom. The face pain scoring system used for children can be usefully applied to adults, particularly if their first language is not English.

Pharmacodynamic Variability

Although there are widespread pharmacokinetic variations among patients in response to administration of opioids, the major reason for variation in opioid sensitivity is pharmacodynamic, i.e. a difference in the inherent sensitivity of opioid receptors.

Using continuous infusions of opioids to achieve equilibrium between receptor drug concentration and plasma concentration, it is possible to define a steady-state plasma concentration of opioid at which analgesia is produced. This is termed the minimum effective analgesic concentration (MEAC); values of MEAC for the commonly available opioids are shown in Table 41.4. MEAC levels vary four- to fivefold among individual patients and are affected by age and differences in psychological profile.

- A binary scale is one of the simplest to use. For example, 'Is your pain at least 50% relieved?', to which the patient answers yes or no.
- A simple numerical scale is often used. For example 0–3, 0 representing no pain and 3 the worst pain ever. The advantage of this scale is that it is easy for the patient to remember the options and easy for nursing staff to record.

All of these scoring systems function best for the patient's subjective feeling of pain intensity at a specific time i.e. present pain intensity. They can be used for pain in the last 24 h or over the last week, but are limited by the patient's memory of pain and altered by other events in the intervening time period.

TREATMENT OF POSTOPERATIVE PAIN

Treatment should aim to fulfil the following criteria:

1. Easy to administer and understand
2. Easy to assess effectiveness and side-effects
3. Be administered using the gastrointestinal tract if possible
4. Easy to train nursing and medical staff to use, monitor, and know of side-effects
5. Cost-effective
6. Efficacious
7. Have few side-effects or side-effects which can be detected and easily reversed
8. Easy to prescribe using standardised prescriptions
9. Easy to place in a flow chart

METHODS OF TREATING POSTOPERATIVE PAIN

See Table 41.5.

Traditional Administration of Opioids

Intramuscular administration of opioids on a *pro re nata* (p.r.n.; as required) basis was traditionally the method used most commonly for prescribing postoperative analgesia. However, for the reasons noted above, this technique leads frequently to inadequate pain relief. Almost 60% of patients report dissatisfaction with the quality of postoperative analgesia administered in this way.

TABLE 41.5
Methods of Treating Postoperative Pain

Traditional administration of opioid
Intramuscular or subcutaneous on-demand bolus

Parenteral administration of opioid
Bolus intravenous administration
Continuous intravenous infusion
Patient-controlled analgesia
Bolus intravenous
Bolus+infusion
Subcutaneous

Non-parenteral administration of opioid
Sublingual
Oral
Transmucosal
Rectal
Transdermal
Nasal
Inhalation
Intra-articular opioids

Local anaesthetic techniques
Spinal/extradural opioids
Entonox
Non-steroidal anti-inflammatory drugs (NSAIDs)
COX-2 selective inhibitors
Paracetamol
NMDA antagonists
α_2-*Adrenergic agonists*
Systemically
Extradurally

Non-pharmacological methods
Cryotherapy
Transcutaneous electrical nerve stimulation (TENS)
Acupuncture
Psychological methods

Intramuscular injection results in variable absorption, particularly in patients with hypothermia, hypovolaemia, hypotension or excessive adipose tissue. This may result in the formation of a depot of opioid, which may be absorbed much later and may add to already adequate plasma concentrations of drug, resulting in toxicity. In addition, there is inevitably a considerable delay between a request for analgesia and subsequent administration while controlled drugs are checked and drawn into a syringe. Although it is customary to prescribe opioids on a 4-hourly p.r.n. basis, there are frequently much longer periods between injections and this may lead to considerable 'breakthrough' pain.

Regular administration of intramuscular opioids provides improved analgesia, although care must be taken to avoid the formation of a depot of opioid as described above, or overdosage in debilitated patients and those at the extremes of age. Each injection should be at a different site to reduce the risk of accumulation in one site and to reduce the risk of changes in the muscle and skin composition.

The advantages and disadvantages of repeated p.r.n. administration of opioids are listed in Table 41.6. The use of pethidine for postoperative pain relief is decreasing because of the potential accumulation of the excitatory metabolite norpethidine with repeated use.

The commonest cause of postoperative nausea and vomiting is the administration of opioids either intraoperatively or in the postoperative period. It should therefore be standard practice to prescribe antiemetic drugs regularly for administration with opioids. Drugs used commonly for postoperative pain and antiemesis are listed in Table 41.7; their pharmacological properties are discussed fully in Chapters 5 and 42.

Subcutaneous Administration of Opioids

Morphine may be given subcutaneously, and patients prefer this to intramuscular injections. A small-gauge

TABLE 41.6

Advantages and Disadvantages of Intramuscular p.r.n. Administration of Opioids

Advantages	Disadvantages
Familiar practice	Fixed dose not related to pharmacovariability
Gradual onset of side-effects	I.m. administration causes profound pharmacovariability
Nursing assessment before administration	Painful injections
Inexpensive	Fluctuating plasma concentrations
	Delayed onset of analgesia

TABLE 41.7

Drugs Used Systemically for Postoperative Pain Relief and Antiemesis

Drug	Dose i.m. or s.c. (Healthy Adult)
Opioids	
Morphine	10 mg 4-hourly
Pethidine	100 mg 3-hourly
Buprenorphine (sublingual)	0.4 mg 6-hourly
Tramadol	50–100 mg 4–6-hourly
Moderate analgesics	
Ketorolac	10–30 mg 6-hourly
Paracetamol	1 g 6-hourly
Dihydrocodeine	50 mg 4-hourly
Antiemetics	
Prochlorperazine	12.5 mg 6-hourly
Cyclizine	50 mg 6-hourly
Metoclopramide	10 mg 6-hourly
Ondansetron	4 mg i.v. 6-hourly

cannula may be inserted subcutaneously and left in place for 2–3 days, avoiding the need for repeated skin punctures. Absorption of morphine from the subcutaneous route is comparable with absorption from the intramuscular route. It is particularly useful in the elderly, in children and in adults with learning difficulties to administer timely opioid analgesia when the other methods described below are inappropriate or impractical.

Algorithms for Opioid Administration

Some acute pain services have constructed algorithms for postoperative intramuscular or subcutaneous opioid administration which other less experienced members of staff may then follow to provide safe and effective pain relief for their patients. Figure 41.5 is an example. Many operating theatre suite postoperative care areas also use algorithms for the intravenous administration of opioids either via single bolus or via a PCA pump. An important aspect of such algorithms is the frequent assessment of the patient to ensure safety and efficacy of the treatment. Clinical assessments include pain (at rest and on movement) and sedation scores, nausea and vomiting scores, respiratory rate, heart rate and arterial blood pressure. The algorithm includes a description of recommended doses and instructions on

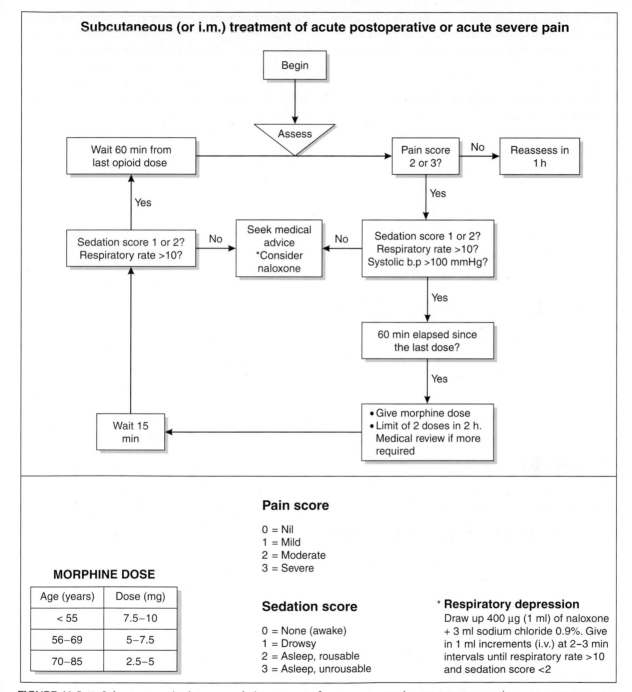

FIGURE 41.5 ■ Subcutaneous (or intramuscular) treatment of acute postoperative or acute severe pain.

how to treat recognized side effects such as respiratory depression. An important feature of such algorithms is that they permit more frequent opioid administration, e.g. '2-hourly p.r.n.'.

Sites of Action and Properties of Morphine and Morphine-Like Drugs

Opioids act supraspinally (nucleus raphe magnus, periaqueductal and periventricular grey areas), in the spinal cord (around C-fibre terminals in lamina I and the substantia gelatinosa, lamina II), and peripherally (opioid receptors are transported peripherally in axons, and are expressed by immune cells at the site of tissue damage). The actions of morphine are:

- analgesia – morphine produces analgesia by binding with opioid receptors, which are present in high concentrations in the periaqueductal area and limbic system of the brain and in the region of the substantia gelatinosa of the spinal cord
- ventilatory depression
- sedation
- cough suppression
- vasodilatation
- release of histamine
- constipation
- nausea and vomiting
- pupillary constriction
- biliary spasm, this is now thought to be clinically insignificant.
- urine retention
- tolerance
- physical dependence (although addiction to opioids is rare when they are used for the relief of acute postoperative pain)
- reduced immune function with prolonged use
- with prolonged use, an adverse affect on the production of sex hormones
- recent animal studies indicate opioid-induced analgesia with increased postoperative pain following intraoperative opiates e.g. remifentanil; the mechanism is thought to be complex, involving central sensitization and numerous systems e.g. NMDA, $5HT_3$, CCK and Substance P.

The most important side effects of morphine are ventilatory depression, and nausea and vomiting. Significant hypoxaemia may occur for several days postoperatively, and supplemental oxygen is recommended for at least the first 48–72 h following major surgery, and in the elderly or high-risk patient regardless of the analgesic method used. Purists advocate that morphine should not be administered to patients with biliary or renal colic (occasionally it may precipitate pain in patients with gallbladder disease when administered as premedication). However, in the clinical setting, it is seldom a problem and morphine is increasingly used as pethidine availability is reduced. Morphine should be used with care in patients with head injury and perhaps in asthmatics. Tramadol is an interesting synthetic analgesic which has both opioid and non-opioid mechanisms of action and may produce analgesia with less respiratory depression, sedation, gastrointestinal stasis and abuse potential. Unfortunately, as with morphine, the use of tramadol is associated with nausea and vomiting. Tramadol does have significant side-effects, particularly in the elderly, and it has a narrow therapeutic window, numbers needed to harm being 9.0 and numbers needed to treat being 3.9.

Parenteral Routes of Opioid Administration

Systemic opioids cannot relieve severe dynamic pain provoked by movement needed to get the patient out of bed or mobilizing bronchial secretions by forceful coughing without causing unacceptable side-effects. Patients and staff treating the patient should be aware of this and, if predicted, it should be alleviated using multimodal techniques and/or local anaesthetic techniques.

Bolus I.V. Administration

It is possible to improve the quality of analgesia in the postoperative period by giving small incremental doses of opioid i.v when required. However, this carries the risk of rapid induction of ventilatory depression and in many hospitals cannot be undertaken by nursing staff in the wards. In general, this technique is employed only by anaesthetists and experienced nursing staff in the immediate recovery period.

Continuous I.V. Infusion

Continuous i.v. infusion (Table 41.8) is employed to provide analgesia in patients receiving artificial ventilation in an intensive therapy unit (ITU). An infusion

TABLE 41.8
Advantages and Disadvantages of Continuous i.v. Infusions

Advantages	Disadvantages
Rapid onset of analgesia Steady-state plasma concentrations	Fixed dose not related to pharmacodynamic variability
Painless	Errors may be fatal
	Expensive fail-safe equipment required
	May result in less frequent assessment by nursing staff

TABLE 41.9
Advantages and Disadvantages of Patient-Controlled Analgesia (PCA)

Advantages	Disadvantages
Dose matches patient's requirements and therefore compensates for pharmacodynamic variability	Technical errors may be fatal Expensive equipment Requires ability to cooperate and understand
Doses given are small and therefore fluctuations in plasma concentration is reduced	
Reduces nurses' workload	
Painless	
Placebo effect from patient autonomy	

rate designed to exceed MEAC in all patients is clearly safe and ventilatory depression is an advantage in this situation.

Continuous infusions have been used in general surgical wards for the provision of postoperative analgesia in spontaneously breathing patients. The dosage rate is determined by the medical attendant on a trial-and-error basis, and a fixed infusion rate prescribed. However, this carries great risks of producing ventilatory depression and cannot be recommended in spontaneously breathing patients outside a high-dependency unit or ITU.

Patient-Controlled Analgesia

The main problem with continuous i.v. infusion is that there is no way of predicting an individual patient's MEAC. With patient-controlled analgesia (PCA), the patient determines the rate of i.v. administration of the drug, thereby providing feedback control.

PCA equipment comprises an accurate source of infusion coupled to an i.v. cannula, and controlled by a patient-machine interface device. Safety features are incorporated to limit the preset dose, the number of doses, which may be administered and the 'lockout' period between doses. Advantages and disadvantages of PCA are listed in Table 41.9.

The drug that has been used most commonly with PCA is morphine. The size of the demand dose is usually 1–2 mg with a lockout period of between 5 and 10 min. Fentanyl (10–20 µg), pethidine (10 mg), oxycodone (0.5–1.0 mg) and hydromorphone (0.2 mg) may also be used for intravenous PCA. Although there may be some theoretical advantage in the use of a continuous low-dose infusion on which the patient may superimpose demand bolus administrations, several clinical investigations have failed to reveal any advantage. Because of the slightly increased risk of overdosage, therefore, it is generally recommended that PCA apparatus be used in the 'bolus alone' mode.

Intravenous PCA is now a standard method of providing postoperative analgesia in many hospitals worldwide. It provides better pain relief than conventional intermittent intramuscular administration. It is essential that monitoring of the patient is not reduced because respiratory depression may occur with this technique and many patients may require antiemetics for nausea. If the pump is being used to deliver morphine via an intravenous infusion, it is essential that a one-way valve is incorporated between the PCA equipment and the infusion giving set in order to prevent morphine collecting in the giving set if the cannula becomes occluded; if this happens, a large bolus may be delivered at a later time, with possible lethal effects.

The effective and safe use of PCA requires frequent monitoring of the patient by nurses who have had in-service training and accreditation in the use of the drugs and devices. There is evidence that PCA is more effective when it is overseen by an acute pain service involving pain nursing staff and pharmacists. Standard PCA prescription orders and drug dilutions may minimize complications. PCA may also be used to deliver opioids subcutaneously or epidurally.

Non-Parenteral Opioid Administration
(see Table 41.10**)**

Sublingual Opioids

Sublingual administration requires cooperation. With buprenorphine, good analgesia may be provided without the need for painful injections, making this route popular with patients and convenient for nursing staff.

This route is confined largely to buprenorphine. Combination with morphine may result in dysphoria and withdrawal phenomena. If this route is chosen, it is preferable to use buprenorphine as the sole opioid in the perioperative period, although, as it is a partial opioid agonist, it has a ceiling effect for analgesia.

Oral Route

All the opioids undergo extensive metabolism in the gut wall and liver (first-pass metabolism) and therefore the bioavailability is relatively low (e.g. 20–30% for morphine). Oxycodone (UK; OxyNorm) undergoes less biotransformation, acts rapidly, and is therefore a useful oral opioid for the relief of severe pain (e.g. 5–10 mg, 2–3-hourly). Oxycodone is also available as a sustained-release preparation and an injectable form. In the immediate postoperative period, there is invariably a reduction in the rate of gastric emptying (caused mainly by the intraoperative or preoperative use of opioids). For this reason, care should be taken if opioids are used orally for pain relief in the postoperative period.

- Absorption may be delayed, with poor analgesia.
- If opioids have been given orally on a regular basis, there is a danger of a large dose being propelled into the upper gastrointestinal tract when gastric motility returns to normal, resulting in overdosage and ventilatory depression.

If normal gastric emptying has resumed, then oral opioids may be used safely and effectively after surgery to provide analgesia without the need for injections.

Transmucosal

Oral transmucosal fentanyl citrate has been prepared as a palatable solid matrix (presented as a lollipop) for use as a pre-anaesthetic medication in children. The time to the onset of pain relief is of the order of 9 min, and both transmucosal (buccal) and gastric routes contribute to the absorption of fentanyl. These are also available for specific acute pain conditions in some hospitals. Recent advances have introduced effervescent fentanyl tablets; the product licence is restricted to cancer pain but they are available in some hospitals for specific acute pain conditions under the

TABLE 41.10			
Analgesics, Route of Administration and Efficacy on Types of Pain			
Analgesic	*Route of Administration*	*Potency*	*Type of Pain*
Paracetamol	Oral, rectal, i.v.	Mild	Nociceptive/inflammatory
Codeine	Oral	Mild	Nociceptive/inflammatory
Paracetamol/codeine combinations	Oral	Mild	Nociceptive/inflammatory
Tramadol	Oral, i.m., i.v.	Moderate	Nociceptive/inflammatory/ neuropathic
NSAIDS	Oral, rectal, i.m., i.v.	Mild	Nociceptive/inflammatory
Oramorph	Oral	Strong	Nociceptive
Morphine	I.v., long-acting oral, i.m., s.c.	Strong	Nociceptive
Fentanyl	I.v., patch, submucosal	Strong	Nociceptive
Oxycodone	I.v., oral	Strong	Nociceptive
Pethidine	I.v., i.m., oral	Strong	Nociceptive
Antiemetics	Oral, i.m., i.v., s.c.	N/A	N/A
Antispasmodics	Oral, i.v., i.m.	N/A	visceral

direct supervision of the Inpatient Pain Team. Side-effects include nausea and vomiting, and hypoxaemia. Fentanyl is highly addictive and should not be used in these formulations over a pronged period of time (for more than 2–3 days) for acute pain, for undiagnosed pain or in patients with a history of drug or alcohol addiction. Advice from the Inpatient Pain Team should be sought before these medications are started.

The Rectal Route

The rectal route may be used as a means of delivering morphine but there is marked variability in the plasma concentrations achieved. Venous blood from the lower part of the rectum drains directly into the systemic circulation, but the upper part drains into the portal circulation. Thus, bioavailability varies according to the site of a suppository within the rectum. However, this route avoids the problems of reduced gastrointestinal motility. Probably the best indication for the rectal route is the treatment of chronic intractable pain, particularly when there is dysphagia.

Inhaled/Intranasal

Intranasal spray devices for fentanyl are now available in some countries. Inhaled opioid preparations are being developed with metered inhalers, improved pulmonary drug delivery systems and lockout times, and in the future they may allow noninvasive PCA administration.

Transdermal

Because of the high lipid solubility and high potency of fentanyl, this drug is absorbed across the skin in sufficient quantities to produce effective plasma concentrations. Transdermal fentanyl patches are available with delivery rates from 12.5 to $100\,\mu g\,h^{-1}$. Because of the difficulty in matching transdermal patches of differing strengths to the pharmacodynamic variability among different patients, this technique is not suitable for management of acute pain, but is used for the relief of cancer or chronic nonmalignant pain.

Intra-Articular and Intraperitoneal

Opioids with or without a local anaesthetic are used to provide postoperative analgesia. The surgeon usually administers these medications after the operative procedure, as the surgery is ending.

REGIONAL ANAESTHESIA AND PAIN MANAGEMENT

Recent literature reviews have indicated that regional techniques are superior to systemic opioids with regard to analgesic profile and adverse effects in the context of a wide variety of surgical procedures. Regional analgesic techniques decrease multisystem comorbidity and mortality following major surgery in high-risk patients. A systematic review in 2000 compared central neuraxial blocks with systemic (mainly opioid-based) analgesia. The review found that the use of central neuraxial blockade was associated with significantly less morbidity and a reduction in mortality of up to one-third. Respiratory complications were reduced by 39%, pneumonia by 59%, deep venous thrombosis was decreased by 44% and pulmonary embolism by 55%.

Local Anaesthetic Techniques

Many local anaesthetic techniques, administered for the purpose of operative surgery or during the course of general anaesthesia, may provide excellent analgesia in the early postoperative period. However, it is usually necessary for the anaesthetist to administer an opioid to the patient before the block regresses to reduce the likelihood of severe pain when the block wears off.

Local anaesthetic techniques may be used for the primary purpose of providing analgesia in the early postoperative period. However, a major disadvantage is that the duration of blockade with a 'single-shot' technique is relatively short. Bupivacaine (0.25% or 0.5%) has been the drug of choice and may produce peripheral nerve blockade lasting for 8–12 h and occasionally for as long as 18 h. The duration of action for epidural nerve block is 4–6 h. Ropivacaine has similar local anaesthetic characteristics to those of bupivacaine, but with less cardiac toxicity. Ropivacaine is available as 2, 7.5 and $10\,mg\,mL^{-1}$ preparations; motor blockade is less at low doses than with bupivacaine. Levobupivacaine is the single 'S' isomer derivative of bupivacaine, has similar local anaesthetic properties, but with the theoretical promise of less cardiotoxicity. Levobupivacaine is available as 2, 5 and $7.5\,mg\,mL^{-1}$ preparations

Adrenaline may be added to a local anaesthetic solution to prolong the block, although this produces

relatively little effect on the duration of analgesia produced by bupivacaine or ropivacaine. The most effective means of prolonging the block is by the use of
a catheter to permit either repeated bolus doses or a
continuous infusion of local anaesthetic. The recent
introduction of elastomeric pumps allowing ambulatory continuous infusion of local anaesthetics has
been a welcome addition to the Inpatient Pain Team
armoury. These pumps give a continuous set rate infusion of local anaesthetic over a preset time; various
preset times and doses are available.

Local anaesthetic blocks in common use are described in Chapter 24. The following blocks represent those which are most useful for postoperative
analgesia.

Spinal Nerve Block

Subarachnoid analgesia rarely lasts more than 3–4 h
with the drugs currently available and is therefore of
limited use for postoperative analgesia, although there
is evidence that intrathecal analgesia may modify the
physiological changes associated with surgery. The
insertion of a catheter into the subarachnoid space is
used in the USA; this is not a popular manoeuvre in
the UK or Australia.

Epidural Block

Epidural block is popular for postoperative analgesia
because of familiarity with the technique and ease of insertion of a catheter. Epidural analgesic techniques can
provide superior postoperative analgesia and modify
the physiological changes associated with some forms
of surgery. Postoperative epidural analgesia can reduce the incidence of pulmonary morbidity. However,
epidural techniques also have uncommon but serious
risks attached to catheter insertion and removal (e.g.
epidural haematoma) and the risk:benefit ratio for
each patient must be considered. Repeated injections
may be made through the catheter or a dilute solution
of local anaesthetic infused continuously (usually 0.1
or 0.125%). Initially, bupivacaine produces analgesia
lasting up to 4 h, but by 24–48 h, some tolerance develops and single-bolus administrations may last for only
2 h. Ropivacaine, in low doses, may offer the advantage
of producing similar sensory block with less motor impairment. Levobupivacaine produces local anaesthetic
effects similar to those of bupivacaine.

Bupivacaine 0.25% injected at L2/3 provides good
analgesia after lower abdominal or perineal surgery,
e.g. hysterectomy or transurethral resection of prostate. Upper abdominal procedures require a higher
block, performed usually in the lower thoracic spine.

For thoracic surgery, an epidural catheter may be
inserted in the thoracic region between T6 and T8, and
volumes of bupivacaine of 6–12 mL may provide excellent postoperative analgesia.

An opioid can be added to the continuous infusion
of local anaesthetic or to bolus doses. Usually, fen-
tanyl $2 \mu g \, mL^{-1}$ or $4 \mu g \, mL^{-1}$ (occasionally $5 \mu g \, mL^{-1}$) is
added to infusion solutions. However, fentanyl has too
short a duration of action for single bolus epidurals
without infusion and diamorphine is preferred. There
is inconclusive evidence in the adult population of effectiveness using other adjuvants such as clonidine,
magnesium and midazolam, and there is some concern regarding neurotoxicity.

Recently, liposomal delivery systems have been developed to provide a reservoir of drug and are used
to prolong the duration of action of the medication.
Liposomes are microscopic lipid vesicles which, when
placed in aqueous suspension, form a central aqueous
central compartment surrounded by a lipid bilayer.
Drugs can be placed either in the central aqueous
compartment or in the lipid bilayer and can diffuse
from one compartment to the other. The liposome
provides a reservoir of drug large enough to prevent
redistribution from the site of injection, reducing the
risk of systemic toxicity because only a fraction of the
drug is bioavailable. Both local anaesthetics and morphine have been used in these systems with promising results. However, the safety of liposomes has yet to
be established, with concerns regarding neurotoxicity
and liposomal breakdown resulting in rapid release of
free drug.

In general, it is recommended that epidural catheter techniques should be used only when the patient is nursed in a High Dependency Unit, because
of the risks of hypotension after epidural injections
and total spinal block if the catheter migrates into
the subarachnoid space. However, in some institutions, continuous infusion epidural techniques are
managed on general wards, but only with the benefit
of adequate medical and nursing staff training and
experience, support from the Inpatient Pain Team

and the existence of clear protocols for monitoring and early detection of side-effects. This is becoming more common due to the increasing complexity of surgery, familiarization with the technique, great demand for high dependency beds and patients' knowledge and expectations of postoperative analgesia. Patient information leaflets have been written by the Royal College of Anaesthetists and the Association of Anaesthetists and are available on their web sites.

Some institutions also allow the use of patient-controlled epidural analgesia (PCEA) on the general wards, often very successfully.

Potential Advantages of Epidural Analgesia
- Superior pain relief.
- Starting analgesia before surgical incision may reduce postoperative pain by decreasing nervous system sensitization.
- Improved postoperative respiratory function.
- Reduction in the stress response to surgery after lower abdominal and lower limb surgery (minimal effect after upper abdominal or thoracic surgery).
- Reduction in the hypercoagulable state after major surgery; there are decreased incidences of deep venous thrombosis and pulmonary embolism after hip surgery.
- Reduced intraoperative blood loss during surgery on the lower part of the body.
- Improved postoperative gut function, facilitating early enteral nutrition.
- Earlier ambulation and potentially reduced hospital stay.
- Several studies have indicated improved quality of life post operatively compared with i.v. PCA.

Potential Complications of Epidural Analgesia
- Dural puncture (0.6–1.3%).
- Epidural haematoma – the risk is increased by impaired haemostasis when the catheter is inserted or removed. Guidelines must be followed for concomitant prophylactic low-molecular weight heparin and low-dose heparin therapy.
- Epidural abscess, meningitis and direct neurological damage.
- Systemic local anaesthetic toxicity.
- Total spinal anaesthesia.
- Sympathetic blockade (haemodynamic effects), urinary retention and motor block.

Haematoma and Abscess after Epidural Analgesia. In recent years, there has been an increase of epidural analgesia alongside the increased use of prophylactic anticoagulation and low-dependency care of patients with indwelling catheters. The Royal College of Anaesthetists carried out a national audit to determine the incidence of these serious complications. The overall risk of permanent injury associated with the use of epidural analgesia was approximately 1 in 20 000. However, there were large differences in the risk depending on the indication for epidural block. In obstetric practice, the risk of permanent injury was about 1 in 200 000, but when epidural analgesia was used after major surgery, the risk was much greater, about 1 in 8000.

Several issues have been raised regarding the detection and management of these complications:

1. Failure of the medical and nursing teams to recognize or appreciate new neurological signs in a patient with an epidural catheter in situ.
2. Failure to perform an MRI scan and act on the results.
3. Failure to have protocols in place for the management of epidural haematoma and epidural abscess on the wards and after discharge.

A possible protocol (adapted from Meikle et al 2008) for the detection of complications in patients with indwelling postoperative epidural catheters and infusions could be:

- assessment of motor block at least every 4 h
- assessment and observations should continue for at least 24 h after removal of the catheter
- a senior designated person should be responsible for investigating signs suggestive of an epidural haematoma or abscess
- in the absence of a recent local anaesthetic bolus, a significant deterioration in motor function should prompt immediate contact of the designated person
- if motor block can possibly be attributed to a local anaesthetic bolus, re-assessment should occur 2 h later
- if an epidural infusion is running it should be turned off and the patient re-assessed 2 h later;

if the motor block has not resolved then epidural haematoma or abscess should be considered until proven otherwise

- once an epidural haematoma or abscess is suspected, an immediate MRI should be organized; a protocol should be agreed in advance with the diagnostic imaging service
- if MRI scanning is not available in the local hospital or there will be delay then the patient should be referred urgently to a neurosurgical unit to be scanned; it may be appropriate to arrange a protocol or patient pathway with the local neurosurgical unit to minimize delays in investigation and treatment.

Caudal Block

Caudal administration of local anaesthetic drugs is useful for child day-case surgery, e.g. circumcision, or in patients undergoing anal or perineal surgery. It is customary to administer only a single dose of local anaesthetic; catheter techniques are unpopular in the UK because of the risk of infection. Suitable doses of local anaesthetic solution for use by the caudal route are shown in Table 41.11.

Other Regional Blocks Used for Postoperative Analgesia

Intercostal nerve blockade. Blocks from T4 to T8 or 9 provide satisfactory analgesia for pain relief after subcostal incision for cholecystectomy, fractured ribs or thoracotomy. Intercostal blocks may be repeated at regular intervals; catheters have been used for repeated administration. Bilateral blockade should not be carried out because of the risk of pneumothorax.

Paravertebral block. This may be used to provide analgesia after thoracic or abdominal surgery. Local anaesthetic solution is injected into the region of the paravertebral space to block the dorsal sensory nerve

roots as they emerge from the vertebral foramina. This technique may be performed using single or repeated injections or with an indwelling catheter.

Interpleural analgesia may be used to provide unilateral analgesia after thoracotomy, breast surgery open cholecystectomy and renal surgery. The use of interpleural analgesia can improve postoperative respiratory function, although the presence of intercostal chest drains or haemothorax may diminish the effectiveness of this procedure.

Brachial plexus analgesia, using a catheter placed close to the plexus and a continuous infusion of local anaesthetic, covers almost all of the upper limb and produces a sympathetic block which may be beneficial following plastic surgery.

Femoral nerve block, using a continuous infusion technique, is useful for relief of pain after knee surgery and may facilitate recovery after knee arthroplasty

Combined ilioinguinal and iliohypogastric nerve block is a safe and effective regional technique for postoperative pain control after inguinal hernia repair.

Wound infiltration after minor or paediatric surgery is an established analgesic technique for pain relief, but the benefit after major surgery is not clear. Portable continuous infusion devices have been developed to allow prolonged administration of local anaesthetics after surgery, e.g. to provide good analgesia after shoulder surgery.

Rectus sheath block is used for diagnostic and interventional laparoscopy. It is more effective for incisions limited to the midline. Large volumes of local anaesthetic should be instilled bilaterally.

Transversus abdominis plane (TAP) block is a relatively new technique with the instillation of 15–20 mL of local anaesthetic into the neurofascial plane between internal oblique and transverses abdominis, either by the surgeon under direct vision or by the anaesthetist using ultrasound guidance. Within this plane run the afferents of T6–L1 which provide sensation to the anterior and lateral abdominal wall. These nerves then form a plexus or directly supply the superficial musculature and skin of the anterior abdominal wall. The two most popular sites to enter the TAP are in the lower abdominal wall, the so-called posterior approach into the triangle of Petit and the subcostal approach in the upper abdominal wall. Both can utilize a single bolus or continuous catheter techniques.

TABLE 41.11
Doses of Bupivacaine (0.25% Plain) for Caudal Analgesia

Adult	Child
0.3–0.4 mL kg⁻¹	0.5–0.7 mL kg⁻¹ (or 0.1 mL year⁻¹ for each segment to be blocked)

N.B. Dosage of bupivacaine should *never* exceed 2 mg kg⁻¹.

Spinal and Epidural Opioids

In recent years, there has been great interest in the use of opioids by the subarachnoid or epidural routes. After injection of opioid into the cerebrospinal fluid (CSF), drug is taken up in the region of the substantia gelatinosa within the dorsal horn. It is thought that opioids act predominantly on the presynaptic enkephalin receptors, although opioid is absorbed from the CSF into the circulation. After epidural administration of opioids, the drug diffuses through the dura into the CSF and produces analgesia by the same mechanism as that associated with subarachnoid injection. However, there is more rapid uptake of opioid into the circulation via the rich network of blood vessels in the epidural space. Consequently, there is a rapid increase in both CSF and blood concentrations of the drug after epidural administration.

Uptake into the dorsal horn and rate of passage through the dura are dependent upon lipid solubility. Thus, the more highly lipid-soluble drugs (e.g. fentanyl) have a more rapid onset and a shorter duration of action. The less lipid-soluble drugs (e.g. morphine) have a slower rate of onset of action; in addition there is a greater dispersion within the CSF because of reduced uptake into the spinal cord and the drug may reach the medulla to cause delayed ventilatory depression.

Subarachnoid Opioids

This route is less popular than the epidural route of administration for opioids because of the production of post-dural puncture headache. However, smaller doses are required than with the epidural route and therefore systemic concentrations are lower. The quality of analgesia is not as good as that achieved with subarachnoid local anaesthetic drugs.

Epidural Opioids

The administration of epidural opioids is more popular because spinal headache is avoided and a catheter technique may be used. It is possible to achieve analgesia without the motor or autonomic block produced by local anaesthetic injected into the epidural space. Thus, postural hypotension and changes in heart rate do not occur. Early ventilatory depression may occur as a result of systemic absorption (e.g. within the first 1–2 h), but late ventilatory depression (8–20 h) is a result of rostral spread of opioid within the CSF to the medulla. Prolonged duration of action of analgesia is produced by a single injection (up to 24 h).

A recent analysis of five randomized trials on epidural morphine determined three main findings:

1. Epidural morphine gives greater patient satisfaction despite relatively high rates of adverse events.
2. Moderate to severe pruritus is more common with i.v. PCA and epidural morphine than i.v. PCA and placebo.
3. Extended-release morphine had lower pain scores with less i.v. PCA opioid.

Side Effects of Epidural Opioids

- Early ventilatory depression occurs more commonly with lipid-soluble agents.
- Late ventilatory depression occurs more commonly with agents of lower lipophilicity.
- Coma occurs relatively late, usually in association with late ventilatory depression, and can be reversed by naloxone.
- Urinary retention.
- Itching is reversed only partially by naloxone.
- Nausea and vomiting.

Epidural opioids are more effective when used in combination with local anaesthetics to produce a synergistic analgesic action. This reduces the necessary dose and the side-effects which would be associated with the local anaesthetic or the opioid alone. For example, continuous epidural infusion of a combined solution of a low concentration of bupivacaine with fentanyl provides a good postoperative analgesia with minimal side-effects. As discussed above, the recent development of liposomal delivery systems may reduce the need for infusions of epidural opioids.

Inhalation of Volatile or Gaseous Anaesthetics

Although volatile anaesthetics were used in the past, the only agent in current use is N_2O. This is administered in the form of Entonox (premixed 50% N_2O, 50% O_2) usually via a demand valve and facemask. Entonox is used extensively in obstetric analgesia, in the field situation (e.g. by ambulance personnel to provide analgesia at the site of an accident) and occasionally in the wards during change of surgical dressings (protocols often exist for its use on general wards). The potential spinal cord and haematological adverse effects of nitrous oxide, via interference with vitamin B_{12} metabolism, may prevent repeated use.

Non-Steroidal Anti-Inflammatory Drugs (NSAIDs) and Selective Cox-2 Inhibitors

The use of NSAIDs (cyclo-oxygenase inhibitors) for postoperative pain relief is now routine practice. NSAIDs may be given orally, rectally (e.g. diclofenac 100 mg) or intravenously (e.g. ketorolac 10 mg, Dyloject 75 mg). NSAIDs produce pain relief without sedation, respiratory depression or nausea and vomiting, but their use is limited by gastric, renal and platelet side-effects. A recent authoritative and extensive review of the published literature concerning NSAIDs drew the following conclusions.

- NSAIDs are not sufficiently effective as the sole analgesic agent after major surgery.
- NSAIDs are often effective after minor or outpatient surgery.
- NSAIDs often decrease opioid requirement by reducing the excretion of the active metabolite morphine-6 glucuronide. Significant reduction in opioid side-effects has been noted in a few studies only.
- The quality of opioid-based analgesia is often enhanced by NSAIDs.
- NSAIDs increase bleeding time and some studies have shown increased blood loss after surgery.

The major adverse effects of NSAIDs for surgical patients are those involving the gastrointestinal system, renal and platelet function, and aspirin-induced asthma in susceptible patients. The adverse effects of NSAIDs are serious, and contraindications (e.g. peptic ulceration, bleeding diathesis, renal impairment, aspirin-induced asthma) must be respected. The incidence and severity of NSAID-related adverse effects are greater in elderly patients. Aspirin is contraindicated in children less than 12 years of age. There have been case reports of sudden renal dysfunction in patients given NSAIDs perioperatively; risk factors for this may include nephrotoxic antibiotics (e.g. gentamicin), raised intra-abdominal pressure during laparoscopy, hypovolaemia and age greater than 65 years.

New drugs have been developed which selectively inhibit the inducible cyclo-oxygenase enzyme, COX-2, and spare the constitutive, COX-1, enzyme. Most conventional NSAIDs in clinical use are nonselective inhibitors of COX-1 and COX-2, and many of the side-effects of the older drugs may be by COX-1 inhibition and disruption of physiological prostaglandin production. COX-2 is induced by tissue damage and inflammation, and selective inhibitors of this enzyme produce analgesia with fewer side-effects. Studies have confirmed that COX-2 inhibitors produce effective analgesia after surgery, similar to that of the NSAIDs. There is encouraging evidence that COX-2 inhibitors have less gastrointestinal side-effects, but the effect on the kidneys is similar to that of conventional NSAIDs. As platelets produce thromboxane for aggregation via COX-1 only, COX-2 inhibitors do not affect platelet function and have been shown to be associated with lower surgical blood loss. The role of COX-2 inhibitors in producing a tendency to thrombosis, by inhibition of endothelial prostacyclin but no antiplatelet effect, is a significant disadvantage which has led to the withdrawal of rofecoxib and restrictions on the use of other agents. There is evidence that COX-2 inhibitors are tolerated well by individuals who suffer from aspirin-induced asthma.

Paracetamol

Paracetamol is a useful adjunct to opioids in the treatment of postoperative pain, with fewer contraindications than the NSAIDs. It is analgesic and antipyretic, but not anti-inflammatory. The mechanism of action is unclear, but may involve the selective inhibition of prostaglandin synthesis in the central nervous system, perhaps by inhibition of another cyclo-oxygenase subtype, COX-3. In adults with normal hepatic and renal function, the recommended dose is 500–1000 mg orally or rectally every 3–6 h when necessary, with a maximum daily dose of 6 g for acute use and 4 g for chronic use. Care must be taken to avoid inadvertent paracetamol overdosage and resultant hepatic and renal toxicity. An intravenous preparation is available and has been shown to be an effective postoperative analgesic.

NMDA Antagonists

The activation by excitatory amino acids (glutamate) of spinal cord dorsal horn N-methyl-D-aspartate (NMDA) receptors is essential for the development of central sensitization. The anaesthetic agent ketamine is a potent NMDA receptor antagonist. Low-dose subcutaneous or intravenous ketamine infusions ($5-15\,mg\,h^{-1}$) produce significant pain relief after surgery. Studies have shown that ketamine added to morphine PCA can decrease opioid hyperalgesia, prevent opioid tolerance and lower morphine consumption. Unfortunately, the side-effects of ketamine, including hallucinations, limit its use. Dextromethorphan is an alternative NMDA receptor antagonist which has been shown to reduce opioid requirements following oral surgery and during abdominal surgery.

Other Drugs

Intravenous lidocaine given intraoperatively and as a postoperative infusion for 24 h has been shown to improve postoperative analgesia, fatigue and bowel function after laparoscopic cholecystectomy.

Oral gabapentin has been shown to reduce morphine use after total abdominal hysterectomy, although the number of trials is small.

Non-Pharmacological Methods

Cryotherapy

This may be applied to intercostal nerves exposed during a thoracotomy. The nerve is surrounded by an ice-ball produced by intense sub-zero temperatures at the end of a probe. The neuronal disruption produced by this method is temporary and sensation returns after some months, although it may be accompanied by unpleasant paraesthesiae and occasionally by persistent neuralgia.

Transcutaneous Electrical Stimulation

A small alternating current is passed between two surface electrodes at low voltage and at a frequency of 0.2–200 Hz. It is thought that the technique acts by increasing CNS concentrations of endorphins. Acupuncture may work in a similar manner. The technique produces only moderate analgesia.

Acupuncture

Acupuncture has been assessed as a technique for postoperative pain relief. There is evidence that acupuncture reduces pain and analgesic consumption after dental and abdominal surgery, although there is some variability in the method of administration. Acupuncture has also been shown to be efficacious in the reduction/prevention of postoperative nausea and vomiting.

PRE-EMPTIVE ANALGESIA

The importance of peripheral and central sensitization in amplifying pain perception has directed research towards preventing these processes. Experimentally, it has been shown that nociceptive stimulation from the periphery causes functional changes in the spinal cord, which lead to enhancement and prolongation of the sensation of pain. It has also been shown that prior administration of analgesics may inhibit the development of the hyperexcitability within the spinal cord. Unfortunately however, in clinical practice, prior administration of analgesics (pre-emptive analgesia) has not been shown to have an important effect on postoperative pain. Further studies are being performed on pre-emptive analgesia, incorporating additional strategies to prevent and modulate the prolonged neuronal input to the spinal cord from the peripheral tissue inflammatory process.

BALANCED (MULTIMODAL) ANALGESIA

The concept of balanced analgesia is analogous to that of balanced anaesthesia. It is possible to block the development of pain by the use of a combination of different drugs acting at different sites: peripherally, on somatic and sympathetic nerves, at spinal cord level and centrally. The benefit of this technique is that not only may superior analgesia be achieved by a combination of drugs but also their individual doses may be reduced, thereby decreasing the incidence of side-effects. For example, after thoracotomy, the addition of an NSAID to a regimen based on intercostal nerve blocks and PCA morphine significantly improves analgesia.

Pain transmission may be blocked clinically at the following sites:

- inhibition of peripheral nociceptor mechanisms using NSAIDs, COX-2 inhibitors, steroids or opioids
- blockade of afferent neuronal transmission using peripheral, epidural or spinal local anaesthetic administration
- interference at both spinal cord level and higher centres using spinal and systemic opioids.

The use of non-opioid analgesics in multimodal analgesia minimizes opioid side-effects, including gastrointestinal stasis. After bowel surgery, multimodal analgesia (an epidural infusion of a low-dose local anaesthetic and opioid mixture, and systemic NSAID) produces excellent pain relief, avoids the need for systemic opioids and speeds the recovery of gastrointestinal function. This facilitates early mobilization of the patient and a more rapid return to enteral nutrition.

Typically, for minor surgery, e.g. hernia repair on a day-case basis, the anaesthetist may employ multimodal or balanced analgesia in the form of:

- preoperative administration of a mild oral analgesic, e.g. paracetamol and an NSAID or a COX-2 inhibitor; this can be achieved using Patient Group Directives allowing nursing staff to administer these drugs preoperatively.
- administration of fentanyl intraoperatively±tramadol
- local anaesthetic block using ilioinguinal and iliohypogastric nerve blocks and wound infiltration
- the use of NSAIDs in the form of a diclofenac suppository 100 mg, or a COX-2 inhibitor.

With this technique, patients frequently do not require supplementary opioids postoperatively and may be managed on a day-case basis using simple oral analgesics in the postoperative period, e.g. paracetamol. Oral tramadol may be useful if stronger postoperative analgesia is required.

NEUROPATHIC PAIN IN THE POSTOPERATIVE PERIOD

The possibility of the development of neuropathic pain should be borne in mind after surgery, as it is often missed in patients with acute pain and may require specific therapy (see Ch 46). A useful definition of neuropathic pain is 'pain associated with injury, disease or surgical section of the peripheral or central nervous system'. One diagnostic clue after surgery is an unexpected increase in opioid consumption, because neuropathic pain often responds poorly to normal doses of opioids. Features suggestive of neuropathic pain include:

- pain without ongoing tissue damage
- sensory loss
- allodynia (pain in response to non-painful stimuli)
- hyperalgesia (increased pain in response to painful stimuli)
- dysaesthesiae (unpleasant abnormal sensations)
- burning, stabbing or shooting pain
- a delay in onset after injury

Patients presenting with these symptoms should be referred to the Inpatient Pain Team for assessment and treatment.

Pre-Anaesthetic Assessment Clinics

Staffed by anaesthetists with a broad knowledge of anaesthesia, surgery and medical conditions, these clinics serve many functions. In the context of pain management, the clinics have several roles:

- Education of the patient on options for postoperative analgesia using discussion and leaflets.
- Explanation of the advantages and risks of more invasive analgesic techniques.
- Answering patient questions.
- Obtaining informed consent for invasive analgesic techniques.

FURTHER READING

McQuay, H., Moore, A. (Eds.), 1998. An evidence-based resource for pain relief. Oxford University Press, Oxford.

Meikle, J., Bird, S., Nightingale, J.J., White, N., 2008. Detection and management of epidural haematomas related to anaesthesia in the UK: a national survey of current practice. Br. J. Anaesth. 101, 400–404.

National Health and Medical Research Council of Australia, 2005. Acute pain management: scientific evidence, second ed. Canberra, Commonwealth of Australia.

Royal College of Anaesthetists, 1998. Guidelines for the use of nonsteroidal anti-inflammatory drugs in the perioperative period. Royal College of Anaesthetists, London.

Royal College of Anaesthetists, 2009. NAP 3: report and findings of the 3rd National Audit Project of the Royal College of Anaesthetists. Royal College of Anaesthetists, London.

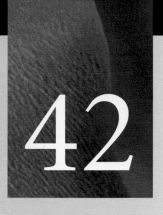

42

POSTOPERATIVE NAUSEA AND VOMITING

I t is estimated that up to 80% of patients experience postoperative nausea and/or vomiting (PONV) within the first 24h after surgery. For most, PONV is easily manageable but for a smaller, 'high risk' cohort, symptoms can be distressing and disabling and, in some cases, have been described as worse than the pain of surgery. It is a common misconception that general anaesthetics are solely responsible for PONV because it is often forgotten that surgical procedures under anaesthesia involve not only a pharmacological but also a physical 'assault' on the patient. Fortunately, the multifactorial aetiology of PONV lends itself to interventions using a variety of different treatment options. Prevention, along with prompt and effective treatment of PONV, decreases the risk of adverse effects, limits the length of inpatient stay and reduces hospital costs. More importantly, successful prevention of PONV greatly improves patient satisfaction.

DEFINITIONS

Nausea is derived from the Greek word *naus* denoting 'ship' and was used originally to describe the feeling of seasickness. Nausea is an unpleasant sensation referred to the upper gastrointestinal tract and pharynx. It is associated with dizziness and a strong urge to vomit. Assessment of nausea is extremely difficult because symptoms are subjective, entirely patient-dependent and often difficult to quantify. For this reason, the incidence of postoperative nausea is frequently underestimated. **Retching** is the involuntary process of 'unproductive vomiting'. It is characterized by the synchronous contraction of diaphragmatic and abdominal

muscles against a closed mouth and glottis. Retching is extremely distressing and is usually accompanied by feelings of intense nausea. **Vomiting** represents the final common pathway of a highly coordinated sequence of events involving gastrointestinal, abdominal, respiratory and pharyngeal muscles which results in the active and rapid expulsion of contents from the stomach and upper intestine. In contrast to the rather subjective assessment of nausea, vomiting is easily identifiable and measurable!

MECHANISMS OF NAUSEA AND VOMITING

Vomiting Centre

The vomiting reflex probably developed as an evolutionary protective mechanism against ingestion of harmful substances or toxins. However, vomiting also occurs in response to a wide range of pathological and environmental triggers including sight, smell, motion and gastrointestinal disturbances. Afferent signals mediated by the vagus, vestibular and higher cortical nerves are carried to discrete areas within the brainstem collectively known as the 'vomiting centre' (Fig. 42.1). Traditionally, the vomiting centre was thought to be a single anatomical entity but there is increasing evidence that it is made up of a disparate group of interconnected cells and nuclei located in the lateral reticular formation of the medulla and the nucleus tractus solitarius (NTS). All information entering the vomiting centre is processed and co-ordinated (via autonomic and motor nerves) into a highly complex series of neuronal signals to initiate the three phases of the vomiting reflex.

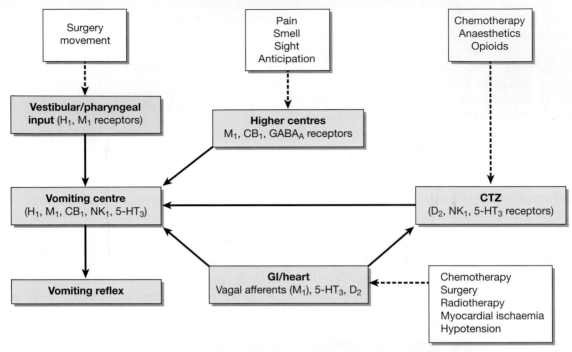

FIGURE 42.1 ■ Schematic diagram of the vomiting reflex. See text for details.

Chemoreceptor Trigger Zone (CTZ)

The so-called 'chemoreceptor trigger zone' consists of several nuclei found within the area postrema at the caudal end of the fourth ventricle. Although the CTZ is anatomically located within the central nervous system, its unusual pattern of endothelial fenestrations allows it to 'sense' chemicals not only within cerebrospinal fluid, but also within circulating peripheral blood. In simple terms, the highly vascularized CTZ utilizes its defective blood brain barrier to detect potentially harmful substances present within the circulation. The CTZ contains an abundance of cholinergic, dopaminergic, histaminergic, serotinergic (5-HT) and opioid receptors which send afferent projections to the vomiting centre. Stimulation of the CTZ contributes significantly to the nausea and vomiting experienced by surgical patients, and pharmacological antagonism of receptor signalling within this important area represents a key strategy in the prevention and treatment of PONV.

Stimulation of the Vomiting Centre

Figure 42.1 outlines the various triggers and neural connections involved in the initiation of the vomiting reflex. The vomiting centre acts as the final processor for all sensory information received from central and peripheral receptors. Although the majority of afferent information from the periphery is relayed through the CTZ, other important causes of emesis are described below.

Gastrointestinal Tract

The normal functioning of the gastrointestinal (GI) tract is dependent on fully integrated neural feedback mechanisms. As part of this dynamic process, numerous mechano- and chemo-receptors send information to the central nervous system via the vagal nerve afferents. Any threat to the integrity of the GI system, e.g. gastric distension, irritation, damage or toxins, triggers an increase in ascending vagal activity which relays directly or indirectly to the vomiting centre. Cholinergic M_1, serotoninergic $5-HT_3$ and dopaminergic D_2 receptors are the principal mediators of signal transduction within the gut mucosa. Stimulation of one or all of these key receptors initiates a key step in the vomiting reflex and pharmacological antagonism at these sites represents a logical approach in the management of nausea and vomiting.

Vestibular System

Motion sickness is an unpleasant side-effect induced by aberrant vestibular or visual activity. Susceptible individuals develop motion sickness in childhood, with the incidence peaking during early adolescence. Fortunately, symptoms diminish with advancing age. Numerous studies report that females are more prone to motion sickness than men. The neurophysiological mechanisms responsible for motion sickness are largely unknown but it is likely that an imbalance between the vestibular-cerebellar-visual axis together with stimulation of higher autonomic nerves triggers activation of the vomiting reflex. Therefore, female patients with a history of motion sickness have two independent predictors of PONV (see below).

Cardiovascular System

Most anaesthetists recognize that nausea may represent an important sign of underlying hypotension, particularly in patients who have just received regional nerve blockade. Myocardial ischaemia leading to infarction is also associated with a high incidence of vomiting. It is likely that retrograde autonomic signalling to the brainstem is responsible for these early warning signs of cardiovascular compromise.

Cortical Inputs

Higher cortical centres (e.g. the limbic system) are intimately involved with initiation and modification of the vomiting reflex. For example, unpleasant sights, sounds or smells induce emetic responses. In this context, cholinergic M_1 antagonists (e.g. hyoscine) may provide some relief. Patients with preconceived expectations or anxiety can be encouraged to modify their behaviour to reduce the incidence of nausea or vomiting. In cases involving anticipatory symptoms (e.g. protracted chemotherapy-induced nausea), anxiolytics may be beneficial.

Gag Reflex

The gag reflex reduces the risk of upper airway obstruction and ingestion of noxious material. The glossopharyngeal nerve (cranial nerve IX) mediates the afferent limb of this reflex, synapsing directly within the nucleus solitarius in the brainstem. The efferent limb is coordinated by the vagus nerve (cranial nerve X). This primitive reflex is one of the strongest triggers of emesis and is particularly active following insertion of oral airway adjuncts in semiconscious patients.

Neural and Muscular Co-ordination During Vomiting

The synchronized events mediating the vomiting reflex are divided into three phases: pre-ejection, ejection and post-ejection.

Pre-Ejection Phase

- Nausea (not a prerequisite to vomiting).
- Gastric smooth muscle relaxes and retrograde peristalsis begins.
- Deep inspiration.
- Glottis closes (to avoid aspiration).

Ejection Phase

- Abdominal and diaphragmatic muscles contract.
- Lower and upper oesophageal sphincters relax.
- Intra-abdominal pressure increases.
- Mouth opens and gastric contents are forcefully expelled.

Post-Ejection Phase

- Autonomic and visceral nerves 'recalibrate'
- Lethargy and weakness.

Increased autonomic activity results in salivation, pallor and tachycardia throughout all phases of the vomiting reflex.

ADVERSE EFFECTS

Some clinicians dismiss PONV as an inevitable consequence of surgery but from the patients perspective PONV is almost always associated with distress and dissatisfaction. Importantly, if nausea or vomiting persist there is a risk of rare, but potentially serious, perioperative morbidity. These complications are summarized in Table 42.1.

Intact laryngeal reflexes ensure glottic closure during vomiting, but in the immediate postoperative phase, laryngeal reflexes may be obtunded due to residual effects of general anaesthesia and centrally acting analgesics. Vomiting can result in aspiration of gastric contents if the upper airway is not protected. The physical act of vomiting may lead to pain, wound dehiscence, haemorrhage, haematoma or possibly oesophageal rupture. If PONV persists, dehydration, reduced oral intake, electrolyte imbalance and delayed mobilization can result

TABLE 42.1
Adverse Affects of PONV
Patient distress and dissatisfaction
Pulmonary aspiration
Postoperative pain

Wound dehiscence/haemorrhage
   Eyes
   Head and neck
   Oesophageal
   Abdominal

Dehydration, electrolyte disturbance and/or requirement for intravenous fluids

Delayed oral input
   Drugs
   Nutrition
   Fluids

Delayed mobilization
Delayed discharge

TABLE 42.2
Factors Which Increase the Risk of PONV
Patient
Female
Non-smoker
History of PONV or motion sickness
Children (age>3 years)
Anaesthetic
Volatile anaesthetics
Opioids
Nitrous oxide
Postoperative pain
Hypotension
Neostigmine >2.5 mg
Surgical
Duration

Type
   Gynaecological
   Squint
   ENT
   Head and neck

in serious medical complications and significantly increased healthcare costs associated with delayed discharge and unplanned admissions.

IDENTIFYING PATIENTS AT RISK

Many different approaches have been adopted in an attempt to stratify patients according to their individual risk of PONV. Risk stratification allows clinicians to optimize prevention and treatment strategies while minimizing the incidence of adverse drug reactions in patients at lower risk of PONV. Indiscriminate use of antiemetics in surgical patients is ill-advised and not cost-effective. A more logical and evidence-based approach involves identifying patients at moderate to high risk of PONV and prescribing appropriately.

Patient Factors

Although it is not possible to identify every patient at risk of PONV, a number of factors contribute to the incidence of nausea and vomiting in the postoperative period. The main factors are shown in Table 42.2. Numerous studies report that smoking habits, female patients and those with a history of PONV or motion sickness are all strong independent predictors for PONV. Delayed gastric emptying, anxiety and obesity may increase the risk of PONV but the evidence for a

statistically significant association is currently lacking. Children over the age of 3 years are also at high risk of developing PONV in comparison to adults. Vomiting, rather than nausea, is often used as an outcome measure in paediatric studies because of the difficulty in assessing and quantifying nausea in young children. Fortunately, the risk of PONV decreases as children reach adolescence.

Anaesthetic Factors

Identifying specific anaesthetic triggers of PONV is difficult because of the large number of drugs given as part of a 'standard' general anaesthetic technique. However, the evidence for opioids and volatile agents inducing PONV is incontrovertible. Opioid administration by whatever route (oral, intramuscular, intravenous, epidural or spinal) is associated with a high incidence of PONV. Activation of peripheral and central opioid receptors by exogenous opioids leads to stimulation of the CTZ, direct activation of the vomiting centre and reduced gastric emptying. Increased sensitivity of the vestibular nerve (possibly as a result of activation of histaminergic H_1 and muscarinic M_1 receptors) may also play a role in the genesis of PONV. This is particularly prevalent during movement in the immediate postoperative phase. Preoperative opioids contribute towards a higher prevalence of PONV, but opioid-based premedication has largely been superseded by the use of non-opioid anxiolytic agents, e.g. benzodiazepines. Ineffective postoperative analgesia and pain can induce significant nausea and vomiting in susceptible individuals. In this situation, a non-opioid based analgesic approach is justified (e.g. simple analgesics and nerve blocks). Alternatively, careful titration of opioids may be appropriate.

Most intravenous anaesthetic induction agents induce PONV, but at subhypnotic concentrations, propofol exhibits some antiemetic activity. It is thought that this beneficial pharmacodynamic action is due to antagonism of dopaminergic D_2 receptors. The increasing popularity of total intravenous anaesthesia (TIVA) techniques exploits the intrinsic antiemetic activity of propofol while avoiding the strong emetogenic stimuli from the volatile agents.

Evidence for the much-maligned nitrous oxide is less compelling. If used as part of a gas and oxygen mixture (e.g. Entonox), nitrous oxide has been shown to induce nausea and vomiting. However, studies using a combination of nitrous oxide with volatile agents do not report a consistently increased incidence of nausea and vomiting, particularly in patients at high risk of PONV.

The nondepolarizing neuromuscular reversal agent neostigmine has been implicated as a possible trigger for PONV. Anticholinesterase activity increases gastrointestinal motility and retrograde vagal nerve activity by activation of M_1 receptors in the gut. However, these effects are normally antagonized by the co-administration of antimuscarinic agents, e.g. glycopyrrolate. It is only when higher doses of neostigmine are required (>2.5 mg) that PONV becomes problematic.

Surgical Factors

Numerous studies have concluded that the type of surgery influences the risk of developing PONV. For example, stimulation of vestibular or pharyngeal nerves after ENT surgery is associated with an increased prevalence of emesis. Similarly, squint correction surgery (usually carried out in children) is reported to have a disproportionately high incidence of PONV. Patients undergoing gynaecological procedures are often recruited into studies to assess the efficacy of antiemetic drugs. However, it has been argued that many female patients are already at high risk of PONV, which places some doubt as to whether gynaecological surgery is an independent risk factor for PONV.

The cumulative doses of volatile agents and opioids are greater after lengthy surgical procedures, and therefore it is not surprising that the duration of surgery directly influences the number of patients experiencing PONV.

Risk Stratification

One of the most widely adopted scoring systems developed by Apfel and colleagues uses four of the independent predictors described in Table 42.2 to determine the likelihood of experiencing PONV. These are:

- female
- non-smokers
- history of PONV or motion sickness
- use of opioids.

Each positive predictor is assigned a score of 1. Using this system, a score of 0, 1, 2, 3 or 4 predicts the chance of developing PONV as approximately 10, 20, 40, 60 or 80%. (Fig. 42.2) Other scoring systems include the duration and type of anaesthesia but these have not been found to have any additional predictive value beyond that of Apfel's simplified version.

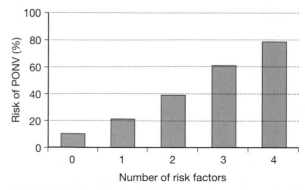

FIGURE 42.2 ■ Relationship between the number of risk factors and the incidence of PONV. *(Derived from Fero et al (2011)).*

Post-Discharge Nausea and Vomiting (PDNV)

Increasing numbers of surgical procedures are now carried out on a day-case basis. Despite meeting strict discharge criteria, many patients experience PDNV after leaving hospital. Of those, up to 35% do not have any symptoms prior to discharge. One reason for this discrepancy relates to the relatively short half-lives of current antiemetic agents. Unfortunately, most patients have limited or no access to antiemetic treatment after discharge, which leads to delayed recovery and patient dissatisfaction. Prescribing antiemetic prophylaxis to every patient is neither beneficial nor cost-effective. Prophylaxis is best targeted towards patients at moderate to high risk of PONV, who should be offered oral antiemetics as part of their 'take home' prescription.

MANAGEMENT

Prevention

Prevention is the key to effective management of PONV. Identifying patients who are at risk of developing symptoms following surgery is the first step in this process. In simple terms, patients can be divided into three groups: low, moderate or high risk. Those at low risk do not require pharmacological intervention. Simply reducing or avoiding key triggers, e.g. opioids and/or volatile agents, may be sufficient to prevent the onset of PONV. Furthermore, prophylaxis for every patient is not necessary and adopting such a blanket approach may lead to adverse drug effects. For those at moderate to high risk, adopting a multimodal strategy, i.e. avoiding key triggers whilst giving one or more antiemetic, helps to reduce the risk of developing symptoms of PONV. For patients at highest risk, a combined approach usually works best, e.g. risk reduction measures in conjunction with increasing number of antiemetics.

Treatment

Despite careful planning and risk reduction, some patients still experience troublesome PONV. If so, it is vital that all possible causes of PONV are ruled out to avoid missing important signs of serious underlying pathology. The commonest causes of PONV are highlighted in Table 42.3. Each patient should be thoroughly assessed to exclude other treatable causes. Only

TABLE 42.3
Important Causes of PONV
Hypotension
Hypoxaemia
Drugs
Opioids
Antibiotics
Intra-abdominal pathology
Psychological factors e.g. anticipation/anxiety
Early mobilization
Fluid intake
Nasogastric tube
Pain

when these have been excluded is it appropriate to consider an antiemetic treatment strategy. If antiemetic prophylaxis has already been given, repeat dosing may be required depending on the pharmacokinetic profile of the initial prophylactic agent(s), while bearing in mind that a second dose may be ineffective and might simply increase the risk of an adverse drug effect.

The next stage in treatment involves the use of various classes of drug targeting a range of different receptors. This logical approach maximizes pharmacodynamic efficacy whilst minimizing the risk of adverse drug events. For example, PONV prophylaxis using a glucocorticoid can be supplemented using one or more of the available D_2, M_1, H_1 or 5-HT_3 receptor antagonists.

PHARMACOLOGY

From an anaesthetist's perspective, the numerous afferent and efferent components of the vomiting reflex lend themselves to pharmacological manipulation at multiple receptor sites within the peripheral and central nervous systems. Antagonism of one or more of the four key neurotransmitters involved in the vomiting reflex (dopamine, histamine, acetylcholine or 5-HT_3) forms the basis of established treatment of PONV. Table 42.4 gives examples of the main classes of drug used worldwide for the treatment of nausea and vomiting. Not all are suitable or have been licensed for the

TABLE 42.4
Drugs Used in Management of PONV

Drug	Routes of Administration	Suggested Timing	Comments	Common Adverse Effects
5-HT$_3$ receptor antagonists				
Ondansetron	i.v./i.m./oral/p.r.	End of surgery		Abnormal liver function, Headache, QT prolongation
Granisetron	i.v./oral	Before induction		
Palonosetron	i.v./oral	–	Not licensed for PONV in the UK	
Tropisetron	i.v.	End of surgery	Not available in the UK	
Dopamine (D$_2$) receptor antagonists				
Benzamides				
Metoclopramide	i.v./i.m./oral	At induction	Severe EPE in children and young adults	Sedation/EPE/ hypotension
Butyrophenones				
Droperidol	i.v.	End of surgery		Sedation/EPE/ hypotension
Domperidone	oral/p.r.	–	Less sedative than phenothiazine	Agitation/EPE/ hypotension
Phenothiazines				
Prochlorperazine	oral/i.m./buccal	Recovery room		Sedation/EPS/ hypotension
Perphenazine	oral	–	Not licensed for PONV in the UK	
Anticholinergics (M$_1$ receptor antagonist)				
Hyoscine	oral/transdermal	Night before surgery	Antispasmodic and useful for motion sickness – Not licensed for PONV in the UK	Sedation/dry mouth/ blurred vision
Antihistamines (H$_1$ receptor antagonists)				
Cyclizine	oral/i.v./i.m.	At induction	Can induce significant tachycardia	Sedation/dry mouth/ blurred vision
Promethazine	oral	–	Useful for motion sickness – Not licensed for PONV in the UK	
Glucocorticoids				
Dexamethasone	i.v./i.m./oral	At Induction	Often used in combination with 5-HT$_3$ antagonists	Perineal stimulation
NK$_1$ antagonists				
Aprepitant	oral	1–3 h prior to induction	Not licensed for PONV in the UK	Headaches/ dizziness/ hiccups
Fosaprepitant (Prodrug of aprepitant)	i.v.	At induction	Not licensed for PONV in the UK	
Cannabinoids				
Nabilone	oral	–	Not licensed for PONV in the UK	Mood changes/Dry mouth/ataxia

EPE, extrapyramidal effects; i.v., intravenous; i.m., intramuscular; p.r., per rectum.

treatment of PONV in the UK but are included in the table to indicate current or potential drug development strategies.

Dopamine D₂ Receptor Antagonists

Peripheral and central dopaminergic D_2 receptors are located within the gastrointestinal tract and the CTZ, respectively. D_2 receptors mediate gastrointestinal activity and dopaminergic neurotransmission within the CTZ. The antiemetic efficacy of D_2 receptor antagonists relates to a combination of increased gut motility and raising the emetogenic threshold within the CTZ. Butyrophenones, phenothiazines and benzamides act primarily as D_2 receptor antagonists although most harbour cross-sensitivity with other receptor systems as shown in Table 42.5.

Butyrophenones

Droperidol was withdrawn from clinical practice in 2001 due to concerns over QTc prolongation following chronic treatment. After successful campaigning (mainly by anaesthetists), droperidol was reintroduced specifically for the acute management of PONV. It acts mainly as a D_2 antagonist but it also has weak α_1-adrenergic blocking activity. Intravenous droperidol administered 30 min before the end of surgery is economical and generally effective at reducing PONV and it can be co-administered with opioids using patient-controlled analgesia (PCA) pumps. Side-effects may limit treatment. These include sedation, extrapyramidal effects and gastrointestinal upset. Droperidol is contraindicated in patients with long QT syndrome.

Although not used routinely, oral domperidone may be prescribed to assist with the management of PONV. It is generally well tolerated and causes less central effects (mainly sedation) than many of the phenothiazines. Side-effects and contraindications are similar to those for droperidol although galactorrhoea and gynaecomastia can occur after chronic administration.

Phenothiazines

Phenothiazines were introduced originally to treat psychotic states including mania and schizophrenia. Subsequently, many were found to have useful antiemetic properties and are now used routinely during treatment of neoplastic disease. The main mechanism of action of the phenothiazines is via antagonism of the D_2 receptor, but it is possible that some of their clinical effects are derived from blockade of other neurotransmitters involved in the vomiting reflex (Table 42.5). Prochlorperazine is used routinely in the treatment of PONV and labyrinthine disorders. It can be administered via intramuscular, oral or buccal routes. Side-effects include sedation, hypotension and extrapyramidal features.

TABLE 42.5
Relative Receptor Specificities

Drug	Serotonin 5-HT₃	Dopamine D₂	Acetylcholine M₁	Histamine (H₁)
5-HT₃ antagonists e.g. ondansetron	++++	−	−	−
Benzamides e.g. metoclopramide	++	+++	+	−
Butyrophenones e.g. droperidol	+	++++	−	+
Phenothiazines e.g. prochlorperazine	−	++++	+	+
Anticholinergics e.g. hyoscine	−	+	++++	+
Antihistamines e.g. cyclizine	−	++	++	+++

Perphenazine is not licensed for treatment of PONV in the UK, but has proved to be useful as an oral antiemetic preparation.

Benzamides

Metoclopramide has been used extensively in the treatment of nausea and vomiting secondary to gastrointestinal disease and chemo-radiotherapy. Surprisingly, there is little evidence for its efficacy in PONV. At standard doses, it blocks D_2 receptors in the gut and CTZ, but at higher doses it also acts as a 5-HT_3 antagonist. Current preparations are available for intravenous, oral and intramuscular administration. Adverse effects include extrapyramidal symptoms, hypotension and sedation. Extrapyramidal symptoms are dose-related and occur most frequently in children and young adults. It is recommended that intravenous administration takes place over 1–2 min to reduce the risk of side-effects.

Histamine H_1 Receptor Antagonists

H_1 receptors are located in the CTZ, vomiting centre and possibly the vestibular apparatus. Most antihistamine drugs display dual activity at histaminergic H_1 and cholinergic M_1 receptors. Increasing doses lead to D_2 receptor blockade. Combined activity at H_1 and M_1 receptors makes antihistamines particularly useful in the treatment of motion sickness. Cyclizine is used routinely for PONV because it has less central sedating effect in comparison with other drugs in its class. It can be administered via oral, intramuscular and intravenous routes. Side-effects include dry mouth, sedation and blurred vision, all of which are related to inherent anticholinergic activity. Rapid intravenous injection of cyclizine induces tachycardia and it should be used with caution in patients with heart failure.

Cholinergic M_1 Receptor Antagonists

Hyoscine (scopolamime) is not specifically indicated for the management of PONV. It is used mainly as an antispasmodic, antisialagogue premedicant and in the prevention of motion sickness. Various preparations are available for administration using intramuscular, intravenous, subcutaneous, oral or transdermal routes. Some centres report a reduction in PONV following perioperative use of a transdermal hyoscine patch. In susceptible individuals, hyoscine causes significant sedation, dry mouth, visual disturbance and, rarely, central anticholinergic syndrome.

Serotonin 5-HT_3 Receptor Antagonists

5-HT_3 antagonists are indicated for use in the management of PONV and in the management of nausea and vomiting induced by chemo-radiotherapy. 5-HT_3 receptors are located in the CTZ, vomiting centre and the gastrointestinal tract. 5-HT_3 plays an important role in detecting and transmitting emetogenic signals from the CTZ to the vomiting centre whereas peripheral 5-HT receptors stimulate vagal afferents in response to damaging stimuli within the gut mucosa. 5-HT is also released in the area postrema in response to increased vagal activity. Therefore, it is likely that the efficacy of 5-HT_3 antagonists is due to a combination of central and peripheral effects.

Ondansetron and granisetron are both licensed for treatment of PONV in the UK. Ondansetron has a shorter half-life than granisetron and can be administered via oral, intramuscular, intravenous or rectal routes. Although other 5-HT_3 receptor antagonists (including topisetron and dolasetron) exist, they are not currently available in the UK. Ondansetron and granisetron are free from sedative and extrapyramidal side-effects, but in susceptible individuals they may induce QTc prolongation and abnormal liver function tests.

Corticosteroids

Dexamethasone is a corticosteroid with high glucocorticoid activity and virtually no mineralocorticoid activity. Its mechanism of action is unknown but it is possible that either direct genomic or indirect non-genomic effects on 5-HT_3 and $GABA_A$ receptors contribute towards its antiemetic activity. Many of the original studies were carried out using 8-10 mg of dexamethasone, but recent evidence suggests that smaller doses (2.5–4 mg) are equally efficacious. Concerns about adrenal suppression and other steroid-induced side-effects following a single dose of dexamethasone are unfounded. The main side-effect of dexamethasone involves intense perineal stimulation following rapid intravenous injection.

Substance P (NK_1) Antagonists

Substance P, neurokinin A (NKA) and neurokinin B (NKB) are genetically related neuropeptides (tachykinins) which activate G-protein-coupled NK_1, NK_2 and

NK_3 receptors within peripheral and central compartments. Substance P is thought to play a key role in the generation of emetogenic stimuli by binding to NK_1 receptors in the gut and also centrally within the nucleus tractus solitarius and area postrema. In theory, blocking substance P activity should be highly effective in the treatment of PONV but NK_1 antagonists are no better (i.e. non-inferior) at reducing postoperative *nausea* than standard ondansetron therapy. In contrast, they can significantly reduce the incidence of postoperative *vomiting*. Further investigation of NK_1 antagonists is needed to determine whether they have a place in the management of PONV. Two NK_1 antagonists (aprepitant and its i.v. formulation, fosaprepitant) are licensed for use in the UK, but both are currently restricted to treatment of chemotherapy-induced nausea and vomiting (CINV). To date, no serious adverse effects have been attributed to the use of NK_1 antagonists.

Cannabinoids

Nabilone is a synthetic cannabinoid which targets endogenous CB_1 and CB_2 cannabinoid receptors. Nabilone's UK licence is restricted to the treatment of CINV although some centres report encouraging results for PONV. Serious side-effects have been reported during treatment with nabilone, including psychosis, behavioural changes and ataxia. Consequently, close supervision is recommended.

Other Techniques

Various non-pharmacological techniques have been used to reduce the incidence of PONV. Acupuncture targeted at the P6 (Neiguan) point between the flexor carpi radialis and the palmaris longus is one of the most effective non-pharmacological options. Symptomatic relief can be achieved for up to 6 h and can be extended if treatment is repeated. In cases of refractory PONV, acupuncture may prove beneficial but availability of suitably trained Chinese therapists is required. Transcutaneous nerve stimulation (TENS) offers an alternative non-pharmacological approach for the management of PONV but the evidence base for this technique is currently lacking.

FURTHER READING

Diemunsch, P., Joshi, G.P., Brichant, J.F., 2009. Neurokinin-1 receptor antagonists in the prevention of postoperative nausea and vomiting. Br. J. Anaesth. 103, 7–13.

Fero, K.E., Jalota, L., Hornuss, C., Apfel, C.C., 2011. Pharmacologic management of postoperative nausea and vomiting. Expert Opin. Pharmacother. 12, 2283–2296.

Gan, T.J., Meyer, T., Apfel, C.C., et al., 2003. Consensus guidelines for managing postoperative nausea and vomiting. Anesth. Analg. 97, 62–71.

Habib, A.S., Gan, T.J., 2004. Evidence-based management of postoperative nausea and vomiting: a review. Can. J. Anaesth. 51, 326–341.

Watcha, M.F., White, P.F., 1992. Postoperative nausea and vomiting. Its etiology, treatment and prevention. Anesthesiology 77, 162–184.

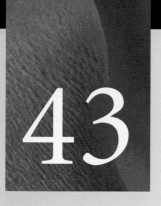

COMPLICATIONS DURING ANAESTHESIA

Complications are unexpected and unwanted events. They occur in approximately 10% of anaesthetics. Only the minority of these complications cause lasting harm to the patient. Death complicates five anaesthetics per million given in the UK (0.0005%). Every complication has the *potential* to cause lasting harm to the patient. Therefore, deviations from the norm must be recognized and managed promptly and appropriately.

The most frequent complications during anaesthesia are arrhythmia, hypotension, adverse drug effects and inadequate ventilation of the lungs. Inadequate ventilation may be caused by poorly managed or difficult tracheal intubation, pulmonary aspiration of gastric contents, breathing system disconnections or gas supply failure. These complications are also the major causes of anaesthetic mortality, preventable intraoperative cardiac arrest and permanent neurological damage. In particular, hypotension and hypoxaemia are implicated consistently in studies of adverse outcome from anaesthesia.

CAUSES OF COMPLICATIONS

Human Error

Human error is a common contributor to anaesthetic complications, often in association with poor monitoring, equipment malfunction and organizational failure. Human error is commonly associated with poor training, fatigue, inadequate experience and poor preparation of the patient, the environment and the equipment. These conditions are, generally, avoidable, and good organization should usually prevent such circumstances. When complications do occur, effective monitoring and vigilance allow a greater period for action before the complication grows in severity. During this 'window', when the complication is apparent but has not yet damaged the patient, the anaesthetist must act with precision. Such precision of action may be obtained through the use of 'action plans' or 'drills' that have been rehearsed previously.

Communication Failure

Failure of communication is frequently implicated in the generation of complications in the perioperative period. Poor working relationships, varying levels of training amongst staff and poor working conditions make such failure more likely. Team training and simulation-based training are effective in reducing the incidence of this type of error.

Equipment Failure

Equipment failure may result in significant risk to the patient. In particular, failures of breathing systems, airway devices and gas supplies have resulted in several deaths in recent years. In addition, malfunction of mechanical infusion pumps and infusion pressurizing devices have caused injury and death in several cases. Meticulous checking of equipment before use is mandatory. The anaesthetist must not only ensure the correct functioning of items of equipment that may be life-saving or of critical importance but must also ensure that alternative devices are available should the primary device fail.

Coexisting Disease

Some complications stem from the deterioration of the patient's medical condition, which may have existed before the anaesthetist's involvement. While such deterioration may be coincidental, it must be recognized that anaesthesia and surgery frequently introduce altered conditions into a patient's finely balanced combination of pathology and compensatory physiology. This may be sufficient to generate instability in the patient's condition and result in sudden worsening of an apparently stable pathology. Typical examples include diabetes mellitus, angina, hypertension and asthma.

Inevitable Complications

There exists a subgroup of complications which may be classed as 'inevitable'. Despite excellent surgical and anaesthetic practice, the patient may still experience a complication that brings morbidity or even death. While we must, at all times, make stringent efforts to save our patients from harm, it is also important to recognize that it is not always necessary to place the blame for a complication on a healthcare provider.

AVOIDANCE OF COMPLICATIONS

The most effective steps in preventing harm from complications are implemented before the complication occurs. Thorough preparation should prevent the majority of complications. This preparation includes:

- preoperative assessment, investigation and counselling of the patient
- preoperative checking of equipment and the assurance of backup equipment
- the availability of an appropriately trained assistant
- preoperative consultation with more experienced personnel, where necessary, regarding the most appropriate anaesthetic technique
- the use of appropriate monitoring techniques.

Experience

Complications occur more commonly in inexperienced hands. Clearly, finite resources exist, and appropriately experienced personnel are not always allocated to appropriate patients and procedures. It is the individual anaesthetist's responsibility to ensure that he or she has adequate training for the task presented. If the anaesthetist does not have the necessary experience, then senior assistance must be sought.

Record-Keeping

The maintenance of accurate records of a patient's treatment and vital signs is of paramount importance in preventing complications. It allows the observation of trends in vital signs, often providing valuable clues to a gradual deviation from a stable physiological state and allowing early intervention before a harmful condition arises. Accurate record-keeping also allows safer sharing of care between anaesthetists, facilitating handover of care during long operations and allowing better teamwork in complex cases in which two anaesthetists are required. It also allows after-the-event investigation and learning – an important system-level mechanism for reducing the impact and incidence of complications.

Redundant Systems

The use of redundant systems helps prevent complications. The availability of at least two working laryngoscopes illustrates this. Should one system fail, another may be put in its place. Other examples include the insertion of two or more intravenous cannulae if significant blood loss is expected, and monitoring of expired volatile agent concentration in addition to depth of anaesthesia monitors to minimize the risk of awareness.

Monitoring

Monitoring systems have been designed to detect and prevent complications during anaesthesia. Aspects of the patient should be monitored that are *likely* to deviate from the norm, or that are *dangerous* if they deviate from the norm. The Association of Anaesthetists of Great Britain and Ireland (AAGBI) has produced guidelines stipulating the acceptable minimum level of intraoperative monitoring (see Ch 16).

Modern monitoring systems have automatically activated alarms, and the anaesthetist chooses the values at which these alarms sound. The default values are not always the optimal choices. Thought should be applied to the values at which the anaesthetist gains useful insight into the patient's deviation from the healthy *status quo*, without generating unnecessary visual and auditory pollution which may detract from the anaesthetist's concentration and reduce the effectiveness of the monitor. In general, alarms should sound before the value in question reaches a potentially damaging level, but should not sound at values that would be considered within the patient's expected range. Clearly, this is different for each patient, whose coexisting disease, age, anaesthesia and surgical procedure vary greatly. The repeated sounding of an alarm should not trigger reflex silencing of the alarm but should cause the anaesthetist to consider if treatment of the patient is required or if the alarm limit should be altered.

MANAGEMENT OF COMPLICATIONS

Generic Management of Complications

The majority of complications that result in serious harm to the patient compromise the delivery of oxygen to tissues. Organs which are damaged most rapidly by a deficiency in oxygen supply include the brain and heart. The liver and the kidneys are less fragile, but potentially at risk from even short interruptions of oxygen supply. Cessation of perfusion results in more rapid damage to organs than low levels of oxygenation while perfusion is maintained. Treatment must be provided rapidly when organ perfusion is threatened or when arterial oxygenation is impaired. The management of virtually any significant complication should include the provision of a high inspired oxygen fraction and the assurance of an adequate cardiac output.

In general, complications should be dealt with through a sequence of:

1. Continual vigilance and monitoring
2. Recognition of the evolution of a problem
3. Creation of a list of differential diagnoses
4. Choice of a *working diagnosis,* which is either the most *likely* or the most *dangerous* possibility
5. Treatment of the *working diagnosis*
6. Assessment of the response of the problem to the treatment administered
7. Refinement of the list of differential diagnoses, especially if the response has not been as expected
8. Confirmation or elimination of the choice of *working diagnosis;* if the response to treatment has been unexpected then replacement with a more *likely* working diagnosis is indicated
9. Go to step 5 and repeat until the problem is resolved.

The Evolving Problem

The early recognition of an evolving problem allows the anaesthetist time to manage a complication before it damages the patient. Appropriate selection of monitoring alarm limits and the anaesthetist's vigilance should allow more time for pre-emptive treatment can be provided to reduce the impact of the complication.

The first response to an emerging complication should be to minimize the potential harm to the patient. Such harm may be produced by the anaesthetist's treatment or by a pathological source. It is important to ensure that an abnormal reading from a monitor is not an artefact; inaccurate information may be displayed if, for example, a pulse oximeter probe is poorly positioned or if an ECG electrode becomes displaced and the anaesthetist should ensure, through rapid clinical assessment of the patient, that the values shown on the monitor screen are consistent with the patient's clinical appearance and the context. For example, a sudden reading of arterial oxygen saturation of 70% when the values have been greater than 96% throughout the procedure should prompt a rapid examination of the patient; if the patient is not cyanosed and ventilation appears to continue uninterrupted, then the position of the pulse oximeter probe should be checked, particularly if the plethysmograph trace is poor.

In most situations in which complications become apparent, the diagnosis is simple and treatment may progress in a linear fashion. Such linear treatment of complications is detailed later in this chapter. However, the causes of some complications, such as hypoxaemia, are not always immediately clear, and several potential aetiologies may exist. Where the differential diagnoses relating to a problem appear equally likely, the anaesthetist should treat the problem that threatens the most harm to the patient. During the management of problems during anaesthesia, the anaesthetist must constantly be reconsidering the list of differential diagnoses, re-arranging them mentally in order of likelihood and treating the most likely and most dangerous possibilities first.

Record-Keeping

Record-keeping, while useful in preventing complications, is also important *during* complications. Trends in a patient's physiological data may become apparent only when charted, and new differential diagnoses may be generated through examination of the recorded data. Review of critical incidents and complications is vitally important in preventing future repetitions of the incident and in providing continuing education to individual practitioners and to Departments of Anaesthesia. Thorough record-keeping is vital in allowing informed review of these cases. Finally, some complications result in harm to the patient and it is very important for the practitioner and the patient that detailed records are available for later review. In a minority of such cases, legal action may result and detailed, legible records are vital in defending the actions of the staff and in providing an adequate explanation to the patient (and possibly to the court) of what happened in the operating theatre.

MEDICOLEGAL ASPECTS OF COMPLICATIONS

A minority of complications result in a formal complaint, but litigation by patients who feel that they have been wronged by the healthcare system is becoming increasingly common. Defensive practice is consequently becoming widespread. Such practice aims to reduce the potential culpability of the anaesthetist should complications arise. In some situations, this may lead to overinvestigation of patients and even to the provision of care which is not necessarily optimal for the patient. The 'culture of blame' in which we now practise dictates that anaesthetists must protect themselves as well as their patients. Meticulous record-keeping, preoperative information and consent, and frank discussion of risks with the patient are vital.

Management of the Medicolegal Aspects of Complications

Complications must be recognized promptly and treated efficiently, with the patient's best outcome the aim of treatment. Record-keeping must continue to be meticulous, even during the occurrence of problems during an anaesthetic. Help should be sought early if there is any doubt about the anaesthetist's ability or experience.

Complaints by patients should be dealt with promptly and professionally. The complaint and the anaesthetist's response must be recorded clearly in the patient's records. The anaesthetist should express

regret and sympathy that the complication has occurred, and explain why. A frank discussion of the difficulties that occurred during an anaesthetic may provide the patient with sufficient information. If human error has occurred, then the anaesthetist should apologize, and assure the patient that further information will be provided when it becomes available. If the anaesthetist is a trainee, then it is prudent to enlist the assistance of a consultant to attend discussions with the patient. The clinical director should be informed of all discussions with the patient. It may be prudent that the clinical director accompanies the anaesthetist during their dealings with the patient. The results and content of all such discussions must be recorded in the patient's medical records.

Any complaint that goes further than an informal conversation should be referred to the hospital's complaints department and the anaesthetist's defence organization should be informed. The defence organization will provide advice on subsequent action. It must be emphasized that throughout this often distressing process, meticulous and professional record-keeping may make the difference between exoneration and condemnation, irrespective of the true source of fault.

COMPLICATIONS

The presentation, causes and management of the most common and most dangerous complications which occur during anaesthesia are described below. Complications are classified, where possible, according to the body system involved. Some complications (such as hypothermia) do not fit easily into this classification and are described separately. This list of complications is not exhaustive and the reader is encouraged to consult the texts listed at the end of the chapter.

Respiratory System

Respiratory Obstruction

Table 43.1 details the common causes of respiratory obstruction during anaesthesia. Obstruction may occur at any point from the gas delivery system through the patient's airway and bronchi to the expiratory parts of the breathing system and the scavenging tubing. It is common and potentially very dangerous. The commonest sites for obstruction are the larynx (e.g. laryngospasm), the tracheal tube (e.g. biting or secretions)

TABLE 43.1
Causes of Respiratory Obstruction During Anaesthesia

Equipment

Breathing system	Valve malfunction, kinking
Tracheal tube	External compression (surgical gag/manipulation, kinking, biting)
	Occlusion of lumen (secretions, blood)
	Cuff (overinflation, herniation)
	Oesophageal or bronchial intubation

Patient

Oropharynx	Soft tissue (oedema from trauma/infection, reduced muscle tone)
	Secretions (blood, surgical packs)
	Tumour
Larynx	Laryngospasm
	Recurrent laryngeal nerve palsy
	Oedema (drug hypersensitivity, pre-eclampsia, infection)
	Tumour
Trachea	Laryngotracheobronchitis
	External compression (surgical, haematoma, thyroid tumour)
	Stricture (radiotherapy, scarring from previous tracheostomy)
Bronchi	Secretions
	Pneumothorax
	Bronchospasm
	Tumour
	Surgical manipulation

and the bronchi (e.g. bronchospasm). Respiratory obstruction causes inadequate ventilation and impaired gas exchange. This causes hypercapnia, hypoxaemia and reduced uptake of volatile anaesthetic agent. Respiratory obstruction prevents the mass inflow of ambient gas which occurs during apnoea and thus produces hypoxaemia more rapidly than does apnoea with an open airway.

Partial obstruction is indicated by noisy breathing or stridor, while complete obstruction is silent. In spontaneously breathing patients, tracheal tug, paradoxical chest and abdominal movement ('see-saw' ventilation) and reduced movement of the breathing system's reservoir bag are other signs. The generation of a large negative intrathoracic pressure during powerful attempts to inhale may cause pulmonary oedema in some patients, particularly young adults. In patients whose lungs are mechanically ventilated, respiratory obstruction may be associated with increased inflation pressure, a prolonged expiratory phase, hypercapnia and alteration of the end-tidal carbon dioxide waveform.

Management. Any significant airway obstruction should be treated by gentle, manual ventilation of the patient's lungs with oxygen. Location of the site of obstruction should be sought urgently. In the absence of a laryngeal mask airway (LMA) or tracheal tube, apposition of the tongue and pharyngeal soft tissue is a common cause of upper airway obstruction. This may be overcome by a jaw lift or neck extension. It may require the use of an oro- or nasopharyngeal airway, although these devices may themselves provoke laryngospasm or pharyngeal abrasion. Absolute obstruction suggests an equipment problem. Easy passage of a suction catheter through the tracheal tube confirms its patency. If obstruction persists and no obvious cause is identified, then the tracheal tube or laryngeal mask may be the site of obstruction and should be replaced.

Suction removes accumulated secretions in the pharynx, but may cause laryngospasm during light anaesthesia. The presence of symmetrical chest movements and breath sounds should be confirmed. Other causes of obstruction such as laryngospasm, bronchospasm, aspiration and pneumothorax should be excluded.

The most common airway complication is partial respiratory obstruction during spontaneous ventilation or during assisted manual ventilation in the absence of a formal (equipment) airway. A gentle jaw thrust, head tilt and chin lift usually clear a partially obstructed airway, and insertion of an oropharyngeal or nasopharyngeal airway resolves almost all of the remainder. In the rare situation of complete inability to ventilate the patient's lungs manually, and after equipment failure has been excluded, the insertion of a laryngeal mask airway or tracheal tube may be necessary. Allowing the patient to awaken is prudent if there is no urgency to proceed with the operation. If it is necessary to continue the operation or if the patient cannot be wakened, and insertion of a laryngeal mask airway and tracheal tube have proved impossible, then it becomes necessary to establish a *surgical airway.* This may take the form of a cricothyroid cannula, a surgical cricothyrotomy or an emergency tracheostomy. These procedures must be learned and practised *before* the occurrence of the incident. They are technically demanding and are themselves potentially life-threatening to the patient if performed inexpertly (see Ch 22).

Laryngospasm

Laryngospasm is a reflex, prolonged closure of the vocal cords. It occurs usually in response to a trigger, and this is often laryngeal stimulation by airway devices, secretions or gastric contents during light anaesthesia. Laryngospasm is most common during induction and emergence. It may also be produced by surgical and visceral stimuli such as skin incision, peritoneal traction and anal or cervical dilatation. Children are particularly prone to laryngospasm. The use of thiopental inhibits laryngeal reflexes to a lesser extent than propofol and increases the risk of laryngospasm. Poor management of laryngospasm may lead to inadequate ventilation with hypoxaemia, hypercapnia and reduced depth of anaesthesia. Crowing inspiratory noises with signs of respiratory obstruction suggest laryngospasm. Complete obstruction caused by severe laryngospasm is silent.

Management. Where possible, airway and surgical stimulation should be avoided during light anaesthesia and the lateral position should be used for control of secretions during extubation and transfer. Surgical stimuli should be anticipated and anaesthetic depth should be adjusted accordingly. The anaesthetist should remove the stimulus to laryngospasm, administer 100% oxygen and provide a clear airway. Gentle pharyngeal suction should be applied. Where appropriate, anaesthetic depth may be increased by administration of an intravenous anaesthetic agent and the lungs ventilated manually, applying continuous positive airway pressure (CPAP). Most episodes of laryngospasm respond to this treatment. If laryngospasm persists and hypoxaemia ensues, a small dose of succinylcholine (e.g. 25 mg in adults) relaxes the vocal cords and allows manual ventilation and oxygenation. A full dose of succinylcholine may be given if tracheal intubation is indicated, but this is usually unnecessary. Doxapram, an analeptic and respiratory stimulant, has also been used successfully in the treatment of laryngospasm.

Bronchospasm

General anaesthesia may alter airway resistance by influencing bronchomotor tone, lung volumes and bronchial secretions. Patients with increased airway reactivity from recent respiratory infection, asthma, atopy or smoking are more susceptible to bronchospasm during anaesthesia. Bronchospasm may be precipitated by the rapid introduction of a pungent volatile anaesthetic agent (e.g. isoflurane, desflurane), the insertion of an artificial airway during light anaesthesia, stimulation of the carina or bronchi by a tracheal tube or by drugs causing β-blockade or release of histamine. Drug hypersensitivity, pulmonary aspiration and a foreign body in the lower airway may also present as bronchospasm. Bronchospasm causes expiratory wheeze, a prolonged expiratory phase (evident from the upwardly sloping end-tidal carbon dioxide plateau) and increased ventilator inflation pressures. Wheezing may occur in association with other causes of respiratory obstruction, such as pneumothorax, and these should be excluded. If bronchospasm is very severe, ventilation may be quiet and wheeze may not be apparent.

Management. Bronchospasm during anaesthesia results in hypercapnia, hypoxaemia and pulmonary gas trapping, which may cause hypotension (through reduction in left ventricular preload). Management is aimed at preventing hypoxaemia, and resolving the bronchospasm. Initially, 100% oxygen should be given, anaesthesia deepened if appropriate and any aggravating factors removed (e.g. the tracheal tube should be repositioned and surgery stopped). If further treatment is necessary, a bronchodilator should be given in increments according to the response. Recommended drugs include intravenous aminophylline (up to 6 mg kg^{-1}) or salbutamol (up to 3 μg kg^{-1}). Volatile anaesthetic agents and ketamine are also effective bronchodilators. Adrenaline is indicated in life-threatening situations and may be given via the tracheal tube. Steroids and H$_1$-receptor antagonists have no immediate effect but may be indicated in the later management of severe cases of bronchospasm.

If hypoxaemia develops in the spontaneously breathing patient, then tracheal intubation and artificial ventilation should be considered. Mechanical ventilation should incorporate a long expiratory phase to prevent the development of high end-expiratory alveolar pressures, which may cause hypotension, alveolar barotrauma and further hypoventilation. Severe gas trapping (intrinsic PEEP) may result in thoracic hyperexpansion, poor ventilation and pulmonary barotrauma. A very long expiratory phase or disconnection from the ventilator for up to 30 s may be necessary to allow thoracic depressurization. Positive end-expiratory pressure (PEEP) and high ventilatory rates should be avoided if bronchospasm is present because these favour the development of gas trapping. Hypercapnia may have to be tolerated in order to avoid gas trapping and barotrauma.

Complications Associated with Tracheal Intubation

Difficult Intubation

Some difficulty is experienced during tracheal intubation in about one in ten patients (10%). Approximately one in ten of these patients (1%) presents significant difficulty in intubation. Intubation is impossible in about one in ten of these patients (0.1%), and both intubation and ventilation are impossible in about one in ten of these (0.01%). In most instances, the cause of difficulty with the airway is difficulty in attaining an adequate view of the laryngeal inlet at laryngoscopy.

Poor management of difficult intubation is a significant cause of morbidity and mortality during anaesthesia. Sequelae include dental and airway trauma, pulmonary aspiration, hypoxaemia, brain damage and death. Table 43.2 shows the commonest causes of difficulty in intubation. The single most important cause is an inexperienced or inadequately prepared anaesthetist and the difficulty is often compounded by equipment malfunction. The anatomical features associated with difficult laryngoscopy are listed in Table 43.3. Of these, the atlanto-occipital distance is the best predictor of difficulty but requires a lateral cervical X-ray. Many of these factors are normal anatomical variations, but extreme abnormalities do occur. A cluster of normal variations in an apparently healthy patient may be sufficient to cause major difficulties in laryngoscopy.

Management. Preoperative examination of the airway (Table 43.4) is essential. Identification of patients with a potentially difficult airway (see Tables 43.2 and 43.3)

TABLE 43.2
Causes of Difficult Intubation

Anaesthetist
Inadequate preoperative assessment
Inadequate preparation of equipment
Inexperience
Poor technique

Equipment
Malfunction
Unavailability
No trained assistance

Patient

Congenital	Syndromes (Down, Pierre Robin, Treacher Collins, Marfan)
	Achondroplasia
	Cystic hygroma
	Encephalocele
Acquired	Reduced jaw movement:
	Trismus (abscess, infection, fracture, tetanus)
	Fibrosis (post-infection, post-radiotherapy, trauma)
	Rheumatoid arthritis
	Ankylosing spondylitis
	Tumours
	Jaw wiring
	Reduced neck movement:
	Arthritis
	Ankylosing spondylitis
	Cervical fracture, instability, fusion
	Airway:
	Oedema (infection, trauma, angio-oedema, burns)
	Compression (goitre, haematoma)
	Scarring (radiotherapy, infection, burns)
	Tumours, polyps
	Foreign body
	Nerve palsy
	Others:
	Morbid obesity
	Pregnancy
	Acromegaly

before anaesthesia allows time to plan an appropriate anaesthetic technique. The Mallampati test is a widely used and simple classification of the pharyngeal view obtained during maximal mouth opening and tongue protrusion (see pp. 455–456). In practice, this test suggests a higher likelihood of difficult laryngoscopy if the posterior pharyngeal wall is not seen. The predictive

TABLE 43.3
Anatomical Factors Associated with Difficult Laryngoscopy

Short, wide, muscular neck

Protruding incisors

High, arched palate

Receding lower jaw

Poor mobility of the mandible

Increased anterior depth of mandible

Increased posterior depth of mandible (reduces jaw opening, requires X-ray)

Decreased atlanto-occipital distance (reduces neck extension, requires X-ray)

TABLE 43.4
Preoperative Assessment of the Airway

General appearance of the neck, face, maxilla and mandible

Jaw movement

Head extension and neck movement

Teeth and oropharynx

Soft tissues of the neck

Recent chest and cervical spine X-rays

Previous anaesthetic records

Mallampati classification

Thyromental distance

value of this test may be strengthened if the thyromental distance (the distance between the thyroid cartilage prominence and the bony point of the chin during full head extension) is less than 6.5 cm.

Premedication with an antisialagogue reduces airway secretions. This is advantageous before inhalational induction and essential for awake fibreoptic laryngoscopy to maximize the effectiveness of topical local anaesthesia. An anxiolytic may also be given (but is contraindicated in patients with airway obstruction, e.g. caused by burns, trauma, tumour or infection affecting the larynx or pharynx). The presence of a trained assistant is essential and the availability of an experienced anaesthetist and a 'difficult intubation' trolley with a range of equipment

such as bougies, a variety of laryngoscopes and tracheal tubes, and cricothyrotomy needles is desirable (see Ch 22).

A variety of options exists for the patient in whom a difficult laryngoscopy is anticipated. If the procedure can be carried out under local or regional anaesthesia, then this technique should be used as the first choice (see Ch 24). However, the patient, anaesthetist and equipment must be prepared for general anaesthesia in case a complication arises.

If general anaesthesia is necessary for the procedure, or if the patient refuses local or regional anaesthesia despite a frank discussion of the risks, then steps must be taken to secure the airway safely. Unless tracheal intubation is essential for airway protection or to enable muscle relaxation and ventilation, the use of an artificial airway such as the laryngeal mask with spontaneous ventilation is usually a safe technique. If intubation is essential, the appropriate anaesthetic technique depends on the anticipated degree of difficulty, the presence or absence of airway obstruction and the risk of regurgitation of gastric fluid. The management of the patient in whom difficulties with airway management are anticipated is detailed in Ch 22.

There is no place for the use of a long-acting muscle relaxant to facilitate tracheal intubation if difficulty is anticipated. Correct positioning of the head and neck is essential and the lungs should be denitrogenated after establishing intravenous access and appropriate monitoring.

The safest anaesthetic technique may usually be chosen from the following clinical examples.

1. *Patients with an increased risk of regurgitation and aspiration (e.g. full stomach, intra-abdominal pathology, pregnancy).* An inhalational induction is inappropriate in these patients. Regional anaesthesia is preferable in the parturient (see Ch 35). Preoxygenation and a rapid sequence induction with succinylcholine can be used if there is little anticipated difficulty. If intubation is unsuccessful, no further doses of neuromuscular blocking drug should be used, the patient allowed to wake and further assistance sought. If there is a high degree of anticipated difficulty, an awake technique is recommended (see below).

2. *Patients with little anticipated difficulty and no airway obstruction (e.g. mild reduction of jaw or neck movement).* After a sleep dose of intravenous induction agent and confirmation of the ability to ventilate the lungs manually by mask, succinylcholine may be given to provide the best conditions for tracheal intubation. If difficulty is encountered, the patient is allowed to wake up and the procedure replanned. Where appropriate, anaesthesia is deepened by spontaneous ventilation using a volatile agent and alternative techniques to facilitate tracheal intubation used (see Ch 22).

3. *Patients with severe anticipated difficulty and no airway obstruction (e.g. severe reduction of jaw or neck movement).* Appropriate techniques include inhalational induction with sevoflurane or the use of fibreoptic laryngoscopy either in the awake patient or after inhalational induction. Neuromuscular blocking drugs must not be used until the ability to ventilate the lungs manually and view the vocal cords is confirmed.

4. *Patients with airway obstruction (e.g. burns, infection, trauma).* An inhalational induction may be used; otherwise an awake technique should be considered. Neuromuscular blocking drugs should not be used until tracheal intubation is confirmed.

5. *Extreme clinical situations.* Tracheostomy performed under local anaesthesia may be the safest technique.

Inhalational Induction

Premedication with an antisialagogue is desirable. Depth of anaesthesia is increased carefully by spontaneous ventilation of increasing concentrations of a volatile anaesthetic agent in 100% oxygen until laryngoscopy may be performed safely. Sevoflurane currently provides the best conditions for this purpose. If the larynx is viewed easily, intubation may be performed with or without a muscle relaxant. If the view is limited, a suitable bougie may be inserted to assist passage of the tracheal tube through the larynx. Correct insertion of the bougie in the trachea may be confirmed by detecting the palpable bumps of the tracheal rings or resistance when the carina is

encountered. The tracheal tube is then passed over the bougie into the trachea. This manoeuvre is facilitated by rotating the tracheal tube 90° as it passes through the glottis. If intubation during direct laryngoscopy is unsuccessful, anaesthesia may be maintained and the use of fibreoptic laryngoscopy, blind nasal intubation or a retrograde technique considered.

Awake Intubation

Fibreoptic laryngoscopy and intubation require special equipment, skill and time. The procedure may be performed by the nasal or oral route after topical anaesthesia has been achieved by spraying the nasal and oropharyngeal mucosa or gargling viscous preparations of local anaesthetic. The injection of 3–5 mL of 2% lidocaine through the cricothyroid membrane induces coughing and anaesthetizes the tracheal and laryngeal mucosa.

Conventional laryngoscopy can also be performed in conscious patients under local anaesthesia. After cricothyroid injection of lidocaine, laryngoscopy is performed in stages. The oropharynx is progressively anaesthetized with lidocaine spray until the patient tolerates deep insertion of the laryngoscope, enabling the larynx to be viewed.

Failed Intubation

The total incidence of failed tracheal intubation is approximately 1 in 1000 (0.1%), but about 1 in 300 (0.3%) in obstetric patients. However, failed intubation in obstetric patients is now a rare event because of the high percentage of obstetric surgical patients operated on under regional anaesthesia.

Most failed intubations result from the anaesthetist failing to insert the tube, but occasionally the tube may be misplaced, most commonly in the oesophagus. This complication has resulted in many deaths since the advent of tracheal intubation. It should be suspected whenever difficulty has been experienced in inserting a tracheal tube, particularly when direct visual confirmation of the passage of the tube into the larynx has not been possible. Auscultation of the chest is recommended, although inflation of the stomach may occasionally mimic breath sounds. Auscultation over the stomach usually detects a bubbling sound if the oesophagus has been intubated.

Observation of a normal capnogram usually provides assurance of tracheal placement of the tube, but cases have been described of patients who have 'expired' carbon dioxide *briefly* despite oesophageal intubation, having ingested carbonated drinks or bicarbonate antacids shortly before anaesthesia. A normal and *persistent* expiratory capnogram should be sought as confirmation of tracheal tube placement.

Fibreoptic bronchoscopy provides an excellent method of assuring the location of the tube, but is not usually available in every operating theatre. The 'Wee' oesophageal intubation detector tests for the free aspiration of air via the tracheal tube into a rubber bulb. The device is cheap, easy to use and accurate, but total reliance should not be placed on this device. The capnogram is the 'gold standard' for confirming correct tracheal intubation.

Poor management of failed intubation is a significant cause of serious morbidity and mortality. The aims of management are to maintain oxygenation and prevent aspiration of gastric contents. The 'failed intubation drill' is now established as an important skill for safe anaesthetic practice. An early decision to use a failed intubation protocol and to call for assistance is essential, because continued attempts at tracheal intubation may result in trauma to the airway, pulmonary aspiration or hypoxaemia (see Ch 22). The obstetric patient is a special case and is considered in Chapter 35.

If the airway is obstructed and ventilation is inadequate during management of a failed intubation, then insertion of an LMA should be considered (see Figs 22.3–22.5). It has been used successfully to provide an airway and allow ventilation when attempts to intubate the trachea and ventilate the lungs by other means have failed. Alternatively, it may be possible to pass a small-diameter tracheal tube or a bougie through the LMA into the trachea; a variant of the LMA, the intubating LMA (ILMA) is designed specifically to facilitate tracheal intubation. The LMA should not be regarded as providing protection against pulmonary aspiration, although it is claimed that the ProSeal™ LMA, which has a rearward port for the downward passage of a gastric tube or the upward passage of gastric contents, is better in this regard. The oesophageal obturator airway and similar devices are alternatives in an emergency, but there are doubts about their efficacy and there have been reports of misplacement and oesophageal rupture associated with their use. A recent innovation is an ILMA which incorporates a video camera and LCD screen, allowing direct visualization of the introduction of a tracheal tube through the larynx.

When consciousness cannot be restored rapidly for pharmacological reasons, then transtracheal ventilation can be life-saving. A cannula or small-diameter tracheal tube may be passed via the cricothyroid membrane. Ventilation through a cannula requires high-pressure, 'jet' ventilation from a Sanders injector or the high-pressure oxygen outlet of the anaesthetic machine. More conventional ventilation is possible through a small-diameter tube placed via the cricothyroid membrane, but the procedure, which requires a transcutaneous scalpel incision, requires some practice and may result in haemorrhage. Both techniques allow adequate oxygenation for many minutes, and should provide time to allow the patient to awaken. Exhalation through a cricothyroid cannula may be inadequate, and if the laryngeal inlet is not patent then inadequate ventilation and barotrauma may result. In this situation, an additional cannula should be inserted to allow gas to escape.

If it is essential that surgery proceeds without the patient awakening then oxygenation and carbon dioxide elimination must be maintained while ensuring an adequate depth of anaesthesia. Any of the rescue techniques described above may be used, but usually the laryngeal mask or the fibreoptic bronchoscope prove most useful.

Unintentional Bronchial Intubation

Bronchial intubation results in the ventilation of one lung and denial of ventilation to the other. This causes hypoxaemia through the inevitably large pulmonary shunt caused by atelectasis and collapse of the unventilated lung. Intubation of the right main bronchus is more common because of its smaller angle with the trachea. This complication is avoided by cutting the tracheal tube to an appropriate length before intubation, observation of the passage of the tube through the vocal cords and adjusting the length of the tube at the patient's incisors, and by confirmation of its position by auscultation after intubation and after changes in position of the patient on the operating table.

Aspiration of Gastric Contents

Regurgitation of gastric contents is common during anaesthesia. Frequently, regurgitation proceeds only as far as the mid-oesophagus, but occasionally gastric contents enter the oropharynx. This is particularly likely in patients with a hiatus hernia or a full stomach. The latter may result from recent eating or drinking or may be the result of gastric outlet or bowel obstruction, pain, stress or drugs which delay gastric emptying, such as morphine and alcohol. Once gastric contents enter the oropharynx, there exists the potential for aspiration into the lungs. This is uncommon, but remains an important cause of morbidity and mortality associated with anaesthesia. Aspiration of oropharyngeal contents is more likely if those contents are allowed to remain in the oropharynx for a significant time, and if laryngeal reflexes are depressed. Aspiration may occur also in the sedated patient, whose laryngeal reflexes are diminished. Aspiration is more common during difficult intubation, emergency cases and in obese or pregnant patients.

Mortality is high after aspiration of large quantities of gastric contents and the aspiration of solids, in particular, is associated with a poor prognosis. The acidity of gastric contents is also important in determining the degree of severity of the pulmonary reaction to aspiration, with highly acid material being particularly inflammatory. Bronchospasm may be the first sign of pulmonary aspiration during general anaesthesia. If a large quantity of gastric material is aspirated, respiratory obstruction, ventilation–perfusion mismatch and intrapulmonary shunting may produce severe hypoxaemia, with later development of chemical pneumonitis and/or infection.

Management. At-risk patients should be managed actively to prevent the aspiration of gastric contents. The volume and acidity of the gastric contents should be reduced as far as possible. Preoperative fasting, histamine H_2-receptor blockers and a gastric prokinetic drug (e.g. metoclopramide) are recommended. If general anaesthesia is essential, then the trachea must be intubated. Most commonly, this is achieved using a rapid-sequence induction with cricoid pressure (see Ch 37), but awake intubation is advisable if difficulty in intubation is predicted. During emergence, the tracheal tube should not be removed until protective airway reflexes are regained when the patient is awake.

If aspiration occurs during anaesthesia, further regurgitation should be prevented by immediate application of cricoid pressure, and the patient should be placed in a head-down position. The left lateral position should also be considered to encourage the drainage of gastric contents out of the mouth. In all but the mildest cases, the trachea should be intubated to facilitate removal of the aspirated material by suction before the use of positive-pressure ventilation. However, ventilation should not be delayed if significant hypoxaemia is present. Bronchodilator therapy may be required and the inspired oxygen concentration should be increased. Positive end-expiratory pressure may be used if hypoxaemia is refractory to increasing inspired oxygen fraction. Non-emergency surgery should be abandoned if significant morbidity develops. Flexible bronchoscopy permits the removal of liquids, although rigid bronchoscopy may be necessary for the removal of solid matter. Intravenous steroids and pulmonary lavage with saline via a flexible bronchoscope may reduce the post-aspiration inflammatory response. A chest X-ray and arterial blood gas measurement help in the assessment of the severity of injury. The patient should be transferred to a critical care unit for further monitoring and respiratory care.

Hiccups

Regular and repeated spasmodic diaphragmatic movements may occur after i.v. induction of anaesthesia and in association with vagal stimulation during light anaesthesia. Anticholinergic premedication reduces the incidence of hiccups. Although difficult to treat, hiccups are of little consequence unless surgery, or rarely oxygenation, is compromised. Persistent hiccups may be abolished by deepening anaesthesia, stimulating the nasopharynx with a suction catheter or administering metoclopramide. Profound muscle relaxation may be justified to stop all diaphragmatic movement if hiccups are causing surgical difficulty.

Hypoxaemia

Hypoxaemia is an inadequate partial pressure of oxygen in arterial blood. Hypoxia is oxygen deficiency at the tissue level. A practical classification of the causes of hypoxaemia is shown in Table 43.5. Hypoxaemia threatens tissues globally and, if allowed to persist, risks permanent damage to those organs most delicately dependent upon continued oxygen supply. The first

TABLE 43.5
Causes of Hypoxaemia During Anaesthesia

Hypoxic Inspired Gas Mixture

Equipment	Oxygen supply (cylinder or pipeline failure, misconnection)
	Flowmeters (inaccurate settings, leak)
	Breathing system (obstruction, leak)

Hypoventilation

Equipment	Ventilator failure, inadequate ventilatory minute volume
	Breathing system (obstruction, leak, disconnection)
	Tracheal tube (obstruction, oesophageal intubation)
Patient	Respiratory depression (spontaneously breathing)
	Obstruction

$\dot{V}/\dot{Q}$ Mismatch

Patient	Inadequate ventilation	Bronchial intubation
		Secretions
		Atelectasis
		Pneumothorax
		Bronchospasm
		Pulmonary aspiration
		Pulmonary oedema
	Inadequate perfusion	Embolus (gas, thrombus, amniotic fluid)
		Low cardiac output

Other

	Methaemoglobinaemia
	Malignant hyperthermia

organs to be damaged, most commonly, are the brain and heart, and any pathological impairment of their blood supply increases the risk of early and permanent damage. There is no categorically *safe* or *unsafe* level of arterial oxygen tension (PaO_2). The risk presented by a level of hypoxaemia is dependent upon the patient's haemoglobin concentration, cardiac output, state of hydration, concurrent disease processes (especially vasculopathic diseases) and the duration of exposure to the lowered PaO_2. In general, few patients are harmed by arterial oxyhaemoglobin saturations of greater than 80%, but clearly, this low level provides very little margin for safety should any other complication occur. Most anaesthetists choose to set the arterial oxygen saturation alarm limits on the pulse oximeter at 92–94%.

Severe hypoxaemia produces tachycardia, sweating, hypertension and arrhythmias, although bradycardia is the commoner response in children. Tachypnoea occurs in spontaneously breathing patients. There may also be clinical signs associated with the cause. As arterial desaturation progresses, bradycardia and hypotension (caused by myocardial depression) develop. Eventually, cardiac arrest occurs, usually in asystole. By this stage, the heart, brain, kidneys and liver may have incurred irreversible ischaemic damage.

Hypoventilation is very common during anaesthesia, but in the presence of an adequate inspired oxygen concentration (i.e. over 30%) must be very severe to cause hypoxaemia. Reduction of the ventilatory minute volume from a normal value of $5\,L\,min^{-1}$ to $2\,L\,min^{-1}$ in the presence of an inspired oxygen concentration of 30% causes arterial oxygen saturation to decrease to only around 90% in an otherwise healthy patient. This represents severe hypoventilation, and produces an arterial carbon dioxide tension of approximately 13 kPa. The pulmonary shunting and atelectasis that can occur during anaesthesia are much more likely to cause hypoxaemia than is hypoventilation.

Management. Hypoxaemia occurring during anaesthesia is almost invariably treatable and its complications are preventable. Cyanosis should seldom be witnessed by the vigilant anaesthetist because the routine use of pulse oximetry allows early detection and treatment of hypoxaemia. If hypoxaemia is detected, the following drill should be instituted.

1. A-B-C. Ensure an adequate airway, ensure adequate ventilation and check for an adequate cardiac output by feeling the carotid pulse.
2. Exclude delivery of a hypoxic gas mixture using an oxygen analyser. Increase the inspired oxygen concentration to 100%.
3. Test the integrity of the breathing system by manual ventilation of the lungs and confirm bilateral chest movement and breath sounds. Blow down the tracheal tube if necessary.
4. Confirm the position and patency of the tracheal tube by assessing the capnogram, passing a suction catheter through the tracheal tube and auscultating the chest.
5. Search for clinical evidence of the causes of $\dot{V}/\dot{Q}$ mismatch with early exclusion of pneumothorax. If atelectasis or reduced functional residual capacity (FRC) is contributory, gentle hyperinflation of the lungs should improve oxygenation. Lung volume may be maintained by applying PEEP.
6. If the diagnosis is difficult, measure core temperature, and consider arterial blood gas analysis and chest X-ray examination.

Apnoea

Apnoea occurs during most anaesthetics. It is eminently treatable, and usually results in no harm to the patient. The occurrence of hypoxaemia, hypercapnia and acidaemia are predictable consequences of prolonged apnoea. The development of hypoxaemia after induction of anaesthesia is often delayed by preoxygenation of the patient's lungs. However, when hypoxaemia becomes evident, it progresses swiftly and inexorably unless oxygenation of the lungs is restored. Rapid progression of hypoxaemia occurs in the presence of airway obstruction, high oxygen consumption and small FRC. Such factors may appear in combination in small children, pregnancy and obesity. Carbon dioxide is retained during apnoea, and $PaCO_2$ increases by 0.4–0.8 kPa min^{-1}, while arterial pH decreases by approximately 1.5 h^{-1} or 0.025 min^{-1}. Atelectasis develops quickly during apnoea under anaesthesia, particularly in obese patients.

As a consequence of its water solubility, very little carbon dioxide enters the lungs during apnoea and the net flow of ambient gas through an open airway and into the alveoli is very nearly equal to the rate of oxygen consumption (i.e. 250 mL min^{-1}). Consequently, adequate oxygenation may be assured for many minutes by the provision of 100% oxygen to the open airway during apnoea. If the airway is obstructed then this mass flow cannot occur and hypoxaemia develops much more quickly. In addition, the intrathoracic pressure may become significantly hypobaric if the airway is obstructed, and this further reduces the alveolar and arterial oxygen tensions.

Management. Unless required for surgery (e.g. during cardiopulmonary bypass or delicate lung surgery), apnoea should not be allowed to persist untreated. Significant atelectasis, hypercapnia and acidaemia may develop silently. If atelectasis develops, then recruitment manoeuvres may be successful in reversing it (see p. 867).

The development of hypoxaemia during apnoea is greatly slowed by the provision of 100% oxygen to an open airway. Therefore, it is mandatory that periods of apnoea (e.g. during rapid-sequence induction) are accompanied by an airway open to a breathing system supplying 100% oxygen. This is of particular importance during periods of high oxygen consumption (e.g. during fasciculations associated with administration of succinylcholine). Following the rescue of an obstructed airway, there is a rapid influx of ambient gas into the previously hypobaric thorax. Provision of 100% oxygen at this point may significantly restore depleted oxygen reserves and arterial oxygen saturation.

Hypercapnia

Hypercapnia is an abnormally high partial pressure of carbon dioxide in arterial blood ($PaCO_2$). Typically, this is indicated by a $PaCO_2$ greater than 6 kPa. Hypercapnia is caused by either inadequate carbon dioxide removal (e.g. caused by hypoventilation or increased pulmonary dead space) or excessive carbon dioxide production. During anaesthesia, hypercapnia may also result from an inadequate fresh gas flow rate into a semiclosed anaesthetic breathing system, or by exhausted carbon dioxide absorbent in a circle system, resulting in rebreathing of carbon dioxide.

Carbon dioxide production increases during pyrexia, malignant hyperthermia and shivering. Inadvertent or excessive carbon dioxide delivery from the anaesthetic machine and absorption of carbon dioxide during laparoscopic procedures are other causes of hypercapnia.

Hypercapnia stimulates activity of the sympathetic nervous system and causes tachycardia, sweating and arrhythmias (usually ectopics or tachyarrhythmias), increased cerebral blood flow, increased intracranial pressure, tachypnoea and alterations in arterial pressure. As anaesthetic drugs suppress autonomic responses, these signs may not occur during anaesthesia until $PaCO_2$ is markedly increased. Acute respiratory acidosis produces an increase in serum potassium concentration.

Management. Mild degrees of hypercapnia are usually tolerated well by spontaneously breathing patients unless there is a contraindication such as head injury. If signs of significant hypercapnia occur, the anaesthetist should control ventilation and provide an appropriate ventilatory minute volume to normalize $PaCO_2$.

Hypocapnia

Hypocapnia is an abnormally low $PaCO_2$ (less than 4.5 kPa). The most common cause is mechanical hyperventilation. Decreased carbon dioxide production may occasionally be responsible if the patient is cold or deeply anaesthetized. Hypocapnia produces respiratory alkalosis with a decrease in serum potassium concentration. There is generalized vasoconstriction and reductions in cerebral blood flow, cardiac output and tissue oxygen delivery. Patients with critical cerebrovascular stenosis may risk cerebral ischaemia, but otherwise hypocapnia tends not to produce significant morbidity. There may be a delay in onset of spontaneous ventilation at the conclusion of anaesthesia in which mechanical ventilation has been used while $PaCO_2$ increases to levels which stimulate ventilation.

Management. Decreasing the ventilatory minute volume or increasing the breathing system dead space reduce removal of carbon dioxide from the blood. It is important to note that the most accessible representation of $PaCO_2$ currently available to anaesthetists is the end-tidal carbon dioxide tension (P_ECO_2). This is usually approximately 0.5–1.0 kPa less than $PaCO_2$ but this gap varies significantly with the site of sampling

of expired gas and with variations in the alveolar dead space fraction. The latter is affected by alterations in arterial pressure, cardiac output, posture and tidal volume. The anaesthetist should not assume, therefore, that a low value of end-tidal carbon dioxide tension necessarily reflects a low $PaCO_2$. Such an assumption could result in significant hypoventilation if the minute volume is reduced inappropriately.

Pneumothorax

The causes of pneumothorax include trauma, central venous cannulation especially via the subclavian route, brachial plexus blockade, cervical and thoracic surgery, and barotrauma. Occasionally, pneumothorax may develop spontaneously in patients with asthma, chronic obstructive pulmonary disease, congenital cystic pulmonary disease or Marfan's syndrome. During anaesthesia, very high mechanically generated peak inspiratory airway pressures greatly increase the risk of pulmonary barotrauma and pneumothorax. Patients with recent chest trauma, asthma or chronic lung disease (particularly with bullae) are most at risk. Pneumothorax significantly reduces ventilation of the affected lung with resultant carbon dioxide retention. Simultaneously, pulmonary shunting often occurs, with resultant hypoxaemia.

Nitrous oxide diffuses into air-filled spaces more rapidly than nitrogen diffuses out, and causes pneumothoraces to expand. Mechanical ventilation forces gas into the pleural space if the lung has been punctured, with a rapid increase in the size of the pneumothorax. Increasing $\dot{V}/\dot{Q}$ mismatch and hypoxaemia follow. If the pneumothorax is under tension, hypoxaemia, mediastinal shift, reduced venous return and impairment of cardiac output may be life-threatening. A pneumothorax should be excluded during anaesthesia if unexplained tachycardia, hypotension, hypoxaemia, hypoventilation (in the spontaneously breathing patient) or high inflation pressures (in the ventilated patient) occur intraoperatively. Examination may reveal unequal air entry, asymmetrical chest movement, wheeze, surgical emphysema, elevated jugular or central venous pressure, or mediastinal shift. Chest X-ray examination provides a definitive diagnosis, but treatment should not be delayed for this investigation if severe hypoxaemia or hypotension exist and a pneumothorax is suspected.

Management. If pneumothorax is suspected prior to anaesthesia, then it should be excluded by chest X-ray. A chest X-ray should be performed preoperatively in all patients who have suffered recent chest trauma and in those in whom a central venous catheter has recently been inserted. Occasionally a chest X-ray fails to show a small pneumothorax which may expand rapidly with the use of nitrous oxide and positive-pressure ventilation. In patients with recent chest trauma, including rib fractures, regional analgesia may be the preferred technique. If tracheal intubation and mechanical ventilation are required in a patient with a pneumothorax, a chest drain should be inserted before induction of anaesthesia. If there is a chest drain *in situ*, its patency and position should be checked before induction of anaesthesia.

If a pneumothorax is suspected intraoperatively, *treatment should not be delayed to confirm the diagnosis by chest X-ray examination.* Administration of nitrous oxide should be discontinued and the lungs ventilated with 100% oxygen, using low inflation pressures. The presence of air in the pleural space may be confirmed by careful aspiration through an intravenous cannula inserted through the chest wall on the suspected side via the second intercostal space in the mid-clavicular line or in the fifth space in the mid-axillary line. If the pneumothorax is under tension, there may be a hiss as air is released. Temporary decompression using one or more large intravenous cannulae may be life-saving. If a pneumothorax is confirmed, the intravenous cannula should be left in place while a formal chest drain is inserted.

The presence of a bronchopleural fistula with substantial air leak may make ventilation ineffective. In this situation, hypoventilation ensues, resulting in carbon dioxide retention. A tension pneumothorax may result. The affected lung may be isolated by insertion of a bronchial tube (either single- or double-lumen) or gas exchange improved by the use of high-frequency ventilation. A chest drain allows decompression of the pneumothorax.

Atelectasis

The reduction in functional residual capacity and the tendency to hypoventilation which occur during general anaesthesia make alveolar collapse, or atelectasis, common. Atelectasis causes impairment of gas exchange and increases the risk of postoperative chest infection. Risk factors for its development include pre-existing lung disease, lengthy anaesthesia, spontaneous ventilation, high abdominal pressures, high inspired oxygen fractions and the head-down position. Extended exposure of the open airway to atmospheric pressure adds significantly to the risk of alveolar collapse. In particular, prolonged apnoea during anaesthesia (e.g. while awaiting the onset of spontaneous ventilation) causes atelectasis.

Management. Atelectasis may be reduced through the use of mechanical ventilation during lengthy operations, the incorporation of nitrogen into the inspired gas mixture, the use of a head-up position where possible and the use of PEEP during mechanical ventilation or continuous positive airways pressure (CPAP) during spontaneous ventilation. If atelectasis is suspected (usually through observation of a gradual downward drift in arterial oxygen saturation or a gradual increase in peak inspiratory pressure during mechanical ventilation), several gentle manual hyperinflations of the lungs usually re-inflate the collapsed alveoli (alveolar recruitment) and result in an increase in arterial oxygen saturation. Inflation for up to 20 s at 40 cmH$_2$O is often required for a successful recruitment manoeuvre. Such a recruitment manoeuvre is probably best performed using a mechanical ventilator.

If atelectasis becomes established during general anaesthesia, then the patient is at increased risk of pulmonary dysfunction postoperatively. In this situation, the provision of good analgesia (to encourage coughing and mobilization), use of the sitting position and physiotherapy reduce postoperative morbidity.

Cardiovascular Complications

Hypertension

Intraoperative hypertension may be defined as an arterial pressure (systolic, mean or diastolic) 25% greater than the patient's preoperative value. Systolic hypertension increases myocardial work by increasing afterload and left ventricular wall tension. It is often associated with tachycardia, which places additional metabolic demands on the myocardium. Patients with ischaemic heart disease or left ventricular hypertrophy may be placed at risk of myocardial ischaemia or infarction. Chronic hypertension is associated with impaired organ perfusion through atherosclerosis. Acute intraoperative hypertension increases the risks of ischaemia, infarction and haemorrhage in other organs, and in particular, the brain.

Table 43.6 shows the commonest causes of hypertension during anaesthesia. In the absence of pre-existing hypertension, the majority of instances of intraoperative hypertension are related to increased activity of the sympathetic nervous system. This may be associated with tachycardia and arrhythmias. The commonest causes of hypertension are inadequate analgesia, light anaesthesia, surgical stimulation and airway manipulation. Drug administration errors are probably under-recognised underlying causes. However, all instances of intraoperative hypertension must prompt exclusion of awareness and malignant hyperthermia as the cause.

Management. Preoperative preparation reduces the incidence of unexpected intraoperative hypertension. Adequate pharmacological treatment of chronic hypertension is essential. Poorly controlled chronic hypertension may result in exaggerated vascular responses during anaesthesia and these patients may suffer greater intraoperative and postoperative morbidity and mortality from arrhythmias and myocardial ischaemia. A calm, relaxed patient is less likely to experience intraoperative hypertension, so consideration should be given to anxiolytic premedication. Where

TABLE 43.6
Causes of Hypertension During Anaesthesia

Pre-Existing

Undiagnosed or poorly controlled hypertension
Pregnancy-induced hypertension
Withdrawal of antihypertensive medication

Increased Sympathetic Tone

Inadequate analgesia
Inadequate anaesthesia
Hypoxaemia
Airway manipulation (laryngoscopy, extubation)
Hypercapnia

Drug Overdose

Vasoconstrictors (noradrenaline, phenylephrine)
Inotropes (dobutamine)
Mixed inotropes/vasoconstrictors (adrenaline, ephedrine)
Ketamine
Ergometrine

Other

Aortic cross-clamping
Phaeochromocytoma
Malignant hyperthermia

possible, surgery should be postponed until adequate control is achieved (e.g. arterial pressure less than 180/110 mmHg) and organ function (e.g. heart and kidneys) assessed. If end-organ damage is found, it should be investigated, treated and the perioperative risk re-assessed. In the absence of such damage, anaesthesia and surgery can usually proceed. There is some evidence that beta blockade, alpha$_2$ agonists or thoracic epidural block may aid cardiovascular stability.

Stimulating events during anaesthesia and surgery cause surges in sympathetic tone, with significant increases in arterial pressure. These events may usually be anticipated and a short-acting opioid (e.g. alfentanil $10 \mu g\, kg^{-1}$), β-blocker (e.g. esmolol $0.5\, mg\, kg^{-1}$), lidocaine ($1\, mg\, kg^{-1}$) or temporary deepening of the anaesthetic may be used to obtund potentially damaging hypertension. Such events include laryngoscopy, surgical incision, extubation and aortic cross-clamping. Hypertension which occurs despite normoxaemia, adequately deep anaesthesia and adequate analgesia should prompt the exclusion of the causes listed in Table 43.6. If no pathological cause is found, the use of an antihypertensive agent such as labetalol or hydralazine may be indicated. The effect of negatively inotropic and vasodilating drugs is potentiated by anaesthetic agents, so careful titration is required.

Hypotension

During anaesthesia, hypotension is usefully defined as a mean arterial pressure 25% less than the patient's usual, resting value. Hypotension may impair perfusion and, consequently, oxygenation of vital organs. During anaesthesia, myocardial and cerebral metabolic rates are reduced significantly, and intraoperative hypotension is less likely to cause permanent damage to these organs than would be the case in the conscious state. However, pathological processes (e.g. atherosclerosis) commonly compromise the arterial supply to organs, and hypotension during anaesthesia occasionally results in critical loss of flow to vital organs. Left ventricular coronary artery flow occurs predominantly in diastole, and diastolic arterial pressure is particularly important in determining myocardial viability in patients with ischaemic heart disease.

Hypotension is caused by decreases in cardiac output or systemic vascular resistance. Table 43.7 shows the common causes of intraoperative hypotension. Most anaesthetic agents cause vasodilatation and have

TABLE 43.7

Causes of Hypotension During Anaesthesia

Decreased Cardiac Output

Decreased preload	Hypovolaemia	Inadequate preoperative resuscitation
		Gastrointestinal fluid loss
		Haemorrhage
	Obstruction	Pulmonary embolus
		Aorto-caval compression (surgery, pregnancy, tumour)
		Pericardial effusion/tamponade
	Raised intrathoracic pressure	Mechanical ventilation, PEEP
		Pneumothorax
	Head-up position	
Myocardial	Reduced contractility	Drugs (most anaesthetic agents, β-blockers, calcium antagonists)
		Acidosis
		Ischaemia/infarction
		Arrhythmias
		Pericardial tamponade

Decreased Afterload

Drugs	Relative or absolute overdose (most anaesthetic agents, antihypertensives)
	Hypersensitivity (drugs, colloids, blood)
	Direct histamine release (morphine, atracurium)
	Central regional blockade (local anaesthetics)
Sepsis/Systemic inflammatory response syndrome	

a negative inotropic effect, and moderate hypotension is very common during anaesthesia, particularly before the start of surgery when there is no physical stimulation to counteract the effects of anaesthetic drugs. Concurrent hypovolaemia caused by preoperative fluid restriction, in combination with haemorrhage or concurrent antihypertensive drugs, may result in decreases in mean arterial pressure during anaesthesia and surgery. A mean arterial pressure of 50 mmHg or less is potentially damaging, even in healthy individuals, and should not be allowed to persist. The patients most at risk from the effects of hypotension are, unfortunately, often the patients most likely to develop it because of concurrent medications, poor myocardial reserve and atherosclerosis. Elderly or hypertensive patients should, therefore, be observed carefully for the development of hypotension, and it should be treated promptly.

Management. Preoperative correction of hypovolaemia helps to avoid excessive reduction in arterial pressure following induction of anaesthesia. The cardiovascular effects of anaesthetic agents are predictable, and judicious doses of drugs should be used.

Artefactual measurements are not uncommon when using oscillometric devices to measure arterial pressure. If intraoperative hypotension occurs and the measurement is validated, then a working diagnosis should be established and treatment should be commenced, aimed at correcting the cause of the hypotension. Most commonly, this involves administering intravenous fluids or decreasing the concentration or infusion rate of anaesthetic agents, although care must be taken to ensure delivery of sufficient anaesthetic agent to avoid awareness. This treatment is effective in most patients. Persistent hypotension, where significant pathological causes (e.g. arrhythmia, anaphylaxis, concealed haemorrhage or pneumothorax) have been excluded, may be treated with a cautious dose of a vasopressor agent (e.g. ephedrine 5 mg or metaraminol 1 mg). Treatment of hypotension should follow the sequence of assess→treat→re-assess. Unexpected responses to treatment should prompt a re-evaluation of the diagnosis and suspected aetiology.

Hypovolaemia

Hypovolaemia is a common intraoperative cause of hypotension. Its common aetiologies are listed in Table 43.8. The additive effects of anaesthesia, positive-pressure ventilation and hypovolaemia may cause sudden and severe hypotension, which may be life-threatening. All patients who are undergoing surgery, and in particular patients who require emergency surgery, should be assessed preoperatively with regard to intravascular fluid volume and fluid balance. Signs of hypovolaemia include thirst, dryness of mucous membranes, cool peripheries, oliguria (urine output $<0.5\,mL\,kg^{-1}\,h^{-1}$), reduced tissue turgor, tachycardia and

---

TABLE 43.8

Causes of Hypovolaemia and Fluid Loss

Preoperative

Haemorrhage
  Trauma
  Obstetric
  Gastrointestinal
  Major vessel rupture (aortic aneurysm)

Gastrointestinal
  Vomiting
  Obstruction
  Fistulae
  Diarrhoea

Other
  Fasting
  Diuretics
  Fever
  Burns

Intraoperative

Haemorrhage

Insensible loss
  Sweating
  Expired water vapour

Third-space loss
  Prolonged procedures
  Extensive surgery
  Prolonged retraction

Drainage of stomach, bowel, or ascites

---

postural hypotension. Patients treated with a β-blocking drug may not develop a compensatory tachycardia despite being hypovolaemic. Fluid deficit and replacement are easily underestimated, especially in patients with intestinal obstruction or concealed haemorrhage. Surgery, unless immediately life-saving, should be delayed to allow adequate fluid resuscitation and restoration of intravascular volume. The response of central venous pressure (CVP) to fluid challenges is a useful guide when assessing and treating patients with significant hypovolaemia. Hypokalaemia and other electrolyte abnormalities are often associated with fluid deficits, particularly when there have been gastrointestinal losses.

In the presence of hypovolaemia, hypotension after induction of anaesthesia is often exaggerated in the elderly and in patients with decreased cardiac reserve or pre-existing hypertension. It is made less likely by fluid preloading and by titration of the induction agent to effect. Etomidate and ketamine produce less cardiovascular depression than do other induction agents.

Blood loss during surgery may be concealed. The anaesthetist must note carefully the total loss in suction jars, swabs and spillage. Body water is lost during anaesthesia and surgery in urine, sweat and exhaled breath. Adequate intraoperative fluid replacement must account for all of these losses. During abdominal surgery, up to $5\,mL\,kg^{-1}\,h^{-1}$ may be required to replace evaporative and third-space losses in addition to maintenance requirements and replacement of blood loss.

Haemorrhage

Haemorrhage is the loss of blood and is inevitable during most forms of surgery. Loss of a significant proportion of the total intravascular volume threatens the patient's well-being. Hypovolaemia causes reduced tissue perfusion, while loss of red cell mass causes reduced oxygen carriage in arterial blood. There is no *safe* degree of haemorrhage, in that patients differ in their ability to tolerate blood loss. Anaemic or hypovolaemic patients are less able to compensate for haemorrhage than healthy patients. Patients with pre-existing compromise of vital organ perfusion (e.g. patients with diabetes mellitus or hypertension) suffer deleterious consequences of haemorrhage sooner than healthy patients. In general, adults who have lost 15% of circulating blood volume may require red blood cell transfusion to maintain oxygen-carrying capacity.

Blood loss can be estimated by weighing swabs, measuring the volume of blood in suction bottles and assessing the clinical response to fluid therapy. Estimation is often difficult if large volumes of irrigation fluid have been used, e.g. during transurethral resection of the prostate. Intraoperative measurement of haemoglobin concentration aids estimation of blood loss and guides therapy. With severe or ongoing haemorrhage, maintenance of intravascular volume is essential. When the cardiac output is preserved, very severe anaemia is often well tolerated for short periods, but low tissue blood flow in the presence of anaemia may produce rapid and irreversible organ damage.

Massive blood loss may require the administration of stored blood, fresh frozen plasma, clotting factors and electrolytes. The problems of massive transfusion are discussed in Chapter 13.

Disturbances of Heart Rate

Bradycardia. Bradycardia is commonly defined as a heart rate less than 60 beat min^{-1}. Heart rate very commonly decreases during anaesthesia because much afferent input is lost and because many anaesthetic agents and opioids have parasympathomimetic actions. Surgical manipulations such as traction on the eye, cervical or anal dilatation and peritoneal traction may increase vagal tone, producing bradycardia and occasionally sinus arrest. Several drugs may cause bradycardia. Succinylcholine may produce a profound decrease in heart rate, especially following repeat doses. Bradycardia occurs in some patients after intravenous injection of rapidly acting opioid analgesics such as remifentanil, alfentanil and fentanyl. There have been several reports of profound bradycardia in association with the use of propofol. Finally, neostigmine and β-blockers may cause profound bradycardia. Anaesthesia-induced bradycardia often leads to an *escape* rhythm, with a wandering suprajunctional pacemaker. Hypothermia and hypothyroidism can also cause bradycardia.

Bradycardia reduces cardiac output, although the longer diastolic filling time and lower afterload may result in a larger ejection fraction. Diastolic pressure usually decreases and, consequently, myocardial perfusion is reduced. The concurrent reduction in myocardial oxygen demand protects against myocardial ischaemia, and myocardial damage caused by

bradycardia is very rare. However, other organs may suffer; in particular, the brain, kidneys and liver may become ischaemic if a very low heart rate is allowed to persist.

Management. Healthy patients usually tolerate a heart rate of 30 beat min^{-1} without organ damage. Patients with impaired organ perfusion or impaired oxygen carriage may not tolerate such low heart rates well. The risk of sinus arrest or asystole is heightened at this low rate, and most anaesthetists treat bradycardia if the heart rate decreases to 40 beat min^{-1} or less. Bradycardia becomes particularly significant if associated with significant hypotension. Bradycardia may be treated by administration of an anticholinergic, antimuscarinic agent such as glycopyrronium or atropine. If bradycardia is refractory to antimuscarinic agents, intravenous isoprenaline or cardiac pacing may be indicated. Atropine or glycopyrronium may be given prophylactically in operations in which surgical stimulation increases the risk of bradycardia (e.g. ophthalmic surgery) or before a second dose of succinylcholine.

Tachycardia. During anaesthesia, tachycardia may be defined as a heart rate greater than 100 beat min^{-1}. Tachycardia is a normal sign of increased sympathetic nervous system activity. It is observed in most patients at some time during the perioperative period. Sympathetic nervous system activity is increased by hypoxaemia, hypercapnia, inadequate anaesthesia, inadequate analgesia, hypovolaemia, hypotension and noxious stimulation such as airway manipulations or surgical incision. Other signs of sympathetic nervous activity may be present, including hypertension. Tachycardia is associated also with an increase in metabolic rate (e.g. fever, sepsis, burns, hyperthyroidism, malignant hyperthermia), or the administration of vagolytic drugs (e.g. atropine, pancuronium) or sympathomimetic drugs (e.g. ephedrine, adrenaline). Isoflurane and desflurane may also increase heart rate, particularly if introduced rapidly in a high concentration. Tachycardia reduces diastolic coronary perfusion and simultaneously increases myocardial work. This may precipitate myocardial ischaemia in patients with coronary artery or hypertensive heart disease.

Management. The cause of the tachycardia should be determined and treated, e.g. by providing additional analgesia, deepening anaesthesia or giving intravenous fluids for hypovolaemia. Sinus tachycardia may be associated with myocardial ischaemia despite exclusion or treatment of other causes. In this situation, the tachycardia may be controlled by careful intravenous titration of a β-blocker such as esmolol.

Arrhythmia. Arrhythmias are not infrequent during anaesthesia, and common causes are listed in Table 43.9. Extracellular potassium concentration has a profound effect on myocardial electrical activity. Hypokalaemia increases ventricular irritability and the risks of ventricular ectopics, tachycardia and fibrillation. This effect is potentiated in patients with ischaemic heart disease and in those receiving digoxin. Hyperventilation alters acid–base balance, with acute transmembrane redistribution of potassium. Serum potassium concentration decreases by approximately

---

TABLE 43.9

Causes of Arrhythmias During Anaesthesia

Cardiorespiratory

Hypoxaemia
Hypotension
Hypocapnia
Hypercapnia
Myocardial ischaemia

Metabolic

Catecholamines:
  Inadequate analgesia
  Inadequate anaesthesia
  Airway manipulation
Sympathomimetics
Hyperthyroidism
Electrolyte disturbance:
  Hypokalaemia/hyperkalaemia
  Hypercalcaemia/hypocalcaemia
Malignant hyperthermia

Surgical

Increased vagal tone (traction on eye, anus, peritoneum)
Direct cardiac stimulation (chest surgery, CVP cannulae)
Dental surgery

Drugs

Vagolytics (atropine, pancuronium)
Sympathomimetics (adrenaline, ephedrine)
Volatile anaesthetic agents (halothane, enflurane)
Digoxin

$1\,mmol\,L^{-1}$ for every 2.5 kPa reduction in $PaCO_2$. Life-threatening hyperkalaemia with atrioventricular conduction block or ventricular fibrillation may occur if succinylcholine is used in patients with burns or denervating injuries. Electrolyte disorders are discussed further in Chapter 12.

Management. Preoperative correction of fluid, electrolyte and acid–base imbalance is essential. Optimization of coronary artery disease and hypertension is also helpful in avoiding intraoperative arrhythmias (Ch 18).

Continuous intraoperative ECG monitoring is mandatory during anaesthesia because arrhythmias are so common. Lead II best demonstrates atrial activity and its use is recommended for routine ECG monitoring. As the ECG gives no indication of cardiac output or tissue perfusion, the detection of an abnormal cardiac rhythm should be followed by rapid assessment of the circulation. An absent pulse, severe hypotension or ventricular tachycardia or fibrillation should be treated as a cardiac arrest. The anaesthetist must exclude hypoxaemia, hypotension, inadequate analgesia and light anaesthesia as possible causes of arrhythmia. Correction of the precipitating factor is often the only treatment required. If the arrhythmia persists and causes a significant decrease in cardiac output, if it is associated with myocardial ischaemia or if it predisposes to ventricular tachycardia or fibrillation, intervention with a specific antiarrhythmic agent or electrical cardioversion is indicated. Serum potassium concentration should be measured if ventricular arrhythmias occur, especially if the patient is receiving digoxin.

Atrial Arrhythmias. These may reduce the atrial contribution to left ventricular filling, resulting in a decrease in cardiac output. Premature atrial contractions and wandering atrial pacemakers are common and of little consequence.

Junctional rhythm is associated usually with the use of halothane. Reduction in concentration or change of volatile agent is indicated. Administration of an anticholinergic drug may be required to restore sinus rhythm.

Accelerated nodal rhythm may be precipitated by an increase in sympathetic tone in the presence of a sensitizing volatile anaesthetic agent. Adjusting the depth of anaesthesia or changing the anaesthetic agent is appropriate treatment.

Supraventricular tachycardia (SVT) may occur at any time during the perioperative period in susceptible patients, such as those with Wolff–Parkinson–White or other 'pre-excitation' syndromes. If attempts to increase vagal tone and terminate the SVT by carotid sinus or eyeball massage are unsuccessful, the treatment of choice is adenosine by rapid intravenous injection. This is safe and effective during haemodynamic instability because its duration of action is less than 60 s. It blocks atrioventricular conduction without compromising ventricular function. Adenosine should not be given to patients with asthma or atrioventricular conduction block. If adenosine is unavailable and the patient is normotensive, intravenous verapamil or esmolol may be given in increments. Verapamil may cause prolonged hypotension and depression of ventricular function, especially in the presence of anaesthetic agents which cause myocardial depression; β-blockers should not be used in conjunction with verapamil because of their unpredictable synergy, which may result in profound bradycardia. DC cardioversion is indicated if the SVT is associated with hypotension and adenosine is unavailable.

Atrial flutter or fibrillation may be observed during anaesthesia *de novo* or as a paroxysmal increase in ventricular rate in patients with pre-existing atrial flutter or fibrillation. After correcting any precipitating factors, rate control with a beta-blocker is the usual first choice. Digoxin may be appropriate for patients with heart failure. Amiodarone may also be used. Immediate cardioversion should be considered if the ventricular rate is fast with a significant reduction in cardiac output.

Ventricular Arrhythmias. *Premature ventricular contractions* (PVCs) are common in healthy patients and may be present preoperatively. If associated with a slow atrial rate (escape beats), increasing the sinus rate by administration of an anticholinergic drug should abolish them. In other situations, an underlying cause should be sought before antiarrhythmic agents are considered, as PVCs rarely progress to more serious arrhythmias unless they are multifocal and frequent or if there is underlying myocardial ischaemia or hypoxaemia. Halothane lowers the threshold for catecholamine-induced ventricular arrhythmias, and

this effect is exacerbated by hypercapnia. Halothane should be used with care in patients receiving sympathomimetic drugs (including local anaesthetics containing adrenaline) and in patients taking aminophylline or drugs that block noradrenaline re-uptake, such as tricyclic or other antidepressants. The maximum recommended dose of adrenaline for infiltration in the presence of halothane is 100 μg (10 mL of 1 in 100 000) during any 10-min period, although the rate of absorption depends on the site of injection. The use of isoflurane carries a much lower risk of development of arrhythmias and sevoflurane has an even lower potential to cause myocardial sensitization to catecholamines.

Heart block. Impulses from the atria may be variably conducted to the ventricles. Degrees of impairment range from a small time delay in onward transmission to complete failure of onward propagation of impulses. Heart block may result in bradycardia and reduced cardiac output. Treatment is seldom necessary during anaesthesia, but minor degrees of atrioventricular block may progress to complete heart block, in which atrial impulses do not reach the ventricles. In this situation, bradycardia is usually severe and the atria no longer assist in filling the ventricles before ventricular systole. Cardiac output may fall to life-threateningly low levels, and immediate treatment is necessary. This includes intravenous isoprenaline and transcutaneous or transvenous cardiac pacing.

Ventricular tachycardia is uncommon during anaesthesia. If it is not causing significant hypotension, current ALS guidelines recommend amiodarone 300 mg i.v. over 20-60 min followed by 900 mg over 24 hr. DC cardioversion may be required if the patient is unstable. Ventricular tachycardia with no cardiac output should be treated according to ALS guidelines for cardiac arrest.

Ventricular fibrillation is very uncommon in association with anaesthesia. It requires immediate DC cardioversion.

Any arrhythmia which causes the loss of a palpable pulse should be treated as for cardiac arrest, with immediate external (or internal, if appropriate) cardiac massage, ventilation of the lungs with 100% oxygen and drug treatment as specified in the appropriate Advanced Life Support protocol (see Ch 47).

Myocardial Ischaemia

The heart has the highest oxygen consumption per tissue mass of almost all the organs (second only to the carotid body). Resting coronary blood flow is $250 \, \text{mL min}^{-1}$ and represents 5% of the cardiac output. The oxygen extraction ratio of the myocardium is 70–80%, compared with an average of 25% for other tissues. Increased oxygen consumption must be matched by an increase in coronary blood flow. Ischaemia results when the oxygen demand outstrips supply. Even very brief reductions in supply result in ischaemia, which may lead rapidly to infarction and permanent loss of muscle function in the affected area.

Myocardial oxygen delivery is the product of arterial oxygen content and coronary artery blood flow. The diastolic pressure time index (DPTI) reflects coronary blood supply. It is the product of the coronary perfusion pressure (predominantly diastolic arterial pressure) and diastolic time. Oxygen demand is represented by the tension time index (TTI), the product of systolic pressure and systolic time.

The ratio of DPTI/TTI is the endocardial viability ratio (EVR) and represents the myocardial oxygen supply–demand balance. The EVR is usually greater than one. A value of less than 0.7 is associated with subendocardial ischaemia. Such a value may be reached in a patient with the data shown in Table 43.10.

It is clear from the above that tachycardia is particularly dangerous in generating myocardial ischaemia, while systolic hypertension and diastolic hypotension may also contribute. Patients with coronary artery disease are most at risk. Intraoperative myocardial ischaemia may manifest clinically as arrhythmia, hypotension or pulmonary oedema. It is diagnosed by ECG ST-segment changes (usually depression), although these are not always detected reliably without computer-assisted analysis. The use of the V5 electrode is recommended for ECG monitoring in susceptible patients (e.g. the CM5 configuration; see Ch 16) because it is the most sensitive ECG lead for the detection of left ventricular ischaemia. When used alone, it may detect up to 85% of the ST abnormalities on a standard 12-lead ECG.

Transoesophageal echocardiography may detect abnormal myocardial wall motion, which is a sensitive indicator of ischaemia and is associated with increased perioperative morbidity. Regional wall dysfunction often persists into the postoperative period without clinical signs. Increased myocardial work during this period (e.g. from pain) may precipitate further ischaemia or infarction in susceptible patients. While the risk of infarction in the general surgical population is low, the overall mortality rate following perioperative myocardial infarction approaches 50%.

Management. Preoperative preparation of the at-risk patient includes optimization of anti-anginal and antihypertensive medication, suppression of anxiety and assurance of normal intravascular volume. During anaesthesia, the risks associated with ischaemia are minimized by the use of an appropriate anaesthetic technique and early detection by the use of appropriate monitoring in susceptible patients.

If ischaemia is detected, arterial oxygen content should be increased by optimizing PaO_2 and haemoglobin concentration. Tachycardia should be controlled by ensuring that analgesia, anaesthesia and intravascular volume are satisfactory. If systolic hypertension, diastolic hypotension or tachycardia exist, then these may be controlled pharmacologically; most commonly, increments of a vasodilator or β-blocker are administered to treat hypertension or tachycardia. If signs of myocardial ischaemia persist, the use of a venodilator such as glyceryl trinitrate by intravenous infusion should be considered.

TABLE 43.10	
Patient Data Generating a Dangerously Low Endocardial Viability Ratio	
Arterial pressure:	180/90 mmHg
Heart rate (HR):	130 beat min^{-1}
LVEDP	10 mmHg
DPTI	= (90 − 10) mmHg × (60s/130 − 0.2 s) = 21 s mmHg
TTI	= 180 mmHg × 0.2 s = 36 s mmHg
EVR	= 0.58

Systolic time is typically fixed at 0.2 s, and diastole occupies the remaining time.

Embolus

An embolus is the passage of a non-blood mass through the vascular system. Venous emboli usually become lodged in the lung, where they impair gas exchange and cause a local inflammatory reaction. Arterial emboli cause obstruction, which may result in distal ischaemia.

Thromboembolus

Embolization of thrombus occurs usually from the deep veins of the legs or pelvis. It is uncommon during anaesthesia. It is often preceded by a period of immobilization, so that patients whose hospital stay is extended or who have suffered major trauma are at highest risk. Other risk factors include malignancy, smoking, pelvic and limb surgery, the oral contraceptive or hormone replacement therapy, and a past history of venous thromboembolism. Venous stasis caused by venous compression, hypovolaemia, hypotension, hypothermia or the use of tourniquets also increases the risk of deep venous thrombosis. Veins may sustain trauma during positioning and surgery, and increased blood coagulability, with a consequent increase in the risk of venous thrombosis, is a consequence of the stress response to surgery.

During anaesthesia, pulmonary thromboembolism may present with tachycardia, hypoxaemia, arrhythmia, hypotension, bronchospasm, an acute decrease in the end-tidal carbon dioxide concentration or cardiovascular collapse.

Management. Patients with risks factors should be managed actively to prevent deep venous thrombosis. The oral contraceptive pill or hormone replacement therapy should be stopped at least 6 weeks before elective surgery in patients at risk. Prophylactic heparin, graduated compression stockings and intraoperative intermittent calf compression reduce the likelihood of new thrombosis. The use of subarachnoid or epidural anaesthesia reduces the risk of postoperative venous thromboembolism in some surgical groups.

If intraoperative pulmonary embolism is suspected, the lungs should be ventilated with 100% oxygen and bronchodilator therapy, fluid loading and inotropic support of the circulation should be considered. In extreme presentations, cardiac arrest protocols should be used. After management of the initial haemodynamic disturbance, thrombolytic therapy (if not contraindicated), anticoagulation and, rarely, surgical removal of the embolus may be indicated.

Gas Embolus

Gas usually enters the circulation through a surgical wound. A subatmospheric venous pressure greatly encourages the entrainment of air into the venous system. Therefore, positions that place the operative site above the right atrium carry an increased risk of air embolism. Such positions include sitting, park bench, knee-chest and head-up. Vascular catheters are another potential route for air entry, particularly during their insertion. Gas embolism (usually carbon dioxide) may also occur during laparoscopy and thoracoscopy.

Clinical presentation varies with the volume and rate of gas entry into the circulation. An entry rate of $0.5\,mL\,kg^{-1}\,min^{-1}$ has been reported to produce clinical signs. If a significant volume of gas enters the right side of the heart, an airlock may develop, preventing ejection of blood and effectively halting cardiac output. A 'millwheel murmur' may be heard via a precordial or oesophageal stethoscope, although this is reported to be a late sign and only occurs with very large emboli. The sudden decrease in right ventricular output results in a rapid decrease in end-tidal carbon dioxide concentration. Hypoxaemia, tachycardia, ECG changes (especially arrhythmia) and an increase in pulmonary artery pressure follow.

Transoesophageal echocardiography and precordial Doppler ultrasound are the most sensitive monitors for gas embolus. Clinical and ECG signs have a low sensitivity for detection of gas embolism. As the foramen ovale is potentially patent in more than 25% of the population, an increase in right heart pressure may open the foramen in these patients. Paradoxical gas embolism via this route or across the pulmonary capillary bed to the coronary or cerebral circulations may cause myocardial or cerebral ischaemia and infarction.

Management. Prevention of intraoperative air embolus requires adjustment of the patient's position and the site of the operative field with respect to the right atrium. If air embolism is detected, further air entry is prevented by flooding the operative site with saline. During head and neck procedures, the venous pressure at the surgical site may be increased by compressing the jugular veins. If possible, the operative site should be lowered relative to the right atrium. The application of PEEP increases venous pressure and reduces further ingress of air.

During insufflation procedures, the surgeon should be instructed to depressurize the insufflated body cavity. If the gas embolus is symptomatic, administration of nitrous oxide should be discontinued to avoid expansion of gas bubbles and the lungs should be ventilated with 100% oxygen. Carbon dioxide is absorbed by tissues much more rapidly than air. Carbon dioxide embolism usually results in transient hypotension or cardiac arrest, whereas air embolism is often fatal.

Occasionally, gas may be aspirated from the right ventricle or atrium via a venous catheter. However, insertion of a catheter is usually impractical and time-consuming, and aspiration is only worth attempting if a catheter is already in place. Expansion of the intravascular fluid volume, inotropic support of the circulation and internal or external cardiac massage may be necessary. Placing the patient in a head-down left lateral position may help by allowing gas from the right ventricle to escape into the atrium and vena cava.

Other Emboli

Fat dislodged from long bone fractures may embolize to the lungs. Patients typically develop sudden mental disturbance, shortness of breath, hypoxaemia, and axillary and subconjunctival petechiae. Onset is usually 2–48 h after the injury. Fat globules may be seen in the urine and sputum, or in the retinal vessels during fundoscopy. There should be a high index of suspicion if unexpected haemodynamic events or hypoxaemia occur in patients undergoing surgery for pelvic or lower limb fractures. Treatment is with intravenous fluids, steroids and ventilatory support as necessary. The use of intravenous albumin to bind free fat is controversial.

Other material which may embolize includes tumour fragments, amniotic fluid and orthopaedic cement. Air or clot may embolize via arterial cannulae and produce distal ischaemia.

Neurological Complications

Awareness

Recall of intraoperative events occurs in 0.03–0.3% of anaesthetics. Such recall may be spontaneous, or may be provoked by postoperative events or questioning.

Awareness during anaesthesia may be a very distressing event for a patient, particularly if it is accompanied by awareness of the painful nature of an operation or the presence of paralysis. However, the majority of recalled events are not painful, and 80–90% of patients recalling intraoperative events have not experienced pain. Awareness may have psychological sequelae including insomnia, depression and post-traumatic stress disorder (PTSD) with distressing flashbacks.

The risk of awareness correlates with depth of anaesthesia. Light anaesthesia, particularly when the patient is paralysed by muscle relaxants, is associated with the highest risk of awareness. Awareness is associated frequently with poor anaesthetic technique. Errors include the omission or late commencement of volatile agent, inadequate dosing or failure to recognize the signs of awareness. Underdosing of anaesthetic agent may occur during hypotensive episodes, when anaesthetic is withheld in an attempt to maintain arterial pressure. Breathing system malfunctions, misconnections and disconnections have been associated with awareness.

The signs of awareness in a paralysed patient arise from activation of the sympathetic nervous system (sweating, tachycardia, hypertension, tear formation), and dilatation and reactivity to light of the pupils. Unparalysed patients experiencing noxious stimulation may move or grimace. Depth of anaesthesia may be assessed through clinical examination, monitoring of the patient's expired volatile agent concentration or using specialized monitoring equipment. Such equipment includes processed electroencephalography such as the bispectral index and auditory evoked potential monitoring systems. If the end-tidal concentrations of inhaled anaesthetic agents summate to a total of greater than about 0.8–0.9 MAC, it is exceptionally unlikely that a patient experiences intraoperative awareness.

Awareness is more likely to occur during emergency and obstetric surgery, during neuromuscular paralysis, during periods of hypotension and in patients treated with a β-blocker (which prevents tachycardia and hypertension). The use of intravenous drugs for maintenance of anaesthesia (e.g. propofol target-controlled infusion) may be associated with an increased risk of awareness compared with the use of inhaled anaesthetic agents. It is not possible currently to monitor, in real time, the concentration of intravenous agents in blood, while it is possible to monitor exhaled volatile agents. Additionally, the scatter about the mean of the minimum inhibitory concentration (MIC) for intravenous agents is greater than the equivalent for inhaled agents (MAC).

Management. If the anaesthetist suspects, intraoperatively, that a patient may be experiencing awareness, anaesthesia should be deepened immediately. If the arterial pressure is low despite an inadequate dose of anaesthetic agent, then the arterial pressure should be supported through the use of intravenous fluids, modification of ventilatory pattern or intravenous administration of a vasopressor, and anaesthesia deepened appropriately. Consideration should be given to the use of an intravenous benzodiazepine (e.g. midazolam 5 mg). Some retrograde amnesia *may* be gained and further recall is made less likely through the anterograde amnesic effect.

If a patient complains in the postoperative period of intraoperative awareness, the anaesthetist should be informed and should visit the patient. The anaesthetist should establish the timing of the episode and try to distinguish between dreaming and awareness. If there is genuine awareness and a clear anaesthetic error, then a prompt apology and explanation should be provided. All details should be recorded in the case notes. The situation may be exacerbated if staff refuse to believe the patient. It is essential to offer follow-up counselling for the patient and to inform the patient's general practitioner. See the *Medicolegal aspects of complications* section above for further detail of dealing with any subsequent formal complaints.

Awareness occasionally occurs despite apparently excellent practice and in the absence of equipment malfunction. Successful defence against litigation requires that the anaesthetist has made thorough records. It is advisable that the anaesthetist always records the timing (absolute and relative to surgery) and dose of anaesthetic agents (inhaled or intravenous).

Neurological Injury

Ischaemia of the Central Nervous System

Transient disruptions of central nervous system (CNS) perfusion and oxygenation are common during anaesthesia. However, prolonged reduction in oxygenation of the CNS may result in ischaemia or infarction. Ischaemic injury varies from minimal, focal dysfunction to stroke or death. The mechanism is related usually to hypoxaemia and/or hypotension. The risk of ischaemic brain damage related to hypotension is increased in patients with atherosclerosis, and, in particular, cerebrovascular disease. A history of previous transient ischaemic attacks or stroke makes CNS injury much more likely during anaesthesia. Rarely, intracerebral haemorrhage may occur during anaesthesia, with consequent local compression and downstream ischaemic injury. Although the risk is increased if arterial pressure has been very high, there have been reports of intracerebral haemorrhage during anaesthesia without episodes of hypertension. It is likely that previously undetected vascular abnormalities were present in these cases.

The cervical spinal cord may be damaged during tracheal intubation and positioning in patients with cervical spine instability from fractures, rheumatoid arthritis or congenital conditions such as Down's syndrome. Extreme rotation, flexion or extension of the neck may cause cerebral ischaemia because of vertebrobasilar insufficiency in susceptible patients. Ischaemic spinal cord injury may also occur during major vascular and spinal surgery, when the local arterial supply may be compromised.

Management. Hypoxaemia and hypotension should not be allowed to persist, particularly in patients at risk of CNS ischaemic injury. Severe hypocapnia should be avoided because of its potential for global cerebral vasoconstriction. Deep anaesthesia results in a greatly lowered cerebral metabolic rate, and this confers some protection against cerebral ischaemia.

Peripheral Nerve Injury

Peripheral nerves may be injured through hypotension and hypoxaemia, but they are far more resistant than is the CNS. Peripheral injuries occur more commonly because of poor positioning or direct injury during nerve blockade or vascular catheter placement. This topic is dealt with in more detail later in this chapter.

Temperature

Hypothermia

Body temperature very commonly decreases during anaesthesia. A decrease to a core temperature below 36 °C represents hypothermia. Hypothermia causes physiological derangement and increases perioperative morbidity (see also Ch 11).

Heat production is decreased during anaesthesia. Anaesthetic agents alter hypothalamic function, reduce metabolic rate, abolish behavioural responses to heat loss and abolish shivering. Heat loss increases during anaesthesia and surgery because of heat redistribution to the peripheries by vasodilatation and increased radiation by the exposure of large, moist surfaces. Evaporative heat loss is increased by ventilation of the lungs with cold dry gas, the use of wet packs and operations on open body cavities. Heat loss is exacerbated by low ambient temperature, and high air flow in the operating theatre promotes convective and evaporative loss. Irrigation and intravenous infusion of cold fluids are also associated with increased heat loss. The risks of hypothermia are greatest in neonates and infants, patients with a low metabolic rate (such as the elderly) and patients with burns.

The effects of hypothermia are dependent upon the change in core temperature. Metabolic rate reduces by approximately 10% for each 1 °C reduction in core temperature. Cardiac output decreases and the affinity of haemoglobin for oxygen is increased, causing a reduction in tissue oxygenation. Significant hypothermia is associated with metabolic (lactic) acidosis, oliguria, altered platelet and clotting function, and reduced hepatic blood flow with slower drug metabolism. The MAC of volatile agents is reduced (also by approximately 10% for each 1 °C decrease) and muscle relaxants have a longer and more variable duration of effect. Postoperative shivering increases oxygen consumption and myocardial work. Peripheral vasoconstriction increases afterload, further increasing the risk of myocardial ischaemia. Hypothermia also increases the risk of postoperative infections because of suppression of function of the immune system.

Management. Ambient temperature and humidity should be maintained as high as is comfortable for staff working in the operating theatre. The patient should be protected from the cool ambient environment during all phases of anaesthesia and during transfers. A convective warming blanket (e.g. Bair Hugger™), which surrounds the patient with a microenvironment of warm air, is particularly effective. The head and any exposed moist viscera lose heat particularly quickly and wrapping these is effective in preventing radiation and evaporative heat loss. Cold intravenous fluids should be warmed where possible, although this should not compromise the administration of adequate volumes. Inspired gases should be warmed and humidified. A heat and moisture exchanging device is very effective in this regard, and is often combined with a microbial filter.

In all but very short operations, the measures described above should be started as soon as possible after induction of anaesthesia, and core temperature should be monitored both to detect hypothermia and to adjust the warming devices to prevent hyperthermia developing. If core temperature remains significantly below 35 °C at the end of surgery, consideration should be given to keeping the patient anaesthetized until temperature is normalized. This applies particularly to patients with cardiovascular or cerebrovascular disease, or metabolic abnormalities.

Induced deep hypothermia (as low as 16 °C) may be used for neurosurgical, aortic or cardiac procedures in which circulatory arrest is required to provide the necessary operating conditions. Large reductions in the metabolic rate reduce tissue oxygen consumption and allow a short period of circulatory arrest. Hypothermia reduces cerebral oxygen consumption and is used in the management of severe head injury or after cerebral hypoxic/ischaemic events.

Hyperthermia

Hyperthermia during anaesthesia may be defined as a core body temperature greater than 37.5 °C and is usually caused by an increase in heat production. Common causes include sepsis and infection, drug reactions (anaphylaxis, incompatible blood transfusion), excessive catecholamine activity (phaeochromocytoma, thyroid storm) and malignant hyperthermia. Elevated metabolic rate may lead to acidosis. Without treatment, sweating and vasodilatation produce hypovolaemia and tissue hypoxia. Seizures and CNS damage may ensue.

Management. General measures include exposure of the body surface, application of ice packs, use of fans and administration of cold intravenous fluids. Specific measures depend on the cause. Paracetamol and non-steroidal anti-inflammatory agents may reduce core temperature if the cause is sepsis-related. The occurrence of any unexplained increase in temperature, especially if temperature is increasing rapidly, must prompt the urgent exclusion of malignant hyperthermia.

Malignant Hyperthermia

Malignant hyperthermia (MH) is an inherited disorder of muscle. The incidence varies geographically from 0.02% to 0.002% (1 in 5000 to 1 in 50 000). MH had a mortality rate of 75% at the time it was identified in 1960. Treatment consisted of cooling the patient and treating complications as they arose. The cause was then unknown, and could not be treated. Currently, mortality is approximately 5%. Increased awareness amongst anaesthetists has resulted in earlier diagnosis and treatment. Since 1979, dantrolene has been available for the treatment of MH and has resulted in the dramatic decline in death and disability from the condition.

Malignant hyperthermia is an inherited disorder. Mutations in the human ryanodine receptor in skeletal muscle (a calcium-release channel with a role in excitation-contraction coupling) are apparent in some families. Predisposition to MH has been identified in only three rare clinical myopathies. Abnormal calcium release and re uptake by the sarcoplasmic reticulum lead to myofibrillar contraction, depletion of high-energy muscle phosphate stores, accelerated metabolic rate, increased carbon dioxide and heat production, increased oxygen consumption and metabolic acidosis. The usual triggering agents are succinylcholine or any volatile anaesthetic agent.

The MH syndrome may present at any time during the perioperative period. The clinical features and their severity vary considerably. The most consistent and early signs are unexplained tachycardia and an increase in the end-tidal PCO_2. Spontaneously breathing patients may present with tachypnoea. MH should be considered in any anaesthetized patient if core temperature increases during anaesthesia. Core temperature increases typically by $2\,^\circ C\ h^{-1}$ and may exceed $40\,^\circ C$. Muscle rigidity is common and usually involves the limbs and jaw. Without treatment, the full MH syndrome may develop, with sweating, cyanosis, mottled skin, hypoxaemia, ventricular arrhythmias and severe metabolic and respiratory acidosis. Muscle injury causes significant potassium release, with ECG signs of hyperkalaemia. Coagulopathy hypocalcaemia, oliguria, myoglobinuria and acute renal failure are other sequelae.

Masseter muscle rigidity (MMR) occasionally complicates anaesthesia, particularly following administration of succinylcholine. This progresses to MH in approximately 10% of cases.

Management. Administration of a volatile anaesthetic agent should be discontinued immediately and the lungs hyperventilated with 100% oxygen. The anaesthetic breathing system should be replaced with an unused (and therefore uncontaminated) system. Anaesthesia should be maintained with an intravenous agent. The trachea should be intubated at the earliest opportunity if a tracheal tube is not already in place. Experienced help should be obtained in both the operating theatre and the laboratory, and the operation must be abandoned as soon as possible. Specific tasks should be allocated (e.g. preparation of dantrolene, monitoring, managing communication with lab etc.). Intravenous dantrolene should be given as an immediate bolus (2.5 mg/kg). Further boluses of 1 mg/kg should be given as required to a maximum of 10 mg/kg until the increase in $P_E'CO_2$ is controlled. Dantrolene is packaged as a powder which takes several minutes to reconstitute. For a 70 kg adult, the intial dose would be 9 vials of dantrolene (20 mg each), mixed with 60 mL sterile water. It is a skeletal muscle relaxant and causes muscle weakness in large doses. The massive increase in metabolic rate commonly produces severe acidosis, and large amounts of intravenous fluids and sodium bicarbonate may be required. Ice packs should be placed around the neck, axillae and groin, and chilled saline should be infused intravenously. If necessary, gastric, rectal and peritoneal lavage with iced saline may be life-saving if hyperthermia is severe. Cardiopulmonary bypass has been used in severe cases.

Core temperature, CVP, direct arterial pressure and urine output should be monitored. Acid–base status, arterial gas tensions, coagulation status and serum electrolyte concentrations should be measured frequently. Hyperkalaemia is common, and should be treated with intravenous glucose and insulin. Arrhythmias usually resolve after treatment of hyperkalaemia and acidosis, but specific antiarrhythmic drugs may be required. Calcium channel blockers should be avoided due to their interaction with dantrolene. Renal hypoperfusion and medullary hypoxia may result rapidly in acute tubular necrosis. Urine output should be maintained by ensuring an adequate circulating blood volume and using intravenous mannitol. Haemofiltration may be required to correct severe biochemical abnormalities or renal dysfunction. The syndrome often persists beyond the initial acute episode, and hyperthermia may return up to 48 h later. The patient should be managed in a high-dependency area and oral dantrolene should be continued during this time.

Following an episode of MH, the patient should be referred to a specialist centre for further assessment. The tests used to identify individuals with MH susceptibility vary among centres. The most common test is halothane- and caffeine-induced contracture of a muscle specimen. Less invasive genetic tests are being developed. First-degree family members should also be screened for MH.

Anaesthesia for the MH-Susceptible Patient

A 'clean' anaesthetic machine is used, and this may be prepared by flushing the machine for 12 h with 100% oxygen and by using a new breathing system. Contact with volatile agents and succinylcholine is absolutely contraindicated. Regional anaesthesia should be used if possible. If general anaesthesia is unavoidable, then total intravenous anaesthesia with propofol is recommended. Dantrolene is not usually used as a premedicant, but should be immediately available throughout the perioperative period. Monitoring of end-tidal carbon dioxide concentration, ECG, arterial pressure, oxygen saturation and core temperature is mandatory.

Equipment Malfunction

About a third of all critical incidents are related to equipment failure and most are preventable. Most equipment problems have implications for the patient and some have been described above (e.g. leaks and disconnections involving the anaesthetic machine and gas delivery system). Meticulous preparation of equipment prevents most malfunctions, while a systematic approach to identifying problems as they arise should prevent most potentially serious complications.

Monitoring equipment may provide inaccurate and misleading data. Non-invasive arterial pressure devices and pulse oximeters often produce inaccurate readings. Movement, diathermy and poor contact with the patient may contribute to artefact in monitored values. Incorrect data may lead to incorrect treatment of the patient, and artefact must always be borne in mind as a cause for a sudden change to a value outside the acceptable range. Data supplied by monitors must always be used in conjunction with clinical examination of the patient and should be considered in context (e.g. type of surgery, patient's pre-existing illnesses).

Drug Reactions

Hypersensitivity

Susceptible patients may display an enhanced immunological reaction to a trigger, which may be a drug or an environmental agent. These *hypersensitivity* reactions may be anaphylactic or anaphylactoid. Some drugs produce histamine release directly, without an immunological basis.

The incidence of anaphylaxis varies according to the antigen involved. Of the intravenous drugs, reactions are most commonly to muscle relaxants (1 in 5000 to 1 in 10 000). Succinylcholine is the most immunogenic, although reactions to all non-depolarizing relaxants have also been reported. The majority of reactions are IgE-mediated. There is significant cross-reactivity between muscle relaxants and other drugs which contain a quaternary ammonium group. Pancuronium appears to be the least likely muscle relaxant to cause anaphylaxis.

Reactions to intravenous induction agents are far less common (1 in 15 000 to 1 in 50 000). Hypersensitivity to benzodiazepines and etomidate is rare and these drugs do not cause direct histamine release.

Hypersensitivity to local anaesthetics is very rare. Reactions are more likely to be the result of dose-related toxicity, sensitivity to the effects of added vasoconstrictor or a reaction to preservatives such as paraben, sulphites and benzoates. Amide local anaesthetic agents are less allergenic than esters.

Antibiotics are frequently implicated in allergic reactions. Penicillins are most often to blame, and there is cross-reactivity with cephalosporin antibiotics in 10% of penicillin-allergic patients.

Latex is emerging as one of the more important causes of anaphylaxis during anaesthesia and surgery. Reactions usually begin 30–60 min following exposure, and may be very severe. Previous frequent exposure to latex (e.g. spina bifida) is a strong risk factor for latex allergy. There is often a history of intolerance to some foods, including banana and avocado. Many medical devices contain latex (e.g. arterial pressure cuffs, surgical gloves), and it is important that all such products are eliminated from the care of latex-susceptible patients.

Anaphylaxis also occurs in response to radiocontrast media, blood products, colloid solutions, protamine, streptokinase, aprotinin, atropine, bone cement and opioids. Allergic reactions to volatile agents are exceptionally uncommon.

Anaphylaxis (type 1 hypersensitivity) is an IgE-mediated reaction to an antigen. Antibodies bind to mast cells, which degranulate, releasing the chemical mediators of anaphylaxis. These include histamine, prostaglandins, platelet-activating factor (PAF) and leukotrienes. The signs produced by the actions of these mediators of anaphylaxis include urticaria, cutaneous flushing, bronchospasm, hypotension, arrhythmia and cardiac arrest. *Only one of these signs may be present*, and it is important to have a high index of suspicion. Anaphylaxis has been reported in patients without apparent previous exposure to the specific antigen, probably because of immunological cross-reactivity. This is true particularly of reactions to muscle relaxants; cosmetics and some foods contain structurally similar compounds.

Anaphylactoid reactions are not IgE-mediated, although the clinical presentation is identical to anaphylaxis. The precise immunological mechanism is not always evident, although many reactions involve complement, kinin and coagulation pathway activation.

Non-immunological histamine release is caused by the direct action of a drug on mast cells. The clinical response depends on both the drug dose and the rate of delivery but is usually benign and confined to the skin. Anaesthetic drugs which release histamine directly include d-tubocurarine, atracurium, doxacurium, mivacurium (all of similar chemical derivation), morphine and pethidine. Clinical evidence of histamine release, usually cutaneous, occurs in up to 30% of patients during anaesthesia. However, some very serious reactions have been reported in association with administration of atracurium and mivacurium.

Hypersensitivity reaction should be considered in the differential diagnosis of any major cardiorespiratory problem during anaesthesia. Reactions are more common in women, and in patients with a history of allergy, atopy or previous exposure to anaesthetic agents. Over 90% of reactions occur immediately after induction of anaesthesia. There is a clinical spectrum of severity from the mildest urticaria to immediate cardiac arrest. Coughing, skin erythema, difficulty with ventilation and loss of a palpable pulse are common early signs. Reactions often involve a single, major physiological system (e.g. bradycardia and profound hypotension without bronchospasm). This may make diagnosis confusing, but every instance of bronchospasm, unexpected hypotension, arrhythmia or urticaria should be considered to be due to anaphylaxis until proved otherwise. Erythema of the skin may be short-lived or absent because cyanosis from poor tissue perfusion and hypoxaemia may occur rapidly and be profound. The conscious patient may experience a sense of impending doom, dyspnoea, dizziness, palpitations and nausea. The differential diagnosis includes anaesthetic drug overdose and other causes of bronchospasm, hypotension or hypoxaemia.

Management. Death may result from tissue hypoxia secondary to inadequate perfusion and/or hypoxaemia. Early recognition and treatment are essential. The aims of management are to obtund the effect of the anaphylaxis mediators and to prevent their further release. A management 'drill' should be used (Table 43.11). The early use of adrenaline is life-saving during severe anaphylactic reactions because it treats the symptoms (through peripheral vasoconstriction, increased cardiac output and bronchodilation) and the cause (through mast cell restabilization). Corticosteroids and histamine H_1-receptor antagonists have a delayed onset of action, but have a role in later management.

Anaphylaxis may persist, despite a promising initial response to management. Therefore, subsequent management should be in a critical care area (e.g. an intensive care unit). An infusion of adrenaline may be required to treat persistent hypotension or bronchospasm, and in the interests of preventing further mast cell degranulation. Progressive oedema involving the airway may develop rapidly and tracheal intubation

TABLE 43.11
Drill for the Management of Major Anaphylaxis

Initial Therapy

Stop administration of drug(s) likely to have caused the anaphylaxis
Call for help and note the time
Maintain airway. Give 100% oxygen
Lay patient supine with feet elevated
Give adrenaline. This may be given intramuscularly in a dose of 0.5 (0.5 of 1:1000) and may be repeated after 5 min according to the arterial pressure and pulse until improvement occurs. Alternatively, adrenaline may be administered intravenously. The dose given depends upon the severity of the reaction. Minor symptoms may be treated with 50 μg boluses, while cardiovascular collapse requires a bolus dose of 1000 μg. Further doses are likely to be required
Start intravascular volume expansion with crystalloid or colloid

Secondary Therapy

Antihistamines (chlorpheniramine 10 mg i.v.)
Corticosteroids (hydrocortisone 200 mg i.v.)
Catecholamine infusions (starting doses:
adrenaline 0.05–0.1 μg kg^{-1} min^{-1}
noradrenaline 0.05–0.1 μg kg^{-1} min^{-1})
Consider bicarbonate (0.5 mmol kg^{-1} i.v.) for acidosis, repeated as necessary
Airway evaluation (before extubation)
Bronchodilators (salbutamol 2.5 mg kg^{-1}) may be required for persistent bronchospasm

and mechanical ventilation of the lungs are recommended until the patient is clinically stable and airway patency guaranteed after a period of observation. Blood coagulation status, serum electrolyte concentrations and arterial gas tensions should also be measured regularly.

Venous blood samples (5–10 mL clotted blood) should be obtained as early in the reaction as possible, but resuscitation should not be delayed to take this sample. The most important sample is 1 h after the beginning of the reaction. A third sample at 24 hours or at the allergy clinic should be taken for 'baseline' tryptase levels. The samples should be separated and stored at −20 °C for subsequent measurement of serum tryptase concentration. Serum tryptase is a specific marker of mast cell degranulation, and has replaced the measurement of serum IgE as the test of choice for confirming a diagnosis of anaphylaxis. If death occurs, the serum tryptase concentration can be measured in blood taken at post mortem examination. This can be very helpful

in identifying the cause of death. However, a negative test does not exclude a hypersensitivity reaction.

The patient should be reviewed at a later date by an appropriate clinician (e.g. a clinical immunologist) and further investigations performed. Skin prick tests are recommended to identify the culpable agent and any associated cross-reactivity. Such cross-reactivity is commonly found when the reaction has been to muscle relaxants, and the patient is frequently allergic to several related compounds. If allergy is confirmed, then a MedicAlert® bracelet should be worn by the patient. The details of the reaction must be recorded in the medical records and reported to the patient's general practitioner and the appropriate adverse drug reactions body (AAGBI National Anaesthetic Anaphylaxis Database in the UK).

Anaesthesia in the Susceptible Patient

Unless the patient is allergic to local anaesthetics, regional anaesthesia should be used if possible. If the patient requires general anaesthesia, the preoperative use of corticosteroids and histamine H$_1$- and H$_2$-receptor antagonists should be considered as prophylaxis. The anaesthetic technique chosen should avoid re-exposure to implicated agents. Drugs should be chosen that have a low potential for hypersensitivity and direct histamine release. Typically safe drugs include volatile agents, etomidate, fentanyl, pancuronium and benzodiazepines. All drugs should be given slowly in diluted form, and resuscitation facilities must be immediately available.

Other Drug Reactions

An idiosyncratic drug reaction is a qualitatively abnormal and harmful drug effect which occurs in a small number of individuals and is precipitated usually by small drug doses. There is often an associated genetic defect and the reaction may be severe or even fatal.

Succinylcholine sensitivity, malignant hyperthermia (see above) and acute intermittent porphyria are important examples of drug idiosyncrasy in anaesthetic practice.

Acute Intermittent Porphyria. Acute intermittent porphyria (AIP) is a rare but serious metabolic disorder caused by an inherited deficiency of an enzyme required for haem synthesis. Porphyrin precursors accumulate and cause acute neuropathy, abdominal pain (mimicking an acute abdomen), delirium and death. These precursors are produced in the liver by δ-amino laevulinic acid synthetase, and this enzyme may be induced by barbiturates, amongst other drugs. If an at-risk patient is identified, porphyrinogenic drugs (including barbiturates) must be avoided. Drugs considered safe include propofol, midazolam, succinylcholine, vecuronium, nitrous oxide, morphine, fentanyl, neostigmine and atropine.

Regional Anaesthesia

Central Techniques

Epidural and subarachnoid anaesthesia are often chosen to reduce the patient's perioperative risk. However, these techniques may pose independent risks.

Hypotension. Arterial and venous dilatation caused by sympathetic pharmacological denervation reduce cardiac afterload and preload. Systemic hypotension results, and may be severe enough to compromise organ perfusion. Signs include tachycardia, low arterial pressure, confusion, nausea and dizziness. Fluid preloading may reduce the incidence of hypotension, and the left lateral position is helpful in pregnant patients. Intravenous titration of a vasopressor agent (e.g. bolus doses of ephedrine 5 mg or metaraminol 1 mg) usually restores arterial pressure rapidly. Directly acting arterial constrictors are more appropriate than indirectly acting sympathomimetics if tachycardia is present and in patients with severe ischaemic heart disease.

Nerve Injury. Nerve injury may result from direct trauma caused by the needle, or through chemical toxicity. It is widely held that epidural and subarachnoid block should be undertaken in the conscious patient to allow early identification of impingement upon a nerve or the spinal cord.

Infection and Haematoma. Spinal abscess presents as sudden, painless loss of motor function, usually several days after performance of the block, and is a devastating complication of central nervous blockade. Meticulous aseptic technique helps to reduce the incidence of this complication but some cases arise spontaneously, probably as a result of bacteraemia caused by surgery and inoculation of a small and otherwise asymptomatic epidural haematoma. Urgent magnetic resonance imaging and referral to a neurosurgeon are indicated if spinal abscess is suspected.

Epidural haematoma is a common complication of epidural catheter placement. The large majority of haematomata are asymptomatic and resolve spontaneously. They may be apparent only upon spinal imaging. Large haematomata may cause permanent nerve injury. Epidural catheters should not be inserted in patients who are receiving warfarin or intravenous heparin, or who have abnormal coagulation for some other reason. Caution should be exercised if a patient is receiving low-dose heparin for thromboprophylaxis. At least 12 h should be allowed to elapse between administration of low-molecular-weight heparin prophylaxis and epidural block. If blood is obtained via the needle or catheter during insertion and the patient is expected to be fully heparinized (e.g. during cardiac or major vascular surgery), the procedure should be postponed for 24 h. As with spinal abscesses, urgent imaging and referral to a neurosurgeon are indicated. Often, imaging is delayed because numbness and weakness are attributed to the effects of the epidural block; low concentrations of local anaesthetic (e.g. 0.1% or 0.125% bupivacaine) do not cause weakness and cause minimal numbness, and there should be a high level of suspicion about the possibility of epidural haematoma if these signs arise in the postoperative period.

Peripheral Nerve Blocks. There is a risk of direct damage to nerves in association with any peripheral nerve block. Paraesthesia or pain in the distribution of a nerve are signs of the proximity of a nerve and should prompt needle withdrawal. Pain during injection of local anaesthetic, failure to abolish the muscular twitch from a nerve stimulator or the requirement for increased injection force may indicate intraneural positioning of the needle and should prompt immediate cessation of injection and withdrawal of the needle.

Local Anaesthetic Toxicity

Local anaesthetic drugs may cause toxic side-effects when excessive serum concentrations are achieved. This is most commonly caused by accidental intravenous injection, excessively rapid absorption or absolute overdosage. Some sites of injection display a much more rapid uptake into the systemic circulation, usually because of local vascularity. Intercostal nerve blocks result in higher serum concentrations than subcutaneous infiltration, which produces higher serum concentrations than plexus blocks.

Cerebral symptoms occur first. Dizziness, drowsiness, confusion, tinnitus, circumoral tingling, anxiety and a metallic taste are common signs of toxicity. Patients should be asked about the presence of these symptoms. In severe toxicity, tonic-clonic convulsions occur. Cardiovascular symptoms include bradycardia with hypotension, although solutions which contain adrenaline may produce tachycardia and hypertension. Cardiovascular collapse occurs usually at 4–6 times the serum concentration at which convulsions occur. Local anaesthetics directly depress the myocardium and cause systemic vasodilatation. Cardiovascular collapse occurs earlier with bupivacaine than with lidocaine because of myocardial binding. Severe and intractable arrhythmias may occur with accidental intravenous injection. The toxicity of local anaesthetics is increased by a rapid rate of increase of serum concentration. Thus, a rapid intravenous injection of a small dose has the potential to cause toxicity.

Management. Intravenous access should be secured and adequate resuscitation equipment and drugs should be immediately available before a local anaesthetic block is undertaken. The patient should be adequately monitored. The lowest dose of the least toxic drug available should be used to achieve the effect required (Table 43.12). The total dose should be reduced in frail patients and in patients otherwise at risk of toxicity (e.g. patients with epilepsy or heart block). Local anaesthetics should always be injected slowly with repeated aspiration for blood, and with constant verbal contact with, and observation of, the patient. Any change in the patient's apparent mental state should prompt immediate cessation of injection. Injection of a test dose of a local anaesthetic which contains adrenaline usually results in sudden tachycardia if intravascular injection has occurred.

The addition of adrenaline reduces the speed of absorption from tissues, allowing larger maximum doses, reducing the potential for toxicity and prolonging the action of the local anaesthetic. Adrenaline (1:200 000) typically reduces the maximum serum concentration by approximately 50%. However, the addition of Adrenaline does not reduce local anaesthetic toxicity following intravenous injection.

If toxicity occurs, the injection must be stopped, assistance summoned and the patient assessed. The airway should be checked and oxygen should be administered; this prevents hypoxaemia, which makes fitting more likely and makes arrhythmias more difficult to control. If hypoventilation or apnoea ensue, the lungs should be ventilated using a self-inflating bag or anaesthetic breathing system. Tracheal intubation is required if the patient is unconscious or unable to maintain an airway. Intravenous fluids and vasopressors (e.g. ephedrine 10 mg) may be required to treat hypotension. Arrhythmias may occur and should be treated appropriately (see above). Severe heart block may require an infusion of isoprenaline or pacing. Chest compressions are required if there is no palpable pulse. Convulsions are very common in significant toxicity and administration of an anticonvulsant (e.g. diazepam 10 mg, thiopental 50 mg) is often necessary. The intravenous administration of lipid emulsion has been shown to reduce the effects of systemic toxicity from local anaesthetics, in the presence of cardiovascular collapse and convulsions (note: propofol is not a suitable substitute for lipid emulsion in this scenario).

An initial of bolus of 1.5 mL kg^{-1} 20% lipid emulsion over 1 min is recommended, followed by an infusion at 15 mL kg^{-1} hr^{-1}.

A maximum of two repeat bolus doses can be given if cardiovascular stability is not restored or deteriorates; 5 min should be left between boluses. The infusion rate can also be doubled to 20 mL kg^{-1} hr^{-1} if necessary. The maximum cumulative dose should be limited to 12 mL kg^{-1} (840 mL for a 70 kg adult).

If lipid has been given, its use should be reported to the international registry at www.lipidregistry.org.

Survival from local anaesthetic toxicity should approach 100%. Good preparation, early recognition and prompt treatment are vital in preventing progression to a situation of poor tissue oxygenation and organ damage.

TABLE 43.12
Maximum Safe Doses of Local Anaesthetics in Common Use

Drug	Maximum Dose
Lidocaine	4 (7) mg kg^{-1}
Bupivacaine	2 (2) mg kg^{-1}
Levobupivacaine	2.5 (2.5) mg kg^{-1}
Prilocaine	6 (8) mg kg^{-1}

Maximum doses in the presence of 1:200 000 adrenaline are given in parentheses.

Injury

Direct physical injury of the patient is a fairly common event in the perioperative period. Most of these injuries are preventable. Tracheal intubation and poor patient positioning are commonly to blame. Nerve, dental and ophthalmic injuries are common causes of litigation against anaesthetists. Thermal and electrical injuries are less common but potentially disastrous. Neurological deficits presenting during the postoperative period have usually been sustained intraoperatively.

Cutaneous and Muscular Injury

Skin is damaged easily by poor or prolonged positioning, the use of highly adhesive tape and incautious movement of the patient. In particular, elderly patients and patients who have been treated with steroids for a prolonged period may have very fragile skin, and this must be protected. These patients also tend to heal very slowly, and an apparently minor skin injury may produce many months of suffering postoperatively. Pressure sores which originate during the intra-operative period are increasingly recognised. Muscle injury is produced most commonly by poor positioning, but tourniquets may also cause direct muscle damage.

Peripheral Nerve Injury

Peripheral nerves may be injured directly, through peripheral nerve blockade or vascular catheter insertion or surgery, indirectly, by poor positioning during anaesthesia, or through ischaemia during severe hypoxaemia or hypotension. Peripheral nerve injury occurs during 0.1% of anaesthetics. The position of the patient during general anaesthesia is the commonest cause of injury. The brachial plexus and superficial nerves of the limbs (ulnar, radial and common peroneal) are the most frequently affected nerves. The usual mechanism of injury to superficial nerves is ischaemia from compression of the vasa vasorum by surgical retractors, leg stirrups or contact with other equipment. Nerve injury may occur as part of a compartment syndrome after ischaemia from poor positioning, particularly when the legs are placed in Lloyd-Davies supports and the patient is positioned head-down. Ischaemic injury is more likely to occur during periods of poor peripheral perfusion associated with hypotension or hypothermia. Nerves may also be injured by traction (e.g. the brachial plexus during excessive shoulder abduction).

Meticulous care is necessary when positioning the patient. Padding should be used beneath tourniquets and to protect pressure points. Extreme joint positions should be avoided. Close surveillance of tourniquet ischaemia times is essential. Although many injuries recover within several months, all patients with a peripheral nerve injury must be referred to a neurologist for assessment and continuing care. Many ulnar nerve palsies occur in patients with an anatomical predisposition, and this may be deduced from a history of numbness after sleep or as a result of posture at work. In these patients, the elbows should not be placed in flexion during surgery.

Injury During Airway Management

Dental damage is the most frequently reported anaesthetic injury and is usually sustained during laryngoscopy. Damage to teeth is much more likely if laryngoscopy is difficult. Most dental injuries result from a rotational force applied to the laryngoscope during attempts to lever the tip of the laryngoscope blade upwards using the upper incisors as a fulcrum. The correct, and much safer, practice is to apply a force upwards and away from the anaesthetist without any leverage on the incisors. Injuries vary from chipped teeth to complete avulsion. The upper incisors are most commonly involved. Preoperative assessment and documentation of dentition are essential. Patients with poor dentition, or in whom a difficult laryngoscopy is anticipated, should be warned of the possibility of dental injury. If a tooth is accidentally avulsed, it should be reimplanted in its socket with minimal interference and a dental surgeon consulted at the earliest opportunity.

Mucosal damage is common during airway management, and mucosal abrasion may be very painful postoperatively. Overinflation of the cuff of a tube in the larynx or trachea may produce local ischaemia, with consequent scarring and stenosis; cuff pressure should be checked regularly, particularly during prolonged surgery and when nitrous oxide is used. Other reported injuries include dislocated arytenoid cartilages (intubation), recurrent laryngeal nerve damage (laryngoscopy), uvular ischaemia (Guedel airway), epistaxis and nasal turbinate fracture (nasal intubation).

Ophthalmic Injury

Retinal ischaemic injury may follow prolonged pressure on the orbit from equipment or the use of the prone position. Permanent blindness may result.

Corneal abrasions are associated with inadequate eye protection, especially during transfer or use of the prone position. The use of adhesive tape to close the eyelids is also a risk factor. Lubricated dressings such as sterile paraffin gauze may be a preferable method of securing the eyelids.

Thermal and Electrical Injury

The high-density electrical current of surgical diathermy is a potential source of injury. If the return current path is interrupted by incorrect application of the diathermy pad, then the ECG electrodes or other points of contact between skin and metal may provide an alternative electrical path, producing serious burns. Failure of thermostatic control on warming devices is a potential source of thermal injury. Warming devices should always be used in accordance with the manufacturer's guidelines. In particular, hot air hoses used to inflate convective warming blankets must never be used alone to blow hot air under the patient's blankets, as serious thermal injury may result. Ignition of alcohol-based surgical preparation solutions is possible, especially if they are not allowed to evaporate fully and if diathermy is used. Airway fires have occurred during laser surgery to the larynx; it is advisable to use a low inspired oxygen fraction and omit nitrous oxide in this situation.

Fires should be extinguished immediately and the area should be soaked in cool saline or covered with saline-soaked swabs. If the burned area is significant, the opinion of a burns surgeon should be sought.

Vascular Injury and Tourniquets

Arterial catheters may produce significant arterial injury, resulting in ischaemia and, potentially, loss of the distal limb. Arterial tourniquets reduce surgical bleeding but also rob the distal tissue of its perfusion. An absolute maximum duration of 2 h should be observed, and inflation pressures should be just high enough to occlude arterial flow. Typically, a pressure of 200–250 mmHg is adequate for the upper limb, and 250–300 mmHg for the lower limb. Vascular occlusion (e.g. during tourniquet use, aortic cross-clamping) risks distal ischaemia and infarction. Assurance of an adequate arterial pressure and oxygen saturation is important in facilitating distal oxygenation via collateral flow. Parts distal to an arterial occlusion should never be warmed, because this raises local metabolic rate and causes the onset of ischaemia to be more rapid.

FURTHER READING

Atlee, J.L. (Ed.), 2006. Complications in anesthesia, second ed. Saunders, New York.

Benumof, J.L., Saidman, L.J. (Eds.), 1999. Anesthesia and perioperative complications, second ed. Year Book Medical Publications, New York.

Contractor, S., Hardman, J.G., 2006. Injury during anaesthesia. CEACCP 6, 67.

Finucane, B.T. (Ed.), 1999. Complications of regional anesthesia. Elsevier, New York.

Gravenstein, N. (Ed.), 2006. Complications in Anesthesia. Lippincott Williams & Wilkins, Philadelphia.

Hardman, J.G., Aitkenhead, A.R., 2005. Awareness during anaesthesia. CEACCP 5, 183.

44 QUALITY AND SAFETY IN ANAESTHESIA

The agenda of quality improvement and patient safety is among the top priorities for individual anaesthetists, departments of anaesthesia and health care organizations. In recent years, since publication of the Institute of Medicine (IOM) report *To Err is Human*, there has been growing realization that a co-ordinated approach involving all layers of organizational management and clinical services is required to improve quality and patient safety.

Patient safety incidents remain a cause for concern in healthcare systems all over the world. According to IOM, as many as 98 000 deaths in the USA can be attributed to medical errors. In the UK, approximately 900 000 incidents and near misses are reported every year, of which around 2000 result in death. It has been estimated that additional hospital stay costs approximately £2 billion a year, and negligence claims amount to an extra £400 million a year.

This chapter addresses current concepts of quality and patient safety. In particular, the following topics will be covered.

- The definition of quality
- The culture of quality and safety
- Can quality and safety be measured?
- Tools for improving quality and patient safety.

QUALITY

Various attempts have been made to define quality in health care systems precisely. In the IOM's 2001 report *Crossing the Quality Chasm*, six aims were proposed to define 'what healthcare should be'. The six aims, i.e. safety, effectiveness, patient-centredness,

timeliness, efficiency and equity, provide components of a working definition of quality in healthcare systems (Table 44.1). The six aims can be used as the attributes of a comprehensive quality care system, which can be continuously monitored and improved. These six aims are the cornerstones for designing and delivering a quality service from which both patients and clinicians are likely to benefit in terms of better patient care, less suffering and increased productivity and satisfaction.

Any attempts to improve quality within an organization and a department, focussing on these attributes of high quality care, should consider whether there is organizational readiness to embrace the quality improvement programme. This will be determined by the existing culture within the organization and/or department. Establishing a quality culture within a department and making it more positive is the key to the success of any quality improvement interventions with regard to their implementation, staff compliance and sustainability.

CULTURE OF QUALITY AND SAFETY

Understanding Generation of Errors: Systems Approach

In health care systems, there is still a prevalence of a 'judicial' approach to errors. After an incident, people are generally quick to make judgements which often result in blaming the individual most obviously associated with the incident. This approach is a big barrier to understanding the nature of adverse events and how they can be prevented. In this regard, the healthcare industry has much to learn from other industries, such

TABLE 44.1

Aims of a High Quality Healthcare System

1. Safe	Prevention of injuries to patients from the care that is intended to help them
2. Effective	Provision of services based on scientific knowledge to all who could benefit, and refraining from providing services to those not likely to benefit
3. Patient-centred	Providing care that is respectful of and responsive to individual patient preferences, needs and values, and ensuring that patient values guide all clinical decisions
4. Timely	Reducing waits and sometimes harmful delays for both who receive care and those who give it
5. Efficient	Avoiding waste, including waste of equipment, supplies, ideas and energy
6. Equitable	Providing care that does not vary in quality because of personal characteristics such as gender, ethnicity, geographic location, and socio-economic status.

as aviation and nuclear power, which now have significant track records of a robust safety culture.

One central message from the IOM report has been that, in general, the cause of preventable deaths in healthcare systems is not incompetent or careless people, but bad systems. In order to reach this level of understanding, it is important to understand the aetiology of an error in complex organizations such as hospitals (Box 44.1). A safety incident should be seen in an organizational framework of latent failures – the conditions which produce

BOX 44.1
TAXONOMY OF ERROR

LATENT FAILURES are factors which exist within an organization or process and which increase the risk of another error causing an incident. They are separated in time and often in place from the occurrence of the incident. Reason described these as organizational influences, unsafe supervision and preconditions for unsafe acts.

Organizational influences may include aspects such as training budgets and curricula, and organizational safety culture.

Unsafe supervision might be reflected by a trainee anaesthetizing a complex case near the limits of their competence without adequate consultant supervision.

Preconditions for unsafe acts include lack of robust checking procedures, near-identical drug ampoules and inadequate rest breaks for staff.

Active errors are unsafe acts which cause (or could cause) an incident. They may be errors of commission (doing the wrong thing) or omission (not doing the right thing). Various categories of active error are often described.

Execution failures: the knowledge and the intent are appropriate, but for a variety of reasons the correct actions do not ensue. These are often referred to as slips (observable actions, related to attention) and lapses (internal events, related to memory failures). They may be failures of Recognition, Attention, Memory and Selection. These are exemplified by drugs errors in anaesthesia: every anaesthetist will be able to recall events where each of these failures has happened in their own practice.

Mistakes: the action proceeds as intended, but the wrong course has been chosen. These may be:

Rule-based: prior knowledge, intuition or a protocol is available for this situation (e.g. failed intubation) but is wrongly applied. This may be by omission, too late, or by applying the wrong rule.

Knowledge-based: an unfamiliar or novel situation requires the 'calculation' of a solution based on the (usually incomplete) evidence. These require thought and are particularly prone to confirmation bias – evidence which supports the current model is sought, and contrary evidence is ignored.

Violations: these are deliberate choices to deviate from agreed practice (formal standing operating procedures (SOPs), or informal custom and practice). Again, these can be subdivided:

Routine violations: corners are routinely cut. This may be at an individual or departmental level. 'Normalization of deviance' may occur, where unacceptable practice becomes accepted practice over time. The risk is that practice becomes further and further away from good practice gradually, such that it is not noticed or dealt with until too late.

Self-serving violations: breaking the rules for personal gratification.

Situational violations: breaking the rules because (correctly) the situation demands it. There will always be circumstances when rules and procedures do not fit. A safety-conscious organization seeks to learn from these incidents.

error and violation – and active failures. This concept is captured in James Reason's model of an organizational accident. It should be emphasized that some active failures (such as simple mistakes, lapse, fall, slip) have only a local context and can be explained by factors related to individual performance and/or the task at hand. However, it is now understood that major incidents evolve over time and involve many factors.

In the generation of an incident, organizational factors are the beginning of the sequence. These create latent failures which result from the negative consequences of management decisions, and organizational strategy and/or planning. The latent failures then permeate through departmental pathways to the workplace (e.g. the operating theatre complex). Here, they create conditions which allow violations and commission of errors. The errors generated in the workplace environment may be prevented by a front-end clinician (near-miss). However, a simple active failure on the part of the clinician at this stage allows the error to produce damaging outcomes. Figure 44.1 illustrates an example: how a medication error can result from a combination of latent failures, conditions contributing to error and violations, and active failure.

In view of this knowledge, in order to facilitate quality and safety culture, it is important that, first, the healthcare organization must accept that in the vast majority of errors/accidents, 'system' failure has a major role to play. Second, the organization needs to be 'open' about it, and this openness and transparency must reflect in all their policies and procedures. Third, the organization's response to these accidents must be 'just', and non-punitive for the individual involved. Finally, there must be mechanisms and forums so that 'learning' can occur at all levels within the organization, and so that systems are continuously improved.

Focus on Safety Behaviour and Non-Technical Skills

In clinical practice, some personal attributes of health care workers naturally render them more safe than others. These attributes are what one might see in a most highly respected member of a department.

- *Conscientiousness.* Being sensible and meticulous, checking the information/drugs/equipment him/herself, ensuring that the job is done properly, and being thorough.

- *Honesty.* Accepting limitations, giving correct and complete information, accepting own mistakes, compliance with procedures and protocols.
- *Humility.* Thanking colleagues, juniors and nurses for their help and contribution, taking and seeking advice from other members of the team.
- *Self-awareness.* Knowing limitations, knowing when tired, sleepy or pre-occupied
- *Confidence.* Knowing capabilities and being confident about them, able to speak up if necessary.

There is now growing realization that these attributes along with non-technical skills are essential among staff to raise quality and safety in an organization. The General Medical Council in the UK makes it clear that doctors are expected to have these personal attributes. Detailed analyses of some of the high-profile incidents in anaesthesia have drawn attention towards non-technical skills. These non-technical skills (NTS) are defined as 'The cognitive, social and personal resource skills that complement technical skills and contribute to safe and efficient task performance. They are not new or mysterious skills but are essentially what the best practitioners do in order to achieve consistently high performance and what the rest of us do on a good day'.

The underlying premise is that:

- the operating theatre is a complex environment with complicated tasks
- many people come together to work in this environment
- there is heightened potential for accidents and disasters in operating theatres, and
- every human has limitations.

In view of these facts, and the recent knowledge about human behaviour under stressful conditions, it is important that health care organizations and workers have commitment to education and practice in non-technical skills. In particular, for the operating theatre environment, the following skills are important:

- communication, sharing of information
- team work
- situational awareness
- anticipation and preparedness
- decision making.

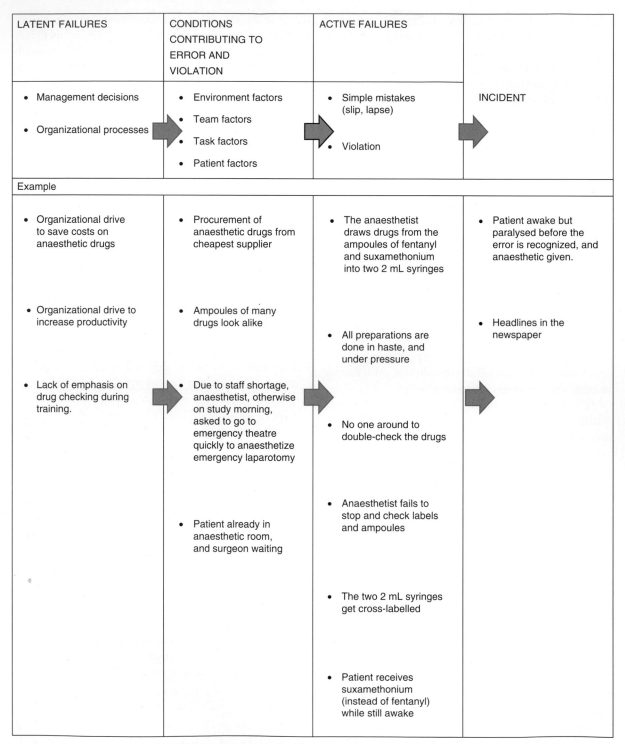

LATENT FAILURES	CONDITIONS CONTRIBUTING TO ERROR AND VIOLATION	ACTIVE FAILURES	
• Management decisions • Organizational processes	• Environment factors • Team factors • Task factors • Patient factors	• Simple mistakes (slip, lapse) • Violation	INCIDENT
Example			
• Organizational drive to save costs on anaesthetic drugs • Organizational drive to increase productivity • Lack of emphasis on drug checking during training.	• Procurement of anaesthetic drugs from cheapest supplier • Ampoules of many drugs look alike • Due to staff shortage, anaesthetist, otherwise on study morning, asked to go to emergency theatre quickly to anaesthetize emergency laparotomy • Patient already in anaesthetic room, and surgeon waiting	• The anaesthetist draws drugs from the ampoules of fentanyl and suxamethonium into two 2 mL syringes • All preparations are done in haste, and under pressure • No one around to double-check the drugs • Anaesthetist fails to stop and check labels and ampoules • The two 2 mL syringes get cross-labelled • Patient receives suxamethonium (instead of fentanyl) while still awake	• Patient awake but paralysed before the error is recognized, and anaesthetic given. • Headlines in the newspaper

FIGURE 44.1 ■ An example of the generation of a medication error.

TABLE 44.2
Components of a Pre-List Briefing

Components	Details	Rationale
Timing	Before the start of the list	
Who	All key members of the team	In a safe team, all members have a contribution. Involving all staff should increase the chance of at least one person speaking up if there is a potential problem
Aspects Covered		
People	Team introductions Who is doing what in the list? Are any other key individuals needed during the day?	Safe teams know who each other are, and what each other's roles and competencies are
Patients	Particular issues for each individual patient	The whole team is aware of issues (or lack of them). Particular requirements are highlighted at a time when solutions can be found
Equipment	Is all necessary equipment available? Anaesthesia, surgery, positioning	Equipment issues are common, frustrating for staff and potentially dangerous
External issues	Emergency work, staffing issues elsewhere	Most operating theatres do not work alone, and resilient departments will have an understanding of wider issues
Debriefing	Issues from previous debriefings	Truly novel problems are unusual. Learning from issues in previous lists is a key aspect of a positive safety culture

Communication and Teamwork

Some of us are better communicators and better team workers than others. However, it is now well known that, if the skills are delineated, if awareness is raised about them and tools of learning are implemented by the organization, everyone can improve these skills beyond their previous level. The best possible scenario would be when all members of the team know each other, have mutual trust, are able to discuss problems and issues openly, learn from each other and work together for a common goal. Team leaders have special responsibility for ensuring that they have complete trust in the other members of their team. Listening to each other is extremely important to gain trust. In an ideal world, team members would respect and trust each other, know each others' strengths and weaknesses, have a low threshold for discussion and learning, and would be able to manage and allocate tasks such that the job at hand is accomplished in the most efficient and safe manner with all members of the team deriving great satisfaction from a job well done. In practice, it is difficult to accomplish this ideal. Therefore, organizations must actively explore and implement tools and training programmes which allow employees to enhance their level of communication and team working.

Pre-list briefings are an important component of this process for the whole operating team. They are tools to foster good communication, planning and learning for the whole team.

Debriefings are a complement to the briefing process (Table 44.2). The concept is that the team reviews its performance each day – did it match the plans made at the start of the day? Good practice is reinforced and areas of improvement are discussed constructively. Information from debriefings should be shared with other team members and necessary actions should be completed and fed back to the team.

Situational Awareness

This term implies broader understanding of 'what is going on', and how events may unfold. The term conveys more than just paying attention to the task. For example, a junior trainee anaesthetist being supervised by a middle-grade anaesthetist on emergency duty might be about to anaesthetize a patient undergoing straightforward minor emergency surgery, but also formulating a plan in the event that he/she is called to attend a cardiac arrest elsewhere in the hospital, bearing in mind that the consultant is dealing with a complicated case in another theatre and the middle-grade is very new to the environment of the hospital. The core elements of situational awareness include:

- continuous information gathering
- anticipation of events which may unfold
- processing current information to interpret the situation in view of anticipated events.

Analyses of major critical events, and experiments in simulated conditions, have shown that, under stress, individuals tend to develop 'task fixation', and lose an overall perspective of the situation. A typical example of task fixation would be an anaesthetist single-handedly making multiple attempts at intubating a patient's trachea while overlooking the facts that the patient has been hypoxic for some time, that the assistant brought the difficult airway trolley into the anaesthetic room some time ago and that a very experienced airway expert and an ENT surgeon are working in close vicinity. Often in the aftermath of an adverse incident, one comes across statements such as 'I had not realized that….', 'we had not anticipated that…..', 'it just took us all by surprise…..'.

Situational awareness refers to the ability to appraise the overall picture, to acquire relevant information quickly by scanning the whole environment and to monitor the environment continuously, in particular for any change. For example, an anaesthetist who is about to anaesthetize a patient with anticipated airway difficulty realizes that the assistant is in conversation with a colleague regarding rota cover for the evening, and the nurse is on the telephone talking to someone about a malfunctioning piece of equipment. The theatre environment, when put under stress, can expose latent conditions which produce errors. The anaesthetist would be wise to wait for a few seconds until these matters are resolved or temporarily postponed, and ensure that all relevant members of staff are not distracted from the task at hand.

Anticipation and Preparedness

Anticipation is the key component of full situational awareness. It involves thinking ahead about all reasonably predictable hazards, e.g. 'what if there is severe bleeding', 'what if I am unable to see larynx', 'what if the blood pressure drops on tourniquet release', 'what if there is power failure'? Having considered what can go wrong, it is useful to mentally try responses, and then work out whether these responses would address the problem. These mental exercises allow the clinician to adjust/prepare the environment to avoid these hazards, and prepare to deal with the hazards, if they were to arise, in a calm, systematic manner.

Decision-Making

This is a sensitive area, because individual decisions can be deeply entangled with the individual's professional capability. To be potentially challenged on the decisions can be intimidating for an individual, and damaging to their self-esteem. In the area of patient safety, where evidence is still emerging, education not established and procedures and protocols still not embedded, decision-making for an individual in a condition of uncertainty can be very challenging.

Decisions may have to be taken based on previous experience, knowledge, intuition and/or good prevailing sense at the time. However, the process of decision-making can be evolved and evaluated using crisis management scenarios in a simulated environment. Here, the decisions do not have clinical consequences and the evaluation can be non-threatening. Examples of training in such scenarios include, among many others, rapid sequence induction, failed intubation, unexpected severe hypotension, cardiac arrest, malignant hyperthermia and anaphylaxis. All anaesthesia departments should have working protocols to deal with crisis situations in order to help clinicians to make logical, systematic decisions under stressful conditions. The scenarios should be practised regularly in teams, and the experience of training should be enhanced by debriefing on team work and individual decisions. It is unlikely that all existing protocols will cover all possible eventualities. Therefore, decisions will still need to be made on individual choices and judgements. A culture of openness within the department should allow healthy discussion on decisions if different options could be considered, and lessons should be learnt to reinforce decision-making skills in a collective manner.

MEASURING SAFETY AND QUALITY

Safety Culture

So far, the measurement of the safety culture within an organization or a department has been mainly the subject of research projects. In the clinical arena, these concepts are now being considered essential for understanding the prevailing conditions and also to monitor the progress and success of various safety and quality initiatives or interventions.

The terms 'safety culture' and 'safety climate' have often been used interchangeably. However, there are differences which are important to understand.

According to one of many definitions, safety culture is 'the product of individual and group values, attitudes, competencies and patterns of behaviour that determine the commitment to, and the style and proficiency of, an organization's health and safety programmes'. In simple terms, safety culture refers to 'the way we do things round here'; the 'here' in this context could be an individual, a group, a team, a department or an organization. One can also think in terms of culture being 'what happens when no-one is watching'. A positive safety culture in an organization is characterized by its individual members respecting and trusting each other, perceiving safety to be important and having confidence that the safety interventions would be effective.

Safety climate refers to 'surface features of safety culture from attitudes and perceptions of individuals at a given point in time', or 'measurable components of safety culture'.

The two terms, safety culture and safety climate, can be differentiated by comparing the 'culture' to an individual's personality, and 'climate' to his/her mood.

The commonest method of measuring safety culture/climate in healthcare involves using quantitative questionnaires. These questionnaires have different dimensions, lengths and reliability on psychometric testing. The most commonly used tools are:

- AHRQ's (Agency for Healthcare Research and Quality) Hospital Survey on Patient Safety Culture
- Safety attitudes questionnaire
- Patient Safety Culture in Healthcare Organizations Survey
- Modified Stanford Patient Safety Culture Survey Instrument

In addition to these quantitative questionnaires, many researchers use qualitative methodology including observations, semi-structured interviews and focus groups to make in-depth assessments. According to the concept of varying models of cultural maturity in healthcare settings, safety culture can be described in terms of five different levels of maturity:

- *Pathological.* 'Who cares so long as we are not caught?'
- *Reactive.* 'We do a lot of 'safety' whenever we have an accident'
- *Calculative.* 'We have systems in place to manage all hazards'
- *Proactive.* 'We anticipate problems before they arise'
- *Generative.* 'Safety is how we do business around here'.

Some safety measurement tools such as the Manchester Patient Safety Framework and the Patient Safety Culture Improvement Tool incorporate the concept of culture maturity, and are therefore useful in assessing changes in culture and its maturity over a period of time.

Measuring Quality

A comprehensive measurement of quality would assess, and somehow measure, all the individual components of the quality matrix, i.e. safety, clinical effectiveness, patient experience, timeliness, efficiency and equity. In 1988, Avedis Donabedian introduced a framework for assessing quality in healthcare (Table 44.3). This framework is based on three core domains – structure, processes and outcomes.

It is important to understand that the three domains of measuring quality are interdependent. Good processes depend upon good structures, and they often lead to good outcomes. Consequently, assessment of only one domain (e.g. outcome - mortality) cannot assess quality, or serve to improve it. It becomes useful only when this assessment is combined with finding the gaps in structure (e.g. staff shortage) and/or processes (e.g. non-adherence to guidelines). At present, much is being written and discussed about what should be measured to assess the existing quality of care, and any improvements. The Donabedian framework can be used to address each component of quality as shown in Table 44.4.

TABLE 44.3	
Donabedian's Framework for Measuring Quality	
Domain	**Description**
Structure	*Set-up for providing care* including: ▪ Material resources ▪ Facilities ▪ Human resources ▪ Technology infrastructure ▪ Equipment ▪ Guidelines and implementation programmes ▪ Teaching programmes ▪ Rotas
Process	*What happens around delivery of care* including: ▪ Patient pathway from evaluation through diagnosis to treatment ▪ Assessment before anaesthesia ▪ Optimization of comorbidities ▪ Adherence to guidelines and teaching programmes ▪ Checklists ▪ Monitoring ▪ Incident reporting and actions ▪ Ongoing audits of different aspects of care delivery ▪ Quality improvement programmes
Outcome	*The effects of care* including: ▪ Morbidity ▪ Mortality ▪ Patient satisfaction ▪ Other clinical outcomes* as decided by the department

*See text for details.

Clinical Outcomes: Real or Surrogate

In anaesthesia, a lot of reliance is put on real clinical outcomes to indicate quality of care, such as incidences of epidural haematoma, nerve damage, brain damage or death. Although this may sound straightforward, there are limitations associated with real outcomes.

- The real outcomes may depend on many factors including the patient's pre-existing condition, population dynamics, surgical factors and individual reactions (e.g. unknown allergies), which may not necessarily indicate quality of care *per se*.

TABLE 44.4	
Measurement of Each Attribute of Quality Care	
Attribute	**Measurement (Examples)**
Safety	▪ Incident reporting ▪ Clustering of incidents ▪ Safety programmes ▪ Safety interventions ▪ Success of implementing safety interventions ▪ Safety culture surveys ▪ Safety climate surveys
Effectiveness	▪ Guidelines, protocols, checklists and adherence to these ▪ Evidence-based treatment ▪ Morbidity and mortality ▪ Complications ▪ Other clinical outcomes as determined by the department/speciality
Patient-centredness	▪ Surveys of patient satisfaction ▪ Complaints and their resolution ▪ Involvement of patients in governance of the hospital ▪ Consent procedures
Timeliness, efficiency, equity	▪ Hospital-wide audits ▪ Data captured by hospital informatics ▪ Annual reports ▪ Business case ▪ Departmental cost savings

- Direct anaesthesia-related mortality is rare, and serious morbidity infrequent. Consequently, measuring anaesthesia-related mortality and morbidity can only be very crude measures and may not provide enough data to monitor quality on a regular basis (monthly or quarterly).

For these reasons, adverse events and near misses are usually taken as surrogate clinical outcomes. By monitoring the surrogates, a comprehensive picture can be obtained of the work flow and processes. Overall, more than 100 outcome measures have been described which can be used to assess the quality of anaesthesia care. It is clear that monitoring all of these will require resources beyond the capacity of many individual departments. Therefore, departments and individuals will be making their own choices about what to measure.

Selecting a Good Quality Indicator

It is clear that no single indicator is sufficient as a quality measure in anaesthesia. It is also clear that recording only major morbidity and mortality has limitations. Surrogate measures give a better picture of work flow and processes, and potential problems, but they do not replace real outcomes. Whatever indicators are chosen, it is important that they have specific characteristics. The indicator should be easy to define and record, but also must have a finite frequency of occurrence so that it can be monitored regularly. In addition, the rate of occurrence must be influenced by quality, and also must indicate something important about the process.

Quality Indicators at Individual Patient Level

There is very little guidance as to what individual departments of anaesthesia should be measuring on a routine basis in every patient as part of their quality improvement programme. A framework is suggested here, which includes sentinel events, adverse events, rate-based outcome indicators and work process quality indicators (Fig. 44.2). Some of these data would be available from existing hospital IT systems; others may have to be collected as part of on-going audit or service evaluation programmes. The framework can also be used by individual anaesthetists to maintain a record of their own activity and quality of care. At the departmental level this can inform, on a continuous basis, the quality of care which the department is providing to its patients, and the effect of any quality improvement programme.

Quality Assessment at Departmental Level

At the departmental level, in addition to the outcome data at individual patient level (Fig. 44.2), quality measures would include structural and process attributes as summarized in Tables 44.3 and 44.4.

Quality Improvement Tools

Requirements for Quality Improvement. The challenge for a department, in addition to collecting all the data at an individual patient level, is to analyse the data systematically, disseminate the findings as widely as possible and identify learning outcomes and areas

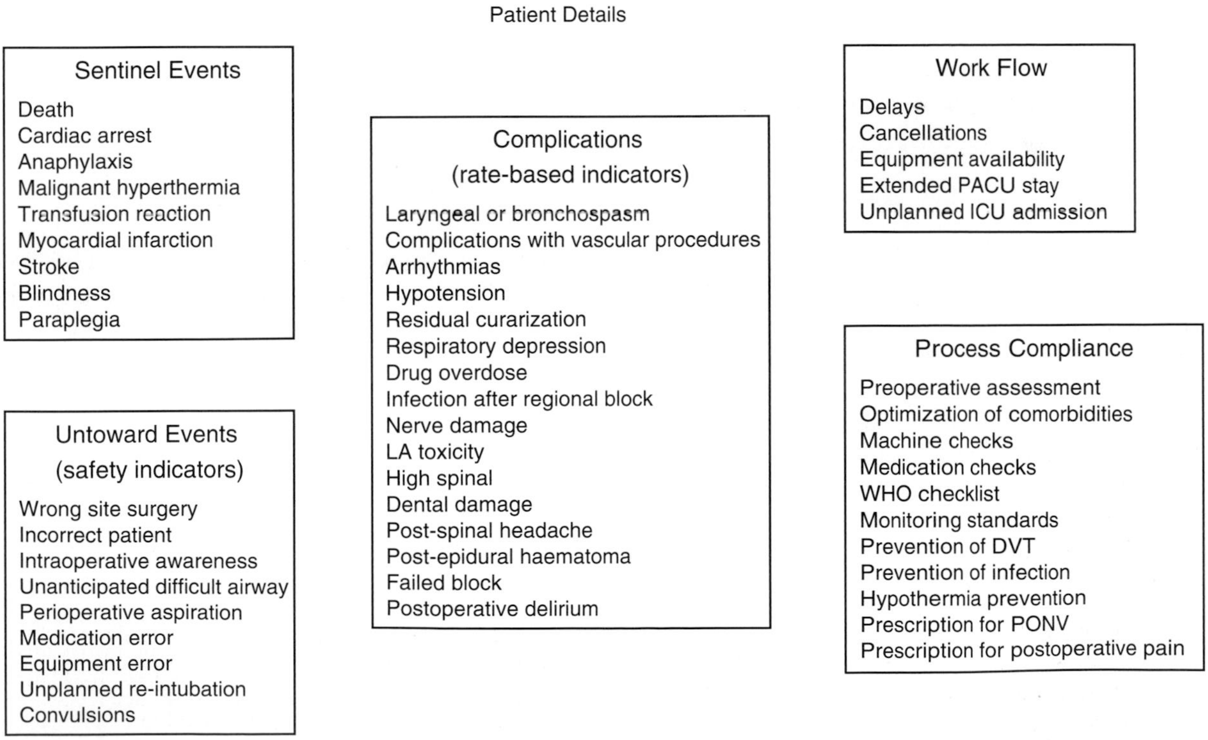

Patient Details

Sentinel Events
Death
Cardiac arrest
Anaphylaxis
Malignant hyperthermia
Transfusion reaction
Myocardial infarction
Stroke
Blindness
Paraplegia

Complications (rate-based indicators)
Laryngeal or bronchospasm
Complications with vascular procedures
Arrhythmias
Hypotension
Residual curarization
Respiratory depression
Drug overdose
Infection after regional block
Nerve damage
LA toxicity
High spinal
Dental damage
Post-spinal headache
Post-epidural haematoma
Failed block
Postoperative delirium

Work Flow
Delays
Cancellations
Equipment availability
Extended PACU stay
Unplanned ICU admission

Untoward Events (safety indicators)
Wrong site surgery
Incorrect patient
Intraoperative awareness
Unanticipated difficult airway
Perioperative aspiration
Medication error
Equipment error
Unplanned re-intubation
Convulsions

Process Compliance
Preoperative assessment
Optimization of comorbidities
Machine checks
Medication checks
WHO checklist
Monitoring standards
Prevention of DVT
Prevention of infection
Hypothermia prevention
Prescription for PONV
Prescription for postoperative pain

FIGURE 44.2 ■ A suggested framework for quality measurement at individual patient level in an anaesthesia department.

for improvement. In order to improve quality, departments will be required to develop interventions targeted at areas for improvement, implement them, and monitor progress and the impact of implementation on outcome measures. For a successful quality improvement programme, it is important for departments to invest in creating leaders and teams. It is vital for the leaders to address and improve the prevailing quality culture within the department. Continuing education and programmes to raise awareness are extremely important. Embedding a culture of incident reporting and learning is vital. Morbidity and mortality meetings and other network opportunities at which all quality issues can be aired and discussed without fear of a punitive outcome are absolutely essential for embedding quality consciousness.

Recent experience with implementing the WHO checklist has presented many challenges and has provided insight into what is required for successful implementation of a quality improvement intervention. Clear demonstration of success of the interventions, with the help of data and its rigorous analysis, is vital for motivating staff and increasing their belief in such interventions. Whilst all failures should be used as learning experiences, the successes must be celebrated. Barriers, facilitators and approaches in engaging staff into quality improvement are summarized in Table 44.5.

Checklists. Although they existed earlier, the modern era of the safety checklist is generally attributed to the crash of the newly designed Model 299 Boeing bomber in 1935. The cause of the crash was straightforward – the elevator lock had been left on. However, two extremely important facts emerged from the investigation. First, the pilot was an extremely experienced and competent pilot. Second, taking the elevator lock off was not an unusual requirement. The pilot would do this normally, but on this occasion, presumably due to distraction by other things, he forgot. The response of pilots was to create a process which ensured that simple things did not get missed, regardless of the situation.

The introduction of the WHO checklist as a strongly encouraged or mandated part of theatre practice has re-focussed attention on the potential benefits and risks of checklists in healthcare, and particularly

TABLE 44.5
Barriers, Facilitators and Approaches to Engage Staff in Quality Improvement

BARRIERS	
	■ Top heavy approach
	■ Lack of involvement at the beginning
	■ Punitive actions
	■ Lack of evidence
	■ Lack of assurance
	■ Lack of control
FACILITATORS	
	■ Role models
	■ Peer pressure
	■ Evidence
	■ Common sense
	■ Good outcomes
	■ Enhancement of professional position
	■ Rewards
APPROACHES	**Science approach**
	■ Safety research
	■ Research into causes of errors
	■ Research into prevention of errors
	■ Research into systems
	■ Safety interventions
	■ Safety measures
	Educational approach
	■ Curriculum
	■ Training
	■ Courses
	■ Cross-learning modules
	■ Faculty
	Management approach
	■ Vision
	■ Strategy
	■ Organizational change
	■ Risk management
	■ Implementation
	■ Professional leadership
	■ Networking

perioperative care. Checklists are not new in anaesthesia. Various national bodies produced anaesthetic machine checklists in the 1980s and 1990s. This was in response to the emerging data that demonstrated a significant number of patient safety incidents which could have been avoided by proper checking of equipment.

The term checklist is used for documents which may have a variety of purposes. Conceptually, they can be thought of as:

- checking
- briefing
- planning.

There is a multitude of checklists in use by anaesthetists and they encompass these different purposes to varying degrees. Some are designed better than others.

Most checklists are tabulations or summaries of accepted best practice. We would hope that anaesthetists would recognize the need to undertake these actions regardless of whether a checklist exists. Their role is therefore about **ensuring** that these actions take place for **every** patient, **every** time. The human memory is fallible and regardless of professional status, cannot be **relied** upon to remember more than about seven items.

There is a substantial body of evidence to show that anaesthetists are not particularly good at completing all the necessary checks. This applies to the anaesthesia machine, drug checking and the WHO checklist. The reasons for this are multifactorial and relate to all aspects of safety and quality discussed in this chapter. Specific barriers to full engagement with checklist processes include the following.

Perceived importance. The rate of incidents related to the items on the checklists is very low and therefore the overwhelming likelihood is that there will be nothing amiss. The anaesthetist may therefore consciously, or subconsciously, choose to prioritize another activity.

Organizational culture. Perceptions of organizational prioritization of efficiency over safety may encourage an individual to save time by shortening or omitting checklists. Conversely, an organization which fails to monitor compliance with checklists, or hold individuals to account when appropriate, sends a message that it does not value them either.

Resistance to standardization. Anaesthetists are highly trained individuals with a large amount of professional autonomy. Checklists, by definition, standardize and consequently restrict practice, and may therefore be resisted. This may manifest itself in 'academic' arguments about the validity of evidence in favour of specific checklists.

'Professional' behaviour and stereotypes. As a result of the three aspects above, senior medical staff may view the checklist process as beneath them, and something to be delegated to more junior staff. This may in turn promote a culture of non-importance.

Checklist design. Undoubtedly, some checklists are badly worded and designed. There may be too many questions, questions asked at the wrong time in the process, or questions which encourage yes/no answers without true engagement. The evolution of the AAGBI Anaesthetic Machine Checklist demonstrates improvements in layout and wording to encourage full compliance.

Human fallibility. However well designed the checklist process, humans will make mistakes. Most commonly reported are automatic responses – answering yes, when the checks have not actually been done, and performing checklists by rote.

WHO Checklist. The WHO checklist is a hybrid checklist. It involves elements of planning, briefing and checking (Table 44.6). The components on the checklist match the WHO Safe Surgery Saves Lives objectives believed to be fundamental to improving outcomes following surgery (Table 44.7).

There are three phases to the checklist:

- Sign-in: is it safe to start anaesthesia?
- Time-out: is it safe to start surgery?
- Sign-out: has surgery been completed safely? Is it safe to hand over to the next phase of care.

Local adaptation is encouraged, both to match local circumstances and to ensure the appropriate questions are asked. For instance, cataract surgery under local anaesthesia is ill-served by questions related to airway management, but may have specific issues around preoperative biometry.

There are other surgical checklists, notably the SURPASS system, pioneered in the Netherlands. The basic principles are the same.

There is reasonable evidence that implementation of the WHO checklist is associated with improvement in outcomes following surgery. The degree of compliance with perioperative checklists appears to be associated with both intraoperative teamwork, and postoperative outcomes. In other words, doing it well is as important as doing it at all.

TABLE 44.6

Examples of Different Purposes of Checklists

Checklist	Purpose	Example	Notes
Anaesthesia machine	Checking	Check that the anaesthetic apparatus is connected to a supply of oxygen and that an adequate reserve supply of oxygen is available from a spare cylinder	Printed cards attached to machine Long-list
Advanced life support 4 Hs and 4 Ts	Checking	Potential causes or aggravating factors for which specific treatment exists must be sought during any cardiac arrest. For ease of memory, these are divided into two groups of four, based upon their initial letter, either H or T: **H**ypoxia **H**ypovolaemia...	Memorization encouraged Time-critical
WHO Checklist	Multiple/hybrid		No explicit differentiation between checking, briefing and planning
WHO Checklist	Checking	Is the anaesthesia machine and medication check complete? (Sign-in) Have the specimens been labelled (including patient name)? (Sign-out)	Refers to another process/SOP
WHO Checklist	Briefing	Are there any critical or unexpected steps you want the team to know about? (Time-out)	A 'stop – go' moment, but mainly a confirmation of adequate staff briefing
WHO Checklist	Planning	Are there any specific equipment requirements or special investigations? (Time-out)	Really a planning question May be too late to solve the problem

TABLE 44.7

WHO Safe Surgery Saves Lives Objectives

	Objective
1.	The team will operate on the correct patient at the correct site.
2.	The team will use methods known to prevent harm from anaesthetic administration, while protecting the patient from pain.
3.	The team will recognize and effectively prepare for life-threatening loss of airway or respiratory function.
4.	The team will recognize and effectively prepare for risk of high blood loss.
5.	The team will avoid inducing an allergic or adverse drug reaction known to be a significant risk to the patient.
6.	The team will consistently use methods known to minimize the risk of surgical site infection.
7.	The team will prevent inadvertent retention of swabs or instruments in surgical wounds.
8.	The team will secure and accurately identify all surgical specimens.
9.	The team will effectively communicate and exchange critical patient information for the safe conduct of the operation.
10.	Hospitals and public health systems will establish routine surveillance of surgical capacity, volume and results.

As with all checklists, lack of engagement, over-familiarity and 'tick-boxing' are significant risks from its continued use.

The WHO checklist is a per patient checklist. Many authorities argue that its safety role is enhanced by broader per list processes such as briefings and debriefings which promote wider team communication and allow problems to be identified and addressed without the pressure of having a patient present.

DESIGNING PROBLEMS OUT OF THE SYSTEM

Human error is inevitable. A key approach to minimizing error is therefore to limit the possibility for human error. In many respects, anaesthesia provides exemplars of how this can be done, although there are many areas in which progress could be made.

Safety by Design

The anaesthetic machine is a device designed to deliver a safe mixture of gases to a patient. Over the years, almost every method of failing to do this has happened, often with tragic consequences. It is now difficult to deliver hypoxic mixtures regardless of human interaction. Specific design features include non-interchangeable screw threads and valves on gas supplies, hypoxic guards and linkages on flowmeters and standardized connections for breathing systems. The same approach can be taken with presetting of infusion protocols for PCAS, epidural infusions, TCI, etc.

Organizational Design

There are theoretical safety (and financial) advantages to limiting the variation in drugs and equipment available to anaesthetists. There is usually little evidence to suggest that one drug or device is better than another, but by limiting choices, individuals are more likely to be familiar with what is available and possibly less likely to confuse one for another. This approach can be seen in the rationalization of anaesthetic drug cupboards to have the same core drugs, laid out in the same way. 'Dangerous' drugs which are used rarely but with potentially catastrophic consequences (e.g. neat KCl) are kept out of routine drug cupboards.

Making it Easy to do the Right Thing

Most individuals will choose the easiest option if there are no other issues to consider. If the system is designed to make the correct option the easiest option, then safety should be enhanced. For instance, providing procedure packs with full sterile protective equipment and drapes is associated with better compliance with sterile precautions and reduction in central line-associated infections. No new equipment or policies are required, simply a redesign of the process.

Understanding Workarounds

Even with these designs, individuals may deliberately circumvent the system. When this occurs, organizations and departments need to understand why this has happened. The answer will often reveal deficiencies in the current design, and a lack of understanding of why processes are designed in the current way. Organizations with proactive and generative safety cultures will seek to address these rather than simply exhorting staff to follow policies and procedures.

Learning from Incidents

A key indicator of a safe organization is its desire and ability to learn from previous incidents and near-misses. To quote Sir Liam Donaldson, a past UK Chief Medical Officer: 'To err is human, to cover up is unforgivable, and to fail to learn is inexcusable.'

There are several key components to learning from incidents and near-misses:

Acknowledging and Recording that they Happen.

Unfortunately, there is still a common perception of punitive responses to incidents which, in part, leads to significant under-reporting. A cultural failure to recognize the importance of incidents and near-misses may result in some organizations simply not reporting incidents which have occurred. There are structural barriers to reporting in many organizations, with cumbersome paper or electronic systems.

Appropriate Analysis of Incidents

Large industrial companies have specific teams trained to collate, analyse and investigate incidents. Such an approach is relatively rare within healthcare. The anaesthetic profession has made significant progress in this area with prospective studies of rare events (such as the UK National Audit Projects investigating complications of neuraxial blocks, airway management and unintentional awareness); analysis of legal claims (US Closed Claims, NHLSA database in the UK); and prospective studies of incidents (AIMS study – Australia). Many countries now have some form of national reporting system (e.g. the National Reporting and Learning System), although these are of course only as good as the data entered.

Analysis of individual incidents and aggregated data is a skill. This requires training to ensure that the correct interpretation of events is made and that any recommendations will reduce the risk of recurrence without introducing new risks.

Departmental morbidity and mortality meetings provide a good opportunity for colleagues to learn from incidents, provided they are facilitated well.

Feedback to Relevant Staff. A common reason why staff choose not to fill in incident reports is that they feel nothing changes anyway. Departments and organizations have to develop processes which allow staff to receive meaningful feedback about incidents without being swamped by an overload of information.

Organizational Memory. Most errors within healthcare have happened before. Sadly, healthcare has too often forgotten the lessons it learnt last time. This happens particularly when events are separated widely in time or geography. National organizations such as the Colleges and Associations have a key role to play in ensuring that the lessons learnt in previous times are passed on to successive generations of anaesthetists.

Models for Implementing Quality Improvement Programmes

Different models used in quality improvement programmes involve identifying an area for improvement, carefully defining an improvement and developing tools which can be used to measure improvement. A multidisciplinary team then considers and develops the interventions aimed at making these improvements; interventions are implemented and progress is monitored. If the intervention leads to improvements, it is then integrated into everyday work flow. A clear understanding of the aims and positive workplace quality culture are required for the success of any such programme, which requires an integrated approach involving all stakeholders at organizational, departmental and individual levels.

Some of the models of quality improvement which are often used in healthcare settings are described below.

Plan-Do-Study-Act (PDSA). The Institute of Healthcare Improvement has used this method widely for rapid cyclical improvements. At the beginning of the cycle, the nature of the problem is determined. The next stage is that of planning for a specific targeted change. The change is then implemented, and data and information collected to study the impact. The last part of the cycle involves taking action by either implementing the change or starting the process again. The overall improvement may require many small and frequent PDSA cycles rather than one big and slow cycle.

Six Sigma. The main aim of this model is to improve processes to minimize or eliminate waste. The improvement is measured by assessing process capability. Before an intervention is designed and undertaken, baseline assessment is carried out to establish how a process is performing. This is done by observing the process and counting the defects or areas of improvement. The defect rate per million is then calculated to a *sigma* metric using statistical tools. Potential solutions for improvement are then designed and piloted. The measurements of the *sigma* metric are undertaken again to quantify improvement in the process. This method is useful mainly for process improvements and the methodology can be undertaken on a regular basis while efforts to improve processes with multiple interventions are being undertaken in an organization.

Lean Production System. This system overlaps with the six sigma methodology, and is similarly aimed at minimizing waste and improving efficiency by simplifying overcomplicated processes and avoiding duplications and rework. The front-line staff are involved throughout the process and the problems are rigorously tracked as the staff experiment with potential improvements. The lean system is driven by the identification of customer needs. With a focus on the needs of the customers, any activity which does not add value (waste) is then removed. Thus, the value-added activities are maximized, waste is removed and efficiency savings are made.

Root Cause Analysis. This methodology is commonly used for improvements at organizational and departmental level. The analysis is triggered by an adverse event. A retrospective systematic analysis is undertaken to tease out the underlying factors which may have caused and/or contributed to the generation of the event. The spirit of analysis is the belief that systems, rather than individual incompetence, are likely to be the root cause of most problems. With an overarching systems approach to understanding the problem in a non-punitive manner, a trained multidisciplinary team investigates the event to ask a series of questions: what happened, why did it happen, what factors caused it, what contributed to it and what system improvements could prevent it. The team then makes recommendations for changes in system improvements.

Failure Modes and Effects Analysis. The methodology and the underlying principles of this analysis are similar to root cause analysis. The difference is that failure modes and effects analysis is undertaken proactively. The processes and systems are observed and analysed for any potential failure by a multidisciplinary team. The team then evaluates a number of options which can mitigate potential failures, and finally makes recommendations for systems improvements.

SUMMARY

The attributes of quality in healthcare include safety, effectiveness, patient-centredness, timeliness, efficiency and equity. In order to achieve delivery of a high quality of care, it is essential that the organizations, departments and individual members of staff develop a positive quality and safety culture. Such a culture promotes openness and learning from everyday events without being punitive. The common understanding in this culture is that the generation of an error involves latent organizational failures, error-facilitating workplace conditions and human error at the front end. Because human error is inevitable, efforts must be directed towards strengthening the systems so that reliance on the front-end of care delivery is minimized. Any quality improvement programme requires systems which measure quality and safety. A number of methods and techniques are available to assess safety culture in the workplace. In addition, specialty-specific outcome measures should be monitored to obtain a comprehensive assessment of quality. These outcome measures should be context-specific and should include clinical outcomes as well as process measures. Sentinel events are important but do not allow continuous outcome monitoring because of their low occurrence rate. Therefore, rate-based indicators, complications and adverse outcomes need to be monitored to obtain an overall sense of the quality of care. Once the areas for improvement have been identified, departments and organizations should hold team meetings to develop and design new interventions which can narrow the gap between the existing state and the desired state of quality. For implementation of these interventions, a number of approaches, e.g. educational, research, social, may be undertaken. The tools and methodologies for implementing improvement programmes include PDSA cycles, six sigma, lean production system, root cause analysis and failure mode and effects analysis.

FURTHER READING

Donabedian, A., 1966. Evaluating quality of medical care. Milbank Q. 44, 166–206.

Leape, L.L., 2009. Errors in medicine. Clin. Chim. Acta 404, 2–5.

Staender, S., Mellin-Oslen, J., Pelosi, P., Van Aken, H., 2011. Safety in anaesthesia. Best Pract. Res. Clin. Anaesthesiol 25, 109–304.

Varkey, P., Peller, K., Resar, R.K., 2007. Basics of quality improvement in healthcare. Mayo Clin. Proc. 82, 735–739.

Vincent, C., 2010. Patient safety, second ed. Wiley-Blackwell, Oxford.

45 THE INTENSIVE CARE UNIT

Historically, critical care medicine can be traced as far back as the Crimean war and Florence Nightingale's pioneering work in monitoring the critically ill patient. The poliomyelitis outbreak in Denmark in the 1950s saw the onset of positive pressure ventilation in specific designated areas, and continued evolution has led to what we recognize as intensive care medicine today. This chapter aims to provide an overview of the provision of general adult intensive care.

The key components of intensive care are resuscitation and stabilization, physiological optimization to prevent organ failure, support of the failing organ systems and recognition of futility of treatment. The Department of Health NHS Executive defines intensive care as 'a service for patients with potentially recoverable conditions who can benefit from more detailed observation and treatment than can safely be provided in general wards or high dependency areas'. Levels of care within the hospital can be described from level 0 (ward-based care) to level 3 (patients requiring advanced respiratory support alone or a minimum of 2 organs being supported) (Table 45.1). There is now a move towards a comprehensive critical care system, where the needs of all patients who are critically ill, rather than just those who are admitted to designated intensive care or high dependency beds, are met with consistency.

In the UK, intensive care beds generally account for 1–2% of the total number of acute beds. The design of ICUs varies from hospital to hospital but they are characterized by being designated areas in which traditionally there is a minimum nurse:patient ratio of 1:1 in addition to a nurse in charge at all times, 24 h cover by resident medical staff (without commitments elsewhere) and the facilities to support organ system failures. High-dependency units (HDUs) are designated areas with a nurse:patient ratio of 1:2 in addition to a nurse in charge at all times, continuous availability of medical staff either from the admitting specialty, or from the ICU, and an appropriate level of monitoring and other equipment. While ICU and HDU may be situated separately in the hospital, all critical care beds should ideally be in adjacent locations.

The physical floor space for each bed in an ICU should be greater than $20 \, m^2$, more than on an ordinary ward because several nurses may need to treat a patient simultaneously and bulky items of equipment often need to be accommodated. Increased bed spacing and the presence of isolated side rooms may help to reduce the risk of nosocomial infection. Each bed area is supplied with piped oxygen, suction, and medical compressed air. The plethora of electronic monitors requires at least 12 electric power sockets (with emergency backup electrical supply) at each bed. Sufficient bedside storage space, at least $5 \, m^2$, is needed for drugs and disposable equipment. Each bed area should be equipped with a self-inflating resuscitation bag to enable staff to maintain artificial ventilation if the mechanical ventilator, gas or electricity supply fails.

STAFFING AN INTENSIVE CARE UNIT

Care of the individual patient in an ICU is increasingly complex and involves contributions from a variety of medical staff, as well as high standards of care from

TABLE 45.1	
Levels of ICU Care	
LEVEL 0	▪ Requires hospitalization
	▪ Patient's needs can be met through normal ward care
LEVEL 1	▪ Patients recently discharged from a higher level of care
	▪ Patients in need of additional monitoring/clinical interventions
	▪ Patients requiring critical care outreach service support, clinical input or advice
LEVEL 2	▪ Patients needing preoperative optimization
	▪ Patients needing extended postoperative care
	▪ Patients stepping down to Level 2 care from Level 3
	▪ Patients receiving single organ support including basic cardiovascular and respiratory support
LEVEL 3	▪ Patients receiving Advanced Respiratory Support alone
	▪ Patients requiring a minimum of 2 organs supported

nurses, physiotherapists, dieticians, pharmacists and other health professionals. Each member of the multidisciplinary team has a broad spectrum of experience and skills and it is worth remembering the value of good teamwork to ensure that high standards of quality patient care are provided. Often the consultant in the specialty under which the patient was admitted may still be nominally in charge, but confusion is minimized if day to day decisions are made through the ICU team, in close liaison with the parent specialty. Good communication is paramount, both within the ICU environment and with the various other teams.

The ICU Consultant

There must be twenty-four hour cover of the ICU by a named consultant who has appropriate experience and competencies. Difficult therapeutic and ethical policy decisions may be required at any time in the ICU and it is essential that they are taken by an individual whose previous experience allows a reasonable assessment of the likely outcome, and whose therapeutic expertise is likely to give the patient the optimal chance of recovery. The ICU consultant, if not physically present in the unit, must always be available by telephone and should not be involved in any activity which precludes his or her attendance there within 30 min. Because of the critical nature of ICU patients' illnesses, the ICU consultant expects to be informed immediately of any significant change in their condition. Similarly they should be informed of any potential admissions and all new patients should be seen

within 12 hours. The consultant's base specialty is less important than appropriate training and experience.

The ICU Resident

The junior medical staff in ICU have a pivotal role in the co-ordination of all aspects of patient care, particularly to maintain good lines of communication between the different teams involved. Because of their continuous presence in the unit, the ICU resident is best informed about the patient's recent diagnostic results, physiological status and therapeutic responses and should attempt to use current knowledge to guide treatment along rational lines. Daily work comprises at least one main ward round, usually in the presence of the multidisciplinary team, whereby clinical decisions are made. Following patient assessment, findings should be documented, the results of relevant investigations reviewed and appropriate actions taken. Because of the potential to change, the patients' clinical state should be frequently reassessed. Other duties may include discussion with relatives, but as with all aspects of intensive care, both clinical and non-clinical duties should fall within the expertise and remit as set by both the junior and consultant. There is a broad range of training opportunities to be had with time spent on the unit, and training in intensive care should be focused on a competency-based programme.

Nursing Staff

It should be appreciated that the nursing staff provide most of the care that patients receive in ICU. ICU nurses have greatly extended roles, experience and responsibility. They have undergone specific training to enable them to perform titration of fluid replacement, analgesia, vasoactive drug therapy and weaning from mechanical ventilation. The route by which complex instructions and information are transmitted between medical and nursing staff is of vital importance. A system in which a relatively junior clinician serves as a 'final common pathway' for all instructions works well in practice, provided that the doctor involved is present within the unit at all times so that the nurses may obtain clarification of instructions, report changes in status and receive immediate help in emergencies. It is essential that a nurse is present and takes part when discussions take place with the patient, or their relatives or friends. The content of such discussions must be recorded accurately in the patient's notes. The resident should remember that the majority of ICU nurses (especially the senior nurses) have an enormous amount of 'bedside' experience with critically ill patients and considerable reliance should be placed on their observations.

Physiotherapists

Physiotherapists provide therapy for clearance of chest secretions and are involved in decisions regarding weaning from mechanical ventilation and tracheostomy decannulation. In addition, physiotherapy is used to help preserve joint and muscle function in the bedbound patient and promote eventual independent ambulation where possible. Their advice on the changing physical status of patients is invaluable.

Pharmacists

Polypharmacy is often a feature in the critically ill and there is great potential for drug interactions and incompatibility of infusions. In addition, many drug doses need to be modified in the presence of critical illness because of altered pharmacodynamics or pharmacokinetics. These changes are likely to be particularly marked in patients with hepatic or renal failure, and can be difficult to predict. Pharmacists have a vital role in checking prescriptions and providing detailed advice on drug therapies.

Dieticians

For all but extremely short ICU stays, the critically ill patient should receive some form of nutrition while in ICU. The role of the dietician is to assess the nutritional status and requirements of the patient and hence provide individually tailored support. They may also be involved in the TPN team.

The Microbiologist

Critically ill patients are immunocompromised as a result of the underlying pathological process, the impact of treatments (such as steroids) and the presence of surgical/traumatic wounds, multiple vascular catheters and other invasive tubing. This predisposes them to hospital-acquired infections. Prolonged use of broad-spectrum antibiotics encourages the development of resistant pathogens and overgrowth of other organisms. In order to effectively treat sepsis and prevent resistance, there is usually a nominated microbiologist, who is familiar with the flora and resistance patterns of the unit, and who visits the ICU daily to advise on microbiology results and antibiotic therapy. It is also essential to adhere to local policies aimed at reducing cross infection and minimizing the number of hospital-acquired infections. The National Patient Safety Agency (NPSA) also has a number of helpful guidelines for personnel working on ICU (www.npsa.nhs.uk).

OUTREACH/FOLLOW-UP

The critical care outreach team collaborates between the ICU and other areas of the hospital. The aims of the outreach team are to identify the deteriorating patient early with the aim of averting ICU admission, to facilitate timely admission to ICU if required, and to assist in the timely and appropriate discharge from ICU. It is important to identify those patients who are unlikely to benefit from further resuscitation or critical care support due to the nature of their acute illness or underlying diseases, to prevent futile interventions and ensure equitable use of scarce ICU resources. By following up patients discharged from ICU/HDU, a level of continuity of care can be provided and in addition critical care skills may be shared between the team and ward-based staff. The team may comprise of senior members of medical, nursing and physiotherapy staff.

A number of scoring systems based on abnormal physiological variables, such as the modified early warning score (MEWS) (Table 45.2), can be recorded

TABLE 45.2
Modified Early Warning System (MEWS)

MEWS Score	3	2	1	0	1	2	3
Pulse		<40	41–50	51–100	101–110	111–130	>131
Respiratory rate		<8		9–14	15–20	21–29	>30
Temperature		<35	35.1–36	36.1–38	38.1–38.5	>38.6	
Urine output	<10 mL/h	<20 mL/h					
Systolic BP	<70	71–80	81–100	101–199		>200	
AVPU	U	P	V	A	New agitation/ confusion		
Glasgow Coma Scale				15	14	9–13	<8

AVPU is a simple assessment where: A, Alert; V, Responds to verbal commands only; P, responds to pain; U, completely unresponsive.

by ward staff; the outreach team can be contacted accordingly once a trigger score has been reached. Care needs to be taken with younger fitter patients, who have good physiological reserve and who may not deteriorate in terms of MEWS score until a peri-arrest situation develops (e.g. in presence of bleeding or severe sepsis). Children, obstetric, neurological, renal and other sub-specialty groups have adapted scores to allow for altered background physiological status.

ADMISSION TO THE INTENSIVE CARE UNIT

The decision to admit a patient to the intensive care unit may be straightforward, but is often difficult and confounded by increasing expectations in an ever increasing elderly population with multiple comorbidities. ICU resources are finite and costs high, so in the face of limited prospects for benefit or survival of an individual patient, a number of complex ethical issues can arise surrounding admission, provision and discontinuation of intensive care therapy. It is therefore necessary that all individual cases are discussed with the ICU consultant, as the decision regarding whether to admit the patient often comes down to multidisciplinary team discussion and clinical expertise. Blanket admission policies may be unhelpful, and decisions should consider the individual patient, taking into account their wishes and values. Senior staff should discuss with the patient (where

possible) and/or their relatives potential treatment options and possible outcomes and alternatives. However, acutely ill patients can rarely discuss details of their care, and relatives may find it difficult to make an objective judgement. If a patient has made an Advance Directive ('Living Will') then its contents must be respected.

In essence, the aim of intensive care is to support patients while they recover. It is not to prolong life when there is no hope of recovery. In many cases, unless the outlook is obviously futile, patients will be admitted for a trial of treatment to see whether they will stabilize and improve over time. Patients with little or no prospect of survival may occasionally be admitted to intensive care. This can facilitate more appropriate terminal care, or to allow the relatives time to visit and the bereavement process to be better managed. In the very short term this is a justifiable and appropriate use of a critical care facility.

Assessment of Patients

When dealing with a newly admitted patient with acute disease, assessment and resuscitation often take place simultaneously and follow the standard pattern of recognizing and dealing with problems in the order of airway, breathing and circulation. The resident should heed all the patient's problems and the responses to the treatments instigated and to do this, it is essential to approach the assessment of the patient in a systematic manner.

History

Often the patient is unable to give a full and accurate history. Information should be obtained from the patient's notes, a thorough handover from referring or transferring staff, old notes (which may need to be retrieved from the referring hospital), and information from the patient's family doctor. Speaking to the patient's relatives gives invaluable insight into the patient's pre-morbid condition; and looking at the intensive care chart allows an assessment of progress regarding ventilation, haemodynamic stability, fluid balance and sedation requirement. It is important that details in the history are not overlooked as it is relatively easy for misinformation to be perpetuated from one shift handover to the next.

Examination

It is imperative to adhere to unit policy regarding infection control. Scrupulous hand hygiene and the use of gloves and aprons are necessary before examination of the patient. A systematic approach is vital. Remember that although the patient may appear to be unconscious, hearing and other senses may still be intact, dignity and respect should be maintained at all times. Below is a guide to examination.

Airway and Respiratory System

Note how the airway has been secured, how long any tube (tracheal/tracheostomy) has been in place, relevant cuff pressures and type and volume of respiratory secretions. In a trauma patient, ensure that the cervical spine is stable. Auscultate the lungs to check for bilateral and equal air entry and added sounds. Check the type and adequacy of ventilation, as well as latest arterial blood gas results, and ensure the most recent and relevant past CXRs have been reviewed. If chest drains are present again ascertain their duration and drainage.

Cardiovascular System

Note the pulse, arterial pressure, JVP, heart sounds, CVP, stroke volume and cardiac output. Clinical examination will reveal whether the patient feels cold and 'shut down' or warm and 'well perfused'. Look for the presence of dependent or peripheral oedema. Venous/arterial catheter sites may reveal evidence of infection. Note the type and dose of positive inotropes or other vasoactive drugs required.

Gastointestinal Tract

Examination of the abdomen will reveal whether it is soft, tender or distended. The absence of bowel sounds may be misleading in a patient who is sedated and undergoing artificial ventilation; bowel activity is better ascertained from the observation chart. It should be noted whether the patient is being fed enterally or parenterally. If enteral feeding is being provided, note whether the patient is absorbing the feed and whether any prokinetic drugs are required; stress ulcer prophylaxis is routine. Other information gained from examination may include recent surgical activity, the function of stomas, appearance of wounds and contents of abdominal drains.

Renal System

The important features are urine output, current/cumulative fluid balance and abnormalities of serum electrolytes or acid–base balance. The patient may be receiving renal replacement therapy so make sure catheters and anticoagulation are adequate.

Central Nervous System

Ascertain the patient's level of consciousness as well as the dose and duration of sedative/analgesic drugs. Scoring systems for sedation are widely used. It is increasingly the practice to perform daily sedation holds unless contraindicated, for example a patient with cerebral oedema after traumatic brain injury. Make a note of evidence of focal neurology/seizures/weakness and whether there are purposeful symmetrical movements to verbal command or painful stimulus. Specialist monitoring may be used to measure intracranial pressure and cerebral perfusion pressure, and to guide management.

Limbs/Skin and Wounds

Look for evidence of adequate perfusion (ensure documentation of primary and secondary surveys after trauma), presence of peripheral pulses, adequate capillary refill and evidence of swelling, tenderness, DVT or compartment syndrome.

Surgical wounds and trauma sites should be inspected for adequate healing or infection.

Lines and Sepsis

All invasive catheters and tubing should be inspected for signs of local exit site infection (they will not show internal infection). Their duration should be noted as well as review of their ongoing requirement. Evidence suggesting catheter-related sepsis should prompt their removal and culture, but they should not be routinely replaced as a method of preventing infection. Note the patient's temperature with changes over time and check against markers of infection such as pulse, WCC, CRP and procalcitonin.

Investigations/Planned Interventions

Once the patient has been reviewed, go back through the chart to make sure nothing has been omitted and review the patient's important haematology, biochemistry and microbiology results. Radiological investigations should also be reviewed.

Documentation should be of a high standard. Many units use a standard proforma for admission documentation and other templates, algorithms or protocols to encourage high standards of clinical care. Prescription charts should be reviewed daily, making particular note of antibiotic requirements and appropriateness of stress ulcer and DVT prophylaxis. Fluid and nutrition charts should also be examined.

Formulating a Plan

Finally an action plan needs to be formulated, with special regard to both active and ongoing problems. A plan for each organ system requiring support should be put into place as well as a ventilation and/or weaning proposal. A review of nutrition, 24 h fluid balance and changes to drug therapy should also be undertaken and any planned procedures/interventions should be discussed with the consultant. Communicate back any change in plans to the relevant nursing staff and bear in mind that relatives appreciate honest, up to date progress reports. It is important to note that patient confidentiality should never be compromised via discussion or documentation. Full assessment and examination should be repeated at least daily even in stable patients, because the physiological state of critically ill patients can change rapidly.

Transfers

If the patient is to undergo transfer, whether to another hospital, CT, theatre or other site, meticulous preparation should be undertaken to ensure the patient at all times has availability to an oxygen supply, venous access, monitoring with power backup and an adequate supply of their necessary infusions and pumps. The accompanying personnel, at least 2 persons, must have experience in transfer of the critically ill patient. Emergency drugs and intubation equipment need to be readily available as a transfer, no matter how short, can rapidly become a hazardous situation.

MONITORING IN ICU

There is a plethora of monitoring equipment in ICU, which may at first be daunting. It is important to know that all equipment is working, and accurate and calibrated correctly. Always question whether additional monitoring is necessary and whether it would safely provide further information.

Basic Non-Invasive Monitoring

Monitoring of ECG and oxygen saturation is routine for all patients. Non-invasive blood pressure measurements may be required if the level of care is stepped down. Capnography confirms intubation of the trachea and connection to the ventilator, the presence of airflow obstruction and a cardiac output. It provides some information about the adequacy of ventilation, but correlates poorly with $PaCO_2$. It is essential monitoring for tracheal intubation, during tracheostomy or other airway interventions and is rapidly becoming standard at all times in ventilated patients.

Invasive Monitoring

Arterial Pressure

Arterial cannulation is used in most ICU patients. It allows continuous measurement of arterial blood pressure and easy serial blood gas and other sampling. Significant respiratory variation in the amplitude of the arterial pressure wave ('respiratory swing') is characteristic of hypovolaemia. This pulse pressure variability (which relates to stroke volume variability caused by changes in venous return) can be formally measured by modern monitoring systems and is described as a percentage. Abnormal arterial waveforms can be seen in hyperdynamic circulations and conditions such as aortic stenosis, aortic regurgitation and left ventricular failure. Normal waveforms give an indication of cardiac output, myocardial contractility and outflow resistance.

Central Venous Pressure

Right heart filling pressures may be measured by central venous catheterization of the superior vena cava (common access sites are the internal jugular, subclavian or femoral vein). The trend in measured pressure provides some indication of haemodynamic status/ cardiac function, but should be interpreted with caution as it can be subject to other influences. Central venous access provides a route for intravenous drug infusion as well as a dedicated route for temporary parenteral nutrition. Strict aseptic technique is required when manipulating the catheter or its connections to minimize the risk of catheter-related sepsis.

Pulmonary Artery Catheter

Pulmonary artery (PA) catheterization was for a number of years considered the 'gold standard' for cardiovascular monitoring in ICU. This technique enabled the measurement of pulmonary artery pressure, pulmonary artery occlusion pressure (wedge pressure, PAOP) and CO, and also allowed many other haemodynamic variables to be derived. The value of pulmonary artery catheters has been questioned and its use has fallen significantly with the introduction of alternative forms of monitoring. Given the controversy regarding its potential advantages, its use should be based on the risk/benefit ratio for each individual patient.

Pulse Contour Analysis. The peripheral arterial pulse waveform is a function of the cardiac output, the peripheral vascular resistance, peripheral vascular compliance and the arterial pressure. If the cardiac output is measured for a given peripheral arterial waveform, then after calibration, changes in the peripheral pulse waveform can be used to calculate changes in the cardiac output. To calibrate the system an indicator is injected into a venous catheter and is detected by an arterial line producing a standard dilutional CO measurement. Systems such as PiCCO and LiDCO use thermodilution and lithium respectively as the indicators. Aside from cardiac output, stroke volume and systemic vascular resistance, other variables available with PiCCO include global end diastolic volume (cardiac preload) and intrathoracic blood volume. Dynamic measures, using heart–lung interactions to predict fluid responsiveness, can also be widely determined using beat to beat cardiac output monitoring.

Oesophageal Doppler

A Doppler ultrasound probe is placed in the oesophagus and directed to obtain a signal from the descending aorta. The signal obtained is displayed on the screen and indicates peak velocity and flow time. By making a number of assumptions about the nature of flow in the aorta, the cross-sectional area of the aorta (estimated from body surface area and age) and the percentage of CO passing down the thoracic aorta, SV and CO can be estimated. Trends in values and response to changes in therapy are more useful than absolute values. It is particularly useful for assessing response to fluid challenges in patients who are sedated but requires precise positioning and is therefore operator dependent.

Other Technologies

Echocardiography

Echocardiography is emerging as a very useful tool in the ICU, especially in the assessment of haemodynamics and response to therapeutic interventions. However, this often can prove challenging in the ICU setting. Focused echocardiography is used to assess myocardial activity, filling or the presence of a pericardial collection, for example in the peri-arrest period. Measurement of IVC diameter can be used to assess venous filling. It is likely that the use of echocardiography in critical care will increase.

Ultrasound Imaging

Ultrasound has an established role in venous and arterial access. It is also increasingly used by intensivists for the assessment of pleural collections (air and fluid), ascites, and joint effusions. Adequate training in this modality is essential.

It remains a useful tool for diagnosis and bedside radiological interventions.

ICP/Jugular Venous Saturation/Compressed Spectral Array/BIS

Indications for ICP monitoring vary between units, but may include any cause of coma, commonly head injury and intracranial head injury. Types of monitoring may include extradural fibreoptic probes, a subarachnoid screw, ventricular drain or intracerebral transducer. ICP monitoring allows calculation of cerebral perfusion pressure; both variables can then be used to guide management.

Jugular venous bulb oxygen saturation is an indirect indicator of cerebral oxygen utilization and provides a measure of global cerebral oxygenation. It involves a catheter being placed retrogradely up the internal jugular vein.

Compressed spectral array and bispectral index (BIS) are computerized assessments of EEG signals, which allow depth of anaesthesia and sedation to be assessed. The former will allow seizure activity to be seen and the presence of burst suppression can be used to indicate a greater depth of anaesthesia consistent with a reduced cerebral oxygen demand.

INSTITUTION OF INTENSIVE CARE

It is impossible to provide a comprehensive review of all the conditions requiring ICU care and their full treatment regimens in one chapter. The following sections are an overview of the management of some common problems presenting to ICU.

The Respiratory System

Respiratory failure is one of the commonest reasons for admission to the ICU (Table 45.3). It may be the primary reason for admission or a feature of a non-respiratory pathological process, e.g. adult respiratory distress syndrome (ARDS) in sepsis. Respiratory failure may encompass hypoxaemia with a normal/low $PaCO_2$ (type 1) or a combination of hypoxaemia and high $PaCO_2$ (type 2).

Type 1 Respiratory Failure – PaO_2 <8 kPa with Normal/Low $PaCO_2$

Lung alveolar function is impaired in a number of pathological processes such as pneumonia, pulmonary oedema and ARDS. The combination of blood flowing through unventilated areas of lung results in ventilation–perfusion mismatch or 'shunt'. The resultant hypoxaemia is initially accompanied by hyperventilation, in a physiological bid to reduce CO_2 tension and increase arterial oxygen saturation. However, this can only usually be sustained for a limited period of time and progressive exhaustion ensues, with a concomitant rise in $PaCO_2$ and fall in PaO_2. Respiratory arrest will occur without intervention.

TABLE 45.3	
Causes of Respiratory Failure	
Reduced central drive	Brainstem injury/CVA
	Drug effects, e.g. opioids
	Metabolic encephalopathy
Airway obstruction	Tumour
	Infection
	Sleep apnoea
	Foreign body
Lung pathology	Asthma
	COPD
	Pneumonia
	Fibrosis
	ALI/ARDS
	Lung contusion
Neuromuscular defects	Spinal cord lesion
	Phrenic nerve disruption
	Myasthenia gravis
	Guillain–Barré syndrome
	Critical illness polyneuropathy
Musculoskeletal	Trauma
	Severe scoliosis

Type 2 Respiratory Failure – PaO_2 <8 kPa and $PaCO_2$ >8 kPa

This occurs when there is hypoxaemia and hypoventilation from a variety of causes, e.g. chronic obstructive pulmonary disease (COPD), reduced central respiratory drive, neuromuscular conditions and chest wall deformity. Although the primary problem is hypercapnia, which may eventually result in progressive carbon dioxide narcosis and respiratory arrest, there is typically accompanying hypoxia. The patient with COPD may have a chronically raised $PaCO_2$, which is well tolerated. The associated reduction in respiratory centre sensitivity is not well understood. Such patients may rely on hypoxia to drive their ventilation and will deteriorate when given enough additional oxygen to correct their hypoxaemia.

Assessment of the Patient with Respiratory Failure

Clinical assessment is often the most rapid way to evaluate the patient with respiratory failure (Table 45.4):

- Can patient talk in sentences?
- Are they awake and orientated?
- What is the pulse, BP and respiratory rate?

TABLE 45.4
Signs of Impending Respiratory Arrest
Marked tachypnoea, or hypoventilation, patient exhausted
Use of accessory muscles
Cyanosis and desaturation, especially if on supplemental oxygen
Tachycardia or bradycardia if peri-arrest
Sweaty, peripherally cool/clammy
Mental changes, confusion and leading to coma in extreme conditions

TABLE 45.5
Indications for Ventilatory Support
Indications for ventilatory support in respiratory failure
■ Reduced conscious level
■ Exhaustion
■ Tachypnoea
■ Reduced PaO_2 despite increasing oxygen therapy
■ Increased $PaCO_2$
■ Acidosis
■ Cardiovascular instability
■ Tachycardia/bradycardia
■ Hypotension

- Is the patient using accessory muscles of respiration?
- Can they cough effectively to clear secretions?
- Are they clammy and sweating?
- Do they appear exhausted? Exhaustion and impending respiratory failure that is likely to require ventilatory support is an end-of-bed diagnosis.

A full history including previous functional status, and physical examination are mandatory. Serial arterial blood gases are required to determine the extent of the respiratory failure and response to any therapy. The chest X-ray and other available investigations such as peak flow will aid evaluation of the patient's condition.

Management of Respiratory Failure

Management is directed at correcting hypoxia/ hypercarbia and reversing the underlying condition if possible. Simple manoeuvres such as supplying supplemental oxygen should be instituted initially. Give oxygen via facemask, preferably humidified. Higher concentrations of oxygen can be achieved with a reservoir system and a fixed performance device (e.g. Venturi) may be preferable in titrating oxygen concentrations in those COPD patients who rely on hypoxia to drive their ventilation. The effect of oxygen therapy should be assessed by pulse oximetry and arterial blood gas analysis after around 30 min.

Other therapies may be useful such as bronchodilators, steroids, diuretics and physiotherapy in the first instance depending on the mechanism of respiratory failure. Many patients may be dehydrated due to poor fluid intake and increased losses and will require IV fluids. If there is no improvement over time, additional respiratory support may be necessary (Table 45.5). Options include:

Continuous Positive Airway Pressure (CPAP). CPAP is provided via a tightly fitting mask or hood. A high gas flow (greater than the patient's peak inspiratory flow rate) is required to keep the positive pressure set by the expiratory valve (+5–10 cmH$_2$O) almost constant throughout the respiratory cycle. CPAP increases functional residual capacity (FRC), reduces alveolar collapse and improves oxygenation but it requires a co-operative patient, with no facial injuries. It does not generally help the patient with type 2 respiratory failure. There is a small risk of aspiration as a result of stomach distension.

Non-Invasive Positive Pressure Ventilation (NIPPV or NIV). Non-invasive techniques have been successfully used to treat acute exacerbations in patients with COPD, in the management of pulmonary oedema and as a weaning aid. Biphasic or bi-level positive airway pressure (BiPAP or BPAP) is a common form where a set inspiratory pressure enhances the patient's own respiratory effort to increase achievable tidal volume and the set expiratory pressure is analogous to CPAP.

If the clinical condition continues to deteriorate in conjunction with worsening arterial blood gases in a patient with potentially reversible pulmonary disease, then invasive mechanical ventilation will be necessary.

Mechanical Ventilation

The usual indication for mechanical ventilation is in patients with potentially reversible pathology who are unable to maintain adequate oxygenation or who develop hypercapnia. In some cases, blood gases may be normal but are predicted to deteriorate because the patient is becoming exhausted.

Tracheal Intubation.

To enable mechanical ventilation to be carried out effectively, a cuffed tube must be placed in the trachea either via the mouth or nose, or directly through a tracheostomy stoma. In the emergency situation, an orotracheal tube is usually inserted. If the patient is conscious, anaesthesia should be induced carefully with an appropriate dose of an i.v. anaesthetic induction agent and neuromuscular blocker. The full range of adjuncts for difficult intubation should be available.

The critically ill patient is often exquisitely sensitive to i.v. anaesthetic drugs, and cardiovascular collapse may occur; consequently, full resuscitation equipment must be immediately available. I.v. fluid resuscitation and vasoactive drug infusions are often required.

If the patient is unconscious, a neuromuscular blocker alone may be necessary (but not obligatory) to facilitate the passage of the tube; however, an i.v. anaesthetic induction agent and neuromuscular blocker should always be used in patients with severe head injury to prevent an increase in intracranial pressure (ICP) during laryngoscopy and tracheal intubation.

Many patients are hypoxaemic, and it is essential that 100% oxygen is administered before tracheal intubation.

- After neuromuscular blockade has been produced, the tube should be inserted by the route which is associated with the least delay.
- If the patient is unconscious and the victim of blunt trauma, when cervical spine injury is a possibility, the cervical spine should be immobilized during intubation using manual in-line immobilization.
- Cricoid pressure should be applied to minimize the risk of aspirating gastric contents.
- A sterile, disposable plastic tube with a low-pressure cuff should be used. The tube should

be inserted such that the top of the cuff lies not more than 3 cm below the vocal cords.
- The head should be placed in a neutral or slightly flexed position (on one pillow) after tracheal intubation and a chest X-ray taken to ensure that the tip of the tube lies at least 5 cm above the carina.

Bronchial intubation is a common complication during mechanical ventilation as the tracheal tube may migrate down the trachea when the patient is moved during normal nursing procedures. Intubation of the right main bronchus cannot be detected reliably by observation of chest movements or by auscultation of the chest because of the exaggerated transmission of breath sounds during IPPV, although absent or asynchronous chest movement may occur when pulmonary collapse has taken place. Bronchial intubation is one of the causes of a sudden decrease in compliance, and restlessness and coughing often occur if the end of the tube irritates the carina. If this is suspected, the tube should be withdrawn gradually by up to 5 cm while lung compliance and chest expansion are observed carefully. The position of the tube should always be confirmed by a chest radiograph.

When the upper airway or larynx is obstructed and conventional tracheal intubation is not possible (e.g. occasional cases of epiglottitis or laryngeal trauma), the emergency airway of choice is cricothyroidotomy.

Tracheostomy is increasingly performed percutaneously on the ICU and is most frequently an elective decision. Indications include:

- to maintain the airway, e.g. reduced level of consciousness, upper-airway obstruction
- to protect the airway, e.g. bulbar palsy, brain injury
- for bronchial toilet, e.g. excessive secretions/inadequate cough
- for weaning from IPPV, e.g. patient comfort, reduction of sedation.

The recently completed Tracman study confirmed no clear benefit from early compared with delayed performance of tracheostomy.

Sedation and Analgesia.

Once tracheal intubation has been performed, some amount of sedative drugs will be required to tolerate the tube and facilitate effective mechanical ventilation. The balance between

TABLE 45.6
Problems and Potential Consequences of Excessive Sedation in ICU

Problem	Potential consequence
Accumulation with prolonged infusion	Delayed weaning from supportive care
Detrimental effect on cardiovascular system	Increased requirement for vasoactive drugs
Detrimental effect on pulmonary function	Increased VQ mismatch
Tolerance	Withdrawal on stopping sedation
No REM sleep	Sleep deprivation and ICU psychosis
Reduced intestinal motility	Impairment of enteral feeding
Potential effects on immune/ endocrine function	Drugs such as opioids may have a role in immunomodulation and risk of infection
Adverse effects of specific drugs	e.g. propofol infusion syndrome, with cardiovascular collapse

TABLE 45.7
Sedation Scoring Using the Ramsay Sedation Scale

Ramsay Sedation Scale

1. Patient anxious, agitated or restless
2. Patient co-operative, orientated and tranquil
3. Patient responds to commands only
4. Patient exhibits brisk response to light forehead tap or loud auditory stimulus
5. Patient exhibits sluggish response to light forehead tap or loud auditory stimulus
6. Patient exhibits no response

providing adequate sedation to permit patient co-operation with organ system support and oversedation, which leads to a number of detrimental effects (Table 45.6) is often difficult. The aims of sedation include patient comfort and analgesia, minimizing anxiety, and to allow a calm co-operative patient who is able to sleep when undisturbed and able to tolerate appropriate organ support. Patients must not be paralysed and awake but the efficiency of supportive care will be reduced in the patient who is agitated and distressed. Clearly the patient's needs for sedation will alter with changes in clinical condition and requirements for care, so regular review and sedation scoring are helpful (Table 45.7).

An Overview of Modes of Ventilation

Different manufacturers used different terms for basically similar modes of ventilation which often cause confusion for the inexperienced.

Volume Controlled Ventilation. The simplest form of volume controlled ventilation is controlled mandatory ventilation (CMV). The patient's lungs are ventilated at a preset tidal volume and rate (for example, tidal volume 500 mL and rate 12 breaths min^{-1}). The tidal volume delivered is therefore predetermined and the peak pressure required to deliver this volume varies depending upon other ventilator settings and the patient's pulmonary compliance. A major disadvantage of CMV is that high peak airway pressures may result and this can lead to lung damage or barotrauma. Therefore it is only really suitable for patients who are heavily sedated and/or paralysed and who are making no respiratory effort.

Pressure Controlled Ventilation. Pressure controlled modes of ventilation are commonly used, and are preferred in patients with poor pulmonary compliance. A peak inspiratory pressure is set and so tidal volume delivered is a function of the peak pressure, the inspiratory time and the patient's compliance. By using lower peak pressures and slightly longer inspiratory times the risks of barotrauma can be reduced. As the patient's condition improves and lung compliance increases, the tidal volume achieved for the same settings will increase and the inspiratory pressure can therefore be reduced. Biphasic or bi-level positive airway pressure (BIPAP) is a variation of pressure controlled ventilation which permits spontaneous breaths by the patient at all times during the ventilator cycle.

Synchronized Intermittent Mandatory Ventilation (SIMV). Modes of ventilation have been developed which allow preservation of the patient's own respiratory efforts by detecting an attempt by the patient to breathe in and synchronizing the mechanical breath with spontaneous inspiration; this technique is termed synchronized intermittent mandatory ventilation (SIMV). If no attempt at inspiration is detected over a period of some seconds then a mandatory breath is delivered to ensure that a safe total minute volume is provided.

Pressure Support Ventilation (PSV)/Assisted Spontaneous Breathing (ASB). Breathing through a ventilator can be difficult because respiratory muscles may be weak and ventilator circuits and tracheal tubes provide significant resistance to breathing. During PSV the ventilator senses a spontaneous breath and augments it by addition of positive pressure. This reduces the patient's work of breathing and increases the tidal volume. Pressure support is usually set at 15–20 cmH_2O in the first instance and can be reduced as the patient's condition improves. It is best not to remove pressure support completely, however, because of the internal resistance of the ventilator and its connections. SIMV and PSV require a method of detecting the patient's own respiratory effort, in order to trigger the appropriate ventilator response. This is achieved by flow sensors detecting small changes in gas flow within the circuit.

Positive End Expiratory Pressure (PEEP). PEEP has the advantage of alveolar recruitment and maintenance of functional residual capacity, which will improve lung compliance. Some patients, e.g. those with expiratory airflow limitation can develop air trapping and a degree of so-called 'intrinsic PEEP'. Modern ventilators are capable of calculating this and it is important to consider it when setting levels of externally applied extrinsic PEEP in this subset of patients, as there is a potential risk of sustained lung hyperinflation if external PEEP is set above the level of intrinsic PEEP. While PEEP is beneficial for the vast majority of mechanically ventilated patients, it can reduce venous return and cardiac output so caution must be exercised at higher levels.

Problems Associated with Mechanical Ventilation

Once the patient's trachea is intubated and lungs ventilated they are crucially dependent on technology to avoid hypoxaemia and hypercarbia. Other important aspects of care include; humidification of gases, regular physiotherapy and tracheal toilet and continuous monitoring of SpO_2, end-tidal CO_2, inspired O_2 concentration, minute volume, and peak airway pressure.

Other constant risks include: tracheal tube dislodgement and difficult re-intubation, laryngeal/tracheal damage with prolonged intubation, ventilator associated pneumonia (see below), needs for sedation, and the haemodynamic effects of positive pressure ventilation and PEEP.

Ventilator associated lung injury (VALI) encompasses a number of components including barotrauma where high pressures are applied to the airway, especially if lung compliance is reduced. This may result in clinically obvious damage like pneumothorax, pneumomediastinum, pneumoperitoneum and subcutaneous emphysema. Volume trauma may occur if excessive tidal volumes are applied and the clinical manifestations are similar to barotrauma. In addition there is considerable experimental evidence for less clinically obvious damage to the lung microstructure even with lower tidal volume positive pressure ventilation, with release of cytokines and other markers of inflammation. There is some evidence that such trauma to the lungs may cause systemic inflammation and have a role in the development of lung damage and multi-organ failure.

Problem Solving in Ventilated Patients

The first priorities are to exclude and, if necessary, correct hypoxaemia or hypercapnia and to detect any adverse effects or complications of ventilation. When a problem arises, consider whether the underlying issue is related to the ventilator (by manually 'bagging' the patient, the ventilator can effectively be excluded), an equipment issue, e.g. function/position/blockage of the tracheal tube or is the problem related to the patient's pathophysiology? Is there progression of the lung problem, e.g. ARDS or development of a new problem, e.g. pneumothorax or bronchospasm? When the problem has been identified, correct management will rectify the situation and is often directed at changes in ventilatory settings and sedation.

Ventilation Strategies. The concept of ventilator-induced lung injury by overdistension, shear stress injury and oxygen toxicity has been increasingly recognized over the past few years and a number of strategies have been put into place to reduce such damage:

- Limiting peak pressure to 35 cmH_2O.
- Limiting tidal volume to 6 mL kg^{-1}.
- Acceptance of higher than normal $PaCO_2$ levels (6–8 kPa), so-called 'permissive hypercapnia'.
- Acceptance of PaO_2 7–8 kPa, SaO_2 >90%.
- Use of higher levels of PEEP to improve alveolar recruitment.
- Use of longer inspiratory times.
- Use of ventilation modes which allow and support spontaneous respiratory effort.
- The acceptable threshold for such values is not known and has to be considered on an individual patient basis.

Other Aspects of Ventilation

In view of the above problems, interest is increasing around other forms of ventilation and adjuncts that improve oxygenation and CO_2 clearance. Examples include high frequency oscillation, use of the prone position, nitric oxide and extracorporeal membrane oxygenation.

High-Frequency Oscillation. In patients with poor compliance, high frequency oscillatory ventilation is a means of reducing transpulmonary pressure while providing adequate gas exchange. Small tidal volumes (lower than deadspace) are generated by an oscillating a diaphragm across the open airway resulting in a sinusoidal or square gas flow pattern. Peak airway pressure is reduced but mean airway pressure is increased allowing for alveolar recruitment and improved oxygenation. Oxygenation certainly improves, but outcomes are currently under study.

Prone Positioning. Another strategy to improve ventilation is to place the patient in the prone position. Recent work has suggested that the improvement is related to changes in regional pleural pressure. This may result partly from the decreased volume of lung compressed by the mediastinal structures when in the prone position. In the prone position, pleural pressure becomes more uniform and reduces ventilation–perfusion mismatch. The technique is very labour-intensive; four people are needed to turn the patient and great care is required to ensure that the airway and vascular catheters/cannulae are not dislodged. A recent multicentre European trial has shown that although oxygenation is improved in responders, the effect does not result in improved survival to discharge.

Nitric Oxide. Nitric oxide (NO) is an ultra-short-acting pulmonary vasodilator. When added to the respiratory gases (5–20 parts per million), it is delivered preferentially to the recruited alveoli and results in pulmonary vasodilation in areas of well ventilated lung. Blood is diverted away from poorly ventilated areas and ventilation–perfusion mismatch is reduced. It is rapidly inactivated by haemoglobin and so vasodilator effects are limited to the pulmonary circulation.

NO at high concentrations (>100 ppm) is highly reactive and toxic, and the delivery system used must conform to rigid safety standards. The dose used should be the lowest which is effective in achieving a 20% improvement in PaO_2:FiO_2 ratio. The concentration of methaemoglobin in the blood and the inspired nitrogen dioxide concentration must be measured. NO therapy is expensive and potentially dangerous. It improves oxygenation in the short term in about 50% of patients but the effect is often transient and no outcome benefits have been shown in clinical trials.

Extracorporeal Membrane Oxygenation. Extracorporeal membrane oxygenation (ECMO) is a possible final option if other conventional techniques of providing ventilatory support have failed. Partial cardiopulmonary venovenous bypass is initiated using heparin-bonded vascular catheters, and extracorporeal oxygenation and carbon dioxide removal are achieved using a membrane oxygenator. A low-volume, low-pressure, low-frequency regimen of ventilation is continued to allow the lungs to recover. Results of a recent trial (CESAR) appear favourable in selected patients but the trial design has been subject to criticism and in the UK the availability of ECMO in adults is limited to very few centres, so the additional risks, benefits and timing of transfer of the severely hypoxaemic patient must be considered. Smaller more portable lung assist devices are under evaluation and may be available for use in the future.

Weaning from Mechanical Ventilation

Weaning is the process by which the patient's dependence on mechanical ventilation is gradually reduced to the point where spontaneous breathing sufficient to meet metabolic needs is sustained. Because of the adverse effects of mechanical ventilation, weaning should be undertaken at the earliest opportunity and the decision to commence weaning is based largely on clinical judgement.

Ideally, before weaning, the condition requiring mechanical ventilation should have resolved and a patient should:

- Be awake and co-operative with intact neuromuscular and bulbar function
- Have stable cardiovascular function with minimal requirements for inotropic or vasopressor drugs
- Not have a marked ongoing respiratory metabolic acidosis
- Have inspired oxygen requirements <50%
- Be able to generate a vital capacity 10 mL kg^{-1}, tidal volumes >5 mL kg^{-1} and a negative inspiratory pressure >20 cmH$_2$O
- Have low sputum production and be able to generate a good cough
- Have adequate nutritional status.

Weaning is a dynamic process and will involve reduction in level of ventilatory support. Pressure support ventilation (PSV) and synchronized intermittent mandatory ventilation (SIMV) are the most commonly used ventilatory modes and these techniques are forms of partial ventilatory support. The degree of support should be gradually weaned so that the patient contributes increasingly to the work of breathing. Introduction of ventilator independence can be rapid, e.g. a T-piece trial. This involves allowing the patient to breath spontaneously through a T-piece circuit, ideally for 30 minutes up to a maximum of 2 hours. If successful the patient can be extubated, and if not a repeat trial can be performed on a daily basis. A gradual form of weaning is to allow a short period of spontaneous breathing without ventilatory assistance (e.g. initially 1 to 5 minutes) with close observation and monitoring of the patient. The duration and frequency of these trials is increased as the patient's condition improves.

It may take from a few hours to several weeks before total independence from ventilatory support is achieved. Weaning may also be facilitated by the use of a tracheostomy tube, which has the advantage of reducing dead space and allowing sedation to be discontinued, as they are much better tolerated than a translaryngeal tube. Patients with a tracheostomy and CPAP or partial ventilatory support may be suitable to be stepped down from an ICU to a suitable location (e.g. HDU).

Outcomes from Lung Injury Requiring Prolonged IPPV

While no specific intervention has been shown to provide a clear benefit in the treatment of ALI and ARDS, there appears to be a trend towards increasing survival rates over the past few years. The mortality from ARDS varies widely in the literature and between countries. In the UK mortality approximates to 35–40%, but recognition that lower tidal volume ventilation and avoidance of VALI, as well as more general measures such as bundling of care, restrictive transfusion protocols, early antibiotic administration and nutritional support may all play a part in enhancing survival. Of those that survive, significant functional impairment often persists (severe disease and duration of mechanical ventilation are predictors of persistent abnormal lung function). Reduced exercise capacity, inability to return to work and health-related quality of life significantly below normal are common problems in survivors.

Cardiovascular System

Shock

Many intensive care patients will require support of the cardiovascular system at some time. Failure of the cardiovascular system to deliver an adequate supply of oxygenated blood to organs and tissues results in shock, which if unchecked will result in organ failure and death. Shock often accompanies conditions such as sepsis, multiple trauma and pneumonia and so is often found in ICU patients.

Common mechanisms of tissue underperfusion include: hypovolaemia (e.g. haemorrhage and burns), septic shock, cardiogenic shock, e.g. myocardial infarction and other rarer causes, e.g. anaphylaxis, neurogenic shock and adrenocortical insufficiency. There may be many elements contributing to shock in an individual patient and common features include hypotension, tachycardia, oliguria, increased serum lactate and metabolic acidosis. As initial compensatory mechanisms fail, multiple organ dysfunction ensues, and renal failure and ARDS are common. Hepatic, gastrointestinal, pancreatic impairment and disseminated intravascular coagulation may occur.

Management should be directed at:

- treatment of the underlying pathology
- optimization of circulating blood volume
- optimization of cardiac output
- optimization of blood pressure
- restoration of vascular tone
- optimization of oxygen delivery
- support of any organ failure.

Basic Applied Cardiovascular Physiology

Monitoring the cardiovascular system plays a key role in optimization and support and allows guidance towards provision of the all important balance between oxygen delivery and oxygen consumption.

Oxygen delivery can be calculated from the multiple of cardiac output and arterial oxygen content. Arterial oxygen content is determined by arterial oxygen saturation and haemoglobin concentration. Oxygen consumption is the total amount of oxygen consumed by the tissues. The difference between the amount of oxygen carried to the tissues (arterial oxygen delivery) and the amount of oxygen returned to the heart (venous oxygen delivery) indicates the total amount of oxygen consumed by the tissues. Mixed venous oxygen saturation reflects the amount of oxygen returning to the pulmonary capillaries, since it was not used by the tissues to support metabolic function. The pulmonary artery is the site where SvO_2 values should be measured. It is important to sample only at this site to allow for adequate mixing of blood from the superior and inferior vena cavae and coronary sinus. Controversies exist as to whether SVC venous oxygen saturation can be used as a surrogate for SvO_2 and although it mainly reflects oxygen supply and demand from the head and neck and upper extremities, it correlates reasonably well with the SvO_2, without the need for pulmonary artery catheterization.

If the SvO_2 is in the normal range (60–80%), then the clinician may assume that there is adequate tissue perfusion. If the SvO_2 falls below 60%, a decrease in oxygen delivery and/or an increase in oxygen consumption has occurred. If the SvO_2 is elevated above 80%, an increase in oxygen supply and/or a decrease in demand has occurred. An increase in oxygen delivery can be caused by an increased FiO_2, Hb, or CO. A decrease in oxygen consumption can be seen in hypothermic states or in patients who are anaesthetized, mechanically ventilated or paralysed. In sepsis, oxygen uptake into the tissues may be decreased.

The volume of oxygen carried by 1 g of haemoglobin is 1.34 mL.

O_2 Delivery:

$$DO_2 = \text{cardiac output} \times \text{arterial } O_2 \text{ content}$$
$$= \text{cardiac output} \times [(SaO_2 \times Hb \times 1.34) + (\text{dissolved } O_2)]$$
$$= 850 - 1200 \text{ mL min}^{-1}$$

O_2 Consumption:

$$VO_2 = \text{cardiac output} \times (\text{arterial } O_2 \text{ content} - \text{mixed venous } O_2 \text{ content})$$
$$= 240 - 270 \text{ mL min}^{-1}$$

Therefore, it can be seen that sufficient oxygen delivery can be achieved with good oxygen saturation, haemoglobin concentration 80–100 g L^{-1} and an adequate cardiac output.

Cardiac output is the product of heart rate and stroke volume. Cardiac index is the cardiac output referenced to the patient's body surface area. In health there is little fluctuation of cardiac output within the normal range of heart rate (60–160 beats per min.). However the critically ill, especially those with pre-existing heart disease and the elderly, tolerate extremes of heart rate much less well.

At low heart rates, cardiac output falls as a function of reduced heart rate, despite the maintenance of stroke volume.

Tachycardia results in reduced available time for the ventricles to fill and a subsequent fall in stroke volume. With an increase in heart rate, myocardial consumption also increases and this, coupled with reduced diastolic coronary artery perfusion, can lead to significant myocardial ischaemia.

Stroke volume is the amount of blood ejected with each heartbeat and is determined by preload, contractility and afterload.

Preload is the pressure that stretches the cardiomyocytes of the right or left ventricle before contraction. It reflects venous return or the extent of ventricular filling and depends on venous tone, circulating volume and the extent of ventricular relaxation. According to the Frank–Starling law of the heart, the force of myocardial contraction is proportional to the degree of ventricular filling, up to a point when over-stretch of the ventricle may result in a fall in stroke volume and heart failure will subsequently develop.

Afterload is the tension developed in the wall of the ventricle during ejection, i.e. the pressure required to eject blood from the left ventricle. The term afterload is sometimes confused with systemic vascular resistance, which is the overall resistance to flow in the systemic circulation. Afterload is determined by the degree of vasomotor tone, the elasticity of the arterial tree and the presence of valvular stenosis or arterial disease. Afterload is usually high in compensated cardiogenic shock or heart failure, and low in sepsis and high spinal cord injury.

Contractility is the intrinsic force generated by the myocardium, independent of preload and afterload.

Optimization of the Cardiovascular Status

The key aim in improving a patient's haemodynamic status is optimal cardiac output and oxygen delivery to allow adequate organ perfusion. The precise management of shock is beyond the scope of this chapter but a rational approach includes ensuring optimal filling status initially (a dynamic form of monitoring may be best – see above). If blood pressure, urine output, tissue perfusion and other measures of cardiac output still remain low, positive inotropic or vasopressor drugs may be required. These should be started at low doses and titrated to effect. There is little evidence base to recommend one drug regimen over another and adverse effects can arise with all agents so caution should be exercised.

If the predominant problem is thought to be loss of systemic vascular resistance due to sepsis or other causes then it is logical to start with a vasoconstrictor to increase arterial pressure. Common agents include noradrenaline and phenylephrine, which both act on

TABLE 45.8	
Positive Inotropic Drugs Commonly Used in ICU	
Drug	*Mode of Action*
Dobutamine	Increases contractility, and produces peripheral vasodilatation.
Dopexamine	Vasodilator at low doses, with reflex tachycardia. Positive inotropic effects seen at higher doses.
Dopamine	Vasodilatation at low doses via dopamine receptors. At higher doses, inotropic and vasoconstrictor effects appear.
Adrenaline	Positive inotropic and vasoconstrictor effects.
Milrinone, Enoximone	Positive inotropic and vasodilator effects by inhibition of phosphodiesterase enzymes.
Levosimendan	Positive inotrope which increases myocardial response to calcium.

α_1 receptors. Vasopressin is often given as second line to help restore vascular reactivity and tone. If cardiac contractility is thought to be a problem then a positive inotrope is used. The vasodilatation produced by some agents may be beneficial in the presence of a high systemic vascular resistance which is seen in cardiogenic shock.

Examples of positive inotropes can be found in Table 45.8 and further details are found in Chapter 8. Initiation of these drugs requires central venous access, although low dose phenylephrine can be infused through a peripheral cannula.

Cardiac rhythm disturbances are common in ICU patients. Ensure that general resuscitation measures are adequate and treat any electrolyte disturbances (especially of potassium and magnesium). Specific treatment may be required, e.g. amiodarone or digoxin for supraventricular tachycardia (see Ch 8). Other cardiovascular conditions to consider include myocardial ischaemia, cardiac failure and cardiogenic shock.

Outcome from Shock States

Mortality from all causes of shock remains high (approx 60% if associated with established multiple organ failure) and the effects of tissue hypoperfusion can persist in the longer term. Vasomotor regulation usually returns to normal quickly, but cardiomyopathy is a well reported feature of septic shock and the non infectious systemic inflammatory response syndrome can also give rise to a similar entity. The aetiology is multifactorial and includes mediators such as cytokines and nitric oxide in the presence of ischaemia. Those patients recovering from critical illness, are often rendered immobile for prolonged periods and cardiac muscle can atrophy resulting in deconditioning and a reduced cardiovascular response to physical activity.

Gastrointestinal System

The gastrointestinal tract is important in the pathophysiology of critical illness. Not only is it a common site for surgical intervention and a frequent source of intra-abdominal sepsis, the gut is a large 'third space' for fluid loss within the lumen of the gut and may also act as a bed for altered blood flow (AV shunting) during shock states. It can become a reservoir for bacteria and endotoxins which may translocate into the portal, lymphatic and systemic circulations, producing the systemic inflammatory response syndrome, sepsis and multiorgan failure, particularly during periods of altered blood flow.

Micro-organisms from the gut can also colonize and infect the respiratory tract, and the gastrointestinal tract itself can be a site for secondary nosocomial infections, e.g. *clostridium difficile* colitis. The maintenance of gastrointestinal integrity and function is therefore of major importance during critical illness and adequate splanchnic blood flow is thought to be crucial. Early resuscitation in shock states is essential and both volume resuscitation and vasopressors should be used early to aid perfusion pressure. In those patients who are adequately resuscitated, early enteral nutrition may also be of value in helping to preserve mucosal integrity and gastrointestinal function.

Manifestations of Gastrointestinal Tract Failure

Gastrointestinal tract failure may present in a number of ways: delayed gastric emptying and failure to absorb feed, ileus, pseudo-obstruction, diarrhoea, stress ulceration, gastrointestinal haemorrhage and ischaemia. All of these may indicate impending or established failure. In addition, acalculous cholecystitis, liver dysfunction and systemic inflammatory response syndrome are seen. Investigation of such dysfunction should in the first instance exclude potential remediable abdominal pathology, which often requires the need for imaging, radiological drainage or surgical exploration (e.g. abscesses, ischaemic bowel, peritonitis).

Nutrition

It is important to provide adequate nutrition during critical illness, especially as many patients are likely to be already nutritionally deficient from pre-existing illness. When providing nutritional support, estimation of energy and nitrogen requirements are made to attenuate the negative effects of the catabolic phase. However, it is generally accepted that underfeeding is better than overfeeding in terms of mortality, but failure to provide at least 25% of calculated requirements results in greater risk of infection and death.

Vitamins, minerals and trace elements are essential for health. Water and fat soluble vitamins are provided in commercially available preparations while folic acid and vitamin B_{12} need to be prescribed independently. Trace elements and minerals such as calcium, magnesium and iron can also be added according to need.

Glutamine, arginine, fish oils, selenium and a variety of anti-oxidants have been the focus of research into immuno-nutrition. Currently there is no clear evidence for an improved outcome (many of the studies involved administration of a cocktail of combined substrates) and some substances may only be of benefit in specific patient sub-groups, with associated higher mortality in alternative groups of patients.

It is usually accepted practice to initiate enteral feeding early, although in the resuscitative phase of critical illness, nutrients may not be utilized efficiently. Enteral feeding should be considered before the parenteral route, but can be associated with significant complications, e.g. under-nutrition and high gastric aspirates. Prokinetic drugs (metoclopramide, erythromycin) and the use of a head-up tilt will promote gastric emptying. Diarrhoea can be a problem and the use of pre- and probiotics may help normalize gut flora. There is a risk of aspiration with enteral feeding and recently there has been increased use of post-pyloric feeding; there is no strong evidence that this reduces aspiration.

Parenteral Feeding. If enteral feeding is contraindicated, e.g. for surgical reasons, or cannot be established successfully, then parenteral (i.v.) feeding is initiated. It requires dedicated central venous access and advice from the nutrition team, so that complications relating to overfeeding, hyperglycaemia, hypertriglyceridaemia, uraemia, metabolic acidosis and electrolyte imbalance can be avoided. Hepatobiliary dysfunction (including derangement of liver enzymes and fatty infiltration of the liver) may also occur and is usually caused by the patient's underlying condition and overfeeding.

Refeeding Syndrome. Refeeding syndrome results from shifts in fluid and electrolytes that may occur when a chronically malnourished patient receives artificial feeding, either parenterally or enterally. It results in hypophosphataemia, but may also feature abnormal sodium and fluid balance as well as changes in glucose, protein and fat metabolism and is potentially fatal. Thiamine deficiency, hypokalaemia and hypomagnesaemia may also be present. Patients at high risk include those chronically undernourished and those who have had little or no energy intake for more than 10 days. Ideally these patients require refeeding at an initially low level of energy replacement alongside vitamin supplementation.

Stress Ulcer Prophylaxis. Early enteral feeding promotes and maintains gastric mucosal blood flow, provides essential nutrients to the mucosa and reduces the incidence of stress ulcers. If enteral feeding cannot be established, alternative prophylactic measures need to be prescribed, commonly ranitidine or omeprazole.

Blood Glucose. Modest (not tight) glucose control is advocated for ICU patients and this is usually achieved by an infusion of insulin running alongside a dextrose-based infusion, to allow titration of blood glucose concentrations. High blood glucose worsens outcomes in brain injury and cardiac ischaemia. However, a recent large study has shown that a regimen of tight glycaemic control results in a worse outcome, thought to be primarily due to high rates of significant hypoglycaemia. Greater emphasis should probably be placed on avoiding glucose variability and easier continuous bedside blood glucose monitoring.

Outcomes of Gastrointestinal Failure

Gut function usually returns to normal unless there is a surgical problem, e.g. ischaemia or obstruction. Ileus and subacute (pseudo) obstruction, constipation and diarrhoea are common and it may take a number of days for gut function to return to normal.

Fluid Balance

Ensuring adequate fluid balance is a fundamental requirement in treating the critically ill patient. Normal approximate intake in a 70 kg man is 1500 mL from liquid, 750 mL in food and 250 mL from metabolism. In health, output matches input, with insensible losses accounting for approximately 500 mL. In addition to providing adequate water, electrolytes should be replaced: normal daily sodium and potassium requirements are 50–100 mmol per day and 40–80 mmol per day, respectively. A typical maintenance regime might be based on a balanced salt solution, e.g. Hartmann's, as longer term administration of 0.9% saline can result in hyperchloraemic acidosis.

Fluid balance is almost invariably disturbed in the critically ill patient. Common causes include widespread capillary leak associated with sepsis and inflammatory conditions leading to peripheral and pulmonary oedema, gastrointestinal dysfunction, fluid sequestration and diarrhoea. Fluid losses occur from burns, fistulae and wounds while increased insensible losses are associated with pyrexia and poor humidification of inspired ventilator gases. High urinary output states such as diabetes insipidus will also result in water loss. Therefore fluid and electrolyte replacement should be dictated by the underlying clinical condition, the overall fluid balance and the serum biochemistry.

Colloids are often preferred to crystalloids when rapid resuscitation, rather than maintenance is required, as a greater proportion remains in the intravascular space following infusion. The SAFE study showed no difference in 28-day outcome of patients admitted to ICU and who were given either albumin or 0.9% saline for fluid resuscitation. Albumin is now used less for volume expansion compared to the relatively cheaper synthetic colloids. However, colloids are associated with an increased incidence of adverse reactions and interference with renal function and coagulation. Blood and blood products should be used in cases of haemorrhage and coagulopathy, guided by local policy and senior advice.

Renal Dysfunction

Renal dysfunction is common in ICU and the cause is often multifactorial. Pre-existing renal disease may be worsened by the patient's new pathology, and some nephrotoxic drugs are still used in ICU. This section will deal predominantly with new onset renal dysfunction.

Acute kidney injury is defined as an abrupt (within 48 hours) reduction in kidney function, with the diagnosis made on the specific changes from baseline in patients who have achieved an optimal state of hydration (Table 45.9).

This classification takes into account the significance of even small increases in serum creatinine, given the recognized associated adverse outcomes. When managing a patient with acute kidney injury, focus the history and examination to distinguish potential causes (Table 45.10). These are classically distinguished as prerenal, renal and postrenal causes, although in many patients the cause of acute kidney injury is multifactorial. A sudden cessation of urine output should be assumed to be caused by obstruction until proved otherwise. Ensure the patient is adequately hydrated.

In most cases of AKI the primary cause is prerenal, but up to 10% of cases will have other significant pathologies. Serial U & Es are essential, while urine tests can be helpful (unless the patient has received

TABLE 45.9		
Diagnosis of Acute Kidney Injury		
AKI Stage	*Serum Creatinine Criteria*	*Urine Output Criteria*
1	Increase in serum creatinine ≥ 0.3 mg dL^{-1} or Increase to ≥ 150–200% from baseline	<0.5 mL kg^{-1} h^{-1} for >6 h
2	Increase in serum creatinine >200–300% from baseline	<0.5 mL kg^{-1} h^{-1} for >12 h
3	Increase in serum creatinine to >300% from baseline (or serum creatinine ≥ 4 mg dL^{-1}) with an acute increase ≥ 0.5 mg dL^{-1}, or receiving renal replacement therapy	<0.3 mL kg^{-1} h^{-1} for 24 h Or anuria for 12 h

diuretics) in distinguishing pre-renal from renal failure (Table 45.11).

Other investigations may be needed as determined by the clinical scenario: creatinine kinase/urinary myoglobin, vasculitic screen, and imaging, e.g. CT or renal ultrasound.

In the case of oliguria (urine output <0.5 mL kg^{-1} h^{-1} for at least 2 consecutive hours), consider a fluid challenge of 500 mL colloid. As renal filtration is pressure

TABLE 45.10		
Causes of Renal Dysfunction or Acute Kidney Injury in the ICU. Several Potential Causes Often Co-Exist in ICU Patients		
Causes of Renal Dysfunction		
Pre-renal	*Renal*	*Post renal*
Dehydration	Reno-vascular disease	Kidney outflow obstruction
Hypovolaemia	Autoimmune disease	Ureteric obstruction
Hypotension	SIRS & sepsis	Bladder outlet obstruction
	Hepato-renal syndrome	(Blocked catheter)
	Crush injury (myoglobinuria)	
	Nephrotoxic drugs	

TABLE 45.11

Differential Diagnosis of Acute Kidney Injury

Distinguishing Features of Pre-Renal and Renal Acute Kidney Injury

	Pre-renal	Renal
Urinary sodium	<10 mmol L^{-1}	>30 mmol L^{-1}
Urinary osmolality	High	Low
Urine: plasma urea ratio	>10:1	<8:1
Urine microscopy	Normal	Tubular casts

dependent, renal perfusion pressure should be maintained. If circulating volume is adequate, consider the early use of vasopressors or inotropes to maintain mean arterial pressure >65 mmHg. If the cause of oliguria remains unclear and there is no response, consider whether any prescribed nephrotoxic drugs need to be stopped. Look for and treat sources of sepsis. Consider loop diuretics if the patient remains oliguric. If cardiac output, mean arterial pressure and renal perfusion pressure have been restored with fluids and drugs and there remains no response to diuretics, renal replacement therapy is likely to be required.

Renal Replacement Therapy (RRT)

Continuous renal replacement therapy is used in intensive care units because the gradual correction of biochemical abnormalities and removal of fluid results in greater haemodynamic stability, compared to intermittent haemodialysis (Table 45.12).

TABLE 45.12

Indications for Renal Replacement Therapy

Classical Indications	Alternative Indications
Volume overload	Endotoxic shock
Hyperkalaemia (K$^+$ >6.5)	Severe dysnatraemia (Na$^+$ <115 or >165 mmol L^{-1})
Metabolic acidosis (pH <7.1)	Plasmapheresis
Symptomatic uraemia (encephalopathy, pericarditis, bleeding)	
Dialysable toxins (lithium, aspirin, methanol, ethylene glycol, theophylline)	

Continuous Venovenous Haemofiltration (CVVHF)

The simplest form of continuous renal replacement is continuous venovenous haemofiltration. As the patient's blood passes through a filter, plasma water, electrolytes and small molecular weight molecules pass through down a pressure gradient. This filtrate is discarded and replaced by a balanced electrolyte solution. Typically 200–500 mL h^{-1} of filtrate are removed and replaced. Overall negative fluid balance can be achieved by replacing less fluid than is removed. As no diasylate is used, solute movement is entirely dependent on convective transport, which is a slower removal process, so clearance of small molecules and solutes is inefficient. This can require large volumes of filtrate to be removed and replaced in order to achieve acceptable creatinine clearance.

Continuous Venovenous Haemodialysis (CVVHD)

Continuous haemodialysis depends on diffusive solute clearance occurring because of the countercurrent flow of dialysate fluid through the haemofilter. Fluids, electrolytes and small molecules can move in both directions across the filter, depending on hydrostatic pressure, ionic binding and osmotic gradients. Overall creatinine clearance is greatly improved compared with haemofiltration alone. In CVVHD, provided the volume of dialysis fluid passing out from the system matches the volume of dialysis fluid passing in, there is no net gain or loss of fluid to the patient. By allowing more dialysate fluid to pass out of the filter than passes in, fluid can be effectively removed from the patient, with removal rates of up to 200 mL per hour possible.

Continuous Venovenous Haemodiafiltration (CVVHDF)

This term is best used for systems that intentionally combine both haemodialysis and haemofiltration. Dialysis fluid is passed across the filter to remove solutes by osmosis but at the same time ultrafiltrate is removed and replaced.

Vascular Access for Renal Replacement Therapy

Renal replacement therapies require dedicated vascular access (using a 10–14 Fr gauge catheter). Veno-venous RRT has replaced arteriovenous RRT, as the latter has greater vascular morbidity and requires an adequate arterial pressure to drive flow. For veno-venous access, a single large vein is cannulated percutaneously with a double-lumen catheter using the Seldinger technique. All catheters have a lumen that functions as the 'arterial' outflow limb of the circuit and a second lumen which functions as the 'venous' inflow limb of the circuit. The 'arterial' port removes blood from holes in the side of the catheter and blood is returned down the 'venous' lumen through a single hole at the catheter tip to minimize recirculation of haemofiltered blood. When not in use, these catheters are at risk of clotting off, and so it is often necessary to fill the deadspace (labelled on catheter) with heparin 1000 units mL^{-1}.

Similarly as blood is passing through an extracorporeal circuit, some form of anticoagulation is required (unless the patient has severe coagulopathy) and either heparin or prostacyclin infusions are run directly into the dialysis circuit. Citrate has also been used as a form of anticoagulation.

Table 45.13

Interest has recently centered upon the role of CVVHF in sepsis. Many patients with AKI have multi-organ dysfunction and most mediators involved in the inflammatory response are water soluble middle-sized molecular weight compounds, such as tumour necrosis factor (TNF), interleukins (IL-1, IL-6, IL-8), platelet activating factor (PAF) and complement. The highly porous synthetic membranes used for convective filtration in CVVHF lend themselves to elimination of such compounds through filtration and adsorption. However, high volume haemofiltration (HVHF), producing ultrafiltration volumes of more than 75 litre day^{-1}, may be required

---

TABLE 45.13
Complications of Continuous RRT

- Heparin associated:
  Bleeding (GIT, catheter site, intraoperative)
  Heparin-induced thrombocytopenia (HIT)
- Catheter related:
  Sepsis
  Thrombosis
  Arterio-venous fistulae
  Arrhythmia
  Pneumothorax
  Pain
  Line disconnection
- Hypothermia
- Anaemia, thrombocytopenia
- Hypovolaemia
- Hypotension, worsening gas exchange in lungs
- Membrane reactions (bradykinin release, nausea, anaphylaxis)
- Electrolyte abnormalities (hypophosphataemia, hypokalaemia)
- Metabolic: acidosis (bicarbonate loss), alkalosis (over-buffering)
- Air embolism
- Drug related (altered pharmacokinetics)

---

to produce significant reductions in plasma mediator concentrations because of their very high generation rate. Recent outcome studies have not supported this approach.

Outcomes After Kidney Injury

Acute kidney injury has three potential outcomes: return to baseline function, the development of chronic kidney disease, or persistent renal failure. Most cases of AKI occurring in ICU return to baseline function over time (acute tubular necrosis pattern, may take up to 6 weeks). The re-establishment of a spontaneous urine output is generally followed by a polyuric phase which gradually settles. However, a proportion of patients may develop chronic kidney disease in previously normal kidneys (e.g. acute cortical necrosis pattern, most commonly in pregnancy). Patients with pre-existing renal disease may have accelerated disease progression and increased risk for end stage disease. The latter two groups of patients will therefore benefit from early referral to renal physicians for longer term management.

Neurological System

Despite the wide range of pathologies that require patients to be admitted to the ICU for specialized neurological support, some specific treatment regimens are common to them all. Recognition of the primary problem and any secondary pathologies (e.g. a secondary brain haemorrhage) is important, as is the prevention of secondary injury due to brain swelling or poor perfusion.

Irrespective of the primary cause of neurological damage, secondary injury may be caused by hypoxaemia, hypotension, hypercapnia, seizures, hyperglycaemia and other metabolic disturbance. In order to prevent this, measures need to be taken and will include securing the airway and instituting mechanical ventilation. These are the main principles underlying neuro-critical care. Ventilatory variables should be set to achieve a $PaCO_2$ of 4–5 kPa. Aggressive hyperventilation needs to be avoided as hypocapnia induces cerebral vasoconstriction and may promote cerebral ischaemia in the context of brain injury. The inspired oxygen concentration needs to be adjusted to sustain a PaO_2 in excess of 12 kPa and appropriate steps taken to maintain blood pressure within the normal range. Ideally mean arterial pressure should be maintained above 70 mmHg as even isolated periods of systolic pressures below 90 mmHg have been shown to be associated with worse outcome in the case of traumatic brain injury. Intravenous administration of glucose should be avoided as hyperglycaemia increases cerebral metabolic rate and i.v. insulin should be infused if the blood glucose concentration exceeds 11 mmol L^{-1}.

The plasma osmolality and serum sodium concentration should be monitored carefully because hypo-osmolality of the plasma creates an osmotic gradient across the blood–brain barrier which can provoke cerebral oedema. Hyperthermia (even mild) should be avoided as this increases cerebral metabolism and worsens outcomes. However the benefits of induced hypothermia are unclear as it affects other systems. For example, hypothermia worsens coagulopathy and could be detrimental in the case of cerebral haemorrhage. Currently induced hypothermia has only been shown to be of benefit after out-of-hospital cardiac arrest, where the primary rhythm was ventricular fibrillation.

Patients with severe head injury (GCS <8) and/or focal signs (which may not necessarily require surgical correction) should be referred to a regional neurosurgical centre, as should patients who require ventilation and ICP monitoring. Discussion and review of CT scans should be undertaken with the neurosurgeons before transfer. Transfer should be in accordance with national guidelines and will include:

- Exclude and treat other life threatening injuries elsewhere (e.g. chest and abdominal bleeding)
- Secure the airway definitively
- Staff should be trained in airway and head injury management
- Large-bore intravenous access
- End-tidal CO_2 should be maintained at 4–4.5 kPa on a transport ventilator
- SpO_2 and arterial gases should be checked to ensure adequate oxygenation
- Blood pressure and adequate fluids and vasopressors should be available
- Brain CT imaging should be completed and hard/electronic copies available
- Transfer should be complete within 4 h – no inappropriate delays, e.g. for central venous access.

In patients with severe head injury and an abnormal admission CT scan, it may be appropriate to monitor cerebral perfusion pressure (CPP) by direct measurement of ICP and mean arterial pressure. ICP should be maintained within the normal range if possible; sudden increases may occur in patients who are restless or hypertensive, and adequate sedation and analgesia are usually important components of therapy. Deep sedation with neuromuscular blockade may be necessary to minimize cerebral metabolism and therapy can be guided using the EEG to attain burst suppression.

CPP can be manipulated with fluid loading and the use of vasopressor agents. However, high arterial pressure should be avoided, because many patients with brain injury have impaired cerebral autoregulation and a high CPP may result in increased cerebral oedema. Hypotension does need to be treated, however, as critical CPP, when ischaemia is likely to occur, is in the order of 30–40 mmHg.

Other useful measures to consider when managing the patient with acute neurological injury include nursing in a head up position to improve venous drainage.

Increasing serum osmolality to 300–310 mOsm L^{-1} using mannitol or hypertonic saline judiciously will reduce brain tissue water and result in a fall in ICP. In addition it is important to control clinical and subclinical seizures as these have a detrimental effect on cerebral metabolism. At all times therapy should be adjusted to maximize oxygen delivery, minimize oxygen consumption, preserve cerebral blood flow and normalize ICP.

Outcomes

Advances have been made in neurological monitoring modalities and some specific treatments have become more common with improved outcomes, e.g. radiological coiling for aneurysms and thrombolysis for acute ischaemic stroke. Others treatments like decompression craniectomy are still under study. However, the majority of neurological conditions requiring intensive care, e.g. traumatic brain injury, have remained static in terms of novel therapies, and mortality and morbidity rates remain high. In the UK severe traumatic brain injury occurs in 11 000 people per year and has a mortality rate approaching 50%. Most of the survivors will have residual disability following severe head injury.

OTHER ASPECTS OF INTENSIVE CARE

Venous Thromboembolism Prophylaxis

An estimated 25 000 people in the UK die from preventable hospital-acquired venous thromboembolism (VTE) every year. Therefore it is a considerable cause of mortality and, in non-fatal cases, morbidity. The critical care population is at higher risk than general medical patients for a number of reasons including: severe physiological upset, maximal inflammatory response, the presence of intravascular catheter devices, injuries specifically implicated in VTE, e.g. pelvic and long bone injuries, and often long periods of immobility. Similarly these patients are also at increased risk from anticoagulation therapy, due to disease process/concurrent interventions and treatment, so pharmacological prophylaxis with low molecular weight heparins can potentially be problematic.

Low-molecular-weight heparins are associated with a lower incidence of haemorrhage and heparin-induced thrombocytopaenia than unfractionated heparin. In addition their use does not require monitoring of activated partial prothrombin time (APTT). Unless contraindicated, mechanical means (such as anti-embolic stockings) of VTE prophylaxis should also be given to all patients.

Where both mechanical and pharmacological prophylaxis are contraindicated and the patient is at high risk, consider the requirement of an inferior venal caval filter. There should be a daily review of the risk of venous thromboembolism, risk of bleeding and therefore thromboprophylaxis. Early mobilization and physiotherapy where possible, and avoiding dehydration can also help reduce the risk of VTE.

ICU-Acquired Muscle Weakness

Neuromuscular abnormalities resulting in skeletal muscle weakness are a common occurrence in the intensive care unit. Some degree of loss of muscle mass is likely in all cases of immobility and critical illness. However, more severe problems are commonly seen and they can be described into two distinct conditions, namely polyneuropathy and myopathy. However, it is likely that these two entities often coexist, and while the exact incidence remains variable amongst studies, their presence is associated with multiple adverse outcomes, including higher mortality, prolonged duration of mechanical ventilation, and increased length of stay.

The pathogenesis of such nerve and muscle damage is not well defined, but probably involves inflammatory injury of nerve and/or muscle that is potentiated by functional denervation and corticosteroids. The latter is a well identified risk factor for developing acquired muscle weakness. Other risk factors include sepsis, hyperglycaemia, neuromuscular blockade and increasing severity of illness. The clinical diagnosis of ICU-acquired neuromuscular disorders is suspected in the presence of unexplained weakness in patients recovering from critical illness. Weakness can be so severe as to be confused with coma. Other metabolic, pharmacologic, and central-nervous-system causes of weakness must be ruled out before establishing the diagnosis. Electrophysiological testing is useful primarily to exclude other (possibly treatable) causes of severe weakness, e.g. Guillain–Barré syndrome or cervical spine problems.

So far the only intervention recognized to reduce the incidence of ICU acquired muscle weakness is intensive insulin therapy and standard measures that reduce the severity and duration of the critical illness episode (e.g. early recognition and treatment of sepsis). Physical rehabilitation may accelerate recovery and the National Institute for Health and Care Excellence has published guidelines recognizing the value of rehabilitation during and post critical care, however more research is required for an improved understanding of this illness.

Healthcare-Associated Infection (HAI)

Unfortunately HAI is common, especially amongst ICU patients where risk factors such as immunocompromise, tracheal intubation, the presence of intravascular and urinary catheters, antimicrobial therapy, stress ulcer prophylaxis and protracted length of stay are frequent. Catheter-related blood stream infections, ventilator-associated pneumonia, *Clostridium difficile* diarrhoea and emergence of antibiotic-resistant bacteria such as methicillin-resistant *Staphylococcus aureus* (MRSA) and vancomycin-resistant enterococcus (VRE) remain important causes of ICU mortality, morbidity and increased financial burden. Routine surveillance of HAI rates is essential to identify problematic pathogens and to develop initiatives to reduce their incidence.

Preventative measures are multifactorial and start with good standards of hospital environmental cleanliness. The EPIC study recognized poor hand hygiene as being a major factor in nosocomial infection and great effort has gone into publicizing good hand hygiene at a national level. Protective garments should be worn with all patient contact, however gloves are not a substitute for hand washing.

Catheter-Related Bloodstream Infection (CRBSI)

CRBSI is common in the ICU and results from venous and arterial catheters becoming coated in plasma proteins following insertion. Bacteria are then able to migrate from the skin and catheter hubs to become embedded in this protein sheath, with both external and endoluminal colonization occurring. There is a direct relationship between the number of organisms colonizing the catheter and the risk of CRBSI and presence of thrombus also increases this risk. Mortality from CRBSI may be as high as 25% and diagnosis is made from a positive blood culture with the same organism grown from the access device.

To reduce rates, the need for invasive catheters should always be considered in the first instance. Consider the site of insertion: the subclavian vein has the least risk of catheter-related bloodstream infection compared to the internal jugular and femoral veins, respectively. Strict aseptic technique should be adhered to on insertion and during all handling of catheters. If the device is to be used for parenteral nutrition, ensure that there is a dedicated line or lumen for this. If there is a suspicion of CRBSI, the catheter should be removed and antibiotic therapy tailored to the culture result. Matching Michigan is a quality improvement project based on a model developed in the United States. It introduced data definitions (infection rates per 1000 catheter days) as well as technical and non-technical interventions in order to reduce catheter-related bloodstream infection and a similar project is underway across the UK.

Antibiotic Therapy

Appropriate antibiotic use is imperative, and local policies as well as advice from the microbiologist are important sources of information. If appropriate empirical therapy is started early, clinical outcomes from serious infection are improved (as per the Surviving Sepsis campaign). De-escalation when a causative pathogen is identified reduces inappropriate use and minimizes superinfection. Rotation of antibiotics has been used but conflicting evidence has suggested that there may be promotion of resistance amongst Gram-negative organisms. Selective decontamination of the digestive tract (SDD) is a technique designed to eradicate aerobic, potentially pathogenic bacteria colonizing the oropharynx and upper gastrointestinal tract, thus eliminating an important risk factor for nosocomial pneumonia. It has not been widely adopted in the UK because of its inconsistent effects on mortality and concerns about the potential for selecting antibiotic-resistant pathogens.

Ventilator-Associated Pneumonia (VAP)

VAP is a common nosocomial infection occurring in ICU patients receiving mechanical ventilation for >48 hours. There is no gold standard for diagnosis, so exact incidence remains difficult to estimate but mortality is in the order of 30%. Aerobic Gram-negative bacilli colonize the oropharynx and upper GI tract (augmented by the use of H_2-receptor antagonists) and these pathogens gain access to the lungs with movement aided by the positive pressure of mechanical ventilation. Clinical suspicion should arise with standard diagnostic features of pneumonia but this is non-specific. Quantitative culture of bronchio-alveolar lavage specimens should aid diagnosis. Treatment is timely administration of appropriate antibiotics and preventative measures include scrupulous hand washing, good oral hygiene, nursing the patient semi-recumbent, ensuring adequate tracheal cuff inflation, improved cuff design, supraglottic suction, the rational use of H_2-receptor antagonists, avoiding the need for re-intubation where possible and potentially SDD.

Psychological Problems on the Intensive Care Unit

Longer stay patients on the ICU can suffer significant psychological morbidity. A combination of the underlying pathology, sedative and analgesic drugs, an environment of loud noise, bright lights, and frequent nursing input can all lead to sensory overload which may result in anxiety, depression, delirium and hallucinations during treatment. Research into the longer term consequences of surviving critical illness has suggested that for a significant number of patients there may not only be continuing physical debilitation, but also a risk of subsequent depression, post traumatic stress disorder and a potential loss of cognitive function. Family dynamics may become altered as can financial security, so it is important to identify patients at risk of physical and non-physical morbidity and work towards short and medium term agreed rehabilitation goals in an attempt to optimize recovery.

Delirium in ICU

Delirium is often under diagnosed, but is associated with increased length of hospital stay and is an independent predictor of increased mortality at 6 months. It is often described as hyperactive, hypoactive or a mixture of both. A validated tool such as the Confusion Assessment Method for the Intensive Care Unit (CAM-ICU) can be used to detect delirium. Preventative measures include avoidance of pharmacological precipitants

where possible (although this may be impossible in practice) and employing non-pharmacological interventions such as clear communication, provision of clocks, calendars, diaries and the patient's own familiar objects. In addition, consistent nursing care, controlling excess noise and creating a day/night cycle are also helpful. Allowing self-care where possible and ensuring that the patient has their own glasses, dentures or personal items can often be as important as treating any organic cause. If preventative measures fail and no organic cause can be found, treatment with haloperidol and other drugs may be helpful.

Care Bundles

There is an increasing interest in the development of 'care bundles' for specific ICU illnesses. They consist of a number, usually up to 5 or so, of evidence-based practices each of which has been shown to improve outcome and is easily achievable. When performed collectively, reliably and continuously these bundles confer a greater probability of survival. The most familiar bundles are the Surviving Sepsis Campaign resuscitation (6 hours) and management (24 hours) bundles and ventilator care bundles. The ventilator care bundle comprises the following components to reduce acute lung injury and ARDS:

- **low tidal volumes** (6 mL per kg predicted body weight)
- **capped plateau airway pressure** (30 cmH$_2$O)
- **sedation holds and use of sedation scores.** The practice of interrupting continuous sedative infusions on a daily basis to allow intermittent decreased sedation, has been shown to reduce length of ICU stay
- **permissive hypercapnia** (accepting a PaCO$_2$ above normal to allow pressure limitation and low plateau airway pressures)
- **semi-recumbent positioning** (head up by 45° unless contraindicated) during ventilation to reduce the incidence of ventilator-induced pneumonia
- **lung recruitment by PEEP** to prevent alveolar collapse at end-expiration
- **avoidance of neuromuscular blocking drugs** *may* reduce the incidence of skeletal muscle weakness associated with critical illness
- **protocol-driven weaning**

Ventilator associated pneumonia rates have been shown to be reduced by combining sedation holds, semi-recumbent nursing, peptic ulcer prophylaxis, DVT prophylaxis and daily oral hygiene with chlorhexidine. Good nursing care should not be underestimated and is an important contributor to good overall outcome.

ETHICAL ISSUES IN ICU

As in all medical practice, four ethical principles can be applied to the ICU patient.

Autonomy relates to the patient's individual dignity and is about respect for the individual and their ability to make decisions with regard to their own health and future. To do this they must be able to understand and believe the information given.

Beneficence is the concept that any action that is performed on the patient should be in that patient's best interest, i.e. doing the greatest good whilst balancing the risks and benefits. The corollary of that is that any action carried out on a patient must not harm that patient, which is the concept of *non-maleficence*. The fourth principle is the notion of *justice*. This relates to fairness, equitable use of resources and equal access to care. Individuals should be similarly treated. When a resource is limited, there is potential for an individual's treatment to affect the wellbeing of someone else.

There are inherent problems with achieving all of these ideals in the ICU situation. For a patient to have the capacity to consent to a treatment, they must be able to understand information relevant to that treatment, retain that information, use or weigh up that information as part of the process of making a decision and finally they must be able to communicate their decision. Thus the majority of patients at some point during their ICU admission will lack capacity. It is important to be able to defend decisions regarding treatment or withholding of treatment so there must be robust evidence that a patient's lack of capacity has undergone assessment. It is prudent to discuss complicated matters with consultant colleagues so that a consensus of opinion can be formalized before difficult treatment decisions are made. With the patient who lacks capacity, management is directed towards the patient's best interests and although there should be documented evidence of involvement of the patient's

family and others close to them, the next of kin does not have a decisive role and cannot formally consent on behalf of a patient who lacks capacity.

OUTCOME AFTER INTENSIVE CARE

Attempts to predict outcome after discharge from critical care has led to the development of a number of scoring systems, which generally involve collection of large quantities of data, stratifying this data to produce a risk score and using this to predict survival for a patient population. However there are flaws with this approach including problems of diagnostic categorization: the initial hospital diagnosis may bear little relation to the subsequent, often multiple pathologies in the individual ICU patient. While scoring systems are helpful in predicting population outcomes, their application to individual cases is limited. Patients may survive discharge from the ICU, but mortality remains high on the wards and at home, so that 6-month or 1-year outcomes of mortality and morbidity may prove better end points than the traditional 28-day mortality.

Assessments of functional disability, quality of life and return to work among patients who have survived an admission to the ICU are more difficult to quantify than death, but the small numbers of studies which have been undertaken suggest that mortality is significantly higher than would be expected in matched individuals for several years. In addition, a significant proportion of patients report impaired quality of life and that many remain unable to work for prolonged periods after discharge. However, the majority of patients who survive can return to a reasonable quality of life.

There are a number of scoring systems in use:

- APACHE II. The Acute Physiology and Chronic Health Evaluation score takes into account pre-existing comorbidities as well as acute physiological disturbance and correlates well with the risk of death in an intensive care population, but not on an individual basis. However, it remains one of the more widely used tools and a score is calculated on:
    - worst physiological derangement occurring within the first 24 hours after admission
    - age
    - chronic health status

Some patients with, for example, diabetic keto-acidosis may score highly and have a perceived high risk of death, but they generally get better quickly. Lead-time bias results from the stabilization of patients in the referring hospital before transfer. This artificially lowers the score for the patient arriving at the referral centre. Finally the Glasgow Coma Scale component may be difficult to interpret, as clearly there is a difference in GCS 3 from head injury compared to GCS 3 from drug induced sedation.

- APACHE III has superseded the APACHE II score, with the variations in the physiological components.
- Simplified Acute Physiology Score (SAPS). This scoring system uses 12 physiological variables assigned a score according to the degree of derangement.
- Therapeutic Intervention Score System (TISS). A score is given for each procedure performed on the ICU, so that sicker patients require more procedures. However, procedures undertaken are both clinician and unit specific and so TISS is less useful for comparing outcomes between different units.
- Sequential Organ Failure Assessment (SOFA). This tracks changes in the patient's condition regarding their respiratory, cardiovascular, hepatic, neurological, renal and coagulation status.

The importance of national collaborative audit and research in improving the practice of critical care is well recognized and the Intensive Care National Audit and Research Centre for England and Wales (ICNARC) collects demographic data, diagnostic criteria, physiological scoring and outcome for the majority of patients admitted to ICU. The case mix programme for April 2008 to April 2009 noted almost 90 000 admissions across 180 general ICUs in the UK. In this dataset, mortality in the intensive care unit was 17%, while acute hospital mortality was almost 26%.

DEATH IN THE ICU

Death is common and is a fundamental part of ICU care. Unfortunately, despite maximal support and care, some patients succumb to the overwhelming nature of the underlying disease process. Few deaths are directly attributable to an unexpected primary cardio-respiratory arrest, once the patient is fully supported on the ICU, hence 'do not resuscitate' (DNR) orders are less relevant to critical care than care on the general ward.

Futility and withdrawal

Approximately 70% of deaths occur on the ICU following withdrawal of support, where continued treatment would be futile; however, legally, the cause of death remains the underlying pathological process. This typically follows a variable period of continued deterioration or a failure to improve, despite maximal appropriate supportive therapy.

A principle of justice in the treatment of intensive care patients is based on the fact that all patients have an equal right to all treatments. Yet some patients with extensive comorbidities or very advanced disease have very little prospect of responding to such treatment. Therefore, to offer them such treatment is futile and unlikely to be in their best interests. Equally, it would be misuse of scarce resource which would be then unavailable to another patient.

There is no legal distinction between the withdrawal of life-sustaining treatment or limiting or withholding treatment. It is important to note that withdrawal of treatment does not equate with withdrawal of all of the basic care given by nurses and doctors including symptom relief. There is a lack of consistency regarding withdrawal, as timing, the actual treatments withdrawn and the manner of withdrawal may vary considerably between intensive care units. In the UK, relatives do not have legal rights of decision making but it is important not to exclude them from honest and timely discussions when withdrawal is being considered.

The process of withdrawal centres upon either setting limits to levels of supportive therapy or a reduction of such interventions, in anticipation that the patient is likely to deteriorate or die without such support. Once the decision is made and an agreement with the family and admitting team has been obtained, support is reduced along the following lines:

- Vasopressor and inotropic drug support are reduced and subsequently discontinued.
- Sedation may be increased and inspired oxygen concentration can be reduced to room air.

- Other supportive treatments such as renal replacement therapy are removed.
- Assisted ventilation may be reduced and tracheal extubation carried out.
- Antibiotics are discontinued.
- Feeding and hydration are generally continued if practical and not requiring extra invasive instrumentation.
- Death may occur quickly or be prolonged over hours or days depending on the clinical situation.

The General Medical Council has a guideline relating to withdrawal of treatment and resolution of potential conflicts that may arise when the decision to withdraw is made.

Dependent on the speed of decline, patients may die on the ICU, or be discharged to ward-based care. Occasionally patients may improve despite all odds and clinicians should be prepared to revisit such clinical decisions over time.

Once a patient has died, confirmation of death is required. Although in the UK there is no actual legal definition of death, it should be identified as the irreversible loss of the capacity for consciousness, combined with the irreversible loss of the capacity to breathe. (See a code of practice for the diagnosis and confirmation of death: www.aomrc.org.uk.)

A death certificate may be issued by a doctor who has provided care during the last illness and who has seen the deceased within 14 days of death. Deaths must be reported to the coroner in the following instances:

- Cause of death is unknown
- Sudden, unexpected, suspicious, violent or unnatural deaths
- Deaths due to alcohol or drugs
- Deaths related to surgery or anaesthesia
- Deaths within 24 hours of admission

Depending on the circumstance, a post mortem may be necessary.

Brainstem Death

In patients with overwhelming brain injury, brainstem death testing allows futile treatments to be withdrawn. Clinical features of brainstem death will include profoundly reduced conscious level, with loss of cranial nerve reflexes. As the brainstem is compressed systemic features may include hypertension and bradycardia (Cushing's reflex), followed by hypotension and vasodilation. Hypothalamic and pituitary function is lost (diabetes insipidus) and reduced thyroid hormone synthesis occurs. Hypothermia is common due to a loss of thermoregulation.

Preconditions for brainstem death testing include:

- the presence of identifiable pathology causing irreversible damage
- the patient must be deeply unconscious (hypothermia, depressant drugs and potentially reversible circulatory, metabolic, endocrine disturbances must all be excluded as a cause of the conscious level)
- the patient must be apnoeic

The tests are undertaken by two medical practitioners, one of whom is a consultant and both of whom have been registered with the General Medical Council for more than 5 years. Two sets of tests are performed and time of death is recorded when the first test indicates brainstem death.

- Pupils must be fixed and not responsive to light (cranial nerves II, III)
- There must be no corneal reflex (cranial nerves V, VII)
- Vestibulo-ocular reflexes are absent, i.e. no eye movement occur following injection of ice cold saline into the auditory meatus (cranial nerves, III, IV, VI, VIII)
- No facial movement will occur in response to supra-orbital pressure (cranial nerves V, VII)
- No gag reflex to posterior pharyngeal wall stimulation (cranial nerve IX)
- No cough or other reflex in response to bronchial stimulation with a suction catheter passed down the tracheal tube (cranial nerve X)
- No respiratory movements will occur when disconnected from the ventilator, hypoxia is prevented with pre-oxygenation and oxygen insufflation via a tracheal catheter and $PaCO_2$ should be $>6.65\,kPa$.

Spinal reflexes may be present or exaggerated.

ORGAN DONATION

Patients who fulfil the criteria for brainstem death should be considered for organ donation. If suitable on medical grounds and permission is given by the patient (by previous expressions of interest) or relatives, then so-called beating heart donation can take place. After careful planning, the patient is taken to theatres and organs removed before or at the time of circulatory arrest.

At the time of writing, nearly 8000 patients are registered and waiting for a transplant in the UK and demand continues to outstrip supply. With this in mind, moves have been made towards increasing the numbers of non-heart beating organ donors (patient pronounced dead on the basis of loss of cardiac function before organ retrieval).

Whether organ retrieval is from heart beating or non-heart beating donation, appropriate consent must be obtained and early liaison with the transplant coordinator is crucial in determining suitability. There will be a donor management protocol that should be followed to ensure optimal organ viability. The whole process takes time and major coordination between the various teams involved.

Other tissues, e.g. corneas, skin, bone and heart valves, can be removed later after death if appropriate.

DISCHARGE FROM INTENSIVE CARE

For those patients that survive, discharge from ICU is appropriate when their condition has improved so that they no longer warrant intensive care support. Careful discussion with the relatives and admitting teams should be undertaken with clear documentation of decisions made in relation to re-escalation of treatment, readmission to intensive care, whether or not to attempt resuscitation and other ongoing management.

Those patients whose levels of care are to be reduced need to be sufficiently fit for discharge so that their underlying disease process is stable and/or improving. Consideration needs to be made regarding where such patients are to be discharged to. Frequently, discharge is to a high dependency unit or if the patient is fit enough, back to a general ward, with outreach review. If the patient has been transferred from another hospital, ideally they should be returned to the referring hospital as soon as possible. Discharges should be made during daytime hours, as discharges made outside these times are more likely to experience deterioration and readmission.

Follow-Up Clinics

Follow-up clinics are an important aspect of continued treatment of a patient's physical and emotional wellbeing, as well as a means of service evaluation and an opportunity for patients to reflect and give feedback on their experience. Following periods of critical illness, patients typically experience impaired physical and mental functioning as a result of the underlying disease processes or complications occurring on the ICU. Commonly seen problems include:

- Critical illness neuropathy/myopathy,
- Respiratory dysfunction – breathlessness is a common symptom
- Cardiac problems – MI or cardiomyopathy
- Swallowing difficulties and tracheal stenosis post-intubation/tracheostomy
- Sexual dysfunction, affective disorders and post traumatic stress disorder
- Quality of life may significantly decrease following illness
- Mobility and joint problems.

In the UK, recommendations have been made to advocate the use of follow-up clinics but its provision as yet remains inconsistent, and cost effectiveness may place restraints on its continued development.

FUTURE DEVELOPMENTS

Few major therapeutic developments have been made with regard to ICU care over the last few years. Published trials which initially showed promise have later been repeated and have not translated well to broad use in the critical care setting. This may partly be due to the heterogeneous nature of the disease and the population but also flaws in study design.

Future focus may well be directed toward better identification of patient populations through genetics and biomarkers, which will aid research into novel therapeutic strategies. Whilst there is already recognition that restoration of haemodynamic variables to normal values is not necessary, better use of functional technology and monitoring tools will help guide resuscitation. There probably will be greater emphasis on bundles of care and perfection of weaning and sedation regimes in addition to computer-led advances.

Demand for critical care resources is likely to continue to grow in the face of an ageing population and ongoing improvement in medical management of cardiorespiratory, cancer and other degenerative diseases. It is likely that some sort of rationing may be used when outcomes in terms of quality life years is likely to be poor. A public and legally accepted recognition of the limitations of what can and should be offered is needed.

Intensive care medicine is an exciting and developing specialty and focused training should continue to aim to attract young clinicians from a variety of primary specialties.

FURTHER READING

Brooks, A., Girling, K., Riley, B., et al., (Eds.), 2005. Critical care for postgraduate trainees. Hodder Arnold, London.

Hillman, K., Bishop, G., 2004. Clinical intensive care, second ed. Cambridge University Press, Cambridge.

Hinds, C.J., Watson, J.D., 2008. Intensive care: a concise textbook, third ed. Saunders, London.

Webb, A.R., Shapiro, M., Singer, M., Suter, P., 1999. Oxford textbook of critical care. Oxford University Press, Oxford.

Whiteley, S., Bodenham, A., Bellamy, M., 2010. Churchill Livingstone's pocketbook of intensive care, third ed. Churchill Livingstone, Edinburgh.

46

MANAGEMENT OF CHRONIC PAIN

R ecent advances in the understanding of the fundamental mechanisms involved in the transmission and modulation of noxious impulses have significantly extended the range of assessment tools and treatments clinicians offer to patients with pain. The majority of medical pain specialists in the UK are anaesthetists. Historically, anaesthetists have been responsible for the relief of pain in the perioperative period and have developed skills in percutaneous neural blockade. This expertise, developed originally with local anaesthetics, was then extended to neurolytic agents. Initially, pain clinics started as nerve-blocking clinics and most pain management clinics continue to be directed by anaesthetists who now have access to a formal training programme supervised by the Faculty of Pain Medicine of the Royal College of Anaesthetists, and specialist recognition. However, with increasing awareness of the complexity of the pain experience, there has been recognition that other healthcare professionals have a significant role in the management of patients with chronic pain. A multidisciplinary approach involving anaesthetists, other healthcare professionals, such as psychologists, physiotherapists, occupational therapists, nurse specialists, and other medical practitioners, is the preferred management model for people with pain. Evidence-based practice is now firmly established in clinical decision-making, particularly in formulating guidelines and consensus documents. Pain management clinics are available in most hospitals in the United Kingdom, with local variation in the services offered. Some offer specialist clinics for specific conditions (e.g. pelvic pain clinic, paediatric pain clinic) or treatments (e.g. spinal cord stimulators).

Current health trends are supporting the delivery of pain management services in primary care and in the community, because many patients can be managed in a primary care setting without needing to be referred to hospital. There is an increasing trend to involve the patient as an active participant of treatment and to include self-management strategies as part of the management plan.

DEFINITIONS OF PAIN AND RELATED TERMS

Pain: 'an unpleasant sensory and emotional experience associated with actual or potential tissue damage, or described in terms of such damage' (The International Association for the Study of Pain, http://www.iasp-pain.org/AM/Template.cfm?Section=Pain_Definitions). This definition emphasizes that pain is not only a physical sensation but also a subjective psychological event. It accepts that pain may occur in spite of negative physical findings and investigations. Pain has sensory, cognitive and motivational-affective dimensions and has been described as a biopsychosocial experience, as illustrated in Figure 46.1. This must be taken into account when assessing and planning a treatment strategy for the patient with pain.

Acute pain: pain associated with acute injury (including surgery) or disease.

Chronic or persistent pain: pain that either occurs in disease processes in which healing does not take place or persists beyond the expected time of healing – arbitrarily 3 months.

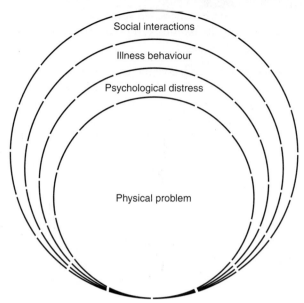

Social interactions

Illness behaviour

Psychological distress

Physical problem

FIGURE 46.1 ■ An illustration of pain as a biopsychosocial phenomenon.

Pain management: a multidisciplinary approach to the assessment and treatment of patients with (acute and chronic) pain.

Pain management programme: a cognitive-behavioural programme for patients with persistent pain and disability.

Pain medicine: the diagnostic and therapeutic activities of medical practitioners.

Chronic pain syndrome: a term used to describe a constellation of pain and other symptoms of complex aetiology associated with Sternbach's 6 Ds:

- Dramatization of complaints
- Drug misuse
- Dysfunction/disuse
- Dependency
- Depression
- Disability.

Chronic pain syndrome can adversely affect the patient in various ways, including depressed mood, fatigue, reduced activity and libido, excessive use of drugs and alcohol, dependent behaviour and disability out of proportion to impairment. It does not respond to the medical model of care and is best managed with a multidisciplinary approach.

THE PARADIGM OF PAIN

Pain management concerns postoperative, acute and chronic pain and cancer-related symptom control in children and adults. A joint report of the College of Anaesthetists and the Royal College of Surgeons of England highlighted the need to improve standards of postoperative pain management and many hospitals have established acute pain teams. However, many hospitalized patients suffer from acute non-postoperative pain. This may be caused by trauma, burns or acutely painful medical conditions (e.g. cardiac pain, osteoporotic vertebral collapse). Some medical conditions may cause recurrent acute painful episodes such as sickle-cell crisis or acute exacerbations of chronic pancreatitis. Unrelieved acute pain may lead to chronic pain. Chronic pain is a complex biopsychosocial phenomenon and a single pathophysiological explanation is not available for many chronic nonmalignant pain states. Palliative care services may refer cancer-related pain problems to the anaesthetist for management as a hospital inpatient, an outpatient, in a hospice or in the home. There are many common areas within the management of acute and chronic pain, and pain is increasingly viewed as a continuum rather than two separate entities, with subsequent merging of management techniques and staff.

Postoperative, acute, recurrent, persistent and cancer-related pain occurs in children. Difficulties in pain assessment and unsubstantiated fears and myths regarding pain and its treatment in children have led to suboptimal management. Recommendations for the management of pain in children have been published.

EPIDEMIOLOGY OF CHRONIC PAIN

The prevalence of chronic pain within the general population has proved difficult to estimate because of variations in the populations studied, the methods used to collect data and the criteria used to define chronic pain. Recent data have suggested that the prevalence of chronic pain in the UK is 13%, i.e. about 1 in 7 of the population. Chronic pain is the presenting complaint in 22% of primary care consultations and is estimated to account for 4.6 million GP visits per year. Patients with persistent pain consult their GPs five times more frequently than those without.

Untreated pain may reduce quality of life for sufferers and carers, resulting in helplessness, isolation, depression and family breakdown. Many patients with persistent pain have significant functional, social and financial consequences. Forty-nine percent take time off from work, 25% lose their jobs, 22% develop depression, 44% have their concentration affected and 56% have disturbed sleep.

Pain is the second commonest cause of days off work through sickness, accounting for 206 million working days lost in the UK in 1999–2000. It is the second commonest reason for people to be given Incapacity Benefit and £3.8 billion is spent per year on Incapacity Benefit for those in pain. The cost of back pain was £12.3 billion (22% of UK health expenditure) – mainly due to work days lost.

Pain is experienced by 20–50% of patients with cancer at the time of diagnosis and by up to 75% of patients with advanced disease.

CLASSIFICATION OF PAIN

Pain may be classified according to its aetiology.

Nociceptive Pain

Nociceptive pain results from tissue damage causing continuous nociceptor stimulation. It may be either somatic or visceral in origin.

Somatic Pain

Somatic pain results from activation of nociceptors in cutaneous and deep tissues, such as skin, muscle and subcutaneous soft tissue. Typically, it is well localized and described as aching, throbbing or gnawing. Somatic pain is usually sensitive to opioids.

Visceral Pain

Visceral pain arises from internal organs. It is characteristically vague in distribution and quality and is often described as deep, dull or dragging. It may be associated with nausea, vomiting and alterations in blood pressure and heart rate. Stimuli such as crushing or burning, which are painful in somatic structures, often evoke no pain in visceral organs. Mechanisms of visceral pain include abnormal distension or contraction of smooth muscle, stretching of the capsule of solid organs, hypoxaemia or necrosis and irritation by algesic substances. Visceral pain is often referred to cutaneous sites distant from the visceral lesion. One example of this is shoulder pain resulting from diaphragmatic irritation.

Hyperalgesia, i.e. increased response to a stimulus which is normally painful, can occur in visceral pain. There are three types:

- Visceral hyperalgesia: increased sensitivity in the painful organ. Pain threshold is lowered in some patients with functional gastrointestinal disease and patients complain of abdominal pain in response to normally innocuous stimuli of the gut.
- Referred hyperalgesia from viscera, in which hypersensitivity is localized in the muscles and often associated with a state of sustained contraction. For example, patients with urinary colic typically display hypersensitivity in the muscles of the lumbar region.
- Viscero-visceral hyperalgesia: pain in one visceral organ can be enhanced by pain in another visceral organ. Women with repeated urinary stones who were also dysmenorrhoeic manifested a higher number of colics than non-dysmenorrhoeic women.

Neuropathic Pain

Neuropathic pain is now defined as 'pain arising as a direct consequence of a lesion or disease affecting the somatosensory system'. It is characteristically dysaesthetic in nature and patients complain of unpleasant abnormal sensations. There may be marked allodynia, i.e. a normally nonpainful stimulus, such as light touch, evokes pain. Pain may be described as shooting or burning and may occur in areas of numbness. Neuropathic pain may develop immediately after nerve injury or after a variable interval. It is often persistent and can be relatively resistant to opioids. There is a tendency for a favourable response to centrally modulating medication, such as anticonvulsants and tricyclic and serotonin-noradrenaline reuptake inhibitor (SNRI) antidepressants.

There are many causes of neuropathic pain. Lesions in the peripheral nervous system include peripheral nerve injuries, peripheral neuropathies, HIV infection, some drugs and tumour infiltration. Central neuropathic pain is associated with lesions of the central nervous system, such as infarction, trauma and demyelination and is very resistant to treatment.

Sympathetically Maintained Pain

Pain which is maintained by sympathetic efferent innervation or by circulating catecholamines is termed sympathetically maintained pain (SMP) and considered a form of neuropathic pain. It may be a

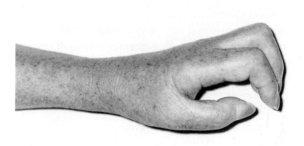

FIGURE 46.2 ■ Complex regional pain syndrome type I following Colles' fracture.

feature of several pain disorders and is not an essential component of any one condition. Sympathetic nerve blocks provide at least temporary reduction of pain, but current thinking is that this does not imply a mechanism for the pain. It is classified into type I (reflex sympathetic dystrophy) and type II (causalgia).

In complex regional pain syndrome (CRPS) type 1, minor injuries, including mild soft tissue trauma or a fracture, precede the onset of symptoms without any overt nerve lesion (Fig. 46.2). CRPS type II develops after injury to a peripheral nerve. Pain is the prominent feature and is characteristically spontaneous and burning in nature and associated with allodynia (abnormal sensitivity of the skin) and hyperalgesia. Autonomic changes may lead to swelling, abnormal sweating and changes in skin blood flow. Atrophy of the skin, nails and muscles can occur and localized osteoporosis may be demonstrated on X-ray or bone scan. Movement of the limb is usually restricted as a result of the pain, and contractures may result. Treatment is directed at providing adequate analgesia to encourage active physiotherapy and improvement of function. In cases with sympathetically maintained pain, sympathetic nerve block may be part of this treatment strategy.

MANAGEMENT OF CHRONIC PAIN

Patients present with pain as a result of many different pathological processes. Some examples of common painful conditions are listed in Table 46.1.

TABLE 46.1
Some Common Painful Conditions

Malignant Aetiology

Primary tumours
Metastases

Nonmalignant Aetiology

Musculoskeletal
  Back pain
  Osteoarthritis
  Rheumatoid arthritis
  Osteoporotic fracture

Neuropathic
  Trigeminal neuralgia
  Postherpetic neuralgia
  Brachial plexus avulsion
  Radicular pain of spinal origin
  Peripheral neuropathy
  Chronic regional pain syndrome (CRPS)

Visceral
  Urogenital pain
  Pancreatitis

Post-surgery
  Phantom pain
  Stump pain
  Scar pain
  Post-laminectomy

Ischaemic
  Peripheral vascular disease
  Raynaud's phenomenon/disease
  Intractable angina

Headaches

Cancer treatment-related: e.g. post-surgery, post-chemotherapy, post-radiotherapy pain

Assessment

Comprehensive assessment of patients with pain is a vital first step. Pain is generally thought of as a symptom rather than a disease in its own right. Efforts should be made to investigate, diagnose and, if possible, treat the underlying cause of the pain before using empirical pain-relieving techniques. However, there is now a growing body of animal and human evidence that chronic pain may involve increased sensitivity of spinal cord neurones and changes in the spinal cord and the brain, which can be responsible for increased pain. Thus, there has been some support for persistent pain to be viewed as a condition in its own right.

Pain History

The key elements of a pain history should be ascertained using a structured interview. The interview includes assessment of the pain, the effect of pain on the patient's mood and also the impact of the pain on quality of life and functioning. Many patients with pain become physically deconditioned and their mood can deteriorate. Both factors may contribute to the pain experience. Assessment can be recorded and audited using tools such as the Brief Pain Inventory.

Key elements in a pain history include:

- mode of onset
- location and radiation, either verbally or graphically using a pain diagram
- frequency
- aggravating factors
- relieving factors
- intensity, e.g. verbal rating scale, visual analogue scale, faces pain scale (children)
- quality, to determine possible somatic or neuropathic aetiology, e.g. burning, shooting; validated screening tools such as The Leeds Assessment of Neuropathic Symptoms and Signs (LANSS) pain scale can be used
- previous treatments
- current medication (analgesics and others)
- concurrent medical illness
- basic psychological assessment to include mood, coping skills, pain beliefs and self-reported disabilities; a Hospital Anxiety and Depression (HAD) scale can assist as a screening tool but if full psychological evaluation is indicated, it should be performed either by a psychiatrist or by a clinical psychologist, preferably one who is an integral member of the pain management team
- patient's own ideas as to causation
- family and social history
- impairment and functionality (Brief Pain Inventory)
- Quality of Life, e.g. EQ-5D as a standardized instrument for use as a measure of health outcome
- expectations of treatment.

Many patients, especially the elderly and those with malignancy, have more than one site of pain and separate histories should be taken for each complaint because their aetiologies may differ. Particular care and skill are needed when taking a pain history from children and the elderly.

Physical Examination

A physical examination relevant to the pain complaint should be performed and may include a full musculoskeletal or neurological assessment. It may involve a vaginal or rectal examination. Signs implicating involvement of the sympathetic nervous system including vasomotor, sudomotor and trophic changes should be considered. Physiotherapy assessment may be part of the initial screening interview.

Investigations

Additional laboratory, radiological and electrophysiological tests may be needed for full evaluation.

Chronic pain affects not only the patient, but also the family. Some patients with chronic pain become depressed and anxious, and lose their job, and financial and social status. Their relationships may deteriorate and it may be important to interview the patient's relatives or significant others with the patient to assess the impact of the pain on family life.

Explanation

Chronic pain is a complex phenomenon and often multifactorial in aetiology. The diagnosis, where possible, is based on the history, examination and the results of any investigations. Classification of the pain aids treatment decisions in some cases but many pains are of a mixed aetiology. The pain complaint and the results of any investigations should be discussed with the patient. This may involve an explanation that there is no obvious structural explanation for the pain, but impressing upon the patient that this is a reflection of our currently inadequate methods for imaging pain and does not imply that the pain is imagined. A patient-led problem list should be formulated and patient expectations for treatment should be explored and, if necessary, rationalized. The limitations of the medical model of disease for some chronic pain complaints should be explained.

Treatment

Total relief of persistent pain is rarely possible. Therefore, it is important that the patient is given information on strategies which can be employed to reduce the impact of the pain on their everyday life. These self-management strategies should include advice about the importance of remaining active, increasing fitness levels, planning and pacing all activities and avoiding over-activity/under-activity cycles. Self-management booklets, such as the Pain Tool-kit, can be given to patients.

A treatment plan should be formulated jointly with the patient after discussion of appropriate treatments, the potential benefits and side-effects of those options and the option of deciding against treatment. Several methods of treatment may be used in the same patient, either concomitantly or sequentially.

The range of interventions for chronic pain is shown in Figure 46.3.

Medication

Many patients in pain are prescribed analgesic drugs. The pharmacology of these agents is discussed fully elsewhere (see Ch 5) and only aspects of particular relevance to their use in chronic pain are mentioned below.

Cancer Pain

Approximately 75% of patients with advanced cancer develop significant pain before death. Most cancer pain responds to pharmacological measures, and successful treatment is based on simple

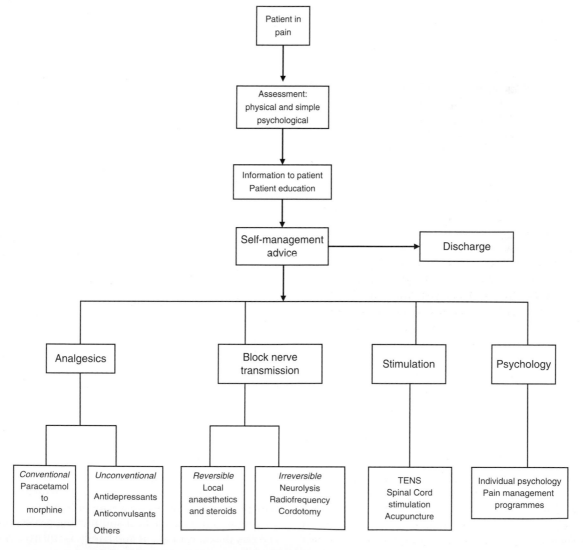

FIGURE 46.3 ■ Management pathway for patient in pain. *(Adapted from Moore et al 2003)*

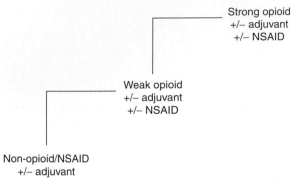

FIGURE 46.4 ■ The WHO analgesic ladder.

principles that have been promoted by the World Health Organization and are extensively validated. Analgesic drugs should be taken 'by mouth', 'by the clock' (i.e. regularly) and 'by the analgesic ladder' (Fig. 46.4). Cancer pain is continuous and medication must be taken regularly. It is given orally unless intractable nausea and vomiting occur or there is a physical impediment to swallowing. The first step on the 'analgesic ladder' is a non-opioid, such as paracetamol, aspirin or a non-steroidal anti-inflammatory drug (NSAID). If this is inadequate, a weak opioid such as codeine is added. The third step is substitution of the weak opioid by a strong opioid. Inadequate pain control at one level requires progression to a drug on the next level, rather than to an alternative of similar efficacy. Adjuvant analgesics, such as tricyclic or SNRI antidepressants, NSAIDs or anticonvulsants, may be used at any stage.

Using these strategies, pain may be controlled successfully in about 90% of patients with cancer pain without resorting to other interventions.

Paracetamol

Paracetamol 4 g daily is a better analgesic than placebo, but probably not as effective as NSAIDs. However, in the elderly patient, paracetamol may be useful because of its low side-effect profile.

Non-Steroidal Anti-Inflammatory Drugs

NSAIDs possess analgesic and anti-inflammatory action and are used widely in the management of mild to moderate pain. They are effective analgesics for pain from osteoarthritis, rheumatoid arthritis, dysmenorrhoea

and bone metastases. NSAIDs are not without adverse effects, the most worrying of which are an increased incidence of gastric ulcers, adverse effect on renal function and a potentially increased thrombotic risk, which has resulted in the European Medicines Agency stating that NSAIDs should be used in the lowest effective dose for the shortest possible duration.

Topical NSAIDs also provide effective pain relief.

Opioid Analgesics

Non-Cancer Pain. Weak opioid drugs, e.g. dihydrocodeine, are useful for moderate pain. However, they may be taken in excess, and often with only little benefit, by the patient with chronic non-malignant pain. Treatment in the pain management clinic may involve weaning the patient off such medication.

The use of strong opioids in non-malignant pain is controversial. There are trials of opioids in non-cancer pain which do show evidence of efficacy of opioids over placebo. However, these studies are often selective with regard to the patient and are short in duration, i.e. up to 3 months. Other studies have concluded that chronic opioid therapy exacerbates psychological distress, impairs cognition and worsens outcome. There is also concern about opioid-induced hyperalgesia, immune function and fertility. The controversy is also compounded by the perceived risk of psychological dependence (addiction) and the poorly understood phenomenon of tolerance. The British Pain Society has published recommendations for the appropriate use of opioids for persistent non-cancer pain and also specific information for patients on this subject.

Opioid Drugs

Morphine is the strong oral opioid of choice. Immediate-release oral morphine, either in liquid or tablet form, is given as often as necessary in increasing dosage until pain is controlled. When the required daily dose has been established, it is usual to convert to sustained-release morphine tablets, which need to be taken only once or twice daily. In addition, immediate-release morphine elixir or tablets should be prescribed for breakthrough cancer pain. The dose of morphine necessary to treat breakthrough cancer pain is one-sixth of the total daily morphine requirement.

Education of the medical and nursing professions, and also the cancer patient and family, is still necessary to ensure that adequate doses of opioids are prescribed and taken. Healthcare professionals often overestimate the side-effects of morphine. Respiratory depression is uncommon when morphine is prescribed for cancer pain. Surveys have shown that patients are concerned about side-effects of morphine, especially tolerance, addiction, constipation and drowsiness. Tolerance does not appear to be a problem clinically. Disease progression may necessitate an increase in dose, but there is no upper limit to the dose of morphine in cancer pain and pain control is usually regained without difficulty. Addiction (psychological dependence) is very uncommon in patients with cancer pain, and if the pain is relieved by other means, such as radiotherapy or a nerve block, many patients will stop taking opioids. Physical dependence always occurs and patients should be warned not to stop opioids precipitously. Nausea and vomiting may occur when treatment with morphine is started and an antiemetic may be prescribed for the first week, but often it may then be stopped. Sedation and cognitive impairment may occur as the dose is increased but these usually resolve. There is no tolerance to the constipating effect of morphine and laxatives need to be taken regularly. A phenomenon of opioid-induced hyperalgesia has been described, in which the patient suffers increasing pain, often of a widespread nature. It is thought that opioid-induced hyperalgesia develops as a result of activation of spinal cord mechanisms. Clinically, tolerance and disease progression need to be ruled out. The treatment of opioid-induced hyperalgesia involves decreasing the dose of opioid, switching to another opioid or the use of centrally acting analgesics such as ketamine.

Efforts should be made to reassure cancer patients and relatives of the efficacy and safety of morphine analgesia in both short and long term to ensure that medication is taken regularly.

Alternative Opioids and Alternative Routes of Administration.

Oxycodone hydrochloride is a semisynthetic congener of morphine. It is available as an immediate-release and a sustained-release preparation. It is approximately twice as potent as morphine (i.e. 5 mg of oxycodone is equivalent to 10 mg of oral morphine). Its advantage in renal failure is the lack of detectable clinically relevant active metabolites, therefore avoiding accumulation. Prolonged release oxycodone is available in combination with prolonged release naloxone to counteract constipation.

Hydromorphone is a semisynthetic opioid with a rapid onset and a shorter duration of action than morphine. It is more potent than morphine, with 1.3 mg of hydromorphone being equivalent to 10 mg of morphine. Immediate-release, sustained-release preparations and parenteral preparations are available.

Methadone is a potent opioid analgesic and also possibly an N-methyl-D-aspartate (NMDA) receptor antagonist. Methadone is absorbed rapidly by the oral route and has a long half-life which may range from 13 to 51 h. Initial dosing must be monitored carefully because relatively small doses of methadone may be needed in comparison with the previous opioid dose. When repeated doses are given, the drug accumulates and after the first few days, the frequency of administration may need to be reduced to two or three times daily. Methadone should be considered a third-line drug indicated for cancer pain which appears poorly responsive to morphine, diamorphine, fentanyl, oxycodone or hydromorphone in spite of dose escalation and the use of adjuvant drugs. Methadone is available as tablets, linctus and injection.

Transdermal Drug Delivery.

If a patient is unable to take medication by mouth, there are various alternative routes for opioid administration. A transdermal drug delivery system has been developed for fentanyl and buprenorphine. Fentanyl patches are applied to the skin and drug from the reservoir diffuses through the rate-controlling membrane and forms a subcutaneous depot from which the drug is taken up into the circulation. There is wide variation in absorption rates and time to steady-state serum concentrations of fentanyl. After removal of the patch, the terminal half-life has been shown to be 17 ± 2.3 h, indicative of the time taken for the drug to clear from the subcutaneous depot. Transdermal fentanyl is available in patches which deliver 12.5, 25, 50, 75 or 100 μg h^{-1} of fentanyl. They should be placed on unbroken skin, usually on the upper body, and need to be changed every 72 h. An appropriate dose of immediate-release morphine or a buccal or transnasal fentanyl preparation should be prescribed for breakthrough pain.

Buprenorphine patches are matrix patches in which buprenorphine is incorporated within an adhesive matrix, allowing constant release of buprenorphine into the systemic circulation at a predetermined rate over a minimum of 72 h. The dose of buprenorphine delivered is dependent upon the amount of drug held in the matrix and the area of the patch. Patch strengths available are 5, 10, 20, 35, 52.5 and 70 µg h^{-1} and patches should be applied either weekly or twice weekly, depending on the dose.

Pharmacokinetic data are of the utmost importance when considering changing medication from an opioid delivered by patch technology to an oral or parenteral opioid or *vice versa*. Patches are suitable for patients who cannot, or prefer not to, take oral medication or who are intolerant of morphine. However, the delay in onset of analgesia makes them unsuitable for treatment of acute pain. A table showing morphine equivalent doses of a variety of patches is available in the British Pain Society booklet 'Opioids for persistent pain'.

Subcutaneous Administration. Continuous subcutaneous administration is another alternative method of administration if oral medication cannot be taken. A small, portable battery-operated syringe driver fitted with a 20 mL syringe containing the total daily opioid dose is usually used. Because of its greater solubility, diamorphine is the drug of choice in the UK for this route of administration. A conversion ratio of 3 mg oral morphine to 1 mg subcutaneous diamorphine is used.

Spinal Administration. Opioids may be administered spinally, either epidurally or intrathecally, for:

- patients whose pain is controlled effectively by oral opioids but who suffer intolerable unacceptable side-effects, such as drowsiness or vomiting
- patients whose pain cannot be controlled by the use of oral or systemic opioids.

Only a small proportion (less than 2%) of patients with cancer pain are candidates for spinal opioids. Much smaller doses of drug are required when given spinally and thus side-effects are minimized. The daily dose of morphine via the epidural route is 1/10 of the oral 24-h dose and the intrathecal dose is 1/10 of the epidural dose. Contraindications to the insertion of a spinal catheter are similar to those in the acute situation. Side-effects, such as respiratory depression, itching and urinary retention which cause such concern in the opioid-naïve patient are rare in cancer patients who have been chronically exposed to systemic opioids.

The field of spinal opioid therapy is sufficiently new that guidelines for selection of route (intrathecal or epidural), choice of drug (opioid or opioid/local anaesthetic combination), administration protocol (intermittent bolus or continuous infusion) and equipment (tunnelled or totally implanted catheter and reservoir) are still being formulated.

Before introducing this technique, it is essential to devise formal protocols and an education programme for hospital, hospice and primary care nurses and doctors to facilitate management of the patient in any of these settings.

Co-Analgesics

These are drugs which have primary indications other than pain but are analgesic in some painful conditions. Full explanation regarding this must be given to the patient. The National Institute for Health and Clinical Excellence (NICE) has recognized the analgesic properties of these drugs.

Anticonvulsants. Anticonvulsants are used in the treatment of neuropathic pain. The precise mechanism of action varies among different anticonvulsants. For example, it is thought that carbamazepine blocks sodium channels and that gabapentin and pregabalin act on the $\alpha_2\delta$ subunit of the calcium channel. Therefore, if one anticonvulsant at maximum dosage is ineffective, then it is worthwhile trying another. Gabapentin, pregabalin, carbamazepine, oxcarbazepine, lamotrigine and phenytoin are used in neuropathic pain and trigeminal neuralgia.

In a variety of neuropathic pains, anticonvulsants have a number needed to treat (NNT) of less than 5 for at least 50% relief of pain, indicating that they are moderately effective for some patients. Data from studies show that for every patient who benefited, one had a minor adverse effect but continued with the treatment. Sedation, ataxia and weight gain are common side-effects of these drugs and may limit dose escalation, especially in the elderly.

Tricyclic and SNRI Antidepressants. Tricyclic and SNRI antidepressants have a role in the management of pain, independent of their effect on mood. Tricyclic drugs and SNRIs are postulated to act as analgesics by reducing the reuptake of the amine neurotransmitters noradrenaline and serotonin into the presynaptic terminal, increasing the concentration and duration of action of these substances at the synapse and thereby enhancing activity in the descending inhibitory pain pathway. Tricyclics also block sodium channels and suppress ectopic neuroma discharge.

Animal models of acute pain have consistently demonstrated the antinociceptive effect of tricyclic drugs. Controlled clinical trials of both tricyclics and SNRI antidepressants have shown beneficial results in postherpetic neuralgia, diabetic neuropathy, atypical facial pain and central pain. The NNT for effectiveness for antidepressants in neuropathic pain ranges from 2.9 for tricyclics to 5.8 for SNRIs. The effective dose of a tricyclic drug for analgesia is usually lower than that required for depression (although a dose response for analgesia has been demonstrated) and analgesia is apparent in 3–4 days compared with 3–4 weeks for antidepressant effects. Amitriptyline is the commonest tricyclic drug prescribed as an analgesic and the normal starting dose is 10–25 mg at night. Side-effects include sedation (which can be beneficial), constipation and a dry mouth. Other tricyclic drugs used as analgesics include imipramine and nortriptyline.

Selective serotonin reuptake inhibitors, such as fluoxetine, appear to be less effective analgesics.

Antiarrhythmic Drugs

Sodium channel blockers may be used to reduce pain caused by nerve damage. Both intraveneous lidocaine (up to $5\,mg\,kg^{-1}$) and oral mexiletine reduce neuropathic pain. Intravenous lidocaine appears effective in fibromyalgia (based on small patient numbers). Unfortunately, the benefits of lidocaine are short-lived and the studies are generally small.

Plasters containing 5% lignocaine have been recommended as another first-line drug for patients with postherpetic neuralgia or focal neuropathy with allodynia, based on three published positive trials. These plasters need to be applied daily for 12 h out of every 24 h.

Ketamine. Ketamine is an NMDA receptor antagonist which has been used successfully as an analgesic via intravenous, subcutaneous and oral routes. Psychometric side-effects may be a problem.

Capsaicin. Capsaicin is an alkaloid derived from chillies. It depletes substance P in local sensory nerve terminals. Local application may alleviate pain in painful diabetic peripheral neuropathy, osteoarthritis, postherpetic neuralgia, intercostobrachial neuralgia and psoriasis.

Recently, a capsaicin 8% plaster has been developed for use in treating neuropathic pain (except diabetic peripheral neuropathy). Although there is evidence of efficacy when used on a three-monthly basis, it is too early to say what its place will be in treating neuropathic pain.

Cannabinoids. Animal studies suggest that cannabinoids reduce hyperalgesia and allodynia in neuropathic, inflammatory and cancer pain. Human trials have also reported modest benefit in neuropathic pain. Cannabinoids act on CB_1 receptors, which are located in the brain, and their CB_2 counterparts found peripherally. Further research is needed to identify which cannabinoids may produce analgesia without psychotropic side-effects.

Oral Corticosteroids. The mechanism by which corticosteroids produce analgesia is unknown. They reduce inflammatory mediators, specifically prostaglandins. They reduce peritumour oedema, thus relieving pain by reducing pressure on adjacent pain-sensitive structures. They are administered for cerebral metastases, spinal cord compression, superior vena caval compression and neural infiltration or compression. In cancer patients, they are also prescribed for their euphoric effect and to stimulate appetite.

Interventional Pain Therapies

Therapeutic interventional therapies in the management of chronic and malignant pain have been performed for many years and include various types of nerve block and minimally invasive surgical procedures. There has been discussion and controversy regarding effectiveness, but significant progress has been made over the last two decades in establishing some evidence base for their use. Such techniques are often included as part of the multidisciplinary management of chronic pain.

Nerve blocks have been performed for many years in the management of pain. A nerve block comprises an injection of a local anaesthetic (sometimes combined with steroid) or a neurolytic agent around a peripheral or central sensory nerve, a sympathetic plexus or a trigger point. Correct use of interventional procedures in the treatment of chronic pain requires an experienced practitioner with a thorough knowledge of anatomy and an understanding of pain syndromes. Interventions should be undertaken in appropriate locations, usually day-case theatre suites, by clinicians who are fully acquainted with the techniques involved and who are competent to manage the complications which may arise. The use of radiological control and contrast media, ultrasound guidance or peripheral nerve stimulation is strongly advocated to confirm accurate needle placement.

Potential sites for neural blockade are shown in Figure 46.5, and indications for neural blockade are listed in Table 46.2. Some comments about commonly performed nerve blocks are made in the section below. For a full description of the techniques of neural blockade, the reader should consult suggested texts in the further reading section.

Agents

Local Anaesthetics. Local anaesthetics block sodium channels and may be used for both diagnostic and therapeutic injections. They have been injected into muscle trigger points for the relief of myofascial pain and it has been shown that prolonged relief of pain may result sometimes from local anaesthetic blocks to peripheral nerves.

Corticosteroids. Corticosteroids have been shown to block transmission in normal unmyelinated C fibres and to suppress ectopic neural discharges in experimental neuromas. They are sometimes added to local

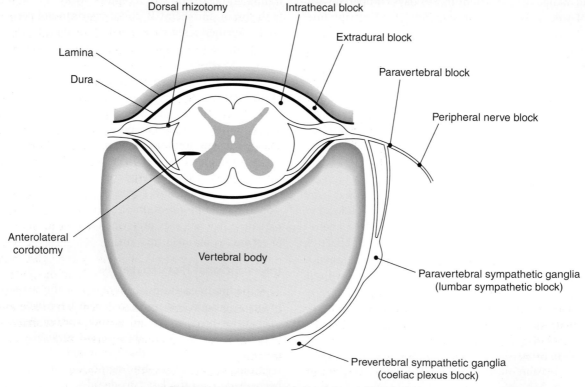

FIGURE 46.5 ■ Potential sites for neural blockade.

TABLE 46.2
Indications for Neural Blockade

Nerve Block	Indications
Trigger point injections	Myofascial pain, scar pain
Somatic nerve block	Nerve root pain, scar pain
Trigeminal nerve block and branches	Trigeminal neuralgia
Stellate ganglion block	SMP, CRPS
Coeliac plexus block	Intra-abdominal malignancy, especially pancreas
Superior hypogastric plexus block	Malignant pelvic pain
Lumbar sympathetic block	Ischaemic rest pain SMP, CRPS Phantom and stump pain
Epidural steroids/root canal injections	Nerve root pain, benign or malignant
Lumbar and cervical medial branch blocks	Back pain Whiplash cervical pain
Intrathecal neurolytics	Malignant pain
Percutaneous cervical cordotomy	Unilateral somatic malignant pain, short life expectancy

SMP, sympathetically maintained pain; CRPS, complex regional pain syndrome.

anaesthetics in nerve blocks and for injection into painful scars.

Botulinum Toxin. Botulinum toxin has been used for the treatment of temporomandibular dysfunction, migraine and vulvodynia. No firm data on effectiveness is available.

Neurolytic Techniques

Neural destruction can be produced by chemical or thermal means. In general, the use of neurolytic techniques has diminished in the last two decades. There are many reasons for this, including the improved use of analgesic drugs, the recognition that the effect of neuroablative procedures is often transient, the development of neurostimulatory techniques and appreciation of the cognitive and behavioural elements of pain. The clinical indications for neurolytic techniques are now limited to patients with cancer pain and a few selected non-cancer conditions. Careful thought with regard to the potential benefits and risks of the procedure, appropriate patient selection and fully informed consent are essential before performing a neurolytic procedure.

Chemical Neurolysis. The commonest neurolytic agents used are phenol and ethyl alcohol. Phenol acts by coagulating proteins and destroys all types of nerves, both motor and sensory. It is available in water or in glycerol. Its most frequent indication is for lumbar sympathetic block for peripheral vascular disease. Large systemic doses cause convulsions followed by central nervous system depression and cardiovascular collapse. Alcohol is the neurolytic agent of choice for coeliac plexus block in patients with intractable abdominal pain due to pancreatic cancer, when the large volume required prohibits the use of phenol. It produces a higher incidence of neuritis than phenol and is not used for other blocks.

Radiofrequency Lesions. Radiofrequency lesioning is indicated for patients in whom non-invasive treatments have failed. A destructive heat lesion is produced by a radiofrequency current generated by a lesion generator. The radiofrequency electrode comprises an insulated needle with a small exposed tip. A high frequency alternating current flows from the electrode tip to the tissues, producing ionic agitation and a heating effect in tissue adjacent to the tip of the probe. The magnitude of this heating effect is monitored by a thermistor in the electrode tip. Damage to nerve fibres sufficient to block conduction occurs at temperatures above 45°C, although in practice most lesions are made with a probe tip temperature of 60–80°C. An integral nerve stimulator is used to ensure accurate positioning of the probe. Whereas the spread of neurolytic solutions is unpredictable, radiofrequency lesions are more precise. The size of the lesion depends on the tip temperature, the duration of the current and the length of the exposed needle tip. Lower-temperature lesions are now being used in an attempt to produce analgesia without nerve destruction in pulsed radiofrequency lesioning.

Radiofrequency lesions of the trigeminal nerve may be used to treat trigeminal neuralgia in the elderly patient whose pain is uncontrolled by anticonvulsant drugs and who is unsuitable for microvascular decompression. Radiofrequency lesions of spinal nerves, including the medial branch of the dorsal ramus, are used in some spinal conditions.

Epidural Steroids

Epidural steroids have been used since 1962 for nerve root pain. A recent meta-analysis of all randomized, controlled trials has concluded that epidural administration of corticosteroids is more effective in reducing lumbosacral radicular pain (in both the short and long term) than placebo. In addition, McQuay and Moore (1998) have addressed the question 'How well do they work?' by investigating the short-term (1–60 days) and long-term (12 weeks–1 year) efficacy of epidural steroids for sciatica. They used the NNT as a measure of clinical benefit. The NNT for short-term, greater than 75% pain relief was just under 7.3. The NNT for long-term (12 weeks–1 year) improvement was 13 for 50% pain relief.

The use of epidural steroids is not without potential hazards and controversy. The most common side-effects relate not to the steroid but to technical aspects of the technique. There have been reports of dural tap (2.5%), transient headache (2.3%) and transient increase in pain (1.9%). As with any spinal injection, an aseptic technique must be used and the usual contraindications observed. Methylprednisolone acetate and triamcinolone are the steroids most commonly used. It has been shown that neither of these preparations is deleterious when injected into the epidural space. However, they may have harmful effects if injected inadvertently into the subarachnoid or subdural spaces.

Before an epidural steroid injection is undertaken, the patient should receive a consultation during which the perceived merits, expectations, risks and possible complications are explained fully. This should include an explanation that the steroid preparation is being used outside its product licence. The doctor should be satisfied that the procedure is indicated, that appropriate neurological examination and investigations have been performed and that there is no contraindication to the procedure. Written consent should be obtained. Arrangements should be made for the outcome to be monitored formally by the doctor or team who prescribed the procedure or the one who performed it.

Provision should be made for an earlier consultation if necessary.

Spinal Endoscopy

Spinal endoscopy is a minimally invasive procedure developed to enable the physician to visualize the epidural space and nerve roots. The epidural space can be accessed with a spinal endoscope and a steerable catheter via the sacral hiatus. This technique allows for a direct visual examination of a specific nerve root and any associated pathology. The catheter is used as a blunt dissector to lyse adhesions which encapsulate the affected nerve root. In addition, irrigation of the nerve root with saline may 'wash away' inflammatory mediators.

Nerve Root Injection

Local anaesthetics and steroids may be injected around a nerve root as it emerges from the intervertebral foramen. This is an alternative to an epidural steroid injection and may be useful when the level of nerve compression is demonstrated by an MR scan. X-ray screening is essential. This technique may be used in the cervical, thoracic and lumbar regions.

Medial Branch Block of the Dorsal Ramus (Lumbar and Cervical Facet Nerve Blocks)

Chronic back and neck pain are common complaints in pain management clinics. Lumbar and cervical facet joints are considered to be potential sources. Injections of local anaesthetic and steroid into both lumbar and cervical facet medial branch nerves are performed commonly, although there is controversy about long-term benefit. Radiofrequency lesions of the facet nerves have been reported to give long-term relief in appropriately selected patients.

Sympathetic Nerve Blocks

Visceral nociceptive afferents travel in the sympathetic nervous system to the spinal cord. Visceral pain tends to be less opioid-sensitive than somatic pain. Percutaneous sympathetic blocks may therefore be useful in the management of severe cancer-related visceral pain which is poorly controlled with opioids or controlled only with intolerable side-effects.

Percutaneous coeliac plexus block using 50% alcohol is one of the most commonly used and effective blocks performed for cancer pain. It is used for pain resulting from upper gastrointestinal neoplasms, in particular carcinoma of the pancreas. Radiological screening, either X-ray or CT, is mandatory, although this does not ensure absence of complications. Hypotension, especially postural hypotension, should be anticipated and managed appropriately. Serious complications are rare, but include paraplegia.

The superior hypogastric plexus innervates the pelvic viscera. Superior hypogastric plexus block with phenol has been used for pelvic pain from cervical, prostatic, colonic, rectal, bladder, uterine and ovarian malignancy, and rectal tenesmus.

Chemical lumbar sympathectomy using phenol is performed for inoperable ischaemic leg pain. Radiological screening using contrast medium is necessary to ensure correct positioning of the needle. The complication rate is low, the most common complication being genitofemoral neuralgia, with a reported incidence varying from 4% to 15%.

Stellate ganglion and lumbar sympathetic block with local anaesthetic are sometimes helpful in the treatment of sympathetically mediated pain, CRPS types I and II, amputation stump and phantom pain.

Intravenous Regional Sympathetic Block with Guanethidine

The intravenous regional guanethidine technique was reported in 1974 and it became a popular method of treating CRPS. The technique is the same as intravenous regional analgesia (IVRA), but with the addition of guanethidine 10–20 mg. However, a recent systematic review of the randomized, controlled studies of intravenous regional guanethidine block in the treatment of CRPS failed to show evidence of effectiveness.

Stimulation-Induced Analgesia

Transcutaneous electrical nerve stimulation, spinal cord stimulation, deep brain stimulation and acupuncture may produce stimulation-induced analgesia.

Transcutaneous Electrical Nerve Stimulation

Transcutaneous electrical nerve stimulation (TENS) has been used widely since Melzack and Wall proposed the gate control theory in 1965. They postulated that large-diameter primary afferents exert a specific inhibitory effect on dorsal horn nociceptive neurones and

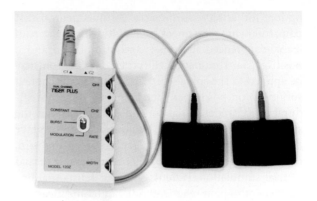

FIGURE 46.6 ■ A transcutaneous electrical nerve stimulator.

that stimulation of these fibres would alleviate pain. Conventional TENS produces high-frequency, low-intensity stimulation which relieves pain in the area in which it produces paraesthesia. Stimulation variables of TENS may be altered to produce low-frequency acupuncture-like TENS, which, unlike conventional TENS, produces analgesia which is antagonized by naloxone.

A small battery-powered unit is used to apply the electrical stimulus to the skin via electrodes (Fig. 46.6). These are placed over the painful area, on either side of it or over nerves supplying the region, and stimulation is applied at an intensity which the patient finds comfortable. Adverse effects are minimal, with allergy to the electrodes being the commonest problem encountered. TENS is used for a variety of musculoskeletal pains and has been advocated recently for refractory angina. Tolerance to TENS does occur sometimes. It may be possible to overcome this by changing stimulation variables.

TENS has been used also for acute postoperative pain and for analgesia for the first stage of labour. However, there is evidence of lack of analgesic effect in both these areas, although women using it as a method of pain relief tend to favour it for future births. Although studies have shown clear benefit from the use of TENS in chronic pain, there is a general lack of evidence for effectiveness of TENS rather than evidence of lack of effect.

Spinal Cord Stimulation

The National Institute for Health and Clinical Excellence (NICE) has produced guidance recommending spinal cord stimulation (SCS) as a treatment option for adults with severe chronic neuropathic pain, following assessment by a multidisciplinary pain team experienced in spinal cord stimulation and a positive trial stimulation. Electrical stimulation may be applied to the spinal cord via electrodes implanted surgically or positioned percutaneously in the epidural space under X-ray control. To be effective, the stimulating electrode must be positioned to produce artificial paraesthesia in the distribution of the pain. It is usual practice for the patient to undergo a period of trial stimulation. Patients showing substantial improvement in pain relief and other outcome measures may be considered for permanent implantation of a battery-driven stimulus generator. The patient uses a magnet to activate the stimulator.

Acupuncture

The Chinese have believed for 4000 years that inserting needles at specific points in the body produces analgesia. According to Chinese philosophy *chi*, the life force, circulates around the body in pathways termed meridians. Injury and illness can block the flow of *chi*, causing pain and disease. Acupuncture is believed to release these blocks and balance the energy of the patient. Traditionally, acupuncture points are stimulated by the insertion of fine needles, which are then rotated manually or stimulated by heat (moxibustion) or electrically.

Acupuncture is widely used for treating chronic pain and yet there is little evidence that it is effective in the long term. Acupuncture may also cause harm, such as infection or pneumothorax.

Psychological Techniques

Pain is not merely a sensation of tissue damage, but a complex interaction of biochemical, behavioural, cognitive and emotional factors. Chronic pain patients become anxious, depressed, distressed, functionally impaired and lose self-esteem. These important aspects should be addressed in the pain management clinic. A clinical psychologist is an essential member of the pain management team. A cognitive and behavioural approach investigates how thoughts (often negative) and behaviours (often maladaptive) reinforce the chronic pain state. Cognitive and behavioural techniques can be used to reduce the helplessness and hopelessness of the pain patient and to increase the level of functioning and emotional well-being in spite of the pain.

Pain Management Programme

A pain management programme is a psychologically based rehabilitative treatment for patients with chronic pain which remains unresolved by currently available medical or other physically based treatments.

The aim of a pain management programme is to reduce the disability and distress caused by chronic pain by teaching sufferers physical, psychological and practical techniques to improve their quality of life. It aims to enable patients to be self-reliant in managing their pain. It differs from other treatment provided in the pain clinic in that pain relief is not the primary goal.

A pain management programme is facilitated by a multidisciplinary healthcare team. Key clinical staff include a doctor with experience in pain management, a clinical psychologist, a physiotherapist and an occupational therapist, all trained in pain management. Information and education about the nature of pain and its management, medication review and advice, psychological assessment and intervention, physical reconditioning, advice on posture and graded return to the activities of daily living are components of pain management programmes.

EVIDENCE-BASED PRACTICE

There is an increasing drive for evidence-based medicine and for offering to patients only those interventions which are known to be effective. For some of the procedures commonly used in the pain management clinic, the evidence of effectiveness is available (e.g. cognitive and behavioural interventions and some medications for specific pain problems) but further work is required to gather this evidence for other interventions.

COSTS OF PAIN MANAGEMENT SERVICES

There is little information on the costs of pain management services. A detailed study of the costs incurred by users of specialty pain clinic services in Canada has shown that users incur less direct healthcare costs than nonusers with similar conditions. Similar results were shown by a small study of NHS pain clinic attendees. This showed that the pain clinic covered its costs by reducing consumption elsewhere and by reducing GP consultations and private treatments.

Advances in knowledge of pain pathophysiology and new methods of brain imaging, such as fMRI and PET scanning, and increasingly close cooperation between scientists and clinicians, have led to a better understanding of mechanisms sustaining chronic pain and an increase in therapeutic options. In addition, the increasing acceptance by the medical profession and the general public of the importance of psychological factors in chronic pain has opened up new treatment opportunities. There is evidence of the effectiveness of many of the treatments used in the management of chronic pain, but further work is needed on those interventions for which information is lacking and in identifying which patients may benefit most from specific treatments.

FURTHER READING

British Pain Society, Opioids for persistent pain. http://www.british-painsociety.org/book_opioid_main.pdf.

British Pain Society, Cancer pain management. http://www.british-painsociety.org/book_cancer_pain.pdf.

Cousins, M.J., Carr, D.B., Horlocker, T.T., Bridenbaugh, P.O. (Eds.), 2008. Neural blockade in clinical anesthesia and pain medicine, fourth ed. Wolters Kluwer, Lippincott, Williams and Wilkins, Philadelphia.

McMahon, S., Koltzenburg, M. (Eds.), 2005. Wall and Melzack's textbook of pain, fifth ed. Elsevier, London.

Moore, A., Edwards, J., Barden, J., McQuay, H., 2003. Bandolier's little book of pain. Oxford University Press, Oxford.

Singh, M.K., Patel, J., Chronic pain syndrome. http://emedicine.medscape.com/article/310834-overview.

Stannard, C.F., Kalso, E., Ballantyne, J. (Eds.), 2010. Evidence-based chronic pain management. John Wiley & Sons Ltd, Chichester.

Twycross, R., Wilcock, A., 2001. Symptom management in advanced cancer. Radcliffe Medical Press, Oxon.

Waldman, S.D., Winnie, A.P., 1996. Interventional pain management. W B Saunders, Philadelphia.

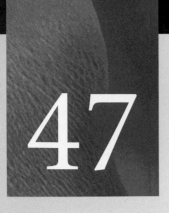

47

RESUSCITATION

INTRODUCTION

Without intervention, cardiac arrest may lead to permanent neurological injury after just three minutes. The interventions that contribute to a successful outcome after a cardiac arrest can be conceptualized as a chain – the Chain of Survival (Fig. 47.1).

The four links in this chain are:

- Early recognition – to potentially enable prevention of cardiac arrest – and call for help
- Early cardiopulmonary resuscitation (CPR)
- Early defibrillation
- Post-resuscitation care.

This chapter includes some background to the epidemiology and the prevention of cardiac arrest. It details the principles of initiating CPR in-hospital, defibrillation, advanced life support (ALS), post-resuscitation care and potential modifications to ALS when cardiac arrest occurs intraoperatively.

SCIENCE AND GUIDELINES

The 2010 International Consensus on Cardiopulmonary Resuscitation and Emergency Cardiovascular Care Science with Treatment Recommendations summarizes all the current science underpinning CPR. The European Resuscitation Council (ERC) and Resuscitation Council (UK) Guidelines for Resuscitation 2010 are derived from the 2010 consensus document and have been used as source material.

EPIDEMIOLOGY

Ischaemic heart disease is the leading cause of death in the world. In Europe, sudden cardiac arrest is responsible for more than 60% of adult deaths from coronary heart disease. In Europe, the annual incidence of emergency medical services (EMS)-treated out-of-hospital cardiopulmonary arrest (OHCA) for all rhythms is 35 per 100 000 population. The annual incidence of EMS-treated ventricular fibrillation (VF) arrest is 17 per 100 000 and survival to hospital discharge is 10.7% for all-rhythm and 21.2% for VF cardiac arrest. There is some evidence that long-term survival rates after cardiac arrest are increasing. On initial heart rhythm analysis, about 25–35% of OHCA victims have VF, a percentage that has declined over the last 20 years. Immediate CPR can double or triple survival from VF OHCA. After VF OHCA, each minute of delay before defibrillation reduces the probability of survival to discharge by about 10%.

The incidence of in-hospital cardiac arrest is difficult to assess because it is influenced heavily by factors such as the criteria for hospital admission and implementation of a do-not-attempt-resuscitation (DNAR) policy. The reported incidence of in-hospital cardiac arrest is in the range of 1–5 per 1000 admissions. Data from the American Heart Association's National Registry of CPR indicate that survival to hospital discharge after in-hospital cardiac arrest is 17.6% (all rhythms). The initial rhythm is VF or pulseless VT in 25% of cases and, of these, 37% survive to leave hospital; after pulseless electrical activity (PEA) or asystole, 11.5% survive to hospital discharge. Preliminary data from the United Kingdom National Cardiac Arrest Audit (NCAA), which includes all individuals receiving chest compressions and/or defibrillation and attended by the hospital-based resuscitation team (or equivalent) in response to a 2222 call, indicates that the survival to hospital discharge after all-rhythm cardiac arrest is 19.5%.

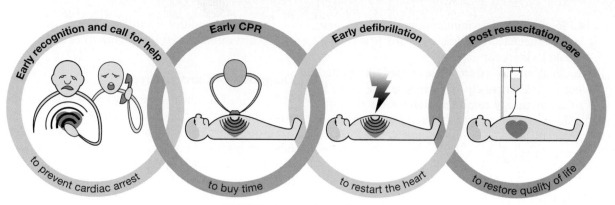

FIGURE 47.1 ■ Chain of survival.

PREVENTION

Out of hospital, recognition of the importance of chest pain enables victims or bystanders to call the EMS and receive treatment that can prevent cardiac arrest.

Cardiac arrest in hospital patients in unmonitored ward areas is not usually a sudden unpredictable event; it is also not usually caused by primary cardiac disease. These patients often have slow and progressive physiological deterioration, involving hypoxaemia and hypotension that has been unnoticed by staff, or recognised but treated poorly. Many such patients have unmonitored arrests, and the underlying cardiac arrest rhythm is usually non-shockable; the preliminary NCAA data show that survival to hospital discharge for this group is just 7%.

Guidelines for Prevention of In-Hospital Cardiac Arrest (Resuscitation Council (UK))

1. Place critically ill patients, or those at risk of clinical deterioration, in areas where the level of care is matched to the level of patient sickness.
2. Monitor such patients regularly using simple vital sign observations (e.g. pulse, blood pressure, respiratory rate, conscious level, temperature and SpO_2). Match the frequency and type of observations to the severity of illness of the patient.
3. Use an early warning score (EWS) system or 'calling criteria' to identify patients who are critically ill, at risk of clinical deterioration or cardiopulmonary arrest, or both.
4. Use a patient vital signs chart that encourages and permits the regular measurement and recording of vital signs and, where used, early warning scores.
5. Ensure that the hospital has a clear policy that requires a timely, appropriate, clinical response to deterioration in the patient's clinical condition.
6. Introduce into each hospital a clearly identified response to critical illness. This will vary between sites, but may include an outreach service or resuscitation team (e.g. medical emergency team (MET)) capable of responding to acute clinical crises. This team should be alerted, using an early warning system, and the service must be available 24 hours a day.
7. Ensure that all clinical staff are trained in the recognition, monitoring, and management of the critically ill patient, and that they know their role in the rapid response system.
8. Empower staff to call for help when they identify a patient at risk of deterioration or cardiac arrest. Use a structured communication tool to ensure effective handover of information between staff (e.g. SBAR – Situation-Background-Assessment-Recommendation).
9. Agree a hospital do-not-attempt-resuscitation (DNAR) policy, based on current national guidance. Identify patients who do not wish to receive

CPR and those for whom cardiopulmonary arrest is an anticipated terminal event for whom CPR would be inappropriate.

10. Audit all cardiac arrests, 'false arrests', unexpected deaths, and unanticipated intensive care unit admissions, using a common dataset. Audit the antecedents and clinical responses to these events. All hospitals should consider joining NCAA (https://ncaa.icnarc.org).

CARDIOPULMONARY RESUSCITATION

The division between basic life support and advanced life support is arbitrary – the resuscitation process is a continuum. The keys steps are that cardiorespiratory arrest is recognized immediately, help is summoned, and CPR (chest compressions and ventilations) is started immediately and, if indicated, defibrillation attempted as soon as possible (ideally, within 3 min of collapse).

The sequence of actions and outcome depends on:

- *Location* – out-of-hospital versus in-hospital; witnessed versus unwitnessed; monitored versus unmonitored.
- *Skills of the responders* – in some public places staff may be trained in CPR and defibrillation. All healthcare professionals should be able to recognize cardiac arrest, call for help, and start resuscitation.
- *Number of responders* – single responders must ensure that help is coming. If other staff are nearby, several actions can be undertaken simultaneously.
- *Equipment available* – AEDs are available in some public places. In hospital, ideally, the equipment used for CPR (including defibrillators) and the layout of equipment and drugs should be standardized throughout the hospital. AEDs should be considered for clinical and non-clinical areas where staff do not have rhythm recognition skills or rarely need to use a defibrillator.
- *Response system to cardiac arrest and medical emergencies* – outside hospital the EMS should be summoned. In hospital, the resuscitation team can be a traditional cardiac arrest team (called when cardiac arrest is recognized) or a MET.

Diagnosis of Cardiac Arrest

Many trained healthcare staff may not be able to assess a patient's breathing and pulse sufficiently reliably to confirm cardiac arrest. Agonal breathing is common in the early stages of cardiac arrest and is a sign of cardiac arrest; it should not be confused as being a sign of life/circulation. Agonal breathing can also occur during chest compressions as cerebral perfusion improves, but is not indicative of a return of spontaneous circulation (ROSC). Delivering chest compressions to a patient with a beating heart is unlikely to cause harm.

High-Quality CPR

The quality of chest compressions is often poor and, in particular, frequent and unnecessary interruptions often occur. Even short interruptions to chest compressions may compromise outcome. The correct hand position for chest compression is the middle of the lower half of the sternum. The recommended depth of compression is at 5–6 cm and the rate is 100–120 compressions min^{-1}. Allow the chest to recoil completely in between each compression. If available, use a prompt and/or feedback device to help ensure high-quality chest compressions. The person providing chest compressions should change about every 2 min, or earlier if unable to continue high-quality chest compressions. This change should be done with minimal interruption to compressions.

During CPR, perfusion of the brain and myocardium is, at best, 25% of normal; successful ROSC is more likely the higher the coronary perfusion pressure (CPP). Chest compressions increase the amplitude and the frequency of the VF waveform and increase the likelihood that attempted defibrillation will be successful. Pauses in chest compressions of just 10 seconds before shock delivery (pre-shock pause) reduce the chances of successful defibrillation. Frequent interruptions in chest compressions reduce survival from cardiac arrest: each time chest compressions are stopped the CPP decreases rapidly and takes time to be restored to the same level once the compressions are restarted.

Starting CPR in Hospital

The sequence of actions for initiating CPR in hospital is shown in Figure 47.2.

ADVANCED LIFE SUPPORT

Arrhythmias associated with cardiac arrest are divided into two groups: shockable rhythms (VF/VT) and non-shockable rhythms (asystole and PEA). The principle difference in management is the need for attempted defibrillation in patients with VF/VT. Subsequent actions, including chest compression, airway management and ventilation, vascular access, injection of adrenaline, and the identification and correction of reversible factors, are common to both groups. The ALS algorithm (Fig. 47.3) provides a standardized approach to the management of adult patients in cardiac arrest.

Shockable Rhythms (VF/VT)

The first monitored rhythm is VF/VT in approximately 25% of cardiac arrests, both in or out of hospital. VF/VT will also occur at some stage during resuscitation in about 25% of cardiac arrests with an initial documented rhythm of asystole or PEA. Having confirmed cardiac arrest, help (including a defibrillator) is summoned and CPR initiated, beginning with chest compressions, with a compression:ventilation (CV) ratio

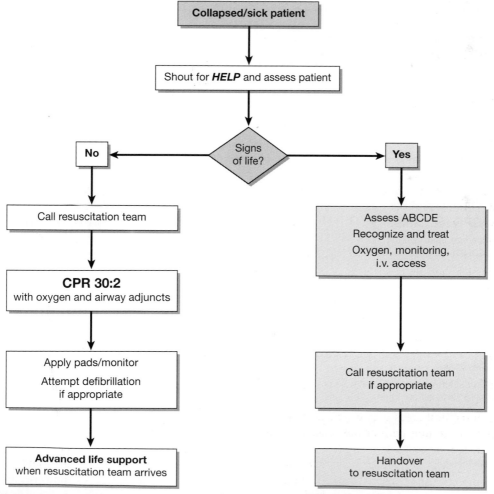

FIGURE 47.2 ■ In-hospital resuscitation algorithm *(adapted from 2010 Resuscitation Guidelines (Resuscitation Council UK))*.

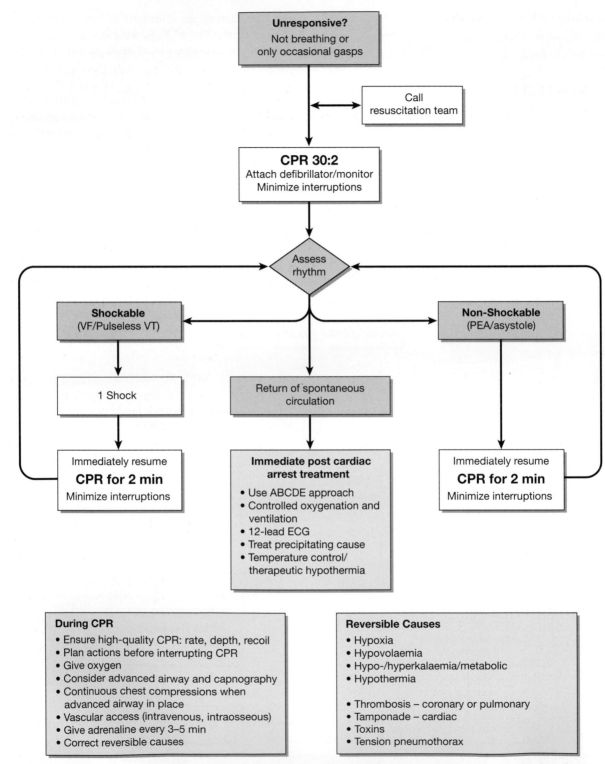

FIGURE 47.3 ■ The advanced life support algorithm *(adapted from 2010 Resuscitation Guidelines (Resuscitation Council UK))*.

of 30:2. When the defibrillator arrives, chest compressions are continued while applying self-adhesive pads. The rhythm is identified and treated according to the ALS algorithm.

Sequence of Actions

- If VF/VT is confirmed, charge the defibrillator while another rescuer continues chest compressions.
- Once the defibrillator is charged, pause the chest compressions, quickly ensure that all rescuers are clear of the patient and then give one shock. The person doing compressions, or another rescuer may deliver the shock. This sequence should be planned before stopping compressions.
- Resume chest compressions immediately (30:2) without reassessing the rhythm or feeling for a pulse.
- Continue CPR for 2 min, then pause briefly to check the monitor:
    - If VF/VT persists:
        - Give a further (2nd) shock and without reassessing the rhythm or feeling for a pulse, resume CPR (CV ratio 30:2) immediately after the shock, starting with chest compressions.
- On completion of CPR for 2 min, pause briefly to check the monitor:
    - If VF/VT persists:
        - Give a further (3rd) shock and without reassessing the rhythm or feeling for a pulse, resume CPR (CV ratio 30:2) immediately after the shock, starting with chest compressions.
- If intravascular (i.v./intraosseous) access has been obtained, give adrenaline 1 mg and amiodarone 300 mg once compressions have resumed. On completion of CPR for 2 min, pause briefly to check the monitor:
    - If VF/VT persists:
        - Give a further (4th) shock; resume CPR immediately and continue for 2 min.
        - Give adrenaline 1 mg with alternate cycles of CPR (i.e. approximately every 3–5 min).
    - If organized electrical activity is seen during this brief pause in compressions, check for a pulse.
        - If a pulse is present, start post-resuscitation care.
        - If no pulse is present, continue CPR and switch to the non-shockable algorithm.

- If asystole is seen, continue CPR and switch to the non-shockable algorithm.

If an organized rhythm is seen during a 2-minute period of CPR, do not interrupt chest compressions to palpate a pulse unless the patient shows signs of life (this may include a sudden increase in end-tidal carbon dioxide $[P_ECO_2]$ if this is being monitored) suggesting ROSC. If there is any doubt about the existence of a pulse in the presence of an organized rhythm, resume CPR. If the patient has ROSC, begin post-resuscitation care.

Precordial Thump

A single precordial thump has a very low success rate for cardioversion of a shockable rhythm and is only likely to succeed if given within the first few seconds of the onset of a shockable rhythm. There is more success with pulseless VT than with VF. Delivery of a precordial thump must not delay calling for help or accessing a defibrillator. It is reasonable to attempt a precordial thump if VF occurs intraoperatively, but do not delay the call for a defibrillator.

Defibrillation Strategy

Pads Versus Paddles. Self-adhesive defibrillation pads have practical benefits over hand-held paddles for routine monitoring and defibrillation and are much preferred to standard defibrillation paddles. Use of self-adhesive pads enables the operator to defibrillate the patient from a safe distance and to deliver a shock more rapidly than with paddles.

Safe Use of Oxygen. In an oxygen-enriched atmosphere, sparks from defibrillator paddles applied poorly can cause a fire. The use of self-adhesive defibrillation pads instead of manual paddles reduces the risk of sparks occurring.

- Remove any oxygen mask or nasal cannulae and place them at least 1 m away from the patient's chest during defibrillation.
- Leave the ventilation bag connected to the tracheal tube or other airway adjunct. Alternatively, disconnect the ventilation bag from the tracheal tube and move it at least 1 m from the patient's chest during defibrillation.

Single Versus Three-Shock Strategy. If defibrillation is attempted immediately after the onset of VF, it is unlikely that chest compressions will improve the already very high chance of ROSC associated with second or third shocks (i.e. myocardial levels of oxygen and adenosine triphosphate are likely to be adequate for the first minute or so). Thus, if VF/VT occurs during cardiac catheterization or in the early post-operative period after cardiac surgery (when chest compressions could disrupt vascular sutures), consider delivering up to three-stacked shocks before starting chest compressions. This three-shock strategy may also be considered for an initial, witnessed VF/VT cardiac arrest if the patient is already connected to a manual defibrillator – this situation will exist perioperatively if defibrillation pads were applied before induction of anaesthesia.

Defibrillation Energy. All modern defibrillators deliver shocks with a biphasic waveform. The initial biphasic shock should be at least 150 J. Because of the lower efficacy of monophasic defibrillators for terminating VF/VT, the recommended initial energy level for the first shock using a monophasic defibrillator is 360 J. If an initial shock has been unsuccessful, deliver the second and subsequent shocks with a higher energy level if the defibrillator is capable of delivering a higher energy. Manufacturers should display the effective waveform energy range on the face of the biphasic device. If you are unaware of the effective energy range of the device, use 200 J for the first shock.

Non-Shockable Rhythms (PEA and Asystole)

Pulseless electrical activity (PEA) is defined as the absence of any palpable pulse in the presence of cardiac electrical activity that would be expected to produce a cardiac output. There may be some mechanical myocardial contractions that are too weak to produce a detectable pulse or blood pressure – this is sometimes described as 'pseudo-PEA'. PEA may be caused by reversible conditions that can be treated if they are identified and corrected. A relative overdose of an induction drug is a well-recognized cause of intraoperative cardiac arrest.

Sequence of Actions for PEA

- Start CPR 30:2 and inject adrenaline 1 mg as soon as intravascular access is achieved.
- Continue CPR 30:2 until the airway is secured, then continue chest compressions without pausing during ventilation.

- Identify and correct any reversible causes of PEA.
- Recheck the patient after 2 min:
  - If there is still **no** pulse and no change in the ECG appearance:
    - □ Continue CPR; recheck the patient after 2 min and proceed accordingly.
    - □ Give further adrenaline 1 mg every 3–5 min (alternate loops).
  - If VF/VT, change to the shockable rhythm algorithm.
  - If a pulse is present, start post-resuscitation care.

Sequence of Actions for Asystole

- Start CPR 30:2.
- Without stopping CPR, check that the leads are attached correctly.
- Give adrenaline 1 mg as soon as intravascular access is achieved.
- Continue CPR 30:2 until the airway is secured, then continue chest compression without pausing during ventilation.
- Identify and correct any reversible causes of asystole.
- Recheck the rhythm after 2 min and proceed accordingly.
- If VF/VT, change to the shockable rhythm algorithm.
- Give adrenaline 1 mg i.v. every 3–5 min (alternate loops).

Whenever a diagnosis of asystole is made, check the ECG carefully for the presence of P waves because the patient may respond to cardiac pacing when there is ventricular standstill with continuing P waves. There is no value in attempting to pace true asystole.

During CPR

During the treatment of persistent VF/VT or PEA/ asystole, there should be an emphasis on giving good-quality chest compressions between defibrillation attempts, whilst recognizing and treating reversible causes (4 Hs and 4 Ts), and whilst obtaining a secure airway and intravascular access. Healthcare providers must practise efficient coordination between CPR and shock delivery. A shock is more likely to be successful if the pre-shock pause is short (less than 10 seconds).

Potentially Reversible Causes

Potential causes or aggravating factors for which specific treatment exists must be sought during any cardiac arrest (Table 47.1).

Minimize the risk of **hypoxia** by ensuring that the patient's lungs are ventilated adequately with 100% oxygen.

Pulseless electrical activity caused by **hypovolaemia** is usually due to severe haemorrhage. Restore intravascular volume rapidly with fluid, coupled with urgent surgery to stop the haemorrhage.

Hyperkalaemia, hypokalaemia, hypocalcaemia, acidaemia, and other metabolic disorders are detected by biochemical tests or suggested by the patient's medical history, e.g. renal failure. A 12-lead ECG may be diagnostic. Intravenous calcium chloride is indicated in the presence of hyperkalaemia, hypocalcaemia, and calcium-channel-blocking drug overdose.

Suspect **hypothermia** in any drowning incident; use a low-reading thermometer.

A **tension pneumothorax** may be the primary cause of PEA and may follow attempts at central venous catheter insertion. Decompress rapidly by needle thoracocentesis or urgent thoracostomy, and then insert a chest drain.

Cardiac **tamponade** is difficult to diagnose because the typical signs of distended neck veins and hypotension are obscured by the arrest itself. Rapid transthoracic echocardiography with minimal interruption to chest compression can be used to identify a pericardial

effusion. Cardiac arrest after penetrating chest trauma is highly suggestive of tamponade and is an indication for resuscitative thoracotomy.

In the absence of a specific history, the accidental or deliberate ingestion of therapeutic or **toxic** substances may be revealed only by laboratory investigations. Where available, the appropriate antidotes should be used, but most often treatment is supportive.

The commonest cause of **thromboembolic** or mechanical circulatory obstruction is massive pulmonary embolus. If cardiac arrest is likely to be caused by pulmonary embolism, consider giving a fibrinolytic drug immediately. Ongoing CPR is not a contraindication to fibrinolysis. Fibrinolytic drugs may take up to 90 min to be effective; give a fibrinolytic drug only if it is appropriate to continue CPR for this duration.

Use of Ultrasound Imaging During Advanced Life Support. Several studies have examined the use of ultrasound during cardiac arrest to detect potentially reversible causes. This imaging provides information that may help to identify reversible causes of cardiac arrest (e.g. cardiac tamponade, pulmonary embolism, ischaemia (regional wall motion abnormality), aortic dissection, hypovolaemia, pneumothorax). When ultrasound imaging and appropriately trained clinicians are available, use them to assist with assessment and treatment of potentially reversible causes of cardiac arrest. The integration of ultrasound into advanced life support requires considerable training to ensure that interruptions to chest compressions are minimized. A sub-xiphoid probe position has been recommended. Placement of the probe just before chest compressions are paused for a planned rhythm assessment enables a well-trained operator to obtain views within 10 seconds.

Resuscitation in the Operating Room

Patients in the operating room are normally monitored fully and there should be little delay in diagnosing cardiac arrest. High-risk patients will often have invasive arterial pressure monitoring, which is invaluable in the event of cardiac arrest. If cardiac arrest is considered a strong possibility, apply self-adhesive defibrillation patches before induction of anaesthesia.

Asystole and VF will be detected immediately but the onset of PEA might not be so obvious – loss of the pulse oximeter signal and end-tidal CO_2 are good

---

TABLE 47.1
Reversible Causes of Cardiac Arrest

- Hypoxia

- Hypovolaemia

- Hyperkalaemia, hypokalaemia, hypocalcaemia, acidaemia, and other metabolic disorders

- Hypothermia

- Tension pneumothorax

- Tamponade

- Toxic substances

- Thromboembolism (pulmonary embolus/coronary thrombosis)

clues and should provoke a pulse check. If asystole occurs intraoperatively, stop any surgical activity likely to be causing excessive vagal activity – if this is the likely cause, give 0.5 mg atropine. Start CPR and immediately look for other reversible causes. The atropine dose can be repeated up to a total of 3 mg. A completely straight line suggests that a monitoring lead has become detached.

In the case of PEA, start CPR while looking quickly for reversible causes. Give fluid unless you are certain the intravascular volume is adequate. Stop giving the anaesthetic. While a vasopressor will be required, in these circumstances 1 mg of adrenaline may be excessive. Give a much smaller dose of adrenaline (e.g. 50–100 μg) or another vasopressor (e.g. metaraminol) initially; if this fails to restore the cardiac output, increase the dose.

Cardiac Arrest in the Prone Position

Cardiac arrest in the prone position is rare but challenging. The risk factors may include cardiac abnormalities in patients undergoing major spinal surgery, hypovolaemia, air embolism, wound irrigation with hydrogen peroxide, poor positioning and occluded venous return. Consider applying self-adhesive defibrillation patches preoperatively to patients deemed at high risk from cardiac arrest. Chest compression in the prone position can be achieved with or without sternal counter-pressure.

Cardiac Arrest Caused by Local Anaesthetic

Systemic toxicity of local anaesthetics involves the central nervous system and the cardiovascular system and occurs when a bolus of local anaesthetic inadvertently enters the circulation, usually during regional anaesthesia. Severe agitation, loss of consciousness, with or without convulsions, sinus bradycardia, conduction blocks, asystole and ventricular tachyarrhythmias can all occur. Patients with cardiovascular collapse or cardiac arrest attributable to local anaesthetic toxicity should be treated with i.v. 20% lipid emulsion in addition to standard ALS. Guidelines for treatment with lipid emulsion have been produced by the Association of Anaesthetists of Great Britain and Ireland (www. aagbi.org): give an initial i.v. bolus of 20% lipid emulsion followed by an infusion at 15 mL kg^{-1} h^{-1}; give up to three bolus doses of lipid at 5-minute intervals

and continue the infusion until the patient is stable or has received up to a maximum of 12 mL kg^{-1} of lipid emulsion.

Airway Management and Ventilation

There are no data supporting the routine use of any specific approach to airway management during cardiac arrest. The best technique depends on the precise circumstances of the cardiac arrest and the competence of the rescuer. During CPR with an unprotected airway, two ventilations are given after each sequence of 30 chest compressions. Once a tracheal tube or supraglottic airway device (SAD) has been inserted, the lungs are ventilated at a rate of about 10 breaths min^{-1} and chest compressions continued without pausing during ventilation.

Several alternative airway devices have been considered for airway management during CPR for those not skilled in tracheal intubation or when attempted intubation fails. There are published studies on the use during CPR of the Combitube, the classic laryngeal mask airway (cLMA), the Laryngeal Tube (LT) and the i-gel, but none of these studies have been powered adequately to enable survival to be studied as a primary endpoint. Currently, the choice of these devices depends entirely on local preference.

Tracheal intubation should be attempted during cardiac arrest only by trained personnel, such as anaesthetists, who are able to carry out the procedure with a high level of skill and confidence. Prolonged attempts at tracheal intubation are harmful; the pause in chest compressions during this time will compromise coronary and cerebral perfusion. No intubation attempt should interrupt chest compressions for more than 10 seconds; if intubation is not achievable within these constraints, bag-mask ventilation is restarted.

Waveform capnography is the most sensitive and specific way to confirm and continuously monitor the position of a tracheal tube in victims of cardiac arrest and should supplement clinical assessment (auscultation and visualization of the tracheal tube passing between the vocal cords). There is concern that low pulmonary blood flow during CPR may not result in detectable exhaled carbon dioxide and that a correctly placed tracheal tube may then be removed in error. However, several studies have indicated that exhaled carbon dioxide is detected reliably during CPR, except after prolonged cardiac arrest (>30 min) when pulmonary flow may be negligible. Existing portable monitors make capnographic initial confirmation and continuous monitoring of tracheal tube position feasible in almost all settings where intubation is performed, including out of hospital, emergency departments, and in-hospital locations.

Assisting the Circulation

Intravascular Access

Peripheral venous cannulation is quicker, easier to perform, and safer than attempting central venous access. Drugs injected peripherally must be followed by a flush of at least 20 mL of fluid. Any attempt at central venous line insertion must be achieved with minimal interruption to chest compressions. If i.v. access cannot be established within the first 2 min of resuscitation, consider gaining intraosseous (IO) access. Intraosseous delivery of resuscitation drugs will achieve adequate plasma concentrations.

Resuscitation drugs can also be given via a tracheal tube, but the plasma concentrations achieved using this route are very variable and generally considerably lower than those achieved by the i.v. or IO routes, particularly with adrenaline. Given the ease of gaining IO access and the lack of efficacy of tracheal drug administration, do not give drugs via the tracheal tube.

Drugs

Adrenaline. Despite the widespread use of adrenaline during resuscitation, and several studies involving vasopressin, there is no placebo-controlled study that shows that the routine use of any vasopressor at any stage during human cardiac arrest increases neurologically-intact survival to hospital discharge. A recent prospective, randomized trial of adrenaline versus placebo for out-of-hospital cardiac arrest has documented higher rates of ROSC with adrenaline for both shockable and non-shockable rhythms. The optimal dose of adrenaline is not known, and there are no data supporting the use of repeated doses. There are few data on the pharmacokinetics of adrenaline during CPR. The optimal duration of CPR and number of shocks that should be given before giving drugs is unknown. On the basis of expert consensus, for VF/VT, adrenaline is given after the third shock once chest compressions have resumed, and then repeated every 3–5 min during cardiac arrest (alternate cycles).

Atropine. Several recent studies have failed to demonstrate any benefit from atropine in out-of-hospital or in-hospital cardiac arrests and its routine use for asystole or PEA is no longer recommended.

Anti-Arrhythmic Drugs. No anti-arrhythmic drug given during human cardiac arrest has been shown to increase survival to hospital discharge, although amiodarone has been shown to increase survival to hospital admission after shock-refractory VF/VT. Based on expert consensus, give amiodarone 300 mg by bolus injection (flushed with 20 mL of 0.9% sodium chloride or 5% dextrose) after the third shock. A further dose of 150 mg may be given for recurrent or refractory VF/VT, followed by an infusion of 900 mg over 24 h. Lidocaine 1 mg kg^{-1} may be used as an alternative if amiodarone is not available, but do not give lidocaine if amiodarone has been given already.

Although the benefits of giving magnesium in known hypomagnesaemic states are recognized, the benefit of giving magnesium routinely during cardiac arrest is unproven. Give an initial i.v. dose of 2 g (= 8 mmol or 4 mL of 50% magnesium sulphate) for refractory VF if there is any suspicion of hypomagnesaemia (e.g. patients on potassium-losing diuretics); it may be repeated after 10–15 min. Other indications are: ventricular tachyarrhythmias in the presence of possible hypomagnesaemia; torsade de pointes VT; digoxin toxicity.

Bicarbonate. Cardiac arrest causes a combined respiratory and metabolic acidosis because pulmonary gas exchange ceases and cellular metabolism becomes anaerobic. The best treatment of acidaemia in cardiac arrest is chest compression; some additional benefit is gained by ventilation. During cardiac arrest, arterial blood gas values may be misleading and bear little relationship to the tissue acid–base state – analysis of central venous blood may provide a better estimation of tissue pH. Giving sodium bicarbonate routinely during cardiac arrest and CPR, or after ROSC, is not recommended. Give sodium bicarbonate 50 mmol if cardiac arrest is associated with hyperkalaemia or tricyclic antidepressant overdose. Repeat the dose according to the clinical condition of the patient and the results of repeated blood gas analysis.

Calcium. There are no data supporting any beneficial action for calcium after most cases of cardiac arrest. High plasma concentrations achieved after injection may be harmful to the ischaemic myocardium and may impair cerebral recovery. Give calcium during resuscitation only when indicated specifically (cardiac arrest caused by hyperkalaemia, hypocalcaemia, or overdose of calcium channel blocking drugs).

Mechanical CPR

At best, standard manual CPR produces coronary and cerebral perfusion that is just 30% of normal. Several CPR techniques and devices may improve haemodynamics or short-term survival when used by well-trained providers in selected cases. However, the success of any technique or device depends on the education and training of the rescuers and on resources (including personnel).

Impedance Threshold Device (ITD). The impedance threshold device (ITD) is a valve that limits air entry into the lungs as the chest recoils during the compression release phase; this decreases intrathoracic pressure and increases venous return to the heart. Recent prospective randomized trials indicate no difference in long term outcome when the ITD is used with standard CPR but one study has documented higher long-term survival rates compared with standard CPR when the ITD is combined with active compression–decompression (ACD) CPR.

Lund University Cardiac Arrest System (LUCAS) CPR. The Lund University cardiac arrest system (LUCAS) is a gas-driven sternal compression device that incorporates a suction cup for ACD-CPR. There are no published randomized human studies comparing LUCAS-CPR with standard CPR although there are two large on-going prehospital studies.

Load-Distributing Band CPR (AutoPulse). The load-distributing band (LDB) is a circumferential chest compression device comprising a pneumatically actu-ated constricting band and backboard. A recent large prehospital randomized trial has shown that LDB-CPR produces similar survival rates to that of high-quality manual CPR.

Mechanical devices have been used to support patients undergoing primary coronary intervention (PCI) and for prolonged resuscitation attempts where rescuer fatigue may impair the effectiveness of manual chest compression.

PERI-ARREST ARRHYTHMIAS

Cardiac arrhythmias are common in the peri-arrest period and treatment algorithms for both tachycardia (Fig. 47.4) and bradycardia (Fig. 47.5) have been de-veloped to enable the non-specialist to initiate treat-ment safely. In all cases, oxygen is given, an i.v. cannula is inserted and the patient is assessed for adverse signs. Whenever possible, record a 12-lead ECG; this will help determine the precise rhythm, either before treat-ment or retrospectively, if necessary with the help of an expert. Correct any electrolyte abnormalities.

The presence or absence of adverse signs or symp-toms will dictate the appropriate treatment for most arrhythmias. The after adverse factors indicate that a patient is unstable because of the arrhythmia:

- Shock – pallor, sweating, cold, clammy extremi-ties, impaired consciousness and hypotension (e.g. systolic blood pressure <90 mmHg).
- Syncope – transient loss of consciousness.
- Heart failure – pulmonary oedema; 3rd heart sound; raised JVP; hepatic congestion; peripheral oedema.
- Myocardial ischaemia – chest pain or evidence of ischaemia on 12-lead ECG.

Depending on the nature of the underlying ar-rhythmia and clinical status of the patient, immedi-ate treatments can be either electrical [cardioversion (tachyarrhythmias) or pacing (bradyarrhythmias)] or pharmacological. If the patient has adverse factors electrical therapy is likely to be appropriate. Drugs usually act more slowly and less reliably than electrical treatments and are usually the preferred treatment for the stable patient without adverse signs.

Tachycardias

If the patient is unstable and deteriorating, synchro-nized cardioversion is the treatment of choice. In pa-tients with otherwise normal hearts, serious signs and symptoms are uncommon if the ventricular rate is <150 min⁻¹. For a broad-complex tachycardia or atrial fibrillation, start with 120–150 J biphasic shock and

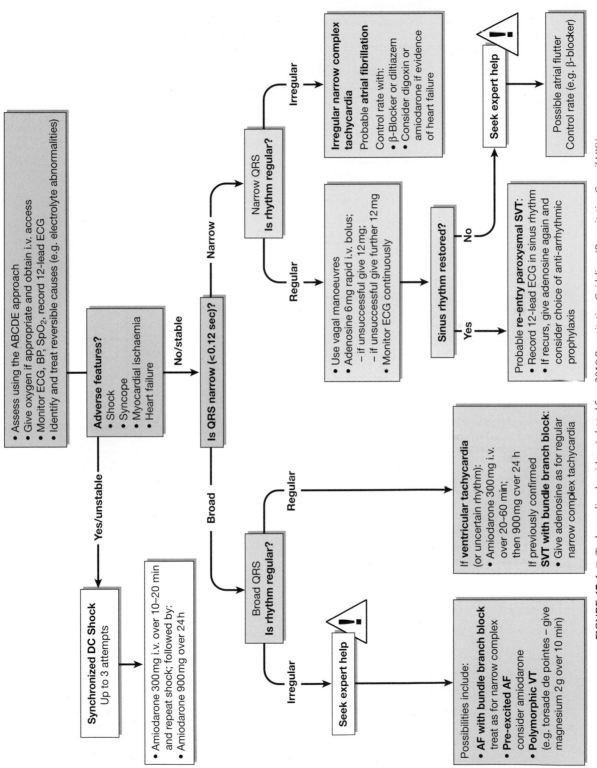

FIGURE 47.4 ■ Tachycardia algorithm *(adapted from 2010 Resuscitation Guidelines (Resuscitation Council UK))*.

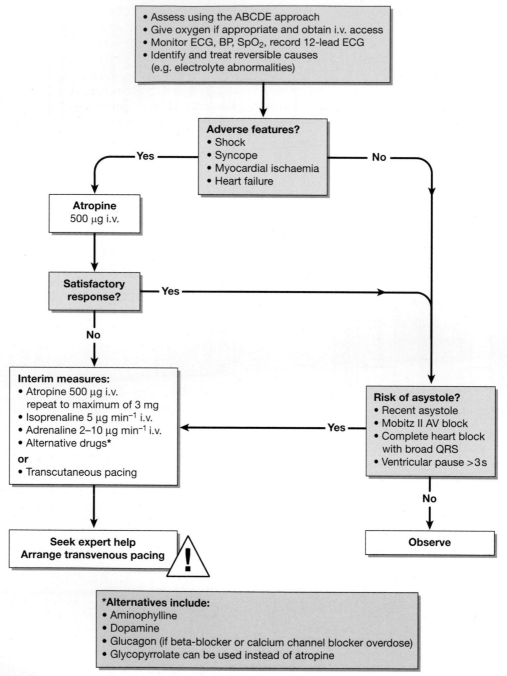

FIGURE 47.5 ▪ Bradycardia algorithm *(adapted from 2010 Resuscitation Guidelines (Resuscitation Council UK))*.

increase in increments if this fails. Atrial flutter and regular narrow-complex tachycardia will often convert with lower energies: start with 70–120 J biphasic. If cardioversion fails to restore sinus rhythm, and the patient remains unstable, give amiodarone 300 mg i.v. over 10–20 min and re-attempt electrical cardioversion. The loading dose of amiodarone can be followed by an infusion of 900 mg over 24 hours.

The treatment for stable tachycardias is outlined in Figure 47.4. A regular broad-complex tachycardia is likely to be VT or a supraventricular rhythm with bundle branch block. In a stable patient, if there is uncertainty about the source of the arrhythmia, give adenosine.

Regular narrow-complex tachycardias include:

- sinus tachycardia;
- AV nodal re-entry tachycardia (AVNRT) – the commonest type of regular narrow-complex tachyarrhythmia;
- AV re-entry tachycardia (AVRT) – due to Wolff–Parkinson–White (WPW) syndrome;
- atrial flutter with regular AV conduction (usually 2:1).

Vagal manoeuvres or adenosine will terminate almost all AVNRT or AVRT within seconds. Failure to terminate a regular narrow-complex tachycardia with adenosine suggests an atrial tachycardia such as atrial flutter. If adenosine is contraindicated, or fails to terminate a regular narrow complex tachycardia without demonstrating that it is atrial flutter, give a calcium-channel blocker, for example verapamil 2.5–5 mg i.v. over 2 min or diltiazem.

An irregular narrow-complex tachycardia is most likely to be AF or sometimes atrial flutter with variable AV conduction. If there are no adverse features, treatment options include:

- rate control by drug therapy;
- rhythm control using drugs to encourage chemical cardioversion;
- rhythm control by electrical cardioversion;
- treatment to prevent complications (e.g. anticoagulation).

In general, patients who have been in AF for more than 48 h should not be treated by cardioversion (electrical or chemical) until they have been fully anticoagulated for at least three weeks, or unless trans-oesophageal echocardiography has shown the absence of atrial thrombus. If cardioversion is required more urgently, give an i.v. bolus injection of heparin followed by a continuous infusion to maintain the activated partial thromboplastin time (APTT) at 1.5 to 2 times the reference control value.

If the aim is to control heart rate, the drugs of choice are beta-blockers, diltiazem (oral only in the UK), or verapamil. Digoxin and amiodarone may be used in patients with heart failure. Magnesium can also been used although the data supporting this are more limited.

If the duration of AF is less than 48 h and rhythm control is considered appropriate, electrical or chemical cardioversion may be attempted. Seek expert help and consider flecainide. Amiodarone may also be used but is less effective.

Bradycardia

If adverse signs are present, give i.v. atropine 500 µg, and, if necessary, repeat every 3–5 min to a total of 3 mg. In the intraoperative setting, stop any surgical activity likely to be causing vagal stimulation.

If treatment with atropine is ineffective, consider second line drugs. These include isoprenaline (5 µg min^{-1} starting dose), adrenaline (2–10 µg min^{-1}) and dopamine (2–10 µg kg^{-1} min^{-1}).

Transcutaneous pacing will be required if there is an inadequate response to drugs. Temporary transvenous pacing should be considered if there is a history of recent asystole; Mobitz type II AV block; complete (third-degree) heart block (especially with broad QRS or initial heart rate <40 min^{-1}) or evidence of ventricular standstill of more than 3 seconds.

POST-RESUSCITATION CARE

The Post-Cardiac-Arrest Syndrome

The post-cardiac-arrest syndrome, which comprises post-cardiac-arrest brain injury, post-cardiac-arrest myocardial dysfunction, the systemic ischaemia/reperfusion response, and persistence of the precipitating pathology, often complicates the post-resuscitation phase. Post-cardiac-arrest brain injury manifests as coma, seizures, varying degrees of neurocognitive dysfunction and brain death. Post-cardiac-arrest brain injury may be exacerbated by microcirculatory failure, impaired autoregulation, hypercarbia, hyperoxia, pyrexia, hyperglycaemia and seizures. Significant myocardial dysfunction is common after cardiac arrest but typically recovers by 2–3 days. The whole body ischaemia/reperfusion that occurs with resuscitation from cardiac arrest activates immunological and coagulation pathways contributing to multiple organ failure and increasing the risk of infection. Thus, the post-cardiac-arrest syndrome has many features in common with sepsis, including intravascular volume depletion and vasodilation.

Airway and Breathing

Hypoxaemia and hypercarbia both increase the likelihood of a further cardiac arrest and may contribute to secondary brain injury. Several animal studies indicate that hyperoxaemia causes oxidative stress and harms post-ischaemic neurones. A clinical registry study documented that post-resuscitation hyperoxaemia was associated with worse outcome, compared with both normoxaemia and hypoxaemia. As soon as arterial blood oxygen saturation can be monitored reliably (by blood gas analysis and/or pulse oximetry), titrate the inspired oxygen concentration to maintain the arterial blood oxygen saturation in the range of 94–98%. Consider tracheal intubation, sedation and controlled ventilation in any patient with obtunded cerebral function. There are no data to support the targeting of a specific arterial $P\text{co}_2$ after resuscitation from cardiac arrest, but it is reasonable to adjust ventilation to achieve normocarbia and to monitor this using the end-tidal $P\text{co}_2$ and arterial blood gas values.

Circulation

Post-cardiac-arrest patients with ST-elevation myocardial infarction (STEMI) should undergo early coronary angiography and percutaneous coronary intervention (PCI). Post-cardiac arrest myocardial dysfunction causes haemodynamic instability, resulting in hypotension, low cardiac index and arrhythmias. If treatment with appropriate fluids and vasoactive drugs is insufficient to support the circulation, an intra-aortic balloon pump may be required. Target the mean arterial blood pressure to achieve an adequate urine output ($1\,\text{mL}\,\text{kg}^{-1}\,\text{h}^{-1}$) and normal or decreasing plasma lactate values, taking into consideration the patient's usual blood pressure (if known).

Disability (Optimizing Neurological Recovery)

Control of Seizures

Seizures occur in 24% of those who remain comatose after out-of-hospital cardiac arrest. Seizures increase cerebral metabolism by up to 3-fold and may cause cerebral injury: treat promptly and effectively with anticonvulsant drugs. Although associated with a poor outcome, the occurrence of seizures does not predict this reliably – in one recent study, 17% of those with seizures ultimately had a good neurological outcome.

Glucose Control

There is a strong association between high blood glucose after resuscitation from cardiac arrest and poor neurological outcome but attempts to control glucose too tightly ($4.5–6.0\,\text{mmol}\,\text{L}^{-1}$) increases the risk of hypoglycaemia and in one large study of general ICU patients increased mortality when compared with conventional glucose control ($\leq 10\,\text{mmol}\,\text{L}^{-1}$). Therefore, after ROSC, maintain blood glucose at $\leq 10\,\text{mmol}\,\text{L}^{-1}$ and avoid hypoglycaemia.

Temperature Control

Treatment of Hyperpyrexia. A period of hyperthermia (hyperpyrexia) is common in the first 48 h after cardiac arrest and this is associated with worse neurological outcome. Treat hyperthermia occurring after cardiac arrest with antipyretics or active cooling.

Therapeutic Hypothermia. Animal and human data indicate that mild hypothermia is neuroprotective and improves outcome after a period of global cerebral hypoxia-ischaemia. Cooling suppresses many of the pathways leading to delayed cell death, including apoptosis (programmed cell death). Hypothermia decreases the cerebral metabolic rate for oxygen by about 6% for each 1 °C reduction in temperature and this may reduce the release of excitatory amino acids and free radicals.

All studies of post-cardiac-arrest therapeutic hypothermia have included only patients in coma. There is good evidence supporting the use of induced hypothermia in comatose survivors of out-of-hospital cardiac arrest caused by VF and there is lower level evidence supporting cooling after cardiac arrest from non-shockable rhythms and after in-hospital cardiac arrest. Cooling should be started as soon as possible after ROSC (pre-ROSC cooling is being investigated) with the aim of maintaining temperature in the range of 32–34 °C for 24 h.

The practical application of therapeutic hypothermia is divided into three phases: induction, maintenance, and rewarming. External and/or internal cooling techniques can be used to initiate cooling. An infusion of 30 mL kg^{-1} of 4 °C 0.9% sodium chloride or Hartmann's solution decreases core temperature by approximately 1.5 °C and can easily be started prehospital. Other methods of inducing and/or maintaining hypothermia include: simple ice packs and/or wet towels; cooling blankets or pads; intranasal cooling; water or air circulating blankets; water circulating gel-coated pads; intravascular heat exchanger; and cardiopulmonary bypass.

In the maintenance phase, a cooling method with effective temperature monitoring that avoids temperature fluctuations is preferred. This is best achieved with external or internal cooling devices that include continuous temperature feedback to achieve a set target temperature. Plasma electrolyte concentrations, effective intravascular volume and metabolic rate can change rapidly during both cooling and rewarming. Control rewarming at 0.25–0.5 °C per hour.

Prognostication

Two thirds of those dying after admission to ICU after out-of-hospital cardiac arrest die from neurological injury. A quarter of those dying after admission to ICU after in-hospital cardiac arrest die from neurological injury. A means of predicting neurological outcome that can be applied to individual comatose patients is required. Many studies have focused on prediction of poor long term outcome (vegetative state or death), based on clinical or test findings that indicate irreversible brain injury, to enable clinicians to limit care or withdraw organ support. The implications of these prognostic tests are such that they should have 100% specificity or zero false positive rate, i.e. no individuals eventually have a 'good' long-term outcome despite the prediction of a poor outcome.

Clinical Examination

There are no clinical neurological signs that predict poor outcome (Cerebral Performance Category [CPC] 3 or 4, or death) reliably less than 24 hours after cardiac arrest. In adult patients who are comatose after cardiac arrest, and who have not been treated with hypothermia and who do not have confounding factors (such as hypotension, sedatives or muscle relaxants), the absence of both pupillary light and corneal reflex at ≥72 hours predicts poor outcome reliably. A GCS motor score of 2 or less at ≥72 hours is less reliable. The presence of myoclonic status is associated strongly with poor outcome but rare cases of good neurological recovery from this situation have been described and accurate diagnosis is problematic.

Biochemical Markers

Serum (e.g. neuronal specific enolase, S100 protein) or cerebrospinal fluid (CSF) biomarkers alone are insufficient as predictors of poor outcomes in comatose patients after cardiac arrest with or without treatment with therapeutic hypothermia.

Neurophysiological Studies

No neurophysiological study predicts outcome for a comatose patient reliably within the first 24 hours after cardiac arrest. If somatosensory evoked potentials (SSEP) are measured after 24 hours in comatose cardiac arrest survivors not treated with therapeutic hypothermia, bilateral absence of the N20 cortical response to median nerve stimulation predicts poor outcome (death or CPC 3 or 4). However, few hospitals in the UK have the resources to enable SSEPs to be measured.

Imaging Studies

Many imaging modalities (magnetic resonance imaging [MRI], computed tomography [CT], single photon emission computed tomography [SPECT], cerebral angiography, transcranial Doppler, nuclear medicine, near infra-red spectroscopy [NIRS]) have been studied to determine their utility for prediction of outcome in adult survivors of cardiac arrest. There are no high-level studies that support the use of any imaging modality to predict outcome of comatose cardiac arrest survivors.

Impact of Therapeutic Hypothermia on Prognostication

There is inadequate evidence to recommend a specific approach to prognosticating poor outcome in post-cardiac-arrest patients treated with therapeutic hypothermia. There are no clinical neurological signs, neurophysiological studies, biomarkers, or imaging modalities that can predict neurological outcome reliably in the first 24 h after cardiac arrest. Potentially reliable prognosticators of poor outcome in patients treated with therapeutic hypothermia after cardiac arrest include bilateral absence of N20 peak on SSEP $\geq$24 h after cardiac arrest and the absence of both corneal and pupillary reflexes three or more days after cardiac arrest. Given the limited data, decisions to limit care should be based on the results of more than one prognostication tool (e.g. clinical examination and EEG). In most cases, treatment withdrawal decisions should be delayed until at least 3 days after return to normothermia.

Organ Donation

Post-cardiac-arrest patients who do not survive represent an opportunity to increase the organ donor pool, either after brain death or as non-heart-beating donors.

DECISIONS RELATING TO CARDIOPULMONARY RESUSCITATION

It is essential to identify patients for whom cardiopulmonary arrest represents an anticipated terminal event and in whom CPR is inappropriate. All institutions should ensure that a clear and explicit resuscitation plan exists for all patients. For some patients this will involve a do-not-attempt-resuscitation (DNAR, also described as DNACPR) decision. National guidelines from the British Medical Association (BMA), Resuscitation Council (UK) and the Royal College of Nursing (RCN), and more recently from the General Medical Council, provide a framework for formulating local policy. The main messages from the BMA/RC(UK)/RCN guidance are:

■ Decisions about CPR must be made on the basis of an *individual* assessment of each patient's case.
■ Advance care planning, including making decisions about CPR, is an important part of good clinical care for those at risk of cardiorespiratory arrest.

■ Communication and the provision of information are essential parts of good quality care.
■ It is not necessary to initiate discussion about CPR with a patient if there is no reason to believe that the patient is likely to suffer a cardiorespiratory arrest.
■ Where no explicit decision has been made in advance there should be an initial presumption in favour of CPR.
■ If CPR would not restart the heart and breathing, it should not be attempted.
■ Where the expected benefit of attempted CPR may be outweighed by the burdens, the patient's informed views are of paramount importance. If the patient lacks capacity, those close to the patient should be involved in discussions to explore the patient's wishes, feelings, beliefs and values.
■ If a patient with capacity refuses CPR, or a patient lacking capacity has a valid and applicable advance decision refusing CPR, this should be respected.
■ A DNAR decision does not override clinical judgement in the unlikely event of a reversible cause of the patient's respiratory or cardiac arrest that does not match the circumstances envisaged.
■ DNAR decisions apply only to CPR and not to any other aspects of treatment.

DNAR Decisions in the Perioperative Period

General or regional anaesthesia may cause cardiovascular or respiratory instability that requires supportive treatment. Many routine interventions used during anaesthesia (for example tracheal intubation, mechanical ventilation or injection of vasoactive drugs) could be considered to be resuscitative measures. The AAGBI has produced guidance for managing DNAR decisions in the perioperative period. The anaesthetist and the surgeon should review DNAR decisions with the patient, or their representative if they lack capacity, as part of the consent process. The DNAR decision can be suspended, modified, or remain valid during the procedure. The DNAR management option would normally apply while the patient remains in the operating room and post anaesthetic care unit.

NATIONAL CARDIAC ARREST AUDIT

All in-hospital cardiac arrests should be reviewed and audited. NCAA is a UK-wide database of in-hospital cardiac arrests and is supported by the RC (UK) and the Intensive Care National Audit & Research Centre (ICNARC). NCAA monitors and reports on the incidence of, and outcome from, in-hospital cardiac arrests in order to inform practice and policy. It aims to improve care delivery and outcomes from cardiac arrest.

ACKNOWLEDGEMENT

Much of this chapter has been adapted, with permission, from the 2010 Resuscitation Council (UK) Guidelines (www.resus.org.uk).

FURTHER READING

Association of Anaesthetists of Great Britain & Ireland, Do not attempt resuscitation (DNAR) decisions in the perioperative period. Available at http://www.aagbi.org/sites/default/files/dnar_09_0.pdf.

British Medical Association, Resuscitation Council (UK) and Royal College of Nursing, 2007. Decisions relating to cardiopulmonary resuscitation. www.resus.org.uk.

Deakin, C.D., Morrison, L.J., Morley, P.T., et al., 2010. Advanced life support chapter collaborators. Part 8. Advanced life support. International consensus on cardiopulmonary resuscitation and emergency cardiovascular care science with treatment recommendations. Resuscitation 81 (Suppl. 1), e93–e174.

Deakin, C.D., Nolan, J.P., Soar, J., et al., 2010. European resuscitation council guidelines for resuscitation 2010 Section 4. Adult advanced life support. Resuscitation 81, 1305–1352.

General Medical Council, 2010. Treatment and care towards the end of life: good practice in decision making. General Medical Council, London, ISBN 978-0-901458-46-9. www.gmc-uk.org.

Nolan, J., Soar, J., Lockey, A., et al., 2011. Advanced life support, sixth ed. Resuscitation Council UK, London, ISBN 978-1-903812-22-8.

Nolan, J.P., 2010. In: Resuscitation guidelines, 2010. Resuscitation Council (UK), London, ISBN 978-1-903812-21-1. www.resus.org.uk.

Nolan, J.P., Hazinski, M.F., Billi, J.E., et al., 2010. Part 1. Executive summary. International consensus on cardiopulmonary resuscitation and emergency cardiovascular care science with treatment recommendations. Resuscitation 81 (Suppl. 1), e1–e25.

Nolan, J.P., Neumar, R.W., Adrie, C., et al., 2008. Post–cardiac arrest syndrome. Epidemiology, pathophysiology, treatment, and prognostication. A consensus statement from the International Liaison Committee on Resuscitation; the American Heart Association Emergency Cardiovascular Care Committee; the Council on Cardiovascular Surgery and Anesthesia; the Council on Cardiopulmonary, Perioperative, and Critical Care; the Council on Clinical Cardiology; and the Stroke Council. Resuscitation 79, 350–379.

Nolan, J.P., Soar, J., Zideman, D.A., et al., 2010. Guidelines writing group. European Resuscitation Council Guidelines for Resuscitation 2010 Section 1. Executive summary. Resuscitation 81, 1219–1276.

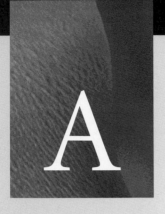

TRAINING AND ASSESSMENT
IN ANAESTHESIA

INTRODUCTION

If you have recently acquired this textbook, you are probably just embarking on a career in anaesthesia. At the outset, this can appear to be a daunting prospect with an apparently overwhelming amount of new knowledge and skills to acquire within a relatively short time-frame. An understanding of the framework of the training scheme, the curriculum which you will follow and the assessment tools (including examinations) against which your progress will be measured will allow you to approach training in your chosen speciality with greater confidence.

This short chapter is designed to illustrate some of the key aspects of postgraduate training and assessment in anaesthesia taking examples from the UK, Irish and Australasian systems. However, the themes discussed will be just as applicable to those training in other healthcare jurisdictions.

BASIC PRINCIPLES

Anaesthesia is a wide-ranging speciality encompassing perioperative management, critical care and pain medicine. Potentially, the anaesthetist has to manage patients of all ages, ranging from the most premature neonate to centenarians. Patients require a diverse range of surgical interventions and can have significant comorbidities which may have implications for the delivery of safe anaesthetic care. Consequently, the anaesthetist needs to have a very broad medical knowledge base, perhaps more so than in any other hospital-based clinical speciality. This knowledge base needs to encompass the basic sciences which

underpin all aspects of anaesthetic practice, general medicine and surgery, and other allied clinical specialities (e.g. radiology), in addition to the specific knowledge and skills related directly to anaesthetic practice.

As well as clinical knowledge and skills, all anaesthetists need to develop the appropriate professional attitudes and behavioural skills which are essential to maintaining good medical practice. Some of these are generic skills which are relevant to any doctor but others are speciality-specific. These affective competencies do not relate to any particular stage of training but should be developed during the training years and continue to be consolidated throughout the doctor's professional life. In the UK training system, these competencies are summarized in 11 domains in a separate annexe of the anaesthetics curriculum document (Table A.1).

Spiral Learning

All anaesthetic training programmes are based on the concept of ensuring that basic principles learnt and understood are repeated, expanded and further elucidated as time in training progresses. To facilitate this approach in most healthcare systems, the training programme is divided into various stages – in the UK system, these are defined as the basic, intermediate, higher and advanced levels of training. The outcome is such that competence within the speciality required to commence independent practice is achieved by the end of training as knowledge, skills, attitudes and behaviours metaphorically spiral upwards.

TABLE A.1

Professionalism and Common Competencies in Medical Practice (from Royal College of Anaesthetists' Certificate of Completion of Training in Anaesthetics 2010, with Permission)

Domain 1: Professional attitudes

- *Commitment*
- *Compassion*
- *Honesty & personal integrity*
- *Respect for others*
- *Community*
- *Competence*

Domain 2: Clinical practice

Domain 3: Team working

Domain 4: Leadership

Domain 5: Innovation

Domain 6: Healthcare management

Domain 7: Education

Domain 8: Safety in clinical practice

Domain 9: Medical ethics and confidentiality

Domain 10: Relationships with patients

Domain 11: Legal framework for practice

Domain 12: Information technology

TABLE A.2

Basis of Anaesthetic Practice Module (from Royal College of Anaesthetists' Curriculum in Anaesthetics 2010, with Permission)

- Preoperative assessment
- Premedication
- Induction
- Intraoperative care
- Postoperative and recovery room care
- Management of cardiorespiratory arrest
- Control of infection
- Introduction to anaesthesia for emergency surgery

Experiential Learning

Research has shown that performance of any skill improves with practice and that up to 200 iterations of a procedure may be required for a learner to approach the standard of performance demonstrated by a truly expert practitioner. Analyses of learning curves reveal that 70–80% of this level of expert performance is achieved after 30 iterations of a skill. In any training system of limited duration, it is unlikely that trainees will achieve mastery in all aspects of anaesthetic practice. Realistically, an anaesthetist can only be regarded as competent in the full range of anaesthetic practice by the end of training and only approach truly expert level of performance in one or two subspecialties at most before becoming a consultant or accredited specialist.

Phases of Training

Although varying in some detail and duration of the component parts, most anaesthetic training systems have similar key phases.

Introduction to Anaesthetic Practice. Doctors come to anaesthetic training with a range of previous medical experience, but for all, there is a steep learning curve to grasp the basic principles of safe anaesthetic practice. This initial phase of training is necessarily heavily supervised and, depending on the individual's aptitude, takes 3–6 months before the trainee is able to work without direct supervision and undertake on-call duties. In the UK system, the anaesthetic curriculum includes a 'basis of anaesthetic practice' module which is designed to guide the trainee through these first few months of training and ensure that they are all introduced in a systematic way to the fundamental concepts sustaining safe practice (Table A.2). Trainees are required to successfully complete all the constituent units of training in this module to progress further in training.

Modular Training. Anaesthetic training both in the UK and Ireland, and elsewhere (e.g. Australasia), is organized on a modular system with trainees focusing on defined areas of anaesthetic practice at different stages of the training programme (Fig. A.1). For some modules, this may require concentrating on one specific area exclusively for an extended period in order to build up a momentum of experience. This is particularly important when being introduced to a new area of practice, e.g. intensive care, pain medicine, paediatric anaesthesia.

There are several subspeciality disciplines in anaesthesia which are regarded as essential components of training in UK/Ireland and Australasia (Table A.3). In the early stages of training, these modules are typically

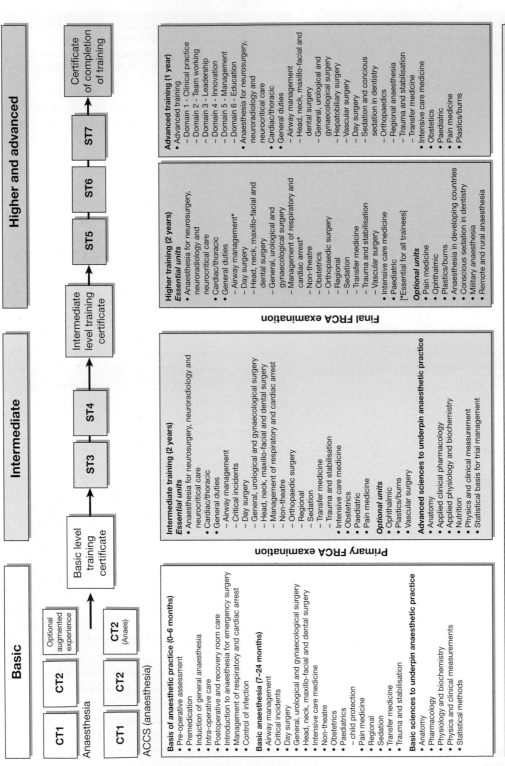

FIGURE A.1 ■ Royal College of Anaesthetists' Certificate of Completion of Training in Anaesthetics modular training programme (with permission).

TABLE A.3
Major Subspeciality Areas of Anaesthetic Practice

- Paediatric anaesthesia
- Obstetric anaesthesia and analgesia
- Pain medicine (acute and chronic)
- Intensive care medicine
- Anaesthesia for cardiac, thoracic and vascular surgery
- Anaesthesia for neurosurgery and neuroradiology

for 1–3 months, but trainees in the later stages of training may spend an extended period in their chosen subspeciality area of practice.

Subspeciality Training. A trainee who has gained experience of a broad range of anaesthetic practice in modular training may decide to focus on a subspeciality area of practice for an extended period (usually at least one year). This phase of training may be accommodated in the trainee's own training programme or, as is becoming increasingly popular, elsewhere in their home country or overseas. Although the essential units of training are the most common options for subspeciality training, other areas of practice including regional anaesthesia, trauma management and academic anaesthesia are also popular choices. It is important to emphasize that organizing subspeciality training outside the trainee's own training scheme (known as 'out of programme training' in the UK) is often a difficult and time-consuming process. It must be approved prospectively by the relevant training supervisors and regulators in the trainee's jurisdiction if the time spent is to be accredited for training purposes.

Less Than Full-Time ('Part-Time') Training. If appointed to a substantive training rotation, trainees in the UK/Ireland and Australasia may apply to train on a less than full-time (LTFT, or 'part-time') basis for the remainder or part of their training programme. However, the overall duration and quality of training must not be lower than that achieved by full-time trainees. The criteria which are accepted as being legitimate grounds to be considered for LTFT training vary among countries but it would be true to say that the most common reason is to accommodate domestic circumstances, particularly those relating to raising a family. All training programmes have an LTFT training

adviser who should be consulted prior to making an application to train on a part-time basis.

Training in Pain Medicine and Intensive Care Medicine

Training in both these major areas of practice is commonly accessed via anaesthesia as the parent speciality in UK/Ireland and Australasia. The duration of training and the assessments, including examinations, required to achieve specialist status successfully in these two areas of practice vary among countries.

Subspeciality training in intensive care medicine (ICM) in the UK is supervised by the Faculty of Intensive Care Medicine of the Royal College of Anaesthetists. All anaesthetists complete a minimum of six months' critical care experience during a standard five-year specialist registrar training programme. In addition, those with a greater commitment to critical care may opt to complete the following training requirements:

Intermediate level ICM training: 4–8 months (usually 6 months) in general adult intensive care medicine in addition to the basic anaesthetic ICM training requirements. Trainees must also complete 10 expanded case summaries as part of intermediate training. This level of training is designed to accommodate those trainees who may have a sessional or on-call commitment to ICM in consultant practice.

Advanced level ICM training: 8–18 months (normally 12 months) of training in ICM undertaken in the final two years of overall training. Up to 50% may be in a specialized ICM unit (e.g. cardiothoracic) and 50% may occur overseas (with prospective approval). This level of training is designed for those who intend a major, full-time commitment to ICM practice.

In addition, 4–8 months (normally 6 months) of speciality level training in acute general medicine is required for both levels of ICM training. Half of the requirement may be met through a suitable post in emergency medicine. A subspeciality examination in ICM is well established in Australasia; a UK Fellowship of the Faculty of Intensive Care Medicine (FFICM) examination was introduced in early 2013.

In the UK, subspeciality training in pain medicine requires a minimum of 12 months in training centres approved by the Faculty of Pain Medicine of the Royal College of Anaesthetists in addition to the basic anaesthetic pain medicine training requirements. A UK subspeciality examination in pain medicine, the Fellowship of the Faculty of Pain Medicine of the Royal College of Anaesthetists (FFPMRCA), began in 2012; subspeciality examinations in pain medicine are already well established in Ireland and Australasia.

ASSESSMENT TOOLS

The knowledge-based aspects of any curriculum are assessed by formal examinations such as the Fellowship of the Royal College of Anaesthetists (FRCA), Fellowship of the College of Anaesthetists of the Royal College of Surgeons of Ireland (FCARCSI) and the Fellowship of the Australian and New Zealand College of Anaesthetists (FANZCA). However, the cognitive, psychomotor and behavioural outcomes require a different set of assessment tools to gauge an individual trainee's competence and therefore progress in these aspects of the curriculum.

In the UK, workplace-based assessments (WPBA) have been developed in recent years to meet this need across all the training years (Table A.4). A similar suite of WPBAs is being developed and will be introduced into the ANZCA training programme. These are already familiar to most doctors who have completed their foundation training in the UK. In addition to the DOPs, A-CEX and CBD, the ALMAT and ACAT have been added, which are similar to tools used in other clinical specialities for the assessment of larger segments of clinical work. They have been adapted to allow the assessment of a whole operating list, pain clinic or ICM shift. A multi-source feedback (MSF), sometimes known as 360° appraisal, is also considered an important assessment tool. It provides a sample of

attitudes and opinions of colleagues (medical, nursing and non-clinical staff, e.g. departmental secretaries) on the clinical performance and professional behaviour of the trainee. It provides data for reflection on performance and gives useful feedback for self-evaluation.

How many WPBAs should trainees undertake? The purpose of these assessments is not to slavishly tick off each individual competence but to provide a series of snapshots from which trainers can infer whether a trainee is making satisfactory progress. In the UK training system, the number of observations is a minimum of one of each assessment type for each major module of training but the final number depends ultimately on the individual trainee's performance.

Usually, a trainee's overall progress in UK training is reviewed on an annual basis by the 'annual review of competence progression' (ARCP). A wide variety of evidence documenting the trainee's progress is available to the ARCP panel (Table A.5). It is the individual trainee's responsibility to present their trainers with evidence of satisfactory progress by assembling a learning portfolio. To facilitate this process, the Royal College of Anaesthetists is developing an e-portfolio which will allow trainees to accumulate the necessary evidence in a secure, paperless environment.

Examinations

Undoubtedly you will already have considerable experience (and success!) in taking examinations from your secondary education and undergraduate years.

TABLE A.4

Workplace-Based Assessment Tools

- Anaesthesia clinical evaluation exercise (A-CEX)
- ICM clinical evaluation exercise (I-CEX)
- Case-based discussion (CBD)
- Direct observation of procedural skills (DOPS)
- Anaesthetic list management tool (ALMAT)
- Acute care assessment tool (ACAT)
- Multi-source feedback (MSF)

TABLE A.5

Evidence to Inform the 'Annual Review of Competence Progression' (ARCP) Process

- Evidence of performance in professional examinations – if applicable
- A log of clinical work undertaken
- A reflective diary of learning experiences
- The results of WPBAs: DOPS, A-CEX, CBD and ALMAT
- The Clinical Supervisors' end of unit Assessment Form(s) [CSAF]
- A record of agreed targets and outcomes from interviews with their educational supervisor
- A multi-source feedback if appropriate
- Specific evidence of performance in areas such as research and education
- Optionally, a record of a School of Anaesthesia appraisal interview

However, compared with your previous experiences, postgraduate examinations pose different challenges. First, you should remember that you will now be working and studying for examinations at the same time. You should not underestimate how fatigued you will feel after a day's clinical work and how this will affect your appetite and receptiveness to learn. In addition, you may now have a partner to consider and perhaps young children and all of the other domestic commitments which inevitably make considerable demands on your non-working time. Furthermore, you may have the stresses of becoming familiar with new working environments, forging new working relationships and coming to grips with the challenges of mastering a whole new skill set in your chosen speciality.

For all these reasons, it is essential that you plan and prepare thoroughly before sitting any postgraduate anaesthetic examinations. At least 4–6 months of preparation is essential to maximize your chances of success. Failure in postgraduate examinations is demoralizing, financially expensive and may jeopardize your future position in a training programme, so working hard to pass first time must be your goal. There now follow some suggestions on how to tackle the different elements of postgraduate anaesthetic examinations. Some of the advice included may seem trite and unnecessary to many readers but the extensive experience of this author has found these basic principles to be ignored by many examination candidates. Full details of the content, timings and marking schemes of the various anaesthetic examinations are available via the relevant College websites.

Multiple-Choice Questions (MCQs). MCQs are a feature of the postgraduate anaesthetic examinations in UK/Ireland and Australasia at Primary and Final levels. The UK uses a combination of multiple true–false (MTF) and single best answer (SBA) questions. SBAs are used widely in undergraduate medicine and by other postgraduate medical examinations both in the UK and internationally. Compared to traditional MTF questions which assess purely factual recall of knowledge, SBAs allow facts to be placed in context, making them suitable for testing the *application* of knowledge and problem solving which is essential in clinical practice.

Preparing for MCQ examinations requires a lot of practice of the appropriate genre of question using practice papers which are as close as possible to the standard encountered in the real examination. Areas of weakness in your knowledge base can then be identified and remedied by focussed reading in that aspect of the curriculum. You should find out the average pass mark for the MCQ paper for your College and ensure that you are able to achieve this level of performance consistently in practice papers under examination conditions before sitting the real examination. All Colleges publish some MCQs from their own question banks and these can be supplemented by the myriad of examination preparation books which populate the market. Speak to your trainers and other more senior trainees for their advice on which books are currently most useful.

Objective Structured Clinical Examination (OSCE). OSCEs feature in the Primary examinations in the UK and Ireland. In the UK, up to 18 stations are utilized, examining resuscitation skills, technical skills, applied anatomy, history taking, physical examination, communication skills, anaesthetic equipment, anaesthetic hazards and radiological interpretation. One of the stations involves the use of a medium-fidelity simulator to assess management of a critical incident.

There are several books on the market which cover the scope of the UK anaesthesia OSCE exam. However, it is advisable that trainees attend at least one full practice OSCE which closely follows the scope and format of the real thing to ensure that they are fully prepared for this element of the examination.

Short Answer Questions (SAQ). Short answer written questions are included in both the Primary and Final FANZCA and the Final examinations in the UK and Ireland. It cannot be emphasized enough that pre-examination practice in writing short answer questions is essential to maximize success. This ensures that trainees focus on the question precisely as phrased by providing in their answer no more and no less than what is asked. Examiners take great care in the wording of questions so when a question asks for a 'List', then a list is what the examiners expect to be produced in the answer. If a question asks for a description of postoperative management, then only that aspect of the patient's care should be discussed in the answer; no credit will be given for material detailing preoperative assessment or intraoperative care, no matter how erudite!

Timing is all-important in written examinations. Trainees should allocate the same amount of time to answering each SAQ and abide strictly to this discipline. The temptation to spend a few extra minutes on some questions should be resisted because it may result in the potentially disastrous consequence of having little or no time to answer the last few questions on the paper. In the UK and Irish examinations, the SAQs are usually broken down into subsections and the percentage marks allocated to each section indicated to allow candidates to allocate their time accordingly.

Structured Oral Examinations (SOE).

SOEs (previously known as *viva voce* examinations) feature in all parts of the anaesthetic postgraduate examinations in the UK, Ireland and Australasia. Although they may assess differing aspects of their respective curricula, the overriding principle being assessed in the oral examinations is the ability to demonstrate *understanding* of the material being discussed rather than the capacity to simply recall facts (factual recall of core knowledge areas is assessed more appropriately by MTF MCQs). It is therefore unlikely that a candidate will be successful in the oral examinations if there is a failure to demonstrate a sound knowledge base, an understanding of the underlying theoretical principles and the ability to apply this knowledge to clinical situations.

With this in mind, it is essential that candidates gain ample coaching in oral examination technique. There is no substitute for having to formulate coherent answers in response to live questioning. Even the most knowledgeable candidates can become tongue-tied, particularly when under stress, and there is no doubt that everyone's performance in oral examinations improves with practice. I tell my trainees that they should aim for 40–50 practice orals before they attempt the real examination. Although your trainers will undoubtedly help you, these practice orals do not all have to be conducted by consultants or involve a lot of personal expense on examination preparation courses. Working in study groups with your peers and taking it in turns to be the examiner can be just as effective.

Asking more senior trainees who have recently passed the relevant examination to help with mock orals is also very useful because they are likely to have a good idea of the standard required to pass.

Learning Resources.

By the time you have entered postgraduate training you will already have a good idea which types of learning resources suit you best. However, in this multimedia age, there is a large range of learning materials at your disposal to aid in preparation for examinations. In addition to the traditional textbooks and examination preparation courses, there are numerous websites devoted to examination preparation. An outstanding example is e-Learning Anaesthesia (e-LA) which is a web-based educational resource produced by the Royal College of Anaesthetists in partnership with e-Learning for Healthcare (e-LfH). Available at no charge to UK anaesthetists practising in the NHS, e-LA delivers the knowledge and key concepts which underpin the anaesthetic curriculum and helps trainees to prepare for the FRCA examination. There are currently over 1000 knowledge and scenario-based sessions covering the first two years of the anaesthetic curriculum. e-LA may be accessed via the Royal College of Anaesthetists' website.

Simulation is becoming a very popular and powerful tool to aid learning. Low, medium and high fidelity simulators are now commonplace and most trainees are able to access these resources at some point in their training. Simulation provides the opportunity to practise technical skills and management of clinical situations (particularly critical incidents) which they may not yet have encountered in real life, in a safe environment. Simulators are also used as an assessment tool in the Primary FRCA OSCE exam, as discussed above.

Working in study groups is a very effective method of examination preparation. It is difficult to judge your own standard of performance and preparedness for postgraduate examinations, particularly in relation to the SOEs, because you are studying in relative isolation from your peers compared to the heavily supervised collegiate approach at undergraduate level. It is reassuring to discuss your worries and concerns about the forthcoming examination in a mutually supportive forum and useful to gauge your knowledge and understanding of topics in discussion with your colleagues.

LIFE-LONG LEARNING AND CPD

Finally, it is worth emphasizing that postgraduate learning does not end with passing College examinations and successfully completing a training programme. Once you have completed training, it is your professional duty to remain up-to-date in all aspects of your clinical practice (including knowledge, skills and professional behaviours) to ensure that you deliver safe, high quality care to your patients throughout your remaining career. From 2012 in the UK, all doctors who are not in training positions have been required to revalidate every five years and this will include a requirement that doctors can demonstrate adequate evidence of continuing professional development (CPD). To facilitate development of a CPD portfolio, the Royal College of Anaesthetists has produced a CPD matrix – a framework of three levels of CPD with specified knowledge and skills which doctors who are not in training grades and who are practising anaesthesia, critical care and pain medicine, need to meet in order to revalidate. The Royal College has introduced an online CPD system which allows all those practising in anaesthesia, critical care and pain medicine to record CPD activity, update their personal development plans and search for CPD-approved events. A similar CPD scheme, including an online CPD portfolio, has also been developed by ANZCA. Full details of both schemes are available via the respective Colleges' websites.

FURTHER READING

Full details of curricula, training programmes and postgraduate examinations relevant to the country in which you are training are available via the respective College or other regulatory authority responsible for postgraduate anaesthetic training. Website addresses for the UK, Irish and Australasian Colleges are as follows:

Royal College of Anaesthetists, www.rcoa.ac.uk.

College of Anaesthetists of Ireland, www.anaesthesia.ie.

Australian & New Zealand College of Anaesthetists, www.anzca.edu.au.

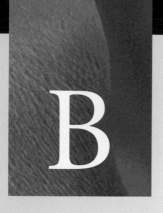

DATA, STATISTICS AND CLINICAL TRIALS

■ ■ ■ ■ ■ ■ ■ ■ ■ ■

S tatistics is the science of learning from data – from collection and organization through to analysis, presentation and dissemination. Like all sciences, it has its own vocabulary and can sometimes appear somewhat impenetrable to the uninitiated. This appendix is intended to give an overview of statistical processes and methods but readers are advised to go to the myriad texts on medical statistics for more detail.

Whenever data are collected, in a more or less systematic fashion, statistics are produced: how many things? What size? How old? The science of statistics is concerned with turning this information into something useful. Generally, this is either to **describe** the things we are measuring or to make some **inference** or **prediction** from them. Often within medicine there is a question attached – commonly of the form: *'Is one group somehow different to another group'*?

TYPES OF DATA

The type of data collected makes a big difference to what can be done with them using statistics.

At the most basic level, it is fairly straightforward to count things. How many patients died? How many were sick after surgery? How many of the patients who were sick were women? Sometimes these are simple categories with no order or value. Apples and oranges are not usually described as 'better' or 'larger' than the other. They are just **categories** or **names** of fruit. Male/female; White British/Indian/Japanese – these are all simple '**categorical**' or '**nominal**' data. The categories may be somewhat arbitrarily defined, with the possibility of overlap. Clear

rules are therefore needed to define what goes in which category.

Sometimes, the categories may have an **order** – mild/moderate/severe pain has a natural order as does easy/difficult/impossible mask ventilation. These are called '**ordinal**' data. Some of these data lend themselves to having numbers attached but these numbers are no more than labels for ordinal data. The Glasgow Outcome Scale has five categories from 1 – Dead, through to 5 – Good recovery. Clearly 1 is a worse outcome than 5, but there is no suggestion that the difference between the numbers is the same. Since the data have an order, the median value has some meaning. The special cases of rating scales (such as pain and anxiety scales) are discussed below.

Data which correspond to measurements of physical constructs are usually amenable to the use of **interval** and **ratio** scales. An interval scale is an ordered sequence of numbers in which there is a constant interval between each point in the scale. For instance, the difference in temperature between 1 and 2 °C is the same as between 101 and 102 °C. However, the zero point is arbitrary, so ratios are not appropriate – 100 °C is not twice as hot as 50 °C.

A ratio scale is a type of interval scale where there is a true zero – negative numbers cannot exist. For example, there is no temperature below 0 Kelvin, and there is no such thing as a negative length. This does allow ratios to be used. 100 Kelvin is twice as hot as 50 Kelvin, and someone who is 2 m tall is twice the height of someone who is 1 m tall. Interval and ratio data can be described using the mean, although this may not always be appropriate.

SUMMARIZING DATA

When describing data, it is often helpful to have some idea of a representative value – the 'average' in common parlance. In statistical terms, this is a value which describes the 'central tendency' of a set of data. In general, there are three types of 'average': mean, median and mode. Within this appendix, the term average is used commonly and deliberately to encompass any of these.

Mode is simply the commonest value. It is used for categorical data.

Median is the middle value (or half way between the two middle values if there is an even number of data points). It is used for ordinal data.

Mean is the representative value used for interval data. The arithmetic mean is most commonly used, but it is only one of three 'Pythagorean means', the other two being the geometric and harmonic means.

Arithmetic mean (AM) is the sum of all the values divided by the number (n) of values $(x_1 \ldots x_n)$. In algebraic notation:

$$AM = \frac{1}{n}\sum_{i=1}^{n} x_i = \frac{x_1 + x_2 + \cdots + x_n}{n}$$

The *geometric mean* (GM) is found by multiplying all the numbers together and then taking the nth root.

$$GM = \sqrt[n]{\prod_{i=1}^{n} x_i} = \sqrt[n]{x_1 x_2 \cdots x_n}$$

The geometric mean is used when factors have a multiplicative effect and we want to find the average effect of these. It is most commonly used in finance (average interest rates) but is used in medicine when the 'mean' of logarithmically transformed values is used.

The *harmonic mean* (HM) is the rather wordy, reciprocal of the arithmetic mean of the reciprocals of the values.

$$HM = \frac{1}{\frac{1}{n}\sum_{i=1}^{n}\frac{1}{x_i}} = \frac{n}{\frac{1}{x} + \frac{1}{x_2} + \cdots + \frac{1}{x_n}}$$

It is the most appropriate mean for comparing rates (such as speeds) or ratios. It is also used when calculating the effect of parallel resistances.

There are some other special means, of which the root mean square (RMS) or *quadratic mean* (QM) is perhaps the most widely quoted.

$$QM = \sqrt{\frac{1}{n}\left(x_1^2 + x_2^2 + \cdots + x_i^2\right)}$$

This is used to describe the average value of a varying quantity such as sine waves – most notably it is the method used to describe the 'average' voltage of an AC current.

The means give some idea of the 'typical' value, but it is usually helpful to have some idea of the **spread** of the values.

At the simplest level, the range or maximum and minimum give an idea of the spread. Similarly, the interquartile range (25th and 75th centiles) describes the middle 50% of the dataset.

The standard deviation is a useful description of the variation around the mean because it can be manipulated in statistical tests. It is defined as the square root of the variance.

If we have data from the whole population (which is relatively uncommon) then the population standard deviation (σ) is:

$$\sigma = \sqrt{\frac{1}{N}\sum_{i=1}^{N}\left(x_i - \mu\right)^2}$$

where N is the number of items in the population, and μ is the population mean.

If we only have a sample, then the sample standard deviation (s) is given by:

$$s = \sqrt{\frac{1}{N-1}\sum_{i=1}^{N}\left(x_i - \overline{x}\right)^2}$$

where $\overline{x}$ is the sample mean.

The use of 'N−1' rather than 'N' is known as Bessel's correction and is needed to account for the fact that the sample standard deviation is less accurate than that of the whole population. Clearly, as the sample becomes larger, the effect of N−1 becomes smaller.

SAMPLING

It is relatively unusual to measure the whole population of interest because it is usually impractical, expensive and unnecessary. In most situations, a sample is taken from the population and the items of interest recorded. Generally, it is hoped that the sample represents the total population as closely as possible. If the sample is a truly random selection from the population then quite robust inferences about the whole population can be made. The randomness of the selection is very important; if the sample is not truly random, then the statistical models used generally do not work well.

PROBABILITY

If an event or measurement is variable, then whenever we measure it, it could have one of a range of values. Probability is simply the proportion of times that the value (or range of values) occurs. Probability is the chance of something occurring and always lies between 1 (always occurs) and 0 (never occurs). If one out of every hundred people is allergic to penicillin then the probability of meeting someone allergic to penicillin is 1 in 100, or 0.01.

The probability of exclusive events are additive, and the sum of all mutually exclusive probabilities must always equal 1. In other words, if the probability of the patients on the emergency theatre list being from gynaecology wards is 0.3 and the probability of them being from general surgical wards is 0.5, then the probability of them being from neither specialty is 0.2 $(1 - (0.3 + 0.5))$.

If probabilities are independent (i.e. the probability of one event is not affected by the outcome of another) then they can be multiplied. For instance, the probability of a general surgical patient being female might be 0.6, in which case the probability of meeting a female general surgical patient on the list would be $0.5 \times 0.6 = 0.3$.

Sometimes, we are interested in relative probabilities; what is the chance of something occurring in one group compared with the chance of something occurring in another group? There are various methods used to describe this, which will be discussed later in this section.

DATA DISTRIBUTIONS

Often, there is apparently random variation in events or processes. If we toss a coin, it falls randomly either heads or tails; similarly, a dice will land on any number between 1 and 6 at random. If we measure the weights of children attending for surgery, they will vary at random around some central value. The probability of any one value, or range of values, is described by the **probability distribution.** Although medicine often refers to the '**normal**' or '**Gaussian**' distribution, this is only one of many possible probability distributions.

Uniform Distributions

The mean value from a 6-sided dice throw is 3.5; if you throw the dice many times and add up the total score and divide by the number of throws, it will be close to 3.5. However, the probability of throwing numbers close to the mean (3 or 4) is the same as the probability of throwing numbers at the extremes (1 or 6). In fact, the probability of any number is the same (1 in 6) – a **uniform distribution.** Uniform distributions are used to generate random numbers – the chance of any particular value is the same. In theory, the probability of being on-call on a particular day is also a uniform distribution, provided there are no special rules.

Non-Uniform Distributions

Most biological data come from non-uniform distributions. Often, these are centred on the average and the probability of a particular value is greater if it is closer to the average. Extreme values are possible but less likely.

The most well-known of these non-uniform distributions is the **normal distribution** - so called because most 'normal' events or processes approximate to it (or can be transformed in some way to approximate it). It is also known as the Gaussian distribution after the polymath Carl Friedrich Gauss (also of Gauss lines in MRI). This distribution is defined mathematically on the basis of two values (parameters) – the mean and standard deviation. The probability frequency distribution is a bell-shaped curve. The mode, median and mean are identical, and the degree of spread is governed by the ratio of the standard deviation (SD) to the mean. It is important to understand that the normal distribution is only one of an infinite number of bell-shaped curves. A bell-shaped probability distribution is not necessarily 'normal'.

The normal distribution has some useful properties, not least that it is possible to calculate the probability of finding a range of values based solely on the standard deviation (Fig. B.1).

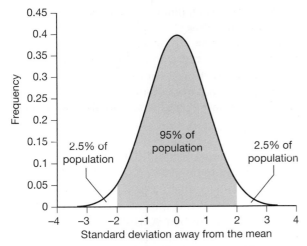

FIGURE B.1 ■ A normal distribution curve, with a mean of zero and standard deviation of one. The unshaded areas which are greater than 1.96 standard deviations above and below the mean each encompass 2.5% of the population. The shaded area (mean±1.96 standard deviations) therefore covers 95% of the population.

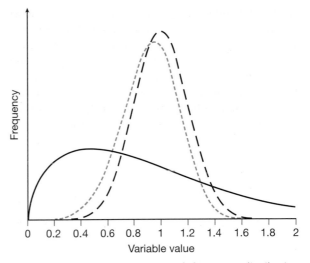

FIGURE B.2 ■ Different types of frequency distribution curve. _____, right/positive skew distribution. _ _ _ _ _ _ _, Weibull distribution. Note that, although it is bell-shaped, it is not a normal distribution. ...., normal distribution.

The 97.5th centile of the normal distribution is 1.96 SD away from the mean. Therefore, the probability of finding a value more extreme than this (there are two sides to the distribution) is 5%. Conversely, 95% of values, if selected at random, would be expected to be found within±1.96 standard deviations of the mean. Similarly, 68.3% of values would be expected to be within 1 standard deviation on either side of the mean.

Sometimes, distributions are skewed – the mean, median and mode are not identical. If the long tail is to the right, this is termed a right-skew (or positive skew), and pulled to the left a left-skew (negative skew). In general, for a left-skew distribution, the mean is less than the median, and both are less than the mode. The converse holds for right-skewed distributions (Fig. B.2).

Skew distributions are not so easy to handle with statistical tests, but often the data can be transformed to create a normal distribution. Commonly, taking the logarithm of the data will transform mildly skewed data into a normal distribution.

Chi-Square Distribution

The chi-square distribution (χ^2) is most commonly seen when used as the basis of comparing proportions of observed versus expected events. However, it is also fundamental to the t-test and analysis of variance (ANOVA). It is defined by only a single number; k is the number of degrees of freedom in the data.

Inferring Information from a Sample

If we were to measure some aspect of a complete population (e.g. the weight of every member of the anaesthetic department) we would be able to state with absolute confidence what the average and spread of that value were. If we measured everyone but one, we would be very confident, but there would be some error in our estimate of the average. If we measured only a few (selected at random) then we would still have an estimate of the average, but we would be less certain still about exactly what it was. Using various statistical tests (see below) we can quantify the degree of confidence that we have in our estimate of the population average.

BIAS

All of the above assumptions about sampling from a population assume that the sample is taken at random and is therefore representative of the whole population. However, there are many sources of bias which can invalidate this assumption. Some of these may be due to the design of the experiment; some may be due to behaviour (conscious or unconscious) of the investigator or the subject of the investigation (e.g. a patient or volunteer). There is no study ever conducted which has no bias somewhere. The role of investigators, regulators, research community, funders and end-users of research is to minimize this bias and account for it as far as possible.

Selection Bias

Topic Selection. The questions asked by researchers are a complex product of their interests and skills, resources available and their ability to attract sufficient funding. It is widely recognized that there is a distortion of research funding by financial resource and equipment. Pharmaceutical companies have a legitimate interest in research in their product areas, but these may not be the most beneficial for patients overall; charities target their resources and government funders may sometimes follow political rather than healthcare imperatives.

Population Selection. Some patient groups are easier to study than others, but the findings in one patient population may not be applicable to others. Within anaesthesia, this is perhaps most evident in the relative lack of pharmacological studies in the very young and the very old.

Similarly, most clinical studies are run from large teaching hospitals, whereas most patients are treated in smaller district general hospitals. Outcomes are not necessarily the same for these groups – although not always better in the larger hospitals.

Inclusion/Exclusion Bias. Even if the appropriate population is studied, there is always a risk that the sample itself will be unrepresentative of the population. Some patients may be more likely to be approached for involvement in a research study, and some may be more likely to consent or refuse.

Methodological Bias. Head-to-head comparisons may be deliberately or accidentally set up to favour one group over another. A study of an adequate dose of a new oral opioid compared with a small dose of paracetamol (acetaminophen) is always going to demonstrate better analgesia with the opioid. Other more subtle biases are common in many anaesthesia and pain research studies.

Outcome Bias

Detection Bias. If an investigator (or patient) has an opinion about the relationship between group membership and outcome then an outcome may be sought, or reported, more readily in one group than another. This may be conscious or unconscious. Most anaesthetists believe that difficult intubation is more common in pregnant women. A simple survey of difficult intubation is likely to reinforce this finding because this is the group in which cases are most likely to be sought. A patient who has received regional anaesthesia may be more likely to report good analgesia than one allocated to receive oral analgesics.

Missing Outcomes. It is not possible to measure every outcome in a study, so the investigator has to make a decision about which ones to choose. If an important variable is not measured, then this may lead to a biased perception of the effects of a treatment.

Reporting Bias. Research with positive results is more likely to be published in high quality journals and negative studies are less likely to be published at all. Some of this is bias from the journals, and some of it is bias by researchers who choose not to submit negative findings. Occasionally, commercial organizations restrict publication of studies which do not portray a favourable view of their product. The effect of this is that there is a bias in the literature in favour of positive studies. To use a coin tossing example, if researchers only ever published data when they got 6 or more heads in a row, the literature would soon be awash with data suggesting that the coins were biased.

More subtle is the non-reporting of measured outcomes. A study which finds a positive effect in a relatively minor outcome may fail to report a neutral or negative effect on a major outcome. This is extremely hard to detect because it relies on transparency from investigators about what they measured.

Outright fraud is still thought to be relatively rare, but there are several high profile cases of anaesthesia researchers fabricating data, publishing studies that never took place or manipulating data to fit their beliefs.

TESTING

Within medicine and anaesthesia, professionals strive to achieve the best outcomes possible for patients. It is therefore very common to ask a question of the form: 'Is the outcome in group A better than in group B?' We already know that if we take a sample from a population (e.g. the total population of group A) we will be able to estimate the true population average. If we do the same for group B, that will provide an estimate for population B. Due to simple random variation, the average value for A and B will always be different, provided we measure them with sufficient precision. What we really want to know is how confident we are that any differences that we see are not just due to chance. As shown in Figure B.3, if the degree of separation of the two groups is small, or the spread of either is relatively large, then there is a reasonable chance that the average estimated for group B could have come from population A. Conversely, if the separation is larger, or the spread is smaller, the chance of the estimated average for B being found in population A is small (but never zero).

This is the fundamental principle behind most statistical testing. What is the probability that the result that has been found has occurred simply by chance? Note that this does not mean that the result could definitely not have occurred by chance, just that it is sufficiently unlikely to support the hypothesis that the groups really are different.

By way of a simple example, the probability of tossing 6 heads in a row with an unbiased coin is 0.5^6 (0.0156), or 1 in 64. This is by definition unlikely, so you would be suspicious of the coin being biased towards heads. However, it is clearly not impossible, and does occur (1 in 64 times on average).

An important principle with statistical testing is the concept of **paired tests**. There is inherent variability between things being measured – people, times, objects. This variability between things increases the spread of values we might measure, making it harder to demonstrate a difference between groups. However, if we measure the difference within an individual then the difference may be easier to find. To take a trivial

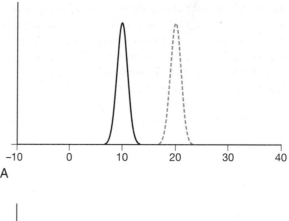

A

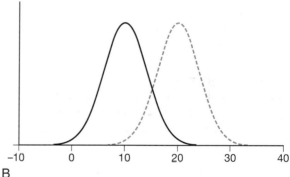

B

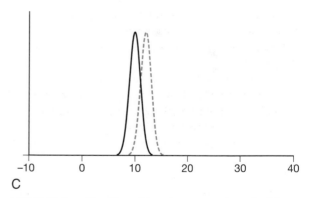

C

FIGURE B.3 ■ The effect of changing mean and standard deviation on overlap of frequency distributions. **A**, solid line – mean 10, standard deviation 1; dotted line – mean 20, standard deviation 1. **B**, solid line – mean 10, standard deviation 4; dotted line – mean 20, standard deviation 4. **C**, solid line – mean 10, standard deviation 1; dotted line – mean 12, standard deviation 1.

example, if we want to see whether fuel consumption is better with one fuel compared with another, we might take 20 cars with one fuel and compare them with 20 cars with another – an **unpaired** test. However, the 40 cars will all have other factors which influence fuel consumption and this variability will hinder our ability to demonstrate a difference. If we take 20 cars and test them with both fuels (choosing at random which fuel to test first) then we have a much better chance of demonstrating a difference. A paired test is one in which the results of some intervention are tested within the individuals in the group, not between groups.

Within anaesthesia, **paired** tests are relatively unusual, because we do not normally have situations in which we can test more than one thing on one individual. There are some examples, such as physiological experiments studying the effects of drugs during anaesthesia.

When data (or their transforms) can be legitimately modelled as coming from a defined probability distribution, they are described as being from a **parametric** distribution. Most commonly, this is the normal distribution, but binomial, Poisson, Weibull, etc. are all defined distributions. Data from undefined probability distributions are **non-parametric.** In general, parametric statistical tests are more **powerful** than non-parametric tests, so should be used **if appropriate**. Non-parametric tests rely on far fewer assumptions and are considered more robust. They can also be used on parametric data.

Before performing any statistical tests, there are a few simple rules and questions which reduce the likelihood of applying the wrong test or misinterpreting the results.

- What question do you want to answer?
- What type of data do you have? Categorical data requires a different approach to ordinal or interval data. Survival analysis, comparison of measurement techniques, etc. will require different approaches.
- Plot the data using scatter plots and frequency histograms. Summary statistics may completely hide a skewed distribution or bimodal data.
- Are there any obvious erroneous data? Transcription errors are fairly common, so always check that the data are accurate.
- Are the data paired or unpaired?
- Can a parametric test be used? If not, can the data be transformed so that a parametric test can be used?
- Is there an element of multiple testing?

A flow-chart suggesting rules to guide selection of tests is shown in Figure B.4. A brief summary of the tests described is given in the next section. The flow chart is not an exhaustive list; there are many other tests and situations not covered, but researchers should always explain if they feel the need to use more recherché approaches.

Chi-Squared Test

This test compares the expected number of events with the actual numbers. Data are tabulated in a **contingency table;** 2×2 tables are the simplest, but larger tables can be used. In general, the number of **degrees of freedom** is the number of columns in the table minus one multiplied by the number of rows minus one. (i.e. for a 2×2 table, the degrees of freedom would be $(2-1) \times (2-1) = 1$.

$$x^2 = \sum_{i=1}^{n} \frac{(O_i - E_i)^2}{E_i}$$

If the expected frequencies are not known (e.g. 50/50 for male/female) the expected value for each cell (E_i) is determined by the number of observed events in that cell's row multiplied by the number of events in that cell's column, divided by the total number of events. An example is shown in Box B.1. The *expected* frequency for cell A is $(A+B) \times (A+C)/N$

The calculated χ^2 statistic is then compared with a table of probability values for χ^2 for each degree of freedom. This gives a probability that the observed frequencies came from the same population as the expected frequencies.

A worked example is shown in Box B.2. The *expected* columns are inserted to show the calculations. The basic table is 2×2. χ^2 is the sum of the $(O - E)^2/E$ values for each cell:

$$\{(15-10.9)^2/10.9\} + \{(40-44.1)^2/44.1\} + \{(6-10.1)^2/10.1\} + \{(45-40.9)^2/40.9\} = 4.0$$

The critical value from the χ^2 tables for $P = 0.05$ and one degree of freedom is 3.84. χ^2 is greater than this, making it unlikely that the distribution of data comes from a single population.

There are some standard assumptions with χ^2 tests. There should be sufficient samples; the expected cell counts should all be >5 in 2×2 tables, or >5 in at least 80% of cells in larger tables. If these conditions are not satisfied, then alternative approaches are used such as Yates' continuity correction or Fisher's exact test.

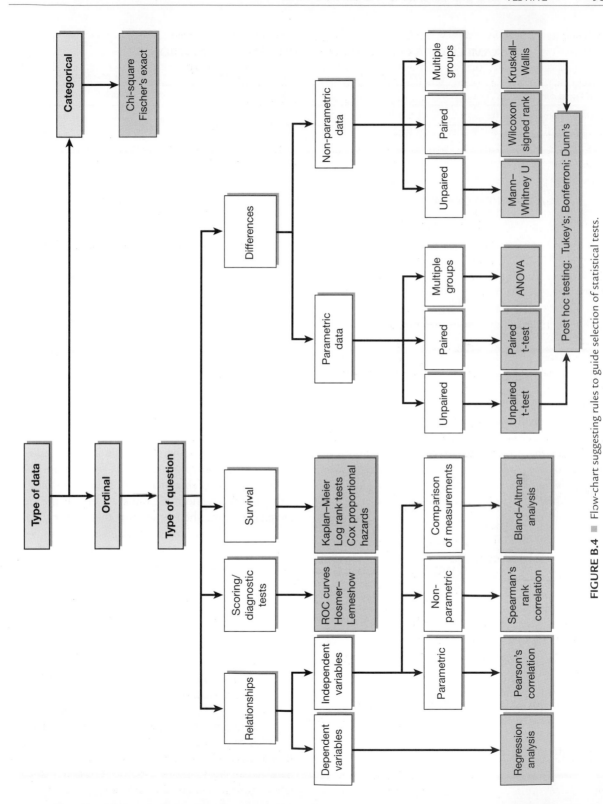

FIGURE B.4 ■ Flow-chart suggesting rules to guide selection of statistical tests.

BOX B.1
EXAMPLE OF A CONTINGENCY TABLE FOR CALCULATION OF χ^2

	With Treatment	Without Treatment	Row Marginals
Good outcome	A	B	E = A + B
Bad outcome	C	D	F = C + D
Column marginals	G = A + C	H = B + D	N (total) = A + B + C + D

BOX B.2
A WORKED EXAMPLE OF A CONTINGENCY TABLE FOR CALCULATION OF χ^2

	WONDER DRUG		PLACEBO		
	Observed	Expected	Observed	Expected	Row Marginals
Lived	15	10.9 (21 x 55)/106	6	10.1 (21 x 51)/106	21
Died	40	44.1 (85 x 55)/106	45	40.9 (85 x 51)/106	85
Column marginals	55		51		106

Rank Tests

If data are ranked in order, then if two groups are sufficiently different, we would expect the sum of these ranks to be much smaller for one group than the other. The bigger the groups, the smaller the difference in the sum of these ranks which we would accept. This concept is the basis for the Wilcoxon signed rank and Mann–Whitney U tests. Essentially, the sum of the ranks, corrected for the sample sizes, is compared with a table of probabilities calculated from the **U-distribution**.

Because these rank tests do not perform any statistical tests on the values themselves, they are robust to the presence of outliers. It does not matter how extreme a particular value is; only its rank is important.

An example is shown in Box B.3. If the null hypothesis is true, the rank sums are equal; the more unequal they are, the less support there is for the null

BOX B.3
A WORKED EXAMPLE OF MANN–WHITNEY U TEST

The first few nausea scores in a trial of cyclizine (group C) and an imaginary anti-emetic NoVom (group N) using a 100 mm visual analogue scale are:

Group C	0	5	12	13	15
Group N	3	6	9	10	12

These scores are ranked and the scores from NoVom are in bold:

Rank order:	0	**3**	5	**6**	**9**	**10**	**12**	12	13	15
Ranking:	1	2	3	4	5	6	7.5	7.5	9	10

The rankings are then summed for each group. Shared scores rank equal, which is why the scores of 12 each rank 7.5:
Group sum of ranks:
Group C = 1 + 3 + 7.5 + 9 + 10 = 30.5
Group N = 2 + 4 + 5 + 6 + 7.5 = 24.5

t-Tests

Provided that the data approximate closely enough to a normal distribution, *t*-tests provide a powerful method for assessing differences between two groups. Unlike the rank tests, the *t*-distribution uses the data values themselves – the calculation uses the mean, standard deviations and sample sizes of the two groups. Again, although it can be done by hand, it is more robust to use one of the myriad statistical software packages available.

Rating scales are extremely popular in anaesthetic research – pain, nausea, satisfaction and anxiety are all commonly measured using verbal, numerical or visual analogue scales. The safest way to analyse these is using non-parametric statistical tests because these avoid any assumptions about the interval between points. However, in practice, many studies assume that the data behave as normally distributed data and analyse them using *t*-tests.

Multiple Testing

Sometimes, we may want to look for differences between multiple groups or at multiple times within groups. In this case, the obvious answer might be to perform multiple tests. However, this leads to a probability problem. If we had three groups (A, B, C) then there would be three comparisons: A–B, A–C and B–C. The chance of finding a 'positive' finding purely by chance is now rather greater. As the number of comparisons increases, the number of 'chance' findings will inevitably increase.

There are numerous approaches to this problem. One is simply to correct the overall *P*-value so that it remains correct by adjusting the *P*-values for the individual tests. This is the principle of the **Bonferroni** correction. This is simple to calculate (the *P*-value for each comparison is approximated by the overall *P*-value divided by the number of comparisons) but it may be too conservative in some situations.

An alternative approach, which is widely used (and abused), is to employ the family of statistical tests known as ANOVA (ANalysis Of VAriance). When properly constructed, ANOVA can provide information about the likelihood of significant variation between or within groups. **ANOVA** requires various assumptions

about the distribution of the data, including normality. The non-parametric equivalent is the **Kruskal–Wallis** test. When applied to two groups, ANOVA is a *t*-test, and Kruskal–Wallis a Mann–Whitney *U*.

If these tests suggest a significant difference, there are various ***post hoc*** tests used to identify where the difference lies, without falling foul of the multiple testing issues described above. Tukey's Honestly Significant Difference is commonly used in medical research.

Relationship Testing

Sometimes, rather than asking the question of whether groups are different, we want to know how certain factors relate to each other. When there are several variables, tests from the family of regression techniques are used, of which **logistic regression** is the best known. Essentially, the strength of association between a set of variables (e.g. age, sex, presence of active malignancy) and an outcome (e.g. length of stay in intensive care) is tested. It is important to note that association does not imply causation and if important variables are left out, then erroneous conclusions can be drawn. For example, yellow staining of the fingers is associated with the diagnosis of lung cancer, but is not the cause.

Sometimes, a more straightforward relationship is sought. How does weight vary with age in children? Correlation statistics give an idea of the strength of such an association – in other words how much scatter around the expected value we might expect. To take the example of children's weight and height, there is a reasonable correlation – hence the various formulae for estimation of children's weight. However, there is considerable scatter due to other factors – nutrition, race, gender – so there is not a perfect correlation.

The most commonly used correlation analysis is **Pearson's** or **least squares correlation**. This gives an estimated equation predicting one variable (y) from another (x) (of the form $y = mx + c$) and a correlation coefficient (R) – a summary statistic of how close the variables lie to this predicted line. Truly random association would have a correlation coefficient of 0, and perfect association 1.

This approach is insensitive to changes in scale of either variable. This is to be expected – the correlation between height and weight should be the same regardless of whether metric or imperial units are used. However, this does mean that correlation can tell us nothing about whether the prediction of one value from another is accurate – only that as one increases, the other increases by a similar relative amount. Second, the statistical interpretation of R^2 is determined by the sample size. A large sample may have low (near zero) R^2 but still have a statistically significant association between the two variables.

The shape of the relationship is important – always look at the data. As seen in Figure B.5, curvilinear relationships may have apparently reasonable correlations.

A similar approach can be taken to correlations between non-parametric data using **Spearman's rank correlation**.

Comparison of Techniques

It is relatively common for anaesthetists to wish to find out whether measurements taken with one device are interchangeable with those from another. For instance, is cardiac output measured by pulse contour analysis equivalent to that obtained by thermodilution? Correlation describes the relationship between two set of measurements – does one increase as the other increases? – but does not adequately describe the accuracy of the technique. This is more appropriately done using the Bland–Altman technique (Fig. B.6).

Paired measurements of the variable of interest are taken, e.g. cardiac output with bolus thermodilution (A) and a new monitor (B). The mean of these values ((A+B)/2) is plotted against the difference (A−B). The mean difference between the measurements is the *bias*. The *limits of agreement* are usually defined as the bias ± 1.96 × the standard deviation of the differences. It should be noted that these *limits of agreement* are purely descriptive. They do not define what is clinically acceptable – that is a matter for the investigator to justify. Often, these limits of agreement are described as percentages of the overall mean value.

Within medicine, there is usually not a true 'gold standard' against which to compare a new device. There is inaccuracy even in the best devices compared to the 'true' value (e.g. real cardiac output). This has important implications for evaluating new devices. A perfect new device would inevitably have some degree of variation compared to current devices. Two devices of equivalent accuracy, when compared with each other, would be expected to have wider limits of agreement than each alone. An example of this is the comparison of thermodilution and other methods of estimating cardiac output. The error for thermodilution against 'true' cardiac

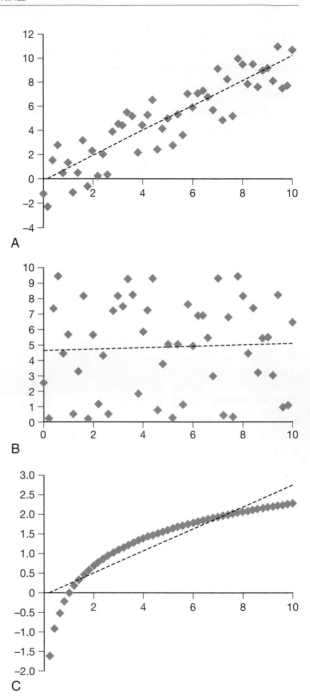

FIGURE B.5 ■ Linear regression. Scatter plots of two possibly related variables. The lines show the calculated regression lines. **A** – shows reasonably well correlated data. $R^2 = 0.8$. **B** – data with no correlation at all. $R^2 \approx 0$. **C** – data which shows reasonable correlation ($R^2 = 0.83$), though in fact is better fitted by a non-linear relationship (logarithmic in this case).

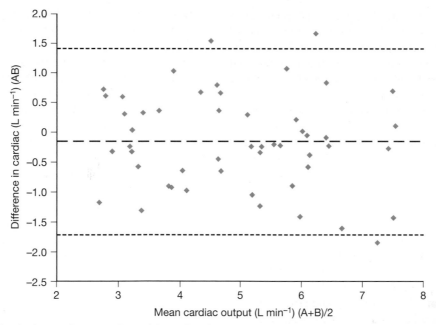

FIGURE B.6 ■ Bland–Altman plot. Hypothetical data of cardiac output measured by two devices (A, B). The dashed line represents the bias (mean difference), the dotted lines represent the upper and lower 95% limits of agreement between the two devices. Note that, in this example, both devices were given a 20% error. The combined limits of agreement are approximately 30%.

output is around 20%. If a new technique has similar accuracy, then the limits of agreement for the two devices compared would be expected to be around 30%.

The Bland–Altman approach was originally designed for single pairs of measurements from multiple subjects. Corrections are required if the approach is used with multiple measurements from the same subject.

PREDICTIVE TESTING AND SCORING SYSTEMS

In clinical practice, anaesthetists often use some form of test to predict the presence or absence of a certain condition, e.g. difficult intubation, malignant hyperthermia or postoperative mortality. In an ideal world, we would have tests available which were completely accurate, cheap, quick and easy to apply in normal practice. Unfortunately, none of the tests we use meets these criteria. The degree to which the available tests match these criteria dictate how we should use them.

Test Accuracy

There are several inter-related characteristics of a diagnostic test. *Sensitivity* is calculated as the proportion of those with a condition (*true positives*) that are correctly identified by the test. Therefore a *sensitive* test identifies all individuals with the condition and if a highly sensitive test is negative it is unlikely that an individual will have the condition. This is usually at the expense of incorrectly identifying individuals who do not actually have the condition (*false positives*). Conversely, *specificity* is calculated as the proportion of those without a condition (*true negatives*) that are correctly identified by the test. Hence a highly *specific* test identifies only those individuals who definitely have the condition of interest – the false positive rate is low; the pay-off is that individuals with the condition may be missed (*false negatives*).

A well-used memory rule for these is 'Spin and Snout' – a positive **SP**ecific test rules an individual **IN** (*they have the condition*); a negative **SeN**sitive test rules them **OUT** (*they don't have the condition*).

The *positive predictive value* (PPV) of a test is the probability that an individual with a positive test result actually has the condition of interest. The *negative predictive value* is the probability that an individual with a negative test is truly free of the condition.

It is extremely important to realize that the positive and negative predictive values of tests are dependent upon the prevalence of the condition in the population as well as the accuracy of the test technique itself. To take an extreme example, over-the-counter pregnancy tests have very high positive and negative predictive values for detecting pregnancy in women of child-bearing age. The negative predictive value is actually higher in men (there are no false negatives), but the positive predictive value is zero (positive tests will occur, but there are no pregnant men). The sensitivity and specificity of the test itself are unchanged. Examples are given in Boxes B.4–6.

Often, diagnostic tests are not truly dichotomous (yes *vs.* no). Rather, some threshold value is used. As this threshold varies, so the sensitivity and specificity of the test varies. To take the pregnancy test example again, the higher the concentration of β-HCG required for a positive test, the greater the specificity, but at the loss of sensitivity.

This trade-off was investigated systematically in the development of radar systems which were monitored by receiver-operators. At one end of the scale, all objects will be identified – aeroplanes and birds – a highly sensitive threshold, but at the cost of a lack of specificity, resulting in a lot of false positives. At the other end of the scale, a positive signal will almost certainly be an aeroplane – very specific, but at the cost of missing quite a few planes. This can be assessed statistically using the so-called 'Receiver-operating characteristic curves' – usually shortened to ROC curves (Fig. B.7).

These plot the false positive rate (1 – specificity) against the true positive rate (sensitivity). A near ideal test would form a right-angle. A test which was no better than tossing a coin would lie on the line of identity. Most tests, of course, lie somewhere in between. Various summary statistics can be derived from ROC curves. The most common is the area under the curve (AUC). A perfect discriminant curve has an AUC of 1; a non-discriminatory test AUC is 0.5. There is no consensus for acceptable AUC, but 0.9–1.0 is considered excellent, 0.8–0.9 good and <0.6 poor.

The point on the curve which is closest to the top left corner (false positive rate 0, true positive rate 1) is sometimes viewed as the best trade-off between sensitivity and specificity, but in practice the thresholds used for diagnostic tests are influenced by wider costs (of the test, of subsequent intervention or further testing and of false negatives).

Risk Scoring

In perioperative medicine, we are often interested in estimating the risk of an event occurring. This is slightly different to diagnostic testing. The question is not whether a person has a certain condition, but what is the risk (probability) of an event (such as death, PONV, morbidity) occurring. Such systems are useful for discussions with patients and relatives, in helping to plan treatments (e.g. critical care, anti-emetics),

---

BOX B.4

SENSITIVITY, SPECIFICITY, POSITIVE (PPV) AND NEGATIVE (NPV) PREDICTIVE VALUES

		DISEASE POSITIVE						
		Yes	No	Totals				
Test positive	Yes	A	B	A+B	Sensitivity	A/(A+C)	PPV	A/(A+B)
	No	C	D	C+D	Specificity	B/(B+D)	NPV	D/(C+D)
	Totals	A+C	B+D	A+B+C+D	Prevalence	(A+C)/ (A+B+C+D)		
Test positive	Yes	True positive	False positive (Type I error)		Sensitivity	True positives/ All disease positive	PPV	True positive/ all test positives
	No	False negative (Type II error)	True Negative		Specificity	True negatives/ All disease negative	NPV	True negative/ all test negatives

BOX B.5
EFFECT OF CHANGING PREVALENCE ON RESULTS. IN THE TWO GROUPS (A – A GENERAL POPULATION; B – A GROUP WITH A KNOWN FAMILY HISTORY OF CHOLINESTERASE DEFICIENCY), THE PREVALENCES OF CHOLINESTERASE DEFICIENCY ARE 1.3% AND 12%. THE TESTS SENSITIVITY AND SPECIFICITY ARE UNCHANGED, BUT THE POSITIVE AND NEGATIVE PREDICTIVE VALUES ARE DIFFERENT

| A: General Population | | TRUE CHOLINESTERASE DEFICIENCY | | | | | | |
		Yes	No	Total				
Cholinesterase activity test	Yes	9	50	59	Sensitivity	0.33	PPV	0.15
	No	18	2000	2018	Specificity	0.98	NPV	0.99
	Totals	27	2050	2077	Prevalence	1.3%		
B: Family History of Cholinesterase Deficiency								
		Yes	No					
Cholinesterase activity test	Yes	9	5	14	Sensitivity	0.33	PPV	0.64
	No	18	200	218	Specificity	0.98	NPV	0.92
	Totals	27	205	232	Prevalence	12%		

BOX B.6
EFFECT OF CHANGING TESTS ON SENSITIVITY AND SPECIFICITY. THESE DATA (FROM ARNÉ ET AL BR J ANAESTH 1998; 80:140–146) SHOW THAT, WITHIN THE SAME POPULATION, SOME TESTS ARE MORE SPECIFIC AND LESS SENSITIVE (PREVIOUS HISTORY OF DIFFICULT INTUBATION) WHEREAS OTHERS MAY BE MORE SENSITIVE (HIGHER MALLAMPATI SCORE)

| | | DIFFICULT INTUBATION | | | | | | |
		Yes	No	Totals				
Previous difficult intubation	Yes	7	2	9	Sensitivity	0.14 (7/ 50)	PPV	0.78 (7/9)
	No	43	1148	1191	Specificity	0.998 (1148/1150)	NPV	0.96 (1148/1191)
	Totals	50	1150	1200				
Mallampati 3–4	Yes	39	168	207	Sensitivity	78	PPV	0.19
	No	11	982	993	Specificity	85	NPV	0.99
	Totals	50	1150	1200				

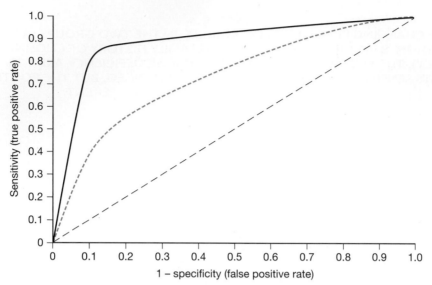

FIGURE B.7 ▪ Receiver-operating characteristic (ROC) curves. The line of identity (i.e. a useless test) is shown as a dashed line. The dotted line shows a moderately discriminatory test (AUC=0.73), whereas the solid line is rather better (AUC=0.88).

benchmarking outcomes against self or others, and in designing research studies.

There are various approaches to creation of such scoring systems. First, predictor variables are chosen, based on some combination of investigator opinion, clinical experience, and previous or ongoing research. The strength of association between the variables and the outcome of interest is assessed, often using logistic regression, in a development cohort. This may then allow creation of a score, whereby relative values (points) are ascribed to each of the variables and summed to create an overall score. The ability of the score to identify risk correctly should then be tested against a separate validation cohort, and ideally against a cohort from outside the original research population.

The commonest method of assessing the *calibration* of scoring systems is to use the *Hosmer–Lemeshow* test. This is an application of the χ^2 test using the observed and predicted outcomes in the population.

Survival Analysis. Rather than looking at events at a specific time interval, we sometimes wish to investigate the effects over time, e.g. disease-free survival following different types of cancer surgery or death following different modes of anaesthesia. These are usually analysed using *Kaplan–Meier* plots (Fig. B.8)

and differences between groups assessed using *log rank* or *Cox proportional hazards* tests.

The number of 'survivors' (as a proportion of the at-risk population) is plotted against time. Note that the 'at-risk' population becomes smaller as the time horizon becomes longer because there are less individuals available for follow-up.

Log rank tests assess the overall difference between survival curves when there are discrete groups (e.g. regional anaesthesia *vs.* general anaesthesia). *Cox proportional hazards* are used for estimating the effect of continuous variables (such as gene expression) on risk.

TYPES OF ERROR

Most statistical questions can be framed with a so-called *null hypothesis.* This is a statement of the form: there is no difference between A and B. Experiments are designed to test this hypothesis. If a set of observations is obtained which is sufficiently unlikely to have occurred if the null hypothesis were true, then the null hypothesis is *rejected.* Conversely, if there is insufficient evidence to reject the null hypothesis, then the experiment has *failed to reject* it. The null hypothesis is never proved. The whole of this chapter has been predicated on the idea that statistics give

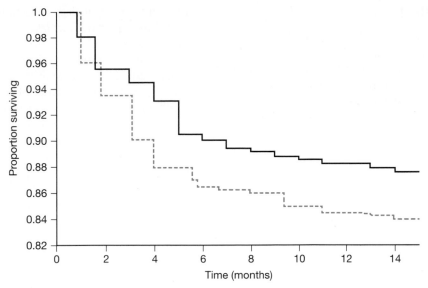

FIGURE B.8 ■ Kaplan–Meier plots. The survival of two groups over time is shown. Each vertical step represents an event. Early on, random variation means that it is not possible to discern the difference in survival between the two groups.

some idea of the probability of an event occurring by chance. This has led statisticians to describe two classical types of statistical error, although more have been proposed.

Type I or **α error** is the probability of a false positive result, falsely rejecting the null hypothesis. It is the '*P*' value used to describe the results and is the type of error most familiar to anaesthetists. For mainly pragmatic reasons within medicine, an accepted type I error rate is 0.05, i.e. 1 in 20.

Type II error or **β error** occurs when the null hypothesis is false, but fails to be rejected. It is directly related to the power of a study (Power = 1 – β). Conventionally, studies have been designed with 80% power, i.e. an 80% chance of rejecting the null hypothesis if it truly should be rejected. More recently, there has been a move to increasing the power of studies. The power of a study is related to the number of participants, the variability in the measurement, the size of difference being sought and the acceptable α error. There is a variety of formulae for estimating the number of participants required for a given power; a simple one is shown below:

$$n = \frac{2\sigma^2 \left(Z_\beta + Z_{\alpha/2} \right)^2}{\Delta^2}$$

n: sample size for each group

σ: standard deviation of outcome variable

Z_β: standardized value based on the desired power (0.84 for 0.8 power)

Z_σ: standardized value based on the desired significance (1.96 for two-sided, α 0.05)

Δ: the clinically significant difference between means

From this, it is straightforward to see that the number of participants needed for a study increases with:

- increasing variability (standard deviation)
- increasing power (Z_β increases as β decreases)
- decreasing type I error (Z_α increases as α decreases)
- smaller clinically significant differences.

Other Categories of Error

Although not part of the traditional Type I and II errors, there are other types of conceptual error – all of which occur within medical research.

- **Type III:** Correctly rejecting the null hypothesis but for the wrong reason
- **Type IV:** Giving the correct answer to the wrong question
- **Type V:** Solving the right problem in the right way, but too late.

CLINICAL TRIALS

'A clinical trial is a carefully and ethically designed experiment with the aim of answering some precisely framed question.' This definition by Sir Austin Bradford Hill, a pioneer of clinical trials, is worth remembering because it encapsulates the fundamentals of good clinical trials. They must be careful, ethical, and with a clear question.

In broad terms, clinical studies can be divided into purely observational studies and interventional studies. Both of these **must** fulfil the requirements listed above.

Observational Studies

These generally answer questions such as:

- Is there an association between factor x and outcome y?
- What is the natural history of a particular condition?

There are three main types of observational study: cohort, case-control and cross-sectional studies.

Cohort studies may be prospective or retrospective. A cohort is a group of people who share a common experience (e.g. all having cancer surgery, first-time labouring women, children under the age of 3 years). Exposures of interest are recorded by the investigators. This cohort is then followed up for sufficient time for the outcome of interest to occur: cancer recurrence; long-term backache; psychological testing at school entry. The relative risk of developing the outcome of interest with and without exposure is then calculated. As with all observational studies, association can be shown but not causality. Confounding factors are a particular issue. To take the three examples: regional anaesthesia may be associated with a lower cancer recurrence rate than general anaesthesia, but this may be due to patient selection or surgical technique; backache may be associated with epidural analgesia, but women requesting epidural analgesia may be those with other reasons to develop post-partum back pain; intellectual ability may be associated with general anaesthetic exposure in childhood, but anaesthesia is always administered in conjunction with surgery or investigations.

Prospective studies take a long time to complete and suffer from loss to follow-up. They have the advantage that the investigators have control over the nature and timing of data collection. They can give information about the *incidence* and *prevalence* of a disease or condition.

Incidence is the **rate** of occurrence of a condition. It is usually expressed relative to the population at risk. For example, the UK incidence of stroke in 2008 was 1.04/1000 person years: in other words, just over one stroke for every 1000 people in one year.

Prevalence is the **proportion** of people with the condition. For example, for the same period, the prevalence of stroke was 7.2/1000 people.

Retrospective studies are sometimes easier to perform, but can suffer from poor quality data collection, bias in data recording and incomplete cohorts.

Case Control Studies

For rare diseases, it may be impractical to identify and follow up a sufficiently large cohort. Instead, 'cases' are identified and matched with 'controls' – individuals without the condition. The odds ratio of exposure for case and controls is then used to estimate risk. The classic example of a case control study is the work of Sir Richard Doll demonstrating the link between tobacco smoking and lung cancer. Within anaesthesia, case control studies have been used to investigate relatively unusual events such as postoperative mortality and failed tracheal intubation. By definition, case control studies are retrospective, because they rely on already identified cases.

Cross-Sectional Studies

Cross-sectional studies involve data collected from a defined population at a single period of time. This is unlike cohort and case-control studies, which involve some collection of data over time. Cross-sectional studies can therefore be used to determine the *prevalence* of conditions. One of the best known cross-sectional studies in perioperative medicine was the EPIC study, which recorded the prevalence of intensive care unit infections in over 1400 units across Europe on a single day.

Interventional Studies

These studies intervene in some way such as:

- using a new/different drug
- delivering care in a different way
- using a different technique.

The 'gold standard' for interventional studies is the multicentre, randomized, controlled, multiply-blinded trial. However, there are many situations in which this cannot occur for ethical, practical and financial reasons, and modifications of the design may be used.

Framing the Question

Before starting any study, an investigator needs to have a clear concept of why the research is needed and how it is to be carried out. There are many structures used to assist in this, but a common device is the **EPICOT** framework. This stands for Evidence, Population, Intervention, Comparison, Outcome and Timeliness. The framework applies to observational studies, interventional studies and systematic reviews.

Evidence. What is the existing research and clinical evidence within the field? Have distinct gaps in knowledge been identified? This requires thorough and systematic searching and appraisal of the literature. Systematic reviews and meta-analyses may already have been done, or if not, may be required.

Population. Many research studies fail to identify clearly the appropriate research population. This needs to be relevant, plausible and accessible to the researcher. For instance, the author's main research interest is in fragility hip fracture. However, there are many studies purporting to be of hip fracture which include sizeable numbers of young patients or patients undergoing elective hip arthroplasty. In the same group, undisplaced intracapsular fractures almost never need blood transfusion, so there is little to be gained from undertaking transfusion-related studies in this group.

Inclusion and exclusion criteria need to be clearly defined and justified for any study. If these are too restrictive, the generalizability of the study may be questioned. Conversely, overly lax criteria reduce the power of the study.

Intervention. Even apparently straightforward drug trials need care in defining the intervention. Consider the previously mentioned hypothetical anti-emetic study of NoVom. What dose should be used? When should it be given? By which route? There is not usually a single perfect answer to these questions, so it is up to the researcher to justify their choices.

Comparison. If the intervention can be hard to pin down, the comparison can be even trickier. Head-to-head drug trials (e.g. cyclizine *vs.* NoVom) usually define two 'intervention' groups, but often the comparator is 'normal' or 'standard' care. If standard care is too loosely defined and practice varies greatly within the comparator groups then it becomes difficult to define exactly what the intervention is being compared with. Conversely, a rigidly defined 'normal' care group may lack relevance to real life.

Outcome. Most clinicians want to know whether something is 'better' than something else. Unfortunately, 'better' is very much in the eye of the beholder. Researchers therefore need to be absolutely clear about the outcome they wish to assess. There is usually a trade-off between practicality of a study and the outcomes of real interest to patients and clinicians. There are myriad studies of intubating devices such as video laryngoscopes. The outcome of interest in these studies is often well defined (e.g. time to successful insertion of tracheal tube) but may not be particularly relevant to patients. Conversely, studies to demonstrate differences in airway-associated mortality would require vast, probably impractical, numbers of participants.

As the research develops from an idea into a full proposal, this section should expand into a fully worked through data collection and statistical analysis plan.

Timeliness. Funders need to know that there is some pressing reason for research to be undertaken now. This may be because practice has changed, new drugs are available or the population has changed.

Regulatory Approvals

All research requires some regulatory approval. There are various legal and ethical requirements set out in guidance and national statutes such as the EU Good Clinical Practice Directive, the Medicines for Human Use (Clinical Trials) Regulations 2004 (and similar legislation internationally) and the Declaration of Helsinki.

Ethical Review. A properly constituted ethical review committee must consider the proposed study and whether the research is ethical and scientifically sound. The role of the ethical review committee is to safeguard the rights, safety, dignity and well-being of people participating in research.

Sponsorship. All research requires a sponsor. This is an organization (or occasionally an individual) which takes responsibility for:

- implementing and maintaining quality assurance and quality control systems
- securing written agreements with all involved parties to ensure direct access to:
  - all trial-related sites
  - source data and documents
  - reports for the purpose of monitoring and auditing by the sponsor and inspection by regulatory agencies
- applying quality control measures to each stage of data handling to ensure that all data are reliable and have been processed correctly.

These responsibilities are usually taken on by pharmaceutical companies, universities or hospitals. In order to meet these responsibilities, the sponsor will have standard operating procedures covering all stages of the research process and regular systematic audit of the research it sponsors.

Local Approvals. The site where the research is to occur needs to approve the research before it can start. This is to ensure that there are adequate facilities and resources to undertake the study in a safe and timely fashion and that there are no undue conflicts with other ongoing studies.

National Approvals. There may be other regulatory bodies which need to be involved, depending on the country and type of research. For instance, in the UK, drug-related studies require approval from the Medicines and Healthcare products Regulatory Agency (MHRA), and gamete and embryo research requires approval from The Human Fertilisation and Embryology Authority (HFEA).

Trial Registration. In an attempt to reduce the risks of selective reporting, most journals now require that clinical trials are registered in publicly accessible trials registries such as Clinicaltrials.gov or the International Standard Randomised Controlled Trial Number (ISRCTN) register.

The intended consequence of these approval processes is that investigators need to comply with a strict framework which should protect the rights and well-being of participants as well as ensuring the quality of research. The ethical review should ensure that research studies are presented to potential participants in open, understandable and unbiased fashion. The research governance frameworks of the sponsor facilitate the design of high quality and efficient research. The undoubted downside is an increase in bureaucracy and costs.

Specific Aspects of Trial Conduct

Informed consent. Involvement in clinical research is a voluntary activity, for which individuals are free to give or withhold their consent. There are strict rules about the amount and type of information which individuals should be given as part of the research process. Investigators must be extremely careful to ensure that potential participants understand the purpose of the research and what it will involve for them, and that they have adequate time to consider the study and discuss it with other people if they wish.

For some areas of research, particularly in perioperative and critical care, it may not be possible to give participants a prolonged period of time to consider inclusion in a study. Wherever possible, investigators should seek to confirm continued consent to study participation at a later date.

There may be occasions on which participants cannot consent for themselves, such as patients who have temporarily lost capacity (such as those unconscious following trauma) or who have longstanding conditions (such as dementia) meaning they are incapable of understanding the information given to them. In these situations, the ethical review committee will consider carefully the balance of risks and benefits to potential participants before granting approval for studies.

Randomization. As discussed earlier in the chapter, a truly random allocation of study participants to treatment groups is very important. Although, in theory, tossing a coin should be adequate, in practice this is a fallible approach, and more and more sophisticated systems have been introduced. Most studies now use some form of computerized system. A good randomization system should ensure several aspects of good trial conduct.

- *A truly random allocation.* Usually the allocations are made with reference to computer-generated random number tables. The investigator has no influence at all on the allocation.
- *An audit trail of randomizations.* It is possible for the sponsor to verify who has been randomized and when.
- *Entry validation.* Screening questions can be included in the randomization process, which ensure that only eligible participants are randomized.
- *Blinding of allocation.* For placebo-controlled studies, the allocation is usually to a pack-number, made up elsewhere, to reduce the risk of the investigator knowing the treatment allocation.

Blinding. In order to reduce investigator and participant bias, ideally all parties would be completely unaware of treatment allocation. The use of the terms single-blind or double-blind are probably best avoided because they do not clearly define who is blinded to what. Such complete blinding is only really possible for drug trials with a placebo or active comparator which has an identical formulation and no easily discerned physiological effects (e.g. bradycardia with β-blockers).

Even though this 'gold standard' is not often achievable, investigators should design their studies in ways to reduce the risk of bias to a minimum. Individuals responsible for data collection should be unaware of treatment allocation, data should be analysed prior to code-breaking as far as possible and clear definitions of outcomes of interest should be provided before data collection starts.

Completeness of Follow-Up. It is extremely important that, as far as possible, data are recorded for all participants in a study. This is to ensure that results are not biased by disproportionate loss of follow-up between groups. Excessive loss to follow-up may raise questions about either the tolerability of the protocol or the adequacy of the research team.

Stages of Drug Trials

Anaesthetists have a professional interest in new drugs. In order to be available for general human use, new drugs have to go through a rigorous process of testing. There are various phases of research outlined in Table B.1. Many drugs fail at the phase 2 stage, often due to unexpected toxicity. Post-marketing surveillance (phases 4 and 5) is an important part of drug development because this is where the real-world effectiveness of the drug is evaluated.

Publication

All research should be disseminated to a wider audience in some way. Traditionally, this has been through the media of scientific conferences and printed publication in peer-reviewed journals. Increasingly, the internet is changing the way in which research results are disseminated. In addition, funders are keen to see their research reaching relevant parties such as patients, non-research clinicians, industry and policy making groups such as charities, medical colleges and associations, and government bodies. The presentation of material for each of these audiences is different – one style does not suit all. Researchers often find it difficult to explain their findings in ways that are meaningful to non-experts and even the most experienced researcher is likely to benefit from lay advice.

Peer-reviewed journals all have their own style, which should be adhered to. However, they all have common core standards. These include the following:

- *Transparency and probity.* Sufficient detail should be given of the research so that others can understand what has been done. There should be no suspicion of hidden data.
- *Intelligible writing.* Published research is wasted if no-one can understand what is being presented.
- *Relevance.* Most journals have a target audience and will not publish material which is unlikely to be of interest to their subscribers.
- *Single publication.* With some exceptions, journals will not tolerate duplicate publication (i.e. publication of a paper that has been previously published elsewhere in whole or in part.) This is partly an issue of honesty, but duplicate publication also distorts the scientific record by exaggerating the results of research.

Publication Checklists. In the same way that the research governance framework should ensure that research is performed well, there are international consensus statements/checklists which journals encourage or require authors to use when submitting.

TABLE B.1

Phases of Drug Development

Phase	Outcomes	Doses Used	Participants (Typical Numbers)	Comments
Preclinical	Mode of action, toxicity, pharmacokinetics, interactions	Wide range	*In vitro* *In vivo* animals Different species and ages	How does the drug work? Is it likely to be safe to use in humans?
Phase 0	Human pharmacodynamics and pharmacokinetics	Very low – sub-therapeutic	Healthy volunteers (10)	Often combined with Phase 1 No information about efficacy or safety. Used to rank candidate drugs to take forward to Phase 1
Phase 1	Dose ranging, safety	Very low and increasing doses. Maximum doses are below toxic doses in animals	Healthy volunteers (20–80)	Is the drug safe to use in phase 2 studies? Single and multiple dosing studies.
Phase 2	Efficacy and more safety data	Range of therapeutic doses	Patients with relevant conditions (100–300)	Does the drug actually work? (2a) What dose should be used? (2b)
Phase 3	Efficacy in trials	Range of therapeutic doses	Patients in clinical trials with relevant conditions (1000–3000)	Does the drug work in patients? Randomized clinical trials and open-label studies.
Phase 4	Post-marketing surveillance	Therapeutic doses	Clinical use (thousands)	Rare side-effects Use in wider populations
Phase 5	Effectiveness research	Therapeutic dose	Clinical use (thousands)	Clinical effectiveness Cost–benefit

CONSORT (Consolidated Standards of Reporting Trials) is a 25-item checklist and flow diagram. It aims to guide authors in reporting all stages of trial design, participant flow, analysis and interpretation (http://www.consort-statement.org/consort-statement/).

STROBE (STrengthening the Reporting of OBservational studies in Epidemiology) is a similar approach for observational studies (http://www.strobe-statement.org/).

Presentation of Results. Journals have their own styles for presentation of summary data and probability values, and these should be followed.

One area of considerable confusion is presentation of the magnitude of effect of a treatment or exposure. Although most of the terms are mathematically interchangeable, the interpretation of each by clinicians, patients and managers may be very different.

Absolute Risk (AR). This is simply the probability of an event occurring without reference to anything else. For instance, the absolute risk of PONV is usually quoted as around 30%. It gives no information about factors which might influence the risk.

Relative Risk (RR). This is the ratio of risk between those with and without exposure. For instance, smokers are about 10 times more likely to get lung cancer than non-smokers so their relative risk is 10. Importantly, the relative risk gives no information about the absolute risk. A doubling of risk for a very rare event still makes the event very rare.

Absolute Risk Reduction (ARR). Absolute risk reduction is the difference in absolute risk between two groups. For instance, in designing the BAG-RECALL study (to compare the incidence of accidental anaesthetic awareness when bispectral index (BIS) or end-tidal gas monitoring was used to regulate depth of anaesthesia), the investigators estimated that the absolute risk of awareness in their two groups would be 0.5% (5 in 1000) in the end-tidal agent monitoring group and 0.1% (1 in 1000) in the (BIS) group. The estimated absolute risk reduction was therefore 0.4% (4 in 1000).

Relative Risk Reduction (RRR). Relative risk reduction is the proportional difference in risk. To take the BAG-RECALL example above, the estimated RRR was 0.4%/0.5% = 80%.

Number Needed to Treat (NNT). The number needed to treat is the number of individuals who would be needed to be treated with the 'new' treatment rather than the old one, for one to benefit. It is the reciprocal of the absolute risk reduction. Again, using the BAG-RECALL example, the estimated NNT was 250 (1/0.04).

Number Needed to Harm (NNH). Given that all drugs have side-effects, the equivalent to the NNT can also be calculated. For instance, a meta-analysis of opioids added to single-shot intrathecal anaesthesia found a NNH for fentanyl-induced pruritus of 3.3. In other words, the absolute risk increase was 30% (1/3.3).

Odds Ratio. In some situations, odds ratios are the appropriate statistical measure, particularly for logistic regression-based techniques. Unfortunately, they are slightly counterintuitive. The odds of an event occurring are the number of events divided by the number of non-events. The odds ratio is simply the ratio of two groups.

The odds ratio overestimates relative risk. This effect becomes smaller as the absolute risk decreases, so for uncommon events the odds ratio **approximates**

BOX B.7
CALCULATION OF ODDS RATIO, ABSOLUTE RISK AND RELATIVE RISK FOR COMPLICATIONS CAUSED BY VENOUS THROMBOEMBOLISM (VTE)

	GA	Neuraxial
Major VTE and VTE-related mortality	73	101
No major VTE and VTE-related mortality	1658	3204
Total	1731	3305
Odds	0.044 (73/1658)	0.032 (101/3204)
Odds ratio	1.4 (0.044/0.032)	
Absolute risk	0.042 (73/1731)	0.031 (101/3305)
Relative risk	1.35 (0.042/0.031)	

relative risk. For example, data from a meta-analysis of type of anaesthesia and thrombotic events after major orthopaedic surgery is shown in Box B.7.

FURTHER READING

Altman, D.G., 2005. Practical statistics for medical research, second ed. Taylor & Francis, London.
Browner, W.S., 1994. A simple recipe for doing it well. Anesthesiology 80, 923.
Cruikshank, S., 1998. Mathematics and statistics in anaesthesia. Oxford University Press, Oxford.
Greenhalgh, T., 2010. How to read a paper – the basis of evidence-based medicine, third ed. BMJ Publishing Group, London.
Rowntree, D., 1991. Statistics without tears. Penguin, London.
Tramèr, M.R. (Ed.), 2003. Evidence-based-resource in anaesthesia and analgesia, second ed. BMJ Publishing Group, London.

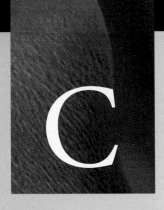

CLINICAL DATA

APPENDIX C (IA): ABBREVIATIONS USED IN TEXT AND APPENDICES

α	adrenoceptor type (after Ahlquist)
ABO	nomenclature for blood groups (after Landsteiner)
ACD	acid citrate dextrose
ACE	angiotensin-converting enzyme
ACh(R)	acetylcholine (receptor)
ACS	Acute coronary syndrome
ACT	activated clotting time
ACTH	adrenocorticotrophic hormone
ADH	antidiuretic hormone
ADP	adenosine diphosphate
AER	auditory evoked response
AIDS	acquired immunodeficiency syndrome
AIP	acute intermittent porphyria
ALS	advanced life support
ALT	alanine aminotransferase
AMP	adenosine monophosphate
AMPA	γ-amino-3-hydroxy-5-methyl-4-isoxazole propionate
ANP	atrial natriuretic peptide
ANS	autonomic nervous system
APACHE	acute physiological and chronic health evaluation
APTT	activated partial thromboplastin time
ARDS	acute respiratory distress syndrome
ASA	American Society of Anesthesiologists
Asp	L-aspartate

AST	aspartate aminotransferase
AT	antithrombin
ATP	adenosine triphosphate
AUC	area under curve
AV	atrioventricular
β	adrenoceptor type (after Ahlquist)
B	bone marrow-dependent (as in B cells)
BM	Boehringer Mannheim (makers of BM Stix blood glucose testing strips)
BP	*British Pharmacopoeia*
BSA	body surface area
BW	body weight
BZ	benzodiazepine
C	cervical or coccygeal vertebra
C	compliance
C	content
°C	degrees Celsius
C_3F_8	perfluoropropane
Ca	calcium
$CaCO_3$	calcium carbonate
cAMP	cyclic adenosine monophosphate
CaO	calcium oxide
CAVG	coronary artery vein graft
CBF	cerebral blood flow
CC	closing capacity
CCU	coronary care unit

CDH	Christiansen Douglas Haldane (effect)		CV	closing volume
CEA	Carotid endarterectomy		CVP	central venous pressure
CEPOD	Confidential Enquiry into Perioperative Deaths (UK)		C_x	clearance of x
			Δ	delta – minimal increment (of)
CEMACE	Centre for Maternal and Child Enquiries		δ	delta opioid receptor
CEMD	Confidential Enquiries into Maternal Deaths		D	dose (of drug)
CFAM	cerebral function analyzing monitor		d	density
CFM	cerebral function monitor		d	deci (one-tenth part)
CGRP	calcitonin gene-related peptide		Da	dalton (measure of atomic weight)
CHO	carbohydrate		D&C	dilatation and curettage (of uterus)
CI	cardiac index (cardiac output/body surface area)		DAP	diastolic arterial pressure
			DBS	double burst stimulation
CK	creatine kinase		DC	direct current
Cl	clearance (of drug)		DCR	dacrocystorhinostomy
cm	centimetre (10^{-2} m; not a unit in the SI system)		DDAVP	desmopressin
			DFP	di-isopropyl fluorophosphonate
cmH_2O	centimetres of water		DIC	disseminated intravascular coagulation
$CMRO_2$	cerebral metabolic rate for oxygen		DNA	deoxyribonucleic acid
CMV	cytomegalovirus		DoH	Department of Health
CNS	central nervous system		Dopa	Deoxyphenylalanine
C_0	concentration at time=0		2,3-DPG	2,3-diphosphoglycerate
CO	cardiac output		dTC	dextrotubocurarine
CO_2	carbon dioxide		DVT	deep vein thrombosis
cp	centipoise		ECC	extracorporeal circulation (heart bypass)
CPAP	continuous positive airways pressure		ECF(V)	extracellular fluid (volume)
CPB	cardiopulmonary bypass		ECG	electrocardiogram
CPD	citrate phosphate dextrose		ECT	electroconvulsive therapy
CPD-A	citrate phosphate dextrose with adenine		EDTA	ethylenediaminetetra-acetic acid
CP(E)X	Cardiopulmonary exercise testing		ED_x	effective dose for x% of population
CPK	creatine phosphokinase		EEG	electroencephalogram
CPP	cerebral perfusion pressure		EF	ejection fraction
CPR	cardiopulmonary resuscitation		EMD	electromechanical dissociation (PEA)
^{51}Cr	chromium atom – isotope weight 51 Da (radiolabelled)		EMG	electromyogram
CSF	cerebrospinal fluid		EMLA®	eutectic mixture of local anaesthetic
C_{ss}	concentration at steady state		ENNS	early neonatal neurobehavioural score
C_t	concentration at time t		ENT	ear, nose and throat
CT	computed tomography		EP	evoked potential
CTM	cricothyroid membrane		EPI	Eysenck personality inventory

EPP	end-plate potential
ERPOC	evacuation of retained products of conception
ESWL	extracorporeal shock wave lithotripsy
EU	European Union
EUA	examination under anaesthesia
EVAR	Endovascular aneurysm repair
EVR	endocardial viability ratio
F	Faraday's constant
FDP	fibrin degradation products
$Fe^{2+(3+)}$	iron ionized – ferrous (ferric) ion
FEV_1	forced expiratory volume (in 1 s)
FF	filtration fraction
FFA	free fatty acid
FFP	fresh frozen plasma
FGF	fresh gas flow
F_IO_2	fractional inspired oxygen concentration
FRC	functional residual capacity
FSH	follicle-stimulating hormone
FVC	forced vital capacity
g	gram
G6PD	glucose-6-phosphate dehydrogenase
GABA	γ-aminobutyric acid
GCS	Glasgow coma score
GFR	glomerular filtration rate
GH	growth hormone
GI	gastrointestinal
Glu	L-glutamate
Gly	glycine
GMP	glutamate monophosphate
GOS	Glasgow outcome score
GTN	glyceryl trinitrate
η	viscosity
h	hour
H^+	hydrogen ion
H_1	histamine – type 1 receptor
H_2	histamine – type 2 receptor
HAFOE	high air flow oxygen enrichment
Hb	haemoglobin

HbA	adult haemoglobin
HbF	fetal haemoglobin
HbNH	carbamino haemoglobin
HBsAg	hepatitis B surface antigen
hCG	human chorionic gonadotrophin
HCO_3^-	bicarbonate ion
H_2CO_3	carbonic acid
Hct	haematocrit
HDU	high-dependency unit
He	helium
HELLP	syndrome of haemolysis, elevated liver enzymes, low platelets
HFJV	high-frequency jet ventilation
HFOV	high-frequency oscillatory ventilation
HFPPV	high-frequency positive-pressure ventilation
HFV	high-frequency ventilation
Hg	mercury
5-HIAA	5-hydroxyindoleacetic acid
HIV	human immunodeficiency virus
HLA	human leucocyte antigen
HOCM	hypertrophic obstructive cardiomyopathy
HPA	hypothalamopituitary axis
hPL	human placental lactogen
HPV	hypoxic pulmonary vasoconstriction
HR	heart rate
5-HT	5-hydroxytryptamine (serotonin)
HTLV	human T cell leukaemia virus
Hz	hertz (cycles per second)
I	infusion rate
IABP	intra-aortic balloon pump
ICF(V)	intracellular fluid (volume)
ICP	isometric contraction period; intracranial pressure
ID	internal diameter
I/E	inspiratory/expiratory
IgA	immunoglobulin type A (γ-globulin A)
IgE	immunoglobulin type E (γ-globulin E, reagin)
IgG	immunoglobulin type G (γ-globulin G)

ILM	intubating laryngeal mask (airway)
i.m.	intramuscular
IMV	intermittent mandatory ventilation
INR	international normalized ratio
IOP	intraocular pressure
IPPV	intermittent positive-pressure ventilation
IRP	isometric relaxation period
ISA	intrinsic sympathomimetic activity
ITU	intensive therapy unit
i.v.	intravenous
IVC	inferior vena cava
IVF	in vitro fertilization
IVRA	intravenous regional anaesthesia
J	joule
κ	kappa – opioid receptor type
K	kelvin
K^+	potassium ion
K_i^+	potassium ion (inside cell)
K_o^+	potassium ion (outside cell)
KCCT	kaolin cephalin clotting time
kg	kilogram
kPa	kilopascal
l	length
L (n)	lumbar vertebra (number n)
LAP	left atrial pressure
LATS	long-acting thyroid stimulator
lb in^{-2}	pounds per square inch
LDH	lactate dehydrogenase
LH	luteinizing hormone
LISS	low ionic strength saline
lm	lumen
LMA	laryngeal mask airway
LMN	lower motor neuron
ln	natural logarithm (to base e)
log	logarithm (to base 10)
LOS	lower oesophageal sphincter
LSCS	lower-segment caesarean section
LVEDP	left ventricular end-diastolic pressure

μ	micro (10^{-6}); mu opioid receptor type
μV	microvolts
m	metre
mA	milliampere
MAC	minimum alveolar concentration (for anaesthesia)
MAHA	Microangiopathic haemolytic anaemia
MAO	monoamine oxidase
MAOI	monoamine oxidase inhibitor
MAP	mean arterial pressure
MC	Mary Caterill (name of proprietary mask)
MCH	Mean corpuscular haemoglobin
MCV	mean corpuscular volume
MEAC	minimum effective analgesic concentration
MEPP	miniature end-plate potential
mg	milligram
Mg^{2+}	magnesium ion
MH	malignant hyperthermia
MI	myocardial infarction
min	minute
mL	millilitre
mm	millimetre
mmHg	millimetres of mercury
MMPI	Minnesota multiphasic personality inventory
MMV	mandatory minute ventilation
mN	millinewton
mol	mole
mosmol	milliosmole
MRI	magnetic resonance imaging
ms	millisecond
MSH	melanocyte-stimulating hormone
mV	millivolt
MVP	mean venous pressure
MW	molecular weight
N	newton (unit of force)
N/A	not available; not applicable
Na	sodium
Na^+	sodium ion

NACS	neurological & adaptive capacity score
Na/K-ATPase	sodium- and potassium-dependent adenosine triphosphatase
NH_3	ammonia
NH_4^+	ammonium ion
NHS	National Health Service (UK)
NMDA	N-methyl-D-aspartate
NO	nitric oxide
N_2O	nitrous oxide
NSAID	non-steroidal anti-inflammatory drug
NTD	neural tube defect
O_2	oxygen
OAA	Obstetric Anaesthetists' Association
ODC	oxyhaemoglobin dissociation curve
ODP	operating department practitioner
osmol	osmole
π	pi (≈ 3.14159)
π_{BC}	oncotic pressure in Bowman's capsule
π_{CAP}	oncotic pressure in capillary
P	wave on ECG (P-wave)
P_{50}	oxygen tension which results in a haemoglobin saturation of 50%
Pa	pascal (unit of pressure)
P_A	alveolar partial pressure (of gas)
P_a	arterial partial pressure (of gas)
PAFC	pulmonary artery flotation catheter
PAH	para-aminohippuric acid
PAP	pulmonary artery pressure
PAOP	pulmonary artery occlusion pressure (= PCWP)
P_B	barometric pressure
P_{BC}	hydrostatic pressure in Bowman's capsule
PCA(S)	patient-controlled analgesia (system)
P_{CAP}	hydrostatic pressure in capillary
PCWP	pulmonary capillary wedge pressure
PDPH	post-dural puncture headache
PE	pulmonary embolus
$P_{\bar{E}}$	mean expired partial pressure

P_E	end-expired partial pressure
PEA	pulseless electrical activity (EMD)
PEEP	positive end-expiratory pressure
PEFR	peak expiratory flow rate
PF	pathological fibrinolysis
PG(X)	prostaglandin type (X)
pH	hydrogen ion activity (negative logarithm to base 10 of the measured hydrogen ion concentration)
P_I	inspired partial pressure
PIFR	peak inspiratory flow rate
pK_a	expression of dissociation constant in an equilibrium (negative logarithm to base 10 of the dissociation constant)
PMGV	piped medical gases and vacuum systems
PONV	postoperative nausea and vomiting
ppm	parts per million
PRN	pro re nata (as needed)
PRP	platelet-rich plasma
PTA	plasma thromboplastin antecedent (factor IX)
PTF	post-tetanic facilitation
PTP	post-tetanic potentiation
P_tCO_2	transcutaneous oxygen partial pressure
PTT(K)	partial thromboplastin time (kaolin)
PVC	polyvinyl chloride; premature ventricular contraction
PVR	pulmonary vascular resistance
$\dot{Q}_t$	total liquid flow in unit time
QRS	complex on ECG (QRS complex)
ρ	rho (= density)
r	radius (of circle or sphere)
R	universal gas constant
RA_x	renal artery concentration of x
RAP	right atrial pressure
RAST	radioallergosorbent test
RBF	renal blood flow
RDS	respiratory distress syndrome
Re	Reynolds number (dimensionless)
REM	rapid eye movement

RH	relative humidity		SVT	supraventricular tachycardia
Rh(x)	Rhesus blood group (major phenotype x)		T	thymus-dependent (T cells)
RLF	retrolental fibroplasia		T	temperature
RNA	ribonucleic acid		$t_{1/2\alpha}$	α half-life (distribution half-life)
RPF	renal plasma flow		$t_{1/2\beta}$	β half-life (elimination half-life)
RPP	rate–pressure product		T_3	tri-iodothyronine
RQ	respiratory quotient		T_4	thyroxine
RSD	reflex sympathetic dystrophy		TA	titratable acid
RV	residual volume		TBG	thyroxine-binding globulin
RV_x	renal vein concentration of x		TBW	total body water
s	second		TEC®	temperature controlled (vaporizer)
S	saturation (of haemoglobin)		TENS	transcutaneous electrical nerve stimulation
SA	sinoatrial		TEPP	tetraethyl pyrophosphate
SAB	subarachnoid block		TFA	trifluoroacetyl
SAGM	saline adenine glucose mannitol		TISS	therapeutic intervention severity score
SAP	systolic arterial pressure		TIVA	total intravenous anaesthesia
s.c.	subcutaneous		TLA	translumbar aortography
SDP	subdural pressure		TLC	total lung capacity
SF_6	sulphur hexafluoride		Tm	tubular maximal reabsorption
SG	specific gravity		TMJ	temporomandibular joint
SH	sulphydryl group		TMP	trimetaphan camsylate
SI	*Système International d'Unités*		TNS	transcutaneous nerve stimulation
SIADH	syndrome of inappropriate antidiuretic hormone secretion		TOF	train of four
			TPR	total (systemic) peripheral resistance
SIIFT	syndrome of inappropriate intravenous fluid therapy		TSH	thyroid-stimulating hormone
			TTP/HUS	Thrombotic thrombocytopaenic purpura/ haemolytic uraemic syndrome
SIMV	synchronized intermittent mandatory ventilation		TURP	transurethral resection of prostate
SNP	sodium nitroprusside		TWC	total water content
SOL	space-occupying lesion		TXA_2	thromboxane A_2
SR	slow release		U	urine concentration
SRS-A	slow-reacting substance of anaphylaxis		UK	United Kingdom
SSRI	selective serotonin reuptake inhibitor		URT(I)	upper respiratory tract (infection)
STOP	surgical termination of pregnancy		USA	United States of America
STP	standard temperature and pressure		V	volt
SV	stroke volume		V	volume
SVC	superior vena cava		$\dot{V}_t$	volume per unit time (gas flow)
SVP	saturated vapour pressure			

v	velocity	VIE	vacuum insulated evaporator
VATS	Video assisted thoracoscopic surgery	VIP	vasoactive intestinal peptide
VC	vital capacity	VT	ventricular tachycardia
V_d	dead space (ventilation); volume of distribution	V_t	tidal volume
$V_{d(ANAT)}$	anatomical dead space	vWF	von Willebrand factor
$V_{d(PHYS)}$	physiological dead space	W	watt
VF	ventricular fibrillation	WHO	World Health Organization

APPENDIX C (IB): SI SYSTEM

The *Système International d'Unités* (SI system) has been developed to reduce the large number of units in everyday physical use to a much smaller number, with standard symbols.

The seven base units are derivatives of the MKS system of physical measurement:		
Length	metre	m
Mass	kilogram	kg
Time	second	s
Electric current	amp	A
Thermodynamic temperature	kelvin	K
Amount of substance	mole	mol
Luminous intensity	candela	cd

Any other units are derived units and may be expressed by multiplication or division of base units:

Volume	cubic metre	m^3		
Force	newton	N	$kg\,m\,s^{-2}$	$= J\,m^{-1}$ (J/m)
Work	joule	J	$kg\,m^2\,s^{-2}$	$= N\,m$
Power (rate of work)	watt	W	$kg\,m^2\,s^{-3}$	$= J\,s^{-1}$ (J/s)
Pressure (force/area)	pascal	Pa	$kg\,m^{-1}\,s^{-2}$	$= N\,m^{-2}$ (N/m^2)

X^{-1} has been used in preference to the solidus (/), either of which is specified in the standard.

Non-standard units such as the litre (L), day hour and minute may be used with SI but are not part of the standard.

VOLUME

The SI unit of volume is the cubic metre, but for medical purposes the litre (L or dm^3) is retained.

TEMPERATURE

A temperature difference of 1 kelvin (1 K) is numerically equivalent to 1 degree Celsius (1 °C). In everyday use the degree Celsius is retained. The Fahrenheit scale is no longer used medically. It is being phased out of use with the general public.

Fraction	SI prefix	Symbol	Multiple	SI prefix	Symbol
10^{-1}	deci	d	10	deca	da
10^{-2}	centi	c	10^2	hecto	h
10^{-3}	milli	m	10^3	kilo	k
10^{-6}	micro	μ	10^6	mega	M
10^{-9}	nano	n	10^9	giga	G
10^{-12}	pico	p	10^{12}	tera	T
10^{-15}	femto	f	10^{15}	peta	P
10^{-18}	atto	a	10^{18}	exa	E

The magnitude of a unit is expressed by the addition of standard prefixes and symbolic prefixes. The magnitude of SI units usually changes by 10^3 per step. It can be seen that the SI handling of 'kilogram' is non-standard; the name of the base unit already contains a preficacial multiple. Names of decimal multiples and submultiples of the unit of mass are formed by attaching prefixes to the word 'gram'.

PRESSURE MEASUREMENTS – CONVERSION FACTORS

Old Units	SI Units	Old to SI (Conversion Factor)	SI to Old (Conversion Factor)
mmHg	kPa	0.133	7.5
bar	kPa	101.3	0.01
cmH_2O	kPa	0.0981	10
lb/sq in	kPa	6.894	0.145

MOLES

Moles = weight in g/molecular weight
   Thus 1 mol H_2O = 18 g/18
   18 g H_2O = 1 mol

For univalent ions, moles and equivalents are numerically equal, but for multivalent ions the number of equivalents must be divided by the valency to obtain the molar value. Thus 10 mEq Ca^{2+} = 5 mmol Ca^{2+}.

MOLES/OSMOLES

Strictly the SI unit of osmolality should be the mole, this representing the calculated number of particles/molecules in solution. However, the osmole is also used; this is the measured osmolality (the number of osmotically active particles per kilogram of solution). Thus, the molar value for osmolality is theoretical, while the osmolar value is empirical.

APPENDIX C (II): INHALATIONAL ANAESTHETIC AGENTS – PHYSICAL PROPERTIES

Name	Formula	MW (Da)	BP (°C)	SVP (kPa, 20°C)	MAC (%)	Flammable in O_2	OSTWALD SOLUBILITY COEFFICIENTS AT 37°C			
							Blood/Gas	Fat/Blood	Oil/Gas	Oil/H_2O
Nitrous oxide	N_2O	44	-88	(5300)	105	0	0.47	2.3	1.4	3.2
Halothane	$CF_3CHClBr$	197	50	32	0.75		2.3	51	224	220
Enflurane	$CHFCl\ CF_2O\ CF_2H$	184.5	56	23	1.7	6	1.9	36	98	120
Isoflurane	$CF_3CHCl\ O\ CF_2H$	184.5	49	32	1.15	6	1.4	45	98	174
Desflurane	$CF_2H\ O\ CFHCF_3$	168	23.5	89	6.0	18–21	0.42	27	18.7	
Sevoflurane	$CH(CF_3)_2O\ CH_2F$	200	58.5	21	2.0		0.68	48	47	
Chloroform	$CHCl_3$	119	61	21.3	0.5		10		260	100
Cyclopropane	$CH_2CH_2CH_2$	42	-33	638	9.2	2–60	0.45		11.5	34.4
Diethyl ether	$C_2H_5\ O\ C_2H_5$	74	35	56.5	1.9	2–82	12	5	62	3.2
Ethyl chloride	C_2H_5Cl	64.5	13	131	2.0	4–67	3.0			
Fluroxene	$CF_3CH_2O\ CHCH_2$	126	43	38	3.5	4	1.4		48	90
Methoxyflurane	$CHCl_2CF_2O\ CH_3$	165	105	3	0.2	5–28	13	38	950	400
Trichloroethylene	$CHClCCl_2$	131	87	8	0.17	9–65	9		960	400

MW, molecular weight; BP, boiling point; SVP, saturated vapour pressure; MAC, minimum alveolar concentration. Drugs listed below the bold line have no product licence in the UK. They are of historical interest only. MAC values are for young adults; MAC is higher in children, and decreases in older adults.

APPENDIX C (III): CARDIOVASCULAR SYSTEM

Appendix III: Cardiovascular System

NORMAL VALUES

Blood Flows	% of Cardiac Output	Flow (mL min⁻¹) (70 kg Man)
Heart	4	200
Brain	14	700
Liver	25	1250
Kidneys	24	1200
Lung	3	150
Muscle	19	950
Skin	5	250
Fat	5	250
Remainder	1	50
Total	**100**	**5000**

ECG times	
P wave	< 0.10 s
PR interval	0.12–0.20 s
QRS time	0.05–0.08 s
QT time	0.35–0.40 s
T wave	< 0.22 s

PRESSURES (mmHg)

	Range	Mean
Central venous pressure (CVP)	0–8	4
Right atrial (RA)	0–8	4
Right ventricular (RV)		
Systolic	14–30	25
End-diastolic (RVEDP)	0–8	4
Pulmonary arterial (PA)		
Systolic	15–30	23
Diastolic	5–15	8
Mean (PAP)	10–20	15
Pulmonary artery wedge (PAWP)		
Mean	5–15	10
Left atrial (LA)	4–12	7
Left ventricular (LV)		
Systolic	90–140	120
End-diastolic (LVEDP)	4–12	7

Derived Haemodynamic Variables

Variable		Typical Value (70 kg)
Cardiac output (CO)	$SV \times HR$	5 Lmin⁻¹
Cardiac index (CI)	$CO \div BSA$	3.2 Lmin⁻¹ m⁻²
Stroke volume (SV)	$(CO \div HR) \times 1000$	80 mL
Stroke index (SI)	$SV \div BSA$	50 mLm⁻²
Systemic vascular resistance (SVR)	$((MAP - CVP) \div CO) \times 80$	1000–1200 dyn s cm⁻⁵ (not SI unit)
Pulmonary vascular resistance (PVR)	$((\overline{PAP} - LAP) \div CO) \times 80$	60–120 dyn s cm⁻⁵ (not SI unit)
Left ventricular stroke work index (LVSWI)	$((1.36 (MAP - LAP)) \div 100) \times SI$	50–60 gm m⁻²
Rate–pressure product (RPP)	$SAP \times HR$	9600
Ejection fraction (EF)	$(ESV - EDV) \div EDV$	> 0.6

BSA, body surface area; HR, heart rate; MAP, mean arterial pressure, CVP, central venous pressure; $\overline{PAP}$, mean pulmonary arterial pressure; LAP, left atrial pressure; SAP, systolic arterial pressure; ESV, end-systolic volume; EDV, end-diastolic volume.

Vasoactive Infusion Regimens

Drug	Diluent	Dilution	Concentration	Infusion Rate	Typical Initial Rate(70 kg Adult)
Amiodarone	5% dextrose	300 mg in 50 mL	6 mg mL^{-1}	Loading dose 5 mg kg^{-1} over 1 h then 900 mg over 23 h	25 mLh^{-1} then 6 mLh^{-1}
Digoxin	5% dextrose 0.9% saline	250 µg in 50 mL 500 µg in 50 mL	5 µg mL^{-1} 10 µg mL^{-1}	250–500 µg over 30-60 min	50 mLh^{-1}
Dobutamine	5% dextrose 0.9% saline	250 mg in 50 mL	5 mg mL^{-1}	0–25 µg kg^{-1} min^{-1}	2 mLh^{-1}
Dopamine	5% dextrose 0.9% saline	200 mg in 50 mL	4 mg mL^{-1}	2–15 µg kg^{-1} min^{-1}	2 mLh^{-1}
Dopexamine	5% dextrose 0.9% saline	50 mg in 50 mL	1 mg mL^{-1}	0.25–1.0 µg kg^{-1} min^{-1}	2 mLh^{-1}
Adrenaline	5% dextrose 0.9% saline	5 mg in 50 mL 10 mg in 50 mL	100 µg mL^{-1} 200 µg mL^{-1}	0.02–0.2 µg kg^{-1} min^{-1}	5 mLh^{-1}
Esmolol	5% dextrose 0.9% saline	2.5 g in 50 mL	50 mg mL^{-1}	50–200 µg kg^{-1} min^{-1}	3 mLh^{-1}
Glyceryl trinitrate	5% dextrose 0.9% saline	50 mg in 50 mL	1 mg mL^{-1}	0.5–12 mgh^{-1}	5 mLh^{-1}
Noradrenaline	5% dextrose 0.9% saline	4 mg in 40 mL 8 mg in 40 mL	100 µg mL^{-1} 200 µg mL^{-1}	0–1.0 µg kg^{-1} min^{-1}	5 mLh^{-1} QMC ITU 0–1 µg kg^{-1} min^{-1}
Sodium nitroprusside	5% dextrose	25 mg in 50 mL	500 µg mL^{-1}	0.3–1.5 µg kg^{-1} min^{-1}	7 mLh^{-1}

APPENDIX C (IVA): CHEMICAL PATHOLOGY – BIOCHEMICAL VALUES

These values are given for example only – each reporting laboratory provides reference values for its own population and method. This is especially true of enzyme assays. No inference should be made about the molecular weight of a substance by reference to US and SI values.

Name	US Units	SI Units
Ammonia	80–110 µg%	<50 µmol L^{-1}
Amylase	80–180 Somogyi units%	70–300 IUL^{-1}
Base excess	± 2 mEq L^{-1}	± 2 mmol L$^-$
Bicarbonate		
Actual	22–30 mEq L^{-1}	22–30 mmol L^{-1}
Standard	21–25 mEq L^{-1}	21–25 mmol L^{-1}
Bilirubin – total	0.3–1.1 mg%	3–18 µmol L^{-1}
Buffer base (pH 7.4, PaCO$_2$ 5.3, Hb 15 g dL^{-1})	48 mEq L^{-1}	48 mmol L^{-1}
Calcium	8.5–10.5 mg% (4.5–5.7 mEq L^{-1})	2.25–2.6 mmol L^{-1}
Total		
Ionized	4–5 mg%	1.0–1.25 mmol L^{-1}
Chloride	95–105 mEq L^{-1}	95–105 mmol L^{-1}
Cholesterol	140–300 mg%	3.6–7.8 mmol L^{-1}
Cholinesterase, plasma (pseudocholinesterase)	Dibucaine number >80% usually normal Dibucaine number <20% usually homozygote for atypical cholinesterase	
Copper	80–150 µg%	13–24 nmol L^{-1}
Urinary copper	15–50 µg per 24 h	0.2–0.8 µmol per 24 h
Cortisol {0900 h radioimmunoassay	9–23 µg L^{-1}	250–635 nmol L^{-1}
{2400 h technique	<7.2 µg%	< 200 nmol L^{-1}
Neonatal (competitive protein-binding technique)	30 µg L^{-1}	200–650 nmol L^{-1} < 200 nmol L^{-1} 330–1700 nmol L^{-1}
Creatine (phospho)kinase (CK)	100 IU L^{-1}– male 60 IU L^{-1} – female	25–200 IU L^{-1} 25–150 IU L^{-1}
Creatinine	0.5–1.4 mg%	45–120 µmol L^{-1}
Adrenaline	100 pg mL^{-1}	0.55 nmol L^{-1}
Fibrinogen	150–400 mg%	1.5–4.0 gL^{-1}
Folate	3–20 ng mL^{-1}	3–20 µg L^{-1} 2.1–27 nmol L^{-1}

Continued

Name	*US Units*	*SI Units*
Glucose		
Fasting	55–85 mg%	4–6 mmol L^{-1}
Postprandial	<180 mg%	<10 mmol L^{-1}
γ-Glutamyl transpeptidase	7–25 IU L^{-1}	male: <50 IU L^{-1}
		female: <30 IU L^{-1}
Hydroxybutyrate dehydrogenase (HBD)		100–240 IU L^{-1}
Iodine – total	3.5–8.0 µg L^{-1}	273–624 nmol L^{-1}
^{131}I uptake	20–50% of administered dose in 24 h	
Iron	80–160 µg%	14–30 µmol L^{-1}
Iron-binding capacity	250–400 µg%	45–69 µmol L^{-1}
Lactate	0.6–1.8 mEq L^{-1}	0.6–1.8 mmol L^{-1}
Lactate dehydrogenase	30–90 IU L^{-1}	100–300 IU L^{-1}
Lead		<1.8 µmol L^{-1}
Magnesium	1–2 mg%	0.7–1.0 mmol L^{-1}
	1.5–2.0 mEq L^{-1}	
Methaemoglobin	<3% of total haemoglobin	
Nitrogen (non-protein) (urea+urate+creatinine+creatine)	18–30 mg%	12.8–21.4 mmol L^{-1}
Noradrenaline	200 pg mL^{-1}	1.25 nmol L^{-1}
Osmolality	280–300 mosmol kg^{-1}	280–300 mmol kg^{-1}
Phosphate	2.0–4.5 mg%	0.8–1.4 mmol L^{-1}
	3.0–6.0 mg% (children)	1.0–1.8 mmol L^{-1} (children)
	<8.1 mg% (neonatal)	<2.6 mmol L^{-1} (neonatal)
Phosphatase		
Acid (total)	1–5 KA units%	1–9 IU L^{-1}
Acid (prostatic)		0–3 IU L^{-1}
Alkaline	3–13 KA units%	17–100 IU L^{-1}
Potassium	3.4–5.3 mEq L^{-1}	3.4–5.3 mmol L^{-1}
Protein		
Total	6.0–8.0 g%	60–80 g L^{-1}
Albumin	3.5–5.0 g%	35–50 g L^{-1}
Globulin	1.5–3.0 g%	15–30 g L^{-1}
Pyruvate	0.4–0.7 mg%	34–80 µmol L^{-1}
Sodium	133–148 mEq L^{-1}	133–148 mmol L^{-1}
Thyroxine (T$_4$)	4.7–11 µg%	52–140 nmol L^{-1}
Transaminase		
aspartate transaminase (AST)	5–40 unit mL^{-1}	5–40 IU L^{-1}
alanine transaminase (ALT)		2–53 IU L^{-1}
Transferrin	220–400 mg%	2.2–4.0 g L^{-1}
Triglycerides (fasting)	71–160 mg%	0.8–1.8 mmol L^{-1}

Name	US Units	SI Units
Tri-iodothyronine (T_3)	90–170 ng%	0.8–2.5 nmol L⁻¹
T_3 uptake	95–117%	95–117%
Urea	15–48 mg%	2.5–8.0 mmol L⁻¹
Urea nitrogen (BUN)	10–20 mg%	7.1–14.3 mmol L⁻¹
Urate		
Men	4–9.5 mg%	225–470 µmol L⁻¹
Women	3–7.5 mg%	180–390 µmol L⁻¹

APPENDIX C (IVB): CONVERSION CHART – HYDROGEN ION CONCENTRATION TO pH

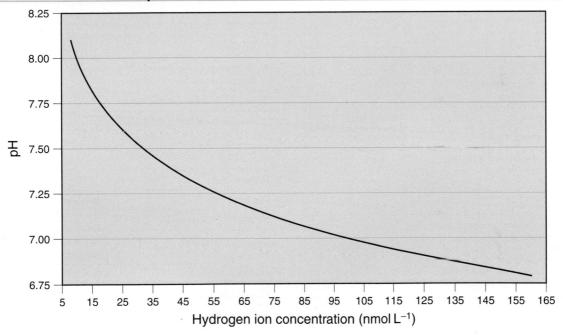

APPENDIX C (V): HAEMATOLOGY

Normal Values

Haemoglobin
Men	13.5–18.0 gd L⁻¹
Women	11.5–16.5 gd L⁻¹
10–12 years	11.5–14.8 gd L⁻¹
1 year	11.0–13.0 gd L⁻¹
3 months	9.5–12.5 gd L⁻¹
Full term	13.6–19.6 gd L⁻¹

Red blood cell count (RBC)
Men	4.5–6.0×10¹² L⁻¹
Women	3.5–5.0×10¹² L⁻¹

White blood cell count (WBC)   4.0–11.0×10⁹ L⁻¹
Neutrophils	40–70%
Lymphocytes	20–45%
Monocytes	2–10%
Eosinophils	1–6%
Basophils	0–1%

Normal Values

Platelet count	$150-400 \times 10^9 \, L^{-1}$
Reticulocyte count	0–2% of RBC
Sedimentation rate	
Men	0–15 mm in 1 h
Women	0–20 mm in 1 h
Plasma viscosity	1.50–1.72 mPas
Packed cell volume (PCV) and haematocrit (Hct)	
Men	0.4–0.55
Women	0.36–0.47
Mean corpuscular volume (MCV)	76–96 fL
Mean corpuscular haemoglobin concentration (MCHC)	31–35 g dL^{-1}
Mean corpuscular haemoglobin (MCH)	27–32 pg

Coagulation Tests

Activated clotting time (ACT; Haemochron type)	80–135 s
Antithrombin III	>80% normal
Bleeding time (platelet function)	2–9 min
Clotting time (largely replaced by ACT)	2–9 min
D dimers	<0.3 mg L^{-1}
Fibrinogen – plasma	1.5–4 g L^{-1}
INR (international normalized ratio warfarin therapy value)	
Therapeutic range for:	
Atrial fibrillation, deep venous thrombosis, pulmonary embolism, tissue heart valves	2–3
Mechanical heart valve	3–4.5
KCCT (also known as PTTK, APTT)	33–41 s
Heparin therapy value	1.5–2.5 × normal
If pregnant	1.5–2.0 × normal
Platelet count	$150-400 \times 10^9 \, L^{-1}$
Prothrombin time	12–14 s
Thrombin time	circa 15 s

KCCT, kaolin cephalin clotting time; PTTK, partial thromboplastin time, kaolin; APTT, activated partial thromboplastin time.

Coagulation Screen

What to check?

- Prothrombin time (PT)
- Kaolin cephalin clotting time (KCCT)
- Thrombin time (TT)
- Fibrinogen
- Platelet count

If all are normal, consider checking bleeding time and, in neonates, factor XIII concentration.
Consider use of thromboelastography or thromboelastometry

When to check?

Elective Patient

- With suspicious history (bleeding after cuts, previous surgery or dental extractions, easy bruising)
- With family history of bleeding problems
- Receiving anticoagulants – warfarin, heparin or aspirin, for example
- With intercurrent illness such as obstructive jaundice, liver disease, uraemia or leukaemia

Emergency or Intraoperative Patient

Tranexamic acid is recommended for patients with major trauma.

With excessive bleeding despite apparent vascular integrity.

What to do?

Possible Cause	Treatment
PT and KCCT Prolonged	
Drug effect (warfarin/ coumarin)	Vitamin K, FFP, coagulation concentrates
Obstructive jaundice	Vitamin K, FFP
Liver disease	Vitamin K, FFP
Haemorrhagic disease of the newborn	Vitamin K
Factor II, V, X deficiency	FFP, coagulation concentrates
If TT is also Prolonged	
Fibrinogen deficiency	Cryoprecipitate, FFP
Are D-dimers Increased?	
Disseminated intravascular coagulation (DIC)	Treat cause, FFP, platelets, ? antithrombin III concentrate

What to do?

Possible Cause	Treatment
Is KCCT Prolonged?	
Heparin therapy	Stop therapy, ? reverse effect with protamine
Factor VIII deficiency – haemophilia	Factor VIII concentrate: high purity
Von Willebrand's disease	Vasopressin, factor VIII concentrate: intermediate purity
Factor IX deficiency	Factor IX concentrate
Factor XI or XII deficiency	FFP
Is PT Prolonged (with normal KCCT)?	
Factor VII deficiency	FFP, factor VII concentrate
Is Platelet Count Decreased ($< 100 \times 10^9 L^{-1}$)?	
Peripheral destruction	
? Immune-mediated	Steroids
? DIC	Treat cause
? TTP or HUS	Platelets, FFP, ? antithrombin III concentrate, plasma exchange
Inadequate production	
Marrow failure	Platelets
Is bleeding time prolonged?	
Von Willebrand's disease	Factor VIII concentrate: intermediate purity, vasopressin
Functional platelet disorder	
Inherited	Platelets
Acquired	Platelets
Uraemia	Dialysis/haemofiltration, cryoprecipitate
Drugs	

Always consult haematology colleague when uncertain.
FFP, fresh frozen plasma; TTP, thrombotic thrombocytopenic purpura; HUS, haemolytic uraemic syndrome.

APPENDIX C (VI): FLUID BALANCE

Fluid composition of body compartments	*Typical Blood Volume*
Infant	$90 \, mL \, kg^{-1}$
Child	$80 \, mL \, kg^{-1}$
Adult male	$70 \, mL \, kg^{-1}$
Adult female	$60 \, mL \, kg^{-1}$

Total water content (TWC)

60% male (55% female) of body weight (18–40 years)

55% male (46% female) of body weight (> 60 years)

Volume of extracellular fluid 35% TWC

Volume of intracellular fluid 65% TWC

Intraoperative Fluid Requirement – Adult

(1) Initial volume	$1.5 \, mL \, kg^{-1} \, h^{-1}$ for duration of preoperative starvation
+ (2) Maintenance	$1.5 \, mL \, kg^{-1} \, h^{-1}$
+ (3) Operative insensible loss	Guided by intra-operative monitoring (e.g. cardiac output); aim for neutral fluid balance
+ (4) Blood loss	Consider replacement with blood and appropriate clotting products when blood loss exceeds 20% of estimated blood volume or $Hb < 8 \, g \, dL^{-1}$

Fluid, Electrolyte and Nutritional Requirements

MINIMUM DAILY REQUIREMENTS PER KILOGRAM FOR ADULTS, AND CHILDREN AND INFANTS. (NEONATES SEE APPENDIX IXB)

	Adults (per kg)	Children and infants (per kg)
Water	30–45 mL	100–150 mL
Energy	30–50 kcal (0.15–0.21 MJ)	90–125 kcal (0.38–0.5 MJ)
Protein	0.7–1.0 g	2.2–2.5 g
Na^+	1–1.4 mmol	1–2.5 mmol
K^+	0.7–0.9 mmol	2 mmol
Ca^{2+}	0.11 mmol	0.5–1 mmol
Mg^{2+}	0.04 mmol	0.15 mmol
Fe^{2+}	1 μmol	2 μmol
Mn^{2+}	0.1 μmol	0.3 μmol
Zn^{2+}	0.7 μmol	1.0 μmol
Cu^+	0.07 μmol	0.3 μmol
Cl^-	1.3–1.9 mmol	1.8–4.3 mmol

Composition of Common Intravenous Fluids

Name	pH	Calculated[a] osmolality	IONS (mmol L^{-1})					CHO (g L^{-1})	Protein (g L^{-1})	MJ L^{-1}
			Na^+	K^+	Cl^-	HCO_3^{-1}	Misc.			
Crystalloids										
Sodium chloride 0.9%	5.0	308	154	0	154	0	0	0	0	0
Glucose 5%	4.0	280	0	0	0	0	0	50	0	0.84
Glucose 4% + saline 0.18%	4.5	286	31	0	31	0	0	40	0	0.67
Glucose 5% + saline 0.45%	4.5	430	77	0	77	0	0	50	0	0.84
Lactated Ringer's (Hartmann's solution)	6.5	280	131	5	112	29 (as lact.)	Mg^{2+} 1 Ca^{2+} 1	0	0	0.038
Plasmalyte 148	4.0–6.5	294	140	5	98	0	Acetate 27 mmol L^{-1} Gluconate 23 mmol L^{-1}			
Sodium bicarbonate 8.4%	8.0	2000	1000	0	0	1000	0	0	0	0

[a]Calculated value, assuming total dissociation of ions.

Name	pH	Oncotic Pressure (mmH$_2$O)	IONIC CONTENT (mmol L^{-1})				CHO (g L^{-1})	Protein (g L^{-1})	MJL^{-1}	Typical Half-Life in Plasma
			Na$^+$	K$^+$	Cl$^-$	Misc.				
Colloids										
Gelatin (polygeline, Gelofusine)	7.4	465	154	0.4	125	Ca^{2+} 0.4 Mg^{2+} 0.4	0	40	0	4 h
Blood products										
Human albumin solution (PPF 4%)	7.4	275	150	2	120					
(20% salt-poor solution also available – ionic content varies with manufacturer)										
Whole blood	> 6.5					Na$^+$ depends on donor values. K$^+$ increases with storage time				
Plasma-reduced blood	> 6.5					Na$^+$ depends on donor value. K$^+$ higher than in whole blood, but total quantity *per unit* is similar				
SAGM blood	> 6.5		150		150	Adenine 0.6%, glucose 2.6%, mannitol 1.6%				
Accepted safe storage times at 4 °C										
Heparinized blood						Only available for special applications				
Acid citrate dextrose						21 days special applications				
Citrate phosphate dextrose						28 days				
Citrate phosphate dextrose adenine						35 days special order e.g. intra-uterine transfusions				
SAGM						35 days				

PPF, plasma protein fraction; SAGM, saline adenine glucose mannitol.

APPENDIX C (VII): RENAL FUNCTION TESTS

Renal Function Tests

Clearance tests

Inulin clearance ≅ glomerular filtration	100–150 mL min^{-1}
Para-aminohippuric acid clearance ≅ renal plasma flow	560–830 mL min^{-1}
Creatinine clearance ≅ glomerular filtration rate (overestimates low glomerular filtration rate)	104–125 mL min^{-1}

Blood tests

Serum/plasma

Osmolality	280–300 mosmol kg^{-1}
Creatinine	45–120 µmol L^{-1}
Urea	2.7–7.0 mmol L^{-1}
Urea nitrogen	1.6–3.3 mmol L^{-1}

Urine tests

Osmolality	300–1200 mosmol kg^{-1}
Creatinine	8.85–17.7 mmol per 24 h
Sodium	50–200 mmol per 24 h

Comparative Urinary Values				
	SG	Osmolality	U/P Urea Ratio	U/P Osmolality
Normal	1000–1040	300–1200	>20:1	>2.0:1
Prerenal failure	>1022	>400	>20:1	>2.0:1
Renal failure	1010	<350	<14:1	<1.7:1
Early			<5:1	<1.1:1
Late				

SG, specific gravity; U, urine; P, plasma

Chronic kidney disease (CKD) stages	eGFR	Description
1	90+	Normal kidney function but urine findings or structural abnormalities or genetic trait point to kidney disease. Observation, control of blood pressure
2	60–89	Mildly reduced kidney function, and other findings (as for stage 1) point to kidney disease Observation, control of blood pressure and risk factors.
3A	45–59	Moderately reduced kidney function. Observation, control of blood pressure and risk factors.
3B	30–44	
4	15–29	Severely reduced kidney function. Planning for endstage renal failure.
5	<15 or on dialysis	Very severe, or endstage kidney failure (sometimes called established renal failure).

APPENDIX C (VIII): PULMONARY FUNCTION TESTS

Commonly Used Abbreviations

Primary Symbols	Secondary Symbols
C=concentration of gas – blood phase	Usually typed as subscripts, capital letters
D=diffusing capacity	indicate gaseous phase; lower-case letters
F=fractional concentration in the dry gas phase	indicate liquid phase.
P=partial pressure – gas	
Q=volume of blood	A=alveolar
R=respiratory exchange ratio	B=barometric
S=saturation of haemoglobin with oxygen or carbon dioxide	D=dead space
V=volume of gas	E=expired
$\dot{X}$ = dot above symbol indicates 'per unit time'	I=inspired
$\overline{X}$ = bar above symbol indicates 'mean value'	T=tidal
Example: PaO_2=partial pressure of arterial oxygen	a=arterial
	c=capillary (pulmonary capillary)
	v=venous
	p=peripleural

Lung Function: Adult and Neonatal Values

Examples	Adult (65 kg)	Neonate (3 kg)
V_D	$2.2\,mL\,kg^{-1}$	$2–3\,mL\,kg^{-1}$
V_T	$7–10\,mL\,kg^{-1}$	$5–7\,mL\,kg^{-1}$
$\dot{V}_E$	$85–100\,mL\,kg^{-1}\,min^{-1}$	$100–200\,mL\,kg^{-1}\,min^{-1}$
Vital capacity	$50–55\,mL\,kg^{-1}$	$33\,mL\,kg^{-1}$
Respiratory rate	$12–18$ breath min^{-1}	$25–40$ breath min^{-1}
PaO_2	12.6 kPa (95 mmHg)	9 kPa (68 mmHg)
$PaCO_2$	5.3 kPa (40 mmHg)	4.5 kPa (33 mmHg)

Lung spirometry

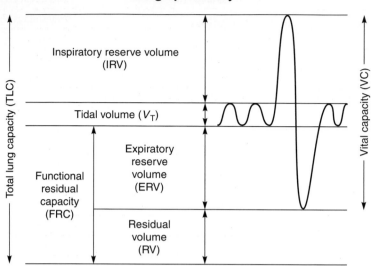

Volumes (mL) in 60kg male

V_T	400–600
IRV	3300–3750
ERV	950–1200
FRC	2300–2600
RV	1200–1700
VC	3800–5000
TLC	5000–6500

FIGURE VIII ■ Lung volumes in an average healthy male adult.

APPENDIX C (IX): PAEDIATRICS

Tracheal and Tracheostomy Tube Size

Age (years)	TT and Tracheostomy Tube Size ID (mm) (cuffed)	TT LENGTH (cm) Oral	Nasal
Premature (by weight)			
1 kg	2.5	7	
2 kg	3.0	8	
3 kg	3.0/3.5	9	
0–3 months	3.0/3.5	10	
3–6 months	3.0/3.5	12	15
6–12 months	3.5/4.5	12	15
2	5.0	13	16
3	5.0	13	16
4	5.5	14	17
5	5.5	14	17
6	6.0	15	18
7	6.0	15	18
8	5.5	16	19
9	5.5	16	19
10	6.0	17	20
11	6.0	17	20
12	6.5	18	21

TT, tracheal tube; ID, internal diameter.
Below 8 years, uncuffed tubes are commonly used.
For children older than 1 year, formulae for estimating tube sizes are:
(Age/4) + 4.5 (uncuffed)
(Age/4) + 3.5 (cuffed)

Dosage of drugs in common anaesthetic usage

Premedication

Atropine	$20\,\mu g\,kg^{-1}$
Hyoscine	$20\,\mu g\,kg^{-1}$
Glycopyrrolate	$5\,\mu g\,kg^{-1}$
Diazepam	$200{-}400\,\mu g\,kg^{-1}$
Alimemazine (Trimeprazine)	$2\,mg\,kg^{-1}$

Intravenous induction

Propofol	$3\,mg\,kg^{-1}$
Thiopental	$5\,mg\,kg^{-1}$
Ketamine	$2\,mg\,kg^{-1}$

Other induction routes

Ketamine intramuscular	$10\,mg\,kg^{-1}$
Thiopental rectal	$30\,mg\,kg^{-1}$

Neuromuscular blocking drugs

Succinylcholine	$2\,mg\,kg^{-1}$
Atracurium	$300{-}500\,\mu g\,kg^{-1}$
Cisatracurium	$80{-}200\,\mu g\,kg^{-1}$
Mivacurium	$250{-}400\,\mu g\,kg^{-1}$
Rocuronium	$500{-}1200\,\mu g\,kg^{-1}$
Vecuronium	$100\,\mu g\,kg^{-1}$
Pancuronium	$80{-}100\,\mu g\,kg^{-1}$

Reversal of neuromuscular blocking drugs

Neostigmine	
Child	$50\,\mu g\,kg^{-1}$
Neonatal	$80\,\mu g\,kg^{-1}$
Atropine	$20\,\mu g\,kg^{-1}$

Analgesics – intravenous/intramuscular

Morphine	$200\,\mu g\,kg^{-1}$
Fentanyl	$0.5{-}1.5\,\mu g\,kg^{-1}$
Alfentanil	$2.5{-}5\,\mu g\,kg^{-1}$

Rectal

Diclofenac	$2\,mg\,kg^{-1}$ (for acute dosage only)

Fluid and Electrolyte Balance

Postoperative fluid and electrolyte requirements in infancy and childhood

Weight	Rate
Up to 10 kg	$100\,mL\,kg^{-1}\,day^{-1}$
10–20 kg	$1000\,mL + (50{\times}[wt\ (kg) - 10])\,mL\,kg^{-1}\,day^{-1}$
20–30 kg	$1500\,mL + (25{\times}[wt\ (kg) - 20])\,mL\,kg^{-1}\,day^{-1}$

Fluid Requirements in the First Week of Life

Day	Rate
1	0
2, 3	$50\,mL\,kg^{-1}\,day^{-1}$
4, 5	$75\,mL\,kg^{-1}\,day^{-1}$
6	$100\,mL\,kg^{-1}\,day^{-1}$
7	$120\,mL\,kg^{-1}\,day^{-1}$

Fluid and Electrolyte Requirements in Infancy and Childhood

	AGE (YEARS)										
	1 wk	1	2	3	4	5	6	7	8	9	10
Weight (kg)	3.5	10	13	15	17	19	21	23	25	28	32
Insensible water loss ($mL\,kg^{-1}\,day^{-1}$)	30	27.5	27	26.5	26	25	24	23	22	21	20
Water requirement ($mL\,kg^{-1}\,day^{-1}$)	120	100	100	90	90	90	70	70	70	70	70
Na^+ requirement ($mmol\,kg^{-1}\,day^{-1}$)	4	3	2.5	2	2	1.9	1.9	1.9	1.8	1.75	1.7
K^+ requirement ($mmol\,kg^{-1}\,day^{-1}$)	2.5	2	2	2	2	1.75	1.75	1.5	1.5	1.5	1.5

These are basal requirements. Additional fluid (10–20%) is required during major surgery, in addition to replacement of overt losses. During the postoperative period, fluid requirements are increased in the presence of pyrexia. Fluid and electrolyte balance should be adjusted after measurement of serum electrolyte concentrations and serum osmolality.

APPENDIX C (X): GAS FLOWS IN ANAESTHETIC BREATHING SYSTEMS

System	Spontaneous Ventilation	Intermittent Positive-Pressure Ventilation
Mapleson A (Lack or Magill)	Minute ventilation (MV; theoretically V_A) 80 mL kg^{-1} min^{-1}	2.5 × MV 200 mL kg^{-1} min^{-1}
Mapleson D (Bain or coaxial Mapleson D)	2–3 × MV 150–250 mL kg^{-1} min^{-1}	70 mL kg^{-1} min^{-1} for $PaCO_2$ of 5.3 kPa 100 mL kg^{-1} min^{-1} for $PaCO_2$ of 4.3 kPa
Mapleson E (Ayre's T-piece)	2 × MV	As Mapleson D Minimum of 3 L min^{-1} fresh gas flow
Mapleson F (Jackson Rees modification of Ayre's T-piece)	As Mapleson E	As Mapleson E

V_A, alveolar minute volume; $PaCO_2$, arterial carbon dioxide tension.

Normal Ventilation Values for Resting Awake Subjects			
Weight (kg)	Minute Volume (mL)	Tidal Volume (mL)	Frequency (Breath min^{-1})
Neonate 2	480	14–16	30–45
3	600	17–24	25–40
10	1680	80	21
20	3040	160	19
30	4080	240	17
40	4800	320	15
50	5200	400	13
60	5280	480	11
70	5600	560	10

INDEX

■ ■

NOTES

Page numbers followed by *f* indicate figures, *t* indicate tables and *b* indicate boxes.

As the subject of this book is anaesthesia, entries have been kept to a minimum under this entry. Readers are advised to look for more specific entries.

Abbreviations

CPB - cardiopulmonary bypass
CPR - cardiopulmonary resuscitation
ECG - electrocardiography
ECT - electroconvulsive therapy
EEG - electroencephalography
ICU - intensive care unit
MRI - magnetic resonance imaging
NSAIDs - non-steroidal anti-inflammatory drugs
PONV - postoperative nausea and vomiting